ADVANCE PRAISE FOR *KETOGENIC DIET AND METABOLIC THERAPIES*

"Publication of this 2nd edition of *Ketogenic Diet and Metabolic Therapies: Expanded Roles in Health and Disease* coincides with the centennial of the first scientific publications introducing this treatment for epilepsy. This is an authoritative compendium of the current state of knowledge of established and emerging uses of ketogenic diets, and their potential mechanisms. It is written by the leading scientists in the field who summarize what is already known and emphasize the gaps in knowledge that need to be filled with further research. This is a must-have reference for anyone who studies or treats epilepsy, or is interested in the interactions between metabolism, human biology and disease." —George B Richerson, MD, PhD; Professor and Chairman, Neurology; Professor, Molecular Physiology & Biophysics; The Roy J Carver Chair in Neuroscience, The University of Iowa

KETOGENIC DIET AND METABOLIC THERAPIES

Expanded Roles in Health and Disease

SECOND EDITION

EDITED BY

SUSAN A. MASINO, PHD

Vernon D. Roosa Professor of Applied Science
Trinity College
Hartford, CT

SECTION EDITORS

DETLEV BOISON, PHD
DOMINIC P. D'AGOSTINO, PHD
ERIC H. KOSSOFF, MD
JONG M. RHO, MD

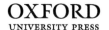

OXFORD
UNIVERSITY PRESS

OXFORD

UNIVERSITY PRESS

Oxford University Press is a department of the University of Oxford. It furthers
the University's objective of excellence in research, scholarship, and education
by publishing worldwide. Oxford is a registered trade mark of Oxford University
Press in the UK and certain other countries.

Published in the United States of America by Oxford University Press
198 Madison Avenue, New York, NY 10016, United States of America.

© Oxford University Press 2022

Library of Congress Cataloging-in-Publication Data
Names: Susan A. Masino, editor.
Title: Ketogenic diet and metabolic therapies : expanded roles in health and disease /
[edited by] Susan A. Masino
Description: Second edition. | New York, NY : Oxford University Press, [2022] |
Includes bibliographical references and index.
Identifiers: LCCN 2021033404 (print) | LCCN 2021033405 (ebook) |
ISBN 9780197501207 (paperback) | ISBN 9780197501221 (epub) |
ISBN 9780197501238 (Digital-Online)
Subjects: MESH: Diet, Ketogenic | Metabolism—physiology |
Metabolic Diseases—diet therapy
Classification: LCC RM237.73 (print) | LCC RM237.73 (ebook) |
NLM WB 427 | DDC 613.2/833—dc23
LC record available at https://lccn.loc.gov/2021033404
LC ebook record available at https://lccn.loc.gov/2021033405

DOI: 10.1093/med/9780197501207.001.0001

3 5 7 9 8 6 4 2

Printed by Marquis, Canada

CONTENTS

CONTRIBUTORS

Jim Abrahams
Charlie Foundation for Ketogenic Therapies
Santa Monica, CA, USA

Csilla Ari, PhD
University of South Florida
Tampa, FL, USA

Stéphane Auvin, MD, PhD
Université de Paris, CHU Robert-Debré, APHP,
Institut Universitaire de France
Paris, France

Ann M. Bergin, MD
Boston Children's Hospital
Boston, MA, USA

A. G. Christina Bergqvist, MD
University of Pennsylvania
Philadelphia, PA, USA

Detlev Boison, PhD
Rutgers Robert Wood Johnson Medical School
New Brunswick, NJ, USA

Karin Borges, PhD
University of Queensland
St Lucia, Australia

Christian-Alexandre Castellano, PhD
University of Sherbrooke
Sherbrooke, Québec, Canada

Mackenzie C. Cervenka, MD
Johns Hopkins School of Medicine
Baltimore, MD, USA

Ning Cheng, PhD
University of Calgary
Calgary, Canada

Stephen C. Cunnane, PhD
Université de Sherbrooke
Sherbrooke, Québec, Canada

Dominic P. D'Agostino, PhD
University of South Florida
Tampa, FL, USA

Nika Danial, PhD
Dana-Farber Cancer Institute, Harvard
Medical School
Boston, MA, USA

Nina Dupuis, PhD
Université Paris Diderot, Sorbonne Paris Cité
Paris, France

Marwa Elamin, MD
UCONN School of Medicine
Farmington, CT, USA

Mélanie Fortier, MSc
Université de Sherbrooke
Sherbrooke, Québec, Canada

Adam L. Hartman, MD
National Institute of Neurological Disorders
and Stroke
Rockville, MD, USA

Cherie L. Herren, MD
University of Oklahoma Health Science Center
Oklahoma City, OK, USA

Peter Hespel, PhD
Bakala Academy-Athletic Performance Center,
Katholieke Universiteit
Leuven, Belgium

David T. Hsieh, MD
Uniformed Services University
Bethesda, MD, USA

Tsuyoshi Inoue, PhD
Okayama University
Okayama, Japan

Damir Janigro, PhD
Case Western Reserve University
Cleveland, OH, USA

Derek Johnson, BS
University of Colorado Anschutz
Medical Campus
Aurora, CO, USA

Emily L. Johnson, MD, PhD
Johns Hopkins School of Medicine
Baltimore, MD, USA

Masahito Kawamura Jr., MD, PhD
The Jikei University School of Medicine
Tokyo, Japan

Shannon L. Kesl, PhD
University of South Florida
Tampa, FL, USA

Sudha Kilaru Kessler, MD, MSCE
University of Pennsylvania
Philadelphia, PA, USA

Joerg Klepper, MD
Klinikum Aschaffenburg-Alzenau
Aschaffenburg, Germany

Kathleen L. Kolehmainen, PhD
University of British Columbia
Vancouver, Canada

Eric Kossoff, MD
Johns Hopkins University
Baltimore, MD, USA

Andrew P. Koutnik, PhD
University of South Florida
Tampa, FL, USA

Zsolt Kovacs, PhD
Eötvös Loránd University, Savaria
University Centre
Szombathely, Hungary

Ann-Katrin Kraeuter, PhD
Northumbria University
Newcastle, UK

Joseph C. LaManna, PhD
Case Western Reserve University
Cleveland, OH, USA

Wendie N. Marks, PhD
University of Calgary
Alberta, Canada

Juan Ramón Martínez-François, PhD
Harvard Medical School
Boston, MA, USA

Susan A. Masino, PhD
Trinity College
Hartford, CT, USA

Sara E. Moss, BS
University of South Florida
Tampa, FL, USA

Chunlong Mu, PhD
University of Calgary
Calgary, Canada

Purna Mukherjee, PhD
Boston College
Chestnut Hill, MA, USA

Madhuvika Murugan, PhD
Rutgers Robert Wood Johnson Medical School
New Brunswick, NJ, USA

Étienne Myette-Côté, PhD
Université de Sherbrooke
Sherbrooke, Quebec, Canada

Rima Nabbout, MD, PhD
Université de Paris
Paris, France

Elizabeth Neal, RD, MSc, PhD
Matthews Friends Charity and Clinics
Lingfield, UK
University College London-Institute of
Child Health
London, UK

Christopher M. Palmer, MD
Harvard Medical School
Belmont, MA, USA

Manisha Patel, PhD
University of Colorado Anschutz
Medical Campus
Aurora, CO, USA

Ward T. Plunet, PhD
University of British Columbia
Vancouver, Canada

Angela M. Poff, PhD
University of South Florida
Tampa, FL, USA

Michelle A. Puchowicz, PhD
The University of Tennessee Health Science Center
Memphis, TN, USA

Jong M. Rho, MD
University of California, San Diego
San Diego, CA, USA

Christopher Q. Rogers, PhD
University of South Florida
Tampa, FL, USA

David N. Ruskin, PhD
Trinity College
Hartford, CT, USA

Paola Sacchetti, PhD
University of Hartford
West Hartford, CT, USA

Nagisa Sada, PhD
Okayama University
Okayama, Japan

Rana R. Said, MD
University of Texas Southwestern Medical Center
Dallas, TX, USA

Zoltán Sarnyai, MD, PhD
James Cook University
Townsville, Queensland, Australia

Morris H. Scantlebury, MD
University of Calgary
Calgary, Canada

Adrienne C. Scheck, PhD
Beshert Alliance Ctr, LLC
Scottsdale, AZ, USA

Oscar Seira, PhD
University of British Columbia
Vancouver, Canada

Aarti Sethuraman, PhD
University of Tennessee Health Science Center
Memphis, TN, USA

Thomas N. Seyfried, MS, PhD
Boston College
Chestnut Hill, MA, USA

Li-Rong Shao, MD
Johns Hopkins University School of Medicine
Baltimore, MD, USA

Jane Shearer, PhD
University of Calgary
Calgary, Canada

Timothy A. Simeone, PhD
Creighton University
Omaha, NE, USA

Carl E. Stafstrom, MD, PhD
Johns Hopkins University School of Medicine
Baltimore, MD, USA

Valérie St-Pierre, MSc
Université de Sherbrooke
Sherbrooke, Québec, Canada

Brianna J. Stubbs, DPhil
Buck Institute for Research on Aging
Novato, CA, USA

Thomas P. Sutula, MD, PhD
University of Wisconsin School of Medicine and
Public Health
Madison, WI, USA

Nelofer Syed, PhD
Imperial College London
London, UK

Fabio C. Tescarollo, PhD
Rutgers University
New Brunswick, NJ, USA

Wolfram Tetzlaff, MD, PhD
University of British Columbia
Vancouver, Canada

Elizabeth A. Thiele, MD, PhD
Harvard Medical School
Boston, MA, USA

Justin Tondt, MD
Eastern Virginia Medical School
Norfolk, VA, USA

Elles J. T. M. van der Louw, RD, PhD
Erasmus MC University Medical Center
Rotterdam, Netherlands

Matthew C. Walker, MA, FRCP, PhD
University College London
London, UK

Eric C. Westman, MD, MHS
Duke University Medical Center
Durham, NC, USA

Emma Williams, MBE
Matthew's Friends
Lingfield, UK

Robin S. B. Williams, BSc, PhD
Royal Holloway University of London
Egham, UK

Kui Xu, MD, PhD
Case Western Reserve University
Cleveland, OH, USA

William S. Yancy, Jr., MD, MHS
Duke University Medical Center
Durham, NC, USA

Ceren Yarar-Fisher, PhD
University of Alabama
Birmingham, AL, USA

Gary Yellen, PhD
Harvard Medical School
Boston, MA, USA

Beth Zupec-Kania, RD, CD
Ketogenic Therapies, LLC
The Charlie Foundation for Ketogenic Therapies
Santa Monica, CA, USA

1

The 100th Anniversary of the Ketogenic Diet

Local and Global Perspectives

Ketogenic diets have been used to treat epilepsy for a century (Wilder, 1921a, 1921b). Finally—no need to say "nearly" 100 years since the ketogenic diet was published in 1921! To many, it feels like a long time, yet we are still at the beginning. It has taken many decades for the potential of ketogenic diet and metabolic therapies in health and disease to be appreciated. Thankfully, good ideas persist. They can, and must, be revisited and retested.

Here, we honor the major milestone of the 100th anniversary of the ketogenic diet with an updated, affordable, full-color second edition of *Ketogenic Diet and Metabolic Therapies: Expanded Roles in Health and Disease*. Many top scientists working in this area have contributed chapters about their latest work—and we acknowledge there is still much we do not know about the relationship between metabolism and health and disease. We do, however, recognize that it is of fundamental importance. It's an exciting time for practitioners and the public to forge or to follow new developments in the field.

The 100th anniversary affirms without reservation the well-established and now expanded power of ketogenic and metabolic therapies in treating seizures in adults and children. It also affirms the rich and expanding landscape of molecular mechanisms, lifestyle changes, metabolic alternatives, and therapeutic opportunities beyond seizures and even well beyond neurologic disorders. It's exciting to see new discoveries alongside those that are truly "back to the future."

Many are aware that the first two reports in the medical literature of metabolic therapy in epilepsy were in July 1921: the reports, written by Dr. R. M. Wilder, were one page each, and they were published on consecutive days in the daily *Mayo Clinic Bulletin*. But these brief initial reports revealed a lot and predicted the future: The first report makes a case for use of a high-fat, low-carbohydrate diet, based on prior successful work with fasting in epilepsy (Wilder, 1921a). The second report consists of case descriptions of three patients who became seizure-free after ketogenic diet treatment (Wilder, 1921b). Interestingly, given that the diet became best known as a treatment for children (and was used almost exclusively in pediatric epilepsy for many decades), two of the three original patients were adults (ages 23 and 31). Furthermore, the brief early papers showed that metabolic therapy could have therapeutic effects that outlasted the administration of the diet—a finding that is now coming to the fore as an exciting research area with many implications.

Taken together, benefits that span age groups and conditions—and persist—were powerful early observations. And while there was a small number of initial patients in 1921, similar outcomes were observed repeatedly for decades. Reports in the next decade highlighted benefits in diabetes (Adams, 1931) and migraines (Baborka, 1930), conditions that are now the objects of major programs in basic and clinical research. Isolated reports decades ago also highlighted improvements in mental illness (Pacheco et al., 1965)—a re-emerging topic for metabolic therapy. Exciting new research areas include cancer, immunology, neurodegeneration, longevity, and much more. Seizures are comorbid in many neurologic disorders; treating them with metabolic approaches has yielded additional insights. Furthermore, there has been rapid progress in developing alternative compounds and supplements that may be able to substitute for, or complement, dietary changes—potentially with increased palatability, efficacy, and applicability.

Improving diet quality has long-term health benefits for anyone, and remarkable success stories in reversing chronic health conditions need careful validation and evidence of a lack of harm. We need more long-term studies, and more that compare effects in women and men. To some extent, increased basic and clinical research in metabolic therapy has been buoyed and fueled by public interest and funded by private donors or foundations. Funding top-notch independent research in metabolic therapy and understanding its impacts on cell signaling, epigenetics, cognition, and behavior remain urgent public policy priorities to ensure sufficient research on fundamental questions and to focus healthcare spending on treatments that are effective and restorative. Despite positive momentum, metabolic approaches remain underutilized. It will continue to take an interdisciplinary scientific village—working together—to understand the relationship between metabolism and health and disease and to continue to make progress.

A horizon of future fundamental discoveries is one of the most exciting aspects of this field. The second edition of *Ketogenic Diet and Metabolic Therapies: Expanded Roles in Health and Disease* is organized into four key subsections spearheaded by leaders in each area: the latest clinical research for treatment of epilepsy (Eric Kossoff, MD), emerging clinical applications (Jong Rho, MD), laboratory research into key mechanisms (Detlev Boison, PhD), and diverse metabolic therapies to treat disease and improve health (Dominic D'Agostino, PhD). The last chapter highlights key nonprofit organizations that continue to play a leading role: the Charlie Foundation for Ketogenic Therapies, established in 1994 in the United States (https://charliefoundation.org), and Matthew's Friends (https://matthewsfriends.org), established in 2004 in the United Kingdom. Together, these foundations are devoted to research, education, outreach, and applications of ketogenic therapies throughout the world. They are always adding to their resources and recipes! An epilogue shares the public announcement of the launch of a new global professional society: International Neurological Ketogenic Society (INKS), at https://neuroketo.org.

As we approached this milestone of the 100th anniversary, we all lost opportunities for in-person celebrations due to the unexpected disruption of a global pandemic. There was a striking link between poor metabolic health and a poor outcome from COVID-19, and clinical trials were mobilized to test the ability of a ketogenic diet to prevent or treat COVID-19 and the associated cytokine storm—perhaps shining a bigger global spotlight on metabolism as the cornerstone of health. In 2021, the Seventh International Symposium on Medical Ketogenic Diet Therapies, postponed from October 2020, became a successful hybrid (online and in-person) meeting in Brighton, United Kingdom (https://globalketo.com).

Early in the production of this second edition we lost a major contributor to the first edition and a titan in ketone research, Dr. Richard "Bud" Veech. Dr. Veech was senior author of two chapters and a leading force in advancing ketone research for many decades. Dr. Veech trained in the Oxford laboratory of Sir Hans Krebs, the winner of the 1953 Nobel Prize for mapping out metabolic reactions central to cellular energy production, commonly referred to as the Krebs cycle. Dr. Veech was focused on the "great controlling nucleotide coenzymes" as key to health and disease, and he found that the ketone body beta-hydroxybutyrate had the unique ability to increase the potential energy of adenosine triphosphate (ATP), the critically important energy-storing nucleotide coenzyme. Dr. Veech's friend and collaborator William Curtis shared this in a tribute:

> Sometimes it takes a prediction coming true to prove a hypothesis. Einstein predicted the gravity of the sun would bend the light from stars. He had to wait for Eddington to take pictures of stars in the background of the sun . . . . Dr. Veech made a bold hypothesis in several papers in 2002 and 2003 that ketones would be important in medicine. An examination of his life's work leads one to ask, "Is there evidence of these predictions? Are ketones becoming important in medicine?" (Curtis, 2020)

As the research shared in this book demonstrates, ketones are beyond "becoming" important—although the pace of change has seemed slow to many. Dr. Veech's unwavering commitment to his research and its potential to change lives kept him working up until age 84. He died in January 2020, shortly after returning home from giving a scientific talk. Dr. Veech's many predictions advanced basic and clinical research significantly.

In the first edition of *Ketogenic Diet and Metabolic Therapies: Expanded Roles in Health and Disease*, I shared that my research program on the ketogenic diet arose organically from a basic science hypothesis about the ketone-based regulation of brain adenosine, an evolutionarily conserved molecule that is a powerful neuromodulator and bioenergetic regulator of brain activity. I started working on adenosine in 1997 with Dr. Tom Dunwiddie, a stellar scientist whose love of the outdoors, particularly rock-climbing, led to his early death in 2001. In recognition of the 20th anniversary of Tom's death, also in July 2021, I thank him for his mentorship and support for testing novel predictions and working across disciplines. It is a gift I carry with me and try to share.

Like the ketogenic diet, adenosine links metabolism and brain activity. The recent recognition that either adenosine or a ketogenic diet can mobilize lasting epigenetic changes offers new ways to think about modifying and preventing disease in a complex biologic system. To this end, the field of metabolic therapy underscores the power of a systems approach—complex systems have many mechanisms for disease, but also many mechanisms for recovering health. Supporting and re-establishing health takes time; every complex system is slightly different. It has become clear to me that the lessons we are learning (and relearning) from ketogenic diets and metabolic therapies have much wider implications and applications.

My PhD is in biology, and I have a deep appreciation for all complex living systems. Complexity emerges and re-emerges through space and time in dynamic natural systems. After publishing the first edition, I began to integrate my work in brain disease and brain health more directly with my long-standing interest in natural ecosystems, particularly forests. Brains are amazing—they govern our thoughts, feelings, memories, and movements—and studying them is a great privilege. In parallel, healthy ecosystems on land and in the water are the lifelines to everything we need, and a natural forest is the most biodiverse land-based ecosystem—emerging over 100 million years before dinosaurs. Spending time in nature, even in a small piece, is a great solace to all people. We need them far more than they need us.

Combining my interests in these complex systems—inside and out—led to a collaboration with a climate scientist and an ecologist on the benefits of proforestation (Moomaw et al., 2019)—simply letting some existing forests grow, accumulate carbon and diversity, and evolve. Contemplating our brains, our bodies, and the staggering diversity of life on Earth is truly awe-inspiring. Many fundamental discoveries in neuroscience were made in the last century—less than a blip in evolutionary time. Together, brains and forests represent many award-winning volumes in the library of evolution, and I am honored to be the spokesperson for Keep the Woods (https://keepthewoods.org/), an interdisciplinary science and education group focused on clean water and natural forest ecosystems.

When I consider the global challenge of neurologic disorders, which becomes so personal and local in every case, I often reflect on what Dr. Thomas Lovejoy, "the godfather of biodiversity," said in an on-site interview with author/journalist Dahr Jamail for his award-winning book titled *The End of Ice* (Jamail, 2019). Lovejoy has studied the Amazon for more than 50 years, and Jamail remarked on how much we must know based on Lovejoy's (and others') life's work. Lovejoy responded, bluntly: "We know nothing." What we do know is that evolution has been solving biologic problems for billions of years, and we continue to discover new species and molecules—potential medicines—around the world. We have a lot to learn about our brains and about the natural world.

Globally, there is no question that we face escalating and interconnected crises in climate, biodiversity, and health. It's an interdisciplinary problem that must be faced with both truth and care. The truth is we need our best brains to meet this challenge, and we need to care for the natural world enough to give it strategic protection at every scale and in every type of landscape: it's our lifeline, our healthline. Our knowledge of nature is woefully short-term and incomplete, and its preciousness is immeasurable.

What we do know is that complex entities like neural systems and ecosystems have catastrophic tipping points: protection and prevention are paramount. It's now indisputable that metabolic therapy alone can prevent, treat, and reverse disease. Similarly, simply protecting and connecting a network of intact nature is the only proven way to protect full native biodiversity — and it has countless and quantifiable short- and long-term benefits. We are part of nature, and patiently and persistently supporting nature wherever possible is akin to a powerful metabolic therapy for the planet: low cost, mobilizes multiple mechanisms, and offers multiple and lasting benefits and resilience.

More than ever, our best health and our best brains are needed to prevent and to solve problems and to face challenges that will disrupt local and global health systems, food systems, economies, and the lives of many. The field of ketogenic diet and metabolic therapies is a network of global citizens who excel at critical thinking and are unafraid to challenge the status quo. We have a track record of success and cross-disciplinary collaboration. I bring up ecology very directly in the introduction to a book about metabolic therapies because it's essential and there are many parallels: protecting and restoring our metabolic health and our healthy intact ecosystems, locally and globally, is urgent, essential, cost-effective, and common sense. Neither has sufficient funding or public education. Neither is the focus of public policies. Both challenge the status quo and suffer from misleading dominant narratives.

Years of basic research on a wonderful molecule called adenosine led me unexpectedly to the ketogenic diet and the most important and exciting translational work of my career. It connected me with a motivated and collaborative global community of researchers, clinicians, patients, and advocates. Combining my interest in healthy brains with my interest in healthy ecosystems has opened a new world of converging experts—climate scientists, ecologists, public health experts, soil scientists, contemporary artists, native peoples, policymakers—and we are all converging on the same conclusion. Prioritize health and intact nature wherever possible. First, do no harm. Collect and share all the data. Protect local communities and their support systems. And apply evidence-based medicine to people and the planet.

Susan A. Masino
Hartford, Connecticut

REFERENCES

Adams, S. F. (1931). The benefit of prolonged low carbohydrate feeding in diabetes: Report of a case. *Mayo Clinic Proceedings, 6*, 534–535.

Baborka, C. J. (1930). Migraine: Results of treatment by ketogenic diet in fifty cases. *Mayo Clinic Proceedings, 5*, 190–191.

Curtis, W. (2020). Richard L. (Bud) Veech: His contribution to science and medicine in simple terms. *KetoNutrition* (blog), February 12, 2020. https://ketonutrition.org/2020-2-11-tribute-to-dr-richard-veech/

Jamail, D. (2019). *The end of ice: Bearing witness and finding meaning in the path of climate disruption.* The New Press.

Moomaw, W. R., Masino, S. A., & Faison, E. K. (2019). Intact forests in the United States: Proforestation mitigates climate change and serves the greatest good. *Frontiers in Forests and Global Change, 2*, 27. https://www.frontiersin.org/articles/10.3389/ffgc.2019.00027/full

Pacheco, A., Easterling, W. S., & Pryer, M. W. (1965). A pilot study of the ketogenic diet in schizophrenia. *American Journal of Psychiatry, 121*, 1110–1111.

Wilder, R. M. (1921a). The effects of ketonemia on the course of epilepsy. *Mayo Clinic Bulletin, 2*, 307.

Wilder, R. M. (1921b). High fat diets in epilepsy. *Mayo Clinic Bulletin, 2*, 308.

SECTION I

Ketogenic Diet for Epilepsy in the Clinic

Overview: Ketogenic Diets and Pediatric Epilepsy

An Update

ERIC KOSSOFF, MD

Now at its 100-year anniversary, the ketogenic diet (KD) has reached an interest level not previously seen. Originally first published in July 1921 by Dr. Russel Wilder at the Mayo Clinic, its creation came at a time in which there were few other options for epilepsy (Wilder, 1921). The KD was widely used for the next several decades in both children and adults, with approximately 50% of patients reporting at least a 50% reduction in seizures in multiple studies. The advent of phenytoin and other modern pharmaceutical antiseizure drugs in the 1940s and afterward, as well as a lack of publications by epilepsy centers, relegated the KD to "alternative" medicine, and it was largely ignored by mainstream neurologists. For many decades it was used only as a last resort in children with intractable epilepsy in very select institutions still implementing it sporadically.

In 1993, one such refractory case prompted renewed interest in dietary therapies. Hollywood producer Jim Abrahams brought his 2-year-old son Charlie to Johns Hopkins Hospital, where Charlie experienced rapid seizure control within days after starting the KD. Abrahams created the Charlie Foundation for Ketogenic Therapies in 1994, which revitalized research efforts, and he produced ". . . First Do No Harm," a TV movie starring Meryl Streep, which promoted the KD. In 1998, the first multicenter prospective study of the KD in children with refractory epilepsy demonstrated that more than half of patients had a greater than 50% reduction in seizure frequency after 6 months (Vining et al., 1998).

In the now 25+ years since the formation of the Charlie Foundation, dietary therapies have experienced a rapid resurgence in research and utilization. The majority of countries have implemented KDs and more than 200 research articles are published yearly (Kossoff et al., 2005). Multiple randomized controlled clinical trials (RCTs), crossover studies, and prospective studies have confirmed a response rate of approximately 50% in children with refractory epilepsy. In 2009, Freeman and colleagues performed the first blinded study of the KD by having all participants consume the KD plus a daily supplement of either saccharin (treatment group) or glucose (to prevent ketosis; control group; Freeman et al., 2009). They found a trend toward improved seizure frequency in the saccharin group, although the effect did not reach statistical significance, possibly due to complex actions of the KD that were not prevented with ingestion of glucose once a day. Neal and colleagues randomized patients to no change in/standard medical management or addition of the KD; they found that patients with refractory epilepsy who were randomized to receive the KD were more likely to have a 50% decrease in seizure frequency than the control group (Neal et al., 2008). Another study, by Sharma et al. in 2013, utilizing a study design similar to Neal's 2008 trial, found the modified Atkins diet to have efficacy in an RCT as well (Sharma et al., 2013). In light of the accumulating evidence to support the efficacy of KDs, the International Ketogenic Diet Study Group, a panel of 26 neurologists and dietitians, recommended that dietary therapies be strongly considered in patients of any age who had failed two antiseizure medications (Kossoff et al., 2009, 2018).

Beyond the formal prospective studies that have proven efficacy, perhaps an even more important factor that has led to the resurgence of dietary therapy has been a combination of flexibility in implementation and recognition of true indications for its use (Kossoff et al., 2018). Treating the appropriate patients (sooner rather than later), as well as considering alternative diets and methods of starting the treatment, has led to widespread availability, willingness of patients and neurologists to consider it in their treatment algorithm, and better (and safer) outcomes. In this section, "Ketogenic Diet for Epilepsy in the Clinic," these factors are discussed in more detail.

First, Elizabeth Neal highlights the many dietary therapies currently being studied, primarily the classic KD, the medium-chain triglyceride (MCT) diet, the low glycemic index treatment (LGIT), and the modified Atkins diet (MAD). The latter two diets have certainly been responsible for the acceptance of dietary therapies by adults, which is discussed by Mackenzie Cervenka and Emily Johnson in their chapter (Cervenka et al., 2013). Flexibility during the initiation week of the classic KD has also revolutionized approaches to the diet by many epilepsy centers, as is outlined by Christina Bergqvist (Bergqvist et al., 2005).

Second, pediatric epilepsy experts discuss the indications for dietary therapy in pediatric patients. Approximately 30 years ago, there was little to no ability to predict which child would be a KD responder. That has radically changed due to research and large cohort studies. The most famous indication, GLUT1 (glucose transporter type 1) deficiency syndrome, uses the KD as its sole, gold-standard therapy and Joerg Klepper has been involved in much of the research on this condition and its response to the KD (Klepper, 2012). Ann Bergin and Elizabeth Thiele then discuss some of the other well-known epilepsy syndromes and genetic indications for dietary therapy, such as infantile spasms, myoclonic-astatic epilepsy, Dravet syndrome, Rett syndrome, tuberous sclerosis complex, and more. These two chapters are followed by contributions by Sudha Kessler and Rima Nabbout highlighting more recent, "novel" indications for dietary therapy, such as absence epilepsy, juvenile myoclonic epilepsy, status epilepticus, and others that have attracted investigators in the last few years (Nabbout et al., 2010). Then, a new chapter in this second edition, by Elles van der Louw, discusses the expanding use of dietary therapy in infancy (van der Louw, 2016).

In the final chapter of this section, Cherie Herren and Rana Said review the latest research on how to identify and treat the adverse effects inherent in dietary therapy as well as how to eventually discontinue treatment when clinically indicated. This important chapter shows how clinical researchers are attempting to make the diet safer for those who require it, especially in the long term. We hope this section gives readers an increased understanding of just how far the clinical use of dietary therapy has come in such a short time.

REFERENCES

Bergqvist, A. G. C., Schall, J. I., Gallagher, P. R., Cnaan, A., & Stallings, V. A. (2005). Fasting versus gradual initiation of the ketogenic diet: A prospective, randomized clinical trial of efficacy. *Epilepsia*, 46, 1810–1819.

Cervenka, M. C., Henry, B., Nathan, J., Wood, S., & Volek, J. S. (2013). Worldwide dietary therapies for adults with epilepsy and other disorders. *Journal of Child Neurology*, 28, 1034–1040.

Freeman, J. M., Vining, E. P., Kossoff, E. H., Pyzik, P. L., Ye, X., & Goodman, S. N. (2009). A blinded, crossover study of the efficacy of the ketogenic diet. *Epilepsia*, 50, 322–325.

Klepper, J. (2012). GLUT1 deficiency syndrome in clinical practice. *Epilepsy Research*, 100, 272–277.

Kossoff, E. H., & McGrogan, J. R. (2005). Worldwide use of the ketogenic diet. *Epilepsia*, 46, 280–289.

Kossoff, E. H., Zupec-Kania, B. A., Amark, P. E., Ballaban-Gil, K. R., Christina Bergqvist, A. G., Blackford, R., . . . Vining, E. P. (2009). Optimal clinical management of children receiving the ketogenic diet: Recommendations of the International Ketogenic Diet Study Group. *Epilepsia*, 50, 304–317.

Kossoff, E. H., Zupec-Kania, B. A., Auvin, S., Ballaban-Gil, K. R., Christina Bergqvist, A. G., Blackford, R., . . . Wirrell, E. C. (2018). Optimal clinical management of children receiving dietary therapies for epilepsy: Updated recommendations of the International Ketogenic Diet Study Group. *Epilepsia Open*, 3, 175–192.

Nabbout, R., Mazzuca, M., Hubert, P., Peudennier, S., Allaire, C., Flurin, V., . . . Dulac, O. (2010). Efficacy of ketogenic diet in severe refractory status epilepticus initiating fever induced refractory epileptic encephalopathy in school age children (FIRES). *Epilepsia*, 51, 2033–2037.

Neal, E. G., Chaffe, H., Schwartz, R. H., Lawson, M. S., Edwards, N., Fitzsimmons, G., . . . Cross, J. H. (2008). The ketogenic diet for the treatment of childhood epilepsy: A randomised controlled trial. *Lancet Neurology*, 7, 500–506.

Sharma, S., Sankhyan, N., Gulati, S., & Agarwala, A. (2013). Use of the modified Atkins diet for treatment of refractory childhood epilepsy: A randomized controlled trial. *Epilepsia*, 54, 481–486.

van der Louw, E., van den Hurk, D., Neal, E., Leiendecker, B., Fitzsimmon, G., Dority, L., . . . Cross, J. H. (2016). Ketogenic diet guidelines for infants with refractory epilepsy. *European Journal of Paediatric Neurology*, 20, 798–809.

Vining, E. P., Freeman, J. M., Ballaban-Gil, K., Camfield, C. S., Camfield, P. R., Holmes, G. L., . . . Wheless, J. W. (1998). A multicenter study of the efficacy of the ketogenic diet. *Archives of Neurology*, 55, 1433–1437.

Wilder, R. M. (1921). The effects of ketonemia on the course of epilepsy. *Mayo Clinic Proceedings*, 2, 307–308.

3

Alternative Ketogenic Diets

ELIZABETH NEAL, RD, MSC, PHD

INTRODUCTION

As the classic ketogenic diet (KD) celebrates its centennial anniversary, the wider ketogenic landscape has expanded considerably both in application and implementation. Although the traditional KD therapy is still extensively used today, it also has been the basis for development of alternative ketogenic protocols. Fifty years after first reports in the 1970s of a KD incorporating medium-chain fatty acids, the KD is used for many children and adolescents, who benefit from the generous carbohydrate allowance facilitated by the increased ketogenic potential of medium-chain triglycerides (MCT). More recently, less restrictive dietary approaches have been developed, including the low-glycemic-index treatment and the modified Atkins diet (MAD). As the advantages of a more liberal KD have been recognized, especially for adults and older children, more liberal approaches are now being used worldwide and are supported by an increasing body of scientific data. This chapter explores the background and evidence for use of the alternative KDs.

THE MCT KD

The predominant fatty acids in the human diet contain 12 or more carbon atoms and originate from animal and plant sources of long-chain triglycerides (LCT), which can be saturated, monounsaturated, or polyunsaturated. The shorter-chain-length medium-chain fatty acids (6 to 12 carbon atoms) originate from MCT, whose main constituents are octanoic (C8) and decanoic (C10) fatty acids. MCT have distinct physical and metabolic differences from LCT, including more efficient digestion and absorption and a mitochondrial transport process facilitating faster metabolism to acetyl CoA. Hepatic ketone body production is primarily determined by the rate of acetyl CoA generation, which led to suggestions by Huttenlocher and colleagues that a KD

replacing LCT with MCT would induce higher ketosis and allow inclusion of significantly more carbohydrate and protein, improving palatability and acceptance. After an initial trial of a KD providing 60% of dietary energy from MCT in 12 children and adolescents with epilepsy (Huttenlocher et al., 1971), further results were reported from 18 patients ages 1.5 to 18 years, of whom 16 had over 50% seizure reduction (Huttenlocher et al., 1976).

Interest in the MCT diet continued, with further studies reported from the United States (Trauner et al., 1985), United Kingdom (Sills et al., 1986), and Taiwan (Mak et al., 1999). A dietary modification with less MCT (30% of energy) was suggested in response to concerns about gastrointestinal side effects of higher MCT intakes (Schwartz et al., 1989). In 2008, researchers based at Great Ormond Street Hospital in London published a trial of classic and MCT KDs in intractable childhood epilepsy in which children 2 to 16 years old were randomized to receive a diet either immediately or after a 3-month delay with no additional treatment changes (control group). After 3 months, seizure frequency was significantly lower in the 54 children in the diet group than in the 49 controls (Neal et al., 2008a). A total of 125 of the children who were randomized received dietary treatment at some stage (61 classic KD and 64 MCT KD). Comparison of the two diet groups using an intention-to-treat analysis found no significant differences; 29% of the MCT group had over 50% seizure reduction at 3 months (Neal et al., 2009). Tolerability and withdrawals were not significantly different at 3 and 6 months, with no evidence that the MCT diet caused more gastrointestinal problems; indeed, a history of vomiting was significantly higher in the children on the classic KD at 12 months. In this trial, the MCT diet was initiated at 40% to 50% energy from the MCT supplement, with the aim of providing the optimal balance between tolerance and good ketosis. However, many children

---

BOX 3.1
MCT DIETARY PROTOCOL

- Starting intake of 40% to 50% of energy as MCT given as prescribed supplement of oil or emulsion divided between all meals and snacks (MCT % can be increased as needed and tolerated during dietary fine-tuning)
- Protein: 10% of energy, increase to ≥ 12% if overall energy needs are low to ensure meeting protein requirements
- Carbohydrate: 15% to 18% of energy (may be lower in older children)
- Remaining 20% to 30% of energy as LCT (from foods)
- Food-choice lists or electronic calculation of recipes, all food weighed
- Stepwise increase to starting MCT dose over 1 to 2 weeks, during which rest of diet can be implemented as above, although may need extra LCT to maintain total energy intake if slower MCT introduction required
- Full vitamin and mineral supplementation
- Carbohydrate-free medications where possible

(Source: Neal, 2012)

---

and adolescents will need a higher intake to achieve optimal seizure control. Christiana Liu reported that in her extensive experience of using the MCT diet in Canada, MCT at 40% to > 70% of energy can be well tolerated without side effects (Liu & Wang, 2013). Prospective follow up of 48 children and adolescents aged 1–18 years on mostly (79%) the MCT diet has recently been reported from Holland. The responder rate was lower; only 17% achieved over 50% seizure reduction after 3 months, with seizure reduction increasing to 23% after 6 months (Lambrechts et al., 2015). A study of 16 Thai children with intractable seizures on the MCT diet reported more positive outcomes: 64% achieved over 50% seizure reduction at 3 months, and 29% were seizure-free (Chomtho et al., 2016).

The MCT diet is implemented using commercially available MCT oil or emulsion products (for example, Liquigen, Nutricia, 50% MCT; Betaquik, Vitaflo, 20% MCT), which in some countries are supplied via medical prescription. The remaining dietary energy is provided by carbohydrate, protein, and LCT. Calculation of this diet is not based on the ketogenic ratio but instead considers the percentage of dietary energy provided by macronutrients (Box 3.1). Total energy intake is controlled, as it is in the classic KD, although it will theoretically depend on the figure applied for energy content of MCT, which is lower than that for LCT (Ranhotra et al., 1995); this is not always

reflected in the conversion factors listed on the products or used for dietary calculation. The MCT diet is strictly prescribed, often with food-choice lists used to develop meal plans, and all food is weighed. The MCT diet is the most generous in carbohydrate of all ketogenic therapies (see Figure 3.1), and many children and adolescents benefit from the flexibility this offers. MCT are included in all meals and snacks, and compliance is improved by encouraging creative incorporation into recipes and ketogenic drinks. The MCT dose is slowly built up over the first week or two of treatment according to tolerance, ketosis, and seizure control.

Recent data indicate there may be specific efficacy benefits of medium-chain fatty acids. Neuronal cell line data from Hughes et al. (2014) suggested that C10 may increase mitochondrial proliferation, and Chang et al. (2013) found C10 significantly outperformed valproic acid in both in vitro and in vivo models of seizure control. These results suggest that MCT could have a more direct influence on seizure activity independent of ketosis, mediated via inhibition of excitatory AMPA receptors and changes in cell energetics through mitochondrial biogenesis (Augustin et al., 2018). The use of an add-on MCT supplement (without a full KD) in adults with epilepsy has been shown to be feasible and well tolerated, with early data suggesting efficacy benefits, although further studies are needed (Borges et al., 2109).

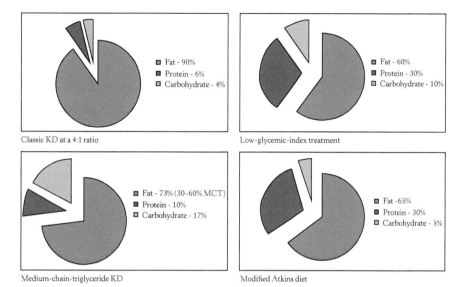

FIGURE 3.1 *Ketogenic Diet Therapies: Comparison of Dietary Energy Contribution from Macronutrients*

THE MAD

In 2003, Kossoff and colleagues at Johns Hopkins Hospital in Baltimore published a brief communication reporting their use of the Atkins diet in six patients with epilepsy (ages between 7 and 52 years); three patients had over 90% seizure reduction, and two of them became seizure free (Kossoff et al., 2003). The Atkins diet, designed in the 1970s as a weight-loss treatment, restricts carbohydrates and encourages fat in a way similar to the classic KD but allows free protein. It was suggested that this could be the basis of a less restrictive KD for epilepsy, the goal being seizure control rather than weight loss. The team at Johns Hopkins went on to trial the MAD in 20 children: 13 children achieved over 50% seizure reduction after 6 months, including four who became seizure-free (Kossoff et al., 2006). In a further study in 30 adults, seizures were reduced by over 50% in 10 patients after 6 months on the MAD (Kossoff et al., 2008a). The advantage of this diet is that it allows free protein and calories, so it can be easier to implement and to comply with than the classic KD. Although the MAD approximates a ketogenic ratio of 1:1 (see Figure 3.1), the only macronutrient strictly controlled on the MAD is carbohydrate. A randomized crossover comparison of daily carbohydrate limits in children suggested that a lower intake (10 g versus 20 g) during the initial 3 months of the MAD was associated with significantly higher likelihood of over 50% seizure reduction at 3 months, after which time carbohydrate could be increased (Kossoff et al., 2007).

The MAD has led the way in a shift of approach to implementation of KD therapy. Previously, the emphasis had been on absolute precision in calculation and accuracy in food weighing, albeit with very successful outcomes in many who followed the strict KD, but with compliance problems in others. As practitioners of the diet, we initially viewed what appeared to be the liberal MAD protocol with caution. Now, over 15 years on, the MAD is being increasingly adopted as an alternative KD that is especially suited to adolescents, adults, and those unable to comply with the stricter classic KD. The MAD is now used worldwide in children and adults (see Table 3.1, which shows studies that were included if they contained five or more subjects) with most centers prescribing the diet as recommended by Eric Kossoff and his team at Johns Hopkins (Box 3.2).

A 2012 review combined data from published MAD studies to examine responder rates. After 3 months of treatment, 54% of 105 children (six studies, both retrospective and prospective) and 34% of 56 adults (three studies, all prospective) had over 50% seizure reduction. Prospective data were available for 82 children (four studies), of whom 52% had over 50% seizure reduction after 3 months (Auvin, 2012). Kossoff and colleagues comprehensively reviewed 10 years of MAD, including all published primary studies in which the MAD was used as first dietary treatment as well as case reports of single patients. Of a combined total of 342 children, 53% had over 50% seizure reduction, with 15% achieving

TABLE 3.1 WORLDWIDE USE OF THE MODIFIED ATKINS DIET

Country	Study	Dietary Prescription—Daily Carbohydrate Allowance*
	Children and Adolescents	
Argentina	Vaccarezza et al., 2014 (Retrospective, $N = 9$)	10% energy
Denmark	Weber et al., 2009 (Prospective, $N = 15$)	10% energy, restricted further to 10 g
	Miranda et al., 2011 (Prospective, $N = 33$)	after 1–2 weeks if poor seizure control (Weber)
		10 g for first 3 months (Miranda)
Egypt	El-Rashidy et al., 2013 (Prospective, $N = 15$)	10 g for first month, then can increase by
	El-Rashidy et al., 2018 (Prospective, $N = 7$)	5-g increments up to 10% energy
France	Porta et al., 2009 (Prospective, $N = 10$)	10 g for first month, then can increase by
		5-g increments up to 10% energy
Germany (Austria & Switzerland)	Wiemer-Krewek et al., 2017 (Retrospective multi-centre, $N = 30$, Doose syndrome)	Mean 13.5 g (range 10–25 g at start, 10–30 g after diet modifications)
India	Sharma et al., 2012 (Prospective, $N = 15$)	10 g (Sharma)
	Sharma et al., 2013 (Randomized controlled trial, $N = 50$ in diet group)	5 g if < 18 months old, 10 g if 18 months to 3 years old (Mehta)
	Sharma et al., 2015 (Retrospective, $N = 25$, Lennox-Gastaut syndrome)	
	Sharma et al., 2016 (Randomized controlled trial of simplified MAD, $N = 41$ in diet group)	
	Mehta et al., 2016 (Prospective, $N = 31$)	
Iran	Tonekaboni et al., 2010 (Prospective, $N = 51$)	10 g
	Barzegar et al., 2010 (Prospective, $N = 21$)	10 g for first month, then increased up to
	Ghazavi et al., 2014 (Retrospective, $N = 20$)	20–30 g daily
Japan	Ito et al., 2011 (Retrospective, $N = 6$)	10 g initially (one child needed 30–20 g
	Kumada et al., 2012 (Prospective, $N = 10$)	step-down start—Kumada)
Korea	Kang et al., 2007 (Prospective, $N = 14$)	10 g for first month, then increase by 5-g
	Kim et al., 2012 (Retrospective, $N = 20$)	increments up to 10% energy*
	Park et al., 2018 (Retrospective, $N = 26$)	
Sweden	Svedlund et al., 2019 (Prospective, $N = 38$)	10–30 g*
United States	Kossoff et al., 2003 (Retrospective, $N = 6$)	10 g for 1–2 months, then increase by 5-g
	Kossoff et al., 2006 (Prospective, $N = 20$)	increments up to 20 g
	Kossoff et al., 2007 (Prospective, $N = 20$)	(20 g initially for five children with
	Kossoff et al., 2010a (Prospective, $N = 5$)	Sturge-Weber syndrome in 2010 paper)
	Kossoff et al., 2011a (Prospective, $N = 30$)	
	Groomes et al., 2011 (Retrospective, $N = 13$)	
	Adults	
Belgium	Carrette et al., 2008 (Prospective, $N = 8$)	20 g
Canada	Smith et al., 2011 (Prospective, $N = 18$)	20 g
Iran	Zare et al., 2017 (Randomized controlled trial, $N = 22$ in diet group)	15 g
Norway	Kverneland et al., 2015 (Prospective, $N = 13$)	16 g
	Kverneland et al., 2018 (Randomized controlled trial, $N = 37$ in diet group)	
United States	Kossoff et al., 2008a (Prospective, $N = 30$)	15 g
	Cervenka et al., 2012 (Prospective, $N = 25$)	20 g
	Kossoff et al., 2013a (Retrospective, $N = 8$)	20 g

* All studies allowed free calories except Kim et al. (2012), who reported using 75% of recommended daily energy requirements and Svedlund et al. (2019), who reported using 80% of recommended energy requirements.

BOX 3.2
MAD DIETARY PROTOCOL

- Carbohydrate for first month: 10 g daily for children, 10 to 15 g daily for adolescents, and 20 g daily for adults (does not include fiber but does include sugar alcohols)
- Encourage high-fat foods, eat with each meal/snack
- Free protein
- Free calories but need to avoid excess weight gain
- Full vitamin and mineral supplementation
- Carbohydrate-free medications
- Ketocal formula (Nutricia) can be used as daily supplement for first month
- After 1 month, daily carbohydrate allowance can be increased by 5 g monthly, with final amount depending on seizure control (generally ~ 20 g for children and 30 g for adults)
- Commercial low-carbohydrate products can be used after 1 month

(Source: Kossoff et al., 2011b)

---

seizure freedom; in a combined total of 92 adults, the response figures were lower, at 30% and 3%, respectively (Kossoff et al., 2013b).

The review included results from Sharma et al. (2013) in India, who published the first randomized trial of the MAD in 102 children (ages 2 to 14 years) with intractable epilepsy. Using a delayed diet-start control group in a design similar to that used by Neal et al. (2008a), Sharma and colleagues found that seizure frequency after 3 months was significantly lower in the 50 MAD-treated children than in the 52 controls (Sharma et al., 2013). Sharma et al. have also published results of a further trial in a similar group of

children using a simplified MAD implemented by household measures and standardized recipes instead of food weighing; seizure frequency at 3 months was again significantly lower in the 41 MAD-treated children than in 40 controls, and the diet was reported to be feasible and well tolerated (Sharma et al., 2016).

There have been two additional randomized trials of the MAD, both in adults. Kverneland et al. reported a significant reduction in seizure frequency in 37 adults with drug-resistant focal epilepsy after 12 weeks on the MAD compared to 38 controls, but only for the over 25% seizure reduction cutoff (Kverneland et al., 2018). Zare

---

BOX 3.3
MKD DIETARY PROTOCOL

- Specific carbohydrate target, usually started at 15 to 30 g daily (~ 5% of energy) and implemented by weighed portion list; may be reduced as needed during fine tuning
- Fat: ~ 65% to 80% of energy with specific targets, usually implemented by weighed portions and choice lists
- Protein: ~ 20% to 25% of energy but usually allowed "free" with no specific targets or portions; may be controlled during fine-tuning if needed
- Free calories but need to avoid excess weight gain
- Full vitamin and mineral supplementation
- Carbohydrate-free medications

(Source: Martin-McGill et al., 2019)

et al. (2017) compared responder rates after 2 months in MAD-treated (*n* = 22) and control (*n* = 32) groups of adults with intractable seizures; significantly better outcome was seen in the diet group (35% had over 50% seizure reduction, compared to no controls).

MODIFIED KETOGENIC DIET

A dietary variant adopted by mainly U.K. and some European centers, and described by Magrath et al. (2012), has been termed the modified KD (MKD). The MKD is distinguished from the MAD by a more generous initial carbohydrate allowance (up to 30 g, with further reduction during fine-tuning depending on seizure control) and a prescribed fat intake using food-choice lists. One study evaluated the feasibility of this approach in adults with refractory epilepsy and reported good tolerance of a 20-g daily carbohydrate, 70% fat energy MKD in 17 patients who started the diet (Martin-McGill et al., 2017). In survey of dietitians from 18 ketogenic centers in UK and Ireland using the MKD, all reported using weighed portion lists for carbohydrate and specific fat targets, and four also included protein targets (Martin-McGill et al., 2019; see Box 3.3). One U.S. study has retrospectively reviewed successful use of this approach in 55 adults on either 15 g or 50 g daily net carbohydrate intake, with personalized protein and fat goals; 60% had over 50% seizure reduction at 3 months, with no significant difference between the two carbohydrate groups, although significantly more of the lower carbohydrate group reported improvement in seizure severity and quality of life (Roehl et al., 2019).

LOW-GLYCEMIC-INDEX TREATMENT

The glycemic index (GI) is based on the blood glucose response to carbohydrate-containing foods (Jenkins et al., 1981). The GI is influenced by the rate of carbohydrate digestion and absorption, with more slowly absorbed foods having a lower GI rating. GI values are compared to a standard reference value of glucose. Other variables influencing the GI of a food include fiber content, cooking methods, processing, ripeness, and the combination of different macronutrients in a meal. Whole grains and other high-fiber foods will lower the meal's GI, as will the addition of fat or protein. Most vegetables and many fruits have a low GI.

BOX 3.4
LGIT DIETARY PROTOCOL

- Dietary goals set for carbohydrate, protein, and fat intake based on a target energy prescription
- Carbohydrate prescribed at 10% of energy (~ 40 to 60 g daily depending on baseline intake). This figure includes dietary fiber. Only carbohydrates with glycemic index < 50 allowed.
- Protein: ~ 30% of energy
- Fat: ~ 60% of energy
- Carbohydrate evenly distributed over the day and always eaten with some fat and/or protein
- Foods not weighed but based on household portion sizes
- Full vitamin and mineral supplementation
- Carbohydrate-free medications

(Source: Pfeifer, 2012)

Blood glucose levels tend to be stable when a person is on the low-carbohydrate KD, and this observation led to the suggestion that a diet based on only low GI carbohydrate (< 50) choices could maintain this glucose stability and facilitate a more liberal KD (see Figure 3.1). This alternative low-GI treatment (LGIT) (Box 3.4) was first tested by researchers from Boston: a preliminary retrospective review of 20 patients found half to have over 90% seizure reduction (Pfeifer & Thiele, 2005). Results were updated in 2009 with a larger review of 76 patients (ages 1.5 to 22 years); half of the patients had over 50% seizure reduction at 3 months, with the number increasing to 66% by 12 months (Muzykewicz et al., 2009). Interestingly, carbohydrate intake ranged from 15 to 150 g daily (mean 53 g at 3 months). Some individuals needed a more restricted amount for seizure control, whereas others were able to relax carbohydrate intake without adverse effect. The same group have successfully used LGIT in children with tuberous sclerosis (Larson et al., 2012), six children with Angelman syndrome studied prospectively (Thilbert et al., 2012), and a more recent retrospective review of 23 children with Angelman syndrome who were on LGIT for an average of 3 years. Most children experienced seizure reduction, and five were completely seizure-free; carbohydrate was prescribed at 45 g daily, while intakes ranged from 27 to 60 g (Grocott et al., 2017).

The LGIT is now used in many centers worldwide. Results in children and adolescents have been reported from Italy, where retrospective data on 15 patients showed more than half of patients with 50% seizure reduction after a mean treatment duration of 14 months (Coppola et al., 2011). In Iran, a prospective study of 42 patients reported over 50% seizure reduction in 74% of patients after 1 month (Karimzadeh et al., 2014). A review of the medical charts of 36 Korean patients (ages 1.5 to 28 years) on LGIT found that 56% had ≥ 50% seizure reduction after 3 months that was maintained by most for a year; two patients became seizure-free after 3 months, and again they maintained that result for a year (Kim et al., 2017). One case study reported a 13-year-old Japanese girl who was able to maintain a 50-g carbohydrate daily LGIT by choosing from specially designed menus that included unpolished rice and natto, which is made from fermented soybeans (Kumada et al., 2013).

A recent systematic review of eight LGIT studies concluded that, although further high-quality studies are needed, the diet had a beneficial effect in epilepsy, with palatability and side-effect advantages over other KDs; meta-analysis was not possible due to differences in outcome time points among the studies (Rezaei et al., 2018).

COMPARING ALTERNATIVE KDS WITH THE CLASSIC KD

With the range of KD therapies available, the initial clinic assessment consultation will include consideration of which diet to choose for an individual patient. A key question for those embarking on ketogenic therapy is which diet could work best to treat the seizures. Will an alternative protocol with potential compliance and tolerance advantages be as effective as the strict classic KD?

The scientific literature has also discussed this question, and certainly review of the many MAD trials shows results comparable to those for the KD (Kossoff et al., 2013b), including long-term follow-up data (Chen & Kossoff, 2012). Direct comparison trials of different KD therapies are limited. Neal et al. found no significant differences in the mean percentage of baseline seizures, or numbers with over 50% or 90% seizure

reduction, between the classic KD and MCT diet groups after 3, 6, and 12 months, and they concluded that the two KDs were comparable in efficacy and tolerability and both had their place in the treatment of childhood epilepsy (Neal et al., 2009).

A number of studies have looked to compare the classic KD and MAD. A retrospective review of children on the classic KD or MAD found significantly more KD children had greater than 50% seizure reduction at 3 months, but not at 6 months (Porta et al., 2009). A prospective evaluation of children on the MAD compared with a previously treated KD group found an initial trend toward greater KD efficacy disappeared when age-adjusted data were used (Miranda et al., 2011). Data from Iran on 40 children prescribed either the classic KD or MAD showed no significant difference in numbers achieving 50% seizure reduction after 1 to 3 months (Ghazavi et al., 2014). Other data suggest there may be benefits of a stricter diet. In a retrospectively analyzed multicenter group of 27 children switched from the MAD to the classic KD, additional seizure reduction was reported in 10, of whom five with Doose syndrome (myoclonic astatic epilepsy) became seizure-free; the authors identified the KD as a "higher dose" of KD therapy than the MAD (Kossoff et al., 2010b). Researchers in Egypt randomly assigned 40 young children (1 to 3 years old) to either classic KD fed by a liquid formula, MAD, or no diet treatment. After 3 months, the classic KD group showed significantly reduced seizure frequency and severity compared to the MAD group; at 6 months, the reduction in seizure frequency was still significant but not the reduction in severity (El-Rashidy et al., 2013).

Kim et al. have reported results of a randomized clinical trial on 104 Korean children and adolescents (ages 1 to 18 years) allocated to either classic KD (N = 51) or MAD (N = 53). The KD group had a lower mean percentage of baseline seizures at 3 months (39% KD versus 48% MAD) and 6 months (34% KD versus 45% MAD), but these differences were not statistically significant. The MAD was better tolerated and had fewer side effects. Significantly more of the 20 children aged 1 to 2 years became seizure-free on the KD (N = 9, 53%) than on the MAD (N = 4, 20%). This difference in seizure freedom was no longer significant at 6 months (N = 9, 53% of KD-treated, versus N = 5, 25% of MAD-treated). The authors concluded that the MAD might be considered as a first diet choice in children, but the classic KD is more suitable in children less than 2 years old (Kim et al., 2016).

A recent systematic review and meta-analysis compared short- and long-term diet efficacy from 70 classic KD and MAD studies in children and adolescents with intractable epilepsy. Pooled efficacy rates (≥ 50% seizure reduction) at 1, 3, 6, and 12 months on classic KD (N = 3,350) were 62%, 60%, 52%, and 42%; on MAD (N = 449) they were 55%, 47%, 42%, and 29%. Two studies were used to compare the classic KD and MAD at 3 months, and three studies were used for comparison at 6 months, with no significant differences in ≥ 50% seizure reduction (Rezaei et al., 2019).

Although one review of published studies on dietary treatment in adults with refractory epilepsy concluded that the classic KD and MAD were equally effective and tolerated (Klein et al., 2014), this was challenged by a meta-analysis of 12 studies on KD therapy in adults. The classic KD was used in six studies, the MAD in five, with one study using both classic and MCT KD. A total of 270 patients were evaluated, and there was a combined efficacy rate of 52% for classic KD and 34% for MAD, as well as an odds ratio for therapeutic success of classic KD relative to MAD of 2.04, a significant difference between the two types of diet. This analysis also examined compliance, which was significantly different between the two diets—38% for the classic KD and 56% for the MAD—which suggests that while the classic KD may be more effective in adults, it is not as well tolerated (Ye et al., 2015).

Suggestions that a stricter diet at the outset of treatment may be more efficacious have been supported by two randomized trials examining the use of different prescriptions within a particular ketogenic therapy. A lower carbohydrate MAD initiation (10 g versus 20 g) was associated with improved efficacy outcome (Kossoff et al., 2007), as was a higher classic KD ketogenic ratio (4:1 versus 3:1; Seo et al., 2007). In both of these studies, the benefits of an initial stricter diet were maintained even after carbohydrate intake was increased later in the course of treatment. Although it is now recognized that ketosis may not be directly linked to seizure control, any correlations between the two seem limited to the first 3 months of dietary treatment (Neal et al., 2009). Researchers at Johns Hopkins found better responder rates in 30 children who were given the 4:1 ratio classic KD supplement Ketocal (Nutricia) daily during the first month of the MAD when compared to published results of MAD alone (Kossoff et al., 2011a). This practice is now regularly implemented at Johns Hopkins (see Box 3.2) However, the same group studied this further in a recent clinical trial of 80 adults on the MAD, who were randomized to start the diet with or without supplemental Ketocal for the first month. There was no significant difference in seizure outcomes between the two groups, although significantly more of the supplemented group stayed on the diet for 6 months or more (McDonald et al., 2018a).

OTHER CONSIDERATIONS IN DIET CHOICE

The question of which diet to use will also consider a patient's age, lifestyle, food preferences, and feeding method. As illustrated in Figure 3.1, alternative dietary protocols have less fat than the classic KD as a proportion of overall dietary energy. The MCT diet is the most generous in carbohydrate, but consideration must be given to the need to incorporate the MCT supplement into all meals and snacks and the use of a strict prescription with food weighing. However, this approach can work well for those who find it too difficult to follow a stricter carbohydrate restriction and need a more structured dietary prescription. Adolescents and adults usually prefer the flexibility of the MAD, with no food weighing and free protein and calories; to maintain ongoing compliance, the MAD or the MKD would routinely be recommended for these age groups. If the patient is unable to adhere to the MAD's stricter carbohydrate restrictions, an alternative would be LGIT. The classic KD is recommended for all ages if the patient is using a feeding tube and for infants less than 2 years old; it may also be preferable for children who have poor appetites and need small meals, for the nutritionally at risk, and for families who require close supervision of meal planning and control of their child's energy intake. In cases where it is clear that both the child and the family would be unable to comply with the high-fat classic KD, the MAD, MKD, and MCT are better options. Prospective follow-up of a small group of Egyptian children who started the MAD after being unable to tolerate the restrictions of a classic KD reported improved growth, seizure control, and maternal quality of life (El-Rashidy et al., 2018).

In view of its reduced demands on time for training and supervision, the MAD is often first choice in centers with fewer dietitians. The MAD's potential for use in resource-poor countries with more limited dietetic support has been identified (Kossoff et al., 2008b; Satte et al., 2017), including the possibility of email-based management in adults (Cervenka et al., 2012). However, the MAD and LGIT require patients or families to design their own meals from the food choices given; in some situations, such as a residential multi-carer setting, this may be more difficult and require greater dietetic input, such as the additional control provided by the MKD.

The stricter classic KD has been recommended in epilepsy syndromes where rapid improvement is needed, such as infantile spasms or status epilepticus (Auvin, 2012) and in glucose transporter type 1 (GLUT1) deficiency syndrome and Doose syndrome (Miranda et al., 2012), although the MAD has been used successfully in both infantile spasms (Sharma et al., 2012) and GLUT1 deficiency syndrome (Ito et al., 2011). Following observed benefits in Doose syndrome children changed from the MAD to classical KD, this switch can be considered in this group if not seizure free after 6 to 12 months on MAD (Kossoff et al., 2010b).

ALTERNATIVE DIETS IN PRACTICE—INITIATION, FOLLOW-UP, AND RISK OF COMPLICATIONS

Medical contraindications to KD therapy are detailed in recommendations for clinical KD management (Kossoff et al., 2009, 2018). The contraindications apply to both classic and alternative KDs and should be excluded prior to initiation using necessary baseline biochemistry. Although some centers hospitalize children upon initiation of the MCT diet, as with the classic KD, it is now generally accepted that the MCT diet can be started at home without any prior fasting period. The daily intake of MCT will be increased stepwise as tolerated (Box 3.1). The MAD, MKD, and LGIT are started on an outpatient basis. All dietary protocols require full vitamin and mineral supplementation to ensure that the requirements for micronutrients are met. Adequate training from the ketogenic team must be given prior to initiation of any KD therapy to ensure that patients and carers understand the dietary prescription and how to manage practicalities at home, including strategies for illness and acute situations.

All diets need careful monitoring to ensure safe implementation. Home monitoring will include regular weight checks, which are important on the MAD, MKD, and LGIT where the calorie content is not strictly prescribed. Traditionally, on the KD ketones were checked

up to twice daily at home because good ketosis was thought to be key to treatment success. This premise has been challenged by alternative diets where ketones are often lower. Regular home testing of blood (or urinary) ketones is recommended on the MCT diet but levels are not as high as those seen on the classic KD (Neal et al., 2009). After the first month of the MAD, with a relaxing of dietary restrictions, ketones will usually be much lower than those seen on the KD, especially in adolescents and adults, and testing frequency can be reduced (Kossoff et al., 2011b), although it has been suggested that consistently high ketones above 3 mmol/L (blood β-hydroxybutyrate) in children on the MAD could be important for maintaining efficacy (Kang et al., 2007). On the LGIT, ketones will usually be very low or even undetectable in some cases; no correlation was seen between ketosis and seizures on this diet (Grocott et al., 2017; Muzykewicz et al., 2009).

Clinic monitoring at regular follow-up visits includes full laboratory studies, growth assessment, review of seizures, diet tolerance, and other diet-related benefits or adverse events. Side effects have been reported with the MCT diet, primarily gastrointestinal and they are usually managed with dietary manipulation (Liu & Wang, 2013; Neal et al., 2009). Gastrointestinal symptoms (including constipation) have also been reported as side effects of the MAD (Auvin, 2012; Chen & Kossoff, 2012; Kang et al., 2007; Sharma et al., 2013). Growth faltering has been reported in children on MCT diets, similar to that seen in children on a classic KD, despite the significantly higher protein intake on the MCT diet (Neal et al., 2008b). A recent prospective 24-month follow-up of 38 children on the MAD did not find any problems with longitudinal growth or bone mass (Svedlund et al., 2019). Raised lipid levels on the MAD have been reported in children (Kang et al., 2007) and adults (Cervenka et al., 2014); the increases were transient and normalized within a year of treatment. The group studying adults further investigated biochemical and vascular markers of cardiovascular health in 20 adult patients on MAD for over a year compared to 21 controls. The MAD group had significantly lower weight, body mass index, waist and hip circumference, percent body fat, and serum triglyceride levels but higher serum levels of small LDL particles; there was no difference in carotid intima-media thickness or in presence of plaques between groups. Although the authors concluded this demonstrated the MAD's cardiovascular safety, they highlighted the importance of monitoring the LDL particles as markers of risk (McDonald et al., 2018b). There are few reports of side effects in LGIT studies; those mentioned include increases in blood urea nitrogen in about a third of patients (Karimzadeh et al., 2014; Muzykewicz et al., 2009). Grocott et al. (2017) noted that nine of their 23 patients with Angelman syndrome experienced side effects on the diet; the patients included two with low carnitine levels that resolved with supplementation, two with diet-induced constipation, and two with possible acidosis.

Fine-tuning of KD therapy aims to alleviate any side effects and to optimize seizure outcomes. Adjustments to prescriptions and micronutrient supplementation will also be needed as a child grows older. The MCT dose may be increased or decreased on the MCT diet, as can carbohydrate intake, with the goal of maximizing benefit. MCT has also been used as an addition to the MAD or MKD, giving a boost to ketosis and seizure control and aiding compliance by facilitating increased carbohydrate allowance. This practice is evidence of a more flexible approach to KD therapy, which involves designing an individualized treatment based primarily on specific dietary and lifestyle requirements, rather than on a rigid diet protocol that is offered by a particular hospital center. The approach may primarily utilize one type of diet, but alternatively may use different aspects of some, or indeed all, of the KD therapies. Well-defined dietary parameters are needed for conducting research studies, but anecdotal reports suggest more dietitians are tending toward this "patient-tailored" prescription of KD therapy in clinical practice (Miranda et al., 2012).

CONCLUSION

As worldwide use of the KD continues to grow, it is clear that alternative dietary protocols have an important place in the treatments offered to children and adults with intractable seizures. The MAD, in particular, has emerged as a KD therapy with great potential for treating not only children with epilepsy, but also adults and those in countries with more limited resources. Further research will enable us to optimize protocols for clinical implementation to ensure the best possible outcome for those embarking on dietary treatment of epilepsy.

REFERENCES

Augustin, K., Khabbush, A., Williams, S., Eaton, S., Orford, M., Cross, J. H., Heales, S. J. R., Walker, M. C., & Williams, R. S. B. (2018). Mechanisms of action for the medium-chain triglyceride ketogenic diet in neurological and metabolic disorders. *Lancet Neurology, 17*(1), 84–93.

Auvin, S. (2012). Should we routinely use modified Atkins diet instead of regular ketogenic diet to treat children with epilepsy? *Seizure, 21*, 237–240.

Barzegar, M., Irandoust, P., & Ebrahimi Mameghani, M. (2010). Modified Atkins diet for intractable childhood epilepsy. *Iranian Journal of Child Neurology, 4*(3), 6.

Borges, K., Kaul, N., Germaine, J., Kwan, P., & O'Brien, T. J. (2019). Randomized trial of add-on triheptanoin vs medium chain triglycerides in adults with refractory epilepsy. *Epilepsia Open, 4*(1), 153–163.

Carrette, E., Vonck, K., de Herdt, V., Dewaele, I., Raedt, R., Goossens, L., Van Zandijcke, M., Wadman, W., Thadani, V., & Boon, P. (2008). A pilot trial with modified Atkins' diet in adult patients with refractory epilepsy. *Clinical Neurology and Neurosurgery, 110*, 797–803.

Cervenka, M. C., Terao, N. N., Bosarge, J. L., Henry, B. J., Klees, A. A., Morrison, P. F., & Kossoff, E. H. (2012). E-mail management of the modified Atkins diet for adults with epilepsy is feasible and effective. *Epilepsia, 53*, 728–732.

Cervenka, M. C., Patton, K., Eloyan, A., Henry, B., & Kossoff, E. H. (2014). The impact of the modified Atkins diet on lipid profiles in adults with epilepsy. *Nutritional Neuroscience, 19*(3), 131–137.

Chang, P., Terbach, N., Plant, N., Chen, P. E., Walker, M. C., & Williams, R. S. (2013). Seizure control by ketogenic diet-associated medium chain fatty acids. *Neuropharmacology, 69*, 105–114.

Chen, W., & Kossoff, E. H. (2012). Long-term follow-up of children treated with the modified Atkins diet. *Journal of Child Neurology, 27*, 754–758.

Chomtho, K., Suteerojntrakool, O., & Chomtho, S. (2016). Effectiveness of medium chain triglyceride ketogenic diet in Thai children with intractable epilepsy. *Journal of the Medical Association of Thailand, 99*(2), 159–165.

Coppola, G., D'Aniello, A., Messana, T., Di Pasquale, F., della Corte, R., Pascotto, A., & Verrotti, A. (2011). Low glycemic index diet in children and young adults with refractory epilepsy: First Italian experience. *Seizure, 20*, 526–528.

El-Rashidy, O. F., Nassar, M. F., Abdel-Hamid, I. A., Shatla, R. H., Abdel-Hamid, M. H., Gabr, S. S., Mohamed, S. G., El-Sayed, W. S., & Shaaban, S. Y. (2013). Modified Atkins diet vs classic ketogenic formula in intractable epilepsy. *Acta Neurologica Scandinavica, 128*, 402–408.

El Rashidy, O. F., Nassar, M. F., El Gendy, Y. G., Deifalla, S. M., & Gaballa, S. (2018). Experience with MAD on children with epilepsy in Egypt after classic KD failure. *Acta Neurologica Scandinavica, 137*(2), 195–198.

Ghazavi, A., Tonekaboni, S. H., Karimzadeh, P., Nikibakhsh, A. A., Khajeh, A., & Fayyazi, A. (2014). The ketogenic and Atkins diets effect on intractable epilepsy: A comparison. *Iranian Journal of Child Neurology, 8*, 12–17.

Grocott, O. R., Herrington, K. S., Pfeifer, H. H., Thiele, E. A., & Thibert, R. L. (2017). Low glycemic index treatment for seizure control in Angelman syndrome: A case series from the Center for Dietary Therapy of Epilepsy at the Massachusetts General Hospital. *Epilepsy & Behavior, 68*, 45–50.

Groomes, L. B., Pyzik, P. L., Turner, Z., Dorward, J. L., Goode, V. H., & Kossoff, E. H. (2011). Do patients with absence epilepsy respond to ketogenic diets? *Journal of Child Neurology, 26*, 160–165.

Hughes, S. D., Kanabus, M., Anderson, G., Hargreaves, I. P., Rutherford, T., O'Donnell, M., Cross, J. H., Rahman, S., Eaton, S., & Heales, S. J. (2014). The ketogenic diet component decanoic acid increases mitochondrial citrate synthase and complex I activity in neuronal cells. *Journal of Neurochemistry, 129*, 426–433.

Huttenlocher, P. R. (1976). Ketonaemia and seizures: Metabolic and anticonvulsant effects of two ketogenic diets in childhood epilepsy. *Pediatric Research, 10*, 536–540.

Huttenlocher, P. R., Wilbourne, A. J., & Sigmore, J. M. (1971). Medium chain triglycerides as a therapy for intractable childhood epilepsy. *Neurology, 1*, 1097–1103.

Ito, Y., Oguni, H., Ito, S., Oguni, M., & Osawa, M. (2011). A modified Atkins diet is promising as a treatment for glucose transporter type 1 deficiency syndrome. *Developmental Medicine & Child Neurology, 53*, 658–663.

Jenkins, D. J., Wolever, T. M., Taylor, R. H., Barker, H., Fielden, H., Baldwin, J. M., Bowling, A. C., Newman, H. C., Jenkins, A. L., & Goff, D. V. (1981). Glycemic index of foods: A physiological basis for carbohydrate exchange. *American Journal of Clinical Nutrition, 34*, 362–366.

Kang, H. C., Lee, H. S., You, S. J., Kang, du C., Ko, T. S., & Kim, H. D. (2007). Use of a modified Atkins diet in intractable childhood epilepsy. *Epilepsia, 48*, 182–186.

Karimzadeh, P., Sedighi, M., Beheshti, M., Azargashb, E., Ghofrani, M., & Abdollahe-Gorgi, F. (2014). Low glycemic index treatment in pediatric refractory epilepsy: The first Middle East report. *Seizure, 23*, 570–572.

Kim, J. A., Yoon, J. R., Lee, E. J., Lee, J. S., Kim, J. T., Kim, H. D., & Kang, H. C. (2016). Efficacy of the classic ketogenic and the modified Atkins diets in refractory childhood epilepsy. *Epilepsia, 57*(1), 51–58.

Kim, S. H., Kang, H. C., Lee, E. J., Lee, J. S., & Kim, H. D. (2017). Low glycemic index treatment in patients with drug-resistant epilepsy. *Brain & Development, 39*(8), 687–692.

Kim, Y. M., Vaidya, V. V., Khusainov, T., Kim, H. D., Kim, S. H., Lee, E. J., Lee, Y. M., Lee, J. S., & Kang, H. C. (2012). Various indications for a modified Atkins diet in intractable childhood epilepsy. *Brain & Development, 34*, 570–575.

Klein, P., Tyrlikova, I., & Mathews, G. C. (2014). Dietary treatment in adults with refractory epilepsy: A review. *Neurology, 83*, 1978–1985.

Kossoff, E. H., Bosarge, J. L., & Comi, A. M. (2010a). A pilot study of the modified Atkins diet for Sturge-Weber syndrome. *Epilepsy Research, 92*, 240–243.

Kossoff, E. H., Bosarge, J. L., Miranda, M. J., Wiemer-Kruel, A., Kang, H. C., & Kim, H. D. (2010b). Will seizure control improve by switching from the modified Atkins diet to the traditional ketogenic diet? *Epilepsia, 51*, 2496–2499.

Kossoff, E. H., Cervenka, M. C., Henry, B. J., Haney, C. A., & Turner, Z. (2013b). A decade of the modified Atkins diet (2003–2013): Results, insights, and future directions. *Epilepsy & Behavior, 29*, 437–442.

Kossoff, E. H., Dorward, J. L., Molinero, M. R., & Holden, K. R. (2008b). The modified Atkins diet: A potential treatment for developing countries. *Epilepsia, 49*, 1646–1647.

Kossoff, E. H., Dorward, J. L., Turner, Z., & Pyzik, P. (2011a). Prospective study of the modified Atkins diet in combination with a ketogenic liquid supplement during the initial month. *Journal of Child Neurology, 26*, 147–151.

Kossoff, E. H., Freeman, J. M., Turner, Z., & Rubenstein, J. E. (2011b). *Ketogenic diets: Treatments for epilepsy and other disorders* (5th ed.). Demos Medical Publishing.

Kossoff, E. H., Henry, B. J., & Cervenka, M. C. (2013a). Efficacy of dietary therapy for juvenile myoclonic epilepsy. *Epilepsy & Behavior, 26*, 162–164.

Kossoff, E. H., Krauss, G. L., McGrogan, J. R., & Freeman, J. M. (2003). Efficacy of the Atkins diet as therapy for intractable epilepsy. *Neurology, 61*, 1789–1791.

Kossoff, E. H., McGrogan, J. R., Bluml, R. M., Pillas, D. J., Rubenstein, J. E., & Vining, E. P. (2006). A modified Atkins diet is effective for the treatment of intractable pediatric epilepsy. *Epilepsia, 47*, 421–424.

Kossoff, E. H., Rowley, H., Sinha, S. R., & Vining, E. P. (2008a). A prospective study of the modified Atkins diet for intractable epilepsy in adults. *Epilepsia, 49*, 316–319.

Kossoff, E. H., Turner, Z., Bluml, R. M., Pyzik, P. L., & Vining, E. P. (2007). A randomized, crossover comparison of daily carbohydrate limits using the modified Atkins diet. *Epilepsy & Behavior, 10*, 432–436.

Kossoff, E. H., Zupec-Kania, B. A., Amark, P. E., Ballaban-Gil, K. R., Bergqvist, A. G., Blackford, R., Buchhalter, J. R., Caraballo, R. H., Cross, J. H., Dahlin, M. G., Donner, E. J., Klepper, J., Jehle, R.

S., Kim, H. D., Liu, Y. M., Nation, J., Nordli Jr, D. J, Pfeifer, H. H., Rho, J. M, . . . Vining, E. P. (2009). Optimal clinical management of children receiving the ketogenic diet: recommendations of the International Ketogenic Diet Study Group. *Epilepsia, 50*, 304–317.

Kossoff, E. H., Zupec-Kania, B. A., Auvin, S., Ballaban-Gil, K. R., Bergqvist, C. A. G., Blackford, R., Buchhalter, J. R., Caraballo, R. H., Cross, J. H., Dahlin, M. G., Donner, E. J., Guzel, O., Jehle, R. S., Klepper, J., Kang, H.-C., Lambrechts, D. A., Liu, Y. M., Nathan, J. K., Nordli Jr., D. R., . . .Wirrell, E. C. (2018). Optimal clinical management of children receiving dietary therapies for epilepsy: Updated recommendations of the International Ketogenic Diet Study Group. *Epilepsia Open, 3*(2), 175–192.

Kumada, T., Hiejima, I., Nozaki, F., Hayashi, A., & Fujii, T. (2013). Glycemic index treatment using Japanese foods in a girl with Lennox-Gastaut syndrome. *Pediatric Neurology, 48*, 390–392.

Kumada, T., Miyajima, T., Oda, N., Shimomura, H., Saito, K., & Fujii, T. (2012). Efficacy and tolerability of modified Atkins diet in Japanese children with medication-resistant epilepsy. *Brain & Development, 34*, 32–38.

Kverneland, M., Molteberg, E., Iversen, P. O., Veierød, M. B., Taubøll, E., Selmer, K. K., & Nakken, K. O. (2018). Effect of modified Atkins diet in adults with drug-resistant focal epilepsy: A randomized clinical trial. *Epilepsia, 59*(8), 1567–1576.

Kverneland, M., Selmer, K. K., Nakken, K. O., Iversen, P. O., & Taubøll, E. (2015). A prospective study of the modified Atkins diet for adults with idiopathic generalized epilepsy. *Epilepsy & Behavior, 53*, 197–201.

Lambrechts, D. A., de Kinderen, R. J., Vles, H. S., de Louw, A. J., Aldenkamp, A. P., & Majoie, M. J. (2015). The MCT-ketogenic diet as a treatment option in refractory childhood epilepsy: A prospective study with 2-year follow-up. *Epilepsy & Behavior, 51*, 261–266.

Larson, A. M., Pfeifer, H. H., & Thiele, E. A. (2012). Low glycemic index treatment for epilepsy in tuberous sclerosis complex. *Epilepsy Research, 99*, 180–182.

Liu, Y. M., & Wang, H. S. (2013). Medium-chain triglyceride ketogenic diet, an effective treatment for drug-resistant epilepsy and a comparison with other ketogenic diets. *Biomedical Journal, 36*, 9–15.

Magrath, G., Leung, M. A., & Randall, T. (2012). The modified Atkins diet. In E. G. Neal (Ed.), *Dietary treatment of epilepsy* (pp. 89–99). Wiley-Blackwell.

Mak, S. C., Chi, C. S., & Wan, C. J. (1999). Clinical experience of ketogenic diet on children with refractory epilepsy. *Acta Paediatrica Taiwan, 40*, 97–100.

Martin-McGill, K. J., Jenkinson, M. D., Tudor Smith, C., & Marson, A. G. (2017). The modified ketogenic diet for adults with refractory epilepsy: An evaluation of a set up service. *Seizure, 52*, 1–6.

Martin-McGill, K. J., Lambert, B., Whiteley, V. J., Wood, S., Neal, E. G., Simpson, Z. R., Schoeler, N. E.; Ketogenic Dietitians Research Network (KDRN). (2019). Understanding the core principles of a 'modified ketogenic diet': A UK and Ireland perspective. *Journal of Human Nutrition and Dietetics, 32*(3), 385–390.

McDonald, T. J. W., Henry-Barron, B. J., Felton, E. A., Gutierrez, E. G., Barnett, J., Fisher, R., Lwin, M., Jan, A., Vizthum, D., Kossoff, E. H., & Cervenka, M. C. (2018a). Improving compliance in adults with epilepsy on a modified Atkins diet: A randomized trial. *Seizure, 60*, 132–138.

McDonald, T. J. W., Ratchford, E. V., Henry-Barron, B. J., Kossoff, E. H., & Cervenka, M. C. (2018b). Impact of the modified Atkins diet on cardiovascular health in adults with epilepsy. *Epilepsy & Behavior, 79*, 82–86.

Mehta, R., Goel, S., Sharma, S., Jain, P., Mukherjee, S. B., & Aneja, S. (2016). Efficacy and tolerability of the modified Atkins diet in young children with refractory epilepsy: Indian experience. *Annals of Indian Academy of Neurology, 19*(4), 523–527.

Miranda, M. J., Mortensen, M., Povlsen, J. H., Nielsen, H., & Beniczky, S. (2011). Danish study of a modified Atkins diet for medically intractable epilepsy in children: Can we achieve the same results as with the classical ketogenic diet? *Seizure, 20*, 151–155.

Miranda, M. J., Turner, Z., & Magrath, G. (2012). Alternative diets to the classical ketogenic diet— Can we be more liberal? *Epilepsy Research, 100*, 278–285.

Muzykewicz, D. A., Lyczkowski, D. A., Memon, N., Conant, K. D., Pfeifer, H. H., & Thiele, E. A. (2009). Efficacy, safety, and tolerability of the low glycemic index treatment in pediatric epilepsy. *Epilepsia, 50*, 1118–1126.

Neal, E. G. (2012). The medium chain ketogenic diet. In E. G. Neal (Ed.), *Dietary treatment of epilepsy* (pp. 78–88). Wiley-Blackwell.

Neal, E. G., Chaffe, H. M., Edwards, N., Lawson, M., Schwartz, R., & Cross, J. H. (2008b). Growth of children on classical and MCT ketogenic diets. *Pediatrics, 122*, e334–340.

Neal, E. G., Chaffe, H. M., Schwartz, R., Edwards, N., Fitzsimmons, G., Whitney, A., & Cross, J. H. (2009). A randomized trial of classical and medium-chain triglyceride ketogenic diets in the treatment of childhood epilepsy. *Epilepsia, 49*, 1–9.

Neal, E. G., Chaffe, H. M., Schwartz, R., Lawson, M., Edwards, N., Fitzsimmons, G., Whitney, A., & Cross, J. H. (2008a). The ketogenic diet in the treatment of epilepsy: A randomised controlled trial. *Lancet Neurology, 7*, 500–506.

Park, E. G., Lee, J., & Lee, J. (2018). Use of the modified Atkins diet in intractable pediatric epilepsy. *Journal of Epilepsy Research, 8*(1), 20–26.

Pfeifer, H. H. (2012). The low glycaemic index treatment. In E. G. Neal (Ed.), *Dietary treatment of epilepsy* (pp. 100–108). Wiley-Blackwell.

Pfeifer, H. H., & Thiele, E. (2005). Low glycemic index treatment: A liberalized ketogenic diet for treatment of intractable epilepsy. *Neurology, 65,* 1810–1812.

Porta, N., Vallée, L., Boutry, E., Fontaine, M., Dessein, A. F., Joriot, S., Cuisset, J. M., Cuvellier, J. C., & Auvin, S. (2009). Comparison of seizure reduction and serum fatty acid levels after receiving the ketogenic and modified Atkins diet. *Seizure, 18,* 359–364.

Ranhotra, G. S., Gelroth, J. A., & Glaser, B. K. (1995). Levels of medium-chain triglycerides and their energy value. *Cereal Chemistry, 72,* 365–367.

Rezaei, S., Abdurahman, A. A., Saghazadeh, A., Badv, R. S., & Mahmoudi, M. (2019). Short-term and long-term efficacy of classical ketogenic diet and modified Atkins diet in children and adolescents with epilepsy: A systematic review and meta-analysis. *Nutritional Neuroscience, 22*(5), 317–334.

Rezaei, S., Harsini, S., Kavoosi, M., Badv, R. S., & Mahmoudi, M. (2018). Efficacy of low glycemic index treatment in epileptic patients: A systematic review. *Acta Neurologica Belgica, 118*(3), 339–349.

Roehl, K., Falco-Walter, J., Ouyang, B., & Balabanov, A. (2019). Modified ketogenic diets in adults with refractory epilepsy: Efficacious improvements in seizure frequency, seizure severity, and quality of life. *Epilepsy & Behavior, 93,* 113–118.

Satte, A., Kossoff, E. H., Belghiti, M., Zerhouni, A., Ouhabi, H., Guerinech, H., & Mounach, J. (2017). Why should modified Atkins diet be encouraged for treating epilepsy in emerging countries? *African Health Sciences, 17*(2), 556–558.

Schwartz, R. H., Eaton, J., Bower, B. D., & Aynsley-Green, A. (1989). Ketogenic diets in the treatment of epilepsy: Short term clinical effects. *Developmental Medicine & Child Neurology, 31,* 145–151.

Seo, J. H., Lee, Y. M., Lee, J. S., Kang, H. C., & Kim H. D. (2007). Efficacy and tolerability of the ketogenic diet according to lipid:nonlipid ratios—Comparison of 3:1 with 4:1 diet. *Epilepsia, 48,* 801–805.

Sharma, S., Goel, S., Jain, P., Agarwala, A., & Aneja, S. (2016). Evaluation of a simplified modified Atkins diet for use by parents with low levels of literacy in children with refractory epilepsy: A randomized controlled trial. *Epilepsy Research, 127,* 152–159.

Sharma, S., Jain, P., Gulati, S., Sankhyan, N., & Agarwala A. (2015). Use of the modified Atkins diet in Lennox Gastaut syndrome. *Journal of Child Neurology, 30,* 576–579.

Sharma, S., Sankhyan, N., Gulati, S., & Agarwala, A. (2012). Use of the modified Atkins diet in infantile spasms refractory to first-line treatment. *Seizure, 21,* 45–48.

Sharma, S., Sankhyan, N., Gulati, S., & Agarwala, A. (2013). Use of the modified Atkins diet for treatment of refractory childhood epilepsy: A randomized controlled trial. *Epilepsia, 54,* 481–486.

Sills, M. A., Forsythe, W. I., Haidukewych, D., MacDonald, A., & Robinson, M. (1986). The medium chain triglyceride diet and intractable epilepsy. *Archives of Disease in Childhood, 61,* 1168–1172.

Smith, M., Politzer, N., MacGarvie, D., McAndrews, M. P., & Del Campo, M. (2011). Efficacy and tolerability of the modified Atkins diet in adults with pharmacoresistant epilepsy: A prospective observational study. *Epilepsia, 52,* 775–780.

Svedlund, A., Hallböök, T., Magnusson, P., Dahlgren, J., & Swolin-Eide, D. (2019). Prospective study of growth and bone mass in Swedish children treated with the modified Atkins diet. *European Journal of Paediatric Neurology, S1090-3798*(18), 30554–3.

Thibert, R. L., Pfeifer, H. H., Larson, A. M., Raby, A. R., Reynolds, A. A., Morgan, A. K., & Thiele, E. A. (2012). Low glycemic index treatment for seizures in Angelman syndrome. *Epilepsia, 53,* 1498–1502.

Tonekaboni, S. H., Mostaghimi, P., Mirmiran, P., Abbaskhanian, A., Abdollah Gorji, F., Ghofrani, M., & Azizi, F. (2010). Efficacy of the Atkins diet as therapy for intractable epilepsy in children. *Archives of Iranian Medicine, 13,* 492–497.

Trauner, D. A. (1985). Medium chain triglyceride diet in intractable seizure disorders. *Neurology, 35,* 237–238.

Vaccarezza, M. M., Toma, M. V., Ramos Guevara, J. D., Diez, C. G., & Agosta, G. E. (2014). Treatment of refractory epilepsy with the modified Atkins diet. *Archivos Argentinos de Pediatria, 112,* 348–351.

Weber, S., Mølgaard, C., Taudorf, K., & Uldall, P. (2009). Modified Atkins diet to children and adolescents with medical intractable epilepsy. *Seizure, 18,* 237–240.

Wiemer-Kruel, A., Haberlandt, E., Hartmann, H., Wohlrab, G., & Bast, T. (2017). Modified Atkins diet is an effective treatment for children with Doose syndrome. *Epilepsia, 58*(4), 657–662.

Ye, F., Li, X. J., Jiang, W. L., Sun, H. B., & Liu, J. (2015). Efficacy of and patient compliance with a ketogenic diet in adults with intractable epilepsy: A meta-analysis. *Journal of Clinical Neurology, 11,* 26–31.

Zare, M., Okhovat, A. A., Esmaillzadeh, A., Mehvari, J., Najafi, M. R., & Saadatnia, M. (2017). Modified Atkins diet in adult with refractory epilepsy: A controlled randomized clinical trial. *Iranian Journal Neurology, 16*(2), 72–77.

4

Ketogenic Diet Therapies in Adults

History, Demand, and Results

EMILY L. JOHNSON, MD, PHD AND MACKENZIE C. CERVENKA, MD

HISTORY

Diet therapy has been used for the treatment of epilepsy since antiquity. Hippocrates wrote of fasting "purifications" as a cure for seizures and reported that some of his contemporaries believed certain foods, such as eel and goat, exacerbated or caused seizures (Hippocrates, c. 400 BC). In the Roman era, drinking gladiators' blood was thought to be a cure for epilepsy (Barborka, 1929).

In modern times, intermittent fasting has been studied for over 100 years. Guelpa and Marie described a cyclical regimen of 4 days of fasting and purges followed by 4 days of a restricted vegetarian diet. Three-quarters of the 20 patients (adults and adolescents) with epilepsy who were studied could not adhere to the diet for more than one cycle. Of the remaining patients, those who followed the diet had significant benefit and in some cases had seizure remission; however, long-term compliance with the diet was limited (in more than one case, noncompliance was caused by friends of the patient who provided foods that were not permitted), and the physicians concluded that their regimen was too difficult for most adults to follow (Guelpa & Marie, 1911).

Geyelin at New York Presbyterian observed a 10-year-old boy with 4 years of refractory epilepsy (under the care of Conklin of Battle Creek) who became cured after intermittent fasting (four fasts over 4 months). Geyelin then treated a 9-year-old boy with a 3-day fast; the boy's multiple daily seizures stopped after the second day. Geyelin went on to treat patients with intermittent fasting of lengthening duration (Geyelin, 1921) and expanded the treatments to adults as well as children. In 22 of 26 patients (ages 3 to 35 years), he observed seizure remission by the tenth day of fasting; 18 of 26 patients (69%) had marked improvement after 1 year of fasting and had no further seizures.

Wilder of the Mayo Clinic, analyzing Geyelin's work, was the first to speculate that

> the benefit . . . may be dependent on the ketonemia which must result from such fasts, and that possibly equal good results could be obtained if a ketonemia were produced by some other means. The ketone bodies, acetoacetic acid and its derivatives, are formed from fat and protein whenever a disproportion exists between the amount of fatty acid and the amount of sugar actually burning in the tissues. . . . It is possible to provoke ketosis by feeding diets which are very rich in fat and low in carbohydrate. It is proposed, therefore, to try the effect of such ketogenic diets on a series of epileptics. (Wilder, 1921)

The Mayo Clinic began treating adults with epilepsy with the "ketogenic diet" (KD) in 1924. Barborka wrote that "epileptic patients have an unusual ability to consume and utilize fat," and hypothesized that the benefits of ketosis may be due to changes in nerve cells, and "decreased irritability of nerves." General wisdom held that the acid–base balance contributed to seizures or seizure protection.

Barborka believed that the KD offered a "ray of hope" and recognized that while the diet was difficult, it was far better to try it than to "merely employ a sedative, and to wait."

Barborka published several articles on the Mayo Clinic experience with the KD. He emphasized the need for patient education and required patients to spend 2 to 3 weeks under strict supervision while learning the diet (Barborka, 1928). The diet was designed to mimic the metabolism of a fasting person in order to produce mild ketosis, using a method originally developed for diabetics. The target maintenance diet was calculated to have sufficient calories to maintain a neutral weight in adults; carbohydrates were limited in order to develop and maintain ketosis. The original diet consisted of six phases with varying amounts of carbohydrates and fat, with a stepwise decrease in the content of carbohydrates and an increase in the amount of fat. Sample menus reveal an emphasis on heavy cream (100 cc of 40% cream with each meal), mayonnaise, and butter (Barborka, 1929). Patients were educated to test their urine for ketosis.

In 1930, Barborka published the experience with a series of 100 adolescent and adult patients (16 to 51 years old) remaining on the diet from 3 months to 5 years. Twelve of the 100 patients achieved complete seizure remission on the KD, and of those, two relaxed to a less strict diet without food weighing and maintained seizure control. Seven patients had at least a 90% reduction in seizures, and 37 additional patients experienced significant benefit, giving a 56% response rate (Barborka, 1930). Of the 44 patients who had no improvement, 23 had not achieved ketosis (although some patients with substantial improvement lacked consistent ketosis as well).

Barborka reported that, in addition to seizure control, patients experienced an improvement in cognition, the "appearance of intelligence, more normal attitude," and decreased irritability.

Twelve of the 56 women in the study had complete cessation of their menses; the seven women who restarted a standard diet had resumption of normal menstrual cycles within a few months. One woman with a history of menorrhagia had normalization of her menstrual cycle.

Across the Atlantic, Bastible studied 29 institutionalized women with epilepsy in Dublin. The women's diet included low-carbohydrate biscuits made with local carrageen moss (*Chondrus crispus*), "an inexpensive seaweed found off the shores of Ireland . . . which gave excellent results." Two of the 29 women became seizure-free. Six of the remaining patients had a 50% to 90% decrease in seizures, and six had an increase in seizures. Bastible concluded that "there is a definite hope of improvement or cure" for adults with epilepsy (Bastible, 1931).

After the 1938 introduction of phenytoin, which was more straightforward to initiate and to maintain, the KD was used and studied less for the next seven decades (Jóźwiak et al., 2011).

DEMAND

Children Transitioning to Adult Epilepsy Providers

The KD for children is widely used and is growing in popularity; in 2013, there were 148 diet centers for children in North America, half of which had been established since 2000 (Jung et al., 2015). The KD is also used in over 40 countries worldwide (Kossoff & McGrogan, 2005). It is now estimated that there are thousands of children currently on the KD. While many children do not continue diet treatments into adulthood, there is a large and growing population of children who will transition to diet therapy as adults.

Not all children who are treated with the KD require transition to adult epilepsy care. Many children become seizure-free on the KD and are successfully weaned off the diet within 2 years; however, there is a risk of seizure recurrence with the change to a less restrictive diet.

At the Johns Hopkins Pediatric Ketogenic Diet Center, Martinez et al. reviewed 557 children who started the KD between 1993 and 2007 (Martinez et al., 2007). Sixty-six children who were seizure-free discontinued the diet (after median 2.1 years, range 0.5 to 8 years). Of those, 20% (13 children) had seizure recurrence up to 5.5 years after discontinuing the diet (median 2.4 years; minimum 0 years). Seven of those patients decided to restart the KD. Risk factors for recurrence included an abnormal MRI and an EEG with epileptiform abnormalities. Parents and patients with a higher risk of recurrence due to MRI and EEG findings may elect to continue diet therapy into adulthood.

Children and adolescents with chronic diseases require thoughtful transition from pediatric to adult specialists, generally at age 18; however, discussions and planning for this transition must take place much earlier. Kossoff et al. identified 10 patients who started the KD or the modified Atkins diet (MAD) as children (the MAD is typically limited to 10 g of net carbohydrates daily in children, with liberal fat intake, and 20 g in adults) in the pediatric epilepsy center, and who remained on diet therapy until at least age 18 (the mean age at initiation was 10.3 years, range 6 to 16). These patients remained on the diet from 4 to 32 years (mean, 15.5 years). All had good to complete seizure control (two with 100% seizure control, eight with 50% to 99% reduction) while on diet therapy. Four patients had previously attempted to reduce the KD ratio or to increase carbohydrates, with immediate seizure worsening. Eight patients transitioned to adult epilepsy clinics; the oldest patients did so at ages 26 and 43 years (after several years of self-management). Four patients switched from KD to MAD (20 g per day net carbohydrate limit as an adult) with no worsening of seizures. All remained on antiseizure drugs (ASDs). Six patients remained on diet therapy, five at the Johns Hopkins Adult Epilepsy Diet Center (AEDC), and maintained good seizure control. At the AEDC, most patients transition to adult providers by age 21 years (Kossoff et al., 2013c).

Children and adolescents with specific genetic or mitochondrial conditions represent a population that requires adult diet therapy as they reach age 18. The KD is frequently helpful for mitochondrial disorders. While mitochondrial disorders with onset in infancy or early childhood may be fatal within a few years, those with onset in later childhood may benefit from the KD and require transitioning to an adult epilepsy provider familiar with the KD (Kossoff et al., 2014).

Glucose transporter type 1 deficiency syndrome (GLUT1DS) is a rare genetic condition caused by impaired glucose transport into the brain and associated with an abnormality in the gene *SLC2A1*. The optimal treatment for GLUT1DS is the KD, which may be prescribed lifelong. It is not known whether patients with GLUT1DS can successfully transition to less restrictive forms of diet therapy, such as the MAD (Kossoff et al., 2014). While it is more commonly diagnosed in childhood, GLUT1DS is also diagnosed in adults. Ninety-one cases of adults with GLUT1DS have been described in the literature, and the KD remains a cornerstone of treatment (Leen et al., 2014).

Juvenile myoclonic epilepsy (JME) is highly treatment responsive, with 90% of patients achieving seizure freedom with appropriate ASDs. However, the remaining 10% have medically resistant seizures. KD therapies have been shown to be effective for JME in a small case series. Eight adolescents and adults (ages 15 to 44 years, mean 24.3) were started on the MAD for treatment of JME. After 1 month, seven remained on the MAD; six patients (75%) had > 50% seizure reduction; after 3 months, five patients had > 50% reduction. Two patients became seizure-free (25%). The mean duration on diet at the time of publication was 13.2 months (range, 0.5 to 40 months). Three patients had increased seizures during brief periods of noncompliance but returned to seizure control when they reinitiated the diet (Kossoff et al., 2013b). Because JME is a diagnosis requiring lifelong treatment, patients with medically refractory JME are a large population of adolescents and adults who could benefit from diet therapy.

Refractory Epilepsy

Worldwide, there are 65 million people with epilepsy; 30% of cases are medically refractory (Moshe et al., 2015), which means there are approximately 19.5 million people in the world with seizures uncontrolled by medications. Many of these patients are not surgical candidates, due to generalized epilepsy (of whom up to 26% may be refractory), multifocal nature, or nonresectable locations of ictal onset.

Patients with seizures resistant to two or more ASDs have a low chance of seizure freedom with additional drugs added. In a longitudinal study of 1,098 newly diagnosed epilepsy patients followed for 2 to 26 years, 49% of patients were seizure-free on the first ASD prescribed; an additional 13.2% became seizure-free with the second drug tried, 3.7% with the third ASD, and 1% with the fourth; with successive ASDs added or attempted, the percent of patients achieving seizure freedom with each additional ASD was less than 1% (Brodie et al., 2012).

In addition to medically refractory epilepsy, the desire to avoid additional ASD side effects also leads patients to pursue KD therapies. Adverse effects from medications (along with psychiatric comorbidities, such as depressive symptoms) are the largest predictors of health-related quality of life in patients with epilepsy, and they are much more strongly predictive of patients' perceived quality of life than seizure frequency. In fact, in a study of 809 adult Italian patients with pharmacoresistant epilepsy, seizure frequency and the presence of generalized tonic-clonic seizures did not significantly affect quality of life, whereas quality of life declined with increased medication side effects (Luoni et al., 2011). In patients without comorbid depression, adverse medication effects are the main determinants of health-related quality of life (Luoni et al., 2011). The KD has the benefit of freedom from many of the adverse effects that can accompany additional medications, particularly cognitive side effects.

Refractory and Super-Refractory Status Epilepticus

Patients with status epilepticus (prolonged seizure lasting more than 5 min, or recurrent seizures without return to baseline) are generally treated with benzodiazepines or other medications; if seizure activity continues despite treatment with intravenous antiepileptic drugs, the condition is termed refractory status epilepticus (RSE), and the patient may be placed in a medically induced coma. If status epilepticus continues after at least 24 hr of general anesthetic medications, it is deemed super-refractory status epilepticus (SRSE), which is associated with high morbidity and mortality, with up to 61% mortality reported (Brophy et al., 2012).

The KD has been used in children for SRSE since 1999 (Baumeister et al., 2004), and it is now used for RSE of different etiologies in children (O'Connor et al., 2014).

In 2008, the first report of KD for SRSE in an adult was published in France (Bodenant et al., 2008). At the University of Pennsylvania, two adults in SRSE were then successfully treated with the KD, after 20 days and 101 days of seizures, respectively, with successful medication weaning at 6 and 11 days after diet initiation, respectively (Wusthoff et al., 2010). Thakur et al. reported on a series of 10 adults (median age, 33 years) at four medical centers who were treated with the KD for SRSE; 70% of the patients had encephalitis. The diet started after a median of 21.5 days (range, 2 to 60 days) and after a median of seven ASDs had been tried (range, 5 to 13 drugs). The status epilepticus ceased in all nine patients who achieved ketosis, in a median of 3 days (Thakur et al., 2014).

A prospective, phase I/II multicenter study of 15 adults with SRSE starting the KD a median of 10 days after SRSE onset (with a median of eight ASDs prior to starting the KD) found that all patients achieved ketosis, and SRSE resolved in 11 patients (79%; Cervenka et al., 2017). In a more recent retrospective study (Francis et al., 2019), the authors started a KD in 11 adults with RSE and found that 10 patients (91%) achieved ketosis in a median of 1 day, and eight patients (73%) had resolution of RSE.

Diet therapy is now used as an adjunct strategy for RSE and SRSE in both children and adults, and in proposed treatment strategies, the recommendation has been made that the KD "should probably be tried in all severe cases" of SRSE (Shorvon & Ferlisi, 2011).

RESULTS

Feasibility, Tolerability, and Adherence

While the KD has been widely used in children in modern times, concerns over adults' ability to tolerate the diet and maintain ketosis have slowed the diet's adoption for use in adults (Barborka, 1930; Swink et al., 1997). Modern studies report a wide range of adherence to the KD in adults, from 22% to 75% at 3 months (Klein et al., 2010; Mosek et al., 2009), with significant variation. The MAD, first published in 2003 as a less restrictive alternative to the classic KD (Kossoff et al., 2003), has had published adherence rates of 56% to 100% at 3 months and 22% to 77.8% at 1 year (Cervenka et al., 2012; Kossoff et al., 2003; Smith et al., 2011). These retention rates are somewhat lower than those seen in add-on drug trials for new ASDs (75% to 80% retention after 12 to 18 weeks; Ben-Menachem et al., 2007; Elger et al., 2007).

The initial decision to begin diet treatment is not undertaken lightly. In some studies, up to two thirds of eligible patients screened decline to participate, due to concerns about restrictiveness or complexity of the diet (Mosek et al., 2009, reported 18 of 27 declined; Klein et al., 2010, reported 23 of 35 declined). However, many people choose to continue diet treatment beyond the initial study periods requested (Carrette et al., 2008; Cervenka et al., 2012; Cervenka et al., 2016a; Kossoff et al., 2013a; Klein et al., 2010;), and some patients have remained on diet therapy as long as 32 years (Kossoff et al., 2013c).

A meta-analysis in 2015 comparing six classic KD studies and five MAD studies concluded that adherence rates are higher in the MAD (combined compliance rate, 56%) than the classic KD (38% adherence; Ye et al., 2015).

Not surprisingly, when diet treatment is effective, patients are motivated to continue treatment. When patients decide to stop diet treatment, the most common reason cited is lack of efficacy, followed by restrictiveness of the diet (Kossoff et al., 2008; Lambrechts et al., 2012; Schoeler et al., 2014). Financial reasons have been cited in a few patients, due to the higher cost of meats compared to processed carbohydrates (Smith et al., 2011).

Efficacy

Adults with pharmacoresistant epilepsy have response rates (defined as a ≥ 50% decrease in seizures) of 33% to 54% with the newer ASDs (Ben-Menachem et al., 2007; Elger et al., 2007; Mbizvo et al., 2012). Rates of seizure freedom with additional agents are much lower, with each additional add-on agent after the second providing a less than 5% chance of seizure freedom (Brodie et al., 2012). Diet therapy compares favorably with these rates in most published studies (Payne et al., 2011), especially because the patients starting diet treatment are typically the most refractory patients, with mean prior ASDs tried ranging from 5.4 to 10.6 (Kossoff et al., 2003; Sirven et al., 1999).

A recent meta-analysis of 16 prospective studies (encompassing the classic KD, MAD, and medium-chain-triglyceride [MCT] diet) with a total of 338 adults found a combined efficacy rate of 13% achieving seizure freedom, with 53% achieving 50% or greater seizure reduction (Liu et al., 2018). So far, two randomized controlled trials have been published; while the trials failed to show a difference in the primary outcome of ≥ 50% seizure reduction between adults starting a KD and adults on standard medical management, both trials lasted less than 6 months, and each trial had individual patients who benefitted greatly (Kverneland et al., 2018; Zare et al., 2017).

In intent-to-treat analysis, classic KD reduces seizures by ≥ 50% in 22% to 55% of patients (Klein et al., 2014; Mosek et al., 2009; Sirven et al.,1999; Table 4.1). Many patients have even higher response rates, with 8% to 27% of patients experiencing > 90% decrease in seizures (Schoeler et al., 2014; Sirven et al.,1999) and seizure freedom achieved in up to 8% (Klein et al., 2010). In a comparison of seizure-free months, Klein and colleagues found an improvement from 20% of months seizure-free at baseline to 56.2% of months seizure-free on the KD (Klein et al., 2010).

The MAD has wider variability in published response rates, ranging from 12% to 67% with ≥ 50% seizure reduction (Kossoff et al., 2008, 2013b, 2013c; Smith et al., 2011) and up to 33% of patients with > 90% reduction (Cervenka et al., 2012; Kossoff et al., 2013b, 2013c; Table 4.1).

Other diet therapies, such as the MCT diet and the low-glycemic-index treatment (Pfeifer & Thiele, 2005), have not been widely studied in adults. In a series of 11 patients on the MCT diet (and four on the classic KD or a combination of MCT/KD during the study), Lambrechts et al. (2012) found that five of 11 patients continued the diet at 1 year, and of those, two had a 50% to 90% reduction in seizures, while the remaining three patients had a < 50% reduction. The mean ASDs used decreased slightly, from 2.7 at baseline to 2.2 at the end of the diet.

Disproving the initial speculations that adults could not maintain ketosis, the majority of adults on KDs have been successful at achieving and maintaining urinary and/or serum ketosis (range of published rates, 58.3% to 87.5%; Klein et al., 2010; Mosek et al., 2009; Sirven et al., 1999), but

levels of ketosis have not been predictive of seizure improvement (Klein et al., 2010; Mosek et al., 2009; Nei et al., 2014).

Kossoff et al. (2008) found a trend toward patients with more frequent seizures at baseline having a larger proportion of ≥ 50% response rates, although this has not been detected in other studies (Mady et al., 2003; Mosek et al., 2009).

With regard to seizure type and response to diet therapies, Nei et al. (2014) detected a trend toward greater seizure reduction in patients with symptomatic generalized epilepsy, with 64% of patients with symptomatic generalized epilepsy having ≥ 50% reduction versus 28% of patients with focal epilepsies. In Mady et al.'s study of 45 adolescents, the patients with multiple seizure types had a greater improvement than those with complex partial or generalized seizure types alone (Mady et al., 2003). As discussed previously, high response rates and seizure freedom were seen in a small series of adolescents and adults with JME, with four of six adults showing > 50% decrease in seizures, with two of six having > 90% decrease, while one of six was seizure-free (Kossoff et al., 2013b).

In patients with GLUT1DS, up to 90% of patients were seizure-free on the KD or MAD, including three adults. One adult had resolution of generalized convulsive seizures but had persistence of likely non-epileptic events; the other two adults were seizure-free (Ramm-Pettersen et al., 2013).

Beyond a reduction in the number of seizures, the severity or duration of seizures reportedly decreased, or the amount of time to recover from a seizure shortened in a subset of patients (Schoeler et al., 2014; Smith et al., 2011).

Some studies have shown that weight loss predicts diet efficacy, with 67% of patients with greater than 0.9 kg/m^2 decrease in body mass index (BMI) having > 50% seizure reduction, compared with 27% of patients with < 0.9 kg/m^2 decrease in BMI ($p = .03$; Kossoff et al., 2008). However, this is not a consistent finding in all studies (Smith et al., 2011), and patients with weight gain can also respond to the diet (Kossoff et al., 2008).

BENEFICIAL EFFECTS

Cognition and Mood

In studies of adults with epilepsy, diet treatment often has positive cognitive and mood effects (Box 4.1). Many patients report improvements in cognition and mood, as well as (or even despite

TABLE 4.1 SUMMARY OF PUBLISHED STUDIES OF THE KETOGENIC DIET AND MODIFIED ATKINS DIET IN ADULTS

Study	Year	Journal	Diet	Number of patients	Improvement ≥ 50%	Improvement ≥ 90%	Retention
Sirven et al.	1999	Epilepsia	KD	11	55% (6/11)	27% (3/11)	7/11 (63.6%) at 8 months
Coppola et al.	2002	Epilepsy Research	KD	5 (18–23)	No age-specific information	No age-specific information	No age-specific information
Mady et al.	2003	Epilepsia	KD	45 adolescents (12–19)	13/28 (46%); no age-specific information	8/28 (28%); no age-specific information	28/45 (62%) at 6 months
Groesbeck et al.	2006	Developmental Medicine & Child Neurology	KD	28	No age-specific information	24/28	No age-specific information
Mosek et al.	2009	Seizure	KD	9	2/9 (22%)		2/9 (22%) at 3 months
Klein et al.	2010	Epilepsy & Behavior	KD	12	5/12 (42%)	2/12 (17%)	9/12 (75%) at 4 months
Lambrechts et al.	2012	Epilepsy & Behavior	KD or MCT	15	2/15 (13%)		5/15 (33%) at 12 months
Nei et al.	2014	Seizure	KD	29 (11–51)	13 (45%)	1/29 (3%)	Mean 9 months
Schoeler et al.	2014	Epilepsy & Behavior	KD	23	9/23 (39%)	2/23 (8%)	9/23 (29%) at 12 months
Kossoff et al.	2003	Neurology	MAD	3 (18–52)	1/3 (33%)	1/3 (33%)	3/3 (100%) at 3 months
Carrette et al.	2008	Clinical Neurology and Neurosurgery	MAD	8	1 (12%)		3/8 (37.5%) at 6 months
Kossoff et al.	2008	Epilepsia	MAD	30	14/30 (47%)	1/30 (3%)	20/30 (67%) at 3 months
Smith et al.	2011	Epilepsia	MAD	18	4/18 (22%)		14/18 (78%) at 6 months
Coppola et al.	2011	Seizure	LGID	3 adults	3/3 (100%)		3/3 (100%) at 2 months
Cervenka et al.	2012	Epilepsia	MAD	22	6 (27%)	4/22 (18%)	14/22 (64%) at 3 months
Kossoff et al.	2013b	Epilepsy & Behavior	MAD	6 adults	4/6 (67%)	2/6 (33%)	5/6 at (83%) 2 months
Ramm-Pettersen et al.	2013	Developmental Medicine & Child Neurology	MAD	3 adults	2/3 (67%)	2/3 (67%)*	1 year (at least)
Kverneland et al.	2015	Epilepsy & Behavior	MAD	13	6 (50%)		46% at 3 months
Cervenka et al.	2016	Epilepsy & Behavior	MAD	168	65 (39%)	37 (22%)	54% at 6 months
Zare et al.**	2017	Iranian Journal of Neurology	MAD	34	12 (35%)		64% at 2 months
Kverneland et al.**	2018	Epilepsia	MAD	37	4 (11%)		85% at 3 months
Roehl et al.	2019	Epilepsy & Behavior	MKD	55	33 (60%)		Variable
Green et al.	2020	Journal of Neurology	MAD, MCT, MKD	42	16 (42%)	5 (13%)	29% at 12 months

Note. KD = ketogenic diet; MAD = modified Atkins diet; MCT = medium-chain-triglyceride diet; MKD = modified ketogenic diet; LGID = low glycemic index diet.
* Suspicion of psychogenic non-epileptic seizure in remaining patient not seizure-free.
** Randomized controlled trial.

BOX 4.1

DIETARY TREATMENT: REPORTED BENEFICIAL EFFECTS (OTHER THAN SEIZURE CONTROL) AND ADVERSE EFFECTS

Reported beneficial effects
Improved cognition
Improved mood
Weight loss (when desired)
Increased alertness
Increased energy
Reduced depression
Improved quality of life
Decreased anxiety
Decreased tension
Decreased length or severity of seizures

Reported adverse effects
Nausea or vomiting
Bloating
Constipation
Temporary lipid elevations
Impaired concentration
Menstrual irregularities
Possible growth restriction
Kidney stones
Skeletal fractures

---

the lack of) improved seizure control; in fact, some patients with no or < 50% improvement in seizure frequency opt to continue diet treatment for the cognitive benefits alone (Coppola et al., 2002; Sirven et al., 1999). The majority of patients in one study of the KD (7 of 11 patients) saw an improvement in mood and cognition, although two of 11 also reported impaired concentration (Sirven et al., 1999). Increased alertness and energy are common findings, seen in 33% to 65% of adults and adolescents on the KD (Lambrechts et al., 2012; Mady et al., 2003; Mosek et al., 2009; Schoeler et al., 2014). One study of the MAD that administered detailed cognitive and depression questionnaires found reduction in depression scores and improved concentration in six of seven patients on the diet for 1 month, and in all three patients who completed 6 months of the study (Carrette et al., 2008). Quality-of-life scores tend to increase rather than decrease on both the MAD

and the KD, although not significantly (Carrette et al., 2008; Klein et al., 2010; Lambrechts et al., 2012). Anxiety, tension, and fatigue may all be improved as well (Lambrechts et al., 2012).

Weight Loss

Weight loss is often a desirable effect of KD therapies. Many patients are able to lose significant amounts of weight and may successfully move from a clinically "obese" BMI to a "normal" or "overweight" BMI. Weight loss is particularly important in the adult population because it is estimated that over one third of adults in the United States are obese (BMI ≥ 30 kg/m^2; Ogden et al., 2014). Obesity can lead to type 2 diabetes, obstructive sleep apnea, and metabolic syndrome, all of which can be combatted with weight loss. In a series of studies investigating weight loss with the MAD, mean weight loss was 7 kg over 3 months (Kossoff et al., 2008) and 10 kg over 6 months (Carrette et al., 2008), including in four of the 11 patients who were obese when they started the diet and who were no longer obese at the conclusion (Kossoff et al., 2008). In a separate study of the KD, mean BMI improved 18%, from 33.8 (obese) to 27.5 (overweight) in 12 adults over 4 months, and the majority of overweight or obese patients had at least a 10% reduction in BMI (Klein et al., 2010).

If patients are of average weight or underweight when starting diet therapy, total calories can be adjusted to prevent or reverse weight loss.

ADVERSE EFFECTS

Gastrointestinal

Gastrointestinal side effects are common, with half to all patients reporting some degree of nausea, constipation, bloating, or vomiting at some point on diet therapy; these complaints generally resolve after the first few days or weeks of treatment with the KD (Coppola et al., 2002; Klein et al., 2010; Sirven et al., 1999). Rarely, patients are unable to continue diet treatment due to intractable nausea or vomiting.

Lipids

Lipids may increase on the KD and should be monitored. Sirven et al. found a significant increase in total fasting cholesterol at 3 and at 6 months on the diet, with an increase of the mean cholesterol from 208 mg/dl (range, 120 to 304 mg/dl) to 291 mg/dl (range, 220 to 395 mg/dl). Triglycerides also increased at 3 months, from a mean of 190 mg/dl (range, 41 to 542 mg/dl) to 203 mg/dl (range, 68 to 417 mg/dl), then plateaued (Sirven et al., 1999). The extension of this study continued to show a significant increase in total cholesterol and in the cholesterol:HDL ratio at the time of diet discontinuation after up to 35 months on diet (Nei et al., 2014). If they are extreme, lipid changes may prompt discontinuation of diet therapy (Mosek et al., 2009). However, elevated lipids are not present in all patients or in all studies, and triglycerides and LDL may not change (Klein et al., 2010).

Lipids increase on the MAD as well (Carrette et al., 2008), although end lipid levels in some studies remained within average cardiovascular risk ranges (Kossoff et al., 2008; Smith et al., 2011). One study of the MAD found a decrease in triglycerides with diet treatment over 12 months (Smith et al., 2011).

Lipids may increase during the initial phase of the diet and then return to baseline: one study of 37 adults on the MAD for at least 3 months found that while total cholesterol and LDL had increased at 3 months, there was no difference from baseline after 1 year ($p = .2$ and $p = .5$, respectively). In the 12 patients followed for $\geq$ 3 years, there were no known cardiac or cerebrovascular events (Cervenka et al., 2016b).

If cholesterol elevation is present, it may be manageable without stopping diet therapy; one patient whose LDL doubled after 3 months continued the MAD, and with carnitine supplementation and the substitution of saturated fats for polyunsaturated fats saw his cholesterol and LDL return to normal (Cervenka et al., 2012). Carnitine supplementation successfully decreased elevated triglycerides in three patients as well (Nei et al., 2014).

Beyond lipid levels, one study comparing 21 diet-naïve patients starting the MAD to 20 patients who had been on a KD for > 12 months found that those on the MAD for > 1 year had lower BMI, lower hip and waist measurements, and less percent of body fat. There was no difference in common carotid artery intima thickness or presence of atherosclerotic plaque in the carotid arteries (McDonald et al., 2018) despite an increased proportion of potentially atherogenic small LDL particles in the MAD group compared to the diet-naïve cohort.

Effects on the Menstrual Cycle
Menstrual irregularities and cessation of menstruation are common in the starvation state.

Given that the KD is designed to mimic starvation, it is not surprising that it can also cause menstrual irregularity. Barborka reported that 12 of 56 women had cessation of their menses during KD treatment; however, in the seven who stopped the diet, normal menstruation resumed (Barborka, 1930). In Sirven et al.'s 1999 study, all nine women developed menstrual irregularities (irregular cycles or cessation of menses) that resolved on diet discontinuation. Menstrual irregularities were also frequent in Mady et al.'s 2003 study of the KD (45% of women). Menstrual irregularities seem to be much less common with the MAD: there were no menstrual irregularities in any of the 19 women in one study (Kossoff et al., 2003) and none reported in nine women in a second study (Smith et al., 2011), and they were present in only one out of 17 women in a third study (Cervenka et al., 2012). Lambrechts et al. (2012) found no irregularities in two women on the KD and two women on the MCT diet.

KDs in Pregnancy
To date, two pregnancies occurring in women on KD therapies have been reported (van der Louw et al., 2017). One occurred while the mother was on the classic KD and resulted in a healthy infant with normal development (up to 1 year at the time of report). One occurred while the mother was on the MAD; the infant had minor malformation of the ears bilaterally, but healthy neurodevelopment (up to 8 months at the time of report). Further safety and long-term side effects remain to be studied.

Other Side Effects
Long-term effects in patients on the KD for 6 years or more (in patients ages 7 to 23 years) included decrease in growth rate: at diet initiation, 14 of 28 (50%) were at or below the tenth percentile for weight, and the number increased to 23 of 28 (82%) at last follow-up (Groesbeck et al., 2006). Growth restriction was not related to degree of ketosis, and it is less of a concern in patients who begin KDs as adults. In one study, one quarter of patients on KDs developed kidney stones, with a median of 2 years after diet onset (Groesbeck et al., 2006). Subsequent studies have shown that urine alkalinization with potassium citrate reduces the risk of kidney stones (Sampath et al., 2007). Kidney stones have not been reported in other studies of adults on diet treatment. Six patients in a long-term study (21%) had skeletal fractures, occurring a median of 18 months

after diet initiation (Groesbeck et al., 2006). One patient had a jaw fracture related to a seizure and stopped the diet (Mosek et al., 2009), but other skeletal fractures have not been reported.

CONCLUSIONS

Diet treatment is feasible in adults and is often highly effective, with seizure reduction rates in medically refractory populations of 33% to 67%, comparable with response rates in children. A significant proportion of patients may become seizure-free. In addition to seizure reduction, patients may also experience improved mood and cognition, as well as intentional weight loss. Lipids should be monitored, but in most cases persistent lipid elevations can be managed with diet adjustments. Diet adherence remains a major challenge for adults.

REFERENCES

Barborka, C. J. (1928). Ketogenic diet treatment of epilepsy in adults. *JAMA*, *91*(2), 73–78.

Barborka, C. J. (1929). The ketogenic diet and its use. *Medical Clinics of North America*, *12*(6), 1639–1653.

Barborka, C. J. (1930). Epilepsy in adults: Results of treatment by ketogenic diet in one hundred cases. *Archives of Neurology & Psychiatry*, *23*, 904–914.

Bastible, C. (1931). The ketogenic treatment of epilepsy. *Irish Journal of Medical Science*, *6*, 506–520.

Baumeister, F. A., Oberhoffer, R., Liebhaber, G. M., Kunkel, J., Eberhardt, J., Holthausen, H., & Peters, J. (2004). Fatal propofol infusion syndrome in association with ketogenic diet. *Neuropediatrics*, *35*, 250–252.

Ben-Menachem, E., Biton, V., Jatuzis, D., Abou-Khalil, B., Doty, P., & Rudd, G. D. (2007). Efficacy and safety of oral lacosamide as adjunctive therapy in adults with partial-onset seizures. *Epilepsia*, *48*, 1308–1317.

Bodenant, M., Moreau, C., Sejourne, C., Auvin, S., Delval, A., Cuisset, J. M., Derambure, P., Destee, A., & Defebvre, L. (2008). Interest of the ketogenic diet in refractory status epilepticus in an adult. *Revue Neurologique (Paris)*, *164*, 194–199.

Brodie, M. J., Barry, S. J., Bamagous, G. A., Norrie, J. D., & Kwan, P. (2012). Patterns of treatment response in newly diagnosed epilepsy. *Neurology*, *78*, 1548–1554.

Brophy, G. M., Bell, R., Claassen, J., Alldredge, B., Bleck, T. P., Glauser, T., LaRoche, S. M., Riviello, J. J., Jr., Shutter, L., Sperling, M. R., Treiman, D., & Vespa, P. M. (2012). Guidelines for the evaluation and management of status epilepticus. *Neurocritical Care*, *17*(1), 3–23.

Carrette, E., Vonck, K., de Herdt, V., Dewaele, I., Raedt, R., Goossens, L., Van Zandijcke, M.,

Wadman, W., Thadani, V., & Boon, P. (2008). A pilot trial with modified Atkins' diet in adult patients with refractory epilepsy. *Clinical Neurology and Neurosurgery*, *110*, 797–803.

Cervenka, M. C., Henry, B. J., Felton, E. A., Patton, K., & Kossoff, E. H. (2016a). Establishing an adult epilepsy diet center: Experience, efficacy and challenges. *Epilepsy & Behavior*, *58*, 61–68.

Cervenka, M. C., Hocker, S., Koenig, M., Bar, B., Henry-Barron, B., Kossoff, E. H., Hartman, A. L., Probasco, J. C., Benavides, D. R., Venkatesan, A., Hagen, E. C., Dittrich, D., Stern, T., Radzik, B., Depew, M., Caserta, F. M., Nyquist, P., Kaplan, P. W., & Geocadin, R. G. (2017). Phase I/II multi-center ketogenic diet study for adult superrefractory status epilepticus. *Neurology*, *88*, 938–943.

Cervenka, M. C., Patton, K., Eloyan, A., Henry, B., & Kossoff, E. H. (2016b). The impact of the modified Atkins diet on lipid profiles in adults with epilepsy. *Nutritional Neuroscience*, *19*, 131–137.

Cervenka, M., Terao, N., Bosarge, J., Henry, B., Klees, A., Morrison, P., & Kossoff, E. (2012). E-mail management of the MAD for adults with epilepsy is feasible and effective. *Epilepsia*, *53*, 728–732.

Coppola, G., D'Aniello, A., Messana, T., Di Pasquale, F., della Corte, R., Pascotto, A., & Verrotti, A. (2011). Low glycemic index diet in children and young adults with refractory epilepsy: First Italian experience. *Seizure*, *20*(7), 526–528.

Coppola, G., Veggiotti, P., Cusmai, R., Bertoli, S., Cardinali, S., Dionisi-Vici, C., Elia, M., Lipsi, M. L., Sarnelli, C., Tagliabue, A., Toraldo, C., & Pascotto, A. (2002). The ketogenic diet in children, adolescents, and young adults with refractory epilepsy: An Italian multicentric experience. *Epilepsy Research*, *48*, 221–227.

Elger, C., Bialer, M., Cramer, J. A., Maia, J., Almeida, L., & Soares-da-Silva P. (2007). Eslicarbazepine acetate: A double-blind, add-on, placebo-controlled exploratory trial in adult patients with partial-onset seizures. *Epilepsia*, *48*, 497–504.

Francis, B. A., Fillenworth, J., Gorelick, P., Karanec, K., & Tanner, A. (2019). The feasibility, safety, and effectiveness of a ketogenic diet for refractory status epilepticus in adults in the intensive care unit. *Neurocritical Care*, *30*, 652–657.

Geyelin, H. R. (1921). Fasting as a method of treating epilepsy. *Medical Record*, *99*, 1037–1039.

Green, S. F., Nguyen, P., Kaalund-Hansen, K., Rajakulendran, S., & Murphy, E. (2020). Effectiveness, retention, and safety of modified ketogenic diet in adults with epilepsy at a tertiary-care centre in the UK. *Journal of Neurology*, *267*, 1171–1178.

Groesbeck, D. K., Bluml, R. M., & Kossoff, E. H. (2006). Long-term use of the ketogenic diet in the treatment of epilepsy. *Developmental Medicine & Child Neurology*, *48*, 978–981.

Guelpa, G., & Marie, A. (1911). La lutte contre l'epilepsie par la desintoication et par la reducation alimentaire. *Revue de Therapeutique Medico-Chirurgicale (Review of Medical and Surgical Therapeutics)*, 78, 8–13.

Hippocrates. (400 BC). *On the sacred disease.* From The Internet Classics Archive, available at: http://classics.mit.edu/Hippocrates/sacred.html

Jóźwiak, S., Kossoff, E. H., & Kotulska-Jóźwiak, K. (2011). Dietary treatment of epilepsy: Rebirth of an ancient treatment. *Neurologia i Neurochirurgia Polska*, 45(4), 370–378.

Jung, D. E., Joshi, S. M., & Berg, A. T. (2015). How do you keto? Survey of North American pediatric ketogenic diet centers. *Journal of Child Neurology*, 30(7), 868–873.

Klein, P., Janousek, J., Barber, A., & Weissberger, R. (2010). Ketogenic diet treatment in adults with refractory epilepsy. *Epilepsy & Behavior*, 19, 575–579.

Klein, P., Tyrlikova, I., & Mathews, G. C. (2014). Dietary treatment in adults with refractory epilepsy: A review. *Neurology*, 18, 1978–1985.

Kossoff, E. H., Krauss, G. L., McGrogan, J. R., & Freeman, J. M. (2003). Efficacy of the Atkins diet as therapy for intractable epilepsy. *Neurology*, 61(12), 1789–1791.

Kossoff, E. H., & McGrogan, J. R. (2005). Worldwide use of the ketogenic diet. *Epilepsia*, 46(2), 280–289.

Kossoff, E. H., Rowley, H., Sinha, S. R., & Vining E. P. (2008). A prospective study of the modified Atkins diet for intractable epilepsy in adults. *Epilepsia*, 49(2), 316–319.

Kossoff, E. H., Cervenka, M. C., Henry, B. J., Haney, C. A., & Turner, Z. (2013a). A decade of the MAD (2003–2013): Results, insights, and future directions. *Epilepsy & Behavior*, 29(3), 437–442.

Kossoff, E. H., Henry, B. J., & Cervenka, M. C. (2013b). Efficacy of dietary therapy for juvenile myoclonic epilepsy. *Epilepsy & Behavior*, 26, 162–164.

Kossoff, E. H., Henry, B. J., & Cervenka, M. C. (2013c). Transitioning pediatric patients receiving ketogenic diets for epilepsy into adulthood. *Seizure*, 22(6), 487–489.

Kossoff, E. H., Veggiotti, P., Genton, P., & Desguerre, I. (2014). Transition for patients with epilepsy due to metabolic and mitochondrial disorders. *Epilepsia*, 55(Suppl. 3), 37–40.

Kverneland, M., Molteberg, E., Iversen, P. O., Veierod, M. B., Tauboll, E., Selmer, K. K., & Nakken, K. O. (2018). Effect of modified Atkins diet in adults with drug-resistant focal epilepsy: A randomized clinical trial. *Epilepsia*, 59, 1567–1576.

Kverneland, M., Selmer, K. K., Nakken, K. O., Iversen, P. O., & Tauboll, E. (2015). A prospective study of the modified Atkins diet for adults with idiopathic generalized epilepsy. *Epilepsy & Behavior*, 53, 197–201.

Lambrechts, D. A., Wielders, L. H., Aldenkamp, A. P., Kessels, F. G., de Kinderen, R. J., & Majoie, M. J. (2012). The ketogenic diet as a treatment option in adults with chronic refractory epilepsy: Efficacy and tolerability in clinical practice. *Epilepsy & Behavior*, 23, 310–314.

Leen, W. G., Taher, M., Verbeek, M. M., Kamsteed, E. J., van de Warrenburg, B. P., & Willemsen, M. A. (2014). GLUT1 deficiency syndrome into adulthood: A follow-up study. *Journal of Neurology*, 261(3), 589–599.

Liu, H., Yang, Y., Wang, Y., Tang, H., Zhang, F., Zhang, Y., & Zhao, Y. (2018). Ketogenic diet for treatment of intractable epilepsy in adults: A meta-analysis of observational studies. *Epilepsia Open*, 3, 9–17.

Luoni, C., Bisulli, F., Canevini, M. P., De Sarro, G., Fattore, C., Galimberti, C. A., Gatti, G., La Neve, A., Muscas, G., Specchio, L. M., Striano, S., & Perruca, E. (2011). Determinants of health-related quality of life in pharmacoresistant epilepsy: Results from a large multicenter study of consecutively enrolled patients using validated quantitative assessments. *Epilepsia*, 52, 2181–2191.

Mady, M. A., Kossoff, E. H., McGregor, A. L., Wheless, J. W., Pyzik, P. L., & Freeman, J. M. (2003). The ketogenic diet: Adolescents can do it, too. *Epilepsia*, 44, 847–851.

Martinez, C. C., Pyzik, P. L., & Kossoff, E. H. (2007). Discontinuing the ketogenic diet in seizure-free children: Recurrence and risk factors. *Epilepsia*, 48(1), 187–190.

Mbizvo, G. K., Dixon, P., Hutton, J. L., & Marson, A. G. (2012). Levetiracetam add-on for drug-resistant focal epilepsy: An updated Cochrane review. *Cochrane Database of Systematic Reviews*, 9. https://www.cochranelibrary.com/cdsr/doi/10.1002/14651858.CD001901.pub2/full

McDonald, T. J. W., Ratchford, E. V., Henry-Barron, B. J., Kossoff, E. H., & Cervenka, M. C. (2018). Impact of the modified Atkins diet on cardiovascular health in adults with epilepsy. *Epilepsy & Behavior*, 79, 82–86.

Mosek, A., Natour, H., Neufeld, M., Shiff, Y., & Vaisam, N. (2009). Ketogenic diet treatment in adults with refractory epilepsy: A prospective pilot study. *Seizure*, 18, 30–33.

Moshe, S. L., Perucca, E., Ryvlin, P., & Tomson, T. (2015). Epilepsy: New advances. *Lancet*, 385, 884–898.

Nei, M., Ngo, L., Sirven, J., & Sperling, M. (2014). Ketogenic diet in adolescents and adults with epilepsy. *Seizure*, 23, 439–442.

O'Connor, S. E., Ream, M. A., Richardson, C., Mikati, M. A., Trescher, W. H., Byeler, D. L., Sather, J. D., Michael, E. H., Urbanik, K. B., Richards, J. L., Davis, R., Zupanc, M. L., & Zupec-Kania, B. (2014). The ketogenic diet for the treatment of pediatric status epilepticus. *Pediatric Neurology*, *50*, 101–103.

Ogden, C. L., Carroll, M. D., Kit, B. K., & Flegal, K. M. (2014). Prevalence of childhood and adult obesity in the United States, 2011–2012. *JAMA, 311*, 806–814.

Payne, N., Cross, J., Sander, J., & Sisodiya, S. (2011). The ketogenic and related diets in adolescents and adults—A review. *Epilepsia, 52*, 1941–1948.

Pfeifer, H. H., & Thiele, E. A. (2005). Low-glycemic-index treatment: A liberalized ketogenic diet for treatment of intractable epilepsy. *Neurology, 65*, 1810–1812.

Ramm-Pettersen, A., Nakken, K., Skogseid, I., Randby, H., Skei, E., Bindoff, L., & Selmer, K. K. (2013). Good outcome in patients with early dietary treatment of GLUT-1 deficiency syndrome: Results from a retrospective Norwegian study. *Developmental Medicine & Child Neurology, 55*, 440–447.

Roehl, K., Falco-Walter, J., Ouyang, B., & Balabanov, A. (2019). Modified ketogenic diets in adults with refractory epilepsy: Efficacious improvements in seizure frequency, seizure severity, and quality of life. *Epilepsy & Behavior, 93*, 113–118.

Sampath, A., Kossoff, E. H., Furth, S. L., Pyzik, P. L., & Vining, E. P. (2007). Kidney stones and the ketogenic diet: Risk factors and prevention. *Journal of Child Neurology, 22*, 375–378.

Schoeler, N., Wood, S., Aldridge, V., Sander, J., Cross, J., & Sisodiya, S. (2014). Ketogenic diet therapies for adults with epilepsy: Feasibility and classification of response. *Epilepsy & Behavior, 37*, 33–81.

Shorvon, S., & Ferlisi, M. (2011). The treatment of super-refractory status epilepticus: A critical review of available therapies and a clinical treatment protocol. *Brain, 134*, 2802–2818.

Sirven, J., Whedon, B., Caplan, D., Liporace, J., Glosser, D., O'Dwyer, J., & Sperling, M. R. (1999). The ketogenic diet for intractable epilepsy in adults: Preliminary results. *Epilepsia, 40*, 1721–1726.

Smith, M., Politzer, N., MacGarvie, D., McAndrews, M., & del Campo, M. (2011). Efficacy and tolerability of the MAD in adults with pharmacoresistant epilepsy: A prospective observational study. *Epilepsia, 52*, 775–780.

Swink, T. D., Vining, E. P., & Freeman, J. M. (1997). The ketogenic diet: 1997. *Advances in Pediatrics, 44*, 297–329.

Thakur, K. T., Probasco, J. C., Hocker, S. E., Roehl, K., Henry, B., Kossoff, E. H., Kaplan, P. W., Geocadin, R. G., Hartman, A. L., Venkatesan, A., & Cervenka, M. (2014). Ketogenic diet for adults in super-refractory status epilepticus. *Neurology, 82*, 665–670.

van der Louw, E. J., Williams, T. J., Henry-Barron, B. J., Olieman, J. F., Duvekot, J. J., Vermeulen, M. J., Bannink, N., Williams, M., Neuteboom, R. F., Kossoff, E. H., Catsman-Berrevoets, C. E., & Cervenka, M. C. (2017). Ketogenic diet therapy for epilepsy during pregnancy: A case series. *Seizure, 45*, 198–201.

Wilder, R. M. (1921). The effect of ketonemia on the course of epilepsy. *Mayo Clinic Proceedings, 2*, 307–308.

Wusthoff, C. J., Kranick, S. M., Morley, J. F., & Christina Berggvist, A. G. (2010). The ketogenic diet in treatment of two adults with prolonged nonconvulsive status epilepticus. *Epilepsia, 51*, 1083–1085.

Ye, F., Li, X. J., Jiang, W. L., Sun, H. B., & Liu, J. (2015). Efficacy of and patient compliance with a ketogenic diet in adults with intractable epilepsy: A meta-analysis. *Journal of Clinical Neurology, 11*, 26–31.

Zare, M., Okhovat, A. A., Esmaillzadeh, A., Mehvari, J., Najafi, M. R., & Saadatnia, M. (2017). Modified Atkins diet in adult with refractory epilepsy: A controlled randomized clinical trial. *Iranian Journal of Neurology, 16*, 72–77.

5

How Do You Implement the Diet?

A. G. CHRISTINA BERGQVIST, MD

INTRODUCTION

The ketogenic diet (KD) has survived and thrived for almost 100 years as an effective treatment for intractable epilepsy. For many years, implementation of the diet remained in large part unchanged from its initial conception by Wilder (Livingston, 1951; Wilder, 1921). Management was based on clinical practice, strongly tied to the diet's history of "fasting [and] calorie and fluid restrictions." As the use of the KD increased locally in the United States and spread across the world, and side effects became better understood, many of the standard practices were questioned and tested, and some were changed or discontinued (Kossoff & McGrogan, 2005). As a result, alternative implementation of the classic KD and creation of newer diets have emerged. Most of the studies published are retrospective chart reviews, but there are now a few randomized trials testing specific implementation practices for their "superiority". Two international consensus statements on the KD have been published that address the differences in management. The updated version was written by 31 contributors from 13 countries and was published in 2018. The documents serve as a basis for future improvements to dietary therapies (Kossoff et al., 2009, 2018). References to the 2018 document are called *International Consensus Statement for Ketogenic Diet* (ICSKD). Multiple publications also detail site-specific implementation practices for the KD (Freeman et al., 2007; Kossoff et al., 2011; Snyder, 2006; Stafstrom et al., 2008). It is not within the scope of this chapter to provide the same detail; instead, the chapter covers the implementation changes that have occurred in the 100-year history of the KD.

NEED FOR A FAMILY-CENTERED TEAM-BASED APPROACH TO DIETARY THERAPIES

The KD is a prescribed diet therapy requiring supervision by a healthcare team. It should never be confused with weight-loss diets that individuals can manage safely themselves. Dietary therapies for epilepsy require periodic physical examination and laboratory testing to remain safe, to promote general health, and to prevent side effects. This is particularly true in children, whose nutritional needs are continuously changing during childhood and adolescence. Technology has changed much of the interaction between the care provider and the KD team and allows for long-distance communication. Communication with the team via phone, email, and electronic medical records (such as EPIC) is necessary for managing the KD. However, ongoing communication is not a replacement for a "in-person" follow-up visit with the KD team including a physical examination.

The ICSKD recommends that patients be evaluated at least four times in the first year of treatment and twice a year thereafter. Younger children, particularly infants, need more frequent (even monthly) evaluations to monitor their nutritional needs.

Composition of the KD Team

The KD is best supervised by a team of experienced healthcare professionals. For a small program, the team comprises, at a minimum, an epileptologist and a dietitian. For truly comprehensive care and for larger programs, the team is expanded to also include a nurse and a social worker. Each team member contributes unique knowledge and skill sets to optimize the patients' care, and the team will grow as the number of patients in the dietary treatment program increases. The latest addition to the team at Children's Hospital of Philadelphia (CHOP) is a chef who assists with creation of recipes in the inpatient KD kitchen (Fenton et al., 2014, 2019; Groveman et al., 2014). Any institution that supports dietary therapies must also provide pharmacy services that can locate medications with the lowest carbohydrate content, a very important task because the carbohydrate content of medication is not routinely reported by industry and is subject to frequent change.

Access to other subspecialties, such as gastroenterology, nutrition, nephrology, urology, endocrinology, a feeding team, and bone health experts, is also essential to provide truly comprehensive care. Children started on the KD today rarely have just treatment-resistant epilepsy; they also have many additional diagnoses, including cerebral palsy, developmental disability, intellectual disability, feeding difficulties (some with G-tube dependencies), behavioral difficulties, autism spectrum disorder, and genetic conditions. Adding the KD to their treatment regimen makes their care truly complex. Parents are important partners, and they are essential to the success of the diet and a keto program. Parents can be effective coaches for new keto parents, assisting them with nonmedical information, and they can also become trained educators as the keto community grows to include schools, nursing agencies, and other therapies (Chee et al., 2014; MacCracken & Scalisi, 1999). Creating a keto community makes it possible to provide comprehensive care.

PRE-KD EVALUATION(S), EDUCATION, AND COUNSELING

For families considering the KD, education about dietary therapies is provided via reading materials, referrals to Internet sites, DVDs, and foundations that advocate for the KD, such as the Charlie Foundation for Ketogenic Therapies (www.charliefoundation.org), Matthew's Friends (https://www.matthewsfriends.org/), and the Epilepsy Foundation (www.efa.org). Some dietary treatment programs offer separate education classes to assist families with their decision about trying dietary therapies (e.g., CHOP, www.chop.edu/treatments/ketogenic-diet).

The KD requires the patient's body to switch from using carbohydrates as the primary energy source to using lipids. There are some disorders for which the use of the KD or fasting can lead to significant morbidity, and even mortality. These disorders include inborn errors of metabolism related to carnitine (mitochondrial transport), β-oxidation defects, pyruvate carboxylase deficiencies, and porphyria (which requires a high-carbohydrate diet). Mitochondrial cytopathies are in their own category because some may benefit from KD therapies, such as pyruvate dehydrogenase deficiency (DiPisa et al., 2012; Weber et al., 2001; Wijburg et al., 1992), while for others the KD would worsen the condition (Bergqvist, 2004;

Horvath et al., 2008; Kang et al., 2007). Obtaining assistance from metabolic or neuromuscular specialists is recommended before attempting the KD in these disorders. A metabolic screen is recommended for any child for whom the KD is considered. ICSKD suggests that the screen include acylcarnitine esters, urinary organic acids, serum amino acids, lactate, and pyruvate. For screening labs that are followed every 3 to 6 months while the patient is on the KD, see the ICSKD.

INITIATION OF THE KD

Initiating the KD can be intimidating to the family, caregiver, and KD team alike. A well-prepared admission and well-educated parents are the best insurance for success. The following section reviews the various initiation methods that have been used and discusses both their benefits and their drawbacks.

Inpatient versus Outpatient Initiation

The classic KD created by Wilder and advocated by Johns Hopkins University (Freeman et al., 2007) is started in the hospital so that the patient can be closely observed, monitored, and treated if needed. Most centers in the United States use an inpatient setting to start the KD because it allows the KD to be advanced relatively quickly and ketosis to be achieved within a few days (Kossoff et al., 2018). The child is closely observed by nursing staff and physicians, and interventions for hypoglycemia, acidosis, dehydration, vomiting, weight loss, or feeding intolerances can be instituted in a timely fashion to minimize any complications. Although seizures more often improve during the admission, they can worsen from the stress of switching metabolic substrate. In this situation, the inpatient setting allows for immediate adjustments in medication and for intensive care unit care, should it be needed. While the family is in the hospital, many hours of direct teaching and "hands-on" education are provided by the KD team. Many centers admit only one child at a time for initiation of the KD. The KD team is on 24/7 permanent call during initiation of the KD. Organization of the admissions on a monthly basis, as well as using a small group setting for teaching, improves efficiency and frees up the team's time to assist with outpatient management. CHOP also provides cooking classes in its keto kitchen as part of starting the KD (Fenton et al., 2019; Groveman et al., 2014). The classes provide hands-on experience with the KD food before the patient leaves the hospital and improve the chances of acceptance of, and success with, the KD at home. Finally, although inborn errors in fatty acid oxidation are rare, the metabolic screening is not infallible. Our center have identified a handful of children with β-oxidation defects during KD admissions since 1994. It is more likely that these children's defects would have been missed and could have resulted in significant morbidity had the diet been started on an outpatient basis.

Outpatient initiation of the KD can be successful, and in some countries it is the standard of care (Neal et al., 2008; Rizzutti et al., 2007; Vaisleib et al., 2004; van der Louw et al., 2019). The outpatient advancement of the KD is in general slower, often taking several weeks before a full KD ratio is achieved. The centers that utilize outpatient initiation of the KD must have a flexible, available staff and the ability to schedule patients for frequent outpatient visits to make sure the diet is proceeding as expected and that the child is safe. Transition into ketosis is not directly observed. Any issues after hours must be directed to the emergency department. The amount of education provided is limited, and KD initiation requires that the family live near the epilepsy center to minimize time traveling. Benefits of outpatient initiation include starting the KD in the comfort of the child's own home and reduced overall cost. However, centers that use outpatient initiation often have a higher dropout rate before the 3-month mark when effectiveness is typically determined (Levy et al., 2012).

THE CLASSIC KD

The classic KD begins with fasting, and only fluids that exclude carbohydrates are consumed. The duration of fasting varies. In the initial protocols used in the 1920s to the 1930s, fasting was commonly extended until 10% of body weight was lost (Linvingston, 1951; Wilder, 1921). The actual time that centers make their patients fast has decreased, but a duration of 12 to 72 hr is often implemented, or "until ketones are large in the urine" Freeman et al. (2007). The KD is then started at the full 90% fat composition and at a third of the calories, and it is advanced daily until the full-calorie meal is tolerated.

Fasting

The KD has a strong historical tie to fasting. The father of medicine, Hippocrates, prescribed fasting for his epilepsy patients. Fasting is also described in the Bible (Mark 9:29) and was used in the early 1900s in a cyclic fashion (for several weeks at a time) as treatment for patients with epilepsy (Wheless, 2008). The KD was created to mimic the metabolic changes that occur during fasting: lowering of the blood glucose and insulin levels, utilization of the body's glycogen stores, slowing of the flux through the glycolytic pathway, and finally utilization of fat stores via β-oxidation (Cahill, 1970; Cahill & Owen, 1970). In the process of breaking down fat, ketone bodies are produced and are transported into the central nervous system for direct use in energy production or to indirectly affect a myriad of metabolic pathways, leading to the "miracle of seizure reduction" (Lutas & Yellen, 2013). Ketone bodies are acidic; therefore, while the patient is fasting or on the KD, the overall acid load is increased. Ketone bodies also suppress the appetite, and it is often difficult to get a lethargic, acidotic, dehydrated child to eat a 90% fat meal without vomiting. For children, particularly young ones, this could become an issue that prolongs admissions and worsens morbidity, and it deters some families from trying the KD. Many centers have used a "kinder, gentler, gradual" advancement without fasting at initiation. Wirrell et al. (2002) first described their success with this approach in a retrospective case series of 14 children. Kim et al. (2004) stopped fasting all of their patients, and instead used the gradual caloric advancement approach of the 4:1 ratio. They reported similar success in seizure reduction at 3 months in 41 patients compared to 81 historical fasting controls. Finally, a randomized prospective trial in 48 patients compared the classic fasting KD with a gradual initiation approach (Bergqvist et al., 2005). Equivalence testing showed the gradual approach (1;1, 2;1, 3;1, 4;1, daily advancement, full-calorie KD) was as effective at reducing seizures at 3 months as the classic KD protocol. Both protocols achieved strong serum ketosis (Betahydroxybutyrate) by the fifth day, the gradual protocol about 1 day later than the fasting. In the gradual protocol, side effects were reduced by about two thirds and interventions were significantly fewer; the protocol was associated with less weight loss, less mild (defined as blood glucose <60 mg/dl and > 45 mg/dl) and severe hypoglycemia(defined as < 45 mg/dl), less dehydration, reduced acidosis, and reduced need for bicarbonate and intravenous fluid administration. Vomiting was not quantified but was reported as present or not, and it occurred in both treatment groups equally. Additional days needed in the hospital were also reduced in the gradual group compared to the fasting group, with a drop-out rate of 4% compared to 8% in the fasting group (very low, overall; Bergqvist et al., 2005). With these data in hand, many centers discontinued the fasting process for routine admissions and use it only when speed of achieving ketosis is of the essence, as with a child in status epilepticus (Cobo et al., 2015). The gradual initiation protocol has been modified and individualized to fit the child better. The CHOP protocol has eliminated the 1:1 ratio, instead using the (2:1, 3:1, 4:1) approach. Many centers do not advance to a full 4;1 ratio, depending on the severity of the child's epilepsy, frequency of seizures, and the response to lower ratios (Seo et al., 2007). The above findings have changed practice, and no centers participating in the ICSKD in 2018 routinely use a fasting initiation, and no one would fast a child younger than 2 years old. A case-by-case decision to fast was used by 28% of the programs. One universal exception where fasting is still considered is status epilepticus, where ketosis must be achieved quickly (Kossoff et al., 2018).

Liquid/Formula versus Food

KD formulas have been created for children who have gastrostomy tubes and for infants. In an attempt to shorten the admission time and to speed up the acceptance of the high-fat KD, some centers use a formula or liquid eggnog to initiate the KD, with similar success. Some centers have reported higher overall seizure reduction in formula-fed children, perhaps due to the decreased risk of noncompliance (Kossoff et al., 2004; Weijenberg et al., 2018). The problem with not modeling a home situation during the admission is that caregivers have had no prior experience or assistance with cooking 90% fat meals that are palatable and have to attempt this by themselves—be it with the support of websites and other keto coaches—once home. A stressful and not easy task for a beginner keto cook. By including hands-on cooking education in the hospital, the caregiver leaves more confident in their abilities to manage the KD at home (Fenton et al., 2019).

Caloric Restriction
Initiation

Caloric restriction was traditionally part of the KD initiation, with the calories gradually advanced during the initiation after the fast (1/3, 2/3, full-calorie 90% fat diet as tolerated). Bansal et al. found better effectiveness at 3 months in 30 children started on full-calorie 4:1 KD without fast, compared to 30 historical controls, but no difference in side effects or interventions, perhaps related to the lack of gradual adjustment to the 90% fat diet in their protocol (Bansal et al., 2014).

Maintenance

Calories are important to a growing child, and caloric needs are continuously changing during infancy and childhood. Calories are controlled on the KD until the dietitian changes the prescription. Clinical practice from KD centers shows that, if a child is given excessive calories and gains weight too quickly, it is associated with less reduction in seizures and lower ketosis until ideal body weight is achieved (Freeman et al., 2007), but this finding has not been tested in any trial. The calories are traditionally determined by a weighed 3-day dietary record provided by parents before the KD is started. This caloric estimate is compared to age and gender RDAs, estimated or measured resting energy expenditure (REE), and an activity factor. Children with epilepsy are less active than healthy children, and those who have additional motor disabilities may need even fewer calories (Wong & Wirrell, 2006). All these factors make it difficult to estimate calories for a KD plan.

Two studies have measured REE (an estimate of the basal metabolic rate) in children treated with the KD. In a short-term 6-month study, the KD did not change REE in 18 children, but change in the respiratory quotient (RQ) correlated with seizure reduction (Tagliabue et al., 2012). In a longer 15-month, prospective trial of 24 children treated with the KD compared to 75 age-matched controls, linear growth status declined while weight status and REE were unchanged; REE remained reduced in children with CP (Groleau et al., 2014). Furthermore, although the children gained weight as calories were adjusted, the weight gain came in the form of a change in body composition and a relative increase in fat mass. That is, the children became what they ate. The increased calories did not prevent the height deceleration seen in these children, a long-term side effect now well established in several prospective studies of the KD (Armeno et al., 2019; Bergqvist et al., 2008; Nation et al., 2014; Spulber et al., 2009; Vining et al., 2002; Williams et al., 2002; see chapter 12 Preventing side effects and diet discontinuation). In summary, calorie restriction is not needed for initiation or maintenance of the KD. Normal growth during the treatment period is encouraged, but the KD appears to alter body composition, and caloric adjustments do not prevent reduction in height velocity (growth failure), which maybe IGF-1 mediated.

WHEN DO WE DETERMINE EFFECTIVENESS OF THE KD?

Almost all efficacy trials related to dietary therapies determine initial effectiveness at 3 months. This is likely due to comparisons with anticonvulsant drug trials, where a 3-month design is standard practice (Sachdeo, 2007; Schmidt et al., 2014). Do patients really need to stay on the diet that long to determine if it works? Can they stop sooner, or should they perhaps stay on the diet longer? To answer these questions, Johns Hopkins University and Children's Memorial Hospital looked at when seizure reduction begins on the KD (Kossoff et al., 2008). In a retrospective analysis of 99 children started on a 4:1 fasting KD or 3–4:1 gradual KD protocol, the median time to first improvement was 5 days, with a range of 1 to 65 days. Reduction in seizures occurred sooner in the children who were fasted than in those who were on a gradual protocol, but long-term effectiveness was not different between the two initiation protocols, confirming prior studies. Five patients did not begin to have any change in their seizures until day 60 or more. Then, four of the five had > 50% to 90% reduction in seizures and one became seizure-free. The investigators concluded that if no change in seizure frequency is seen by 2 months, the KD can be discontinued. However, the data could also be interpreted to confirm the use of a 3-month minimal trial period of the KD. A significant improvement, including seizure freedom, in a 5% treatment-resistant epilepsy cohort is not unsignificant!

SEIZURE FREEDOM

Seizure freedom is the goal for the majority of patients trying the KD. In short-term randomized trials, it has been reported in 15% to 24% of patients (Martin et al., 2016). In longer-term studies, the data analyzed are not always continuous variables; instead, data are often obtained just prior to the time of interest, thereby artificially inflating the percentage reported as seizure-free. This makes it difficult to interpret the data and to counsel families appropriately. Taub et al. (2014) undertook a retrospective chart review of 275 patients started on the KD, of which 65 children (24%) achieved seizure freedom (defined as no seizure for 28 days). All children had daily seizures before starting the KD. The median time to

becoming seizure-free was 1.5 months, and 72% became seizure-free before 3 months (considered early seizure-free), while 28% became seizure-free after 3 months (considered late seizure-free). The longest time to becoming seizure- free was 18 months in one patient. Seizure recurrence (defined as any seizure after having been seizure-free for 28 days) occurred in 84%, and median time to recurrence was 3 months. However, 60% of those who experienced recurrence still had less than one seizure per month. The authors also looked at the timed effect of discontinuing Anti Seizure Medications (ASM) before or after 3 mo of KD treatment and found that timing of discontinuation of the ASM did not affect return of seizures. In general, in those who became seizure-free and experienced recurrence, the seizures did not return to their pre-diet frequency. The chance of remaining seizure-free at 18 months was only 3%. Families should be counseled that seizure freedom may occur at some point during KD treatment, most often in the first few months. If it happens, recurrence is more common than complete remission. In general, seizures remain greatly improved and do not return to the pre-KD frequency.

RATIOS: DO THEY MATTER?

As the KD practices were questioned and clinical protocols changed, less restrictive diets emerged: the modified Atkins diet (MAD, or unlimited protein diet, as it is called in Europe; Kossoff et al., 2003) and the low-glycemic-index diet (Pfeifer & Thiele, 2005). These diets have become popular alternatives to the KD because of their less strict nature, less need for resources, possibly milder side effects, and similar effectiveness to the KD. Some practitioners have even suggested that the modified diets should replace the formal KD for the majority of treatment-resistant patients (Auvin, 2013; Miranda et al., 2012). What data support this idea? Both alternative diets are lower ratio than the KD: MAD has at most a 2:1 ratio if tightly controlled and LGIT has a 1–1.5:1 ratio.

Animal data to date suggest that higher ratios are more effective in controlling seizures, although the ratios used in rodent models (4–6.3:1) are often much higher than what would be used in humans (Bough et al., 1999, 2000; Nylen et al., 2005). Some clinical studies to compare ratios have been randomized but not blinded. Seo et al. (2007) compared a 3:1 KD to a 4:1 KD in 76 randomized patients, and seizure reduction was measured at 3 months. The investigators found that the 4:1 KD reduced seizures more effectively and that there were significantly more seizure-free patients in the 4:1 group than in the 3:1 group. At 3 months, the researchers crossed the two protocols for an additional 3-month extension. Children who were seizure-free at the 3-month mark on the 4:1 KD maintained their seizure freedom on the lower ratio, indicating that perhaps a lower ratio can be used later in KD treatment without sacrificing effectiveness. El-Rashidy et al. (2013) studied 40 patients with symptomatic treatment-resistant epilepsy randomized to MAD, 4:1 KD formula, and standard diet with continued medical treatment. They found that the 4:1 formula resulted in better seizure reduction at 3 and 6 months than the MAD and regular diet. Raju et al. (2011) randomized 38 children to a 4:1 versus 2.5:1 KD and measured effectiveness at 3 months. There were no significant differences in responders or seizure freedom rate at 3 months (58% versus 63% and 26% versus 21%).

Kossoff et al. (2011) evaluated MAD versus MAD with liquid 4:1 supplement in the first month and found that the liquid supplement (i.e., higher ratio) was associated with a better reduction in seizures at 3 months. In a multicenter study, 27 patients from several countries were identified who had not responded completely to the MAD and were switched to the KD. Ten had further improvement, 11 did not. Children with myoclonic astatic epilepsy appeared to particularly improve with the formal KD (Kossoff et al., 2010).

Kim et al. (2016) compared the classic KD with the MAD in a prospective study of 104 patients. The patients were randomized, 51 to KD and 53 to MAD, but the groups tested were not homogeneous, since there was a lower baseline seizure count in the KD group. The researchers did not find a difference in responders (> 50% reduction in seizures) and seizures freedom between the diets at 3 and 6 months, except in children less than 2 years old, in whom the classic KD resulted in better seizure control (53% responders with KD versus 20% with MAD; p = 0.047).

In summary, current data from animal and human-based studies, some prospective and randomized but none blinded, suggest that higher ratios and the formal KD are more effective at reducing seizures than the modified diets, at least in the short term. It is premature to routinely discard the KD in favor of the modified diets, which are better tolerated. No diet will work if the patient cannot be compliant. There are situations where the modified diets are more appropriate (see chapter on modified diets). When choosing the MAD, families should be counseled that the less restrictive diets can take longer to work and may come at the expense of less reduction in seizures. A large, blinded, randomized trial of ratios and KD versus alternatives, with long-term follow-up to assess retention of seizure control and seizure freedom rate, is needed.

PREDICTORS OF RESPONSE

The KD appears to work particularly well in some electroclinical epilepsy syndromes. However, many patients do not fit into one of these categories; therefore, a predictor of response to the dietary therapies would be very helpful in guiding parents about staying on the KD or not. In the multiple observational studies published, there were no demographic parameters that predicted response (such as age, gender, or seizure type).

The electroencephalogram (EEG) appears to be a helpful tool. In a prospective blinded study of 37 patients on the fasting or gradual KD initiation protocol, Kessler et al. (2011) assessed the routine EEG at baseline, at 1 month of KD treatment, and at 3 months into KD treatment. The EEGs were analyzed for background slowing, interictal epileptiform discharges (IED), power spectrum analysis, and manual spike index. The researchers found that 70% of the patients became responders, with 27% becoming seizure-free. Over time, the EEG background slowing improved and there was an overall increase in beta frequencies, but this change did not predict responder status. IED were reduced by 65% by the 1-month EEG, and the 1-month reduction in IED strongly predicted response status to KD, with odds ratio of 4.8 (95% CI 1.1–21.3, p = 0.03). The authors concluded that the routine EEG is an excellent predictor of response and can assist neurologists when counseling parents about staying with the KD in the first 3 months of therapy (Kessler et al., 2011). Ebus et al. (2014) confirmed these findings in 34 patients via 24-hr video-EEG at baseline and at 6 weeks and 3 months into the KD. The patients had a low response rate overall, only 26%, but Ebus and colleagues did notice that a proportional reduction in IEDs of 30% during sleep strongly predicted reduction in seizures or better response status.

DURATION OF TREATMENT

The KD was initially created for a 2-year treatment period and a 6- to 12-month wean. However, there is no definitive treatment period, and the KD can be individualized based on the child's underlying condition and response. In some electroclinical epilepsy syndromes, such as infantile spasms, if the patient responds and becomes seizure-free, the diet treatment period may be shortened to 6 to 12 months, particularly if the EEG has normalized (Kossoff et al., 2002). For others, the KD has resulted in such extraordinary improvement in the child's overall quality of life—not only reduction in seizures, but also removal of all or most medications—that the family chooses to continue the KD longer (Hallböök et al., 2007). Most centers have a few patients who have been on the KD for > 15 years (Kossoff et al., 2007). Often, the ratios of the KD in this group of patients have been weaned to the lowest ratio that successfully maintains seizure control, but attempts to come off the KD have resulted in return of seizures. Continued use of dietary therapies must be weighed against the risk and complications and long-term side effects of a high-fat diet (Zupec-Kania & Zupanc, 2008; see chapter 12, Preventing side effects and diet discontinuation. Patients who are on the KD for life due to an underlying inborn error of metabolism, such as GLUT1 deficiency syndrome or pyruvate dehydrogenase disorder, require particular care in management of their diets (see chapter 6, GLUT1 Deficiency Syndrome and the Ketogenic Dietary Therapies).

REFERENCES

Armeno, M., Verini, A., Del Pino, M., Araujo, M. B., Mestre, G., Reyes, G., & Caraballo, R. H. (2019). A prospective study on changes in nutritional status and growth following two years of ketogenic diet (KD) therapy in children with refractory epilepsy. *Nutrients, 11*(7), 1–9.

Auvin, S. (2012). Should we routinely use modified Atkins diet instead of regular ketogenic diet to treat children with epilepsy? *Seizure, 21*(4), 237–240.

Bansal, S., Cramp, L., Blalock, D., Zelleke, T., Carpenter, J., & Kao, A. (2014). The ketogenic diet: Initiation at goal calories versus gradual caloric advancement. *Pediatric Neurology, 50*(1), 26–30.

Bergqvist, A. G. C. (2004). Indications and contraindications of the ketogenic diet. In C. E. Stafstrom & J. M. Rho (Eds.), *Epilepsy and the ketogenic diet* (pp. 115–117). Humana Press.

Bergqvist, A. G. C, Schall, J. I., Gallagher, P. R., Cnaan, A., & Stallings, V. A. (2005). Fasting versus gradual initiation of the ketogenic diet: A prospective, randomized clinical trial of efficacy. *Epilepsia, 46*(11), 1810–1819.

Bergqvist, A. G., Schall, J. I., Stallings, V. A., & Zemel, B. S. (2008). Progressive bone mineral content loss in children with intractable epilepsy treated with the ketogenic diet. *American Journal of Clinical Nutrition, 88*(6), 1678–1684.

Bough, K. J., Chen, R. S., & Eagles, D. A. (1999). Path analysis shows that increasing ketogenic ratio, but not beta-hydroxybutyrate, elevates seizure threshold in the Rat. *Developmental Neuroscience, 21*(3-5), 400–406.

Bough, K. J., Yao, S. G., & Eagles, D. A. (2000). Higher ketogenic diet ratios confer protection from seizures without neurotoxicity. *Epilepsy Research, 38*(1), 15–25.

Cahill, G. F., Jr. (1970). Starvation in man. *New England Journal of Medicine, 282*(12), 668–675.

Cahill, G. F., Jr., & Owen, O. E. (1970). Body fuels and starvation. *International Journal of Psychiatry in Clinical Practice, 7*(1), 25–36.

Chee, C., Rice, C., Fenton, C., Groveman, S., & Bergqvist, A. G. C. (2014). School personnel understanding of ketogenic diet. (Abstract) Global symposium for dietary treatments of epilepsy and other neurological disorders, Liverpool, England.

Cobo, N. H., Sankar, R., Murata, K. K., Sewak, S. L., Kezele, M. A., & Matsumoto, J. H. (2015). The ketogenic diet as broad-spectrum treatment for super-refractory pediatric status epilepticus: Challenges in implementation in the pediatric and neonatal intensive care units. *Journal of Child Neurology, 30*(2), 259–266.

Di Pisa, V., Cecconi, I., Gentile, V. DiPietro, E., Marchiani, V., Verrotti, A., & Franzoni, E. (2012). Case report of pyruvate dehydrogenase deficiency with unusual increase of fats during ketogenic diet treatment. *Journal of Child Neurology, 27*(12), 1593–1596.

Ebus, S.C., Lambrechts, D. A., Herraets, I. J. T., Majoie, M. J. M., deLouw, A. J., Boon, P. J., Aldenkamp, A. P., & Arends, J. B. (2014). Can an early 24-hour EEG predict the response to the ketogenic diet? A prospective study in 34 children and adults with refractory epilepsy treated with the ketogenic diet. *Seizure, 23*(6), 468–474.

El-Rashidy, O. F., Nassar, M. F., Abdel-Hamid, I. A., Gabr, S. S., Mohamed, S. G., El-Sayed, W. S., & Shaaban, S. Y. (2013). Modified Atkins diet vs classic ketogenic formula in intractable epilepsy. *Acta Neurologica Scandinavica, 128*(6), 402–408.

Fenton, C., Groveman, S., Chee, C. M., & Bergqvist, A. G. C. (2019). Benefits of a ketogenic teaching kitchen. *Journal of Child Neurology, 34*(14), 886–890.

Fenton, C., Groveman, S., Chee, C., Rice, C., & Bergqvist, A. G. C. (2014). Establishing a ketogenic teaching kitchen in the acute care setting. (Abstract) Global symposium for dietary treatments of epilepsy and other neurological disorders, Liverpool, England.

Freeman, J. M., Kossoff, E., & Freeman, M. T. K. (2007). *The ketogenic diet: A treatment for children and others with epilepsy* (4th ed.). Demos Medical Publishing.

Groleau, V., Schall, J. I., Stallings, V. A., & Bergqvist, C. A. (2014). Long-term impact of the ketogenic diet on growth and resting energy expenditure in children with intractable epilepsy. *Developmental Medicine and Child Neurology*, 56(9), 898–904.

Groveman, S., Fenton, C., Chee, C., Rice, C., & Bergqvist, A. G. C. (2014). Use of a ketogenic teaching kitchen in acute care setting. (Abstract) Global symposium for dietary treatments of epilepsy and other neurological disorders, Liverpool, England.

Hallb öö k, T., Lundgren, J., & Rosen, I. (2007). Ketogenic diet improves sleep quality in children with therapy-resistant epilepsy. *Epilepsia*, 48(1), 59–65.

Horvath, R., Gorman, G., & Chinnery, P. F. (2008). How can we treat mitochondrial encephalomyopathies? Approaches to therapy. *Neurotherapeutics*, 5(4), 558–568.

Kang, H. C., Lee, Y. M., Kim, H. D., Lee, J. S., & Slama, A. (2007). Safe and effective use of the ketogenic diet in children with epilepsy and mitochondrial respiratory chain complex defects. *Epilepsia*, 48(1), 82–88.

Kessler, S. K., Gallagher, P. R., Shellhaas, R. A., Clancy, R. R., & Bergqvist, A. G. C. (2011). Early EEG improvement after ketogenic diet initiation. *Epilepsy Research*, 94(1-2), 94–101.

Kim, D. W., Kang, H. C., Park, J. C., & Kim, H. D. (2004). Benefits of the nonfasting ketogenic diet compared with the initial fasting ketogenic diet. *Pediatrics*, 114(6), 1627–1630.

Kim, J. A., Yoon, J. R., Lee, E. J., Kee, J. S., Kim, H. D., & Kang, H. C. (2016). Efficacy of the classic ketogenic and the modified Atkins diets in refractory childhood epilepsy. *Epilepsia*, 57(1), 51–58.

Kossoff, E. H., Bosarge, J. L., Miranda, M. J., Wiemer-Kruel, A., Kang, H. C., & Kim, H. D. (2010). Will seizure control improve by switching from the modified Atkins diet to the traditional ketogenic diet? *Epilepsia*, 51(12), 2496–2499.

Kossoff, E. H., Dorward, J. L., Turner, Z., & Pyzik, P. L. (2011). Prospective study of the modified Atkins diet in combination with a ketogenic liquid supplement during the initial month. *Journal of Child Neurology*, 26(2), 147–151.

Kossoff, E. H., Freeman, J. M., Turner, Z., & Rubenstein, J. E. (2011). *Ketogenic diets: Treatments for epilepsy and other disorders* (5th ed.). Demos Medical Publishing.

Kossoff, E. H., Krauss, G. L., McGrogan, J. R., & Freeman, J. M. (2003). Efficacy of the Atkins diet as therapy for intractable epilepsy. *Neurology*, 61(12), 1789–1791.

Kossoff, E. H., Laux, L. C., Blackford, R., Morrison, P. F., Oyzik, P. L., Hamdy, R. M., Turner, Z., & Nordli, D. R. (2008). When do seizures usually improve with the ketogenic diet? *Epilepsia*, 49(2), 329–333.

Kossoff, E. H., & McGrogan, J. R. (2005). Worldwide use of the ketogenic diet. *Epilepsia*, 46(2), 280–289.

Kossoff, E. H., McGrogan, J. R., & Freeman, J. M. (2004). Benefits of an all-liquid ketogenic diet. *Epilepsia*, 45(9), 1163.

Kossoff, E. H., Pyzik, P. L., McGrogan, J. R., Vining, E. P., & Freeman, J. M. (2002). Efficacy of the ketogenic diet for infantile spasms. *Pediatrics*, 109(5), 780–783.

Kossoff, E. H., Turner, Z., & Bergey, G. K. (2007). Home-guided use of the ketogenic diet in a patient for more than 20 years. *Pediatric Neurology*, 36(6), 424–425.

Kossoff, E. H., Zupec-Kania, B. A., Amark, P. E., Ballaban-Gill, K. R., Bergqvist, A. G. C., Blackford, R., Buchhalter, J. R., Cross, H. J., Dahlin, M. G., Donner, E. J., Klepper, J., Jehle, R. S., Kim, H. D., Liu, C. Y. M., Nation, J., Nordli Jr, D. R., Pfeifer, H. H., Rho, J. M., Stafstrom, C. E., . . . Practice Committee of the Child Neurology Society; International Ketogenic Diet Study Group (2009). Optimal clinical management of children receiving the ketogenic diet: Recommendations of the International Ketogenic Diet Study Group. *Epilepsia*, 50(2), 304–317.

Kossoff, E. H., Zupec-Kania, B. A., Auvin, S., Ballaban-Gil, K. R., Bergqvist, A. G. C., Blackford, R., Buckhalter, J. R., Caraballo, R. H., Cross, H. J., Dahlin, M. G., Donner, E. J., Orkide, G., Jehle, R. S., Klepper, K., Kang, H. C., Lambrechts, D. A., Liu, Y. M. C., Hathan, J. K., Nordli Jr, D. R., . . . Practice Committee of the Child Neurology Society. (2018). Optimal clinical management of children receiving dietary therapies for epilepsy: Updated recommendations of the International Ketogenic Diet Study Group. *Epilepsia Open*, 3(2), 175–192.

Levy, R. G., Cooper, P. N., & Giri, P. (2012). Ketogenic diet and other dietary treatments for epilepsy. *Cochrane Database of Systematic Reviews*, 3, CD001903.

Livingston, S. (1951). The ketogenic diet in the treatment of epilepsy in children. *Postgrad Med. 10*(4), 333–336.

Lutas, A., & Yellen, G. (2013). The ketogenic diet: Metabolic influences on brain excitability and epilepsy. *Trends in Neuroscience*, 36(1), 32–40.

MacCracken, K. A., & Scalisi, J. C. (1999). Development and evaluation of a ketogenic diet program. *Journal of the Academy of Nutrition and Dietetics 99*(12), 1554–1558.

Martin, K., Jackson, C. F., Levy, R. G., & Cooper, P. N. (2016). Ketogenic diet and other dietary treatments for epilepsy. *Cochrane Database of Systematic Reviews*, Feb 9; *2*: CD001903. doi:10.1002/14651858.CD001903.pub3

Miranda, M. J., Turner, Z., & Magrath, G. (2012). Alternative diets to the classical ketogenic diet—Can we be more liberal? *Epilepsy Research, 100*(3), 278–285.

Nation, J., Humphrey, M., MacKay, M., & Boneh, A. (2014). Linear growth of children on a ketogenic diet: Does the protein-to-energy ratio matter? *Journal of Child Neurology, 29*(11), 1496–1501.

Neal, E. G., Chaffe, H., Schwartz, R. H., Lawson, M. S., Edwards, N., Fitzsimmons, G., Whitney, A., & Cross, J. H. (2008). The ketogenic diet for the treatment of childhood epilepsy: A randomised controlled trial. *Lancet Neurology, 7*(6), 500–506.

Nylen, K., Likhodii, S., Abdelmalik, P. A., Clarke, J., & Burnham, W. M. (2005). A comparison of the ability of a 4:1 ketogenic diet and a 6.3:1 ketogenic diet to elevate seizure thresholds in adult and young rats. *Epilepsia, 46*(8), 1198–1204.

Pfeifer, H. H., & Thiele, E. A. (2005). Low-glycemic-index treatment: A liberalized ketogenic diet for treatment of intractable epilepsy. *Neurology, 65*(11), 1810–1812.

Raju, K. N., Gulati, S., Kabra, M., Agarwala, A., Sharma, S., Pandey, R. M., & Kalra, V. (2011). Efficacy of 4:1 (classic) versus 2.5:1 ketogenic ratio diets in refractory epilepsy in young children: A randomized open labeled study. *Epilepsy Research, 96*(1-2), 96–100.

Rizzutti, S., Ramos, A. M., Muszkat, M., & Gabbai, A. A. (2007). Is hospitalization really necessary during the introduction of the ketogenic diet? *Journal of Child Neurology, 22*(1), 33 37.

Sachdeo, R. (2007). Monotherapy clinical trial design. *Neurology, 69*(24, Suppl. 3), S23–27.

Schmidt, D., Friedman, D., & Dichter, M. A. (2014). Anti-epileptogenic clinical trial designs in epilepsy: Issues and options. *Neurotherapeutics, 11*(2), 401–411.

Seo, J. H., Lee, Y. M., Lee, J. S., Kang, H. C., & Kim, H. D. (2007). Efficacy and tolerability of the ketogenic diet according to lipid:nonlipid ratios—Comparison of 3:1 with 4:1 diet. *Epilepsia, 48*(4), 801–805.

Snyder, D. (2006). *Keto kids.* Demos Medical Publishing.

Spulber, G., Spulber, S., Hagenas, L., Amark, P., & Dahlin, M. (2009). Growth dependence on insulin-like growth factor-1 during the ketogenic diet. *Epilepsia, 50*(2), 297–303.

Stafstrom, C. E., Zupec-Kania, B., & Rho, J. M. (2008). Epilepsia: Ketogenic diet and treatments; Introduction/perspectives. *Epilepsia, 49*(Suppl. 8), 1–2.

Tagliabue, A., Bertoli, S., Trentani, C., Borrelli, P., & Veggiotti, P. (2012). Effects of the ketogenic diet on nutritional status, resting energy expenditure, and substrate oxidation in patients with medically refractory epilepsy: A 6-month prospective observational study. *Clinical Nutrition, 31*(2), 246–249.

Taub, K. S., Kessler, S. K., & Bergqvist, A. G. C. (2014). Risk of seizure recurrence after achieving initial seizure freedom on the ketogenic diet. *Epilepsia, 55*(4), 579–583.

Vaisleib, I. I., Buchhalter, J. R., & Zupanc, M. L. (2004). Ketogenic diet: Outpatient initiation, without fluid or caloric restrictions. *Pediatric Neurology, 31*(3), 198–202.

van der Louw, E., Olieman, J., Poley, M. J., Wesstein, T., Vehmeijer, F., Catsman-Berrevoets, C., & Neuteboom, R. (2019). Outpatient initiation of the ketogenic diet in children with pharmacoresistant epilepsy: An effectiveness, safety and economic perspective. *European Journal of Paediatric Neurology, 23*(5), 740–748.

Vining, E. P., Pyzik, P., McGrogan, J., Hladky, H., Anand, A., Kriegler, S., & Freeman, J. M. (2002). Growth of children on the ketogenic diet. *Developmental Medicine and Child Neurology, 44*(12), 796–802.

Weber, T. A., Antognetti, M. R., & Stacpoole, P. W. (2001). Caveats when considering ketogenic diets for the treatment of pyruvate dehydrogenase complex deficiency. *Journal of Pediatrics, 138*(3), 390–395.

Weijenberg, A., van Rijn, M., Callenbach, P. M. C., de Koning, T. J., & Brouwer, O. F. (2018). Ketogenic diet in refractory childhood epilepsy: Starting with a liquid formulation in an outpatient setting. *Child Neurology Open, 5,* 2329048X18779497.

Wheless, J. W. (2008). History of the ketogenic diet. *Epilepsia, 49*(Suppl. 8), 3–5.

Wijburg, F. A., Barth, P. G., Bindoff, L. A., Birch-Machin, M. A., van der Blij, J. F., Ruitenbeek, W., Turnbull, D. M., & Schutgens, R. B. (1992). Leigh syndrome associated with a deficiency of the pyruvate dehydrogenase complex: Results of treatment with a ketogenic diet. *Neuropediatrics, 23*(3), 147–152.

Wilder, R. M. (1921). The effect of ketonemia on the course of epilepsy. *Mayo Clinic Bulletin, 2,* 307–308.

Williams, S., Basualdo-Hammond, C., Curtis, R., & Schuller, R. (2002). Growth retardation in children with epilepsy on the ketogenic diet: a retrospective chart review. *Journal of the American Dietetic Association, 102*(3), 405–407.

Wirrell, E. C., Darwish, H. Z., Williams-Dyjur, C., Blackman, M., & Lange, V. (2002). Is a fast necessary when initiating the ketogenic diet? *Journal of Child Neurology, 17*(3), 179–182.

Wong, J., & Wirrell, E. (2006). Physical activity in children/teens with epilepsy compared with that in their siblings without epilepsy. *Epilepsia, 47*(3), 631–639.

Zupec-Kania, B., & Zupanc, M. L. (2008). Long-term management of the ketogenic diet: Seizure monitoring, nutrition, and supplementation. *Epilepsia, 49*(Suppl. 8), 23–26.

6

GLUT1 Deficiency Syndrome and the Ketogenic Dietary Therapies

JOERG KLEPPER, MD

GLUT1 DEFICIENCY SYNDROME

In the fed state, the human brain relies entirely on glucose for energy metabolism. Glucose entry into the brain is exclusively mediated by the facilitated glucose transporter protein type 1 (GLUT1). Impaired glucose transport into the brain resulting from GLUT1 deficiency (GLUT1DS, OMIM 606777; De Vivo et al., 1991) will cause a cerebral "energy crisis," particularly in the young, because the developing brain requires three to four times more energy than the adult brain. Clinical features of GLUT1DS are global developmental delay, early-onset epilepsy, and a complex movement disorder (Alter et al., 2015; Klepper, 2007, 2020). In fact, the disease mechanism of GLUT1DS is intriguingly straightforward:

1. The GLUT1 defect results in low cerebrospinal fluid (CSF) glucose concentrations, termed hypoglycorrhachia.
2. Hypoglycorrhachia results in the characteristic clinical features: seizures, developmental delay, and movement disorders.
3. GLUT1DS is treatable by means of a ketogenic diet (KDT), which provides ketones as an alternative fuel for brain energy metabolism (Figure 6.1).

An international expert group has developed a consensus statement summarizing the current knowledge on GLUT1DS as well as recommendations for its diagnosis and treatment (Klepper, 2020).

CLINICAL PRESENTATION

In general, the clinical presentation of GLUT1DS depends on the patient's age, the type of genetic mutation, and early initiation of ketogenic diet therapies (KDT). Classic GLUT1DS presents with nonspecific developmental delay associated with early-onset epilepsy, a complex movement disorder, and paroxysmal non-epileptic events. Any combinations of these features are possible (Figure 6.2; Pearson et al., 2013). In early infancy, seizures and distinctive paroxysmal eye–head movements are the initial features of GLUT1DS (Pearson et al., 2017). Seizure type may vary from cyanotic attacks and staring spells in early infancy to early childhood absence epilepsy and myoclonic/generalized grand mal seizures in later childhood. Certain epilepsy syndromes, such as early-onset absence epilepsy (onset before the age of 4 years) and myoclonic astatic epilepsy (Doose syndrome), are also associated with GLUT1DS (Mullen et al., 2010; Suls et al., 2008). The epilepsy of GLUT1DS often stabilizes, whereas the movement disorder and paroxysmal events increase with age and seem to be the major problems in adolescence and adulthood (Alter et al., 2015; Klepper, 2020; Klepper & Leiendecker, 2007).

The complex movement disorder in GLUT1DS features ataxia and spastic gait abnormalities, action limb dystonia, mild chorea, cerebellar action tremor, myoclonus, and dyspraxia (Pons et al., 2010). Secondary microcephaly may reflect the impairment of the developing brain. About 75% of patients describe paroxysmal events that increase with age, particularly paroxysmal exertion-induced dystonia (PED; Klepper et al., 2016). Uncommon features described in single patients include writer's cramp, intermittent ataxia, total body paralysis, Parkinsonism, nocturnal painful muscle cramps in the legs, alternating hemiplegia of childhood, hemiplegic migraine, cyclic vomiting, and strokelike episodes with paroxysmal hemiparesis, dysarthria, or aphasia (Klepper, 2020). Stomatin-associated cryohydrocytosis, a rare form of hemolytic anemia, has been identified as allelic disease associated with *SLC2A1*

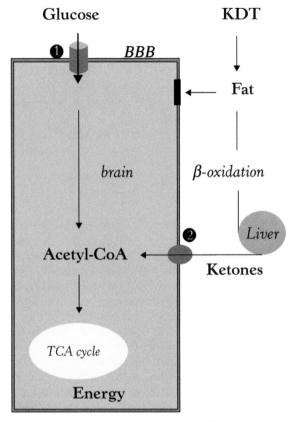

FIGURE 6.1 *The Metabolic Concept of GLUT1 Deficiency Syndrome (GLUT1DS)*

❶ The defect of the GLUT1 transporter at the blood–brain barrier (BBB) results in cerebral energy failure.

❷ Ketones derived from either body fat (fasting) or nutritional fat (KDT) serve as an alternative fuel to restore cerebral energy.

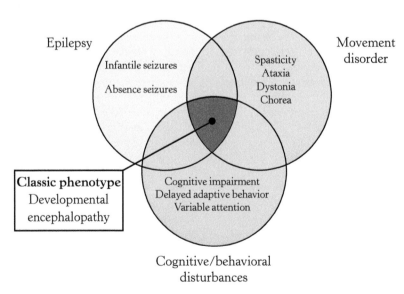

FIGURE 6.2 *The Complex Phenotype of GLUT1 Deficiency Syndrome (GLUT1DS)*

Reproduced with permission from Pearson et al. (2015).

pathogenic variants (Flatt et al., 2011; Weber et al., 2008).

DIAGNOSIS

The diagnosis of GLUT1DS is based on three principal criteria: (1) characteristic clinical features, (2) low glucose concentrations in CSF (hypoglycorrhachia), determined by a fasting lumbar puncture, and (3) *SLC2A1* pathogenic variants. Depending on the number of positive criteria, the diagnosis is rated as confirmed, probable, possible, or negative (Klepper, 2020).

The lumbar puncture should be performed in a metabolic steady state following a 4- to 6-hr fast. In GLUT1DS, CSF glucose concentrations usually are below 50 mg/dl. A CSF/plasma glucose ratio below 0.45 is helpful to determine hypoglycorrhachia, and CSF lactate should always be low to normal (for age-dependent reference values of CSF glucose and lactate, see Leen et al., 2013). Patients with milder phenotypes have CSF glucose values in the range of 41 to 50 mg/dl and never normal values (De Vivo & Wang, 2008). Mild or borderline hypoglycorrhachia associated with missense mutations is often present in extended phenotypes and indicates that a *SLC2A1* analysis should

be performed in addition to a diagnostic lumbar puncture. In approximately 85% to 90% of cases, the condition can be confirmed by heterozygous *SLC2A1* pathogenic variants. Inheritance is predominantly autosomal dominant, and pathogenic variants are mostly de novo (Wang et al., 1993). The type of genetic mutation often correlates with phenotypic severity. Specific pathogenic *SLC2A1* variants affecting functional domains of GLUT1 have been identified (Raja & Kinne, 2020). Familial autosomal dominant and autosomal recessive inheritances have been reported in individual families (Brockmann et al., 2001; Klepper et al., 2001, 2009). Prenatal testing is available if the disease-causing mutation has been identified. Of note, the absence of *SLC2A1* pathogenic variants does not exclude GLUT1DS: pathogenic mechanisms may involve noncoding RNA genes and GLUT1 translation, transcription, processing, activation, and trafficking (Klepper, 2013). *SLC2A1*-negative patients are diagnosed on the basis of distinctive clinical features, hypoglycorrhachia, and favorable response to KDT (Klepper, 2020).

Neuroimaging is generally uninformative, but PET scanning has been reported to show

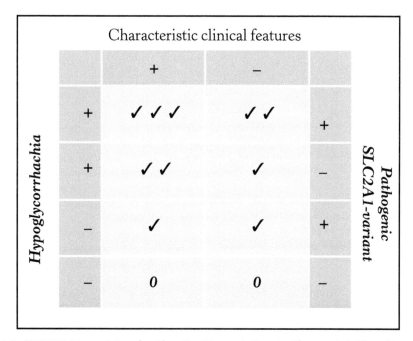

FIGURE 6.3 *GLUT1DS Diagnosis Based on Three Key Diagnostic Criteria: Characteristic Clinical Features, Definite Hypoglycorrhachia, and Pathogenic SLC2A1 Variants*

GLUT1DS = GLUT1 deficiency syndrome; PED = paroxysmal exercise-induced dystonia; CSF = cerebrospinal fluid; KDT = ketogenic diet therapies; MAD = modified Atkins diet

From Klepper et al. (2020).

a distinctive metabolic footprint in the brain (Akman et al., 2015; Pascual et al., 2002). Recently, a blood test that reveals reduced GLUT1 expression by flow cytometry analysis of GLUT1 surface expression on circulating red blood cells has been reported to be of diagnostic value (Gras et al., 2017). Additional techniques, such as assays of glucose uptake into erythrocytes or into oocytes, are available on a research basis only (Klepper, 2020).

KDT IN GLUT1DS

Currently, the only treatment available for GLUT1DS is the KDT. The metabolic concept of the KDT is to mimic the metabolic state of fasting and thus to "refuel" the brain by generating ketones (Figure 6.1). The antiseizure mechanisms described for KDT in drug-resistant childhood epilepsy (Masino & Rho, 2012; Rho, 2017) also contribute to seizure control in GLUT1DS patients. KDT also generate nonspecific positive effects, such as improved physical endurance, improved attention span, and increased alertness (Lambrechts et al., 2012; Ramm-Pettersen et al., 2014), and have a substantial positive impact on the associated movement disorder (Leen et al., 2013).

The practical approach to KDT in GLUT1DS does not differ substantially from KDT for intractable childhood epilepsy (Klepper, 2012). Clinical management of KTD, such as initiation, supplementation, and maintenance, follows established guidelines (Kossoff et al., 2018). In theory, any KDT providing measurable ketosis may be used in GLUT1DS according to age, clinical presentation, and compliance. In practice, long-chain and medium-chain KDT and the MAD are established therapies for GLUT1DS, whereas the low-glycemic-index treatment is not (Klepper, 2020). As summarized in a recent consensus on GLUT1DS diagnosis and treatment (Klepper, 2020), the use of KDT for GLUT1DS differs from the use of KDT in drug-resistant childhood epilepsy. The major differences are:

- Ketones in GLUT1DS provide an alternative fuel for the brain, restoring the cerebral energy deficit. The higher the ketosis, the more energy is provided for the developing brain. Accordingly, the KDT providing the highest ketosis is best for the patient.
- The timing of the introduction of the KDT correlates with outcome. Consequently, KDT should be started as early as possible, even in very young infants, to meet the energy demands of the developing brain.
- KDT in GLUT1DS should be continued throughout childhood into adolescence to provide ketones as an alternative fuel for adequate brain development. Discontinuation of KDT after approximately 2 years, as discussed for drug-resistant childhood epilepsy, is not recommended in GLUT1DS.
- In contrast to the efficacy of KDT in the treatment of drug-resistant childhood epilepsy, the majority of patients with GLUT1DS show immediate and continuing seizure control with KDT (Klepper, 2020; Kossoff et al., 2018). This is even considered a diagnostic tool: if KDT is ineffective, reconsider the diagnosis.

Long-term adverse effects of KDT, such as growth retardation, prolonged QT interval on ECG, selenium deficiency, renal stones, elevated serum lipids, and cardiovascular disease, are serious concerns, and long-term data are only just emerging (Heussinger et al., 2018). Follow-up at regular intervals should include a clinical examination, basic blood parameters with fasting lipids, EEG, and a renal ultrasound (Klepper, 2020). Additional tools can be a DEXA scan for bone density (Bergqvist et al., 2008) and ultrasound of the carotid arteries for atherosclerosis (Coppola et al., 2014; Heussinger et al., 2018; Kapetanakis, 2014). In puberty, maintaining KDT is particularly difficult, and achieving compliance after years on KDT often is the most important practical problem in this age group. Transition programs for GLUT1DS adolescents into adult medicine are essential, but rare—originally considered an exclusively pediatric disorder, GLUT1DS has now arrived in adult neurology (Cervenka et al., 2016; Leen et al., 2014).

When paroxysmal movement disorders prove to be unresponsive to KDT, acetazolamide and L-dopa have been described as beneficial in single cases. Novel compounds, such as ketone esters, are currently being considered to supplement or even replace KDT in childhood epilepsy and metabolic disease. Despite encouraging initial reports, clinical trials of triheptanoin (UX007) for the treatment of seizures and movement disorders in GLUT1DS did not show beneficial effects (Clinical Trials.gov Identifier: NCT01993186; NCT02960217).

OPEN QUESTIONS

GLUT1 not only mediates glucose transport across the blood–brain barrier, but also plays a major role in other energy-dependent tissues, such as retina, muscle, placenta, and heart (Mueckler & Thorens, 2013). The potential involvement of these organs in GLUT1DS remains an unaddressed concern. Accordingly, no sufficient data on pregnancy and KDT are currently available (van der Louw et al., 2017). GLUT1DS is a treatable entity, and neurological outcome correlates with the timing of KDT initiation—neonatal screening would be beneficial but is currently not established due to lack of sufficient methods.

For reasons as yet unclear, a subgroup of GLUT1DS patients do not achieve sufficient seizure control with KDT (Bekker et al., 2019). Also, in a substantial number of patients, KDT fail to control movement disorders, especially PED, sufficiently, highlighting the need for additional therapies, such as supplemental metabolites to compensate for neuroglycopenia. Current research focuses on individual *SLC2A1* variants that may destabilize or generate novel interactions, trigger protein misfolding, or enhance protein aggregation (Raja & Kinne, 2020). *SLC2A1*-negative GLUT1DS may be caused by variations in noncoding RNA genes as well as by downstream defects in GLUT1 translation, transcription, processing, activation, and trafficking (Tang et al., 2019). Novel approaches aim to restore GLUT1 protein content and function via upregulation of the normal *SLC2A1* allele using small-molecule or gene-transfer strategies, because preclinical experiments with gene replacement in GLUT1DS model mice using AAV9 vectors have been shown to be effective (Nakamura et al., 2018; Tang et al., 2017).

CONFLICTS OF INTEREST

The author has received speaker honoraria and travel funds from Nutricia GmbH, SHS, Heilbronn, Germany, and Vitaflo, Steinbach, Germany. He has received project support from the parent support group Glut1-Förderverein, Bremen, Germany.

REFERENCES

Akman, C. I., Provenzano, F., Wang, D., Engelstad, K., Hinton, V., Yu, J., Tikofsky, R., Ichese, M., & De Vivo, D. C. (2015). Topography of brain glucose hypometabolism and epileptic network in glucose transporter 1 deficiency. *Epilepsy Research, 110*, 206–215.

Alter, A. S., Engelstad, K., Hinton, V. J., Montes, J., Pearson, T. S., Akman, C. I., & De Vivo, D. C. (2015). Long-term clinical course of Glut1 deficiency syndrome. *Journal of Child Neurology, 30*(2), 160–169.

Bekker, Y. A. C., Lambrechts, D. A., Verhoeven, J. S., van Boxtel, J., Troost, C., Kamsteeg, E. J., Willemsen, M. A., & Braakman, H. M. H. (2019). Failure of ketogenic diet therapy in GLUT1 deficiency syndrome. *European Journal of Paediatric Neurology, 23*(3), 404–409.

Bergqvist, A. G., Schall, J. I., Stallings, V. A., & Zemel, B. S. (2008). Progressive bone mineral content loss in children with intractable epilepsy treated with the ketogenic diet. *American Journal of Clinical Nutrition, 88*(6), 1678–1684.

Brockmann, K., Wang, D., Korenke, C. G., von Moers, A., Ho, Y. Y., Pascual, J. M., Kuang, K., Yang, H., Ma, L., Kranz-Eble, P., Fischbarg, J., Hanefeld, F., & De Vivo, D. C. (2001). Autosomal dominant Glut-1 deficiency syndrome and familial epilepsy. *Annals of Neurology, 50*(4), 476–485.

Cervenka, M. C., Henry, B. J., Felton, E. A., Patton, K., & Kossoff, E. H. (2016). Establishing an adult epilepsy diet center: Experience, efficacy and challenges. *Epilepsy & Behavior, 58*, 61–68.

Coppola, G., Natale, F., Torino, A., Capasso, R., D'Aniello, A., Pironti, E., Santoro, E., Calabro, R., & Verrotti, A. (2014). The impact of the ketogenic diet on arterial morphology and endothelial function in children and young adults with epilepsy: A case-control study. *Seizure, 23*(4), 260–265.

De Vivo, D. C., Trifiletti, R. R., Jacobson, R. I., Ronen, G. M., Behmand, R. A., & Harik, S. I. (1991). Defective glucose transport across the blood-brain barrier as a cause of persistent hypoglycorrhachia, seizures, and developmental delay. *New England Journal of Medicine, 325*(10), 703–709.

De Vivo, D. C., & Wang, D. (2008). Glut1 deficiency: CSF glucose. How low is too low? *Revue Neurologique (Paris), 164*(11), 877–880.

Flatt, J. F., Guizouarn, H., Burton, N. M., Borgese, F., Tomlinson, R. J., Forsyth, R. J., Baldwin, S. A, Levinson, B. E., Quittet, P., Aguilar-Martinez, P., Delaunay, J, Stewart, G. W., & Bruce, L. J. (2011). Stomatin-deficient cryohydrocytosis results from mutations in *SLC2A1*: A novel form of GLUT1 deficiency syndrome. *Blood, 118*(19), 5267–5277.

Gras, D., Cousin, C., Kappeler, C., Fung, C. W., Auvin, S., Essid, N., Chung, B. H., Da Costa, L., Hainque, E., Luton, M.-P., Petit, V., Vuillaumier-Barrot, S., Boespflug-Tanguy, O., Roze, E., & Mochel, F. (2017). A simple blood test expedites the diagnosis of glucose transporter type 1 deficiency syndrome. *Annals of Neurology, 82*(1), 133–138.

Heussinger, N., Della Marina, A., Beyerlein, A., Leiendecker, B., Hermann-Alves, S., Dalla Pozza,

R., & Klepper, J. (2018). 10 patients, 10 years—Long term follow-up of cardiovascular risk factors in Glut1 deficiency treated with ketogenic diet therapies: A prospective, multicenter case series. *Clinical Nutrition, 37*(6, Part A), 2246–2251.

Kapetanakis, M., Liuba, P., Odermarsky, M., Lundgren, J., & Hallböök, T. (2014). Effects of ketogenic diet on vascular function. *European Journal of Paediatric Neurology, 18*(4), 489–494.

Klepper, J. (2012). GLUT1 deficiency syndrome in clinical practice. *Epilepsy Research, 100*(3), 272–277.

Klepper, J. (2013). Absence of *SLC2A1* mutations does not exclude Glut1 deficiency syndrome. *Neuropediatrics, 44*(4), 235–236.

Klepper, J. (2020). Glut1 deficiency syndrome (Glut1DS): State of the art in 2020 and recommendations of the international Glut1DS study group. *Epilepsia Open,5*(3), 354–365.

Klepper, J., & Leiendecker, B. (2007). GLUT1 deficiency syndrome—2007 update. *Developmental Medicine & Child Neurology, 49*(9), 707–716.

Klepper, J., Leiendecker, B., Eltze, C., & Heussinger, N. (2016). Paroxysmal nonepileptic events in Glut1 deficiency. *Movement Disorders Clinical Practice, 3*(6), 607–610.

Klepper, J., Scheffer, H., Elsaid, M. F., Kamsteeg, E. J., Leferink, M., & Ben-Omran, T. (2009). Autosomal recessive inheritance of GLUT1 deficiency syndrome. *Neuropediatrics, 40*(5), 207–210.

Klepper, J., Willemsen, M., Verrips, A., Guertsen, E., Herrmann, R., Kutzick, C., Flörken, A., & Voit, T. (2001). Autosomal dominant transmission of GLUT1 deficiency. *Human Molecular Genetics, 10*(1), 63–68.

Kossoff, E. H., Zupec-Kania, B. A., Auvin, S., Ballaban-Gil, K. R., Christina Bergqvist, A. G., Blackford, R., Buchhalter, J. R., Caraballo, R. H., Cross, J. H., Dahlin, M. G., Donner, E. J., Guzel, O., Jehle, R. S., Klepper, J., Kang, H.-C., Nordli, D. R., Jr., . . . Practice Committee of the Child Neurology Society. (2018). Optimal clinical management of children receiving dietary therapies for epilepsy: Updated recommendations of the International Ketogenic Diet Study Group. *Epilepsia Open, 3*(2), 175–192.

Lambrechts, D. A., Bovens, M. J., de la Parra, N. M., Hendriksen, J. G., Aldenkamp, A. P., & Majoie, M. J. (2012). Ketogenic diet effects on cognition, mood, and psychosocial adjustment in children. *Acta Neurologica Scandinavica, 127*(2), 103–108.

Leen, W. G., Mewasingh, L., Verbeek, M. M., Kamsteeg, E. J., van de Warrenburg, B. P., & Willemsen, M. A. (2013). Movement disorders in GLUT1 deficiency syndrome respond to the modified Atkins diet. *Movement Disorders, 28*(10), 1439–1442.

Leen, W. G., Taher, M., Verbeek, M. M., Kamsteeg, E. J., van de Warrenburg, B. P., & Willemsen, M. A.

(2014). GLUT1 deficiency syndrome into adulthood: A follow-up study. *Journal of Neurology, 261*(3), 589–599.

Leen, W. G., Wevers, R. A., Kamsteeg, E. J., Scheffer, H., Verbeek, M. M., & Willemsen, M. A. (2013). Cerebrospinal fluid analysis in the workup of GLUT1 deficiency syndrome: A systematic review. *JAMA Neurology, 70*(11), 1440–1444.

Masino, S. A., & Rho, J. M. (2012). Mechanisms of ketogenic diet action. In J. L. Noebels, M. Avoli, M. A. Rogawski, R. W. Olsen, & A. V. Delgado-Escueta (Eds.), *Jasper's* basic mechanisms of the epilepsies (4th ed.). National Center for Biotechnology Information.

Mueckler, M., & Thorens, B. (2013). The SLC2 (GLUT) family of membrane transporters. *Molecular Aspects of Medicine, 34*(2-3), 121–138.

Mullen, S. A., Suls, A., De Jonghe, P., Berkovic, S. F., & Scheffer, I. E. (2010). Absence epilepsies with widely variable onset are a key feature of familial GLUT1 deficiency. *Neurology, 75*(5), 432–440.

Nakamura, S., Muramatsu, S. I., Takino, N., Ito, M., Jimbo, E. F., Shimazaki, K., Onaka, T., Ohtsuki, S., Terasaki, T., Yamagata, T., & Osaka, H. (2018). Gene therapy for Glut1-deficient mouse using an adeno-associated virus vector with the human intrinsic GLUT1 promoter. *Journal of Gene Medicine, 20*(4), e3013.

Pascual, J. M., Van Heertum, R. L., Wang, D., Engelstad, K., & De Vivo, D. C. (2002). Imaging the metabolic footprint of Glut1 deficiency on the brain. *Annals of Neurology, 52*(4), 458–464.

Pearson, T. S., Akman, C., Hinton, V. J., Engelstad, K., & De Vivo, D. C. (2013). Phenotypic spectrum of glucose transporter type 1 deficiency syndrome (Glut1 DS). *Current Neurology and Neuroscience Reports, 13*(4), 342.

Pearson, T. S., Pons, R., Engelstad, K., Kane, S. A., Goldberg, M. E., & De Vivo, D. C. (2017). Paroxysmal eye-head movements in Glut1 deficiency syndrome. *Neurology, 88*(17), 1666–1673.

Pons, R., Collins, A., Rotstein, M., Engelstad, K., & De Vivo, D. C. (2010). The spectrum of movement disorders in Glut-1 deficiency. *Movement Disorders, 25*(3), 275–281.

Raja, M., & Kinne, R. K. H. (2020). Mechanistic insights into protein stability and self-aggregation in GLUT1 genetic variants causing GLUT1-deficiency syndrome. *Journal of Membrane Biology, 253*(2), 87–99.

Ramm-Pettersen, A., Stabell, K. E., Nakken, K. O., & Selmer, K. K. (2014). Does ketogenic diet improve cognitive function in patients with GLUT1-DS? A 6- to 17-month follow-up study. *Epilepsy & Behavior, 39*, 111–115.

Rho, J. M. (2017). How does the ketogenic diet induce anti-seizure effects? *Neuroscience Letters, 637*, 4–10.

Suls, A., Dedeken, P., Goffin, K., Van Esch, H., Dupont, P., Cassiman, D., Kempfle, J., Wuttke, T. V., Weber, Y., Lerche, H., Afawi, Z., Vandenberghe, W., Korczyn, A. D., Berkovic, S. F., Ekstein, D., Kivity, S. Ryvlin, P., Claes, L. R. F., Deprez, L., . . . Van Paesschen, W. (2008). Paroxysmal exercise-induced dyskinesia and epilepsy is due to mutations in *SLC2A1*, encoding the glucose transporter GLUT1. *Brain, 131*(Part 7), 1831–1844.

Tang, M., Gao, G., Rueda, C. B., Yu, H., Thibodeaux, D. N., Awano, T., Engelstad, K. M., Sanchez-Quintero, M.-J., Yang, H., Li, F., Li, H., Su, Q., Shetler, K. E., Jones, L., Seo, R., McConathy, J., Hillman, E. M., Noebels, J. L., De Vivo, D. C., & Monani, U. R. (2017). Brain microvasculature defects and Glut1 deficiency syndrome averted by early repletion of the glucose transporter-1 protein. *Nature Communications, 8*, 14152.

Tang, M., Park, S. H., De Vivo, D. C., & Monani, U. R. (2019). Therapeutic strategies for glucose transporter 1 deficiency syndrome. *Annals of Clinical and Translational Neurology. 6*(9), 1923–1932.

van der Louw, E. J., Williams, T. J., Henry-Barron, B. J., Olieman, J. F., Duvekot, J. J., Vermeulen, M. J., Bannink, N., Williams, M., Neuteboom, R. F., Kossoff, E. H., Catsman-Berrevoets, C. E., & Cervenka, M. C. (2017). Ketogenic diet therapy for epilepsy during pregnancy: A case series. *Seizure, 45*, 198–201.

Wang, D., Pascual, J. M., & De Vivo, D. (1993). Glucose transporter type 1 deficiency syndrome. In M. P. Adam, H. H. Ardinger, R. A. Pagon, S. E. Wallace, L. J. H. Bean, K. Stephens, et al. (Eds.), GeneReviews®.

Weber, Y. G., Storch, A., Wuttke, T. V., Brockmann, K., Kempfle, J., Maljevic, S., Margari, L., Kamm, C., Schneider, S. A., Huber, S. M., Pekrun, A., Roebling, R., Seebohm, G., Koka, S., Lang, C., Kraft, E., Blazevic, D., Salvo-Vargas, A., Fauler, M., . . . Lerche, H. (2008). GLUT1 mutations are a cause of paroxysmal exertion-induced dyskinesias and induce hemolytic anemia by a cation leak. *Journal of Clinical Investigation, 118*(6), 2157–2268.

Ketogenic Diet in Established Epilepsy Indications

ANN M. BERGIN, MD

INTRODUCTION

Arising from biblical anecdote and early 20th century explorations of the effect of fasting for seizure management, the ketogenic diet (KD) developed alongside medical knowledge of the biochemistry of fasting/starvation and ketosis (Wheless, 2014). Falling into relative disuse with the arrival of phenytoin and subsequent anticonvulsant medications, it continued to be used mainly in pediatrics, and primarily under the auspices of Freeman and colleagues at Johns Hopkins University. After the development of waves of new anticonvulsant medications that were associated with reduction in toxicity but not with greater efficacy in patients with refractory epilepsy, interest in the KD re-emerged. Over the years, multiple case series, describing cases achieving remarkable and sustained efficacy in a substantial proportion of children with the most intractable epilepsies (> 400 seizures/month) have been published by the Johns Hopkins group (Hemingway et al., 2001). With the renewed interest in the KD, a multicenter group showed that other centers using the same protocol could achieve similar results (Vining et al., 1998), and finally a randomized controlled study was conducted in London, again supporting the efficacy of this treatment in children with refractory epilepsies (Neal et al., 2008) This chapter reviews diet treatment in epilepsies where its use is well established—refractory nonsurgical epilepsies, epileptic encephalopathies (including infantile spasms), Lennox-Gastaut syndrome, myoclonic-atonic epilepsy (Doose syndrome), and severe myoclonic epilepsy of infancy (Dravet syndrome).

REFRACTORY NONSURGICAL EPILEPSY

Refractory nonsurgical epilepsy is a broad group of disorders, defined by their nonsuitability for potentially curative surgery, and includes lesional, nonlesional, focal, multifocal, and secondary generalized epilepsies. Etiologies include remote symptomatic injuries (pre-, peri-, and postnatal brain injuries of hypoxic, traumatic, infectious, and hemorrhagic origin), developmental brain malformations, genetic/metabolic disorders causing epilepsy as their primary problem or resulting in symptomatic epilepsy, primary and secondary epileptic encephalopathies, and progressive/degenerative epilepsies. In the modern era of molecular specificity, it seems counterintuitive to dwell on such a heterogeneous group. Indeed, increasing surgical prowess and the advancing ability to define specific genetic etiologies and to offer individualized molecularly based therapies have, and will continue, to "chip away" at this broad group. However, it is in precisely such a heterogeneous group that the efficacy of the KD was first described. And, in epilepsy practice, patients presenting with refractory epilepsy constitute exactly this mixed group of patients.

In treatment of epilepsy, serially trialed anti-seizure medication (ASM), after initial failure, are known to have diminishing likelihood of achieving seizure freedom, with only 14% of patients achieving seizure freedom with a second or third agent and only 3% becoming seizure-free with a combination of two drugs (Kwan & Brodie, 2000). Alternative approaches, such as surgery for patients with amenable lesions, and neurostimulation and/or diet manipulation for others, are available in this setting. "Drug-resistant epilepsy may be defined as failure of adequate trials of two tolerated and appropriately chosen and used AED schedules (whether as monotherapies or in combination) to achieve sustained seizure freedom" (Kwan et al., 2010). Once epilepsy is identified as refractory, nonpharmacologic approaches are appropriately considered. Among the options, resective epilepsy surgery offers the possibility of "cure" of epilepsy, and in certain cases it is the best chance of seizure-free, and even medication-free, survival. Consideration of surgical candidacy is therefore important at this point. There are multiple reasons for patients' ineligibility for epilepsy surgery, including the inability to lateralize or localize the seizure focus, presence of multiple foci, high risk of injury to eloquent cortex, and patient/family preference. In this setting, as well as in those for whom epilepsy surgery has already failed, dietary manipulation is an important treatment option.

For many years, evidence of diet efficacy was in the realm of expert opinion, in a narrow community of experts familiar with the diet, who reported retrospective reviews of mixed groups of patients with highly refractory epilepsies (Hemingway et al., 2001; Kinsman et al., 1992; Prasad et al., 1996). Studies included etiologies and seizures of all kinds in children across a broad range of ages, often with very high seizure frequency. Reported efficacy was surprisingly good, comparable to industry standards for efficacy of new drugs today. Their retrospective nature and lack of blinding and control groups limited the interpretability of these studies. Following media exposure in 1994 in a *Dateline NBC* review of the diet and in 1997 after release of the film "First Do No Harm," there was a tidal wave of interest in the diet among parents of children with refractory epilepsy. Parents pressured their providers to provide, or to refer them for a trial of, diet treatment. In this setting, the first prospective studies emerged: a multicenter study (Vining et al., 1998) and a single-institution report (Freeman et al., 1998) described the diet's efficacy in patients with average seizure frequencies of 230/month and 410/month, respectively. The multicenter study assured the community of pediatric epileptologists that the efficacy of the Johns Hopkins protocols could be reproduced in other hands. At this point, in 2000, a review of 11 reports on diet efficacy, including the two cited prospective studies, co-sponsored by BlueCross and Blue Shield, stated, "It is unlikely that this degree of benefit can result from a placebo response and/or spontaneous remission," and therefore concluded, "The evidence is sufficient to determine that the KD is efficacious in reducing seizure frequency in children with refractory epilepsy" (Lefevre & Aronson, 2000). Finally, in 2008, a randomized, controlled but unblinded study of diet in a mixed group of children with refractory epilepsy revealed a statistically significant improvement in seizure control in the group of children treated with KD immediately, compared to a matched group treated with KD 3 months later, a finding

improving the quality of evidence in support of diet efficacy (Neal et al., 2008).

These studies have the great benefit of generalizability to the real world of refractory epilepsy. Therefore, as might be expected, subsequent studies from around the world in similar case series have reported roughly similar efficacy, which can be broadly stated as ~ 50% of refractory epilepsy patients starting the KD can expect to be responders (i.e., have > 50% seizure reduction), 25% to 30% will experience > 90% seizure reduction, and approximately half of the latter will be seizure-free (Hallbrook et al., 2015; Henderson et al., 2006; Kossoff & McGrogan, 2005; Kossoff et al., 2012; Nathan et al., 2009).

Diet therapy in epilepsy is rigorous, requiring precision in preparation and careful attention to administration by caregivers. Formula-fed and tube-fed infants are easiest to initiate and maintain on the diet, and the approach for these patients usually uses the classic KD at a ratio sufficient to induce ketosis with plasma beta-hydroxybutyrate ≥ 4 mmol/L or seizure freedom, whichever comes first. The children are not troubled by dietary restriction and poor palatability the way older, orally fed children are; older patients are accustomed to making dietary choices, have preferences that may not be diet-compliant, and may refuse diet-appropriate foods and fluids. Reduced GI motility may worsen esophageal reflux and constipation in all patients, resulting in discomfort. Diet therapy is not without a variety of systemic adverse effects, and although they occur at low frequency (Kang et al., 2004; Kossoff et al., 2009), they are at least comparable in range and significance to those associated with anticonvulsant medications. Yet, a significant advantage of the KD is its lack of sedating and/or behavioral adverse effects.

It would be extremely helpful to be able to predict which patients are most likely to respond to diet therapy, instead of having to anticipate ~ 50% failure to achieve a useful seizure reduction. Unfortunately, although many studies and reports have attempted to identify predictors, small study size, lack of control groups, heterogeneous diagnostic groups, and the rarity of specific epilepsy syndromes have all limited the ability to reliably identify these factors. Schoeler et al. (2013) published an extensive review of the articles providing data on effectiveness and putative predictive factors. Twenty-one factors were examined. For each factor, the predominance of evidence in favor of an effect, the relative strength of evidence against an effect of that factor, and the number of patients in the cohorts "for" and "against" that factor were considered. No factor had strong evidence for a positive or negative response to diet. Strong evidence for absence of effect was also lacking, except in the case of gender and intellectual ability, which appear to have no effect on diet response. There were "mixed" findings (effect on response was reported in approximately half of reported cases) for epilepsy cause/syndrome, seizure type, and biochemical markers other than ketosis and plasma glucose. "Weak evidence" for an effect on diet response (effect reported in less than half of reported cases) existed for age of seizure onset, age at diet initiation, time from seizure onset to diet initiation, seizure frequency, diet type, ratio, levels of ketosis (beta-hydroxybutyrate, acetone), EEG parameters, AEDs (individual or number/combinations), and body mass index (BMI). Presence or absence of an effect of blood glucose, genetics, and imaging findings could not be assessed because of a limited number of studies reporting and patients reported. Assessment of predictive factors in this way is complicated by interactions among factors, which cannot be resolved in small, uncontrolled, retrospective studies. Ideally, in the future there will be development of consortia of expert centers devoted to analysis of greater numbers of patients managed prospectively and in a standard manner, which will allow dissection of factors predictive of successful treatment. Better understanding may also illuminate potential mechanisms for further study and manipulation.

Patients started on the KD may have a seizure response within 14 days, but most will continue a trial of diet for at least 3 months, assuming no exacerbation of seizures occurs beyond the initial initiation period (Kossoff et al., 2009). Discontinuation after successful treatment is usually attempted after 2 years, although there are no data determining this to be the optimal time. Rarely, diet initiation is associated with persistent exacerbation of seizures beyond the initiation itself. Diet withdrawal is appropriate in this setting. Early diet discontinuation (< 3 months) is usually due to lack of efficacy. Growing intolerance of dietary restriction can be problematic in young patients able to make diet choices.

Barriers to provision of the KD continue to include lack of access to clinical expertise in diet treatment, the cost of high-grade protein and high-fat foods in some communities, individual feeding/dietary preferences, medical complexity and fragility concerning tolerance of the stress of dietary conversion, and side effects.

In summary, for patients falling into the heterogeneous category of nonsurgical epilepsy, KD therapy should be considered once drug resistance and ineligibility for surgery have been established. In general, patients can expect a better chance of efficacy with the KD than with trial of another AED (Kwan & Brodie, 2000).

Many conditions for which the KD can be particularly beneficial have been identified. Several are epilepsy syndromes with refractory generalized seizures. This chapter covers the four most common conditions for which there are sufficient data to recommend the KD as very helpful.

INFANTILE SPASMS

Infantile spasms (IS) are an age-dependent seizure type, occurring typically in children between 6 and 24 months old, and are clinically characterized by clusters of serial body jerks, often at the interfaces of waking and sleep. IS represent the most common type of epileptic spasms. They are often, but not always, associated with a characteristic EEG pattern known as hypsarrhythmia, a chaotic waking pattern of asynchronous, high-voltage, irregular slowing with superimposed multifocal spikes, and a more synchronous pattern and more discontinuous background activity in sleep. When spasms are associated with developmental regression and hypsarrhythmia, the triad constitutes West syndrome. IS can be idiopathic (cause unknown) or associated with genetic or structural disorders or pre-existing brain injuries. Etiology is the strongest predictor of long-term developmental outcome.

High-dose steroids/ACTH and vigabatrin are first-line treatments for this epileptic encephalopathy, which is refractory to initial therapies in 30% to 40% overall (Lux et al., 2005; Pellock et al., 2010). Refractory IS are associated with serious delay in development in most survivors. Early and effective treatment of IS is considered the best chance for normal developmental outcome. With first-line treatment, high-dose steroids/ACTH in most cases (except in tuberous sclerosis-related IS, when vigabatrin is more effective), elimination of clinical spasms by 14 days of treatment is the first marker of successful treatment. Resolution of hypsarrhythmia is also considered an indication of successful treatment of IS, and the EEG is usually assessed first at 14 days, with evaluation for maintenance of improvement in a further 28 days.

Because of the developmental impact of IS, the primary outcome goal should be the seizure-free rate, with EEG resolution of underlying hypsar-rhythmia of equal importance. Complicating the assessment of efficacy of any treatment of IS is the known occurrence of spontaneous remission of IS in untreated cases, which can occur as early as 1 month after onset, and cumulatively in 10% to 15% at 6 months and in up to 25% of patients at 1 year (Hrachovy et al., 1991). (Notably, in Hrachovy and colleagues' retrospective cohort of untreated infants, ~ 90% suffered moderate to severe developmental impairment at follow-up, an average of 80 months later.) There is also a significant relapse rate during treatment with first-line agents. Frequency of relapse is another key outcome measure in assessing any treatment for IS.

The KD is among the options considered after failure of first-line treatments, or if their use is contraindicated for any reason. Most of the studies of KD in IS are retrospective and involve small numbers of patients who are heterogeneous with respect to important baseline characteristics, such as etiology, numbers of prior treatments, and duration of spasms before KD, as well as EEG documentation and duration of follow-up. The general impression from these studies is of moderate efficacy and tolerability, providing the basis for use of KD in a second-line position. A systematic review of studies of the KD in IS yielded a median spasm-free rate of ~ 35% and a long-term median seizure-free rate of ~ 10% (Prezioso et al., 2018).

Interest in KD treatment of IS was stimulated when Nordli et al. (2001) described six of 12 affected infants who attained seizure freedom among a larger group (N = 32) of infants with refractory seizures. Additional studies supported the tolerability of diet intervention in IS infants but not the degree of efficacy. Of 23 children with IS, three were seizure-free at 6 and 12 months (13%), with 13 remaining on diet at 12 months (Kossoff et al., 2002). Hong et al. (2010) reported on 104 infants with IS who were treated with KD after exposure to a mean of 3.6 AEDs, including steroids or vigabatrin in > 70%: 38 infants (36%) were spasm-free after 2.4 months on the diet, and 30 (29%) achieved long-term spasm freedom. Overall, there was a 64% > 50% responder rate in this relatively large group. In a prospective case study of 20 patients with epileptic spasms, 70% and 72% were responders at 3 and 6 months, respectively, and three infants (15%) maintained seizure freedom for at least 6 months (Kayyali et al., 2014). Improvement in spasms was noted within 1 month of starting diet treatment. EEG

improved in 12 (60% of patients) when assessed at 3 to 6 months, and in five of six infants with hypsarrhythmia, the pattern resolved and did not recur up to 12 months after diet initiation. Pires et al. (2013) reported that six of 17 KD-treated patients (35%) were seizure-free at 1 month after failing vigabatrin and hydrocortisone. Eleven of the 17 patients (65%) were seizure-free at 3 months, one after the addition of felbamate. The addition of felbamate to their regimen brought five more into the responder (> 50% reduction) group. In a retrospective, cross-sectional study comparing early (< 1.5 years) with late diet initiation, Dressler et al. included 59 infants with IS in their population of 115 infants. Nineteen (32%) were seizure-free at 3 months (Dressler et al., 2015a). Numis et al. (2011) had nine of 26 patients (32%) seizure-free at 1 to 3 months. They noted an association of spasm response and "other seizure" response in the patients (p = 0.02).

Recently, a prospective study with complex design—a randomized controlled study (RCT) with an additional parallel control group (PC)—compared KD and high-dose ACTH treatment (Dressler et al., 2019). Electroclinical remission at 28 days (the primary outcome) was similar for both treatments for both the RCT patients (N = 32, 62% KD, 69% ACTH) and PC group (N = 69, 41% and 38%). Relapse rate was higher overall for ACTH-treated patients (43%, versus 16% for KD-treated patients). Adverse effects were recorded at a high rate in both groups (79% of KD-treated patients and 94% of ACTH-treated in the combined study groups), but adverse effects requiring acute intervention were more frequent in the ACTH group (94%, versus 30% in the KD-treated). Long-term seizure freedom was similar for both treatments in the RCT (37% KD, 44% ACTH). Vigabatrin appeared to affect treatment outcomes. In infants not treated with vigabatrin, ACTH was significantly more effective in attaining the primary outcome (KD 47%, ACTH 80%, p = 0.02), although relapse rates were higher for the ACTH-treated group, leading finally to similar long-term seizure freedom for both treatment groups. In vigabatrin-treated infants, KD was more effective at 28 days (48% versus 25%), and relapse rates again were higher in the ACTH group, so that long-term seizure freedom was better in the KD group (48% KD, 21% ACTH, p = 0.05). Low power and complex design limited the strength of conclusions from this first prospective comparison study from a single institution, highlighting the need for multicenter cooperation for treatment studies in IS patients.

Diet therapy is relatively easy to provide to infants due to the readily available ketogenic formula and infants' lack of independent choice of dietary intake. Nonetheless, aside from lack of efficacy, difficulty managing the diet protocol (3 of 20 caregivers) can also result in discontinuation (Kayyali et al., 2014). Diet-related side effects, including gastrointestinal intolerability, can also limit utilization of the KD in this population. In an Asian population, nine of 43 patients discontinued diet due to "unacceptable" complications, and seven due to intolerability. An additional nine (21%) discontinued due to insufficient efficacy (Eun et al., 2006). In contrast, Numis et al. (2011) reported that six of 26 patients (23%) had side effects, none serious enough to cause discontinuation of the diet. In this group, five of the 26 discontinued the diet by ∼ 1 year, either due to lack of efficacy or due to difficulty maintaining the diet.

In these young patients, concerns regarding weight gain and appropriate growth were amenable to adjustment downward in ratio for increased protein intake (Hong et al., 2010). Numis et al. (2011) described no significant differences between responders and nonresponders in terms of weight-for-height z scores, although the best responders (> 90% seizure reduction) had lower weight-for-height z scores at all points.

Among the 104 patients described by Hong et al., 10 of the 18 in whom diet was used as the first-line treatment became seizure-free, had normal EEGs within 2 months, and were maintained on the diet for 6 months, after which the diet was withdrawn without relapse (Hong et al., 2010). The same group reported a retrospective case-controlled study of diet versus ACTH as initial therapy for new-onset spasms (Kossoff et al., 2008). Eight of 13 patients on diet therapy (62%) became seizure-free at a median of 6.5 days of treatment, compared to 18 of 20 (90%) treated with high-dose ACTH who were spasm-free at a median of 4 days ($p = 0.06$). One of the eight relapsed (12.5%), versus six (33%) of the 18 ACTH responders ($p = 0.23$). EEG normalization was more likely in the ACTH group (1 of 11 versus 9 of 17, $p = 0.02$) at 1 month, although the EEG normalized in all eight spasm-free patients by 5 months of diet treatment. Adverse effects were significantly less likely in the KD group ($p = 0.006$). There was no difference in developmental outcome between the treatment groups at their last examination at a median of 12 months.

Predicting efficacy of diet has been difficult. Eun et al. associated underlying etiology with efficacy, with "cryptogenic" cases responding at a higher rate than "symptomatic" cases (87.5% seizure-free versus 46% in symptomatic cases, $p = 0.037$), but no other predictor emerged from their series (Eun et al., 2006). No significant predictive factor of diet efficacy was identified in the small diet group in the case-control comparison with ACTH (Kossoff et al., 2008). Numis et al. (2011) reported 11 of 18 males and one of eight females were responders ($p = 0.04$) but cited low sample size and skewed distribution of etiologies as potential biases. This gender difference has not been reported in other studies (Prezioso et al., 2018).

A final area of interest is the possibility of synergistic effects of a combination of the KD with other treatments for IS. Ville and colleagues' study of epileptic encephalopathies (IS, Lennox-Gastaut syndrome/other generalized epilepsies, Continuous Spikes and Waves in Slow sleep (CSWS)) examined the efficacy of KD added to steroid therapy when seizures are not controlled by the initial steroid treatment (Ville et al., 2015). Patients were on a mean of 3.5 mg/kg/day of hydrocortisone (1–10 mg/kg/day). Ketonuria was achieved in all but one case with status epilepticus (SE), and no diet adjustment was made to maintain ketonuria. Plasma ketones were not measured. There were 23 IS cases in the total of 42 patients with epileptic encephalopathies. Twenty were steroid-resistant, and three were steroid-dependent. The data presented did not allow specific analysis with respect to IS, but overall, five of 27 (18.5%) steroid-resistant cases and nine of 15 (60%) steroid-dependent cases were considered responders. More recently another combination therapy, vigabatrin with hormonal therapy, has proven more effective than hormonal monotherapy in achieving early (between 14 and 42 days) spasm freedom in the large ICISS study (O'Callaghan et al., 2017) although developmental and epilepsy outcomes to date (18 months) have been similar in the two treatment strategies (O'Callaghan et al., 2018). Combination of diet and vigabatrin therapy may also be worth investigating, particularly in light of the potential interaction between these therapies identified in the recent Dressler study.

In summary, studies of modest quality indicate that KD is a moderately effective therapy for refractory IS and is generally safe and tolerable in this young population. As a first-line treatment, it has better efficacy for seizure freedom over time, but it may not be as quickly effective as traditional first-line treatments, in particular

ACTH, although the relapse rate may be lower with KD. Patients experiencing improvement do so within 1 month, and definitely by 3 months. There continues to be interest in improving outcomes for IS by combining therapies, rather than progressing through them serially, and it remains to be seen in what setting the KD might be most efficacious. Ideally, large, collaborative study groups will provide answers to these important questions.

LENNOX-GASTAUT SYNDROME (LGS)

LGS is characterized by peak onset between 3 and 5 years of age and rarely presents after 10 years of age. It is associated with a very refractory pleomorphic epilepsy, tonic seizures being most characteristic, particularly in sleep, and also includes atypical absences as well as atonic and myoclonic seizures (Arzimanoglou et al., 2009). Focal seizures with altered consciousness may also occur. Seizures may be very frequent, occurring multiple times per day. Episodes of SE, convulsive and/or nonconvulsive, often prolonged, are common. LGS may occur de novo, or in ~ 20% of patients it develops following West syndrome, but it may also follow other remote symptomatic brain injuries (e.g., hypoxic ischemic encephalopathy). If there is not pre-existing developmental delay, cognitive regression occurs and at least moderate intellectual disability (ID) is expected: in a retrospective review of 68 adult patients followed for a mean of almost 20 years, Kim et al. (2014) described 95% of patients as having moderate to profound ID. Virtually all individuals were dependent in adulthood, with only ~ 40% being independent for basic activities of daily living—eating, bathing, toileting, etc. (Kim et al., 2014). In LGS, the EEG is characterized by slow (1.5–2 Hz) spike-and-wave activity, often with multifocal spikes, and bursts of 10-Hz fast activity during sleep. Slow spike-and-wave activity may wane over the years. Treatment with broad-spectrum anticonvulsant drugs is the mainstay of treatment but is rarely effective in achieving seizure control. Side effects—lethargy and drowsiness—are particularly damaging because they are associated with increased seizures. Nonpharmacologic treatments, including surgical approaches (corpus callosotomy, vagus nerve stimulation) and diet therapies, offer nonsedating adjunctive therapies that, if successful, may allow reduction of medication burden and a resultant improvement in seizures and quality of life.

The early reports of KD efficacy in the most refractory epilepsies typically included patients with LGS, and this subgroup of patients were found to respond to diet with a > 50% reduction in seizures within 5 days of diet initiation with 36 hr of fasting and the development of ketosis (Freeman & Vining, 1999). A blinded crossover study of 20 LGS patients, initiated on diet and subsequently, in a blinded manner, given either 60 g glucose with saccharin to abort diet or saccharin only (allowing continued ketosis) failed to show a significant difference in outcome, but this was likely due to the failure to eliminate ketosis in the glucose + saccharin (control) group (Freeman et al., 2009). Lemmon et al. (2012) reported that, in the literature up to 2012, 88 of 189 (47%) LGS patients had responded to the KD. Using an intention-to-treat analysis, they retrospectively reviewed 71 patients from their institution, Johns Hopkins Hospital, of whom 36 (51%) achieved a > 50% reduction in seizures and 16 (23%) a > 90% reduction, while one patient was seizure-free. The results were similar at 12 months. Caraballo et al. reported similar results in a smaller prospectively studied group of 20 LGS patients started on diet and followed for a minimum of 16 months, with retention of 75% of patients on diet, and two of 20 (15%) seizure-free and 25% with 50% to 99% reduction in seizures (Caraballo et al., 2014). Five children discontinued the diet in this study, three because of lack of efficacy within 3 months, and two because of persistent vomiting, one of whom was also hypoglycemic. LGS patients have also been reported to respond with similar efficacy to the modified Atkins diet (MAD; Sharma et al., 2015). Twelve of 25 were responders and two (8%) were seizure-free.

Zhang et al. (2016) included assessment of EEG background and epileptiform activity in a retrospective study of 47 patients with LGS on KD. They showed a possible association between improvement in the EEG characteristics and response to diet. Limitations of the study identified by the authors as affecting robustness of this association included the fact that the EEG readers were unblinded to case deposition, the lack of a control group, and the lack of ketone measurements. That said, the possibility that improvement in EEG characteristics at 3 months could represent a biomarker of diet efficacy is of interest and would bear further investigation.

In summary, LGS patients, some of the most refractory pediatric epilepsy patients, respond well to KD therapies. With KD efficacy, medication reduction or withdrawal provides special benefit to these patients by reducing sedation and associated seizures, thereby improving quality of life even further. Diet therapy should be considered early, once the LGS diagnosis is clear and refractoriness is established.

DRAVET SYNDROME (DS; SEVERE MYOCLONIC EPILEPSY OF INFANCY, SMEI)

DS/SMEI is a clinical syndrome characterized by initial febrile seizure, often febrile SE, and/or hemiclonic febrile seizures in the first year of life, in the setting of initially normal development. The syndrome occurs in 1 in 20,000 to 40,000 individuals. Febrile and afebrile seizures are quickly recurrent and are associated with subsequent developmental stagnation or regression. The epilepsy is pleomorphic (with multiple seizure types—myoclonic, focal, generalized absences, and generalized motor seizures) and pharmacoresistant. Fever/hyperthermia continues to provoke seizures. Subsequent to seizure onset, ataxia, pyramidal signs, and interictal myoclonus are seen. Early EEGs are normal, but later, generalized spike and polyspike-waves, as well as multifocal spikes, are seen. Historically, many children thought to have pertussis vaccine-related encephalopathy with long-term cognitive sequelae were found to have underlying DS (Berkovic et al., 2006). Up to 80% of DS cases are associated with a heterozygous mutation in the sodium channel gene SCN1A, although not all SCN1A mutations result in DS. Other genetic and/or environmental factors play an unclear role in evolution of the syndrome. Development generally stabilizes, but at least a moderate degree of intellectual disability is the rule. The temporal relationship between seizure onset and developmental impairment suggests a relationship between seizures, SE, and developmental impairment. However, clinical studies in humans and animal studies do not find a correlation between severity of epilepsy and/or SE and cognitive impairment. Instead, sodium-channel-related dysfunction of GABAergic interneurons and glutamatergic neurons is likely responsible. Nonetheless, as described in a recent consensus report, the goal of treatment is to decrease the frequency especially of prolonged seizures and convulsive and nonconvulsive SE (Wirrell et al., 2017). The same consensus report indicated strong support for first- (valproic acid and/or clobazam) and second-line treatments (stiripentol, topiramate, KD). There is a higher mortality in children with DS (Genton et al., 2011),

due to a variety of factors (sudden unexpected death in epilepsy, SE, accident), further motivating efforts to control convulsive seizures. A *Scn1a* mutant mouse model of DS showed decreased latency to seizure onset after an epileptogenic challenge compared to wild-type litter mates. Feeding the mutant mouse a KD increased latency to seizures to levels that were not significantly different from the levels in wild-type litter-mates (Dutton et al., 2011).

Caraballo (2011) reported experience with 59 DS patients, of whom 24 were treated with a 4:1 KD and followed for at least 2 years. Of the 16 patients who remained on the diet at 2 years, two (12.5%) were seizure-free, 10 (62.5%) had 75% to 99% reduction in seizures, and another four (25%) had 50% to 74% reduction in seizures. All five patients with SE responded to diet and had no additional SE during follow-up. Medication reduction, even in those without dramatic KD-related seizure efficacy, resulted in improvement in quality of life. Ten of 15 patients followed by Nabbout et al. (2011) achieved a >75% reduction in seizures. All these patients were already receiving triple combination therapy (valproic acid, stiripentol, clobazam). However, efficacy was lost in ~ 50% by 1 year. Behavioral improvements were noted in all responders.

Laux et al. (2013) followed a subgroup of 20 of 48 DS patients on KD at their center, all of whom remained on the diet at least 6 months, with 17 continuing for at least 18 months. The researchers found that 65% of patients achieved > 50% reduction in seizures and 30% achieved > 90% reduction. They noted that the KD appeared to reduce the frequency of all seizure types, although quantification of myoclonic and absence seizures was not robust.

In a retrospective cross-sectional study, 10 of 32 mutation-positive patients (31 SCN1A mutations and one GABRG mutation) with DS were treated with KD (Dressler et al., 2015b) for at least 3 months. Seven of 10 patients were responders at 3 months, and six at 6 months and 12 months. One child became seizure-free on KD. A striking finding in this group was the lack of SE in the eight patients who had previously suffered this seizure type. No child on KD, responder or not, had SE while on the diet. Given that excess mortality in this syndrome is partly related to SE, this is a notable finding, which has also been reported by Ni et al. (2018) in 20 DS patients with refractory convulsive seizures on KD, all of whom had a history of generalized tonic-clonic seizures (GTCs) ≥ 5 min in duration, and 15 had a history of SE. In this group (Ni et al., 2018), there were 17 responders at 6 months and none experienced an episode of SE or GTC ≥ 5 min in duration during the study. In this study, subjective caregiver assessment indicated improved cognition (alertness, attention, memory) in 80% of responders, despite all but one patient remaining on stable AED doses.

An interesting aspect of the Dressler study is the comparison with other treatments (Dressler et al., 2015b). There was no significant difference in responder rates between the gold standard treatment—a combination of stiripentol, valproic acid, and clobazam (89%)—bromide (78%), KD 70%, valproic acid monotherapy 48%, topiramate 35%, and Vagus Nerve Stimulator (VNS) 37%. KD was more effective than levetiracetam. The conclusions are limited by small numbers but appear worthy of further study.

With respect to positive interaction with other treatments, seven of 16 diet responders were on topiramate in Caraballo's updated group, and three of seven of Dressler's responders were as well.

At the time of writing, novel antiseizure medications (ASMs) are being evaluated in DS patients (Cross et al., 2019). Cannabidiol, recently available in a pharmaceutical-grade formulation, was considered "moderately" effective by the North American consensus group (Wirrell et al., 2017). Fenfluramine is possibly even more promising in early studies and community experience. Therefore, while the North American consensus group as well as a recent authoritative review (Cross et al., 2019) place KDs among second-line treatments, the order of recommended treatments is likely to be revised again. Nonetheless, KD appears effective in decreasing especially prolonged convulsive seizures and SE, while conferring behavioral and cognitive benefits that are likely in part related to the opportunity to reduce ASM burden. The KD therefore remains a useful option in pharmacoresistant DS-related epilepsy, especially in the setting of medication adverse effects. Trial of MAD in older DS patients may offer improved palatability and can be advanced to a more rigorous traditional/classic diet if a trial of more profound ketosis is required.

A still unanswered question is whether early use of the KD, with its lack of cognitive side effects and prominent effect on SE, might ameliorate the developmental stagnation/regression associated with early seizure onset in this disorder. Better understanding of such an effect may help clarify

the KD's position among the available treatment options.

DOOSE SYNDROME (MYOCLONIC ATONIC EPILEPSY, MAE)

MAE is a genetic generalized epilepsy, initially described by Doose (Doose et al., 1970) and distinguished from other causes of myoclonic epilepsy in childhood (SMEI, LGS), although the underlying genetic abnormality is not yet known. MAE occurs in previously normal children, with onset, sometimes explosive, possible as early as the latter half of the first year of life, but more typically between 2 and 5 years of age. There is a high rate of preceding febrile seizures and a family history of epilepsy. It is characterized by frequent myoclonic and myoclonic astatic/atonic seizures, as well as absences, with or without myoclonia, generalized tonic-clonic, clonic, and/or tonic seizures. The occurrence of nocturnal tonic seizures is thought by some to indicate a poor outcome. With extremely frequent seizures, often absences interspersed with myoclonias, nonconvulsive SE or an epileptic encephalopathy can develop. Seizure-related falls are a major component of associated morbidity, and these children are at risk of injury. Many need to wear helmets for protection. The epilepsy is often highly pharmacoresistant, and adverse effects of medication add to the impact of the disorder on cognitive performance and behavior regulation. EEG, initially normal, is associated with generalized spike- and polyspike-wave activity, ranging from 2 to 5 Hz, and this pattern also underlies the myoclonic seizures. Prominent theta activity is a feature of the interictal EEG, as may be the persistence of normal posterior dominant rhythm and sleep architecture in many (Kelley et al., 2010). Among refractory childhood epilepsies, MAE is uniquely responsive to the KD. This has led to exploration of the relationship of the disorder to defects of the glucose transporter type 1 (GLUT1), a possibility that would provide an explanation for its particular responsiveness to ketosis. However, only 0% to 5% of cases have been shown to be associated with a mutation in the responsible gene, *SLC2A1* (Larsen et al., 2015; Mullen et al., 2011). Abnormalities in a number of other genes (*SLC6A1*, *CHD2*, *CACNA1H*, and others) have been found in isolated cases (Routier et al., 2019) but without so far providing an understanding of the pathogenesis of the disorder. Long-term cognitive outcome is normal in about 60% of patients. Continued active seizures are correlated with cognitive decline, with varying degrees of intellectual disability, ranging from mild to moderate severity.

Using the International League Against Epilepsy (ILAE) criteria for diagnosis, Oguni et al. (2002) reported treatment outcome in a group of 81 patients with MAE. Seizure freedom for > 2 years was achieved in 55 patients (65%) by 50 months (± 16 months). Later recurrence of GTCs occurred in 14% up to 18 years later but were then easily controlled, while 18% continued to have refractory epilepsy. Among the treatments used in this group, KD was used for 26 patients, of whom 15 (58%) became free of myoclonic seizures (MS) and atonic seizures (AS), while nine more had > 50% reduction in these seizures. This efficacy was better than that of ACTH ($N = 22$, 36% MS/AS free, 23% > 50% decreased), ethosuximide ($N = 32$, 32% MS/AS free, 32% > 50% decreased), the best of the conventional AEDs used, and was better than that of valproic acid ($N = 57$, 12% MS/AS free, 28% > 50% decreased). Generalized motor seizures gradually decreased thereafter in these patients.

Caraballo et al. (2006) reported on 30 MAE patients, 11 of whom were treated with diet. Six of the patients remained on the diet at 18 months, and two of them (18.2%) were seizure-free, while two each had 75% to 99% reduction and 50% to 74% reduction. EEG was improved in all six and was normal in the seizure-free patients at 18 months. Five patients discontinued the diet within the first 3 months, four for lack of efficacy and one for persistent vomiting. The authors remarked the good response to diet and concluded that for this disorder, it should be considered earlier in the course.

Kilaru et al. (2007) reported the order of exposure to various treatments and their efficacy in 23 MAE patients. KD was tried last in 10 patients and was the most effective treatment in achieving seizure remission. It was initiated an average of 17 months (range 2 to 58 months) after seizure onset, and after an average of five AED trials. Five patients (50%) became seizure-free, three within 1 month, one by 7 months, and the last by 19 months after diet initiation. Three of these patients remained seizure-free for > 6 months. Ethosuximide (25%) and topiramate (23%) were the next most effective in achieving remission of seizures. In this group, steroids (prednisone and ACTH) were ineffective.

Kilaru et al. (2007) noted the possibility of spontaneous remission in this disorder. In this setting, late-used treatments may appear more effective than those used early, when spontaneous remission is less likely. Stenger et al. (2017) reported on 50 severe MAE cases that suggested that efficacy is maintained or improved with early use of KD in the disorder. This was a multicenter, retrospective cohort treated with KD after failure of at least three AEDs, some patients having been treated with more than five AEDs. Long-term (> 6 months) outcome included 27 (54%) with clinical remission, of whom 20 also had EEG normalization. Twenty-five had normal development at the end of observation, 17 (35%) had mild deficits, and eight had severe deficits. Factors correlating with remission were early KD introduction (after no more than three AEDs; $p = 0.028$) and short duration of explosive stage ($p = 0.04$). Early KD was also significantly associated with good cognitive outcome ($p < 0.01$), as was achieving remission ($p = 0.002$). Analysis of the possible interaction between early KD introduction and shorter explosive stage and/or achievement of remission was not reported.

Perhaps because MAE seems especially responsive to the KD, use of a lower ratio, as in the MAD, has been considered as an option for treatment—with the potential of seeing efficacy with a less rigorous, more palatable diet. There is little information available about efficacy in comparison to the classic KD. Simard-Tremblay et al. (2015) used MAD in six, and KD in three, of nine patients after a median of four AEDs. They reported seven of nine patients achieved seizure remission, with one patient on KD and one on MAD failing to respond. One patient advanced from MAD to 4:1 KD and achieved seizure freedom. A more recent study (Wiemer-Kruel et al., 2017) described 30 MAE patients with refractory epilepsy (mean of six AEDs, range 2 to 15) treated with a 10-g carbohydrate MAD in a multicenter, retrospective cohort, with 25 (83%) responders (≥ 50% reduction in seizures), of whom 14 (47%) were seizure-free—achieved in from 2 days to 11 months on diet. There was no benefit noted in 5 patients. Three patients discontinued the diet after 2 years of seizure freedom. Three discontinued because of lack of efficacy, a further two with loss of initial efficacy, and only two for noncompliance. Measures of ketosis were not reported. In a study by Kossoff et al. (2010), when 27 patients were switched from MAD to KD, there was improvement (additional 10% decrease in seizures) in 10 (37%). There were nine MAE patients in this group, of whom seven improved with the change to KD, five of them achieving seizure freedom. These reports suggest that starting treatment with MAD, with the possibility of advancing to a classic KD if needed, may be a reasonable strategy in MAE.

In summary, MAE appears to be more responsive to KDs than other epilepsies, with approximately 50% of patients achieving seizure freedom, allowing medication withdrawal in many and ultimately diet withdrawal also. Assessment of efficacy is complicated by a possible but poorly defined spontaneous remission rate. Diet therapy is being offered as an earlier option more frequently in light of the reports described here. It will be fascinating to discover the relative roles of underlying molecular/genetic milieu and treatment decisions in determining epilepsy and cognitive outcomes.

CONCLUSION

In conclusion, there is general agreement in the literature that patients with the four epilepsies infantile spasms, Lennox-Gastaut syndrome, Dravet syndrome, and myoclonic-astatic epilepsy may benefit from a trial of diet therapy once their epilepsy has become refractory to medication. The quality of the data for individual epilepsy syndromes is modest, at best. These diagnoses are rare, so that only multicenter studies are likely to produce more robust data, comparing diet therapy to other treatments in a controlled manner, and/or establishing the best timing of diet trials. There is also very little information on the efficacy of diet treatment as first-line therapy. The difficulty of administration of diet therapy is likely to limit its acceptance as first-line treatment unless it becomes possible to induce ketosis without diet restrictions (i.e., via a supplement or pill). Future multicenter collaborative studies will be necessary to examine these possibilities.

REFERENCES

Arzimanoglou, A., French, J., Blume, W. T., Cross, J. H., Ernst, J. P., Feucht, M., Genton, P., Guerrini, R., Kluger, G., Pellock, J. M., Perrucca, E., & Wheless, J. W. (2009). Lennox-Gastaut syndrome: A consensus approach on diagnosis, assessment, management, and trial methodology. *Lancet Neurology, 8*, 82–93.

Berkovic, S. F., Harkin, L., McMahon, J. M., Pelekanos, J. T., Zuberi, S. M., Wirrell, E. C., Gill, D. S., Iona, X., Mulley J. C., & Scheffer, I. E. (2006). De-novo mutations of the sodium channel gene *SCN1A* in alleged vaccine encephalopathy: A retrospective study. *Lancet Neurology, 5*, 488–492.

Caraballo, R. H., Fortini, S., Fresler, S., Armeno, M., Ariela, A., Cresta, A., Mestre, G., & Escobal, N. (2014). Ketogenic diet in patients with Lennox-Gastaut syndrome. *Seizure, 23*, 751–755.

Caraballo, R. H. (2011). Nonpharmacologic treatments of Dravet syndrome: Focus on the ketogenic diet. *Epilepsia, 52*(Suppl. 2), 79–82.

Caraballo, R. H., Cersósimo, R. O., Sakr, D., Cresta, A., Escoba, N., & Fejerman, N. (2006). Ketogenic diet in patients with myoclonic-astatic epilepsy. *Epileptic Disorders, 8*, 151–155.

Cross, J. H., Caraballo, R. H., Nabbout, R., Vigevano, F., Guerrini, R., & Lagae, L. (2019). Dravet syndrome: Treatment options and management of prolonged seizures. *Epilepsia, 60*(S3), S39–S48.

Doose, H., Gerken, H., Leonhardt, R., Völzke, E., Völz, C. (1970). Centrencephalic myoclonic-astatic petit mal: Clinical and genetic investigation. *Neuropaediatrie, 2*, 59–78.

Dressler, A., Benninger, F., Trimmel-Schwahofer, P., Gröppel. G., Porsche, B., Abraham, K., Mühlebner, A., Samueli, S., Male, C., & Feucht, M. (2019). Efficacy and tolerability of the ketogenic diet versus high-dose adrenocorticotropic hormone for infantile spasms: A single-center parallel-cohort randomized controlled trial. *Epilepsia, 60*, 441–451.

Dressler, A., Trimmel-Schwahofer, P., Reithofer, E., Gröppel, G., Mühlebner, A., Samueli, S., Grabner, V., Abraham, K., Benninger, F., & Feucht, M. (2015a). The ketogenic diet in infants—Advantages of early use. *Epilepsy Research, 116*, 53–58.

Dressler, A., Trimmel-Schwahofer, P., Reithofer, E., Mühlebner, A., Gröppel, G., Reiter-Fink, R., Benninger, F., Grassl, R., & Feucht, M. (2015b). Efficacy and tolerability of the ketogenic diet in Dravet syndrome—Comparison with various standard antiepileptic drug regimen. *Epilepsy Research, 109*, 81–89.

Dutton, S. B., Sawyer, N. T., Kalume, F., Jumbo-Lucioni, P., Borges, K., Catterall, W. A., & Escayg, A. (2011). Protective effect of the ketogenic diet in *Scn1a* mutant mice. *Epilepsia, 52*, 2050–2056.

Eun, S. H., Kang, H. C., Kim, D. W., & Kim, H. D. (2006). Ketogenic diet for treatment of infantile spasms. *Brain & Development, 28*, 566–571.

Freeman, J. M., & Vining, E. P. (1999). Seizures decrease rapidly after fasting: Preliminary studies of the ketogenic diet. *Archives of Pediatric and Adolescent Medicine, 153*, 946–949.

Freeman, J. M., Vining, E. P., Kossoff, E. H., Pyzik, P. L., Ye, X., & Goodman, S. N. (2009). A blinded, crossover study of the efficacy of the ketogenic diet. *Epilepsia, 50*, 322–325.

Freeman, J. M., Vining, E. P., Pillas, D. J., Pyzik, P. L., Casey, J. C., & Kelly, L. M. (1998). The efficacy of the ketogenic diet: A prospective evaluation of intervention in 150 children. *Pediatrics, 102*, 1358–1363.

Genton, P., Velizarova, R., & Dravet, C. (2011). Dravet syndrome: The long-term outcome. *Epilepsia, 52*(Suppl. 2), 44–49.

Halbrook, T., Sjolander, A., Armak, P., Miranda, M., Bjurulf, B., & Dahlin, M. (2015). Effectiveness of the ketogenic diet used to treat resistant childhood epilepsy in Scandinavia. *European Journal of Paediatric Neurology, 19*, 29–36.

Hemingway, C., Freeman, J. M., Ribbs, D. J., & Pyzik, P. L. (2001). The ketogenic diet: A 3–6 year follow up of 150 children prospectively enrolled. *Pediatrics, 108*, 898–905.

Henderson, C. B., Filloux, F. M., Alder, S. C., Lyon, J. L., & Caplin, D. A. (2006). Efficacy of the ketogenic diet as a treatment option for epilepsy: Meta-analysis. *Journal of Child Neurology, 21*, 193–198.

Hong, A. M., Turner, Z, Hamdy, R. F., & Kossoff, E. H. (2010). Infantile spasms treated with the ketogenic diet: Prospective single-center experience in 104 consecutive infants. *Epilepsia, 51*, 1403–1407.

Hrachovy, R. A., Glaze, D. J., & Frost, J. D., Jr. (1991). A retrospective study of spontaneous remission and long-term outcome in patients with infantile spasms. *Epilepsia, 32*, 212–214.

Kang, H. C., Cheung, D. E., Kim, D. W., & Kim, H. D. (2004). Early and late onset complications in the ketogenic diet for intractable epilepsy. *Epilepsia, 45*, 1116–1123.

Kayyali, H. R., Gustafson, M., Myers, T., Thompson, L., Williams, M., & Abdelmoity, A. (2014). Ketogenic diet efficacy in the treatment of intractable epileptic spasms. *Pediatric Neurology, 50*, 224–227.

Kelley, S. A., & Kossoff, E. H. (2010). Doose syndrome (myoclonic-astatic epilepsy): 40 years of progress. *Developmental Medicine & Child Neurology, 52*, 988–993.

Kilaru, S., & Bergqvist, A. G. C. (2007). Current treatment of myoclonic astatic epilepsy: Clinical experience at the Children's Hospital of Philadelphia. *Epilepsia, 48*, 1703–1707.

Kim, H. J., Kim, H. D., Lee, J. S., Heo, K., Kim, D.-S., & Kang, H.-C. (2014). Long-term prognosis of patients with Lennox-Gastaut syndrome in recent decades. *Epilepsy Research, 110*, 10–19.

Kinsman, S. L., Vining, E. P., Quaskey, S. A., Mellits, D., & Freeman, J. M. (1992). Efficacy of the ketogenic diet for intractable seizure disorders: Review of 58 cases. *Epilepsia, 33*, 1132–1136.

Kossoff, E. H., Bosarge, J. L., Miranda, M. J., Wiemer-Kruel, A., Kang, H. C., & Kim, H. D. (2010). Will seizure control improve by switching from the modified Atkins diet to the traditional ketogenic diet? *Epilepsia, 51*, 2496–2499.

Kossoff, E. H., Caraballo, R. H., du Toit, T., Kim, H. D., MacKay, M. T., Nathan, J. K., & Philip, S. G. (2012). Dietary therapy: A worldwide phenomenon. *Epilepsy Research, 100*, 205–209.

Kossoff, E. H., Hedderick E. F., Turner, Z., & Freeman, J. M. (2008). A case-control evaluation of the ketogenic diet versus ACTH for new-onset infantile spasms. *Epilepsia, 49*, 1504–1509.

Kossoff, E. H., & McGrogan, J. R. (2005). Worldwide use of the ketogenic diet. *Epilepsia, 46*, 280–289.

Kossoff, E. H., Pyzik, P. L., McGrogan, J. R., Vining, E. P., & Freeman, J. M. (2002). Efficacy of the ketogenic diet for infantile spasms. *Pediatrics, 109*, 780–783.

Kossoff, E. H., Zupec-Kania, B. A., Amark, P. E., Ballaban-Gil, K. R., Bergqvist, C. A. G., Blackford, R., Buchhalter, J. R., Caraballo, R. H., Cross, H. J., Dahlin, M. G., Donner, E. J., Klepper, J., Jehle, R. S., Kim, H. D., Christiana Liu, Y. M., Nation, J., Nordli, D. R. Jnr., Pfeifer, H. H., Rho, J. M., . . . Vining, E. P. (2009). Optimal clinical management of children receiving the ketogenic diet: Recommendations of the International Ketogenic Diet Study Group. *Epilepsia, 50*, 304–317.

Kwan, P., Arzimanoglou, A., Berg, A. T., Brodie, M. J., Hauser, A. W., Mathern, G., Moshe, S. L., Perucca, E., Wiebe, S., & French, J. (2010). Definition of drug-resistant epilepsy: Consensus proposed by the ad hoc task force of the ILAE Commission on Therapeutic Strategies. *Epilepsia, 52*, 1069–1077.

Kwan, P., & Brodie, M. J. (2000). Early identification of refractory epilepsy. *New England Journal of Medicine, 342*, 314–319.

Larsen, J., Johannesen, K. M., Ek, J., Tang, S., Marini, C., Blichfeldt, S., Kibæk, M., von Spiczak, S., Weckhuysen, S., Frangu, M., Neubauer, B. A., Uldall, P., Striano, P., Zara, F., MAE working group of the EuroEPINOMICS RES Consortium, Kleiss, R., Simpson, M., Muhle, H., Nikanorova, M., . . . Moller, R. S. (2015). The role of *SLC2A1* mutations in myoclonic astatic epilepsy and absence epilepsy, and the estimated frequency of GLUT1 deficiency syndrome. *Epilepsia, **, 1–6.

Laux, L., & Blackford, R. (2013). The ketogenic diet in Dravet syndrome. *Journal of Child Neurology, 28*, 1041–1044.

Lefevre, F., & Aronson, N. (2000). Ketogenic diet for the treatment of refractory epilepsy in children: A systematic review of efficacy. *Pediatrics, 105*, E46.

Lemmon, M. E., Terao, N. N., Ng, Y.-T., Reisig, W., Rubenstein, J. E., & Kossoff, E. H. (2012). Efficacy of the ketogenic diet in Lennox-Gastaut syndrome: A retrospective review of one institution's experience and summary of the literature. *Developmental Medicine & Child Neurology, 54*, 464–468.

Lux, A. L., Edwards, S. W., Hancock, E., Johnson, A. L., Kennedy, C. R., Newton, R. W., O'Callaghan,

F. J. K., Verity, C. M., Osborne, J. P., & the trial steering committee on behalf of participating investigators. (2005). The United Kingdom Infantile Spasms Study (UKISS) comparing hormone treatment with vigabatrin on developmental and epilepsy outcomes to age 14 months: A multicentre randomised trial. *Lancet Neurology*, *4*, 712–717.

Mullen, S. A., Marini, C., Suls, A., Mei, D., Della Giustina, E., Buti, D., Arsov, T., Damiano, J., Lawrence, K., De Jonghe, P., Berkovic, S. F., & Scheffer, I. E. (2011). Glucose transporter 1 deficiency as a treatable cause of myoclonic astatic epilepsy. *Archives of Neurology*, *68*, 1152–1155.

Nabbout, R., Copioli, C., Chipaux, M., Chemaly, N., Desguerre, I., Dulac, O., & Chiron, C. (2011). Ketogenic diet also benefits Dravet syndrome patients receiving stiripentol: A prospective pilot study. *Epilepsia*, *52*, e54–e57.

Nathan, J. K., Purandare, A. S., Parek, Z. B., & Manohar, H. V. (2009). Ketogenic diet in Indian children with uncontrolled epilepsy. *Indian Pediatrics*, *46*, 669–673.

Neal, E. G., Chaffe, H., Schwartz, R. H., Lawson, M. S., Edwards, N., Fitzsimmons, G., Whitney, A., & Cross, J. H. (2008). The ketogenic diet for the treatment of childhood epilepsy: A randomized controlled trial. *Lancet Neurology*, *7*, 500–506.

Ni, Y., Wang, X.-H., Zhang, L.-M., Chai, Y.-M., Li, W.-H., Zhou, Y.-F., & Zhou, S.-J. (2018). Prospective study of the efficacy of a ketogenic diet in 20 patients with Dravet syndrome. *Seizure*, *60*, 144–148.

Nordli, D. R., Jr., Kuroda, M. M., Carroll, J., Koenigsberger, D. Y., Hirsch, L. J., Bruneri, H. J., Seidel, W. T., & De Vivo, D. C. (2001). Experience with the ketogenic diet in infants. *Pediatrics*, *108*, 129–133.

Numis, A. L., Yellen, M. B., Chu-Shore, C. J., Pfeifer, H. H., & Thiele, E. A. (2011). The relationship of ketosis and growth to the efficacy of the ketogenic diet in infantile spasms. *Epilepsy Research*, *96*, 172–175.

O'Callaghan, F. J. K., Edwards, S. W., Alber, F. D., Borja, M. C., Hancock, E., Johnson, A. L., Kennedy, C. R., Likeman, M., Lux, A. L., Mackay, M., Mallick, A. A., Newton, R. W., Nolan, M., Pressler, R., Rating, D., Schmitt, B., Verity, C. M., Osborne, J. P., on behalf of the ICISS investigators. (2018). Vigabatrin with hormonal treatment versus hormonal treatment alone (ICISS) for infantile spasms: 18-month outcomes of an open-label, randomized controlled trial. *Lancet Child & Adolescent Health*, *2*, 715–725.

O'Callaghan, F. J. K., Edwards, S. W., Alber, F. D., Hancock, E., Johnson, A. L., Kennedy, C. R., Likeman, M., Lux, A. L., Mackay, M., Mallick, A. A., Newton, R. W., Nolan, M., Pressler, R., Rating, D., Schmitt, B., Verity, C. M., & Osborne, J. P., on behalf of the participating investigators. (2017). Safety and effectiveness of hormonal treatment versus hormonal treatment with vigabatrin for infantile spasms (ICISS): A randomized, multicentre, open-label trial. *Lancet Neurology*, *16*, 33–42.

Oguni, H., Tanaka, T., Hayashi, K., Funatsuka, M., Sakauchi, M., Shirakawa, S., & Osawa, M. (2002). Treatment and long-term prognosis of myoclonic-astatic epilepsy of early childhood. *Neuropediatrics*, *33*, 122–132.

Pellock, J. M., Hrachovy, R., Shinnar, S., Baram, T. Z., Bettis, D., Dlugos, D., Gaillard, W. D., Gibson, P. A., Holmes, G. L., Nordli, D. R., et al. (2010). Infantile spasms: A U.S. consensus report. *Epilepsia*, *51*, 2175–2189.

Pires, M. E., Ilea, A., Bourel, E, Bellavoinea, V., Merdariua, D., Berquin, P., & Auvin, S. (2013). Ketogenic diet for infantile spasms refractory to first-line treatments: An open prospective study. *Epilepsy Research*, *105*, 189–194.

Prasad, A. N., Stafstrom, C. F., & Holmes, G. L. (1996). Alternative epilepsy therapies: The ketogenic diet, immunoglobulins, and steroids. *Epilepsia*, *37*(Suppl. 1), S81–S95.

Prezioso, G., Carlone, G., Zaccara, G., & Verotti, A. (2018). Efficacy of ketogenic diet for infantile spasms: A systematic review. *Acta Neurologica Scandinavica*, *137*, 4–11.

Routier, L., Verny, F., Barcia, G., Chemaly, N., Desguerre, I., Colleaux, L., & Nabbout, R. (2019). Exome sequencing findings in 27 patients with myoclonic-atonic epilepsy: Is there a major genetic factor? *Clinical Genetics*, *96*, 254–260.

Schoeler, N. E., Cross, J. H., Sander, J. W., & Sisodiya, S. M. (2013). Can we predict a favourable response to ketogenic diet therapies for drug-resistant epilepsy? *Epilepsy Research*, *106*, 1–16.

Sharma, S., Jain, P., Gulati, S., Sankhyan, N., & Agarwala, A. (2015). Use of the modified Atkins diet in Lennox Gastaut syndrome. *Journal of Child Neurology*, *30*, 576–579.

Simard-Tremblay, S., Berry, P., Owens, A., Cook, W. B., Sittner, H. R., Mazzanti, M., Huber, J., Warner, M., Shurtleff, H., & Saneto, R. P. (2015). High-fat diets and seizure control in myoclonic-astatic epilepsy: A single center's experience. *Seizure*, *25*, 184–186.

Stenger, E., Schaeffer, M., Cances, C., Motte, J., Auvin, S., Ville, D., Maurey, H., Nabbout, R., & Saint-Martin, A. (2017). Efficacy of a ketogenic diet in resistant myoclono-astatic epilepsy: A French multicenter retrospective study. *Epilepsy Research*, *131*, 64–69.

Ville, D., Chiron, C., Laschet, J., & Dulac, O. (2015). The ketogenic diet can be used successfully in combination with corticosteroids for epileptic encephalopathies. *Epilepsy & Behavior*, *48*, 61–65.

Vining, E. P, Freeman, J. M., Ballaban-Gil, K., Camfield, C. S., Camfield, P. R., Holmes, G. L., Shinnar, S., Shuman, R., Trevathan, E., & Wheless, J. W. (1998). A multicenter study of the efficacy of the ketogenic diet. *Archives of Neurology, 55*, 1433–1437.

Wheless, J. W. (2004). *History and origin of the ketogenic diet.* In C. E. Stafstrom & J. M. Rho (Eds.), *Epilepsy and the ketogenic diet* (pp. 31–50). Humana Press.

Wiemer-Kruel, A., Haberlandt, E., Hartmann, H., Wohlrab, G., & Bast, T. (2017). Modified Atkins diet is an effective treatment for children with Doose syndrome. *Epilepsia, 58*, 657–662.

Wirrell, E. C., Laux, L., Donner, E., Jette, N., Knupp, K., Meskis, M. A., Miller, I., Sullivan, J., Welborn, M., & Berg, A. T. (2017). Optimizing the diagnosis and management of Dravet syndrome: Recommendations from a North American consensus panel. *Pediatric Neurology, 68*, 18–34.

Zhang, Y., Wang, Y., Zhou Y., Zhang, L., Yu, L., & Zhou, S. (2016). Therapeutic effects of the ketogenic diet in children with Lennox-Gastaut syndrome. *Epilepsy Research, 128*, 176–180.

8

Ketogenic Diet for Other Epilepsies

DAVID T. HSIEH, MD AND ELIZABETH A. THIELE, MD, PHD

As discussed in other chapters, the ketogenic diet (KD) is the treatment of choice for epilepsy in certain disorders of brain metabolism, in particular glucose transporter type 1 (GLUT1) deficiency (GLUT1DS) and pyruvate dehydrogenase deficiency (PDHD). An understanding of the underlying metabolic pathophysiology of these genetic disorders has been coupled with successful clinical efficacy of the KD in patients with GLUT1DS or PDHD. However, there are also several other genetic disorders that manifest with epilepsy for which dietary therapies appear to be especially effective, but for which the underlying metabolic mechanisms are not as clearly delineated. The International Ketogenic Diet Study Group has listed several other conditions (Box 8.1) for which the KD has been reported as being consistently more beneficial (>70%) than the average 50% response (defined as > 50% seizure reduction; Kossoff et al., 2009a, 2018). Whether efficacy in these conditions is due in part to the broad-spectrum efficacy of the KD or due to mechanisms specific to these conditions is still under investigation. Furthermore, patient populations who are often fed with gastrostomy tubes, such as patients with Rett syndrome, may be especially good candidates for the KD in liquid form, due to the relative ease of administration. This chapter covers the use of dietary therapies for the treatment of epilepsy in certain genetic disorders, such as tuberous sclerosis complex and Angelman syndrome, as listed by the International Ketogenic Diet Study Group, and in addition the chapter discusses the use of epilepsy dietary therapies in patients with Rett syndrome and Sturge-Weber syndrome.

TUBEROUS SCLEROSIS COMPLEX

Tuberous sclerosis complex (TSC) is an autosomal dominant neurocutaneous disorder characterized by hamartomatous growths in multiple organ systems, including the skin, central nervous system, eyes, kidneys, heart, and lungs. Mutations in the *TSC1* and *TSC2* genes, which encode hamartin and tuberin, are present in over 85% of cases, resulting in hamartomatous growths caused by unregulated activation of the mammalian target of rapamycin (mTOR) pathway (Napolioni et al., 2008). The most common lesions found in the brain include cortical tubers, subependymal nodules, subependymal giant cell astrocytomas, and radial migration lines. Epilepsy occurs in up to 85% of TSC patients and is a significant factor in neurologic morbidity. Seizures begin within the first year of life in 63% of patients and before they

---

BOX 8.1

CONDITIONS LISTED BY THE INTERNATIONAL KETOGENIC DIET STUDY GROUP AS HAVING CONSISTENTLY MORE BENEFIT (> 70%) THAN THE AVERAGE 50% KD RESPONSE (DEFINED AS > 50% SEIZURE REDUCTION)

Angelman syndrome
Complex I mitochondrial disorders
Dravet syndrome
Doose syndrome
Glucose transporter type 1 deficiency
Febrile infection-related epilepsy syndrome
Formula-fed (solely) infants and children
Infantile spasms
Ohtahara syndrome
Pyruvate dehydrogenase deficiency
Super-refractory status epilepticus
Tuberous sclerosis complex

are 3 years old in 83% (Chu-Shore et al., 2010a). The majority of patients have multiple seizure types, with the most common being complex partial seizures, followed by infantile spasms, generalized tonic-clonic seizures, and atypical absence (Chu-Shore et al., 2010a). The treatment of epilepsy in TSC usually starts with the use of standard anticonvulsant medications, but the seizures are medication-refractory in 30% to 60% of patients (Chu-Shore et al., 2010a; Vignoli et al., 2013). Patients with TSC who have medication-refractory epilepsy are often considered early for epilepsy surgery, with cortical tubers and abnormal surrounding cortex usually the targets of interest. When surgical candidates are chosen carefully, good outcomes with seizure freedom can be achieved in about 60% (Zhang et al., 2013). For those patients who are not surgical candidates, or for whom the family does not wish to pursue surgical management, alternative epilepsy treatment options, such as dietary therapy, should be considered.

TSC is listed by the International Ketogenic Diet Study Group as a condition for which the KD has been reported as being consistently more beneficial than average. In a published case series of 12 children with TSC between the ages of 8 months and 18 years and treated with the KD, at 6 months, 92% had at least a 50% reduction in seizures, and 67% had at least a 90% reduction (Kossoff et al., 2005). In this series, five children had at least a 5-month seizure-free response. The authors recommended the KD in patients with TSC for whom medications fail and in whom no clear epileptogenic tuber is identified. In another case series of three children with TSC and medication-refractory seizures who were followed for 12 months on the KD, two of the patients became seizure-free, and the third patient experienced a decrease in his drop seizures (Coppola et al., 2006). In a larger series of 71 patients with TSC, six were started on the KD, and two of the six had a 50% decrease in seizures (Overwater et al., 2015).

When the KD is effective, the possibility of weaning off the KD can be considered after 2 years. Unfortunately, TSC is a risk factor for seizure recurrence in patients weaned from the KD after 2 or more years of seizure freedom. In one published series, all three patients with TSC who were weaned off the KD after becoming seizure-free had a recurrence of seizures, and only one regained full control with reinitiation of the KD (Martinez et al., 2007). The authors concluded that patients with TSC may need to be treated for

longer than 2 years, or possibly indefinitely if seizure control is achieved.

There is also evidence that low-glycemic-index treatment (LGIT) can be effective in reducing seizures, and is better tolerated, in patients with TSC. In a case series of 15 patients with TSC started on the LGIT, 47% had a 50% or greater reduction in their seizures (Larson et al., 2012). Many of these patients had been unable to tolerate the KD. In addition, there is a report of a Japanese patient with TSC and Lennox-Gastaut syndrome who responded to the LGIT, achieved using Japanese ethnic foods (Kumada et al., 2013).

It has now been well characterized that the manifestations in TSC are largely due to dysfunctional regulation of the mTOR pathway. It is unclear, however, whether there is a similar underlying mechanism to explain why patients with TSC respond well to dietary therapies. There is some bench evidence that markers of the mTOR pathway, including pS6 and pAkt, are reduced in the hippocampus and liver of rats fed the KD (McDaniel et al., 2011). However, in a series of five patients with TSC who were treated with KD, three of the five patients had progression of known tumors (renal angiomyolipomas or subependymal giant cell astrocytomas) or developed new tumors while being treated with the KD (Chu-Shore et al., 2010b). Thus, if there is some mTOR inhibition provided by the KD, in the small sample studied, it does not appear to provide the same level of tumor regression effects in TSC as better studied mTOR inhibitors, such as sirolimus and everolimus.

ANGELMAN SYNDROME

Angelman syndrome (AS) is neurogenetic disorder characterized by cognitive and language impairment, epilepsy, ataxia, tremorous movements, and sleep disturbances, with patients also tending to have an apparent happy demeanor. AS is maternally inherited, with four possible known genetic mechanisms resulting in reduced expression of the ubiquitin-protein ligase E3A (*UBE3A*) gene, most commonly from a deletion in the 15q11.2-13.1 region (70%; Jiang et al., 1999). Epilepsy is present in over 85% of patients with AS (Laan et al., 1997; Thibert et al., 2009), with the onset of epilepsy in 50% by 1 year of age, and in over 75% by 3 years of age (Valente et al., 2006). The etiology of epilepsy in AS is not clear, but there are known differences in epilepsy genotype–phenotype correlations: AS patients with maternal deletions have higher rates of epilepsy (90%) than those without (55%–75%; Thibert et al., 2009), have an earlier onset, and have a more severe epilepsy phenotype (Minassian et al., 1998; Valente et al., 2005). It has been hypothesized that there may be other related factors in patients with maternal deletions specifically associated with 15q11-13 deletions, such as the genes coding for subunits of the GABA$_A$ receptor complex in this region (Minassian et al., 1998). Epilepsy in AS typically manifests with multiple seizure types, including myoclonic, atypical absence, generalized tonic-clonic, and atonic seizures, and patients with AS commonly have frequent or prolonged seizures (Thibert et al., 2009). Most patients' seizures are medication-refractory, with up to 77% of patients requiring combination medication therapy (Laan et al., 1997; Thibert et al., 2009). Patients with AS and epilepsy are unlikely to be candidates for epilepsy surgery, thus alternative therapies like dietary therapies are often considered.

Several examples of successful treatment of epilepsy in AS with the KD have been published. In one series of 19 patients with genetically confirmed AS and medication-refractory epilepsy, the KD was described as "effective" for all four patients it was initiated in (Valente et al., 2006). In a case report of an infant with AS, the KD produced a rapid and significant reduction in seizures, from hundreds a day to nearly complete control, and was accompanied by increased alertness and smiling (Stein et al., 2010). In another report, a 5-year-old with AS became seizure free within 2 months on the KD and was able to discontinue two of her three anticonvulsant medications (Evangeliou et al., 2010). This patient also had an improvement in her sleep pattern and reduced hyperactivity. In a large electronic survey sent through the Angelman Syndrome Foundation to 461 family members of patients with AS, 11% reported trying dietary therapy, including the KD in 8% and the LGIT in 2%. Of those trying the KD, 36% reported that the KD was the best overall treatment, although only 19% reported still being on the KD (Thibert et al., 2009). Finally in a series of six children with AS followed prospectively on the LGIT for 4 months, five of six of the patients had at least an 80% reduction in seizures, with five remaining on the LGIT for over a year (Thibert et al., 2012). In a follow-up retrospective review at the same institution, of 23 patients with AS who utilized the LGIT, 22% maintained seizure freedom, 43% maintained seizure freedom except in the setting of illness or nonconvulsive status, and 30% had a decrease in seizure frequency (Grocott et al., 2017).

It is uncertain if there are underlying mechanisms explaining the efficacy of dietary therapies in patients with AS. The anticonvulsant effects of the KD are probably multiple (Bough et al., 2007). It has been reported that children on the KD have an increase in GABA, taurine, serine, and glycine in their cerebrospinal fluid (Dahlin et al., 2005); therefore, a possible specific action partly explaining the efficacy of dietary therapies in patients could be the increase of GABA synthesis in the brain.

Specifically for AS, as mentioned, there are genes encoding for the GABA$_A$ receptor within the region of the maternal 15q deletions associated with AS (Minassian et al., 1998), thus it has been hypothesized that increasing GABA levels through the KD may be an important component in its effectiveness in patients with AS.

RETT SYNDROME

Rett syndrome (RTT) is an X-linked dominant neurogenetic disorder characterized clinically by developmental regression around 12 to 18 months of age, specifically with regression of purposeful hand use and spoken language, as well as development of a gait abnormality and hand stereotypies, such as hand wringing (Neul et al., 2010). RTT is associated with mutations in the methyl-CpG-binding protein 2 (*MECP2*) gene at Xq28, which are detected in 95% to 97% of typical RTT patients (Neul et al., 2010). Epilepsy occurs in about 70% of patients with RTT, with a median onset of 3 to 4 years (Nissenkorn et al., 2010, 2015).

Seizure semiology includes all types, with generalized tonic-clonic seizures occurring more frequently than complex partial and secondarily generalized seizures (Cardoza et al., 2011). The treatment of epilepsy in RTT usually involves the use of standard anticonvulsant medications, but about a third of patients have medication-refractory seizures (Pintaudi et al., 2010). Patients with RTT are usually not typical candidates for epilepsy surgery, thus RTT patients with medication-refractory epilepsy are often considered for nonmedication treatments, such as dietary therapy.

RTT is listed by the International Ketogenic Diet Study Group as a condition for which the KD has been reported as being moderately beneficial, defined as not better than the average dietary therapy response or limited to single-center case reports (Kossoff et al., 2018). In a published case series of seven girls with clinical RTT and medication-refractory epilepsy, the KD was initiated in, and tolerated by, five of the patients (Haas et al., 1986). Of these five patients, four had a 50% or better decrease in seizures, including one with 75% decrease and one patient with a 100% decrease. All five of the patients who were able to tolerate the diet also had reported slight behavioral improvements. In another published case of an 8-year-old girl with genetically confirmed RTT and medication-refractory seizures, a 70% reduction in seizures was achieved on the KD (Liebhaber et al., 2003). This patient was able to tolerate the diet for over 4 years and also had improvement reported in her behavior on the KD. Additionally, in a 10-year-old girl with genetically confirmed RTT and medication-refractory seizures, the KD significantly decreased seizure frequency, and the patient was also reported to concurrently became "more communicative" with her family members (Giampietro et al., 2006).

It is uncertain whether there is a specific underlying metabolic process in patients with RTT that would provide the physiologic benefit during treatment with the KD. Some researchers have noted that many patients with RTT have serum markers suggestive of defects in energy metabolism, including serum lactate or pyruvate elevations (Haas et al., 1995) or cerebrospinal fluid lactate elevations (Matsuishi et al., 2011). It has been hypothesized that the KD alters energy metabolism in a favorable direction in patients with RTT (Haas et al., 1986; Mantis et al., 2009), but further research is needed to better understand the implications of the KD in patients with RTT.

STURGE-WEBER SYNDROME

Sturge-Weber syndrome (SWS) is a sporadic neurocutaneous disorder characterized by capillary malformations in the distribution of the trigeminal nerve, glaucoma, and cerebral venous malformations. SWS is associated with a somatic mutation in the GNAQ gene, which plays a key role in cell proliferation (Shirley et al., 2013). Epilepsy is an especially common manifestation of SWS, occurring in over 85% of patients (Pascual-Castroviejo et al., 2008), with onset by 1 year of age in up to 75% (Kossoff et al., 2009b; Sujansky et al., 1995). Most seizures are focal, but generalized seizures can also occur (Ewen et al., 2007), with seizures commonly occurring in a pattern of clustering, with intense seizures followed by prolonged seizure-free periods (Kossoff et al., 2009b). Seizure control in SWS is particularly important because of radiographic evidence of hypoperfusion that can occur ictally in some patients and that may contribute to progressive cortical atrophy (Aylett et al., 1999). The treatment of epilepsy

in SWS usually starts with the use of standard anticonvulsant medications. SWS patients with medication-refractory epilepsy are often given an epilepsy surgical assessment to evaluate them for either a lesionectomy or a hemispherectomy (Arzimanoglou et al., 2000; Kossoff et al., 2002). Hemispherectomy can result in seizure freedom in 81% of patients (Kossoff et al., 2002), without significant postoperative hemiparesis or worsening of cognitive functioning (Arzimanoglou et al., 2000).

Successful implementation of the KD has been reported in a 4-year-old patient with SWS, although a recurrence of seizures occurred 4 months into treatment (Petit et al., 2008). There is a theoretical risk in SWS with the KD due to the fasting and fluid restrictions implemented during the initiation of the KD, which could possibly provoke the strokelike events that patients with SWS are prone to (Kossoff et al., 2010). Thus, the use of less restrictive dietary therapies has been proposed for patients with SWS. In 2010, Kossoff et al. published a case series of the modified Atkins diet (MAD) in five children with SWS: three of the patients had at least a 50% reduction in seizures, including one having a 90% reduction and one becoming seizure-free (Kossoff et al., 2010). Only one patient had a strokelike event on the MAD, although this patient had a prior history of strokelike events prior to initiation of the MAD.

CONCLUSIONS

In conclusion, dietary therapies are effective for a wide spectrum of epilepsy types, and this chapter presents examples of genetic epilepsy syndromes that have been reported to respond well to dietary therapies. Whether efficacy in these conditions is due in part to the broad-spectrum efficacy of the KD or due to mechanisms specific to these conditions is still under investigation. If the specific pathways affected in particular genetic syndromes are better characterized, this may improve understanding of the underlying pathophysiologic mechanisms contributing to the efficacy of dietary therapies in epilepsy.

DISCLOSURES

The view(s) expressed herein are those of the author(s) and do not reflect the official policy or position of Brooke Army Medical Center, the U.S. Army Medical Department, the U.S. Army Office of the Surgeon General, the United States Air Force, the Department of the Army and Department of Defense or the U.S. Government.

REFERENCES

Arzimanoglou, A. A., Andermann, F., Aicardi, J., Sainte-Rose, C., Beaulieu, M. A., Villemure, J. G., Olivier, A., & Rasmussen, T. (2000). Sturge-Weber syndrome: Indications and results of surgery in 20 patients. *Neurology, 55,* 1472–1479.

Aylett, S. E., Neville, B. G., Cross, J. H., Boyd, S., Chong, W. K, & Kirkham, F. J. (1999). Sturge-Weber syndrome: Cerebral haemodynamics during seizure activity. *Developmental Medicine & Child Neurology, 41,* 480–485.

Bough, K. J., & Rho, J. M. (2007). Anticonvulsant mechanisms of the ketogenic diet. *Epilepsia, 48,* 43–58.

Cardoza, B., Clarke, A., Wilcox, J., Gibbon, F., Smith, P. E., Archer, H., Hryniewiecka-Jaworska, A., & Kerr, M. (2011). Epilepsy in Rett syndrome: Association between phenotype and genotype, and implications for practice. *Seizure, 20,* 646–649.

Chu-Shore, C. J., Major, P., Camposano, S., Muzykewicz, D., & Thiele, E. A. (2010a). The natural history of epilepsy in tuberous sclerosis complex. *Epilepsia, 51,* 1236–1241.

Chu-Shore, C. J., & Thiele, E. A. (2010b). Tumor growth in patients with tuberous sclerosis complex on the ketogenic diet. *Brain & Development, 32,* 318–322.

Coppola, G., Klepper, J., Ammendola, E., Fiorillo, M., della Corte, R., Capano, G., & Pascotto, A. (2006). The effects of the ketogenic diet in refractory partial seizures with reference to tuberous sclerosis. *European Journal of Paediatric Neurology, 10,* 148–151.

Dahlin, M., Elfving, A., Ungerstedt, U., & Amark, P. (2005). The ketogenic diet influences the levels of excitatory and inhibitory amino acids in the CSF in children with refractory epilepsy. *Epilepsy Research, 64,* 115–125.

Evangeliou, A., Doulioglou, V., Haidopoulou, K., Aptouramani, M., Spilioti, M., & Varlamis, G. (2010). Ketogenic diet in a patient with Angelman syndrome. *Pediatrics International, 52,* 831–834.

Ewen, J. B., Comi, A. M., & Kossoff, E. H. (2007). Myoclonic-astatic epilepsy in a child with Sturge-Weber syndrome. *Pediatric Neurology, 36,* 115–117.

Giampietro, P. F., Schowalter, D. B., Merchant, S., Campbell, L. R., Swink, T., & Roa, B. B. (2006). Widened clinical spectrum of the Q128P MECP2 mutation in Rett syndrome. *Child's Nervous System, 22,* 320–324.

Grocott, O. R., Herrington, K. S., Pfeifer, H. H., Thiele, E. A., & Thibert, R. L. (2017). Low glycemic index treatment for seizure control in Angelman syndrome: A case series from the Center for Dietary Therapy of Epilepsy at the Massachusetts General Hospital. *Epilepsy & Behavior, 68,* 45–50.

Haas, R. H., Light, M., Rice, M., & Barshop (1995). Oxidative metabolism in Rett synd 1. Clinical studies. *Neuropediatrics, 26,* 90–9

Haas, R. H., Rice, M. A., Trauner, D. A., & Merritt A. (1986). Therapeutic effects of a ketogenic d in Rett syndrome. *American Journal of Medica Genetics, 24,* 225–246.

Jiang, Y., Lev-Lehman, E., Bressler, J., Tsai, T. F., & Beaudet, A. L. (1999). Genetics of Angelman syndrome. *American Journal of Human Genetics, 65,* 1–6.

Kossoff, E. H., Borsage, J. L., & Comi, A. M. (2010). A pilot study of the modified Atkins diet for Sturge-Weber syndrome. *Epilepsy Research, 92,* 240–243.

Kossoff, E. H., Buck, C., & Freeman, J. M. (2002). Outcomes of 32 hemispherectomies for Sturge-Weber syndrome worldwide. *Neurology, 59,* 1735–1738.

Kossoff, E. H., Ferenc, L., & Comi, A. M. (2009b). An infantile-onset, severe, yet sporadic seizure pattern is common in Sturge-Weber syndrome. *Epilepsia, 50,* 2154–2157.

Kossoff, E. H., Thiele, E. A., Pfeifer, H. H., McGrogan, J. R., & Freeman, J. M. (2005). Tuberous sclerosis complex and the ketogenic diet. *Epilepsia, 46,* 1684–1686.

Kossoff, E. H., Zupec-Kania, B. A., Amark, P. E., Ballaban-Gil, K. R., Bergkvist, A. G. C., Blackford, R., Buchhalter, J. R., Caraballo, R. H., Cross, J. H., Dahlin, M. G., Donner, E. J., Klepper, J., Jehle, R. S., Kim, H.-D., Liu, Y. M. C., Nordli, D. R., Jr., Pfeifer, H. H., Rho, J. M., Stafstrom, C. E., . . . International Ketogenic Diet Study Group. (2009a). Optimal clinical management of children receiving the ketogenic diet: Recommendations of the International Ketogenic Diet Study Group. *Epilepsia, 50,* 304–317.

Kossoff, E. H., Zupec-Kania, B. A., Auvin, S., et al. (2018). Optimal clinical management of children receiving dietary therapies for epilepsy: Updated recommendations of the International Ketogenic Diet Study Group. *Epilepsia Open, 3,* 175–192.

Kumada, T., Hiejima, I., Nozaki, F., Hayashi, A., & Fujii, T. (2013). Glycemic index treatment using Japanese foods in a girl with Lennox-Gastaut syndrome. *Pediatric Neurology, 48,* 390–392.

Laan, L. A., Renier, W. O., Arts, W. F., Buntinx, I. M., vd Burgt, I. J., Stroink, H., Beuten, J., Zwinderman, K. H., van Dijk, J. G., & Brouwer, O. F. (1997). Evolution of epilepsy and EEG findings in Angelman syndrome. *Epilepsia, 38,* 195–199.

Larson, A. M., Pfeifer, H. H., & Thiele, E. A. (2012). Low glycemic index treatment for epilepsy in tuberous sclerosis complex. *Epilepsy Research, 99,* 180–182.

Liebhaber, G. M., Riemann, E., & Baumeister, F. A. (2003). Ketogenic diet in Rett syndrome. *Journal of Child Neurology, 18,* 74–75.

Mantis, J. G., Fritz, C. L., Marsh, J., Heinrichs, S. C., & Seyfried, T. N. (2009). Improvement in motor and exploratory behavior in Rett syndrome mice with restricted ketogenic and standard diets. *Epilepsy & Behavior, 15*, 133–141.

Martinez, C. C., Pyzik, P. L., & Kossoff, E. H. (2007). Discontinuing the ketogenic diet in seizure-free children: Recurrence and risk factors. *Epilepsia, 48*, 187–190.

Matsuishi, T., Yamashita, Y., Takahashi, T., & Nagamitsu, S. (2011). Rett syndrome: The state of clinical basic research, and future perspectives. *Brain & Development, 33*, 627–631.

McDaniel, S. S., Rensing, N. R., Thio, L. L., Yamada, K. A., & Wong, M. (2011). The ketogenic diet inhibits the mammalian target of rapamycin (mTOR) pathway. *Epilepsia, 52*, e7–e11.

Minassian, B. A., DeLorey, T. M., Olsen, R. W., Philippart, M., Bronstein, Y., Zhang, Q., Guerrini, R., Van Ness, P., Livet, M. O., & Delgado-Escueta, A. V. (1998). Angelman syndrome: Correlations between epilepsy phenotypes and genotypes. *Annals of Neurology, 43*, 485–493.

Napolioni, V., & Curatolo, P. (2008). Genetics and molecular biology of tuberous sclerosis complex. *Current Genomics, 9*, 475–487.

Neul, J. L., Kaufmann, W. E., Glaze, D. G., Christodoulou, J., Clarke, A. J., Bahi-Buisson, N., Leonard, H., Bailey, M. E. S., Schanen, N. C., Zappella, M., Renieri, A., Huppke, P., Percy, A. K., & RettSearch Consortium. (2010). Rett syndrome: Revised diagnostic criteria and nomenclature. *Annals of Neurology, 68*, 944–950.

Nissenkorn, A., Gak, E., Vecsler, M., Reznki, H., Menascu, S., & Ben Zeev, B. (2010). Epilepsy in Rett syndrome—The experience of a National Rett Center. *Epilepsia, 51*, 1252–1258.

Nissenkorn, A., Levy-Drummer, R. S., Bondi, O., Renieri, A., Villard, L., Mari, F., Mencarelli, M. A., Lo Rizzo, C., Meloni, I., Pineda, M., Armstrong, J., Clarke, A., Bahi-Buisson, N., Mejaski, B. V., Djuric, M., Craiu, D., Djukic, A., Pini, G., Bisgaard, A. M., . . . Ben-Zeev, B. (2015). Epilepsy in Rett syndrome—Lessons from the Rett networked database. *Epilepsia, 56*, 569–576.

Overwater, I. E., Bindels-de Heus, K., Rietman, A. B., Ten Hoopen, L. W., Vergouwe, Y., Moll, H. A., & de Wit, M. C. (2015). Epilepsy in children with tuberous sclerosis complex: Chance of remission and response to antiepileptic drugs. *Epilepsia, 56*, 1239–1245.

Pascual-Castroviejo, I., Pascual-Pascual, S. I., Velazquez-Fragua, R., & Viano, J. (2008). Sturge-Weber syndrome: Study of 55 patients. *Canadian Journal of Neurological Sciences, 35*, 301–307.

Petit, F., Auvin S., Lamblin, M. D., & Vallee, L. (2008). Myoclonic astatic seizures in a child with Sturge-Weber syndrome. *Revue Neurologique, 164*, 953–956.

Pintaudi, M., Calevo, M. G., Vignoli, A., Parodi, E., Aiello, F., Baglietto, M. G., Hayek, Y., Buoni, S., Renieri, A., Russo, S., Cogliati, F., Giordano, L., Canevini, M., & Veneselli, E. (2010). Epilepsy in Rett syndrome: Clinical and genetic features. *Epilepsy & Behavior, 19*, 296–300.

Shirley, M. D., Tang, H., Gallione, C. J., Baugher, J. D., Frelin, L. P., Cohen, B., North, P. E., Marchuk, D. A., Comi, A. M., & Pevsner, J. (2013). Sturge-Weber syndrome and port-wine stains caused by somatic mutation in *GNAQ. New England Journal of Medicine, 368*, 1971–1979.

Stein, D., Chetty, M., & Rho, J. M. (2010). A "happy" toddler presenting with sudden, life-threatening seizures. *Seminars in Pediatric Neurology, 17*, 35–38.

Sujansky, E., & Conradi, S. (1995). Sturge-Weber syndrome: Age of onset of seizures and glaucoma and the prognosis for affected children. *Journal of Child Neurology, 10*, 49–58.

Thibert, R. L., Conant, K. D., Braun, E. K., Bruno, P., Said, R. R., Nespeca, M. P, & Thiele, E. A. (2009). Epilepsy in Angelman syndrome: A questionnaire-based assessment of the natural history and current treatment options. *Epilepsia, 50*, 2369–2376.

Thibert, R. L., Pfeifer, H. H., Larson, A. M., Raby, A. R., Reynolds, A. A., Morgan, A. K., & Thiele, E. A. (2012). Low glycemic index treatment for seizures in Angelman syndrome. *Epilepsia, 53*, 1498–1502.

Valente, K. D., Fridman, C., Varela, M. C., Koiffmann, C. P., Andrade, J. Q., Grossman, R. M., Kok, F., & Marques-Dias, M. J. (2005). Angelman syndrome: Uniparental paternal disomy 15 determines mild epilepsy but has no influence on EEG patterns. *Epilepsy Research, 67*, 163–168.

Valente, K. D., Koiffmann, C. P., Fridman, C., Varella, M., Kok, F., Andrade, J. Q., Grossman, R. M, & Marques-Dias, M. J. (2006). Epilepsy in patients with Angelman syndrome caused by deletion of the chromosome 15q11-13. *Archives of Neurology, 63*, 122–128.

Vignoli, A., La Briola, F., Turner, K., Scornavacca, G., Chiesa, V., Zambrelli, E., Piazzini, A., Savini, M. N., Alfano, R. M., & Canevini, M. P. (2013). Epilepsy in TSC: Certain etiology does not mean certain prognosis. *Epilepsia, 54*, 2134–2142.

Zhang, K., Hu, W. H., Zhang, C., Meng, F. G., Chen, N., & Zhang, J. G. (2013). Predictors of seizure freedom after surgical management of tuberous sclerosis complex: A systematic review and meta-analysis. *Epilepsy Research, 105*, 377–383.

The Ketogenic Diets in Genetic Generalized Epilepsy Syndromes

SUDHA KILARU KESSLER, MD, MSCE

INTRODUCTION

The ketogenic diet (KD) and related dietary therapies, which are characterized by carbohydrate restriction, are now widely accepted as a treatment option for epilepsies that are resistant to medications. Although many studies have demonstrated the efficacy of the KD in severe epilepsies with generalized seizure types, including infantile spasms, Dravet syndrome, Doose syndrome (myoclonic astatic epilepsy), and Lennox-Gastaut syndrome, the KD is perhaps less often considered for Genetic Generalized Epilepsy (GGE) syndromes, also known as genetic generalized epilepsies, which include childhood absence epilepsy, juvenile absence epilepsy, juvenile myoclonic epilepsy, and generalized epilepsy with generalized tonic-clonic seizures (GE-GTC). This chapter discusses the use of the KD in these syndromes. The discussion specifically addresses IGE. The epilepsy associated with GLUT1 (glucose transporter type 1) deficiency syndrome is not discussed, although one of its phenotypes is early-onset absence epilepsy, because this syndrome is discussed in Chapter 6 GLUT1 Deficiency Syndrome and the Ketogenic Dietary Therapies.

CHILDHOOD ABSENCE EPILEPSY

Childhood absence epilepsy (CAE) is the most common pediatric epilepsy syndrome, accounting for 10% of all cases of epilepsy in children (Berg et al., 2000). Onset occurs between 4 and 8 years of age in an otherwise neurologically normal child. Typical seizures are staring spells, lasting only seconds, occurring many times daily, and characterized on EEG by 3-Hz generalized spike-and-wave activity with a normal background. CAE has classically been considered a benign epilepsy syndrome that responds to medication, remits with time, and does not affect neurodevelopmental outcome. Now it appears that treatment response and remission rates are not as high as once assumed, and long-term psychosocial difficulties are common (Masur et al., 2013; Nickels, 2015; Wirrell et al., 1997). Juvenile absence epilepsy (JAE) presents later in childhood, typically between 11 and 17 years of age, and carries a higher risk of treatment resistance and a lower rate of eventual remission. The occurrence of generalized tonic-clonic (GTC) seizures is more common in JAE than in CAE, but in both syndromes, GTC seizures portend a poorer prognosis for remission.

Ethosuximide is the first-line treatment for CAE. Valproic acid is also efficacious but has a greater impact on tests of attention than does ethosuximide (Glauser et al., 2010). Lamotrigine is efficacious in a smaller proportion of patients. Second-line therapies are broad-spectrum antiseizure medications (ASM), such as topiramate, zonisamide, clobazam, or conventional benzodiazepines, such as clonazepam (Kessler & McGinnis, 2019). Antiseizure medications for focal mechanisms of action in epilepsy, including the sodium channel blockers, are avoided because they may exacerbate seizures with generalized mechanisms of action. Thus, treatment choices are limited when first-line drugs fail.

Unfortunately, the published literature on KD-related therapies for absence epilepsy is quite limited. One study from Johns Hopkins University specifically evaluated the efficacy of the KD and the modified Atkins diet (MAD) in children with treatment-resistant absence epilepsy, and the article also included a review of the literature that included studies of absence epilepsy patients (Groomes et al., 2011). In the Johns Hopkins University cohort, eight patients with absence epilepsy were treated with the KD, and 13 patients with absence epilepsy were treated with the MAD. Of the combined 21 patients, only two had a history of GTC seizures in addition to absence, but eight patients had early-onset absence with seizures beginning before the children were 4 years old. Diet initiation occurred 1 to 12 years after seizure onset, and the median number of antiepileptic medications used was four (range 2 to 10). After 3 months of dietary therapy, 18 children (82%) had > 50% seizure reduction, and four (19%) were seizure-free. Too few patients underwent EEG before and during dietary therapy to determine the effect on spike-wave discharges.

The same paper also included a summary of 17 previously published KD studies dating from 1922 to 2008 that included patients with childhood or juvenile absence epilepsy. Of the 133 children with absence epilepsy and documented outcomes (with responses recorded at 3 days to 3 months), more than two thirds reported a greater than 50% seizure reduction and one third experienced periods of seizure freedom. What is not known from this historical review is the proportion of patients presenting with a CAE-like syndrome due to GLUT1 deficiency, which is expected to respond well to the KD.

A case report described a 7-year-old girl with absence epilepsy who became seizure-free with the paleolithic KD, which consists entirely of meat, offal, fish, eggs, and animal fats without calorie restriction, and which the child apparently tolerated well (Clemens et al., 2013). Of note, dietary therapy was used as first-line antiepileptic treatment because of parental concerns about the potential for medication side effects. Also of note, the child had other neurologic abnormalities (developmental delays, social withdrawal, and a history of febrile seizures) and thus was atypical for classic CAE. Whether the child underwent diagnostic testing for GLUT1 deficiency is not reported. After an immediate and gradual decline in seizure frequency, the patient became seizure-free by 6 weeks of therapy. At 3 months, carbohydrates were reintroduced, in the form of low-glycemic-index vegetables. The patient had no evidence of epileptiform discharges on long-term video-EEG monitoring and continued to be seizure-free 20 months after diet initiation.

Several large single-center studies of KD effectiveness included no patients with absence epilepsy (Dressler et al., 2010; Hallböök et al., 2015; Sharma et al., 2009; Wibisono et al., 2015). In a single-center series from Australia that included 61 patients initiating the KD, the 29 patients who were responders at 3 months included two with

treatment-resistant CAE, both of whom continued to be responders at 12 months (Thammongkol et al., 2012). In another single-center series from Argentina that included 216 patients starting the KD, the single patient who had an IGE syndrome (epilepsy with myoclonic absence) experienced > 75% reduction in seizure frequency (Caraballo et al., 2011). In a case series of 29 adolescents and adults with refractory epilepsy, four patients had IGE (syndrome was not noted) and one of these had > 90% reduction in absence seizures specifically but was not seizure-free (Nei et al., 2014).

JUVENILE MYOCLONIC EPILEPSY

Juvenile myoclonic epilepsy (JME) is another GGE syndrome infrequently appearing in KD series. JME is a common and highly recognizable epilepsy syndrome with onset in adolescence or young adulthood (Dreifuss, 1989). The hallmarks of the syndrome are myoclonic seizures (brief bilateral jerks with persevered awareness), often clustering in the morning and sometimes triggered by photic stimulation, and 4-Hz or faster generalized spike-and-wave or polyspike-and-wave discharges on EEG. Many patients initially come to medical attention not when the myoclonic jerks begin, but when the first GTC seizure occurs. Absence seizures occur in a subset of patients and may be a marker of worse long-term seizure prognosis (Senf et al., 2013).

Because valproic acid is efficacious in most patients with JME, it has long been considered the treatment of choice (Dreifuss, 1989). However, growing concerns about the long-term side effects and teratogenic potential of valproic acid have made it a less desirable choice, particularly in young women (Tomson et al., 2015; Wheless et al., 2005). In addition, treatment resistance, even to valproic acid, does occur in JME. Thus, dietary therapy may be considered in this population as well.

Very little published literature has specifically addressed the use of KD-related therapies in JME. In 2013, Kossoff and colleagues described the use of the MAD in eight JME patients ages 15 to 44 years, six of whom were female (Kossoff et al., 2013). Except for one patient who was medication naïve, all others were treatment-resistant to four or more AEDs, and all but three patients had tried valproate. Of note, the mean age of seizure onset was 10.5 years, which is atypically young for JME. Seven of the eight remained on the diet at 1 month and achieved at least moderate urinary ketosis. After 3 months, five (63%) reported > 50% drop in seizure frequency, and two became seizure-free. At the time the paper was published, patients had remained on the diet 0.5 to 40 months. Two patients were able to reduce medications, but none had stopped all AEDs.

Just as for CAE, many of the larger single-center long-term follow-up studies of the KD included no patients with JME. The case series from Australia discussed above also included a single patient with JME, who was a responder at 3 months (no 12-month follow-up was reported; Thammongkol et al., 2012). A study from Norway prospectively evaluated 13 adults with IGE, ages 16 to 57 years, initiating the MAD (Kverneland et al., 2015). The majority, nine, had JME, while two had CAE, one had Jeavons syndrome (absence epilepsy with eyelid myoclonia), and one had an GGE not otherwise specified. Nine patients continued the MAD for at least 4 weeks, and only six reached the 12-week time point. Four patients achieved a 50% or greater reduction in seizure frequency—in one, frequent GTC seizures stopped. Lack of motivation and lack of adherence to the diet were the reasons most frequently cited for dropping out of the study.

While the reason for referral for KD treatment for most IGE patients may be treatment-resistant seizures, the KD has other potential advantages over antiseizure medications besides efficacy. Though specific cognitive and behavioral challenges have been noted (for example, inattention in CAE, impulsivity and other frontal lobe dysfunction in JME), patients with IGE syndromes typically have normal intelligence at baseline—thus, cognitive adverse effects of antiseizure medications may have a substantial impact on function, particularly for those on polytherapy. Although rigorous controlled studies are still lacking, the potentially beneficial effects of the KD on cognition have been repeatedly noted. Therefore, for IGE patients who are experiencing cognitive side effects from one or more antiseizure medications, the KD may be a desirable alternative, or a strategy for reducing the number of antiseizure medications.

Key challenges for dietary epilepsy therapy in patients with IGE are the feasibility and tolerability of the diet at a time when food choices are typically made more autonomously than in early childhood. In addition, maintaining the minimum protein requirements in an adolescent or adult in the context of a protein- and carbohydrate-restricted, but normal calorie-level, KD can be difficult. The modified Atkins diet (MAD), which is a high-fat and low-carbohydrate diet, but less stringent in protein restriction, may be more feasible and tolerable than a classic KD in these patients. However, adult patients may find even the MAD difficult to carry out consistently (Kverneland et al., 2015). There are no reports of the use of two other KD-related therapies, the low-glycemic-index treatment (LGIT) and the MCT oil diet, in GGE syndromes specifically. The available series on LGIT include patients with generalized seizure types, but specific syndrome information has not been reported (Muzykewicz et al., 2009; Pfeifer & Thiele, 2005).

In conclusion, patients with pharmacoresistant idiopathic (genetic) generalized epilepsies are not frequently started on the KD, as evidenced in large KD case series, but there is some evidence that carbohydrate-restriction diets may have some efficacy in this population. However, feasibility and tolerability continue to be major barriers. Further investigations of the long-term outcomes of IGE treated with dietary treatments are needed.

REFERENCES

Berg, A. T., Shinnar, S., Levy, S. R., Testa, F. M., Smith-Rapaport, S., & Beckerman, B. (2000). How well can epilepsy syndromes be identified at diagnosis? A reassessment 2 years after initial diagnosis. *Epilepsia*, 41, 1269–1275.

Caraballo, R., Vaccarezza, M., Cersósimo, R., Rios, V., Soraru, A., Arroyo, H., Agosta, G., Escobal, N., Demartini, M., Maxit, C., Cresta, A., Marchione, D., Carniello, M., & Paníco, L. (2011). Long-term follow-up of the ketogenic diet for refractory epilepsy: Multicenter Argentinean experience in 216 pediatric patients. *Seizure*, 20(8), 640–645.

Clemens, Z., Kelemen, A., Fogarasi, A., & Tóth, C. (2013). Childhood absence epilepsy successfully treated with the paleolithic ketogenic diet. *Neurology and Therapy*, 2, 71–76.

Dreifuss, F. E. (1989). Juvenile myoclonic epilepsy: Characteristics of a primary generalized epilepsy. *Epilepsia*, 30(Suppl. 4), S1–S7; discussion S24–S27.

Dressler, A., Stöcklin, B., Reithofer, E., Benninger, F., Freilinger, M., Hauser, E., Reiter-Fink, E., Seidl, R., Trimmel-Schwahofer, P., & Feucht, M. (2010). Long-term outcome and tolerability of the ketogenic diet in drug-resistant childhood epilepsy—The Austrian experience. *Seizure*, 19, 404–408.

Glauser, T. A., Cnaan, A., Shinnar, S., Hirtz, D. G., Dlugos, D., Masur, D., Clark, P. O., Capparelli, E. V., & Adamson, P. C. (2010). Ethosuximide, valproic acid, and lamotrigine in childhood absence epilepsy. *New England Journal of Medicine*, 362, 790–799.

Groomes, L. B., Pyzik, P. L., Turner, Z., Dorward, J. L., Goode, V. H., & Kossoff, E. H. (2011). Do patients with absence epilepsy respond to ketogenic diets? *Journal of Child Neurology, 26,* 160–165.

Hallböök, T., Sjölander, A., Åmark, P., Miranda, M., Bjurulf, B., & Dahlin, M. (2015). Effectiveness of the ketogenic diet used to treat resistant childhood epilepsy in Scandinavia. *European Journal of Paediatric Neurology, 19,* 29–36.

Kessler, S. K., & McGinnis, E. (2019). A practical guide to treatment of childhood absence epilepsy. *Pediatric Drugs, 21*(1), 15–24.

Kossoff, E. H., Henry, B. J., & Cervenka, M. C. (2013). Efficacy of dietary therapy for juvenile myoclonic epilepsy. *Epilepsy & Behavior, 26,* 162–164.

Kverneland, M., Selmer, K. K., Nakken, K. O., Iversen, P. O., & Taubøll, E. (2015). A prospective study of the modified Atkins diet for adults with idiopathic generalized epilepsy. *Epilepsy & Behavior, 53,* 197–201.

Masur, D., Shinnar, S., Cnaan, A., Shinnar, R. C., Clark, P., Wang, J., Weiss, E. F., Hirtz, D. G., & Glauser, T. A. (2013). Pretreatment cognitive deficits and treatment effects on attention in childhood absence epilepsy. *Neurology, 81,* 1572–1580.

Muzykewicz, D. A., Lyczkowski, D. A., Memon, N., Conant, K. D., Pfeifer, H. H., & Thiele, E. A. (2009). Efficacy, safety, and tolerability of the low glycemic index treatment in pediatric epilepsy. *Epilepsia, 50,* 1118–1126.

Nei, M., Ngo, L., Sirven, J. I., & Sperling, M. R. (2014). Ketogenic diet in adolescents and adults with epilepsy. *Seizure, 23*(6), 439–442.

Nickels, K. (2015). Seizure and psychosocial outcomes of childhood and juvenile onset generalized epilepsies: Wolf in sheep's clothing, or well-dressed wolf? *Epilepsy Currents, 15,* 114–117.

Pfeifer, H. H., & Thiele, E. A. (2005). Low-glycemic-index treatment: A liberalized ketogenic diet for treatment of intractable epilepsy. *Neurology, 65,* 1810–1812.

Senf, P., Schmitz, B., Holtkamp, M., & Janz, D. (2013). Prognosis of juvenile myoclonic epilepsy 45 years after onset: Seizure outcome and predictors. *Neurology, 81,* 2128–2133.

Sharma, S., Gulati, S., Kalra, V., Agarwala, A., & Kabra, M. (2009). Seizure control and biochemical profile on the ketogenic diet in young children with refractory epilepsy—Indian experience. *Seizure, 18,* 446–449.

Thammongkol, S., Vears, D. F., Bicknell-Royle, J., Nation, J., Draffin, K., Stewart, K. G., Scheffer, I. E., & Mackay, M. T. (2012a). Efficacy of the ketogenic diet: Which epilepsies respond? *Epilepsia, 53,* e55–e59.

Tomson, T., Marson, A., Boon, P., Canevini, M. P., Covanis, A., Gaily, E., Kälviäinen, R., & Trinka, E. (2015). Valproate in the treatment of epilepsy in girls and women of childbearing potential. *Epilepsia, 56,* 1006–1019.

Wheless, J. W., Clarke, D. F., & Carpenter, D. (2005). Treatment of pediatric epilepsy: Expert opinion, 2005. *Journal of Child Neurology, 20*(Suppl. 1), S1–S56; quiz S59–S60.

Wibisono, C., Rowe, N., Beavis, E., Kepreotes, H., Mackie, F. E., Lawson, J. A., & Cardamone, M. (2015). Ten-year single-center experience of the ketogenic diet: Factors influencing efficacy, tolerability, and compliance. *Journal of Pediatrics, 166,* 1030–1036.e1.

Wirrell, E. C., Camfield, C. S., Camfield, P. R., Dooley, J. M., Gordon, K. E., & Smith, B. (1997). Long-term psychosocial outcome in typical absence epilepsy: Sometimes a wolf in sheeps' clothing. *Archives of Pediatrics and Adolescent Medicine, 151,* 152–158.

10

Ketogenic Diet Therapy for Infants

*ELLES J. T. M. VAN DER LOUW, RD, PHD, STÉPHANE AUVIN, MD, PHD,
AND J. HELEN CROSS, MD, PHD*

INTRODUCTION

Ketogenic diet therapy (KDT) is a nonpharmacologic treatment for children with pharmacoresistant epilepsy and/or metabolic diseases. The efficacy of KDT has been established by several multicenter studies and one randomized controlled trial. The randomized trial that further established the efficacy of KDT was conducted in children and adolescents 2 to 16 years old (Neal et al., 2008a). The diet may be administered in one of several ways, and each may be valid. An international protocol for its implementation and subsequent follow-up management in children has been published (Kossoff et al., 2009) and recently was updated (Kossoff et al., 2018).

For a long time, the KDT was not recommended for use in infancy (in children < 2 years old) because this is such a crucial period in development and the risk of nutritional inadequacies was considered too great. This was based on the immaturity of lipase activity, liver function, and lipid metabolism and the difficulty of achieving and maintaining ketosis. Moreover, the possible long-term adverse effects are not well identified yet. Nevertheless, a KDT infant formula is now available, making the diet easier to administer in this group.

In 2016, an international group of experts in the KDT field published evidence-based guidelines on how the diet should be administered and in whom (van der Louw et al., 2016), with the aim to set out optimal practice in the care of an infant being treated with KDT.

KDT is usually used in infants with drug-resistant epilepsy syndromes. Nordli et al. (2001) first reported their retrospective experience with treating 32 children < 2 years old with KDT. They concluded that KDT was efficacious in infantile drug-resistant epilepsy as well as safe to use in infants. The use of KDT in infants has been increasingly reported in recent years, allowing better appreciation of the efficacy and safety of this nonpharmacologic treatment in this age group (Table 10.1). Particular attention should be given to growth parameters, as well as the risk of kidney stones, which might be higher than in older children (Herzberg et al., 1990).

EPILEPSY SYNDROMES IN INFANCY WHERE KDT IS BENEFICIAL

Management of epilepsy in infancy is challenging based on the characteristics of the epilepsy and its impact on neurodevelopment of the child. This implies that early, aggressive, and optimal treatment is warranted. First-line treatment of infantile spasms is pharmacologic management with high-dose adrenocorticotrophic hormone (ACTH) or steroids combined with, or followed by, the antiseizure medication (ASM) vigabatrin (Wilmshurst et al., 2015).

As a nonpharmacologic treatment, KDT is currently used in infants with drug-resistant epilepsy syndromes (see Table 10.1), such as infantile spasms (West syndrome) resistant to first-line medication (Dressler et al., 2015; Eun et al., 2006; Hong et al., 2010; Kayyali et al., 2014; Pires et al., 2013), Ohtahara syndrome (Ishii et al., 2011; Sivaraju et al., 2015; Su et al., 2018; Turkdogan et al., 2019), epilepsy of infancy with migrating seizures (Caraballo et al., 2015; Mori et al., 2016), and resistant epilepsy with focal seizures awaiting epilepsy surgery.

There are also other conditions for which KDT is the treatment of choice, such as glucose transporter type 1 (GLUT1) deficiency (Klepper, 2012) and pyruvate dehydrogenase complex (PDHC) deficiency (Prasad et al., 2011; Sofou et al., 2017). Box 10.1 lists epilepsy syndromes specifically seen in infancy.

TABLE 10.1 OVERVIEW OF EFFICACY* IN STUDIES OF KDT IN INFANCY

Study	Population		Outcomes	
Prospective studies		Months	Seizure-free	> 50% seizure reduction
Eun et al., 2006	43	3	15 (34.9%)	15 (34.9%)
		6	17 (39.5%)	8 (18.6%)
Hong et al., 2010	104	3	19 (18.2%)	47 (45.1%)
		6	29 (27.8%)	38 (39.5%)
Pires et al., 2013	17	3	11 (64.7%)	4 (23.5%)
		6	9 (52.9%)	5 (29.4%)
Kayyali et al., 2014	20	3	—	14 (70.0%)
		6	3 (17.6%)	13 (65.0%)
Hirano et al., 2015	6	3	1 (16.6%)	4 (66.7%)
		6	—	—
Hussain et al., 2016	22	3	1 (4.5%)	6 (27.3%)
		6	1 (4.5%)	5 (22.7%)
Dressler et al., 2019a	53	3	25 (47.2%)	—
		Last visit	21 (39.6%)	—
Retrospective studies			Seizure-free	> 50% seizure reduction
Nordli et al., 2001	34	3	0	4 (11.7%)
		6	6 (17.6%)	7 (20.5%)
Kossoff et al., 2002	23	3	3 (13.0%)	11 (47.8%)
		6	3 (13.0%)	10 (43.5%)
Kossoff et al., 2008a	13	3	8 (61.5%)	7 (53.8%)
		6	—	—
Caraballo et al., 2011	12	3	—	—
		18	5 (41.6%)	4 (33.3%)
Numis et al., 2011	26	3	9 (34.6%)	12 (46.1%)
		6	—	11 (42.8%)
Ville et al., 2015	23	3	4 (17.4%)	6 (26.0%)
		6	—	—
Dressler et al., 2015	115	3	31 (26.9%)	39 (33.9%)
		6	29 (25.2%)	34 (29.5%)
Dressler et al., 2019b	79	3	29 (36.7%)	54 (68.3%)
		6	—	—
Kim et al., 2019**	109	3	20 (18.0%)	22 (19.8%)
		6	—	—
Le Pichon et al., 2019	9	3	3 (33.3%)	3 (33.3%)
		Last visit	4 (44.4%)	3 (33.3%)

*Based on intention-to-treat analysis.
**Includes cohort of Nordli et al. (2001).

When to Start

Starting KDT in infants is indicated when there is insufficient seizure control after steroids and/or AED use. However, the retrospective case-control study by Nizamuddin et al. (2008) comparing KDT and ACTH as first-line treatment showed that KDT was highly effective, stopping spasms in 62% of the 20 patients within 1 month. Although ACTH had a higher spasm-free outcome after 1 month of therapy, a higher relapse rate and higher incidence of side effects were seen with ACTH than with KDT (Kossoff et al., 2008a). The outcomes of the first RCT by Dressler et al. (2019), which compared ACTH and KDT as first-line treatment in infantile spasms, are in line with these findings, allowing the cautious conclusion that, overall, the KD is as effective as ACTH in the long term and should, therefore, be considered as an additional early treatment option for infantile spasms. A study in a larger cohort than

BOX 10.1
EPILEPSY SYNDROMES IN INFANCY

- West syndrome (infantile spasm sydrome)
- Ohtahara syndrome (Neonatal developmental epileptic encephalopathy)
- Epilepsy of infancy with migrating focal seizures
- Drug-resistant epilepsy with focal seizures
- Drug-resistant unclassified epilepsy syndrome (after exclusion of contraindication for KDT)
- Epilepsy associated with gene-related encephalopathies

Based on van der Louw et al. (2016).

the reported 53 patients is needed to confirm this conclusion.

Although the study by Ville et al. (2015) using the classic KD 4.0:1 ratio in 42 patients resulted in moderate ketonuria (0.8–1.6 g/L) when combined with hormone therapy suggested to be successful in epileptic encephalopathies (e.g., continuous spike-waves in slow sleep, CSWS), in a subgroup of patients with infantile spasms ($N = 23$) the number of responders and nonresponses to KD were equal between the groups of steroid-dependent and non-steroid-dependent patients (Ville et al., 2015). There currently are no studies of KDT combined with corticosteroid in infants.

KETOGENIC DIET THERAPY IN CLINICAL PRACTICE

Which Diet to Choose and How to Initiate

KDT is a high-fat (71% to 90% of energy) and carbohydrate-restricted (5% to 19% of energy) diet that contains an adequate amount of protein to support growth. Clinical practice shows the classic version of KDT with a 3:1 ratio is routinely used in infants in order to meet protein requirements. This means that for every 3 g of fat there is 1 g of combined protein and carbohydrate. The use of KDT ratios range from 2.5 to 4;1, with respect to tolerance and ketosis, have been reported (Dressler et al., 2015; Eun et al., 2006;

Kayyali et al., 2014; Pires et al., 2013). The classic KDT can be used for both bottle feeding and enteral feeding.

A KDT with medium-chain triglycerides (MCT) consists of 71% to 75% of energy from fat, of which 50% to 60% is MCT and 11% to 25% is long-chain triglycerides (LCT). This version of KDT provides more protein (10% of energy) and carbohydrates (15% to 19% of energy) but is not generally used in infants, who have poor tolerance of high amounts of MCT.

More liberal versions of the traditional KD are the modified Atkins diet (10–30 g of carbohydrates, with free fat and protein intake) and the low-glycemic-index diet (60% of energy from fat, 30% of energy from protein, and 40 to 60 g of carbohydrates with a glycemic index of 50 or lower). These diets are not suitable for infants due to the high amount of protein and the need for strict control.

Information in the literature on how KDT should be initiated in infants is scarce. Raju et al. (2011) showed in a randomized trial of 38 infants that a KDT with a 2.5:1 ratio was as effective as a KDT with a 4:1 ratio, with fewer side effects. Pires et al. (2013) showed in a prospective trial of 17 infants receiving a KDT during hospitalization that a 3:1 (some 4:1) ratio was very effective and well tolerated. Diet initiation used a nonfasting protocol with daily steps of increasing calories and ratio (Pires et al., 2013).

In light of infants' being a vulnerable group of patients, KDT is usually initiated during an admission of at least 3 to 5 days in a specialist hospital setting, which makes close monitoring of side effects possible. In older infants (> 1 year old), initiation at home maybe possible with close communication to, and support from, the multidisciplinary KD team and after thorough education of parents/caregivers.

Using a Ketogenic Formula and/or Breast Milk

While on KDT, the infant can continue bottle feeding. In daily practice, most infants with severe epilepsy have feeding difficulties and may need an enteral tube feed at diet initiation to achieve their requirements.

The KD formula Ketocal 3:1® is specially developed for infants and (young) children to meet their nutritional requirements. Ketocal 3:1® is based on the classic KD and is well tolerated by infants.

It is possible to continue using a limited amount of expressed breast milk combined/mixed with ketogenic formula (Ketocal 3:1®). In cases where there is no expressed breast milk, a limited amount of standard infant formula can be used to combine/mix with the ketogenic formula. This may be given by bottle and/or tube. If using breast milk, it is recommended to start combined use with Ketocal 3:1®. Using Ketocal 4:1® may not fully match with requirements, and careful calculation on an individual basis is highly recommended. When calculated carefully, the protein and vitamin/mineral requirements of the infant can be supplied. In some cases (i.e., the young infant) breast milk on demand may be possible, but this greatly depends on the level of ketosis that is needed to achieve adequate seizure reduction. Studies have shown it is indeed possible. Le Pichon et al. (2019) reported the outcomes of a small study of nine infants who continued breast milk (in a mixture of Ketocal 4:1® formula with expressed breast milk) during KD for at least 1 month and who achieved ketosis before discharge (> 1 mmol/L); the regimen was highly effective after 3 months (> 50% seizure reduction in four of the nine infants, > 90% seizure-free in four of nine). Moreover, Dressler et al. (2020) reported in a retrospective study that 16 of 79 infants treated with KDT and receiving breast milk (median volume 90 ml/day; IQR 53-203) achieved relevant ketosis (> 2 mmol/L) within 47 hr. After 3 months, there was no significant difference in seizure reduction between the infants with, and the infants without, included breast milk (Dressler et al., 2020).

Introduction of Solid Food

To stimulate oral motor activity and to avoid feeding aversion behavior, solid foods may be introduced when infants are 4 to 6 months old (sometimes at 9 months due to developmental delay).

Combination of ketogenic formula with solid food is possible while maintaining the classic diet. Recipes can be calculated based on the original diet ratio (3:1), which is suitable for most infants.

When infants are 9 to 12 months old, when more carbohydrate-containing foods are introduced (such as bread and potatoes), a more liberal KDT version with a low dose of MCT is also possible and well tolerated. The MCT is mixed with a (low-fat) milk product and is gradually increased (for examples, see the Appendix).

The full MCT KD (50% to 60% of energy from MCT) allows a generous amount of protein and carbohydrates but is not recommended because it is poorly tolerated in infancy.

In summary, the international guideline recommends all young infants (< 12 months old) be admitted to hospital for diet initiation. Diet initiation should be undertaken without fasting and with a stepwise start commencing with a 1:1 ratio. Building up to a classic KD with a 3:1 ratio is recommended. The diet can be adjusted to a lower ratio (2.5 or 2:1) or higher ratio (3.5 or 4:1) based on level of ketosis and tolerance. A KD formula with a 3:1 ratio can be used purely or combined with breast milk. The approach to solid food introduction should be individualized to the infant.

Careful calculation to check that individual requirements are met is highly recommended, especially when a 4:1 ratio is applied (van der Louw et al., 2016).

DIETARY PRESCRIPTION

Infants are a vulnerable group of patients with specific nutritional requirements. In order to prevent serious side effects (see Table 10.4), either in the short term or the long term, and to ensure adequate growth and development, the diet has to be calculated securely and adjusted frequently.

In General

- The KDT is introduced via an individually designed step-by-step plan based on full energy intake and without initial fasting.
- The recommended daily allowances (RDA) are recommendations for groups of healthy children, making them less suitable for the individual with epilepsy.
- The ideal weight/age or weight/height has to be used for adequate diet calculation. If the infant has gained a large amount of weight, it is important to determine the most adequate weight/age or weight/height to be used.
- The diet must be adjusted frequently (sometimes on a weekly basis) based on weight gain.
- KDT is done without fluid restriction; moreover, fluid restriction might add to the development of kidney stones.
- The classic KD contains insufficient micronutrients (Christodoulides et al., 2012; Papandreou et al., 2006). Ketocal 3:1® is fully supplemented based on infants' requirements and should be first choice. Ketocal 4:1® may

be used when calculated carefully on an individual level.

- Monitoring the potential carbohydrate content of vitamin/mineral supplements and medications requires close cooperation with a pharmacist.
- Some anticonvulsants interact with some minerals and vitamins; for example, the drugs can influence the absorption of folic acid and the metabolism of calcium and vitamin D (Homer, 2003).

Based on evidence from the literature combined with experience from clinical practice, recommendations on requirements for energy, protein, fat, carbohydrates, fluid, and vitamins/minerals are formulated in the international guideline for KDT of infants with drug-resistant epilepsy (van der Louw et al., 2016). Table 10.2 shows an overview of these recommendations.

MONITORING DURING DIET INITIATION

Glucose

There is a risk of hypoglycemia during diet initiation, although it is uncommon in the absence of a metabolic disease. During admission, blood glucose should be checked twice daily (or more, based on symptoms of hypoglycemia), and frequency must be adjusted based on tolerance. Glucose levels of 2 to 2.5 mmol/L (approximately 40 mg/dl) should be treated immediately with 2 to 4 g carbohydrates by adding a small amount of breast milk, or normal infant formula, or glucose 10% solution (young infants < 4 months old). Older infants (> 4 months old) can be given other sources of rapidly absorbed carbohydrate, such as a couple of tablespoons (30–60 ml) of pure fruit juice. Infants with blood glucose > 3 mmol/L but showing symptoms of hypoglycemia (see Box 10.2) should also be treated in the same way. Blood glucose should be rechecked 15 to 20 min after treatment; if it is not improved, a further dose of breast milk or formula is given (or fruit juice if appropriate).

Ketones

During transition to a ketogenic feeding regime or ketogenic food, the level of ketone bodies in the blood will increase. Monitoring of ketones will ensure a therapeutic level is reached without risking symptoms of excess ketosis (see Box 10.3). Ketones can be measured in blood or urine. Blood testing using a ketometer is recommended during diet initiation because this is more accurate and is unaffected by urine dilution or any possible alterations in water homeostasis that may occur in very young infants. Blood ketones should be checked once or twice daily using a finger or heel prick.

Medical advice should always be sought for persistent hypoglycemia or excess ketosis.

Growth

During diet initiation, weight should be checked daily, with a baseline measure of height.

TABLE 10.2 OVERVIEW OF RECOMMENDATIONS FOR DIET CALCULATION

Age of patient	Energy (kcal)	Fat (type, ratio)	Protein (g/kg/day)*	Carbohydrates (g/kg/day)*	Fluid (ml/kg/day)	Vitamins/ minerals
1–3 months	100–95	LCT MCT: 10%–25% of energy Ratio 3.0:1 (range, 2.0–4.0)	2.0–1.6 1.77–1.36 (WHO/FAO)**	Individually determined	150–140	100% RDA
4–6 months	95–85	As above	1.5–1.3 1.24–1.12 (WHO/FAO)**	Individually determined	120–110	100% RDA
7–12 months	85–80	As above	1.2–1.1 1.12–0.86 (WHO/FAO)**	Individually determined	100–90	100% RDA

*Use the ideal weight/age or weight/height for calculation.
** Check if amount is above the minimal WHO/FAO recommendation.

```
┌─────────────────────────────────────┐
│              BOX 10.2               │
│    SYMPTOMS OF HYPOGLYCEMIA         │
│           IN INFANTS                │
├─────────────────────────────────────┤
│ Jittery                             │
│ Poor body tone, lethargy, pallor    │
│ Poor feeding                        │
│ Low body temperature, cold and clammy │
│ Cyanosis                            │
└─────────────────────────────────────┘
```

Adverse Effects of KDT in Infants During Diet Initiation
General

When the amount of fat is increased gradually, the risk of adverse effects will be limited.

Glucose/Ketones

There is a risk of hypoglycemia, acidosis, dehydration, and high levels of ketones during initiation of the KDT (Kang et al., 2004), and there is increased risk of excess ketosis and metabolic acidosis with concurrent use of carbonic anhydrase inhibitors (for example, topiramate or zonisamide; Takeoka et al., 2002).

Gastrointestinal Complaints

Gastrointestinal problems, such as vomiting, nausea, diarrhea, and abdominal discomfort, are common side effects of KDT (Kang et al., 2004; Schwartz et al., 1989); however, they can usually be alleviated with dietary manipulation and by altering the step-by-step plan.

There is a risk that children with pre-existing gastroesophageal reflux will have symptoms

```
┌─────────────────────────────────────┐
│              BOX 10.3               │
│   SYMPTOMS OF HYPERKETOSIS          │
│           IN INFANTS                │
├─────────────────────────────────────┤
│ Rapid breathing, increased heart rate │
│ Facial flushing                     │
│ Irritability                        │
│ Vomiting                            │
│ Lethargy                            │
│ Poor feeding                        │
└─────────────────────────────────────┘
```

exacerbated by a high-fat regime in view of delayed gastric emptying. Optimization of antireflux medication will help alleviate the symptoms.

Constipation is the most common reported complication of KDT and may already be present prior to diet initiation. Despite dietary changes to help lessen the problem, many children need additional treatment with medication.

DIET FINE-TUNING

Over time, the KDT has to be adjusted on a regular basis (fine-tuning of the diet). This is done to meet the development needs (e.g., introduction of solid foods) of the child, to manage side effects (e.g., gastrointestinal), or during occurrence of frequent intercurrent illnesses without compromising the level of ketosis and/or efficacy of the KDT.

When ketosis doesn't reach an adequate range (2 to 5 mmol/L in blood) within 2 weeks after diet initiation and careful calculation, it is important to adjust the diet (ratio) to maximize the efficacy of the diet for seizure reduction. It is also important to use sugar-free formulations (including IV therapies) where possible.

MONITORING DURING FOLLOW-UP

Follow-Up Schedule

- After the infant's discharge from hospital, phone or email contact by the dietitian or nurse ensures a high level of communication for the first 2 weeks, then at least once (or twice) a week as needed.
- After the first 2 to 4 weeks on the diet, the need for regular communication may diminish and will be determined according to the infant's age, dietary tolerance and/or side effects, family circumstances, and speed with which the diet can be fine-tuned to provide the optimal prescription.
- Clinical reviews by the neurologist and diet team should occur 2 weeks after diet initiation for first review, then at 6 weeks and 3 months after initiation, and then every 3 months until the infant is 2 years old (more frequent follow-up visits are recommended if an infant has medical or nutritional needs that need review). After 2 years, children can be seen every 6 months.
- Recommendations for monitoring during follow-up are summarized in Table 10.3.

TABLE 10.3 RECOMMENDATIONS FOR MONITORING DURING FOLLOW-UP KDT

Investigation	Frequency of monitoring
General	
Epilepsy (seizure diary) frequency and type of seizures	Daily registration
Ketone levels	Daily
Medication	During follow-up visit
Kind and dose of medication	
Nutrition	During follow-up visit
• tolerance	
• intake	
• appetite	
• way of feeding	
Growth	Weekly
• weight	
• height	
Gastrointestinal system	During follow-up visit
• constipation	
• diarrhea	
• vomiting	
Alertness	During follow-up visit
Sleep pattern	During follow-up visit
Biochemical monitoring	
Essential checks	
Blood:	
Full blood count	6 weeks, 3 months, 6 months, then every 6 months
Renal profile (includes sodium, potassium, urea, creatinine, bicarbonate, and albumin)	6 weeks, 3 months, 6 months, then every 6 months
Liver profile	6 weeks, 3 months, 6 months, then every 6 months
Calcium, phosphate, magnesium	6 weeks, 3 months, 6 months, then every 6 months
Glucose	6 weeks, 3 months, 6 months, then every 6 months
Vitamin D	After 3 months, 6 months, then every 6 months
Lipid profile (repeat with fasting if elevated)	After 3 months, 6 months, then every 6 months
Free and acylcarnitine profile	After 3 months, 6 months, then every 6 months
Urine:	
Calcium:creatinine ratio, hematuria	6 weeks, 3 months, 6 months, then every 6 months
Recommended checks	
Blood:	
Vitamins A, E, B_{12}	6 months, then every 12 months
Zinc, selenium, copper	6 months, then every 12 months
Folate, ferritin	6 months, then every 12 months

Adverse Effects of KDT During Follow-Up

Adverse Effects Specific to Infants

Table 10.4 summarizes the incidence of adverse events reported in the literature on KDT in infants. Most commonly seen are gastrointestinal disturbances, especially constipation and reflux, altered lipid levels, renal stones, and acidosis. Most side effects are transient and can be controlled without diet withdrawal by the high level of monitoring recommended in Table 10.3.

However, Eun et al. (2006) reported that 37% of their group of 43 infants discontinued KDT due to complications.

Most studies are based on retrospective data, which implies a lower quality of data on the assessment of side effects.

Gastrointestinal Effects

Gastrointestinal problems, such as vomiting, nausea, diarrhea, and abdominal discomfort, are common ongoing side effects of KDT; however, they can usually be alleviated with dietary manipulation (Kang et al., 2006; Schwartz et al., 1989).

Growth Effects

Besides a case report (Goyens et al., 2002), several prospective studies reported that children treated with KDT for 1 year are at risk for growth retardation (Groleau et al., 2014; Neal et al., 2008b; Peterson et al., 2005; Vining et al., 2002; Williams et al., 2002). The studies concerned groups of children in different age groups and with different etiologies for their seizures. Growth retardation appears to be a problem in children on both classic and MCT KDs despite the latter's providing a significantly higher protein intake (Neal et al., 2008b). However, the study by Nation et al. (2014) in 39 children (of whom 12 were infants) suggested that linear growth is negatively affected by a caloric intake and/or protein intake < 80% of RDA. A prescribed protein:energy ratio of at least 1.5 g protein/100 kcal has been suggested to help prevent growth faltering during KDT (Nation et al., 2014). No correlation has been found between the caloric or protein content of KDT and the best fit line of weight and/or height curve (Neal et al., 2008b). Moreover, long-term follow-up of children treated with KDT in the past suggests that although growth improves after KDT is discontinued, height gain can still be below expected (Kim et al., 2013; Patel et al., 2010). Outcomes from previous studies concerning predictive factors for adequate growth and catch-up growth were not conclusive. Furthermore, because the previous studies were mainly based on small cohorts of patients and were not specified for infants, additional research in a larger cohort of this specific patient group is needed to identify variables influencing long-term growth (6 to 12 months) both during KDT and after KDT has been stopped.

Nutritional Deficiencies

Several studies have reported deficiency of specific vitamins and/or minerals during KDT: levels of vitamin D (Bergqvist et al., 2007), selenium (Bergqvist et al., 2003), and magnesium (Kang et al., 2004) may be especially a problem in children on the classic KD despite micronutrient supplementation (Christodoulides et al., 2012). Vitamin C deficiency has been reported in one child on

KDT (Willmott & Bryan, 2008). Decreased carnitine levels have been seen in children and young adults during the first few months of KDT, in some cases requiring supplementation (Berry-Kravis et al., 2001a), although levels tended to normalize with time on diet therapy. Data from previous studies are not specified for infants.

Although the KD formula Ketocal 3:1® is specially developed for infants and (young) children to meet the nutritional requirements, careful calculation of daily vitamin/mineral intake is essential to prevent deficiencies.

Cardiovascular Effects

Plasma lipid levels can often be elevated by KDT, and significant increases in atherogenic apoB-containing lipoproteins have been reported in children after 6 months on KDT (Kwiterovich et al., 2003). Although there is evidence of a trend back toward normal with time on KDT (Nizamuddin et al., 2008), dyslipidemia raises concern about long-term adverse effects on vascular function. Studies suggest that while arterial stiffness may increase initially (Coppola et al., 2014), the changes in arterial function observed within the first year of KDT are not significant after 24 months and appear to be reversible (Kapetanakis et al., 2014).

Kidney Stones

The use of KDT in infants may increase their risk of kidney stones in comparison to the risk in older children on KDT. In addition to age, the presence of hypercalciuria also increases the risk for the development of kidney stones (Furth et al., 2000). Uric acid, calcium oxalate, calcium phosphate, or mixed-composition stones have been reported in up to 7% of children on KDT (Furth et al., 2000; Herzberg et al., 1990; Kielb et al., 2000). Risk may be higher with long-term treatment (Groesbeck et al., 2006) and concurrent use of carbonic anhydrase inhibitors (Paul et al., 2010). Daily oral intake of citrate potassium, which theoretically alkalinizes the urine and solubilizes urine calcium, can be used to prevent kidney stones, particularly in patients with cumulating risk factors. A retrospective study comparing patients treated by KDT with and without daily potassium citrate supplement has suggested a preventive effect (McNally et al., 2009). Previous studies contain no data specified for infants. Studies by Dressler et al. (2015, 2019b) have reported a low incidence of kidney stones in infants—3 in 58 infants (5%) and 1 in 79 (1%), respectively—at 3-month follow-up of KDT.

Other Side Effects

Other reported, but rare, side effects of KDT are increased infection risk, bruising, raised serum uric acid, fractures, pancreatitis, lipid-aspiration pneumonia, and cardiac abnormalities (Bank et al., 2008; Berry-Kravis et al., 2001b; Best et al., 2000; Kang et al., 2004; Stewart et al., 2001). Again, the data are not specific for infants.

Table 10.4 summarizes the reported side effects of KDT in infants.

ILLNESS

During infancy, intercurrent illness often occurs, and illness can be accompanied by vomiting, nausea, and/or GI complaints. In line with this, intolerance of nutrition might lead to an inadequate

TABLE 10.4 REPORTED ADVERSE EFFECTS OF KDT IN INFANTS

Study	Infant population	Adverse effects
Nordli et al., 2001 (Retrospective review)	32 infants < 24 months Mean age at KD initiation, 14 months	6/32 (19%): Coma due to hypoglycemia and acidosis after initiation ($N = 1$) Vomiting ($N = 1$) Renal stone ($N = 1$) Gastrointestinal bleed (erosive esophagitis from NG tube; $N = 1$) Hyperlipidemia ($N = 1$) Ulcerative colitis ($N = 1$)
Goyens et al., 2002 (Single case report)	KD initiated at 13 days in GLUT1DS neonate	Weight loss and malnutrition associated with low lipase activity, treated with pancreatic enzymes and use of MCT
Eun et al., 2006 (Retrospective review)	43 infants 6 to 42 months old with infantile spasms Mean age at KD initiation, 19 months	24/43 (56%): Gastrointestinal disturbances ($N = 8$), 1 within 4 weeks Serious infectious disease ($N = 4$) Severe dehydration ($N = 3$), 2 within 4 weeks Pneumonia ($N = 3$), 1 lipoid aspiration, 2 within 4 weeks Renal stone ($N = 2$) Hematuria with hypercalciuria ($N = 1$) Reflux esophagitis ($N = 1$) Erosive gastritis ($N = 1$) Fatty liver ($N = 1$)
Kossoff et al., 2008 (Retrospective review)	13 infants < 12 months old, treated with KD as first-line therapy for infantile spasms Median age of spasms onset, 5 months	4/13 (31%): Gastroesophageal reflux ($N = 1$) Constipation ($N = 1$) Poor tolerance of formula ($N = 1$) Weight loss ($N = 1$)
Hong et al., 2010 (Prospective study)	104 infants with infantile spasms Mean age at KD initiation, 1.2 years	34/104 (33%): Dyslipidemia ($N = 17$) Constipation ($N = 7$) Gastroesophageal reflux ($N = 6$) Behavioral problems ($N = 3$) Hematuria ($N = 3$) Diarrhea ($N = 3$) Renal stone ($N = 3$) Acidosis ($N = 3$) Hair thinning ($N = 2$) Hypercalcemia ($N = 2$) Dry skin ($N = 1$) Pica ($N = 1$)

(continued)

TABLE 10.4 CONTINUED

Study	Infant population	Adverse effects
Numis et al., 2011 (Retrospective review)	26 infants with infantile spasms Mean age at KD initiation, 19 months	6/26 (23%): Irritability, lethargy, decreased appetite, persistent hypoglycemia, renal stone, vitamin D deficiency (numbers not specified)
Pires et al., 2013 (Prospective study)	17 infants with infantile spasms, 16 < 12 months old Mean age at KD initiation, 9 months	Weight loss and dyslipidemia (raised triglycerides) in some infants
Kayyali et al., 2014 (Prospective study)	20 infants with infantile spasms Mean age at KD initiation, 1.2 years (range, 0.3 to 2.9 years)	12/20 (60%): Constipation ($N = 7$) Acidosis ($N = 4$) Minor dyslipidemia ($N = 3$) Diarrhea ($N = 1$) Urinary sediment ($N = 1$)
Dressler et al., 2015 (Retrospective study)	58 infants < 18 months old (42 < 9 months old) Mean age at KD initiation, 0.68 years (range, 0.15 to 1.5 years)	29/58 (50%): Carnitine deficiency ($N = 4$) Kidney stones ($N = 3$) Minor dyslipidemia ($N = 21$) Weight gain ($N = 1$) Growth deficiency ($N = 3$) High cholesterol ($N = 2$)
Wirrell et al., 2018 (Retrospective study)	29 infants, age range 2.5 weeks to 23 months	No side effects/mild vomiting/constipation in 75% Biochemical side effects in 38% • hypervitaminosis E • hypercholesterolemia • zinc deficiency
Le Pichon et al., 2019 (Retrospective study)	9 infants, age range 1 to 13 months	4/9 (44%): Vomiting ($N = 1$) Dehydration and metabolic acidosis ($N = 1$) Constipation ($N = 1$) Metabolic acidosis ($N = 1$)
Dressler et al., 2019b (Retrospective study)	79 infants Mean age at KD initiation, 6.2 months (range, 14.6 days to 12 months)	13/16 (81%) in breastfeeding group 63/79 (79%) in control group In total: Tiredness ($N = 6$) Hypoglycemia ($N = 3$) Hyperketosis ($N = 15$) Vomiting ($N = 7$) Food refusal ($N = 23$) Hypertriglyceridemia ($N = 22$) Hypercholesterolemia ($N = 3$) Constipation ($N = 27$) Diarrhea ($N = 4$) Cholecystolithiasis ($N = 2$) Infections ($N = 9$) Carnitine deficiency ($N = 2$) Kidney stones ($N = 1$) Weight gain ($N = 2$) Growth deficiency ($N = 9$)

TABLE 10.4 CONTINUED

Study	Infant population	Adverse effects
Dressler et al., 2019a	101 infants, 53 on KDT Mean age unknown	42/53 (79%): Hypertriglyceridemia ($N = 16$) Constipation ($N = 14$) Hyperketosis ($N = 13$) Solid food refusal ($N = 9$) Infections ($N = 6$) Diarrhea ($N = 6$) Hypercholesterolemia ($N = 5$) Growth deficit ($N = 5$) Cholecystolithiasis ($N = 5$) Tiredness at start ($N = 3$) Hypoglycemia ($N = 3$) Carnitine deficiency ($N = 3$) Weight loss ($N = 3$) Refusal of liquids ($N = 3$) Weight gain ($N = 1$)

intake. It is expected that the KD will have to be adjusted frequently during illness to prevent dehydration and malnutrition. The incidence of adverse effects, such as hypoglycemia and/or hyperketosis, may also be higher during illness, another circumstance that emphasizes the importance of close monitoring and adequate dietary adjustments.

In an infant established on KDT who needs to be NPO (nil by mouth) during illness and who requires hydration intravenously for this or other reasons, solutions containing glucose should be avoided for a limited period (max 6 hr); 0.45% or 0.9% saline or Ringer's lactate should be utilized only with close monitoring of blood sugar and ketone levels.

If an infant has an enteral feeding tube or PEG and is thought to be absorbing nutrients, then a liquid KD based on Ketocal® 3:1 (e.g., temporarily diluted with water) can be utilized as tolerated.

Attention needs to be given to the avoidance of aspiration. An enteral tube feed can also be utilized in an infant with status epilepticus who has failed first- and second-line therapy.

EVALUATION

The overall aim of treatment is to reduce, if not control, epileptic seizures. To monitor this, it is important for seizures to be documented in the form of a seizure diary. Additional gains that may be aimed for include reduction of AEDs and increased alertness and attention, although neither of these outcomes can be predicted.

For infantile spasms, the aim of treatment varies according to the course of the disease. Infantile spasms are the most common seizure type in the first year of life. When KDT is used as first-, second-, or third-line treatment for infantile spasms, the aim remains to achieve seizure freedom. After 1 month on KDT, the patient should be evaluated by a neurologist for use of an AED in addition to KDT (Hong et al., 2010). When KDT is used in drug-resistant infantile spasms, the overall aims are similar to those for other drug-resistant epilepsy syndromes (seizure reduction as well as the reduction of AEDs).

A recently published scientific review of the efficacy of KDT in infants included 341 infants from 13 observational studies for analysis. Almost 65% of patients experienced spasm reduction > 50%, and 35% of patients reached seizure freedom. Patients with infantile spasms of unknown etiology seemed to have an increased probability of achieving freedom from seizures. Moreover, long-term follow-up data revealed a median seizure-free rate of 9.5% (Prezioso et al., 2018). There are strong indications that reaching seizure freedom in infancy is a predictor of long-term outcome (Auvin et al., 2012; O'Callaghan et al., 2011, 2018). This important finding has to be confirmed in larger cohorts of patients.

Cognitive or psychomotor improvement is frequently observed and has been reported in several studies using KDT in infants (Hong et al., 2010; Nordli et al., 2001; Pires et al., 2013; Pulsifer et al., 2001). This outcome requires further evaluation in the future. The current data are limited by the small size of the groups in uncontrolled studies and by the fact that improvements were based on the report of parents during clinic visits or on a questionnaire. The use of validated scales of neurodevelopment or standardized tests that can be repeated to evaluate alertness or attention would permit better assessment in future studies.

Evaluation Period

A formal evaluation of the effectiveness of KDT can be made by the ketogenic team (including neurologist and dietitian) in discussion with the family at any time, depending on the severity of the epilepsy and the number of other treatment options that have previously been tried. Consideration should also be given to diet tolerance and the parent's or caregiver's ability to comply fully with the dietary restrictions.

Only one study has reported on the timing of when the seizures improve in responding patients on KDT (Kossoff et al., 2008b). This retrospective study evaluated the time to seizure reduction in 118 epilepsy patients who started on KDT, of whom 84% had a seizure reduction. The first sign of improvement was observed after a mean time of 5 days (range, 1 to 65 days). Seventy-five percent had improvement within the first 14 days on the diet, and 90% within 23 days (Kossoff et al., 2008b).

Based on this study, we suggest that KDT should be maintained for 2 to 3 months to comprehensively evaluate the efficacy of KDT. During this time, a degree of fine-tuning of the diet may be required.

As mentioned, the delay in seizure control by KDT has been described as a prognostic factor in infantile spasms. The patient with infantile treated by KDT as a first-, second-, or third-line treatment (with the aim of seizure freedom) should be evaluated by the neurologist after 1 month of KDT for consideration of an additional treatment.

Diet Discontinuation

KDT is usually continued for at least 2 years in children who have experienced effective seizure control. There is evidence that seizure control can be maintained after a return to a normal diet in children who have a positive response to diet therapy (Martinez et al., 2007). Children with GLUT1 deficiency or PDHC deficiency usually do not discontinue KDT because the diet treats the underlying metabolic defect as well as any presenting seizures. However, there is evidence that these children may tolerate a reduced ratio in the longer term. In the case of infantile spasms, a study randomizing the seizure-free patients to discontinuation of the diet in either the short term (8 months) or long term (2 years) showed no difference in the rate of seizure relapse between the two groups (Kang et al., 2011). Considering the possible occurrence of side effects, including growth consequences, a shorter duration of KDT in patients with infantile spasms might be considered. Further studies are required to confirm or refute this.

Weaning from KDT back to normal diet should be undertaken gradually, using a stepwise approach over weeks or months. The longer a child has been on KDT, the longer the period of withdrawal advised; if the child is seizure-free, the process may take 3 to 4 months. The ketogenic ratio will be slowly reduced: for example, by 0.25, 0.5, or 1.0 every few days or weeks, or more slowly, such as every month. However, if there has been no benefit from the diet, a full wean within 2 weeks is possible, especially in the young infant who needs to move quickly to the next treatment option. Ketone levels can be monitored during this time, and once ketones are no longer present in blood or urine, the transition to normal diet can be made more quickly. The diet discontinuation process can be an anxious time for parents or caregivers, who may need reassurance and support. If at any point there is deterioration in seizure control, the child can return to the diet at the last ratio used. Concentrated sources of refined carbohydrate should be reintroduced cautiously, and only once the child is fully established on a normal diet without ill effects.

CONCLUSION

Ketogenic Diet Therapy is now a proven, safe, and effective treatment option for infantile spasms after failure of two or three AEDs. KDT appears to have beneficial effects with early use and continued use after the child reaches seizure freedom. Infants are a vulnerable group of patients with specific nutritional requirements, but KDT's side effects are known and manageable, and the evidence-based recommendations for KDT in infants (van der Louw et al., 2016) can be a helpful tool for diet initiation, calculation, and monitoring. Close monitoring by a multidisciplinary team is essential to prevent side effects' becoming a reason for diet termination.

Future prospective intervention studies should focus on fine-tuning the dietary recommendations to the needs of infants, to enable them to reach their developmental milestones, to improve cognitive outcomes, and to limit the side effects (e.g., growth retardation) in the longer term.

APPENDIX

EXAMPLE KDT BASED ON THE CLASSIC KD, WITH FULL BOTTLE FEEDING

Infant 4–6 months old

Weight: ± 6.5 kg
Energy requirement: 540 kcal
Protein requirement: 7.8–9.1 g
Fluid requirement: 715–780 ml

Composition of the bottle feeding

77 g of Ketocal 3:1® powder
Water up to 780 ml

Portions

6 × 130 ml
or
5 × 155 ml bottle feeding

Calories per day — 538 kcal (83 kcal/kg)
Protein g/day (9% of energy) — 12g (1.8 g/kg)
Fat (LCT) g/day (87% of energy) — 52 g
Carbohydrates g/day (4% of energy) — 5.5 g
Fluid per day — 780 ml (120 ml fluid/kg/day)
Ratio — 3:1

EXAMPLE KDT BASED ON BOTTLE FEEDING, INTRODUCTION OF SOLID FOOD BASED ON CLASSIC DIET

Infant 4–6 months old

Weight: ± 6.5 kg
Energy requirement: 540 kcal
Protein requirement: 7.8–9.1 g
Fluid requirement: 715–780 ml

Composition of the bottle feeding

77 g of Ketocal 3:1® powder
Water up to 780 ml

Portions

4 × 155 ml bottle feeding
1 small meal (vegetables*), compensated with fifth bottle (if the infant eats half portion, a 75-ml bottle feeding is used to compensate)

Calories per day — 538 kcal (83 kcal/kg)
Protein g/day (9% of energy) — 12 (1.8 g/kg)
Fat (LCT) g/day (87% of energy) — 52 g
Carbohydrates g/day (4% of energy) — 5.5 g
Fluid per day — 780 ml (120 ml/kg/day)
Ratio — 3:1

* Vegetable/double cream/margarine/oil calculated with same nutritional composition of 1 bottle (= 107 kcal, 2.4 g protein, 10 g fat, 1 g carbohydrates).

EXAMPLE KDT WITH INTRODUCTION OF ORAL FOOD BASED ON CLASSIC DIET

Infant 6–9 months old

Weight: ± 8.5 kg
Energy requirement: ± 705 kcal
Protein requirement: ± 10.2 g
Fluid requirement: ± 765–850 ml

Composition of the bottle feeding

	70 g of Ketocal 3:1® powder
	10 ml Calogen® without flavor
	Water up to 800 ml
Portions	3 × 200 ml bottle feeding
	2 × 100 ml bottle feeding

Beside the bottle feeding

Fruit	2.5 g carbohydrates*
	25 g crème fraiche (35 g fat/100 g cream)
Dinner	Vegetables at 1 g carbohydrates*
	10 g chicken meat
	8 g oil

* According to variation list or ketogenic calculation program.

Calories per day	721 kcal (85 kcal/kg)
Protein g/day (8% of energy)	14 g (1.7 g/kg)
Fat (LCT) g/day (87% of energy)	70 g
Carbohydrates g/day (5% of energy)	9 g
Fluid per day	850 ml (100 ml/kg/day)
Ratio	3:1

EXAMPLE KDT WITH INTRODUCTION OF A SMALL AMOUNT OF MCT EMULSION

Infant 9–12 months old	Weight: ± 9.5 kg
	Energy requirement: ± 800 kcal
	Protein requirement: ± 11.4 g
	Fluid requirement: ± 850–950 ml
Breakfast	200 ml bottle ketogenic formula
Morning snack	Fruit at 2.5 g of carbohydrates*
	25 g crème fraiche (35 g fat/100 g cream)
	65 ml bottle ketogenic formula
	75–100 ml carbohydrate-free drink
Supper	11 g brown bread
	8 g diet margarine (≥ 70 g fat/100 g spread)
	10 g 48+ cheese (spread) or fatty meat products*
	65 ml bottle ketogenic formula 75–100 ml carbohydrate-free drink
Dinner	Potato and vegetables with 5 g carbohydrates*
	15 g meat
	8 g oil
	65 ml bottle ketogenic formula
	75–100 ml carbohydrate-free drink
In the evening	200 ml bottle ketogenic formula

Composition of the bottle feeding

	50 g Ketocal 3:1® powder
	30 ml Liquigen®
	Water up to 600 ml
Portions	2 × 200 ml bottle feeding
	3 × 65 ml bottle feeding

* According to variation lists or ketogenic calculating program.

Calories per day	806 kcal (85 kcal/kg)
Protein g/day (7% of energy)	15 g (1.6 g/kg)
Total fat g/day (84% of energy)	75 g
LCT g/day (67% of energy)	60 g
MCT g/day (17% of energy)	15 g
Carbohydrates g/day (8% of energy)	17 g
Fluid per day	900 ml (95 ml/kg/day)
Ratio	2.7:1

EXAMPLE KDT WITH A SMALL AMOUNT OF MCT

Infant 12 months old	Weight: ± 10–11 kg
	Energy requirement: ± 900 kcal
	Protein requirement: ± 13 g
	Fluid requirement: ± 1,000 ml

Breakfast	15 g brown bread
	8 g diet margarine (≥ 70 g fat /100 g spread)
	10 g 48+ cheese (spread) or fatty meat products*
	or
	Porridge prepared from:
	60 ml full-fat milk
	17 ml double cream (≥ 35 g fat/100 g cream)
	5 g cereal (Bambix® fine grains)
	17 ml Liquigen® + 10 ml yogurt drink (0% fat, sugar-free)
	Carbohydrate-free drink
Morning snack	Fruit at 2.5 g carbohydrates*
	25 g crème fraiche (35 g fat/100 g cream)
	Carbohydrate-free drink
Lunch	15 g brown bread
	8 g diet margarine (≥ 70 g fat/100 g spread)
	10 g 48+ cheese (spread) or fatty meat products*
	17 ml Liquigen® + 10 ml yogurt drink (0% fat, sugar-free)
	Carbohydrate-free drink
Afternoon snack	1 small keto-muffin
	Carbohydrate-free drink
	or
	Bottle ketogenic formula feeding made of:
	15 g of Ketocal 3:1 powder + 100–150 ml water
Dinner	Potato and vegetables with 7.5 g carbohydrates*
	20 g meat
	10 g oil
	17 ml Liquigen® + 10 ml yogurt drink (0% fat, sugar-free)
	Carbohydrate-free drink
In the evening	Bottle of ketogenic formula feeding made of 15 g Ketocal 3:1® powder + 100–150 ml water

* According to variation lists or ketogenic calculating program

Calories per day	925 kcal (85 kcal/kg)
Protein g/day (8% of energy)	18 g (1.6 g/kg)
Total fat g/day (79% of energy)	82 g

LCT g/day (55% of energy)	56 g
MCT g/day (25% of energy)	26 g
Carbohydrates g/day (12% of energy)	28 g
Fluid per day	1,000 ml (95 ml/kg/day)
Ratio	1.8:1

REFERENCES

Auvin, S., Hartman, A. L., Desnous, B., Moreau, A. C., Alberti, C., Delanoe, C., Romano, A., Terrone, G., Kossoff, E. H., Del Giudice, E., & Titomanio, L. (2012). Diagnosis delay in West syndrome: Misdiagnosis and consequences. *European Journal of Pediatrics, 171*, 1695–1701.

Bank, I. M., Shemie, S. D., Rosenblatt, B., Bernard, C., & Mackie, A. S. (2008). Sudden cardiac death in association with the ketogenic diet. *Pediatric Neurology, 39*, 429–431.

Bergqvist, A. G., Chee, C. M., Lutchka, L., Rychik, J., & Stallings, V. A. (2003). Selenium deficiency associated with cardiomyopathy: A complication of the ketogenic diet. *Epilepsia, 44*, 618–620.

Bergqvist, A. G., Schall, J. I., & Stallings, V. A. (2007). Vitamin D status in children with intractable epilepsy, and impact of the ketogenic diet. *Epilepsia, 48*, 66–71.

Berry-Kravis, E., Booth, G., Sanchez, A. C., & Woodbury-Kolb, J. (2001a). Carnitine levels and the ketogenic diet. *Epilepsia, 42*, 1445–1451.

Berry-Kravis, E., Booth, G., Taylor, A., & Valentino, L. A. (2001b). Bruising and the ketogenic diet: Evidence for diet-induced changes in platelet function. *Annals of Neurology, 49*, 98–103.

Best, T. H., Franz, D. N., Gilbert, D. L., Nelson, D. P., & Epstein, M. R. (2000). Cardiac complications in pediatric patients on the ketogenic diet. *Neurology, 54*, 2328–2330.

Caraballo, R., Noli, D., & Cachia, P. (2015). Epilepsy of infancy with migrating focal seizures: Three patients treated with the ketogenic diet. *Epileptic Disorders, 17*, 194–197.

Caraballo, R., Vaccarezza, M., Cersosimo, R., Rios, V., Soraru, A., Arroyo, H., Agosta, G., Escobal, N., Demartini, M., Maxit, C., Cresta, A., Marchione, D., Carniello, M., & Paníco, L. (2011). Long-term follow-up of the ketogenic diet for refractory epilepsy: Multicenter Argentinean experience in 216 pediatric patients. *Seizure, 20*, 640–645.

Christodoulides, S. S., Neal, E. G., Fitzsimmons, G., Chaffe, H. M., Jeanes, Y. M., Aitkenhead, H., & Cross, J. H. (2012). The effect of the classical and medium chain triglyceride ketogenic diet on vitamin and mineral levels. *Journal of Human Nutrition and Dietetics, 25*, 16–26.

Coppola, G., Natale, F., Torino, A., Capasso, R., D'Aniello, A., Pironti, E., Santoro, E., Calabro, R., & Verrotti, A. (2014). The impact of the ketogenic diet on arterial morphology and endothelial function in children and young adults with epilepsy: A case-control study. *Seizure, 23*, 260–265.

Dressler, A., Benninger, F., Trimmel-Schwahofer, P., Groppel, G., Porsche, B., Abraham, K., Muhlebner, A., Samueli, S., Male, C., & Feucht, M. (2019). Efficacy and tolerability of the ketogenic diet versus high-dose adrenocorticotropic hormone for infantile spasms: A single-center parallel-cohort randomized controlled trial. *Epilepsia, 60*, 441–451.

Dressler, A., Hafele, C., Giordano, V., Benninger, F., Trimmel-Schwahofer, P., Groppel, G., Samueli, S., Feucht, M., Male, C., & Repa, A. (2020). The ketogenic diet including breast milk for treatment of infants with severe childhood epilepsy: Feasibility, safety, and effectiveness. *Breastfeeding Medicine, 15*(2), 72–78.

Dressler, A., Trimmel-Schwahofer, P., Reithofer, E., Groppel, G., Muhlebner, A., Samueli, S., Grabner, V., Abraham, K., Benninger, F., & Feucht, M. (2015). The ketogenic diet in infants—Advantages of early use. *Epilepsy Research, 116*, 53–58.

Eun, S. H., Kang, H. C., Kim, D. W., & Kim, H. D. (2006). Ketogenic diet for treatment of infantile spasms. *Brain & Development, 28*, 566–571.

Furth, S. L., Casey, J. C., Pyzik, P. L., Neu, A. M., Docimo, S. G., Vining, E. P., Freeman, J. M., & Fivush, B. A. (2000). Risk factors for urolithiasis in children on the ketogenic diet. *Pediatric Nephrology, 15*, 125–128.

Goyens, P., De Laet, C., Ranguelov, N., Ferreiro, C., Robert, M., & Dan, B. (2002). Pitfalls of ketogenic diet in a neonate. *Pediatrics, 109*, 1185–1186.

Groesbeck, D. K., Bluml, R. M., & Kossoff, E. H. (2006). Long-term use of the ketogenic diet in the treatment of epilepsy. *Developmental Medicine and Child Neurology, 48*, 978–981.

Groleau, V., Schall, J. I., Stallings, V. A., & Bergqvist, C. A. (2014). Long-term impact of the ketogenic diet on growth and resting energy expenditure in children with intractable epilepsy. *Developmental Medicine and Child Neurology, 56*, 898–904.

Herzberg, G. Z., Fivush, B. A., Kinsman, S. L., & Gearhart, J. P. (1990). Urolithiasis associated with the ketogenic diet. *Journal of Pediatrics, 117*, 743–745.

Hirano, Y., Oguni, H., Shiota, M., Nishikawa, A., & Osawa, M. (2015). Ketogenic diet therapy can improve ACTH-resistant West syndrome in Japan. *Brain & Development, 37*, 18–22.

Homer, C. (2003). Nutrition management of seizure disorders. In N. L. Nevin-Folino (Ed.), *Pediatric manual of clinical dietetics* (pp. 423–449). American Dietetic Association.

Hong, A. M., Turner, Z., Hamdy, R. F., & Kossoff, E. H. (2010). Infantile spasms treated with the ketogenic diet: Prospective single-center experience in 104 consecutive infants. *Epilepsia, 51*, 1403–1407.

Hussain, S. A., Shin, J. H., Shih, E. J., Murata, K. K., Sewak, S., Kezele, M. E., Sankar, R., & Matsumoto,

J. H. (2016). Limited efficacy of the ketogenic diet in the treatment of highly refractory epileptic spasms. *Seizure*, 35, 59–64.

Ishii, M., Shimono, M., Senju, A., Kusuhara, K., & Shiota, N. (2011). The ketogenic diet as an effective treatment for Ohtahara syndrome. *Brain & Development*, 43, 47–50.

Kang, H. C., Chung, D. E., Kim, D. W., & Kim, H. D. (2004). Early- and late-onset complications of the ketogenic diet for intractable epilepsy. *Epilepsia*, 45, 1116–1123.

Kang, H. C., Kim, H. D., & Kim, D. W. (2006). Short-term trial of a liquid ketogenic milk to infants with West syndrome. *Brain & Development*, 28, 67.

Kang, H. C., Lee, Y. J., Lee, J. S., Lee, E. J., Eom, S., You, S. J., & Kim, H. D. (2011). Comparison of short- versus long-term ketogenic diet for intractable infantile spasms. *Epilepsia*, 52, 781–787.

Kapetanakis, M., Liuba, P., Odermarsky, M., Lundgren, J., & Hallbook, T. (2014). Effects of ketogenic diet on vascular function. *European Journal of Paediatric Neurology*, 18, 489–494.

Kayyali, H. R., Gustafson, M., Myers, T., Thompson, L., Williams, M., & Abdelmoity, A. (2014). Ketogenic diet efficacy in the treatment of intractable epileptic spasms. *Pediatric Neurology*, 50, 224–227.

Kielb, S., Koo, H. P., Bloom, D. A., & Faerber, G. J. (2000). Nephrolithiasis associated with the ketogenic diet. *Journal of Urology*, 164, 464–466.

Kim, J. T., Kang, H. C., Song, J. E., Lee, M. J., Lee, Y. J., Lee, E. J., Lee, J. S., & Kim, H. D. (2013). Catch-up growth after long-term implementation and weaning from ketogenic diet in pediatric epileptic patients. *Clinical Nutrition*, 32, 98–103.

Kim, S. H., Shaw, A., Blackford, R., Lowman, W., Laux, L. C., Millichap, J. J., & Nordli, D. R., Jr. (2019). The ketogenic diet in children 3 years of age or younger: A 10-year single-center experience. *Scientific Reports*, 9, 8736.

Klepper, J. (2012). GLUT1 deficiency syndrome in clinical practice. *Epilepsy Research*, 100, 272–277.

Kossoff, E. H., Hedderick, E. F., Turner, Z., & Freeman, J. M. (2008a). A case-control evaluation of the ketogenic diet versus ACTH for new-onset infantile spasms. *Epilepsia*, 49, 1504–1509.

Kossoff, E. H., Laux, L. C., Blackford, R., Morrison, P. F., Pyzik, P. L., Hamdy, R. M., Turner, Z., & Nordli, D. R., Jr. (2008b). When do seizures usually improve with the ketogenic diet? *Epilepsia*, 49, 329–333.

Kossoff, E. H., Pyzik, P. L., McGrogan, J. R., Vining, E. P., & Freeman, J. M. (2002). Efficacy of the ketogenic diet for infantile spasms. *Pediatrics*, 109, 780–783.

Kossoff, E. H., Zupec-Kania, B. A., Amark, P. E., Ballaban-Gil, K. R., Bergqvist, A. G. C., Blackford, R., Buchhalter, J. R., Caraballo, R. H., Helen Cross, J., Dahlin, M. G., Donner, E. J., Klepper, J., Jehle, R. S., Kim H. D., Liu, Y. M. C., Nation, J., Nordli, D. R., Pfeiter, H. H., Rho, M. R., . . . Vining, E. P. G. (2009). Optimal clinical management of children receiving the ketogenic diet:

Recommendations of the International Ketogenic Diet Study Group. *Epilepsia*, 50, 304–317.

Kossoff, E. H., Zupec-Kania, B. A., Auvin, S., Ballaban-Gil, K. R., Bergqvist, A. G. C., Blackford, R., Buchhalter, J. R., Caraballo, R. H., Cross, J. H., Dahlin, M. G., Donner, E. J., Guzel, O., Jehle, R. S., Klepper, J., Kang, H. C., Lambrechts, D. A., Liu, Y. M. C., Nathan, J. K., Nordli, D. R., . . . Wirrell, E. C. (2018). Optimal clinical management of children receiving dietary therapies for epilepsy: Updated recommendations of the International Ketogenic Diet Study Group. *Epilepsia Open*, 3, 175–192.

Kwiterovich, P. O., Jr., Vining, E. P., Pyzik, P., Skolasky, R., Jr., & Freeman, J. M. (2003). Effect of a high-fat ketogenic diet on plasma levels of lipids, lipoproteins, and apolipoproteins in children. *JAMA*, 290, 912–920.

Le Pichon, J. B., Thompson, L., Gustafson, M., & Abdelmoity, A. (2019). Initiating the ketogenic diet in infants with treatment refractory epilepsy while maintaining a breast milk diet. *Seizure*, 69, 41–43.

Martinez, C. C., Pyzik, P. L., & Kossoff, E. H. (2007). Discontinuing the ketogenic diet in seizure-free children: Recurrence and risk factors. *Epilepsia*, 48, 187–190.

McNally, M. A., Pyzik, P. L., Rubenstein, J. E., Hamdy, R. F., & Kossoff, E. H. (2009). Empiric use of potassium citrate reduces kidney-stone incidence with the ketogenic diet. *Pediatrics*, 124, e300–e304.

Mori, T., Imai, K., Oboshi, T., Fujiwara, Y., Takeshita, S., Saitsu, H., Matsumoto, N., Takahashi, Y., & Inoue, Y. (2016). Usefulness of ketogenic diet in a girl with migrating partial seizures in infancy. *Brain & Development*, 38, 601–604.

Nation, J., Humphrey, M., MacKay, M., & Boneh, A. (2014). Linear growth of children on a ketogenic diet: Does the protein-to-energy ratio matter? *Journal of Child Neurology*, 29, 1496–1501.

Neal, E. G., Chaffe, H. M., Edwards, N., Lawson, M. S., Schwartz, R. H., & Cross, J. H. (2008b). Growth of children on classical and medium-chain triglyceride ketogenic diets. *Pediatrics*, 122, e334–e340.

Neal, E. G., Chaffe, H., Schwartz, R. H., Lawson, M. S., Edwards, N., Fitzsimmons, G., Whitney, A., & Cross, J. H. (2008a). The ketogenic diet for the treatment of childhood epilepsy: A randomised controlled trial. *Lancet Neurology*, 7, 500–506.

Nizamuddin, J., Turner, Z., Rubenstein, J. E., Pyzik, P. L., & Kossoff, E. H. (2008). Management and risk factors for dyslipidemia with the ketogenic diet. *Journal of Child Neurology*, 23, 758–761.

Nordli, D. R., Jr., Kuroda, M. M., Carroll, J., Koenigsberger, D. Y., Hirsch, L. J., Bruner, H. J., Seidel, W. T., & De Vivo, D. C. (2001). Experience with the ketogenic diet in infants. *Pediatrics*, 108, 129–133.

Numis, A. L., Yellen, M. B., Chu-Shore, C. J., Pfeifer, H. H., & Thiele, E. A. (2011). The relationship of ketosis and growth to the efficacy of the ketogenic diet in infantile spasms. *Epilepsy Research*, 96, 172–175.

O'Callaghan, F. J., Edwards, S. W., Alber, F. D., Cortina Borja, M., Hancock, E., Johnson, A. L.,

Kennedy, C. R., Likeman, M., Lux, A. L., Mackay, M. T., Mallick, A. A., Newton, R. W., Nolan, M., Pressler, R., Rating, D., Schmitt, B., Verity, C. M., & Osborne, J. P. (2018). Vigabatrin with hormonal treatment versus hormonal treatment alone (ICISS) for infantile spasms: 18-month outcomes of an open-label, randomised controlled trial. *Lancet Child & Adolescent Health, 2*, 715–725.

O'Callaghan, F. J., Lux, A. L., Darke, K., Edwards, S. W., Hancock, E., Johnson, A. L., Kennedy, C. R., Newton, R. W., Verity, C. M., Osborne, J. P. (2011). The effect of lead time to treatment and of age of onset on developmental outcome at 4 years in infantile spasms: Evidence from the United Kingdom Infantile Spasms Study. *Epilepsia, 52*, 1359–1364.

Papandreou, D., Pavlou, E., Kalimeri, E., & Mavromichalis, I. (2006). The ketogenic diet in children with epilepsy. *British Journal of Nutrition, 95*, 5–13.

Patel, A., Pyzik, P. L., Turner, Z., Rubenstein, J. E., & Kossoff, E. H. (2010). Long-term outcomes of children treated with the ketogenic diet in the past. *Epilepsia, 51*, 1277–1282.

Paul, E., Conant, K. D., Dunne, I. E., Pfeifer, H. H., Lyczkowski, D. A., Linshaw, M. A., & Thiele, E.A. (2010). Urolithiasis on the ketogenic diet with concurrent topiramate or zonisamide therapy. *Epilepsy Research, 90*, 151–156.

Peterson, S. J., Tangney, C. C., Pimentel-Zablah, E. M., Hjelmgren, B., Booth, G., & Berry-Kravis, E. (2005). Changes in growth and seizure reduction in children on the ketogenic diet as a treatment for intractable epilepsy. *Journal of the American Dietetic Association, 105*, 718–725.

Pires, M. E., Ilea, A., Bourel, E., Bellavoine, V., Merdariu, D., Berquin, P., & Auvin, S. (2013). Ketogenic diet for infantile spasms refractory to first-line treatments: An open prospective study. *Epilepsy Research, 105*, 189–194.

Prasad, C., Rupar, T., & Prasad, A. N. (2011). Pyruvate dehydrogenase deficiency and epilepsy. *Brain & Development, 33*, 856–865.

Prezioso, G., Carlone, G., Zaccara, G., & Verrotti, A. (2018). Efficacy of ketogenic diet for infantile spasms: A systematic review. *Acta Neurologica Scandinavica, 137*, 4–11.

Pulsifer, M. B., Gordon, J. M., Brandt, J., Vining, E. P., & Freeman, J. M. (2001). Effects of ketogenic diet on development and behavior: Preliminary report of a prospective study. *Developmental Medicine and Child Neurology, 43*, 301–306.

Raju, K. N., Gulati, S., Kabra, M., Agarwala, A., Sharma, S., Pandey, R. M., & Kalra, V. (2011). Efficacy of 4:1 (classic) versus 2.5:1 ketogenic ratio diets in refractory epilepsy in young children: A randomized open labeled study. *Epilepsy Research, 96*, 96–100.

Schwartz, R. M., Boyes, S., & Aynsley-Green, A. (1989). Metabolic effects of three ketogenic diets in the treatment of severe epilepsy. *Developmental Medicine and Child Neurology, 31*, 152–160.

Sivaraju, A., Nussbaum, I., Cardoza, C. S., & Mattson, R. H. (2015). Substantial and sustained seizure reduction with ketogenic diet in a patient with Ohtahara syndrome. *Epilepsy & Behavior Case Reports, 3*, 43–45.

Sofou, K., Dahlin, M., Hallbook, T., Lindefeldt, M., Viggedal, G., & Darin, N. (2017). Ketogenic diet in pyruvate dehydrogenase complex deficiency: Short- and long-term outcomes. *Journal of Inherited Metabolic Disease, 40*, 237–245.

Stewart, W. A., Gordon, K., & Camfield, P. (2001). Acute pancreatitis causing death in a child on the ketogenic diet. *Journal of Child Neurology, 16*, 682.

Su, D. J., Lu, J. F., Lin, L. J., Liang, J. S., & Hung, K. L. (2018). *SCN2A* mutation in an infant presenting with migrating focal seizures and infantile spasm responsive to a ketogenic diet. *Brain & Development, 40*, 724–727.

Takeoka, M., Riviello, J. J., Jr., Pfeifer, H., & Thiele, E. A. (2002). Concomitant treatment with topiramate and ketogenic diet in pediatric epilepsy. *Epilepsia, 43*, 1072–1075.

Turkdogan, D., Thomas, G., & Demirel, B. (2019). Ketogenic diet as a successful early treatment modality for *SCN2A* mutation. *Brain & Development, 41*, 389–391.

van der Louw, E., van den Hurk, D., Neal, E., Leiendecker, B., Fitzsimmon, G., Dority, L., Thompson, L., Marchio, M., Dudzinska, M., Dressler, A., Klepper, J., Auvin, S., & Cross, J. H. (2016). Ketogenic diet guidelines for infants with refractory epilepsy. *European Journal of Paediatric Neurology, 20*, 798–809.

Ville, D., Chiron, C., Laschet, J., & Dulac, O. (2015). The ketogenic diet can be used successfully in combination with corticosteroids for epileptic encephalopathies. *Epilepsy & Behavior, 48*, 61–65.

Vining, E. P., Pyzik, P., McGrogan, J., Hladky, H., Anand, A., Kriegler, S., & Freeman, J. M. (2002). Growth of children on the ketogenic diet. *Developmental Medicine and Child Neurology, 44*, 796–802.

Williams, S., Basualdo-Hammond, C., Curtis, R., & Schuller, R. (2002). Growth retardation in children with epilepsy on the ketogenic diet: A retrospective chart review. *Journal of the American Dietetic Association, 102*, 405–407.

Willmott, N. S., & Bryan, R.A. (2008). Case report: Scurvy in an epileptic child on a ketogenic diet with oral complications. *European Archives of Paediatric Dentistry, 9*, 148–152.

Wilmshurst, J. M., Gaillard, W. D., Vinayan, K. P., Tsuchida, T. N., Plouin, P., Van Bogaert, P., Carrizosa, J., Elia, M., Craiu, D., Jovic, N. J., Hirtz, D., Wong, V., Glauser, T., Mizrahi, E. M., & Cross, J. H. (2015). Summary of recommendations for the management of infantile seizures: Task Force Report for the ILAE Commission of Pediatrics. *Epilepsia, 56*, 1185–1197.

Wirrell, E., Eckert, S., Wong-Kisiel, L., Payne, E., & Nickels, K. (2018). Ketogenic diet therapy in infants: Efficacy and tolerability. *Pediatric Neurology, 82*, 13–18.

11

Ketogenic Diet in Status Epilepticus

RIMA NABBOUT, MD, PHD

INTRODUCTION

Status epilepticus (SE) is defined by continuous seizures with alteration of consciousness. The incidence of SE is 3 to 41 per 100,000 individuals per year (Chin et al., 2006; Dham et al., 2014; Raspall-Chaure et al., 2007), and SE is the second most common neurologic emergency in adults and the first most common in children. The duration of SE was long debated, and an operational definition proposed for tonic-clonic SE defines T1 as the time that emergency treatment should be started and T2 as the time at which long-term consequences in the brain might be expected (Trinka et al., 2015). For instance, T1 is ≥ 5 min and T2 is over 30 min (Trinka et al., 2015). Of patients with SE, 12% to 43% fail to respond to first- and second-line therapy, and they are then classified as having refractory SE (RSE) after 2 hr from the onset of SE. Super-refractory SE (SRSE) is defined by the persistence of SE over 24 hr (Ferlisi & Shorvon, 2012). Overall, ~ 15% of SE cases admitted to the hospital become SRSE (DeLorenzo et al., 1995; Ferlisi & Shorvon, 2012; Krumholz, 1999).

In adults, SRSE has a high mortality rate of > 60% (Ferlisi & Shorvon, 2012). Although the risk of death is low in the pediatric population, the risk of subsequent neurologic morbidity and cognitive problems is high (Scott, 2009). The therapeutic intervention aims to reduce SRSE duration, mortality, and short- and long-term comorbidities.

SE can be tonic-clonic, tonic, or myoclonic. It can be associated with acute or chronic brain disease or can occur in patients with known epilepsy. It may occur at the onset or in the course of the disease (Trinka et al., 2015). SE can occur during the course of epilepsy syndromes; tonic-clonic or clonic SE in Dravet syndrome, and tonic SE in Lennox-Gastaut syndrome. In epilepsy with myoclonic atonic seizures (Doose syndrome), myoclonic SE might occur at onset or during the first months. Myoclonic nonconvulsive SE is frequent

in some genetic syndromes, such as Angelman syndrome, and in mitochondrial diseases (Trinka et al., 2015).

Identifying a possible underlying cause and addressing it are important steps in the treatment of SE. An etiology-targeted therapy should be instituted as soon as the etiology is identified (antibiotics for CNS infections, antiviral agents for encephalitis, immune therapy for autoimmune encephalitis).

Benzodiazepines are the first-line therapy for SE, with different molecules used and different routes of administration (buccal, nasal, intrarectal, or intramuscular). If benzodiazepines fail to stop the SE, phenytoin (or fosphenytoin) is usually the second-line drug. The use of other anti-seizure medication (ASM) with IV formulations is the usual next step after the failure of phenytoin (Shorvon & Ferlisi, 2011). Barbiturate anesthesia is the most common third-line approach. Propofol and ketamine can be also used, but for limited times (Ferlisi et al., 2015). The failure rate of anesthetic barbiturates and the frequent recurrence after withdrawal, with associated high mortality and morbidity, make it essential to develop other therapies for medication-resistant SE.

The ketogenic diet (KD) has reported efficacy in SE (Kossoff & Nabbout, 2013). The multiple mechanisms of action of KD, lack of interactions with drugs, and both enteral and parenteral administration possibilities make it a good choice for RSE. The inherent combination of these mechanisms can mimic AED polytherapy, an approach that is suggested to be a good choice for RSE (Gama et al., 2015; Löscher, 2015; Lusardi et al., 2015).

KD IN CONVULSIVE SE

The first report of efficacy of KD in a series of patients with highly recurrent seizures was by Villeneuve et al. (2009). The authors reported KD response in a retrospective pediatric series of patients with focal pharmacoresistant epilepsies. The efficacy of KD was higher in patients who presented with SE or recent worsening of seizure frequency (Villeneuve et al., 2009). In this first series, efficacy was reported in different etiologies, such as Sturge-Weber syndrome, FIRES (febrile infection-related epilepsy syndrome), and cryptogenic focal SE (Villeneuve et al., 2009). A second paper in 2010 reported an international series of nine patients with SRSE due to FIRES, with seven of nine responders to KD (Nabbout et al., 2010). The KD was well tolerated via nasogastric tube in the pediatric ICU setting. Ketosis was achieved mostly within 24 hr, and SE stopped during the first days of the diet, as well as in all responders within the first week (Nabbout et al., 2010).

Other reports of SE due to FIRES or similar immune entities were further reported in the literature, for both pediatric (Nam et al., 2011; O'Connor et al., 2014; Sort et al., 2013; Vaccarezza et al., 2012) and adult patients (Cervenka et al., 2017; Thakhur et al., 2014). The pathophysiology of FIRES, based on activation of an inflammatory cascade (Nabbout et al., 2011), makes this syndrome a possible specific target for KD. Most patients reported had RSE due to inflammatory etiologies. This trend is confirmed by the largest pediatric series with FIRES (Nabbout et al., 2010) and in adult series (Thakur et al., 2014). In this last series of 10 patients, four patients presented with NORSE, two with anti-NMDA encephalitis, and one with LGI1 encephalitis.

However, other etiologies, involving the inflammation cascades or not, were reported as a possible indication for KD in SE, and the overrepresentation of these inflammatory etiologies might be due to their frequency in SRSE. Response in patients with Rasmussen syndrome, an encephalitis involving the activation of the T-cell pathway, was reported for a few pediatric (Villeneuve et al., 2009) and adult patients (Wusthoff et al., 2010).

Patients with SE in mitochondrial diseases, such as in Alpers disease with POLG1 mutations (Martikainen et al., 2012) and with stroke-like episodes, as in MELAS syndrome (Steriade et al., 2014), are good candidates for KD to be introduced early, at onset (Desguerre et al., 2014). Other small series of patients with focal SE due to structural lesions were also reported as responders to KD, in both pediatric (Caraballo et al., 2014; Lin et al., 2015; Villeneuve et al., 2009) and adult studies (Bodenant et al., 2008).

Since the first edition of this book, there have been several publications demonstrating success of the KD for SRSE. One of the largest in pediatrics was published in 2018 by the Pediatric Status Epilepticus Research Group (pSERG) and reported success with the KD in 71% of 14 children, mostly with SE of unknown etiologies (Arya et al., 2018). Many of the current studies continue to show excellent results with the KD for SRSE due to FIRES. Another large prospective study demonstrated dietary efficacy in 11 of 15 adults (79%), with resolution of SRSE (Cervenka et al., 2017). Additional prospective trials are underway.

KD IN NONCONVULSIVE SE

The efficacy of KD is not restricted to convulsive SE. The efficacy of KD was reported in myoclonic SE of mitochondrial diseases and POLG mutations (Desguerres et al., 2014; Martikainen et al., 2012) and of myoclonic astatic epilepsy, or Doose syndrome (Caraballo et al., 2013; Kelley & Kossoff, 2010), and in patients with myoclonic SE from unknown etiologies (Caraballo et al., 2015). KD efficacy was also reported in patients with electrical SE of sleep (ESES; Kelley & Kossoff, 2016; Reyes et al., 2015; Veggiotti et al., 2012).

CHALLENGES OF KD USE IN SE

The challenges of the KD could raise some concerns that limit its widespread use for SE in ICUs. Implementation of the diet could be a complex issue in ICUs, especially in centers lacking KD teams. The availability of a KD team and daily communication among the neurologists, child neurologists, dietitians, and ICU teams are strongly recommended, enabling initiation of the diet under optimal conditions. The daily communication makes it possible to respect the follow-up of the KD, thus avoiding any additional glucose load from fluids and concomitant medications. Enteral feeding should be privileged, since parenteral feeding cannot achieve a high-ratio KD. Enteral feeding is usually well tolerated in our experience, especially when initiated with continuous infusion and slowly increasing the feeding rate to achieve the total caloric intake within 48 to 72 hr. The major steps for successful implementation in the ICU are summarized in Figure 11.1.

Another factor limiting the use of the diet might be the time lag for efficacy. In the reported series, ketosis appears within 24 to 72 hr and seizure reduction within the first week. This time lag is difficult to accept in a severe condition like SE, especially when AEDs are available to try. Although many studies confirmed the main role

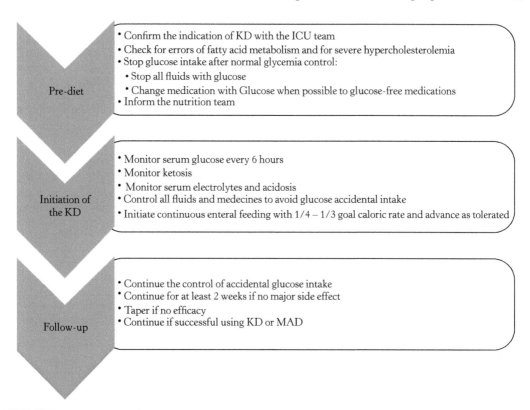

FIGURE 11.1 *Steps to Implement the KD in an ICU*

From S. A. Masino (Ed.). (2017). *Ketogenic Diet and Metabolic Therapies: Expanded Roles in Health and Disease* (1st ed.).

of underlying etiology in the cognitive outcome of SE, the long duration of SE might also negatively impact the long-term outcome (Kilbride et al., 2013). However, after the first- and second-line therapies for SE, treatment alternatives are scarce and the use of an anesthetic agent is usually the main strategy remaining (Ferlisi & Shorvon, 2012). Anesthetic agents are potent seizure suppressors and might help to shorten the SE, but their use is based on expert opinion and not on evidence-based medicine. In addition, some concerns have been raised about possible worsening of the outcome of RSE after the use of anesthetic agents (Ferlisi et al., 2015; Sutter & Kaplan, 2015; Sutter et al., 2014). Limiting use of dextrose-containing IV fluids early during SE after blood glucose has been controlled and initiating the diet as soon as inborn errors of fat metabolism are ruled out may help to shorten the delay of ketosis and improve the efficacy of KD. Along these lines, some medications used in the setting of SE and RSE, such as steroids, can delay ketosis. They should be avoided when they are medically unnecessary (Nabbout et al., 2010). Additionally,

there has been recent use of ketogenic total parenteral nutrition (TPN), usually on a short-term basis (van der Louw et al., 2020). In the 2020 guideline, recommendations are available for how best to implement the KD in this manner. It is also important to have a plan ready for success: if KD stops SRSE and the patient needs to stay on it (for months to years), is there a KD center willing and able to continue to manage the KD, or does the patient need to be transferred elsewhere?

The reports of KD in SE are mainly retrospective, with small numbers of individuals treated and rarely referring to patients where the diet failed. In addition, co-medication and changing doses of co-medication within the possible time to achieve efficacy of the diet might make causal attribution debatable. Finally, the reports lack the long-term follow-up that evaluates cognitive and neurologic outcomes, which are, apart from mortality, the major endpoints of any treatment of RSE. Indeed, KD reports share the same weakness of all third-line therapies in RSE, where no drug or therapy has achieved a high level of evidence-based medicine (Ferlisi & Shorvon, 2012).

The KD is well tolerated in the ICU setting, with low rates of side effects in the short and long term, as detailed in different reports. The increasing number of reports worldwide demonstrate the KD's possible implementation in ICUs. Its efficacy in inflammatory SE or in SE from other etiologies, convulsive and nonconvulsive, should make it a therapeutic option in the treatment of RSE. Furthermore, a few data on possible improvement of cognitive outcome have been gathered from patients with FIRES (Kramer et al., 2011; Singh et al., 2014).

A prospective, randomized controlled trial is necessary to validate the KD treatment option, as is true for all third-line therapies for RSE. This is important for physicians—at least one patient has died after the KD was stopped after seizure arrest because "this indication was not considered . . . good clinical practice" (Nabbout et al., 2010). The trial should evaluate the KD's efficacy and tolerance, which would be mandatory for the acceptance of KD by physicians and by health authorities and institutions. Outcomes should be evaluated in the short term—aiming for control of SE—and in the long term (at a few months or longer) to evaluate seizure control as well as cognitive outcomes. Pending the results of such a trial, KD should be available in ICUs and be part of the treatment arsenal for RSE, a critical situation where evidence-based medicine is dramatically lacking to date.

REFERENCES

Arya, R., Peariso, K., Gainza-Lein, M., Harvey, J., Bergin, A., Brenton, J. N., Burrows, B. T., Glauser, T., Goodkin, H. P., Lai, Y. C., Mikati, M. A., Fernández, I. S., Tchapyjnikov, D., Wilfong, A. A., Williams, K., Loddenkemper, T., Pediatric Status Epilepticus Research Group (pSERG), et al. (2018). Efficacy and safety of ketogenic diet for treatment of pediatric convulsive refractory status epilepticus. *Epilepsy Research*, 144, 1–6.

Bodenant, M., Moreau, C., Sejourné, C., Auvin, S., Delval, A., Cuisset, J. M, Derambure, P., Destée, A., & Defebvre, L. (2008). Interest of the ketogenic diet in a refractory status epilepticus in adults. *Revue Neurologique (Paris)*, 164(2), 194–199.

Caraballo, R. H., Chamorro, N., Darra, F., Fortini, S., & Arroyo H. (2013). Epilepsy with myoclonic atonic seizures: An electroclinical study of 69 patients. *Pediatric Neurology*, 48(5), 355–362.

Caraballo, R. H., Flesler, S., Armeno, M., Fortini, S., Agustinho, A., Mestre, G., Cresta, A., Buompadre, M. C., & Escobal, N. (2014). Ketogenic diet in pediatric patients with refractory focal status epilepticus. *Epilepsy Research*, 108(10), 1912–1916.

Caraballo, R. H., Valenzuela, G. R., Armeno, M., Fortini, S., Mestre, G., & Cresta A. (2015). The ketogenic diet in two paediatric patients with refractory myoclonic status epilepticus. *Epileptic Disorders*, 17(4), 491–495.

Cervenka, M. C., Hocker, S., Koenig, M., Bar, B., Henry-Barron, B., Kossoff, E. H., Hartman, A. L., Probasco, J. C., Benavides, D. R., Venkatesan, A., Hagen, E. C., Dittrich, D., Stern, T., Radzik, B., Depew, M., Caserta, F. M., Nyquist, P., Kaplan, P. W., & Geocadin, R. G. (2017). Phase I/II multicenter ketogenic diet study for adult super-refractory status epilepticus. *Neurology*, 88(10), 938–943.

Chin, R. F., Neville, B. G., Peckham, C., Bedford, H., Wade, A., & Scott, R.C; NLSTEPSS Collaborative Group. (2006). Incidence, cause, and short-term outcome of convulsive status epilepticus in childhood: Prospective population-based study. *Lancet*, 368(9531), 222–229.

DeLorenzo, R. J., Pellock, J. M., Towne, A. R., & Boggs, J. G. (1995). Epidemiology of status epilepticus. *Journal of Clinical Neurophysiology*, 12(4), 316–325.

Desguerre, I., Hully, M., Rio, M., & Nabbout, R. (2014). Mitochondrial disorders and epilepsy. *Revue Neurologique (Paris)*, 170(5), 375–380.

Dham, B. S., Hunter, K., & Rincon, F. (2014). The epidemiology of status epilepticus in the United States. *Neurocritical Care*, 20(3), 476–483.

Ferlisi, M., & Shorvon, S. (2012). The outcome of therapies in refractory and super-refractory convulsive status epilepticus and recommendations for therapy. *Brain*, 135(Part 8), 2314–2328.

Ferlisi, M., Hocker, S., Grade, M., Trinka, E., & Shorvon, S.; International Steering Committee of the StEp Audit. (2015). Preliminary results of the global audit of treatment of refractory status epilepticus. *Epilepsy & Behavior*, 49, 318–324.

Gama, I. R., Trindade-Filho, E. M., Oliveira, S. L., Bueno, N. B., Melo, I. T., Cabral-Junior, C. R., Barros, E. M., Galvão, J. A., Pereira, W. S., Ferreira, R. C., Domingos, B. R., de Rocha Ataide, T. (2015). Effects of ketogenic diets on the occurrence of pilocarpine-induced status epilepticus of rats. *Metabolic Brain Disease*, 30(1), 93–98.

Kelley, S. A., & Kossoff, E. H. (2010). Doose syndrome (myoclonic-astatic epilepsy): 40 years of progress. *Developmental Medicine & Child Neurology*, 52(11), 988–993.

Kelley, S. A., & Kossoff, E. H. (2016). How effective is the ketogenic diet for electrical status epilepticus of sleep? *Epilepsy Research*, 127, 339–343.

Kilbride, R. D., Reynolds, A. S., Szaflarski, J. P., & Hirsch, L. J. (2013). Clinical outcomes following prolonged refractory status epilepticus (PRSE). *Neurocritical Care, 18*(3), 374–385.

Kossoff, E. H., & Nabbout, R. (2014). Use of dietary therapy for status epilepticus. *Journal of Child Neurology, 28*(8), 1049–1051.

Kramer, U., Chi, C. S., Lin, K. L., Specchio, N., Sahin, M., Olson, H., Nabbout, R., Kluger, G., Lin, J. J., & van Baalen, A. (2011). Febrile infection-related epilepsy syndrome (FIRES): Pathogenesis, treatment, and outcome; A multicenter study on 77 children. *Epilepsia, 52*(11), 1956–1965.

Krumholz, A. (1999). Epidemiology and evidence for morbidity of nonconvulsive status epilepticus. *Journal of Clinical Neurophysiology, 16*(4), 314–322; discussion 353.

Lin, J. J., Lin, K. L., Chan, O. W., Hsia, S. H., & Wang, H. S.; CHEESE Study Group. (2015). Intravenous ketogenic diet therapy for treatment of the acute stage of super-refractory status epilepticus in a pediatric patient. *Pediatric Neurology, 52*(4), 442–445.

Löscher, W. (2015). Single versus combinatorial therapies in status epilepticus: Novel data from preclinical models. *Epilepsy & Behavior, 49*, 20–25.

Lusardi, T. A., Akula, K. K., Coffman, S. Q., Ruskin, D. N., Masino, S. A., & Boison, D. (2015). Ketogenic diet prevents epileptogenesis and disease progression in adult mice and rats. *Neuropharmacology, 99*, 500–509.

Martikainen, M. H., Päivärinta, M., Jääskeläinen, S., & Majamaa, K. (2012). Successful treatment of POLG-related mitochondrial epilepsy with antiepileptic drugs and low glycaemic index diet. *Epileptic Disorders, 14*(4), 438–441.

Nabbout, R., Mazzuca, M., Hubert, P., Peudennier, S., Allaire, C., Flurin, V., Aberastury, M., Silva, W., & Dulac, O. (2010). Efficacy of ketogenic diet in severe refractory status epilepticus initiating fever induced refractory epileptic encephalopathy in school age children (FIRES). *Epilepsia, 51*(10), 2033–2037.

Nabbout, R., Vezzani, A., Dulac, O., & Chiron, C. (2011). Acute encephalopathy with inflammation-mediated status epilepticus. *Lancet Neurology, 10*(1), 99–108.

Nam, S. H., Lee, B. L., Lee, C. G., Yu, H. J., Joo, E. Y., Lee, J., & Lee, M. (2011). The role of ketogenic diet in the treatment of refractory status epilepticus. *Epilepsia, 52*(11), e181–184.

O'Connor, S. E., Ream, M. A., Richardson, C., Mikati, M. A., Trescher, W. H., Byler, D. L., Sather, J. D., Michael, E. H., Urbanik, K. B., Richards, J. L., Davis, R., Zupanc, M. L., Zupec-Kania, B. (2014). The ketogenic diet for the treatment of pediatric status epilepticus. *Pediatric Neurology, 50*(1), 101–103.

Raspall-Chaure, M., Chin, R. F., Neville, B. G., Bedford, H., & Scott, R. C. (2007). The epidemiology of convulsive status epilepticus in children: A critical review. *Epilepsia, 48*(9), 1652–1663.

Reyes, G., Flesler, S., Armeno, M., Fortini, S., Ariela, A., Cresta, A., Mestre, G., & Caraballo, R. H. (2015). Ketogenic diet in patients with epileptic encephalopathy with electrical status epilepticus during slow sleep. *Epilepsy Research, 113*, 126–131.

Scott, R. C. (2009). Status epilepticus in the developing brain: Long-term effects seen in humans. *Epilepsia, 50*(Suppl. 12), 32e3.

Shorvon, S., & Ferlisi, M. (2011). The treatment of super-refractory status epilepticus: A critical review of available therapies and a clinical treatment protocol. *Brain, 134*(Part 10), 2802–2818.

Singh, R. K., Joshi, S. M., Potter, D. M., Leber, S. M., Carlson, M. D., & Shellhaas, R. A. (2014). Cognitive outcomes in febrile infection-related epilepsy syndrome treated with the ketogenic diet. *Pediatrics, 134*(5), e1431–1435.

Sort, R., Born, A. P., Pedersen, K. N., Fonsmark, L., & Uldall, P. (2013). Ketogenic diet in 3 cases of childhood refractory status epilepticus. *European Journal of Paediatric Neurology, 17*(6), 531–536.

Steriade, C., Andrade, D. M., Faghfoury, H., Tarnopolsky, M. A., & Tai, P. (2014). Mitochondrial encephalopathy with lactic acidosis and stroke-like episodes (MELAS) may respond to adjunctive ketogenic diet. *Pediatric Neurology, 50*(5), 498–502.

Sutter, R., & Kaplan, P. W. (2015). Can anesthetic treatment worsen outcome in status epilepticus? *Epilepsy & Behavior, 49*, 294–297.

Sutter, R., Marsch, S., Fuhr, P., Kaplan, P. W., & Rüegg, S. (2014). Anesthetic drugs in status epilepticus: Risk or rescue? A 6-year cohort study. *Neurology, 82*(8), 656–664.

Thakur, K. T., Probasco, J. C., Hocker, S. E., Roehl, K., Henry, B., Kossoff, E. H., Kaplan, P. W., Geocadin, R. G., Hartman, A. L., Venkatesan, A., Cervenka, M. C. (2014). Ketogenic diet for adults in super-refractory status epilepticus. *Neurology, 82*(8), 665–670.

Trinka, E., Cock, H., Hesdorffer, D., Rossetti, A. O., Scheffer, I. E., Shinnar, S., Shorvon, S., & Lowenstein, D. H. (2015). A definition and classification of status epilepticus: Report of the ILAE Task Force on Classification of Status Epilepticus. *Epilepsia, 56*, 1515–1523.

Vaccarezza, M., Silva, W., Maxit, C., & Agosta, G. (2012). Super-refractory status epilepticus: Treatment with ketogenic diet in pediatrics. *Revue Neurologique, 55*(1), 20–25.

van der Louw, E., Aldaz, V., Harvey, J., Roan, M., van den Hurk, D., Cross, J. H., & Auvin, S. (2020).

Optimal clinical management of children receiving ketogenic parenteral nutrition: A clinical practice guide. *Developmental Medicine & Child Neurology, 62*(1), 48–56.

Veggiotti, P., Pera, M. C., Teutonico, F., Brazzo, D., Balottin, U., & Tassinari, C. A. (2012). Therapy of encephalopathy with status epilepticus during sleep (ESES/CSWS syndrome): An update. *Epileptic Disorders, 14*(1), 1–11.

Villeneuve, N., Pinton, F., Bahi-Buisson, N., Dulac, O., Chiron, C., & Nabbout, R. (2009). The ketogenic diet improves recently worsened focal epilepsy. *Developmental Medicine & Child Neurology, 51*(4), 276–281.

Wusthoff, C. J., Kranick, S. M., Morley, J. F., & Christina Bergqvist, A. G. C. (2010). The ketogenic diet in treatment of two adults with prolonged nonconvulsive status epilepticus. *Epilepsia, 51*(6), 1083–1085.

Preventing Side Effects and Diet Discontinuation

CHERIE L. HERREN, MD AND RANA R. SAID, MD

INTRODUCTION

In general, the ketogenic diet (KD) is well tolerated. On average, 60% of patients remain on the diet for over 6 months. Those who stop the diet typically do so due to its lack of efficacy rather than its intolerability (Keene et al., 2006). Adverse effects of KD therapy can be divided into common and serious side effects. They can also be categorized according to their timing during KD therapy (during initiation, during maintenance, or during discontinuation). Common side effects include constipation, vomiting, acidosis, and vitamin/mineral deficiencies. More significant side effects are rare, but include pancreatitis, hepatitis, kidney stones, and cardiomyopathy. During initiation, transient side effects can include dehydration, hypoglycemia, acidosis, vomiting, and refusal to eat. Children need to be monitored closely during initiation so that adverse effects can be avoided and treated. Fasting and fluid restriction may aggravate side effects and are not uniformly implemented in KD programs. Fluid restriction contributes to dehydration and metabolic acidosis, which subsequently can cause vomiting and lethargy. With appropriate monitoring and supplementation, adverse effects can be minimized, so that the patient can remain on the diet as long as indicated. In addition, there may be social issues, including refusal to eat and problems managing special occasions and holidays. With support and resources, most families can overcome these obstacles. When patients come off dietary therapy, discontinuation must be done gradually and with close supervision, because there may be an increase in seizures. Patients must be provided support and direction on how to safely discontinue the diet.

SCREENING

One of the most important steps in avoiding potential side effects (especially those that are potentially severe or life-threatening) is proper screening of patients. Patients with disorders of fat metabolism could present with severe and potentially fatal complications if started on the KD, because the diet will require a shift from carbohydrate metabolism to fat metabolism for energy. All patients should have a thorough metabolic assessment prior to initiation of dietary therapy. The screening should include electrolytes, blood counts, lipids, acylcarnitine panel, serum amino acids, urine organic acids, liver and kidney function tests, urinalysis, and urine calcium and creatinine assays (Kossoff et al., 2009). Patients with disorders of fat metabolism with impaired fatty acid transport and oxidation should not be started on the KD. There are other specific diagnoses for which the KD should not be used, and they are listed in Table 12.1.

TABLE 12.1 CONTRAINDICATIONS TO THE USE THE KETOGENIC DIET (KOSSOFF ET AL, 2008)

Absolute
Carnitine deficiency (primary)
Carnitine palmitoyltransferase (CPT) I or II deficiency
Carnitine translocase deficiency
β-oxidation defects
   Medium-chain acyl dehydrogenase deficiency
    (MCAD)
   Long-chain acyl dehydrogenase deficiency (LCAD)
   Short-chain acyl dehydrogenase deficiency (SCAD)
   Long-chain 3-hydroxyacyl-CoA deficiency
   Medium-chain 3-hydroxyacyl-CoA deficiency.
Pyruvate carboxylase deficiency
Porphyria
Relative
Inability to maintain adequate nutrition
Surgical focus identified by neuroimaging and video
   EEG monitoring
Parent or caregiver noncompliance

SOCIAL ASPECTS

To avoid complications, it is imperative to screen patients both medically and socially. Patients and families, including all caregivers, should be adequately educated about what to expect while on the diet and the follow-up that will be needed (typically every 3 to 6 months). For those unwilling or unable to comply with the needed follow-up, careful consideration should be given to whether the diet is an appropriate treatment option. Once patients are started on the diet, good social support can be beneficial to families to maintain adherence and can increase the likelihood that they continue the diet. This support often comes from medical staff, including neurologists, dietitians, and nursing personnel, who are well educated about the diet and the demands it places on families. Engagement and education of teachers and schools are vital to the success of KD therapy in school-age children. Reassurance and encouragement can also come from support groups designed specifically for families and from KD-specific functions, such as Halloween parties. Special occasions tend to be especially difficult, but families may take comfort in knowing there are numerous recipes available for everything from ice cream to birthday cake! Some centers also utilize parent coaches, who can help families navigate issues like food refusal and menu ideas in real life. Online resources are also available, including The Charlie Foundation, Matthew's Friends, and the Epilepsy Foundation. However, parents should be cautioned about unreliable online information forums, because "ketogenic diet" has become popularized as a nonmedical fad diet.

SIDE EFFECTS

Vomiting

Vomiting is a common side effect seen in patients on the KD and is estimated to occur in 5% of patients (Keene et al., 2006). Vomiting most commonly occurs during the initiation phase of the diet. Metabolic acidosis may contribute to vomiting, and in turn, vomiting may worsen acidosis, creating a worsening cycle of symptoms. In many cases, reversing metabolic acidosis will alleviate nausea and vomiting. In patients who are experiencing vomiting, maintaining proper hydration, either enterally or intravenously, is an important factor in breaking the cycle. Initiation is a common time for patients to experience vomiting related to the diet itself; however, vomiting can occur for other reasons (infections, etc.) at any time while on the diet. Families and providers should be watchful for vomiting and have a low threshold for providing intervention. In those patients who cannot adequately maintain oral hydration due to vomiting or in those who have increasing lethargy, intravenous (IV) fluids may be required. Monitoring for constipation is also important, because children with constipation may be predisposed to vomit.

Families often are concerned about whether to re-dose antiseizure medications (ASMs) with emesis; we advise parents to repeat the dose if vomiting occurred less than 30 min from dose administration. Management of constipation with polyethylene glycol (Miralax®) is well tolerated. Some children require slower delivery of feeds, either with more frequent, smaller meals or, if they are gastrostomy tube fed, with slower rates of infusion with a feeding pump. For short-term vomiting around times of illness, use of Gatorade Zero®, Powerade Zero®, or Propel Zero® can provide hydration and electrolytes, without carbohydrates. In instances of more prolonged feeding intolerance, half-strength Pedialyte® to provide a source of calories is usually well tolerated, without significant reduction in ketosis.

Acidosis

Metabolic acidosis can be found in patients on the KD and can be associated with lethargy and vomiting. Acidosis will typically present during initiation and can be minimized with the use of buffering agents, such as sodium bicarbonate or Polycitra K®(Cypress Pharmaceuticals, Madison, Mississippi). Practitioners should be aware of medications that could worsen acidosis, especially common ASMs, such as topiramate and zonisamide. In some cases, it may be necessary to decrease these medications in order to manage acidosis. During initiation, acidosis should be treated with aggressive hydration and use of oral alkalinizing agents. Rarely would IV alkalinization be indicated. Once the patient is on a stable diet ratio, with adequate doses of alkalinizing agents, acidosis becomes less problematic. However, during times of illness, with decreased oral intake and/or with vomiting, acidosis can again become problematic and typically can be managed with hydration.

Constipation

Given the composition of the KD, an increase in constipation is not unexpected. Constipation is common and occurs in up to 65% of patients (Wibisono et al., 2015). It can be particularly problematic in those who had pre-existing constipation, and for those who have impaired mobility. Increased hydration may help with symptoms, but many patients will require medications to manage their constipation. Polyethylene glycol (Miralax®) is a common choice for treatment because it is not significantly absorbed in the gut and is safe for patients on the KD. Glycerin suppositories, increased dietary fiber, medium-chain triglyceride (MCT) oil, or mineral oil could also be considered.

Hypoglycemia

Like many other potential side effects, hypoglycemia tends to occur during the initiation phase of the diet. If patients have severe hypoglycemia (< 30 mg/dl) or symptomatic hypoglycemia (< 40 mg/dl with lethargy, vomiting, diaphoresis, seizures, or shakiness), small amounts of juice (10–20 ml) or dextrose (D5W infusion until blood glucose is > 60 mg/dl) can be given to correct the blood sugar. If hypoglycemia is a persistent problem, a reduction in ratio should be considered. Once the patient is stable on the diet, blood glucose tends to be on the low end of normal (50–70 mg/dl) but is overall very stable. Fasting prior to initiation of KD therapy may increase the chances of hypoglycemia (Bergqvist et al., 2005); therefore, close glucose monitoring is recommended in these patients.

Kidney Stones

Renal calculi have been reported in 3% to 7% of children on the KD (Kielb et al., 2000). The stones typically form, on average, after 18 months of KD therapy. However, there have been reports of development of urolithiasis after just 1 month on the diet. The majority of calculi are uric acid stones; however, calcium oxalate, calcium phosphate, and mixed calcium/uric acid stones are seen.

Approximately 50% of stones are uric acid stones (Kielb et al., 2000), probably because the KD lowers urinary pH, which facilitates formation of uric acid crystals since the solubility of uric acid decreases as pH drops. The KD also has been associated with uric acidemia and increased urinary uric acid, which further predispose the patient to the development of uric acid stones. This risk can be compounded by fluid restriction, which produces a more acidic urine and decreased urine flow, with precipitation of urate crystals.

The KD has also been associated with hypercalciuria, which can result in calcium crystal formation. Hypocitraturia also occurs due to chronic metabolic acidosis. Urinary citrate is an inhibitor of calcium crystal formation; therefore, low urinary levels increase the risk of calcium stone formation. Again, fluid restriction increases the risk.

Children typically present with gross or microscopic hematuria; therefore, they require regular screening urinalysis. They may also, less commonly, have gritty urine or pain. There may be a role for periodically checking serum uric acid and urinary calcium:creatinine ratios. Renal ultrasound is necessary if there is evidence of hematuria. Children with family histories of kidney stones who are receiving carbonic anhydrase inhibitors (topiramate, zonisamide, or acetazolamide) are also at higher risk for stones (Furth et al., 2000). Treatment includes fluid liberalization and urinary alkalinization with bicarbonate. In children with a higher risk for kidney stone formation, prophylactic treatment with Polycitra K® has been shown to reduce the incidence of kidney stones in this susceptible population (McNally et al., 2009).

Increased Infections

Several studies have reported increased infections rates in up to 2% to 4% of children on the KD (Summ et al., 1996; Vining et al., 1998; Woody et al., 1989). Woody et al. assessed neutrophil function in nine children on the KD, demonstrating that while these patients were ketotic, they had significantly less bacterial phagocytosis and killing. The effects were reversible, with resolution when the diet was discontinued (Woody et al., 1989). Other conditions associated with ketosis, such as diabetes mellitus, alcoholism, glycogen storage disease, protein-calorie malnutrition, certain carbohydrate-restricted diets, and intralipid infusions, have also been reported to cause impairments in neutrophil function. The exact mechanism is not well understood, but it is likely related to serum metabolites that affect early processes in phagocytosis (Woody et al., 1989). Interestingly, only one of the Woody group's patients experienced serious bacterial infections.

Vitamin Deficiencies

Due to the restrictive nature of the KD (with limited vegetables and grains), the diet is known to be deficient in several vitamins and minerals, especially B vitamins, calcium, and vitamin D. The International Ketogenic Study Group

(Kossoff et al., 2009) made it a universal recommendation that all patients on the KD should be on a multivitamin with minerals and receive calcium with vitamin D supplements. In the study, some suggested that additional supplementation may be needed for zinc, magnesium, selenium, and phosphorus, but this was not a universal recommendation, and supplementation may be considered on an as-needed basis depending on laboratory values. Care should be taken to select a carbohydrate-free or low-carbohydrate multivitamin, such as NanoVM® (Solace Nutrition, Rockville, Maryland), FruitiVits® (Vitaflo, Alexandria, Virginia), Centrum® (Wyeth, Madison, New Jersey), or Bugs Bunny Sugar Free® (Bayer, Morristown, New Jersey). Vitamin levels should be monitored on a routine basis during follow-up, and early supplementation is optimal to avoid deficiencies.

Electrolyte Imbalances

Electrolytes like calcium, magnesium, sodium, potassium, and phosphorus are often depleted or deficient in a child on KD therapy. Laboratory values must be monitored closely, and electrolytes must be adequately supplemented. In children on KD formulas, many electrolytes may be included in the formula. However, children on solid diets will often need additional supplements, which can be in the form of dietary supplements (such as Morton's Lite Salt®) or by prescription (K-Phos Neutral®).

Hyperlipidemia

Studies show that between 30% and 60% of patients on the KD develop hypercholesterolemia (Nizamuddin et al., 2008; Wibisono et al., 2015). Nizamuddin and colleagues found the cholesterol level increased 25% from pre-initiation (baseline) level. Notably, patients eating a solid diet had a greater risk for developing high cholesterol than patients who consumed a formula-based diet, likely secondary to an increase in saturated fats in solid foods compared to the liquid formulation. The dyslipidemia improved spontaneously and without intervention in about half of patients, a finding suggesting that patients are better able to metabolize the fat over time (Nizamuddin et al., 2008). It is unclear if the dyslipidemia seen with the diet has any long-term cardiovascular or atherosclerotic effects, but, given the temporary use of the diet, such effects appear unlikely, and the benefit of the diet outweighs the potential risk. Currently, there are no universal recommendations for intervention for elevated cholesterol or triglyceride levels in children.

Pancreatitis

Hyperlipidemia and hypertriglyceridemia are risk factors for development of pancreatitis, which is also a potential complication of KD therapy. Concomitant therapy with valproic acid (VPA) may increase this risk. There has been a case report of a 9-year-old who died from acute hemorrhagic pancreatitis while on KD therapy. The development of pancreatitis while on the KD would necessitate coming off the diet (Stewart et al., 2001). Parenteral KD therapy with intralipids also places children at high risk for developing pancreatitis and should be used judiciously.

Hepatitis

While rare, hepatitis is a potentially significant side effect of the KD. It has been suggested that concomitant use of VPA may increase the risk of hepatitis; however, Kang et al. (2004) did not find a statistically significant increase in hepatitis among patients on VPA, compared to those not taking this medication. Decreased carnitine levels may also increase the risk for liver dysfunction, but the risk appears to be low (Berry-Kravis et al., 2001). Nonetheless, routine monitoring of serum carnitine and carnitine supplementation are recommended (Neal et al., 2009). Regular monitoring of liver enzymes is recommended, and in the event that elevations are noted, hepatic ultrasound and co-management with gastroenterology should be considered, including possible diet discontinuation.

Cardiac Side Effects

Cardiac complications have been reported in children on the KD, including cardiomyopathy and prolonged QT interval. These risks may be related to carnitine and selenium deficiencies associated with the KD. Bergqvist et al. (2003) reported a child with cardiomyopathy in association with selenium deficiency and other children who had lowering of selenium levels while on the KD. In a study of 20 children on the KD, 15% (3 children) had prolongation of the QTc interval. Of these three children, two had pre-initiation electrocardiograms (ECGs), which confirmed that the QTc abnormalities developed while they were on the diet. Two of the patients had left atrial and left ventricular enlargement and one had severe ventricular dilatation and dysfunction, with associated symptoms of heart failure. Interestingly, all the patients in this series had normal selenium levels. It was postulated that higher beta-hydroxy-butyrate levels and more significant metabolic acidosis may be associated with the development of cardiac complications.

There are also reports of two children who developed severe dilated cardiomyopathy while on the KD (Ballaban-Gil et al.,1999). In these cases, the cardiomyopathy resolved after discontinuation of the KD. It is suggested that baseline ECGs and echocardiograms be completed prior to initiation of the KD and while the patient is on the diet, along with monitoring of carnitine and selenium levels. Supplementation with carnitine and selenium should be strongly considered.

Growth Effects

There are conflicting reports of how the KD affects growth—both linear and weight—in children on the diet. Williams et al. (2002) retrospectively reviewed 21 children treated with the KD for 9.6 months to 2 years, specifically looking at linear growth velocity. Eighteen children (86%) had a drop from their original height percentiles while on the diet. This was independent of mean age, duration on the diet, protein intake, or calories consumed per kg body weight while on the diet. The investigators concluded that decreased linear growth may be secondary to poor nutritional status. While the children received the recommended intake of protein, calories were typically restricted to 75% of recommended daily intake. The authors postulated that dietary protein was needed to fill the calorie gap for energy and gluconeogenesis, resulting in relative protein insufficiency to support growth (Williams et al., 2002).

Vining et al. prospectively reviewed the growth of 237 children treated with the KD. They found that older children grew taller "almost normally," but younger children fell more than 2 standard deviations below the mean in height (Vining et al., 2002). However, Couch et al. (1999) retrospectively evaluated the nutritional status and growth of 21 children on the KD for 6 months. They found a statistically significant increase in both height and weight after 6 months on the diet. Six children had a decrease in mean percentile standard weight for height, but no child fell below their pre-KD height-for-age percentile after 6 months on the diet. However, the study was limited by the short duration of follow-up (Couch et al.,1999).

Children on the KD need to be monitored closely for adequate protein intake and growth

parameters. Often, children with intractable epilepsy become more physically active as seizures improve, and energy needs must be recalculated. Protein intake must be adequate, and regular laboratory studies to assess protein, albumin, and pre-albumin are necessary. Lack of weight gain is commonly seen; however, inadequate or slowed growth (which is more problematic in infants) and inappropriate weight loss occur less frequently.

Osteopenia

Baseline bone mineral content may be low in patients starting the KD, with only an estimated 54% to 63% of patients receiving adequate calcium and vitamin D through their pre-initiation diet (Bergqvist et al., 2008). The poor bone health seen may be secondary to ASM use, which can interfere with calcium and vitamin D metabolism and directly impacts the cells of bone formation and absorption. Despite adequate supplementation with calcium and vitamin D, and an overall reduction in ASMs, once patients were started on the KD, there was further decline in bone mineral content. Chronic acidosis may contribute to the decline in bone health, and buffering agents, such as sodium bicarbonate or sodium citrate/citric acid, may be beneficial in reducing the risk of osteopenia and fractures. Bone density scans may not be indicated for all patients but could be considered in those at higher risk (younger non-ambulatory patients) or for those who have experienced pathologic fractures.

Food Refusal

Tolerability of the KD is the single most important factor limiting individual acceptance for initiation; however, 60% of children who start the KD are still on it at 6-month follow-up (Table 12.2). The most common reason for discontinuation of the diet is not food refusal or concerns with palatability of the diet, but lack of efficacy.

Food refusal is typically related to a limited repertoire of foods. Families are encouraged to keep several menus on rotation to minimize food fatigue. Even changing the presentation of meals can help with tolerability; for example, one family used a child's tea service, with its smaller plates, to make meals more enjoyable. Close communication with the KD registered dietitian is vital, because dietitians have a wealth of suggestions for improved food intake. Parent KD coaches are also a tremendous resource. Food refusal may also represent a food intolerance; changing

TABLE 12.2 (KEENE, 2006) TIME PATIENT REMAINS
ON KETOGENIC DIET

Author	Total Sample	% Sample at 3 Months	% Sample at 6 Months	% Sample at 12 Months
DiMario [2]	48	?	50	37
Coppola [3]	56	75	38	7
Maydell [4]	147	80	66	48
Hassan [5]	52	68	39	13
Kankirawatana [6]	35	62	57	12
Kang [7]	199	88	61	27
Vining [9]	51	88	69	47
Freeman [10]	150	83	71	55
Ruthenstein [13]	13	85	77	50
Kossoff [11]	23	91	78	56

to a lactose-free formula may be helpful. If food refusal becomes a significant battle, reducing the KD ratio or changing to the MCT-based diet to increase amounts of carbohydrates may be necessary. At times, changing to another dietary therapy, such as the modified Atkins diet or low-glycemic-index therapy, is warranted.

SPECIAL POPULATIONS
Studies have demonstrated that overall the KD is well tolerated in infants. However, certain matters must be considered, including the increased risk for dehydration and hypoglycemia during initiation. Acidosis should be tracked closely during this period, and supplemental bicarbonate, fluid resuscitation, and glucose may be indicated. Accordingly, inpatient initiation is strongly recommended (Wirrell et al., 2018).

In the adult population on the KD, adverse effects were considered mild. The most common short-term adverse effects were gastrointestinal, including nausea, vomiting, bloating, diarrhea, and constipation. Long-term effects, including kidney stones and excessive weight loss, were more common; however, most adverse effects were preventable and treatable. Careful supervision by an experienced neurologist and dietitian may mitigate these adverse effects, thereby improving compliance and efficacy (Liu et al., 2018).

DISCONTINUING THE KD
There are many reasons why the KD is discontinued, the most common being lack of efficacy after 3 to 6 months or worsening of seizures. After 2 years of effective use of the KD, most neurologists consider its discontinuation. The typical approach is gradually lowering the ratio

of fat to protein and carbohydrate, then relaxing the weighing of ingredients, and finally adding new carbohydrate foods while keeping calories constant. This is followed by relaxation of calorie restriction, then gradual introduction of carbohydrate-containing foods. The ideal speed of weaning from the KD is not clear, specifically as it pertains to the risk of increased seizures. Worden et al. (2011) retrospectively reviewed 183 children who discontinued the KD. There was no significant difference in the incidence of seizure worsening among immediate (< 1 week), quick (1 to 6 weeks), or slow (> 6 weeks) rates. However, there was an increased risk of seizure worsening specifically in the patients with a 50% to 99% seizure reduction and those who were receiving more ASMs (Worden et al., 2011).

Approximately 80% of children will remain seizure-free when tapered off the KD if they have completely responded to diet therapy and are medication-free. Factors associated with a higher risk of recurrence include an epileptiform electroencephalogram (EEG), focal abnormalities on neuroimaging, and tuberous sclerosis complex. Approximately 50% of children with seizure recurrence have seizures that are difficult to control once again, even with resumption of the KD (Martinez et al., 2007).

CONCLUSION
While the KD is an effective therapy for refractory epilepsy and certain metabolic disorders, there are potential adverse effects. Providers must be aware of these risks and engage in proper monitoring of patients and counseling of families. Often, adverse effects can be minimized with appropriate monitoring by experienced neurologists and dietitians.

Like all medical therapies, the KD has potential risks that are weighed against its benefits.

REFERENCES

Ballaban-Gil, K. R. (1999). Cardiomyopathy associated with the ketogenic diet. *Epilepsia,* 40(Suppl. 7), 129.

Berry-Kravis, E., Booth, G., Sanchez, A. C., & Woodbury-Kolb, J. (2001). Carnitine levels and the ketogenic diet. *Epilepsia,* 42, 1445–1451.

Bergqvist, A. G. C., Schall, J. I., Gallagher, P. R., Cnaan, A., & Stallings, V. A. (2005). Fasting versus gradual initiation of the ketogenic diet: A prospective, randomized clinical trial of efficacy. *Epilepsia,* 46, 1810–1819.

Bergqvist, A. G. C., Chee, C. M., Lutchka, L., Rychik, J., & Stallings, V. A. (2003). Selenium deficiency associated with cardiomyopathy: A complication of the ketogenic diet. *Epilepsia,* 44, 618–620.

Bergqvist, A. G. C., Schall, J. I., Stallings, V. A., & Zemel, B. S. (2008). Progressive bone mineral loss in children with intractable epilepsy treated with the ketogenic diet. *American Journal of Clinical Nutrition,* 88, 1678–1684.

Couch, S. C., Schwarzman, F., Carroll, J., Koeniqsberger, D., Nordli, D. R., Deckelbaum, R. J., & DeFelice, A. R. (1999). Growth and nutritional outcomes of children treated with the ketogenic diet. *Journal of the American Dietetic Association,* 99, 1573–1575.

Furth, S. L., Casey, J. C., Pyzik, P. L., Neu, A. M., Docimo, S. G., Vining, E. P., Freeman, J. M., & Fivush, B. A. (2000). Risk factors for urolithiasis in children on the ketogenic diet. *Pediatric Nephrology,* 15, 125–128.

Kang, H. C., Chung, D. E., Kim, D. W., & Kim, H. D. (2004). Early and late-onset complications of the ketogenic diet for intractable epilepsy. *Epilepsia,* 45, 1116–1123.

Keene, D. L. (2006). A systematic review of the use of the ketogenic diet in childhood epilepsy. *Pediatric Neurology,* 35, 1–5.

Kielb, S., Koo, H. P., Bloom, D. A., & Faerber, G. J. (2000). Nephrolithiasis associated with the ketogenic diet. *Journal of Urology,* 164, 464–466.

Kossoff, E. H., Zupec-Kania, B. A., Amark, P. E., Ballaban-Gil, K. R., Christina Bergqvist, A. G., Blackford, R., Buchhalter, J. R., Caraballo, R. H., Helen Cross, J., Dahlin, M. G., Donner, E. J., Klepper, J., Jehle, R. S., Kim, H. D., Christiana Liu, Y. M., Nation, J., Nordli Jr, D. R., Pfeifer, H. H., Rho, J. M., . . . Vining, E. P. (2009). Optimal clinical management of children receiving the ketogenic diet: Recommendations of the International Ketogenic Diet Study Group. *Epilepsia,* 50, 304–317.

Liu, H., Yang, Y, Wang, Y., Tang, H., Zhang, Y., & Zhao, Y. (2018). Ketogenic diet for treatment of intractable epilepsy in adults: A meta-analysis of observational studies. *Epilepsia Open,* 3(1), 9–17.

Martinez, C. C., Pyzik, P. I., & Kossoff, E. H. (2007). Discontinuing the ketogenic diet in seizure-free children: Risk factors and recurrence. *Epilepsia,* 48, 187–190.

McNally, M. A. Pyzik, P. L., Rubenstein, J. E., Hamdy, R. F., & Kossoff, E. H. (2009). Empiric use of potassium citrate reduces kidney stone incidence with ketogenic diet. *Pediatrics,* 124, e300–e304.

Neal, E. G., Zupec-Kania, B., & Pfeifer, H. H. (2012). Carnitine, nutritional supplementation and discontinuation of ketogenic diet therapies. *Epilepsy Research,* 100, 267–271.

Nizamuddin, J., Turner, Z., Rubenstein, J. E., Pyzik, P. L., & Kossoff, E. H. (2008). Management and risk factors of dyslipidemia with ketogenic diet. *Journal of Child Neurology,* 23, 758–761.

Stewart, W. A., Gordon, K., & Camfield, P. (2001). Acute pancreatitis causing death in a child on the ketogenic diet. *Journal of Child Neurology,* 16, 682

Summ, M., Woch, M. A., & McNeil, T. (1996). Success and complications of the ketogenic diet for intractable childhood epilepsy. *Epilepsia,* 37(Suppl. 5), 109.

Vining, E. P., Freeman, J. M., Ballaban-Gil, K., Camfield, C. S., Holmes, G. L., Shinnar, R., Trevathan, E., & Wheless, J. W. (1998). A multicenter study of the efficacy of the ketogenic diet. *Archives of Neurology,* 55, 1433–1437.

Vining, E. P., Pyzik, P., McGrogan, J., Hladky, H., Anand, A., Kriegler, S., & Freeman, J. M. (2002). Growth of children on the ketogenic diet. *Developmental Medicine & Child Neurology,* 44, 796–802.

Wibisono, C., Rowe, N., Beavis, E., Kepreotes, H., Mackie, F. E., Lawson, J. A., & Cardamone, M. (2015). Ten-year single-center experience of the ketogenic diet: Factors influencing efficacy, tolerability, and compliance. *Journal of Pediatrics,* 166, 1030–1036.

Williams, S., Basualdo-Hammond, C., Curtis, R., & Schuller, R. (2002). Growth retardation in children with epilepsy on the ketogenic diet: A retrospective chart review. *Journal of the American Dietetic Association,* 102, 405–407.

Wirrell, E., Wong-Kisiel, L., Payne, E., Nickels, K., & Eckert, S. (2018). Ketogenic diet therapy in infants: Efficacy and tolerability. *Pediatric Neurology,* 82, 13–18.

Woody, R. C., Steele, R. W., Knapple, W. L., & Pilkington, N. S., Jr. (1989). Impaired neutrophil function in children with seizures treated with the ketogenic diet. *Journal of Pediatrics,* 115, 427–430.

Worden, L. T., Turner, Z., Pyzik, P. L., Rubenstein, J. E., & Kossoff, E. H. (2011). Is there an ideal way to discontinue the ketogenic diet? *Epilepsy Research,* 95, 232–236.

SECTION II

Ketogenic Diet

Emerging Clinical Applications and Future Potential

13

Overview

Expanded Uses of Ketogenic Therapies

JONG M. RHO, MD

The ketogenic diet (KD) is now a proven therapy for drug-resistant epilepsy (Neal et al., 2008; Vining et al., 1998), and while the mechanisms underlying its antiseizure efficacy remain unclear (Boison, 2017; Masino & Rho, 2012; Rogawski et al., 2016), there is growing experimental evidence for the neuroprotective properties of the KD's metabolism-based treatment (Baranano & Hartman, 2008; Gano et al., 2014; Maalouf et al., 2009). In this regard, while definitive clinical evidence for the KD's use outside of epilepsy (and even in non-neurologic conditions) is presently lacking, there has nevertheless been a virtual explosion in planned and ongoing human clinical trials (www.ClinicalTrials.gov; search using the term *ketogenic diet*) assessing whether ketogenic therapy can ameliorate symptoms and even the disease processes themselves (Stafstrom & Rho, 2012). Much of the experimental evidence has been converging on the notion that the broad efficacy of the KD is due in major part to normalization of aberrant energy metabolism (Boison, 2017; Masino & Rho, 2019). The concept that multiple brain-related disorders are pathophysiologically linked to energy dysregulation (Masino & Rho, 2019; Pathak et al., 2013) has been strengthened by numerous studies evaluating brain bioenergetics and provides a solid rationale for how dietary treatments that ameliorate underlying dysfunction can treat or even prevent disease symptomatology.

In this section, "Ketogenic Diet—Emerging Clinical Applications and Future Potential," leading investigators in the field of ketogenic therapies provide updated and newly crafted reviews summarizing the evidence that the ketogenic diet may prove useful in the treatment of neurologic, and even psychiatric, conditions. Seyfried, Scheck, and colleagues put forward a compelling case for cancer as being in part a metabolic (and perhaps more specifically, a mitochondrial) disorder, and that the KD should be strongly considered as adjunctive treatment for malignant brain tumors. These chapters are followed by a comprehensive review by Cheng and coauthors of metabolic treatments for autism spectrum disorder, whose prevalence has been rising rapidly throughout the world and which remains bereft of medical treatments that mitigate core behavioral deficits. Next, Cunnane and collaborators provide a unique translational perspective on brain metabolism—using novel positron emission tomography techniques to make the case that nutritional ketosis, achieved through several currently available strategies, can correct the underlying problem of declining brain fuels during aging. Tetzlaff and coauthors then review the evidence that the KD (and especially, ketone bodies) can prevent the metabolic, oxidative, and inflammatory cascades that ensue after spinal cord injury and traumatic brain injury. In the next chapter, Ruskin and colleagues review the mounting evidence that the KD possesses anti-inflammatory properties, relevant not only to the pathophysiology of pain syndromes and multiple sclerosis, but also to other neurologic disorders as well. New to the current second edition of the present volume, Palmer and coauthors review the scientific rationale for using the KD to treat schizophrenia. Finally, Shearer and colleagues review the growing literature on the effects of the KD on the gut microbiome—a topic that has received tremendous attention from the epilepsy community since 2018.

For all these apparently distinct neurologic (and even psychiatric) conditions, it should become clear to the reader that metabolic derangements are now considered key to the pathophysiology of the disorders, and that a dietary treatment like the KD can potentially benefit patients afflicted with perhaps all brain-related conditions. It is also the hope of all authors and editors that those curious about how altered metabolism can both induce and mitigate neurodegeneration and brain dysfunction will be compelled to pursue further laboratory and/or clinical research in this growing and fascinating area of translational neurosciences.

REFERENCES

Barañano, K. W., & Hartman, A. L. (2008). The ketogenic diet: Uses in epilepsy and other neurologic illnesses. *Current Treatment Options in Neurology, 10*(6), 410–419.

Boison, D. (2017). New insights into the mechanisms of the ketogenic diet. *Current Opinion in Neurology, 30*(2), 187–192.

Gano, L. B., Patel, M., & Rho, J. M. (2014). Ketogenic diets, mitochondria, and neurological diseases. *Journal of Lipid Research, 55*(11), 2211–2228.

Maalouf, M., Rho, J. M., & Mattson, M. P. (2009). The neuroprotective properties of calorie restriction, the ketogenic diet, and ketone bodies. *Brain Research Reviews, 59*(2), 293–315.

Masino, S. A., & Rho, J. M. (2012). Mechanisms of ketogenic diet action. In J. L. Noebels, M. Avoli, M. A. Rogawski, R. W. Olsen, & A. W. Delgado-Escueta (Eds.), *Jasper's basic mechanisms of the epilepsies* (4th ed.) [Internet]. National Center for Biotechnology Information (US).

Masino, S. A., & Rho, J. M. (2019). Metabolism and epilepsy: Ketogenic diets as a homeostatic link. *Brain Research, 1703,* 26–30.

Neal, E. G., Chaffe, H., Schwartz, R. H., Lawson, M. S., Edwards, N., Fitzsimmons, G., Whitney, A., & Cross, J. H. (2008). The ketogenic diet for the treatment of childhood epilepsy: A randomised controlled trial. *Lancet Neurology, 7*(6), 500–506.

Pathak, D., Berthet, A., & Nakamura, K. (2013). Energy failure: Does it contribute to neurodegeneration? *Annals of Neurology, 74*(4), 506–516.

Rogawski, M. A., Löscher, W., & Rho, J. M. (2016). Mechanisms of action of antiseizure drugs and the ketogenic diet. *Cold Spring Harbor Perspectives in Medicine, 6*(5), a022780.

Stafstrom, C. E., & Rho, J. M. (2012). The ketogenic diet as a treatment paradigm for diverse neurological disorders. *Frontiers in Pharmacology, 3,* 59.

Vining, E. P., Freeman, J. M., Ballaban-Gil, K., Camfield, C. S., Camfield, P. R., Holmes, G. L., Shinnar, S., Shuman, R., Trevathan, E., & Wheless, J. W. (1998). A multicenter study of the efficacy of the ketogenic diet. *Archives of Neurology, 55*(11), 1433–1437.

14

Metabolism-Based Treatments for Managing Cancer

Scientific Rationale

THOMAS N. SEYFRIED, MS, PHD, PURNA MUKHERJEE, PHD,
AND CHRISTOS CHINOPOULOS, MD, PHD

INTRODUCTION

Cancer has long been recognized as a genetic disease involving mutations in oncogenes and tumor suppressor genes that reside in the tumor cell nucleus. The nuclear gene mutations found in nearly all types of tumors are considered the primary cause of the cancer's hallmarks, which include sustained proliferative signaling, evasion of growth suppressors, resistance to cell death, replicative immortality, enhanced angiogenesis, and activation of invasion and metastasis (Hanahan & Weinberg, 2000, 2011). The somatic driver mutations in tumor cells arise randomly during DNA replication in normal nontumorigenic stem cells and are thought to be the origin of cancer (Tomasetti & Vogelstein, 2015; Vogelstein et al., 2013). The somatic mutation theory (SMT) is the most widely accepted explanation for the origin of cancer and is the justification for developing targeted or personalized therapies for managing the various forms of the disease (Hou & Ma, 2014; McLeod, 2013; Seyfried, 2015; Vaux, 2011; Weller & Le Rhun, 2019). There are, however, a growing number of serious inconsistencies that challenge the SMT as a credible explanation for the origin of cancer. Some of the major inconsistencies include:

1. The absence of gene mutations and chromosomal abnormalities in some cancers (Baker, 2015; Bayreuther, 1960; Braun, 1970; Kiebish & Seyfried, 2005; Pitot, 1966; Soto & Sonnenschein, 2004). Specifically, Greenman et al. (2007) found no mutations following extensive sequencing in 73 of 210 cancers, whereas Parsons et al. (2008) found that only some patients with glioblastoma had mutations in the P53, the PI3K, or the RB1 pathways, and that a tumor tissue sample (Br20P)

of one glioblastoma patient had no mutations. According to the SMT, if cancer is due to gene mutations, these tissue samples should not exist.

2. The identification and clonal expansion of numerous cancer "driver" gene mutations in a broad range of normal human tissues (Chanock, 2018; Martincorena & Campbell, 2015; Martincorena et al., 2018; Yizhak et al., 2019; Yokoyama et al., 2019). The targeting of these mutations could produce significant adverse effects in normal tissues. No clear explanation has been presented on how the SMT can account for malignant tumors that have no mutations or for normal cells and tissues that express cancer driver mutations but do not develop tumors.

3. The rarity of cancers in chimpanzees despite their having about 98.5% gene and protein sequence identity with humans, even at the *BRCA1* locus (Huttley et al., 2000; Lowenstine et al., 2016; Puente et al., 2006; Varki & Varki, 2015). Although breast cancer accounts for about 30% of all human female cancers (Seyfried et al., 2020b), breast cancer has not yet been documented in a female chimpanzee, suggesting that environmental factors (diet and lifestyle), rather than genetic mutations, are largely responsible for the disease (Kopp, 2019; Varki & Varki, 2015). Because DNA replication would be similar in normal tissue stem cells of chimpanzees and humans, the rarity of cancer in all chimpanzee organs undermines the "bad luck" hypothesis of Tomasetti and Vogelstein, which posits that cancer risk is due to random mutations arising during DNA replication in normal, noncancerous stem cells (Tomasetti & Vogelstein, 2015).

4. It is also interesting that Theodor Boveri, the person most recognized as the originator of the SMT (Barrett, 1993; Knudson, 2002), never directly studied cancer and was highly apologetic for his general lack of knowledge about the disease (Boveri, 2008). He also did not exclude the possibility that cancer could arise from defects in the cytoplasm.

5. The most compelling evidence against the SMT comes from the nuclear/cytoplasm transfer experiments showing that normal cells and tissues can be produced from tumorigenic nuclei, as long as the tumorigenic nuclei are localized in cytoplasm containing normal mitochondria (Seyfried, 2012c, 2015). Moreover, recent studies show that normal mitochondria can downregulate multiple oncogenic pathways and growth behavior in glioma, melanoma, and metastatic breast cancer cells (Chang et al., 2019; Fu et al., 2019; Kaipparettu et al., 2013; Ma et al., 2010; Sun et al., 2019). These findings demonstrate that normal mitochondrial function can suppress tumorigenesis regardless of the gene or chromosomal abnormalities that might be present in the tumor nucleus. When

viewed collectively, these findings suggest that the somatic mutations found in many cancers are not the primary cause of the disease and seriously challenge the SMT as a credible explanation for the origin of cancer. Figure 14.1 summarizes the data from the cytoplasm/nuclear transfer experiments.

Despite these serious inconsistencies, the SMT continues to be presented as if it were dogma in most current college textbooks of genetics, biochemistry, and cell biology, and it is the mainstay of the National Cancer Institute (NCI) statement that, "Cancer is a genetic disease—that is, it is caused by changes to genes that control the way our cells function, especially how they grow and divide" (http://www.cancer.gov/cancertopics/what-is-cancer; Seyfried, 2015). It should be recognized, however, that there is no place in science for epistemologic dogmatism, as dogma tranquilizes creative thinking and blocks consideration of viable alternatives (Rous, 1959; Seyfried et al., 2017; Sonnenschein & Soto, 2000). It is not clear how long it may take before NCI comes to recognize this information.

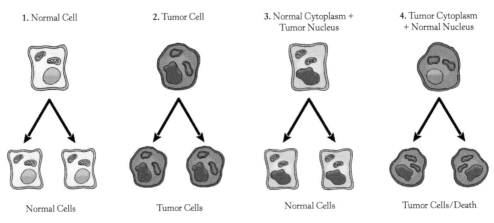

1. Normal Cell   2. Tumor Cell   3. Normal Cytoplasm + Tumor Nucleus   4. Tumor Cytoplasm + Normal Nucleus

Normal Cells   Tumor Cells   Normal Cells   Tumor Cells/Death

FIGURE 14.1 *Role of the Nucleus and Mitochondria in the Origin of Tumors*

Summary of a role of the mitochondria in the origin of tumorigenesis, as previously described (Seyfried, 2015). Normal cells are shown in green, with nuclear and mitochondrial morphology indicative of normal gene expression and respiration, respectively. Tumor cells are shown in red, with abnormal nuclear and mitochondrial morphology indicative of genomic instability and abnormal OxPhos respiration, respectively.

1) Normal cells beget normal cells. 2) Tumor cells beget tumor cells. 3) Transfer of a tumor cell nucleus into a normal cytoplasm begets normal cells, despite the presence of the tumor-associated genomic abnormalities. 4) Transfer of a normal cell nucleus into a tumor cell cytoplasm begets dead cells or tumor cells, but not normal cells. The results suggest that nuclear genomic defects alone cannot account for the origin of tumors, and that normal mitochondria can suppress tumorigenesis. (Seyfried, 2012c)

The collective experiments supporting these conclusions, which involved a broad range of tumor types, animal species, and experimental techniques, present the strongest evidence to date indicating that cancer is a mitochondrial metabolic disease and not a genetic disease according to the somatic mutation theory (Seyfried, 2015). Original diagram reproduced from Jeffrey Ling and Thomas N. Seyfried, with permission.

CANCER AS A MITOCHONDRIAL METABOLIC DISEASE

As an alternative to the SMT, prior and emerging evidence indicates that cancer is primarily a mitochondrial metabolic disease (Bartesaghi et al., 2015; Fosslien, 2008; Galluzzi et al., 2010; Hu et al., 2012; John, 2001; Pedersen, 1978; Poljsak et al., 2019; Roskelley et al., 1943; Seyfried, 2015; Seyfried et al., 2014; Seyfried & Shelton, 2010; Verschoor et al., 2013; Wishart, 2015). The consideration of cancer as a mitochondrial metabolic disease originated from the experiments of Otto Warburg (Burk et al., 1967; Warburg, 1956a, 1956b). According to Warburg's theory, respiratory insufficiency is the origin of cancer. All other phenotypes of the disease, including the somatic mutations and aerobic fermentation, arise either directly or indirectly from insufficient respiration (Seyfried, 2012a; Seyfried et al., 2014; Warburg, 1956a). Warburg's metabolic theory was also in line with the concepts of others showing that cancer is largely a cytoplasmic mitochondrial disease (Darlington, 1948; Seeger, 1959; Seyfried, 2012a, 2015; Seyfried & Shelton, 2010; Woods & du Buy, 1945). Advocates of the SMT, however, consider the abnormal energy metabolism of tumor cells as simply another phenotype that "is programmed by proliferation-inducing oncogenes and defective tumor suppressor genes" (Hanahan and Weinberg, 2011; Seyfried, 2015). This view, however, is inconsistent with the data obtained from the nuclear-cytoplasm transfer experiments mentioned above and in Figure 14.1.

Viewed in the light of Warburg's central theory, the nuclear-cytoplasm transfer experiments show that cancer originates from damage to the *mitochondria* in the cytoplasm rather than from damage to the genome in the nucleus (Seyfried, 2015). The genomic instability seen in tumor cells follows, rather than precedes, the disturbances in cellular respiration. The common pathophysiologic mechanism underlying cancer—"the oncogenic paradox"—is explained when cancer is considered as a mitochondrial metabolic disease rather than a genetic disease (Seyfried, 2012d; Seyfried et al., 2014; Seyfried & Shelton, 2010). We have clearly outlined how all roads to the origin and progression of cancer pass through the mitochondria (Chinopoulos & Seyfried, 2018; Seyfried, 2015; Seyfried et al., 2014, 2020b). Hence, novel therapeutic strategies for management and prevention emerge when cancer is recognized as a mitochondrial metabolic disease (Seyfried et al., 2017).

CANCER CELL METABOLISM

Reduced oxidative phosphorylation (OxPhos) efficiency in cancer cells can arise from any type of defect in the number, structure, or function of mitochondria (Arismendi-Morillo et al., 2017; Arismendi-Morillo & Castellano-Ramirez, 2008; Elliott et al., 2012; Feichtinger et al., 2010, 2015; Kiebish et al., 2008; Pedersen, 1978; Seyfried et al., 2014; Singh et al., 2015; Srinivasan et al., 2016; Weber et al., 2019; Yuan et al., 2020). Mitochondrial structure is linked directly to mitochondrial function (Cogliati et al., 2016; Hackenbrock, 1968; Lehninger, 1964; Putignani et al., 2012; Stroud & Ryan, 2013). Although some mouse brain tumors have OxPhos defects in the absence of mitochondrial mutations (Kiebish et al., 2008; Kiebish & Seyfried, 2005), recent studies show that that the majority of human cancers express mtDNA mutations that compromise OxPhos function (Yuan et al., 2020). The mtDNA mutations found in cancers are also considered secondary causes, rather primary causes, because no common gene mutation has been detected in all cells of any cancer type (Seyfried et al., 2020b). Hence, most malignant tumor tissues from cancer patients contain mitochondria that express some degree of abnormality in number, structure, or function.

Abnormalities in mitochondria number, structure, and function will cause tumors to increase fermentation metabolism. It is well known that lactate fermentation is the common metabolic malady seen in most, if not all, cancer cells (Seyfried et al., 2014; Warburg, 1931, 1956a, 1956b, 1969; Yu et al., 2019). Indeed, lactate fermentation can be detected even in the slowest growing tumors (Burk & Schade, 1956; Burk et al., 1967). The greater the lactate production is, the greater is the rate of tumor malignancy (Yu et al., 2019). In addition to expressing robust fermentation in hypoxic environments, cancer cells also ferment lactate in aerobic environments. Although "aerobic" fermentation is not unique to tumor cells, "anaerobic" fermentation is unique, as normal mammalian cells cannot survive for long periods in hypoxia (Barron, 1930; Warburg, 1956a, 1956b). Lactate production is greater in cancer cells than in normal cells because glucose carbons are required for cell proliferation. Although Warburg and others thought that ATP synthesis through glycolysis could compensate for reduced ATP synthesis through OxPhos, accumulating evidence shows that this might not be the case. Most tumor cells express the glycolytic pyruvate kinase M2 (PKM2) isoform, which produces much less ATP than the PKM1 isoform (Chinopoulos & Seyfried, 2018; David et al., 2010; Dong et al., 2016; Israelsen et al., 2013; Mazurek et al., 2005; Seyfried et al., 2020b; Vander Heiden, 2010; Yu et al., 2019). If ATP synthesis through glycolysis cannot compensate for reduced energy through OxPhos in most tumor cells due to the predominance of the PKM2 isoform, then where would the tumor cells obtain their energy for growth?

In addition to a reliance on glucose, cancer cells also rely heavily on glutamine for growth and survival (DeBerardinis & Cheng, 2010; Yuneva, 2008). Glutamine is the second major fermentable fuel that can compensate for OxPhos deficiency in cancer cells (Chen et al., 2018; Chinopoulos & Seyfried, 2018; Seyfried et al., 2020a). Because Q is the letter designation for glutamine, we have described this phenomenon as the Q-effect to distinguish it from that involving the aerobic fermentation of glucose, the Warburg effect (Chinopoulos & Seyfried, 2018). Both the Warburg effect and the Q-effect arise from compromised OxPhos. Glutamine provides ATP synthesis through the process of mitochondrial substrate-level phosphorylation (mSLP) in the glutaminolysis pathway (Chinopoulos & Seyfried, 2018; Seyfried et al., 2020a, 2020b; Figure 14.2). Substrate-level phosphorylation occurs at the succinyl-CoA synthase reaction (Step 5) of the citric acid cycle or TCA cycle. Only those cells that can make a protracted transition in their energy production from OxPhos to substrate-level phosphorylation through glycolysis in the cytoplasm and through mSLP can become tumor cells. Cells that cannot make this transition will die and can

never become tumor (Warburg, 1956a). Because substrate-level phosphorylation is less efficient in producing ATP than OxPhos is, cancer cells must consume greater amounts of fermentable fuels (glucose and glutamine) than normal cells in order to maintain a $\Delta G'$ ATP hydrolysis in the narrow range of –56 to –59 kJ/mole. This energy of ATP hydrolysis is the endpoint of both genetic and metabolic processes that are required for "life" (Seyfried et al., 2020a; Seyfried & Shelton, 2010; Veech et al., 2019). Because the default state of metazoan cells is proliferation, not quiescence (Sonnenschein & Soto, 2000; Soto & Sonnenschein, 2004), unbridled proliferation is the consequence when fermentation replaces respiration in cancer cells (Seyfried, 2015; Seyfried et al., 2019; Szent-Gyorgyi, 1977). Indeed, unbridled proliferation was the dominant growth phenotype of all organisms before oxygen entered the atmosphere about 2.5 billion years ago (Szent-Gyorgyi, 1977). Hence, the dysregulated growth of cancer cells arises from the gradual replacement of OxPhos with fermentation metabolism in the cytoplasm and in the mitochondria.

Although the evidence supporting mitochondrial abnormalities and OxPhos insufficiency in cancer is now overwhelming, some metabolic studies on cultured tumor cells can be inconsistent with the findings from intact tumor tissue. The unnatural conditions of the in vitro growth environment (Crabtree effect) can make some cancer cells appear to have normal respiration despite their continued production of lactate. The information on tumor cell energy metabolism obtained from in vitro studies, however, is sometimes at odds with the data from in vivo

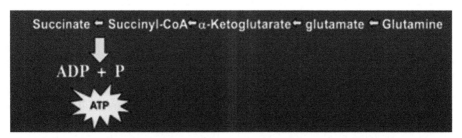

FIGURE 14.2 *The Glutaminolysis Pathway Supports ATP Synthesis Through Mitochondrial Substrate-Level Phosphorylation (mSLP)*

The succinyl-CoA ligase reaction, metabolizing succinyl-CoA to succinate, produces high-energy phosphates (ATP) in the absence of oxidative phosphorylation through the process of substrate-level phosphorylation in the mitochondrial matrix. Provision of succinyl-CoA by the α-ketoglutarate dehydrogenase complex is crucial for maintaining the function of succinyl-CoA ligase, thus preventing the adenine nucleotide translocase from reversing (Seyfried et al., 2020a). Succinate contributes to inflammation and stabilizes HIF-1α, a key transcription factor that contributes to the aerobic fermentation (Chouchani et al., 2014; Selak et al., 2005; Semenza, 2017; Tannahill et al., 2013). Reprinted from Seyfried et al. (2020b) and distributed under a Creative Commons license.

studies (Poteet et al., 2013). The results from many in vitro studies suggest that mitochondrial energy metabolism is similar in normal cells and tumor cells (Cairns, 2015; Koppenol et al., 2011; Moreno-Sanchez et al., 2007). If abnormalities in mitochondrial structure and function are seen in the majority of tumor cells of cancerous tissues, then how is it possible that mitochondria and OxPhos could be normal in cultured cells from the tumors? We recently addressed how oxygen consumption rates could be misinterpreted as a marker for normal OxPhos in cultured tumor cells (Chinopoulos & Seyfried, 2018; Seyfried et al., 2014, 2020a, 2020b). Confusion regarding OxPhos function in cancer cells can come from assuming that oxygen consumption rate (OCR), using the Seahorse instrument, is linked to ATP synthesis through OxPhos in cultured cells. However, the instrument can infer only that ATP flux is linked to OCR. The instrument is presently incapable of distinguishing ATP synthesis arising either from mSLP or from OxPhos (Seyfried et al., 2020a). As normal mitochondrial function is also necessary for obtaining energy from fatty acids and ketone bodies, abnormalities in mitochondrial number, structure, and function would also prevent tumor cells from using fatty acids and ketone bodies for energy (Arismendi-Morillo et al., 2017; Chinopoulos & Seyfried, 2018; Ji et al., 2020; Seyfried et al., 2020a, 2020b). Previous studies showed, however, that fatty acids are potent swelling and uncoupling agents that can stimulate insulin secretion and glucose/glutamine consumption, thus making it appear as if tumor cells can metabolize fatty acids for energy (Giudetti et al., 2019; Lehninger, 1964; Samudio et al., 2009; Vozza et al., 2014). Caution should therefore be used in linking in vitro studies with the situation in the living condition.

The waste products of glucose fermentation (lactic acid) and glutamine fermentation (succinic acid) will acidify the tumor microenvironment, thus increasing inflammation and angiogenesis, which ultimately increases tumor progression. Succinate, produced through glutamine fermentation (Chinopoulos, 2019; Hochachka et al., 1975), can also contribute to microenvironment acidification and inflammation (Tannahill et al., 2013). Succinate stabilizes the *HIF-1α* oncogene, thus enhancing fermentation metabolism in the presence or absence of oxygen. The dependency of tumor cells on glycolysis and glutaminolysis will also make them resistant to apoptosis, damage induced by reactive oxygen species (ROS), and chemotherapy drugs (Xu et al., 2005). Hence,

most cancer characteristics can be linked directly to mitochondrial dysfunction coupled with increased glucose and glutamine fermentation.

Several byproducts of amino acid fermentation can also accumulate in the tumor microenvironment, including acetate, glutamate, alanine, succinate, and ammonia. Although acetate has been considered a potential fuel for supporting tumor cell growth (Comerford et al., 2014; Hosios & Vander Heiden, 2014), acetate levels are generally low in the circulation (Ballard, 1972). Jaworski et al. (2016) provided a comprehensive discussion on the potential role of acetate in tumor metabolism. It should be recognized that, with the exception of glucose and glutamine, none of the other potential fuels for tumor cell metabolism would be present in sufficiently high quantities to maintain robust tumor cell growth (Chinopoulos & Seyfried, 2018). Hence, the restriction of glucose and glutamine becomes of prime importance for targeting tumor cell growth and survival.

CALORIE RESTRICTION

Calorie restriction (CR) with adequate nutrition or underfeeding has been long known to limit tumor growth and to improve general health (Hursting et al., 2010; Kritchevsky, 2001; Mukherjee et al., 1999; Raffaghello et al., 2008; Tannenbaum, 1942). CR targets several of cancer's hallmarks, including angiogenesis, inflammation, edema, proliferation, and distal invasion (Jiang & Wang, 2013; Mukherjee et al., 1999; Mulrooney et al., 2011; Shelton et al., 2010; Thompson et al., 2004; Woolf et al., 2015). Numerous studies have linked rapid tumor growth to elevated blood glucose or hyperglycemia (Barba et al., 2012; de Beer & Liebenberg, 2014; Decker et al., 2019; McGirt et al., 2008; Meyerhardt et al., 2012; Seyfried et al., 2003). CR lowers the level of circulating glucose, thus limiting the prime fermentable fuel for driving tumor growth (Seyfried et al., 2003). In addition, CR or therapeutic fasting elevates the level of circulating ketone bodies, D-β-hydroxybutyrate (βHB) and acetoacetate. Ketone bodies serve as a nonfermentable super fuel for functional mitochondria that also reduce ROS while increasing the delta G' of ATP hydrolysis and metabolic efficiency (Seyfried et al., 2003, 2014; Veech, 2004). Based on these observations, Cahill and Veech (2003) characterized ketone bodies as "good medicine." In contrast to normal cells, which transition to ketone bodies for energy when glucose becomes limiting, tumor cells cannot use ketone bodies effectively for energy (Fredericks & Ramsey, 1978; Magee et al., 1979;

Maurer et al., 2011; Tisdale, 1984). Indeed, ketone bodies can even be toxic to some tumor cells (Fine et al., 2009; Ji et al., 2020; Magee et al., 1979; Poff et al., 2015; Sawai et al., 2004; Skinner et al., 2009; Vallejo et al., 2020). Shimazu et al. (2013) suggested that high-dose βHB could act as a histone deacetylase inhibitor. The multiple defects in mitochondrial structure and function are considered responsible for the failure of tumor cells to effectively use ketone bodies for energy (Seyfried & Mukherjee, 2005; Seyfried & Shelton, 2010; Seyfried et al., 2017, 2020b).

It is important to mention that the therapeutic benefit of a 40% CR for managing cancer in rodents would not be the same as for managing cancer in humans. The basal metabolic rate in humans is about seven times less than that in mice (Terpstra, 2001). Consequently, water-only therapeutic fasting for 2 to 3 weeks would be predicted to produce a benefit similar to that seen in rodents under a 40% CR (Mahoney et al., 2006). As a ketogenic diet can sometimes replicate the physiologic conditions of therapeutic fasting (Seyfried et al., 2009), it might be easier for most cancer patients to use a ketogenic diet than to use therapeutic fasting for tumor management. A recent human case report, however, showed that therapeutic fasting used together with a ketogenic diet was effective in the long-term management of metastatic thymoma (Phillips et al., 2020).

KETOGENIC METABOLIC THERAPY

Ketogenic metabolic therapy (KMT) is a nutritional intervention involving ketogenic or low-glycemic diets for managing a broad range of cancers (Klement, 2019; Phillips et al., 2020; Schwartz et al., 2018; Seyfried et al., 2020b; Weber et al., 2019; Winter et al., 2017). The ketogenic diet (KD) is a low-carbohydrate high-fat diet that is widely used to reduce refractory epileptic seizures in children (Freeman & Kossoff, 2010; Kossoff & Hartman, 2012). KDs are also effective in managing symptoms of a wide range of neurologic and neurodegenerative diseases. The KD is also gaining recognition as an effective therapy for any cancer that expresses the Warburg effect, which includes most metastatic cancers (Yu et al., 2019). The anticancer mechanism of action for the KD is embarrassingly simple. The KD lowers the prime fermentable fuel (glucose) needed for driving metabolite synthesis and lactic acid fermentation, while producing therapeutic levels of nonfermentable blood ketone bodies.

As OxPhos defects are ultimately responsible for the reliance of tumor cells on fermentation, the KD targets the Warburg effect and tumor cell energy metabolism. The KD can more effectively reduce glucose and elevate blood ketone bodies than can CR alone, making the KD potentially more therapeutic against tumors than CR. There are no anticancer drugs presently known that can target tumor cells while enhancing the metabolic efficiency of normal cells the way the KD can.

It is important to mention, however, that in some strains of mice the unrestricted feeding of KDs can cause weight gain, insulin insensitivity, and dyslipidemia, leading to elevated blood levels of insulin and glucose (Meidenbauer et al., 2014). Dyslipidemia from excessive consumption of KD can occur despite the very low amounts of carbohydrate in the diet. This could account in part for our failure to detect a therapeutic benefit against either naturally occurring seizures in EL mice, or against astrocytoma growth in mice that were fed KDs in unrestricted amounts (Mantis et al., 2004; Seyfried et al., 2003; Zhou et al., 2007). Reduced blood glucose is considered essential for managing either epileptic seizures or cancer. Because high-fat diets will elevate the appetite suppressor hormone cholecystokinin, it is possible that dyslipidemia might not occur in most cancer patients on a KD. A therapeutic KD should lower glucose, cholesterol, and triglycerides while elevating ketone bodies and high-density lipoprotein (Meidenbauer et al., 2014).

In contrast to the weight loss associated with cachexia or toxic cancer therapies, which is pathologic, the body weight loss associated with KMT is therapeutic. Cachexic weight loss is associated with elevations of blood glucose and insulin insensitivity that can stimulate tumor growth (Kotler, 2000). These blood elevations are opposite to those seen in KMT, which reduces circulating glucose and insulin levels. High-dose steroids (e.g., dexamethasone), which elevate blood glucose levels, are often given to cancer patients under chemotherapy to reduce nausea and to improve weight gain. It is clear from an understanding of cancer metabolism that steroid administration for improved weight gain would not be in the best interest of the cancer patient (Seyfried et al., 2019, 2020b; Wong et al., 2015). Hence, fundamental metabolic differences exist between the therapeutic weight loss associated with a KMT and the pathologic weight loss associated with cachexia and toxic cancer therapies.

The KD differs from Atkins-type diets in having less protein and more fat than the Atkins diets. This is important, because several amino acids found in proteins can be deaminated to form pyruvate, which is then metabolized to form glucose through gluconeogenesis (Burt et al., 1982). The fats in KDs also contain more saturated medium-chain triglycerides than do Atkins diets. Consequently, blood glucose levels will be lower and ketone body levels will be higher with KDs than with Atkins-type diets. The caprylic acid (octanoic, C8) content of the KD is also important, as caprylic acid not only is effective in elevating ketone bodies, but also has anticancer and neuroprotective properties (Altinoz et al., 2020). Hence, the macro- and micronutrient composition of the KD is important for therapeutic efficacy.

We developed the Glucose/Ketone Index calculator (GKIC) to assess the potential therapeutic effects of various low-carbohydrate diets and KDs for cancer management (Meidenbauer et al., 2015; Seyfried et al., 2017). The GKIC is a simple tool that measures the ratio of blood glucose to blood ketones and can help monitor the efficacy of metabolic therapy in preclinical animal models and in clinical trials for malignant brain cancer or for any cancer that expresses aerobic fermentation. This instrument was used recently to monitor the therapeutic benefit of KMT on a range of human cancers (Elsakka et al., 2018; Hagihara et al., 2020). The GKI can therefore serve as a biomarker to validate the therapeutic efficacy of various diets in targeting cancer cell energy metabolism.

THE FUTURE OF KMT FOR CANCER MANAGEMENT AND PREVENTION

Reduced glucose with therapeutic ketosis, achieved through low-carbohydrate ketogenic diets, can serve as an alternative or complimentary approach to cancer management (Elsakka et al., 2018; Hagihara et al., 2020; Iyikesici, 2019; Iyikesici et al., 2017; Klement, 2019; Phillips et al., 2020; Schwartz et al., 2015, 2018; Seyfried et al., 2017, 2020b; Weber et al., 2019). Evidence also suggests that the therapeutic efficacy of the KMT against tumor growth can be enhanced when it is combined with certain drugs and procedures under a "press-pulse" paradigm, as previously mentioned (Mukherjee et al., 2019; Seyfried et al., 2017). For example, therapeutic synergy was seen in combining the calorie-restricted KD with the

glycolysis inhibitor 2-deoxyglucose for management of gliomas (Marsh et al., 2008; Vallejo et al., 2020), and in combining the KD with hyperbaric oxygen therapy and ketone esters for the management of systemic metastatic management of the syngeneic VM-M3 tumor (Poff et al., 2013, 2015). The KD might also act synergistically to some degree with radiation therapy for glioma management (Klement & Sweeney, 2016; Panhans et al., 2020). The therapeutic effects of KMT seen with preclinical brain tumor models (Ji et al., 2020; Martuscello et al., 2016; Mukherjee et al., 2019), have been corroborated in preclinical studies for several other cancer models, including neuroblastoma, lung cancer, prostate cancer, breast cancer, and ovarian cancer (Allen et al., 2013; Lv et al., 2014; Mavropoulos et al., 2009; Morscher et al., 2015; Weber et al., 2019; Zhuang et al., 2014). These preclinical studies are also motivating case reports and pilot studies in humans with brain cancer and other cancers (Champ et al., 2013, 2014; Maroon et al., 2015; Rieger et al., 2014; Schmidt et al., 2011; Zuccoli et al., 2010). It is clear from these studies, and from the original observation of Linda Nebeling and colleagues (Nebeling et al., 1995), that treatment of cancer patients with KDs is generally well tolerated, which is consistent with decades of research obtained from evaluation of children treated with KDs for epilepsy management. An important question for future research is whether cancer management is more effective in using KMT with nontoxic drugs and procedures or in using KMT with current toxic standards of care.

In recognizing cancer as a mitochondrial metabolic disease, we suggested that protecting cellular mitochondria from toxic or metabolic stress could best prevent cancer (Seyfried, 2012b). Calorie-restricted KDs and therapeutic fasting are excellent ways to reduce oxidative stress in mitochondria. Metabolism of βHB maintains the coenzyme Q couple in an oxidized state, thus reducing the production of damaging ROS (Veech, 2004; Veech et al., 2019). Therapeutic water-only fasting or restricted KDs reduce tissue inflammation (Mulrooney et al., 2011; Youm et al., 2015). Chronic inflammation is known to produce mitochondrial stress and cancer (Bissell & Hines, 2011; Coussens & Werb, 2002; Fosslien, 2008; Kamp et al., 2011). It is our view that glucose:ketone ratios (GKI values) of 1.0 or below could help reduce systemic inflammation (Seyfried et al., 2017). The GKI might therefore serve as an effective biomarker, along with

C-reactive protein, for determining systemic inflammation and for reducing mitochondrial stress to prevent cancer. Further studies will be needed to validate this prediction.

KMT AND GLOBAL BUDGETING FOR CANCER

Cancer kills over 1,600 people in the United States each day (Siegel et al., 2019). The continued high death rate for cancer can be attributed in large part to the misguided belief that cancer is a genetic disease. This misunderstanding underlies the continued development of ineffective precision medicine, much of which is directed at cancer management (Joyner et al., 2018; Shin et al., 2017). Many of the new cancer immunotherapies are associated with unacceptable toxicities that can lead to hyperprogressive disease and rapid patient death (Borcoman et al., 2019; Ferrara et al., 2018; Fojo, 2018). In addition to physical toxicity, many of the new cancer drugs are so massively overpriced that they cause a new type of adverse effect called financial toxicity (McGinnis, 2019). Financial toxicity involves an increased likelihood that cancer patients will experience bankruptcy, relationship problems, and even mortality. It has not escaped our attention that KMT could have significant impact on global budgeting contracts for patient care. It is now recognized that global budget contracts with quality incentives encourage changes in practice patterns that can help reduce spending and improve quality of general health (Prager et al., 2018; Song et al., 2014). KMT is well positioned to serve as a low-cost, nontoxic alternative in both the prevention and the management of cancer. In addition to its use in cancer, therapeutic ketosis could be effective for the management and prevention of a broad range of chronic inflammatory diseases, including obesity, type 2 diabetes, cardiovascular disease, epilepsy, Alzheimer's disease, Parkinson's disease, and traumatic brain injury (Seyfried, 2014). Hence, KMT could have utility for improving health and reducing costs for many of the most challenging diseases seen in Western societies.

ACKNOWLEDGMENTS

This work was supported in part by NIH Grants (HD-39722, NS-108055195, and CA-102135) and by grants from the American Institute of Cancer Research, the Foundation for Metabolic Cancer Therapies, CrossFit Inc., the Nelson and Claudia Peltz Foundation, the Kenneth Rainin Foundation, Children with Cancer UK, Joseph C. Maroon, Edward Miller, and the Boston College Research Expense Fund.

REFERENCES

Allen, B. G., Bhatia, S. K., Buatti, J. M., Brandt, K. E., Lindholm, K. E., Button, A. M., Szweda, L. I., Smith, B. J., Spitz, D. R., & Fath, M. A. (2013). Ketogenic diets enhance oxidative stress and radio-chemotherapy responses in lung cancer xenografts. *Clinical Cancer Research, 19,* 3905–3913.

Altinoz, M. A., Ozpinar, A., & Seyfried, T. N. (2020). Caprylic (octanoic) acid as a potential fatty acid chemotherapeutic for glioblastoma. *Prostaglandins, Leukotrienes and Essential Fatty Acids, 159,* 102142.

Arismendi-Morillo, G. J., & Castellano-Ramirez, A.V. (2008). Ultrastructural mitochondrial pathology in human astrocytic tumors: Potentials implications pro-therapeutics strategies. *Journal of Electron Microscopy (Tokyo), 57,* 33–39.

Arismendi-Morillo, G., Castellano-Ramirez, A., & Seyfried, T. N. (2017). Ultrastructural characterization of the mitochondria-associated membranes abnormalities in human astrocytomas: Functional and therapeutics implications. *Ultrastructural Pathology, 41,* 234–244.

Baker, S. G. (2015). A cancer theory kerfuffle can lead to new lines of research. *Journal of the National Cancer Institute, 107*(2).

Ballard, F. J. (1972). Supply and utilization of acetate in mammals. *American Journal of Clinical Nutrition, 25,* 773–779.

Barba, M., Sperati, F., Stranges, S., Carlomagno, C., Nasti, G., Iaffaioli, V., Caolo, G., Mottolese, M., Botti, G., Terrenato, I., Vici, P., Serpico, D., Giordano, A., D'Aiuto, G., Crispo, A., Montella, M., Capurso, G., Delle Fave, G., Fuhrman, B., Botti, C., & De Placido, S. (2012). Fasting glucose and treatment outcome in breast and colorectal cancer patients treated with targeted agents: Results from a historic cohort. *Annals of Oncology, 23,* 1838–1845.

Barrett, J. C. (1993). Mechanisms of multistep carcinogenesis and carcinogen risk assessment. *Environmental Health Perspectives, 100,* 9–20.

Barron, E. S. (1930). The catalytic effect of methylene blue on the oxygen consumption of tumors and normal tissues. *Journal of Experimental Medicine, 52,* 447–456.

Bartesaghi, S., Graziano, V., Galavotti, S., Henriquez, N. V., Betts, J., Saxena, J., Minieri, V. A. D., Karlsson, A., Martins, L. M., Capasso, M., Nicotera, P., Brandner, S., De Laurenzi, V., & Salomoni, P. (2015). Inhibition of oxidative metabolism leads to p53 genetic inactivation and transformation in neural stem cells. *Proceedings of the National Academy of Sciences of the United States of America, 112,* 1059–1064.

Bayreuther, K. (1960). Chromosomes in primary neoplastic growth. *Nature, 186*, 6–9.

Bissell, M. J., & Hines, W. C. (2011). Why don't we get more cancer? A proposed role of the microenvironment in restraining cancer progression. *Nature Medicine, 17*, 320–329.

Borcoman, E., Kanjanapan, Y., Champiat, S., Kato, S., Servois, V., Kurzrock, R., Goel, S., Bedard, P., & Le Tourneau, C. (2019). Novel patterns of response under immunotherapy. *Annals of Oncology, 30*, 385–396.

Boveri, T. (2008). Concerning the origin of malignant tumours by Theodor Boveri. Translated and annotated by Henry Harris. *Journal of Cell Science, 121*(Suppl. 1), 1–84.

Braun, A. C. (1970). On the origin of the cancer cells. *American Scientist, 58*, 307–320.

Burk, D., & Schade, A. L. (1956). On respiratory impairment in cancer cells. *Science, 124*, 270–272.

Burk, D., Woods, M., & Hunter, J. (1967). On the significance of glucolysis for cancer growth, with special reference to Morris rat hepatomas. *Journal of the National Cancer Institute, 38*, 839–863.

Burt, M. E., Gorschboth, C. M., & Brennan, M. F. (1982). A controlled, prospective, randomized trial evaluating the metabolic effects of enteral and parenteral nutrition in the cancer patient. *Cancer, 49*, 1092–1105.

Cahill, G. F., Jr., & Veech, R. L. (2003). Ketoacids? Good medicine? *Transactions of the American Clinical and Climatological Association, 114*, 149–161; discussion 162-143.

Cairns, R. A. (2015). Drivers of the Warburg phenotype. *Cancer Journal, 21*, 56–61.

Champ, C. E., Mishra, M. V., Showalter, T. N., Ohri, N., Dicker, A. P., & Simone, N. L. (2013). Dietary recommendations during and after cancer treatment: Consistently inconsistent? *Nutrition and Cancer, 65*, 430–439.

Champ, C. E., Palmer, J. D., Volek, J. S., Werner-Wasik, M., Andrews, D. W., Evans, J. J., Glass, J., Kim, L., & Shi, W. (2014). Targeting metabolism with a ketogenic diet during the treatment of glioblastoma multiforme. *Journal of Neuro-Oncology, 117*, 125–131.

Chang, J. C., Chang, H. S., Wu, Y. C., Cheng, W. L., Lin, T. T., Chang, H. J., Kuo, S. J., Chen, S. T., & Liu, C. S. (2019). Mitochondrial transplantation regulates antitumour activity, chemoresistance and mitochondrial dynamics in breast cancer. *Journal of Experimental & Clinical Cancer Research, 38*, 30.

Chanock, S. J. (2018). The paradox of mutations and cancer. *Science, 362*, 893–894.

Chen, Q., Kirk, K., Shurubor, Y. I., Zhao, D., Arreguin, A. J., Shahi, I., Valsecchi, F., Primiano, G., Calder, E. L., Carelli, V., Denton, T. T., Beal, M. F., Gross, S. S., Manfredi, G., & D'Aurelio, M. (2018). Rewiring of glutamine metabolism is a bioenergetic adaptation of human cells with mitochondrial DNA mutations. *Cell Metabolism, 27*, 1007–1025 e1005.

Chinopoulos, C. (2019). Succinate in ischemia: Where does it come from? *International Journal of Biochemistry & Cell Biology, 115*, 105580.

Chinopoulos, C., & Seyfried, T. N. (2018). Mitochondrial substrate-level phosphorylation as energy source for glioblastoma: Review and hypothesis. *ASN NEURO, 10*, 1759091418818261.

Chouchani, E. T., Pell, V. R., Gaude, E., Aksentijevic, D., Sundier, S. Y., Robb, E. L., Logan, A., Nadtochiy, S. M., Ord, E. N. J., Smith, A. C., Eyassu, F., Shirley, R., Hu, C. H., Dare, A. J., James, A. M., Rogatti, S., Hartley, R. C., Eaton, S., Costa, A. S. H., . . . Murphy, M. P. (2014). Ischaemic accumulation of succinate controls reperfusion injury through mitochondrial ROS. *Nature, 515*, 431–435.

Cogliati, S., Enriquez, J. A., & Scorrano, L. (2016). Mitochondrial cristae: Where beauty meets functionality. *Trends in Biochemical Sciences, 41*, 261–273.

Comerford, S. A., Huang, Z., Du, X., Wang, Y., Cai, L., Witkiewicz, A. K., Walters, H., Tantawy, M. N., Fu, A., Manning, H. C., Horton, J. D., Hammer, R. E., McKnight, S. L., & Tu, B. P. (2014). Acetate dependence of tumors. *Cell, 159*, 1591–1602.

Coussens, L. M., & Werb, Z. (2002). Inflammation and cancer. *Nature, 420*, 860–867.

Darlington, C. D. (1948). The plasmagene theory of the origin of cancer. *British Journal of Cancer, 2*, 118–126.

David, C. J., Chen, M., Assanah, M., Canoll, P., & Manley, J. L. (2010). HnRNP proteins controlled by c-Myc deregulate pyruvate kinase mRNA splicing in cancer. *Nature, 463*, 364–368.

de Beer, J. C., & Liebenberg, L. (2014). Does cancer risk increase with HbA1c, independent of diabetes? *British Journal of Cancer, 110*, 2361–2368.

DeBerardinis, R. J., & Cheng, T. (2010). Q's next: The diverse functions of glutamine in metabolism, cell biology and cancer. *Oncogene, 29*, 313–324.

Decker, M., Sacks, P., Abbatematteo, J., De Leo, E., Brennan, M., & Rahman, M. (2019). The effects of hyperglycemia on outcomes in surgical high-grade glioma patients. *Clinical Neurology and Neurosurgery, 179*, 9–13.

Dong, G., Mao, Q., Xia, W., Xu, Y., Wang, J., Xu, L., & Jiang, F. (2016). PKM2 and cancer: The function of PKM2 beyond glycolysis. *Oncology Letters, 11*, 1980–1986.

Elliott, R. L., Jiang, X. P., & Head, J. F. (2012). Mitochondria organelle transplantation: Introduction of normal epithelial mitochondria into human cancer cells inhibits proliferation and increases drug sensitivity. *Breast Cancer Research and Treatment, 136*, 347–354.

Elsakka, A. M. A., Bary, M. A., Abdelzaher, E., Elnaggar, M., Kalamian, M., Mukherjee, P.,

& Seyfried, T. N. (2018). Management of glioblastoma multiforme in a patient treated with ketogenic metabolic therapy and modified standard of care: A 24-month follow-up. *Frontiers in Nutrition, 5*, 20.

Feichtinger, R. G., Weis, S., Mayr, J. A., Zimmermann, F. A., Bogner, B., Sperl, W., & Kofler, B. (2016). Alterations of oxidative phosphorylation in meningiomas and peripheral nerve sheath tumors. *Neuro Oncology, 18*, 184–194.

Feichtinger, R. G., Zimmermann, F., Mayr, J. A., Neureiter, D., Hauser-Kronberger, C., Schilling, F. H., Jones, N., Sperl, W., & Kofler, B. (2010). Low aerobic mitochondrial energy metabolism in poorly- or undifferentiated neuroblastoma. *BMC Cancer, 10*, 149.

Ferrara, R., Mezquita, L., Texier, M., Lahmar, J., Audigier-Valette, C., Tessonnier, L., Mazieres, J., Zalcman, G., Brosseau, S., Le Moulec, S., Leroy, L., Duchemann, B., Lefebvre, C., Veillon, R., Westeel, V., Koscielny, S., Champiat, S., Ferte, C., Planchard, D., . . . Caramella, C. (2018). Hyperprogressive disease in patients with advanced non-small cell lung cancer treated with PD-1/PD-L1 inhibitors or with single-agent chemotherapy. *JAMA Oncology, 4*, 1543–1552.

Fine, E. J., Miller, A., Quadros, E. V., Sequeira, J. M., & Feinman, R. D. (2009). Acetoacetate reduces growth and ATP concentration in cancer cell lines which over-express uncoupling protein 2. *Cancer Cell International, 9*, 14.

Fojo, T. (2018). Desperation oncology. *Seminars in Oncology, 45*, 105–106.

Fosslien, E. (2008). Cancer morphogenesis: Role of mitochondrial failure. *Annals of Clinical & Laboratory Science, 38*, 307–329.

Fredericks, M., & Ramsey, R. B. (1978). 3-Oxo acid coenzyme A transferase activity in brain and tumors of the nervous system. *Journal of Neurochemistry, 31*, 1529–1531.

Freeman, J. M., & Kossoff, E. H. (2010). Ketosis and the ketogenic diet, 2010: Advances in treating epilepsy and other disorders. *Advances in Pediatrics, 57*, 315–329.

Fu, A., Hou, Y., Yu, Z., Zhao, Z., & Liu, Z. (2019). Healthy mitochondria inhibit the metastatic melanoma in lungs. *International Journal of Biological Sciences, 15*, 2707–2718.

Galluzzi, L., Morselli, E., Kepp, O., Vitale, I., Rigoni, A., Vacchelli, E., Michaud, M., Zischka, H., Castedo, M., & Kroemer, G. (2010). Mitochondrial gateways to cancer. *Molecular Aspects of Medicine, 31*, 1–20.

Giudetti, A. M., De Domenico, S., Ragusa, A., Lunetti, P., Gaballo, A., Franck, J., Simeone, P., Nicolardi, G., De Nuccio, F., Santino, A., Capobianco, L., Lanuti, P., Fournier, I., Salzet, M., Maffia, M., & Vergara, D. (2019). A specific lipid metabolic profile is associated with the epithelial mesenchymal transition program. *Biochimica et Biophysica Acta-Molecular and Cell Biology of Lipids, 1864*, 344–357.

Greenman, C., Stephens, P., Smith, R., Dalgliesh, G. L., Hunter, C., Bignell, G., Davies, H., Teague, J., Butler, A., Stevens, C., O'Meara, S., Vastrik, I., Schmidt, E. E., Avis, T., Barthorpe, S., Bhamra, G., Buck, G., Choudhury, B., . . . Stratton, M. R. (2007). Patterns of somatic mutation in human cancer genomes. *Nature, 446*, 153–158.

Hackenbrock, C. R. (1968). Ultrastructural bases for metabolically linked mechanical activity in mitochondria. II. Electron transport-linked ultrastructural transformations in mitochondria. *Journal of Cell Biology, 37*, 345–369.

Hagihara, K., Kajimoto, K., Osaga, S., Nagai, N., Shimosegawa, E., Nakata, H., Saito, H., Nakano, M., Takeuchi, M., Kanki, H., Kagitani-Shimono, K., & Kijima, T. (2020). Promising effect of a new ketogenic diet regimen in patients with advanced cancer. *Nutrients, 12*.

Hanahan, D., & Weinberg, R. A. (2000). The hallmarks of cancer. *Cell, 100*, 57–70.

Hanahan, D., & Weinberg, R. A. (2011). Hallmarks of cancer: The next generation. *Cell, 144*, 646–674.

Hochachka, P. W., Owen, T. G., Allen, J. F., & Whittow, G. C. (1975). Multiple end products of anaerobiosis in diving vertebrates. *Comparative Biochemistry & Physiology Part B: Biochemical and Molecular Biology, 50*, 17–22.

Hosios, A. M., & Vander Heiden, M. G. (2014). Acetate metabolism in cancer cells. *Cancer & Metabolism, 2*, 27.

Hou, J. P., & Ma, J. (2014). DawnRank: Discovering personalized driver genes in cancer. *Genome Medicine, 6*, 56.

Hu, Y., Lu, W., Chen, G., Wang, P., Chen, Z., Zhou, Y., Ogasawara, M., Trachootham, D., Feng, L., Pelicano, H., Chiao, P. J., Keating, M. J., Garcia-Manero, G., & Huang, P. (2012). K-ras(G12V) transformation leads to mitochondrial dysfunction and a metabolic switch from oxidative phosphorylation to glycolysis. *Cell Research, 22*, 399–412.

Hursting, S. D., Smith, S. M., Lashinger, L. M., Harvey, A. E., & Perkins, S. N. (2010). Calories and carcinogenesis: Lessons learned from 30 years of calorie restriction research. *Carcinogenesis, 31*, 83–89.

Huttley, G. A., Easteal, S., Southey, M. C., Tesoriero, A., Giles, G. G., McCredie, M. R., Hopper, J. L., & Venter, D. J. (2000). Adaptive evolution of the tumour suppressor BRCA1 in humans and chimpanzees: Australian Breast Cancer Family Study. *Nature Genetics, 25*, 410–413.

Israelsen, W. J., Dayton, T. L., Davidson, S. M., Fiske, B. P., Hosios, A. M., Bellinger, G., Li, J., Yu, Y., Sasaki, M., Horner, J. W., Burga, L. N., Xie, J., Jurczak, M. J., DePinho, R. A., Clish, C. B., Jacks, T., Kibbey, R. G., Wulf, G. M., Di Vizio, D., Mills,

G. B., Cantley, L. C., & Vander Heiden, M. G. (2013). PKM2 isoform-specific deletion reveals a differential requirement for pyruvate kinase in tumor cells. *Cell, 155*, 397–409.

Iyikesici, M. S. (2019). Feasibility study of metabolically supported chemotherapy with weekly carboplatin/paclitaxel combined with ketogenic diet, hyperthermia and hyperbaric oxygen therapy in metastatic non-small cell lung cancer. *International Journal of Hyperthermia, 36*, 446–455.

Iyikesici, M. S., Slocum, A. K., Slocum, A., Berkarda, F. B., Kalamian, M., & Seyfried, T. N. (2017). Efficacy of metabolically supported chemotherapy combined with ketogenic diet, hyperthermia, and hyperbaric oxygen therapy for stage IV triple-negative breast cancer. *Cureus, 9*, e1445.

Jaworski, D. M., Namboodiri, A. M., & Moffett, J. R. (2016). Acetate as a metabolic and epigenetic modifier of cancer therapy. *Journal of Cellular Biochemistry, 117*, 574–588.

Ji, C. C., Hu, Y. Y., Cheng, G., Liang, L., Gao, B., Ren, Y. P., Liu, J. T., Cao, X. L., Zheng, M. H., Li, S. Z., Wan, F., Han, H., & Fei, Z. (2020). A ketogenic diet attenuates proliferation and stemness of glioma stemlike cells by altering metabolism resulting in increased ROS production. *International Journal of Oncology, 56*, 606–617.

Jiang, Y. S., & Wang, F. R. (2013). Caloric restriction reduces edema and prolongs survival in a mouse glioma model. *Journal of Neuro-Oncology, 114*, 25–32.

John, A. P. (2001). Dysfunctional mitochondria, not oxygen insufficiency, cause cancer cells to produce inordinate amounts of lactic acid: The impact of this on the treatment of cancer. *Medical Hypotheses, 57*, 429–431.

Joyner, M. J., Boros, L. G., & Fink, G. (2018). Biological reductionism versus redundancy in a degenerate world. *Perspectives in Biology and Medicine, 61*, 517–526.

Kaipparettu, B. A., Ma, Y., Park, J. H., Lee, T. L., Zhang, Y., Yotnda, P., Creighton, C. J., Chan, W. Y., & Wong, L. J. (2013). Crosstalk from non-cancerous mitochondria can inhibit tumor properties of metastatic cells by suppressing oncogenic pathways. *PLOS ONE, 8*, Article e61747.

Kamp, D. W., Shacter, E., & Weitzman, S. A. (2011). Chronic inflammation and cancer: The role of the mitochondria. *Oncology (Williston Park), 25*, 400–410, 413.

Kiebish, M. A., Han, X., Cheng, H., Chuang, J. H., & Seyfried, T. N. (2008). Cardiolipin and electron transport chain abnormalities in mouse brain tumor mitochondria: Lipidomic evidence supporting the Warburg theory of cancer. *Journal of Lipid Research, 49*, 2545–2556.

Kiebish, M. A., & Seyfried, T. N. (2005). Absence of pathogenic mitochondrial DNA mutations in mouse brain tumors. *BMC Cancer, 5*, 102.

Klement, R. J. (2019). The emerging role of ketogenic diets in cancer treatment. *Current Opinion in Clinical Nutrition and Metabolic Care, 22*, 129–134.

Klement, R. J., & Sweeney, R. A. (2016). Impact of a ketogenic diet intervention during radiotherapy on body composition: I. Initial clinical experience with six prospectively studied patients. *BMC Research Notes, 9*, 143.

Knudson, A. G. (2002). Cancer genetics. *American Journal of Medical Genetics, 111*, 96–102.

Kopp, W. (2019). How Western diet and lifestyle drive the pandemic of obesity and civilization diseases. *Diabetes, Metabolic Syndrome and Obesity: Targets and Therapy, 12*, 2221–2236.

Koppenol, W. H., Bounds, P. L., & Dang, C. V. (2011). Otto Warburg's contributions to current concepts of cancer metabolism. *Nature Reviews Cancer, 11*, 325–337.

Kossoff, E. H., & Hartman, A. L. (2012). Ketogenic diets: new advances for metabolism-based therapies. *Current Opinion in Neurology, 25*, 173–178.

Kotler, D. P. (2000). Cachexia. *Annals of Internal Medicine, 133*, 622–634.

Kritchevsky, D. (2001). Caloric restriction and cancer. *Journal of Nutritional Science and Vitaminology, 47*, 13–19.

Lehninger, A. L. (1964). *The mitochondrion: Molecular basis of structure and function.* W. A. Benjamin.

Lowenstine, L. J., McManamon, R., & Terio, K. A. (2016). Comparative pathology of aging great apes: Bonobos, chimpanzees, gorillas, and orangutans. *Veterinary Pathology, 53*, 250–276.

Lv, M., Zhu, X., Wang, H., Wang, F., & Guan, W. (2014). Roles of caloric restriction, ketogenic diet and intermittent fasting during initiation, progression and metastasis of cancer in animal models: A systematic review and meta-analysis. *PLOS ONE, 9*, Article e115147.

Ma, Y., Bai, R. K., Trieu, R., & Wong, L. J. (2010). Mitochondrial dysfunction in human breast cancer cells and their transmitochondrial cybrids. *Biochimica et Biophysica Acta, 1797*, 29–37.

Magee, B. A., Potezny, N., Rofe, A. M., & Conyers, R. A. (1979). The inhibition of malignant cell growth by ketone bodies. *Australian Journal of Experimental Biology and Medical Science, 57*, 529–539.

Mahoney, L. B., Denny, C. A., & Seyfried, T. N. (2006). Caloric restriction in C57BL/6J mice mimics therapeutic fasting in humans. *Lipids in Health and Disease, 5*, 13.

Mantis, J. G., Centeno, N. A., Todorova, M. T., McGowan, R., & Seyfried, T. N. (2004). Management of multifactorial idiopathic epilepsy in EL mice with caloric restriction and the ketogenic diet: Role of glucose and ketone bodies. *Nutrition & Metabolism, 1*, 11.

Maroon, J. C., Seyfried, T. N., Donohue, J. P., & Bost, J. (2015). The role of metabolic therapy in treating glioblastoma multiforme. *Surgical Neurology International*, 6, 61.

Marsh, J., Mukherjee, P., & Seyfried, T. N. (2008). Drug/diet synergy for managing malignant astrocytoma in mice: 2-Deoxy-D-glucose and the restricted ketogenic diet. *Nutrition & Metabolism*, 5, 33.

Martincorena, I., & Campbell, P. J. (2015). Somatic mutation in cancer and normal cells. *Science*, 349, 1483–1489.

Martincorena, I., Fowler, J. C., Wabik, A., Lawson, A. R. J., Abascal, F., Hall, M. W. J., Cagan, A., Murai, K., Mahbubani, K., Stratton, M. R., Fitzgerald, R. C., Handford, P. A., Campbell, P. J., Saeb-Parsy, K., & Jones, P. H. (2018). Somatic mutant clones colonize the human esophagus with age. *Science*, 362, 911–917.

Martuscello, R. T., Vedam-Mai, V., McCarthy, D. J., Schmoll, M. E., Jundi, M. A., Louviere, C. D., Griffith, B. G., Skinner, C. L., Suslov, O., Deleyrolle, L. P., & Reynolds, B. A. (2016). A supplemented high-fat low-carbohydrate diet for the treatment of glioblastoma. *Clinical Cancer Research*, 22, 2482–2495.

Maurer, G. D., Brucker, D. P., Baehr, O., Harter, P. N., Hattingen, E., Walenta, S., Mueller-Klieser, W., Steinbach, J. P., & Rieger, J. (2011). Differential utilization of ketone bodies by neurons and glioma cell lines: A rationale for ketogenic diet as experimental glioma therapy. *BMC Cancer*, 11, 315.

Mavropoulos, J. C., Buschemeyer, W. C., III, Tewari, A. K., Rokhfeld, D., Pollak, M., Zhao, Y., Febbo, P. G., Cohen, P., Hwang, D., Devi, G., Demark-Wahnefried, W., Westman, E. C., Peterson, B. L., Pizzo, S. V., & Freeland, S. J. (2009). The effects of varying dietary carbohydrate and fat content on survival in a murine LNCaP prostate cancer xenograft model. *Cancer Prevention Research (Philadelphia, Pa.)*, 2, 557–565.

Mazurek, S., Boschek, C. B., Hugo, F., & Eigenbrodt, E. (2005). Pyruvate kinase type M2 and its role in tumor growth and spreading. *Seminars in Cancer Biology*, 15, 300–308.

McGinnis, A. D. (2019). On the origin of financial toxicity for cancer patients. *eScholarship@BC*, 1-26.

McGirt, M. J., Chaichana, K. L., Gathinji, M., Attenello, F., Than, K., Ruiz, A. J., Olivi, A., & Quinones-Hinojosa, A. (2008). Persistent outpatient hyperglycemia is independently associated with decreased survival after primary resection of malignant brain astrocytomas. *Neurosurgery*, 63, 286–291.

McLeod, H. L. (2013). Cancer pharmacogenomics: Early promise, but concerted effort needed. *Science*, 339, 1563–1566.

Meidenbauer, J. J., Mukherjee, P., & Seyfried, T. N. (2015). The glucose ketone index calculator: A simple tool to monitor therapeutic efficacy for metabolic management of brain cancer. *Nutrition & Metabolism*, 12, 12.

Meidenbauer, J. J., Ta, N., & Seyfried, T. N. (2014). Influence of a ketogenic diet, fish-oil, and calorie restriction on plasma metabolites and lipids in C57BL/6J mice. *Nutrition & Metabolism*, 11, 23.

Meyerhardt, J. A., Sato, K., Niedzwiecki, D., Ye, C., Saltz, L. B., Mayer, R. J., Mowat, R. B., Whittom, R., Hantel, A., Benson, A., Wigler, D. S., Venook, A., & Fuchs, C. S. (2012). Dietary glycemic load and cancer recurrence and survival in patients with stage III colon cancer: Findings from CALGB 89803. *Journal of the National Cancer Institute*, 104, 1702–1711.

Moreno-Sanchez, R., Rodriguez-Enriquez, S., Marin-Hernandez, A., & Saavedra, E. (2007). Energy metabolism in tumor cells. *FEBS Journal*, 274, 1393–1418.

Morscher, R. J., Aminzadeh-Gohari, S., Feichtinger, R. G., Mayr, J. A., Lang, R., Neureiter, D., Sperl, W., & Kofler, B. (2015). Inhibition of neuroblastoma tumor growth by ketogenic diet and/or calorie restriction in a CD1-Nu mouse model. *PLOS ONE*, 10, Article e0129802.

Mukherjee, P., Augur, Z. M., Li, M., Hill, C., Greenwood, B., Domin, M. A., Kondakci, G., Narain, N. R., Kiebish, M. A., Bronson, R. T., Arismendi-Morillo, G., Chinopoulos, C., & Seyfried, T. N. (2019). Therapeutic benefit of combining calorie-restricted ketogenic diet and glutamine targeting in late-stage experimental glioblastoma. *Communications Biology*, 2, 200.

Mukherjee, P., Sotnikov, A. V., Mangian, H. J., Zhou, J. R., Visek, W. J., & Clinton, S. K. (1999). Energy intake and prostate tumor growth, angiogenesis, and vascular endothelial growth factor expression. *Journal of the National Cancer Institute*, 91, 512–523.

Mulrooney, T. J., Marsh, J., Urits, I., Seyfried, T. N., & Mukherjee, P. (2011). Influence of caloric restriction on constitutive expression of NF-kappaB in an experimental mouse astrocytoma. *PLOS ONE*, 6, Article e18085.

Nebeling, L. C., Miraldi, F., Shurin, S. B., & Lerner, E. (1995). Effects of a ketogenic diet on tumor metabolism and nutritional status in pediatric oncology patients: Two case reports. *Journal of the American College of Nutrition*, 14, 202–208.

Panhans, C. M., Gresham, G., Amaral, J. L., & Hu, J. (2020). Exploring the feasibility and effects of a ketogenic diet in patients with CNS malignancies: A retrospective case series. *Frontiers in Neuroscience*, 14, 390.

Parsons, D. W., Jones, S., Zhang, X., Lin, J. C., Leary, R. J., Angenendt, P., Mankoo, P., Carter, H., Siu, I. M., Gallia, G. L., Olivi, A., McLendon, R., Rasheed, B. A., Keir, S., Nikolskaya, T., Nikolsky, Y., Busam, D. A., Tekleab, H., Diaz, L. A., Jr., . .

. Kinzler, K. W. (2008). An integrated genomic analysis of human glioblastoma multiforme. *Science, 321*, 1807–1812.

Pedersen, P. L. (1978). Tumor mitochondria and the bioenergetics of cancer cells. *Progress in Experimental Tumor Research, 22*, 190–274.

Phillips, M. C. L., Murtagh, D. K. J., Sinha, S. K., & Moon, B. G. (2020). Managing metastatic thymoma with metabolic and medical therapy: A case report. *Frontiers in Oncology, 10*, 578.

Pitot, H. C. (1966). Some biochemical aspects of malignancy. *Annual Review of Biochemistry, 35*, 335–368.

Poff, A. M., Ari, C., Seyfried, T. N., & D'Agostino, D. P. (2013). The ketogenic diet and hyperbaric oxygen therapy prolong survival in mice with systemic metastatic cancer. *PLOS ONE, 8*, Article e65522.

Poff, A. M., Ward, N., Seyfried, T. N., Arnold, P., & D'Agostino, D. P. (2015). Non-toxic metabolic management of metastatic cancer in VM mice: Novel combination of ketogenic diet, ketone supplementation, and hyperbaric oxygen therapy. *PLOS ONE, 10*, Article e0127407.

Poljsak, B., Kovac, V., Dahmane, R., Levec, T., & Starc, A. (2019). Cancer etiology: A metabolic disease originating from life's major evolutionary transition? *Oxidative Medicine and Cellular Longevity, 2019*, 7831952.

Poteet, E., Choudhury, G. R., Winters, A., Li, W., Ryou, M. G., Liu, R., Tang, L., Ghorpade, A., Wen, Y., Yuan, F., Keir, S. T., Yan, H., Bigner, D. D., Simpkins, J. W., & Yang, S. H. (2013). Reversing the Warburg effect as a treatment for glioblastoma. *Journal of Biological Chemistry, 288*, 9153–9164.

Prager, G. W., Braga, S., Bystricky, B., Qvortrup, C., Criscitiello, C., Esin, E., Sonke, G. S., Martinez, G. A., Frenel, J. S., Karamouzis, M., Strijbos, M., Yazici, O., Bossi, P., Banerjee, S., Troiani, T., Eniu, A., Ciardiello, F., Tabernero, J., Zielinski, C. C., . . . Ilbawi, A. (2018). Global cancer control: responding to the growing burden, rising costs and inequalities in access. *ESMO Open, 3*, Article e000285.

Puente, X. S., Velasco, G., Gutierrez-Fernandez, A., Bertranpetit, J., King, M. C., & Lopez-Otin, C. (2006). Comparative analysis of cancer genes in the human and chimpanzee genomes. *BMC Genomics, 7*, 15.

Putignani, L., Raffa, S., Pescosolido, R., Rizza, T., Del Chierico, F., Leone, L., Aimati, L., Signore, F., Carrozzo, R., Callea, F., Torrisi, M. R., & Grammatico, P. (2012). Preliminary evidences on mitochondrial injury and impaired oxidative metabolism in breast cancer. *Mitochondrion, 12*, 363–369.

Raffaghello, L., Lee, C., Safdie, F. M., Wei, M., Madia, F., Bianchi, G., & Longo, V. D. (2008). Starvation-dependent differential stress resistance protects normal but not cancer cells against high-dose chemotherapy. *Proceedings of the National Academy of Sciences of the United States of America, 105*, 8215–8220.

Rieger, J., Bahr, O., Maurer, G. D., Hattingen, E., Franz, K., Brucker, D., Walenta, S., Kammerer, U., Coy, J. F., Weller, M., & Steinbach, J. P. (2014). ERGO: A pilot study of ketogenic diet in recurrent glioblastoma. *International Journal of Oncology, 44*, 1843–1852.

Roskelley, R. C., Mayer, N., Horwitt, B. N., & Salter, W. T. (1943). Studies in cancer. VII. Enzyme deficiency in human and experimental cancer. *Journal of Clinical Investigation, 22*, 743–751.

Rous, P. (1959). Surmise and fact on the nature of cancer. *Nature, 183*, 1357–1361.

Samudio, I., Fiegl, M., & Andreeff, M. (2009). Mitochondrial uncoupling and the Warburg effect: Molecular basis for the reprogramming of cancer cell metabolism. *Cancer Research, 69*, 2163–2166.

Sawai, M., Yashiro, M., Nishiguchi, Y., Ohira, M., & Hirakawa, K. (2004). Growth-inhibitory effects of the ketone body, monoacetoacetin, on human gastric cancer cells with succinyl-CoA:3-oxoacid CoA-transferase (SCOT) deficiency. *Anticancer Research, 24*, 2213–2217.

Schmidt, M., Pfetzer, N., Schwab, M., Strauss, I., & Kammerer, U. (2011). Effects of a ketogenic diet on the quality of life in 16 patients with advanced cancer: A pilot trial. *Nutrition & Metabolism, 8*, 54.

Schwartz, K., Chang, H. T., Nikolai, M., Pernicone, J., Rhee, S., Olson, K., Kurniali, P. C., Hord, N. G., & Noel, M. (2015). Treatment of glioma patients with ketogenic diets: Report of two cases treated with an IRB-approved energy-restricted ketogenic diet protocol and review of the literature. *Cancer & Metabolism, 3*, 3.

Schwartz, K. A., Noel, M., Nikolai, M., & Chang, H. T. (2018). Investigating the ketogenic diet as treatment for primary aggressive brain cancer: Challenges and lessons learned. *Frontiers in Nutrition, 5*, 11.

Seeger, P. G. (1959). Cell respiration and cancer. *Das Deutsche Gesundheitswesen, 14*, 893–898.

Selak, M. A., Armour, S. M., MacKenzie, E. D., Boulahbel, H., Watson, D. G., Mansfield, K. D., Pan, Y., Simon, M. C., Thompson, C. B., & Gottlieb, E. (2005). Succinate links TCA cycle dysfunction to oncogenesis by inhibiting HIF-alpha prolyl hydroxylase. *Cancer Cell, 7*, 77–85.

Semenza, G. L. (2017). Hypoxia-inducible factors: Coupling glucose metabolism and redox regulation with induction of the breast cancer stem cell phenotype. *EMBO Journal, 36*, 252–259.

Seyfried, T. N. (2012a). *Cancer as a metabolic disease: On the origin, management, and prevention of cancer.* John Wiley & Sons.

Seyfried, T. N. (2012b). Cancer prevention. Chapter 19. In *Cancer as a metabolic disease: On the origin, management, and prevention of cancer* (pp. 375–386). John Wiley & Sons.

Seyfried, T. N. (2012c). Mitochondria: The ultimate tumor suppressor. Chapter 11. In *Cancer as a metabolic disease: On the origin, management, and prevention of cancer* (pp. 195–205). John Wiley & Sons.

Seyfried, T. N. (2012d). Mitochondrial respiratory dysfunction and the extrachromosomal origin of cancer. Chapter 14. In *Cancer as a metabolic disease: On the origin, management, and prevention of cancer* (pp. 253–259). John Wiley & Sons.

Seyfried, T. N. (2014). Ketone strong: Emerging evidence for a therapeutic role of ketone bodies in neurological and neurodegenerative diseases. *Journal of Lipid Research, 55*, 1815–1817.

Seyfried, T. N. (2015). Cancer as a mitochondrial metabolic disease. *Frontiers in Cell and Developmental Biology, 3*, 43.

Seyfried, T. N., Arismendi-Morillo, G., Mukherjee, P., & Chinopoulos, C. (2020a). On the origin of ATP synthesis in cancer. *iScience, 23*, 101761.

Seyfried, T. N., Flores, R. E., Poff, A. M., & D'Agostino, D. P. (2014). Cancer as a metabolic disease: Implications for novel therapeutics. *Carcinogenesis, 35*, 515–527.

Seyfried, T. N., Mantis, J. G., Todorova, M. T., & Greene, A. E. (2009). Dietary management of epilepsy: Role of glucose and ketone bodies. In P. A. Schwartzkroin (Ed.), *Encyclopedia of basic epilepsy research*, Vol. 2 (pp. 687–693). Academic Press.

Seyfried, T. N., & Mukherjee, P. (2005). Targeting energy metabolism in brain cancer: Review and hypothesis. *Nutrition & Metabolism, 2*, 30.

Seyfried, T. N., Mukherjee, P., Iyikesici, M. S., Slocum, A., Kalamian, M., Spinosa, J. P., & Chinopoulos, C. (2020b). Consideration of ketogenic metabolic therapy as a complementary or alternative approach for managing breast cancer. *Frontiers in Nutrition, 7*, 21.

Seyfried, T. N., Sanderson, T. M., El-Abbadi, M. M., McGowan, R., & Mukherjee, P. (2003). Role of glucose and ketone bodies in the metabolic control of experimental brain cancer. *British Journal of Cancer, 89*, 1375–1382.

Seyfried, T. N., Shelton, L., Arismendi-Morillo, G., Kalamian, M., Elsakka, A., Maroon, J., & Mukherjee, P. (2019). Provocative question: Should ketogenic metabolic therapy become the standard of care for glioblastoma? *Neurochemical Research, 44*, 2392–2404.

Seyfried, T. N., & Shelton, L. M. (2010). Cancer as a metabolic disease. *Nutrition & Metabolism, 7*, 7.

Seyfried, T. N., Yu, G., Maroon, J. C., & D'Agostino, D. P. (2017). Press-pulse: A novel therapeutic strategy for the metabolic management of cancer. *Nutrition & Metabolism, 14*, 19.

Shelton, L. M., Huysentruyt, L. C., Mukherjee, P., & Seyfried, T. N. (2010). Calorie restriction as an anti-invasive therapy for malignant brain cancer in the VM mouse. *ASN Neuro, 2*, e00038.

Shimazu, T., Hirschey, M. D., Newman, J., He, W., Shirakawa, K., Le Moan, N., Grueter, C. A., Lim, H., Saunders, L. R., Stevens, R. D., Newgard, C. B., Farese, R. V., Jr., de Cabo, R., Ulrich, S., Akassoglou, K., & Verdin, E. (2013). Suppression of oxidative stress by beta-hydroxybutyrate, an endogenous histone deacetylase inhibitor. *Science, 339*, 211–214.

Shin, S. H., Bode, A. M., & Dong, Z. (2017). Precision medicine: The foundation of future cancer therapeutics. *NPJ Precision Oncology, 1*, 12.

Siegel, R. L., Miller, K. D., & Jemal, A. (2019). Cancer statistics, 2019. *CA: A Cancer Journal for Clinicians, 69*, 7–34.

Singh, L., Nag, T. C., & Kashyap, S. (2015). Ultrastructural changes of mitochondria in human retinoblastoma: Correlation with tumor differentiation and invasiveness. *Tumour Biology, 37*(5), 5797–5803.

Skinner, R., Trujillo, A., Ma, X., & Beierle, E. A. (2009). Ketone bodies inhibit the viability of human neuroblastoma cells. *Journal of Pediatric Surgery, 44*, 212–216.

Song, Z., Rose, S., Safran, D. G., Landon, B. E., Day, M. P., & Chernew, M. E. (2014). Changes in health care spending and quality 4 years into global payment. *New England Journal of Medicine, 371*, 1704–1714.

Sonnenschein, C., & Soto, A. M. (2000). Somatic mutation theory of carcinogenesis: Why it should be dropped and replaced. *Molecular Carcinogenesis, 29*, 205–211.

Soto, A. M., & Sonnenschein, C. (2004). The somatic mutation theory of cancer: Growing problems with the paradigm? *Bioessays, 26*, 1097–1107.

Srinivasan, S., Guha, M., Dong, D. W., Whelan, K. A., Ruthel, G., Uchikado, Y., Natsugoe, S., Nakagawa, H., & Avadhani, N. G. (2016). Disruption of cytochrome c oxidase function induces the Warburg effect and metabolic reprogramming. *Oncogene, 35*, 1585–1595.

Stroud, D. A., & Ryan, M. T. (2013). Mitochondria: Organization of respiratory chain complexes becomes cristae-lized. *Current Biology, 23*, R969–971.

Sun, C., Liu, X., Wang, B., Wang, Z., Liu, Y., Di, C., Si, J., Li, H., Wu, Q., Xu, D., Li, J., Li, G., Wang, Y., Wang, F., & Zhang, H. (2019). Endocytosis-mediated mitochondrial transplantation: Transferring normal human astrocytic mitochondria into glioma cells rescues aerobic respiration and enhances radiosensitivity. *Theranostics, 9*, 3595–3607.

Szent-Gyorgyi, A. (1977). The living state and cancer. *Proceedings of the National Academy of Sciences of the United States of America, 74*, 2844–2847.

Tannahill, G. M., Curtis, A. M., Adamik, J., Palsson-McDermott, E. M., McGettrick, A. F., Goel, G., Frezza, C., Bernard, N. J., Kelly, B., Foley, N. H., Zheng, L., Gardet, A., Tong, Z., Jany, S. S., Corr, S. C., Haneklaus, M., Caffrey, B. E., Pierce, K., Walmsley, S., . . . O'Neill, L. A. (2013). Succinate is an inflammatory signal that induces IL-1beta through HIF-1alpha. *Nature, 496*, 238–242.

Tannenbaum, A. (1942). The genesis and growth of tumors: II. Effects of caloric restriction per se. *Cancer Research, 2*, 460–467.

Terpstra, A. H. (2001). Differences between humans and mice in efficacy of the body fat lowering effect of conjugated linoleic acid: Role of metabolic rate. *Journal of Nutrition, 131*, 2067–2068.

Thompson, H. J., McGinley, J. N., Spoelstra, N. S., Jiang, W., Zhu, Z., & Wolfe, P. (2004). Effect of dietary energy restriction on vascular density during mammary carcinogenesis. *Cancer Research, 64*, 5643–5650.

Tisdale, M. J. (1984). Role of acetoacetyl-CoA synthetase in acetoacetate utilization by tumor cells. *Cancer Biochemistry Biophysics, 7*, 101–107.

Tomasetti, C., & Vogelstein, B. (2015). Cancer etiology: Variation in cancer risk among tissues can be explained by the number of stem cell divisions. *Science, 347*, 78–81.

Vallejo, F. A., Shah, S. S., de Cordoba, N., Walters, W. M., Prince, J., Khatib, Z., Komotar, R. J., Vanni, S., & Graham, R. M. (2020). The contribution of ketone bodies to glycolytic inhibition for the treatment of adult and pediatric glioblastoma. *Journal of Neuro-Oncology, 147*, 317–326.

Vander Heiden, M. G. (2010). Targeting cell metabolism in cancer patients. *Science Translational Medicine, 2*, 31ed31.

Varki, N. M., & Varki, A. (2015). On the apparent rarity of epithelial cancers in captive chimpanzees. *Philosophical Transactions of the Royal Society B: Biological Sciences, 370*, 1–7.

Vaux, D. L. (2011). In defense of the somatic mutation theory of cancer. *Bioessays, 33*, 341–343.

Veech, R. L. (2004). The therapeutic implications of ketone bodies: The effects of ketone bodies in pathological conditions; Ketosis, ketogenic diet, redox states, insulin resistance, and mitochondrial metabolism. *Prostaglandins, Leukotrienes and Essential Fatty Acids, 70*, 309–319.

Veech, R. L., Todd King, M., Pawlosky, R., Kashiwaya, Y., Bradshaw, P. C., & Curtis, W. (2019). The "great" controlling nucleotide coenzymes. *IUBMB Life, 71*, 1–15.

Verschoor, M. L., Ungard, R., Harbottle, A., Jakupciak, J. P., Parr, R. L., & Singh, G. (2013). Mitochondria and cancer: Past, present, and future. *BioMed Research International, 2013*, 612369.

Vogelstein, B., Papadopoulos, N., Velculescu, V. E., Zhou, S., Diaz, L. A., Jr., & Kinzler, K. W. (2013). Cancer genome landscapes. *Science, 339*, 1546–1558.

Vozza, A., Parisi, G., De Leonardis, F., Lasorsa, F. M., Castegna, A., Amorese, D., Marmo, R., Calcagnile, V. M., Palmieri, L., Ricquier, D., Paradies, E., Scarcia, P., Palmieri, F., Bouillaud, F., & Fiermonte, G. (2014). UCP2 transports C4 metabolites out of mitochondria, regulating glucose and glutamine oxidation. *Proceedings of the National Academy of Sciences of the United States of America, 111*, 960–965.

Warburg, O. (1931). *The metabolism of tumours.* Richard R. Smith Inc.

Warburg, O. (1956a). On the origin of cancer cells. *Science, 123*, 309–314.

Warburg, O. (1956b). On the respiratory impairment in cancer cells. *Science, 124*, 269–270.

Warburg, O. (1969). Revised Lindau Lectures: The prime cause of cancer and prevention—Parts 1 & 2. In D. Burk (Ed.), Meeting of the Nobel-Laureates (pp. 1–9). K. Triltsch.

Weber, D. D., Aminzadeh-Gohari, S., Tulipan, J., Catalano, L., Feichtinger, R. G., & Kofler, B. (2019). Ketogenic diet in the treatment of cancer—Where do we stand? *Molecular Metabolism, 33*, 102–121.

Weller, M., & Le Rhun, E. (2019). Immunotherapy for glioblastoma: Quo vadis? *Nature Reviews Clinical Oncology, 16*, 405–406.

Winter, S. F., Loebel, F., & Dietrich, J. (2017). Role of ketogenic metabolic therapy in malignant glioma: A systematic review. *Critical Reviews in Oncology/Hematology, 112*, 41–58.

Wishart, D. S. (2015). Is cancer a genetic disease or a metabolic disease? *EBioMedicine, 2*, 478–479.

Wong, E. T., Lok, E., Gautam, S., & Swanson, K. D. (2015). Dexamethasone exerts profound immunologic interference on treatment efficacy for recurrent glioblastoma. *British Journal of Cancer, 113*, 232–241.

Woods, M. W., & du Buy, H. G. (1945). Cytoplasmic diseases and cancer. *Science, 102*, 591–593.

Woolf, E. C., Curley, K. L., Liu, Q., Turner, G. H., Charlton, J. A., Preul, M. C., & Scheck, A. C. (2015). The ketogenic diet alters the hypoxic response and affects expression of proteins associated with angiogenesis, invasive potential and vascular permeability in a mouse glioma model. *PLOS ONE, 10*, Article e0130357.

Xu, R. H., Pelicano, H., Zhou, Y., Carew, J. S., Feng, L., Bhalla, K. N., Keating, M. J., & Huang, P. (2005). Inhibition of glycolysis in cancer cells: A novel strategy to overcome drug resistance associated with mitochondrial respiratory defect and hypoxia. *Cancer Research, 65*, 613–621.

Yizhak, K., Aguet, F., Kim, J., Hess, J. M., Kubler, K., Grimsby, J., Frazer, R., Zhang, H., Haradhvala,

N. J., Rosebrock, D., Livitz, D., Li, X., Arich-Landkof, E., Shoresh, N., Stewart, C., Segre, A. V., Branton, P. A., Polak, P., Ardlie, K. G., & Getz, G. (2019). RNA sequence analysis reveals macroscopic somatic clonal expansion across normal tissues. *Science, 364.*

Yokoyama, A., Kakiuchi, N., Yoshizato, T., Nannya, Y., Suzuki, H., Takeuchi, Y., Shiozawa, Y., Sato, Y., Aoki, K., Kim, S. K., Fujii, Y., Yoshida, K., Kataoka, K., Nakagawa, M. M., Inoue, Y., Hirano, T., Shiraishi, Y., Chiba, K., Tanaka, H., . . . Ogawa, S. (2019). Age-related remodelling of oesophageal epithelia by mutated cancer drivers. *Nature, 565,* 312–317.

Youm, Y. H., Nguyen, K. Y., Grant, R. W., Goldberg, E. L., Bodogai, M., Kim, D., D'Agostino, D., Planavsky, N., Lupfer, C., Kanneganti, T. D., Kang, S., Horvath, T. L., Fahmy, T. M., Crawford, P. A., Biragyn, A., Alnemri, E., & Dixit, V. D. (2015). The ketone metabolite beta-hydroxy-butyrate blocks NLRP3 inflammasome-mediated inflammatory disease. *Nature Medicine, 21,* 263–269.

Yu, M., Chen, S., Hong, W., Gu, Y., Huang, B., Lin, Y., Zhou, Y., Jin, H., Deng, Y., Tu, L., Hou, B., & Jian, Z. (2019). Prognostic role of glycolysis for cancer outcome: Evidence from 86 studies. *Journal of Cancer Research and Clinical Oncology, 145,* 967–999.

Yuan, Y., Ju, Y. S., Kim, Y., Li, J., Wang, Y., Yoon, C. J., Yang, Y., Martincorena, I., Creighton, C. J., Weinstein, J. N., Xu, Y., Han, L., Kim, H. L., Nakagawa, H., Park, K., Campbell, P. J., Liang, H., & Pcawg Consortium. (2020). Comprehensive molecular characterization of mitochondrial genomes in human cancers. *Nature Genetics, 2*(3), 342–352. doi:10.1038/s41588-019-0557-x. Epub 2020 Feb 5.

Yuneva, M. (2008). Finding an "Achilles' heel" of cancer: The role of glucose and glutamine metabolism in the survival of transformed cells. *Cell Cycle, 7,* 2083–2089.

Zhou, W., Mukherjee, P., Kiebish, M. A., Markis, W. T., Mantis, J. G., & Seyfried, T. N. (2007). The calorically restricted ketogenic diet, an effective alternative therapy for malignant brain cancer. *Nutrition & Metabolism, 4,* 5.

Zhuang, Y., Chan, D. K., Haugrud, A. B., & Miskimins, W. K. (2014). Mechanisms by which low glucose enhances the cytotoxicity of metformin to cancer cells both in vitro and in vivo. *PLOS ONE, 9,* Article e108444.

Zuccoli, G., Marcello, N., Pisanello, A., Servadei, F., Vaccaro, S., Mukherjee, P., & Seyfried, T. N. (2010). Metabolic management of glioblastoma multiforme using standard therapy together with a restricted ketogenic diet: Case report. *Nutrition & Metabolism, 7,* 33.

Ketogenic Diet as Adjunctive Therapy for Malignant Brain Cancer

ADRIENNE C. SCHECK, PHD AND NELOFER SYED, PHD

INTRODUCTION

Human malignant glioma is a uniformly fatal disease, in part due to the limitations of currently available treatments, which include surgery, chemotherapy, and radiation therapy. The average survival of patients with glioblastoma multiforme (GBM) is 1.5 years. Therefore, it is of paramount importance that new therapeutic strategies for brain cancer be developed, especially strategies that can enhance the efficacy of current treatment options without damaging normal brain tissue. Advances in our understanding of the biology of brain tumors have led to an increase in the number of targeted therapies in preclinical and clinical trials (Alexandru et al., 2020; Bi et al., 2020; Cahill et al., 2016; Chen et al., 2016; Gwak & Park, 2017; Miller & Wen, 2016; Mondesir et al., 2016; Rodríguez-Hernández et al., 2020; Ryall et al., 2020; Shahcheraghi et al., 2020; Wanigasooriya et al., 2020; Weathers & Gilbert, 2016; Yang et al., 2020). While these therapies may prove somewhat effective, the heterogeneity of brain tumors and their genomic instability often precludes the targeted molecules from being found on all cells in the tumor, thus reducing the efficacy of targeted treatments. In contrast, one trait shared by virtually all tumor cells is altered metabolism.

TUMOR METABOLISM

Alterations in the metabolism of cancer cells, what is called the Warburg effect or aerobic glycolysis, was first described by Otto Warburg in 1927 (Warburg et al., 1927). Cancer cells are capable of using glycolysis to provide energy and biomolecules regardless of the availability of oxygen. This results in the production of fewer ATP molecules per molecule of glucose, and thus tumor cells require large amounts of glucose. The shift toward increased glycolytic flux in the cytosol and away from the tricarboxylic acid cycle and

oxidative phosphorylation in the mitochondria can occur very early in tumorigenesis. This allows for rapid cell proliferation even under conditions of hypoxia and in the presence of dysfunctional mitochondria. Since Warburg's discovery, metabolism has been of interest in the cancer field, but for many years it was overshadowed by discoveries of oncogenes, tumor suppressor genes, growth factor pathways, molecular subtypes of cancers, etc. There is a resurgence of interest in metabolism as a central theme in cancer, and altered metabolism is known to be a hallmark of cancer (Cantor & Sabatini, 2012; Hanahan & Weinberg, 2011; Ward & Thompson, 2012) in addition to being involved in virtually all of the cancer hallmarks described in the seminal paper by Hanahan and Weinberg (Hanahan & Weinberg, 2011; Lewis & Abdel-Haleem, 2013). We now know that metabolic pathways are inexorably intertwined with key components of tumor initiation, progression, and therapy response (Bi et al., 2020; Masui et al., 2015, 2016, 2019; Nijsten & van Dam, 2009; Venneti & Mischel, 2015; Wolf et al., 2010). For example, the tumor suppressor protein p53, which has long been known to play a pivotal role in the cellular responses to hypoxia, DNA damage, and oncogene activation, is now known to participate in modulation of anabolic and catabolic pathways to maintain cell survival under conditions of metabolic stress (Alexandru et al., 2020; Barker et al., 2020; Bi et al., 2020; Cahill et al., 2016; Chen et al., 2016; Gwak & Park, 2017; Kung et al., 2017; Labuschagne et al., 2018; Miller & Wen, 2016; Mondesir et al., 2016; Rodríguez-Hernández et al., 2020; Ryall et al., 2020; Weathers & Gilbert, 2016). It has been shown to regulate glycolysis and assist in maintaining mitochondrial integrity (Branco et al., 2016; Puzio-Kuter, 2011) and to regulate lipid metabolism (Parrales & Iwakuma, 2016), as well as helping cells adapt to depletion of a variety of nutrients, including glucose (Faubert et al., 2015; Jones et al., 2005; Khan et al., 2017; Mai et al., 2017), glutamine (Reid et al., 2013), and some amino acids, such as serine (Ou et al., 2015).

The term *metabolic remodeling* has been used to describe the far-reaching metabolic changes that can occur in cancer cells (Lorito et al., 2020; Masui et al., 2019; Obre & Rossignol, 2015), perhaps due to our increased knowledge of the complexity of alterations that can occur. The metabolic alterations found in cancer involve a great deal more than just the Warburg effect, and cancer cells increase their intracellular stores of macromolecules, such as lipids, amino acids, and nucleotides, through a variety of mechanisms (Bi et al., 2020; Masui et al., 2015, 2019, 2020; Venneti & Mischel, 2015). Perhaps more importantly, metabolic remodeling is an adaptive process wherein the cancer cell not only demonstrates altered metabolism due to its own genetics, but also adapts to nutrient availability and other signals from the cell's microenvironment (Badr et al., 2020; Costa et al., 2014; Jing et al., 2019; Jung & Le, 2018; Justus et al., 2015; Läsche et al., 2020; McLaughlin et al., 2020; Moldogazieva et al., 2020; Molon et al., 2016; Peck & Schulze, 2019; Scanlon & Glazer, 2015; Syn et al., 2016). This may include adjacent tumor cells with a different genetic profile due to tumor heterogeneity, or interactions with neighboring or infiltrating normal cells. Thus, when looking at altered metabolism in gliomas, particularly with regards to its use as a target for therapeutic intervention, it may also be useful to look not only at the genetics of the tumor, but also at the individual's metabolism, the nutrigenomic profile, and the metabolic profile of adjacent normal tissue, since this affects the tumor's microenvironment and may provide additional therapeutic targets (Le Rhun et al., 2019). In fact, Gargini et al. (2020) even suggested that classification of gliomas should include characterization of the microenvironment. Just as advances in our ability to study aberrant gene sequence and expression led to increased understanding of the tumor's genetic profile and potential therapeutic targets, we are now seeing improvements in the tools available to study glioma metabolism, both in vitro and in vivo. Metabolomics provides information on not only the steady-state levels of macromolecules and metabolites, but also metabolite flux, through the use of radiolabeled compounds. Positron emission tomography (PET) and magnetic resonance spectroscopy (MRS) allow non-invasive imaging of tumor metabolism and of surrounding normal brain in preclinical models

and in patients (Berrington et al., 2019). Indeed, we can now even use genomic profiling to interrogate an individual's normal genetics with respect to nutritional response. The clinical utility of these types of data is rapidly expanding (Bordoni & Gabbianelli, 2019). An in-depth discussion of glioma metabolism and effects of the microenvironment is beyond the scope of this chapter and can be found in excellent reviews (Bader et al., 2020; Baltazar et al., 2020; Bi et al., 2020; Casey et al., 2015; Coleman et al., 2020; Costa et al., 2014; Desbats et al., 2020; Giannone et al., 2020; Jing et al., 2019; Jung & Le, 2018; Justus et al., 2015; Larionova et al., 2020; Läsche et al., 2020; Lee & Griffiths, 2020; Li et al., 2016; Marchiq & Pouyssegur, 2016; Masui et al., 2020; McLaughlin et al., 2020; Nazemi & Rainero, 2020; Ordway et al., 2020; Ramalho et al., 2020; Sanegre et al., 2020; Turdo et al., 2020). This chapter focuses on aspects of glioma metabolism that may be affected by therapeutic ketosis, particularly as it relates to glioma therapy.

MOLECULAR ALTERATIONS IN GLIOMA CELLS AND THERAPEUTIC VULNERABILITIES

Amplification and/or gain of function of receptor tyrosine kinase receptors, such as epidermal growth factor receptor (EGFR) and the alpha subunit of platelet-derived growth factor (PDGFRα), as well as mutations in components of these signaling pathways, such as PI3K and PTEN (phosphatase and tensin homolog), are common in gliomas (Alexandru et al., 2020; Delgado-López et al., 2020; Duchatel et al., 2019; Sun et al., 2020). In fact, approximately 50% of gliomas have amplification and/or an activating mutation of EGFR. We now know that these growth factor pathways are intertwined with metabolic signaling pathways (Courtnay et al., 2015; Dibble & Cantley, 2015; Iurlaro et al., 2014; Kinnaird & Michelakis, 2015; Moldogazieva et al., 2020; Nadeem Abbas et al., 2019; Paddock et al., 2019; Poli & Camporeale, 2015; Rizzo et al., 2016; Roberts & Miyamoto, 2015; Seystahl et al., 2016; Stine et al., 2015; Tan et al., 2016). Activation of these pathways leads to activation of the PI3K/AKT/mTOR signaling pathway, which has been closely linked to metabolism. This also causes a number of downstream effects, including enhanced utilization of glucose and acetate, enhanced lipogenesis, MYC activation, and epigenetic reprogramming, to name a few (Bi et al., 2020; Gozzelino et al., 2020;

Masui et al., 2019, 2020; Shahcheraghi et al., 2020; Wanigasooriya et al., 2020).

One of the most important effects is overexpression of MYC, because it acts as a "hub" for metabolic reprogramming (Bi et al., 2020; Dong et al., 2020; Duffy & Crown, 2020; Yoshida, 2020). Overexpression of MYC occurs in a wide variety of cancers, and c-MYC is amplified in subgroup 3 medulloblastomas, the most aggressive of the four subgroups (Lhermitte et al., 2018; Menyhárt et al., 2019). MYC is a multifunctional transcription factor, and the list of its target genes includes those involved in both cell proliferation and cell metabolism (Miller et al., 2012). In addition to stimulating glycolysis, c-MYC has been found to activate glutaminolysis (Munksgaard Thorén et al., 2017) and lipid synthesis (Guo et al., 2014) from citrate (Obre & Rossignol, 2015). It increases intratumoral glutamine in GBMs and is involved in NAD^+ biosynthesis (Bi et al., 2020). Another important "hub" linking metabolism and cancer is hypoxia-inducible factor 1α (HIF-1α; Bacigalupa & Rathmell, 2020; Chakraborty, 2020; Fuchs et al., 2020; Ghoneum et al., 2020; Moldogazieva et al., 2020; Nagao et al., 2019; Shen et al., 2020; Wang et al., 2020a). HIF-1α expression is activated by hypoxia, which is typically found in high-grade gliomas and other cancers. HIF-1α is a heterodimeric transcription factor that induces the transcription of a variety of genes involved in angiogenesis (vascular endothelial growth factor [VEGF] and other cytokines) in an attempt to improve tissue perfusion. This results in the formation of abnormal blood vessels that can increase inflammation and edema in brain tumors, as well as induction of the transcription of a variety of genes that promote invasion, migration, and tumor growth (Fischer et al., 2002; Fujiwara et al., 2007; Hayashi et al., 2007; Horing et al., 2012; Justus et al., 2015; Kaur et al., 2005; Masson & Ratcliffe, 2014; Mou et al., 2010; Proescholdt et al., 2012; Yang et al., 2012). In addition to specific actions that relate to the tumor cell's response to oxygen availability, HIF-1α interacts with the PI3K/AKT signaling path to act as a regulator of cancer metabolism, proliferation, and glycolysis (Courtnay et al., 2015; Justus et al., 2015; Pore et al., 2006; Wei et al., 2013). It also affects the activation of nuclear factor-κB (NF-κB), a transcriptional activator that is central to the regulation of various signal transduction pathways and to transcriptional activation events that mediate inflammation, cell proliferation, cell migration, and angiogenesis. HIF-1α may, at least in part, provide the molecular basis

for the Warburg effect by "reprogramming" cellular metabolism in response to oxygen availability (Corbet & Feron, 2015; Courtnay et al., 2015). HIF-1α also is a central figure in alterations to the tumor microenvironment, which affect not only tumor cell growth, but also response to therapy (Amberger-Murphy, 2009; Azzi et al., 2013; Bayley & Devilee, 2010; Bruzzese et al., 2014; Casey et al., 2015; Danhier et al., 2013; Dewhirst, 2009; Hattingen et al., 2011; Horing et al., 2012; Hu et al., 2011; Jing et al., 2019; Joon et al., 2004; Justus et al., 2015; Marie & Shinjo, 2011; Masson & Ratcliffe, 2014; Metallo et al., 2011; Semenza, 2013; Shweiki et al., 1995; Stegeman et al., 2014; Wei et al., 2011; Yamada et al., 1999; Yang et al., 2012).

The molecular background of a tumor cell can also affect the regulation of the pathways described above. Loss of function of PTEN enhances proliferation and increases glycolysis (Blouin et al., 2010). Mutation of PTEN and mutation of p53 also increase HIF-1α, as does the accumulation of reactive oxygen species (ROS). ROS are multifaceted effector molecules involved in numerous cellular pathways, including those regulating autophagic/apoptotic responses to genotoxic stress, hypoxia, and nutrient deprivation. Cancer cells often have increased levels of ROS (Fruehauf & Meyskens, 2007), and ROS have been implicated in angiogenesis induction and tumor growth through the regulation of VEGF and HIF-1α (Weinberg & Chandel, 2009).

When discussing the molecular alterations present in glioma one must go beyond genetics to include epigenetic alterations. Such alterations are common features of cancer, and it has been proposed that cancer is in fact a three-step process that starts with epigenetic alteration of stem cells followed by mutation in a gatekeeper gene, leading to genetic instability during tumor progression that is the basis of the epigenetic progenitor model (Feinberg et al., 2006). Epigenetic signatures are used to classify gliomas into subtypes in much the same way as genetic alterations (Gusyatiner & Hegi, 2018; Lee et al., 2018). Epigenetic mechanisms include DNA methylation, histone modification, nucleosome remodeling, and expression of noncoding RNAs. Such modifications are influenced by changes in metabolism, and the two are closely linked, where metabolic intermediates are utilized by components of the epigenetic machinery. Thus, changes in intracellular metabolism can alter the expression of epigenetic enzymes and confer widespread variations in epigenetic modification patterns (Venneti & Thompson, 2013). Metabolic remodeling by cancer cells can alter the epigenome to affect changes in tumor growth and therapy response, and conversely epigenetic changes can alter the tumor cell's response to metabolic alterations in the tumor microenvironment (Becker et al., 2020; Ciechomska et al., 2020; Dong & Cui, 2019; Larionova et al., 2020; Masui et al., 2019, 2020; Rodrigues et al., 2017; Venneti & Thompson, 2017). Genetic changes in the tumor can also play into this. For example, another link between metabolism, oncogenesis, and epigenetic alterations is seen in tumors with mutations of isocitrate dehydrogenase (IDH1 and IDH2). This occurs in 80% to 90% of low-grade gliomas. IDH1 and 2 are NADP$^+$-dependent enzymes that catalyze the conversion of isocitrate to α-ketoglutarate (αKG) in the cytosol and mitochondria, respectively. Mutant IDH causes the conversion of αKG to 2-hydroxyglutarate (2HG), which affects the activity of a number of αKG-dependent enzymes, ultimately affecting mTOR signaling, response to hypoxia, and epigenetic regulation. Thus, one of the downstream effects of this is aberrant DNA and histone methylation, and tumors with mutated IDH are said to have a CpG-island methylator phenotype (G-CIMP).

A burgeoning field linking metabolism and glioma growth and therapy is the study of the microbiome. The microbiome plays a role in the tumor microenvironment and alterations in tumor metabolism and therapeutic response, particularly in regard to immunotherapy. In preclinical studies using the GL261 mouse model of glioma, it has been shown that alterations in the intestinal microbiota can cause reduced cytotoxic natural killer (NK) cell subsets and altered expression of inflammatory and homeostatic proteins in microglia. Moreover, both mice and humans exhibit similar changes in the gut microbiome when fed a ketogenic diet (KD). Changes in the microbiome may even play a role in the proposed antidepressant effects of the KD (Ricci et al., 2020). Studies of the microbiome and ways to alter it to enhance therapeutic efficacy are a hot vein of current research (Chan, 2020; Giannone et al., 2020; Golonka et al., 2020; Huang et al., 2020; Inamura, 2021; Ke et al., 2020; Klement & Pazienza, 2019; Mehrian-Shai et al., 2019; Ramalho et al., 2020; Singh et al., 2020, 2021; Suraya et al., 2020).

It is clear that cancer cell metabolism is far more complex than originally thought. A number of cancer-associated mutations affect metabolism, and mitochondrial defects are seen in cancer that also link metabolism with cancer initiation and progression. Although some of these interactions are mentioned above, in-depth discussion of all of the interactions that occur between cancer and metabolism is beyond the scope of this chapter, and the reader is referred to reviews on these subjects (Badr et al., 2020; Bi et al., 2020; Cantor & Sabatini, 2012; Cassim et al., 2020; Faubert et al., 2020; Gatenby & Gillies, 2004; Gaude & Frezza, 2014; Gray et al., 2020; Kanarek et al., 2020; Kang, 2020; Larionova et al., 2020; Läsche et al., 2020; Masson & Ratcliffe, 2014; Masui et al., 2020; Moldogazieva et al., 2020; Nazemi & Rainero, 2020; Obara-Michlewska & Szeliga, 2020; Pavlova & Thompson, 2016; Ramalho et al., 2020; Robey et al., 2015; Semenza, 2013; Shingler et al., 2019; Tajan & Vousden, 2020; Turdo et al., 2020; Vander Heiden et al., 2009; Ward & Thompson, 2012; Zam et al., 2021; Zou et al., 2020). The fact that metabolic dysregulation is seen in virtually all tumor cells has led to suggestions that a promising therapeutic strategy may be to exploit this feature. One potential way to achieve this goal is through the use of the therapeutic KD or physiologically similar methods, such as caloric restriction (CR) or intermittent fasting.

THE KD

The KD is more correctly referred to as "metabolic therapy" rather than a "diet." This high-fat, low-carbohydrate, adequate-protein regimen is used to treat medically refractory epilepsy in children, and more recently in some adults (Cross, 2013; Kim & Rho, 2008). The KD is not without side effects; however, these are typically readily managed when the patient has appropriate supervision by a multidisciplinary team (i.e., dietitian, nurse, and physician) skilled in its use. The KD has been shown to have neuroprotective effects and there are now studies to determine its efficacy for several neurologic disorders, including Alzheimer's disease, traumatic brain injury, autism, and amyotrophic lateral sclerosis, to name a few (deCampo & Kossoff, 2019; Hartman & Patel, 2020; Kraeuter et al., 2020; Maalouf et al., 2009; Stafstrom & Rho, 2012).

The original hypothesis regarding the use of a KD for glioma was that the reduction in glucose that results from the KD would essentially "starve" the tumor cells and thus inhibit their growth (Baranano & Hartman, 2008; Bozzetti & Zupec-Kania, 2016; Freedland et al., 2008; Klement, 2013; Maroon et al., 2015; Seyfried et al., 2009, 2015; Simone et al., 2013; Wallace et al., 2010). The KD increases blood ketones and decreases blood glucose by simulating the physiologic response to fasting, thus leading to high rates of fatty acid oxidation and an increase in the production of acetyl coenzyme A (acetyl-CoA). When the amount of acetyl-CoA exceeds the capacity of the tricarboxylic acid cycle to utilize it, there is an increase in the production of the ketone bodies β-hydroxybutyrate (βHB) and acetoacetate (ACA), which can be used as an energy source in the normal brain (Cahill & Veech, 2003; Gasior et al., 2006; Morris, 2005; Vanitallie & Nufert, 2003; Veech et al., 2001). Since normal cells readily use ketones as an alternate energy source, they are unlikely to be adversely affected by reduced glucose. In contrast, the metabolic alterations found in cancer cells are generally thought to reduce their ability to be "flexible" regarding their primary energy source, and therefore they typically require glucose (Fredericks & Ramsey, 1978; Maurer et al., 2011; Seyfried, 2012; Seyfried et al., 2011; Seyfried & Mukherjee, 2005; Tisdale & Brennan, 1983; Zhou et al., 2007). Thus, when used as a therapy, the KD can take advantage of the Warburg effect. We now know that glioma cells are not limited strictly to glucose as an energy source (Bi et al., 2020; Masui et al., 2019; Tanaka et al., 2015); however, the KD can still be an effective adjuvant therapy, as the effects of the KD on glioma cells go far beyond energetics (Augustin et al., 2018; Bandera-Merchan et al., 2020; Jagust et al., 2019; Jung & Le, 2018; Li et al., 2020; Newman & Verdin, 2014a, 2014b; Schwartz et al., 2018; Shingler et al., 2019).

In addition to the effects mediated by glucose reduction, the KD can exhibit antitumor effects even in the absence of glucose reduction. We demonstrated the effect of adding ketones to media containing glucose in vitro using the AO2V4 cell line (Scheck et al., 2012). This cell line was derived from a recurrent human glioblastoma and is grown in Waymouth's MAB 87/3 media containing 28 mM glucose and supplemented with 20% fetal calf serum. When 5 mM βHB plus 5 mM ACA were added to complete media, cell growth was significantly inhibited. When 1,3-bis(2-chloroethyl)-1-nitrosourea (BCNU, carmustine; one of the chemotherapeutic agents given to this patient prior to tumor recurrence) was used in addition to ketones, there was more growth inhibition than with either ketones or BCNU alone. More recent work has shown that the ketones themselves exert antitumor effects separate from the effects of reduced blood glucose (Magee et al., 1979; Scheck et al., 2012; Skinner et al., 2009). The ketone βHB has been shown to inhibit histone deacetylases

(HDACs), which can result in epigenetic suppression of the expression of a variety of genes (Newman & Verdin, 2014a, 2014b; Shimazu et al., 2013). Thus, ketones may provide an additional link between metabolism and tumorigenesis, although the precise nature of these changes is as yet unknown (Newman & Verdin, 2014a, 2014b; Sassone-Corsi, 2013; Shimazu et al., 2013). The remainder of this chapter addresses the utility of increasing blood ketones and reducing blood glucose for the treatment of brain tumors.

PRECLINICAL EVIDENCE OF THE EFFICACY OF THE KD FOR TREATMENT OF GLIOMAS

The KD and similar diets used as a monotherapy have a pluripotent effect on the growth of tumors in vivo and tumor cells in vitro. This may depend, at least in part, on the model system, the specific metabolic intervention, and the molecular underpinnings of the tumor itself (Caso et al., 2013; Freedland et al., 2008; Hao et al., 2015; Kim et al., 2012b; Klement et al., 2016; Lv et al., 2014; Martuscello et al., 2016; Mavropoulos et al., 2009; Otto et al., 2008; Poff et al., 2013, 2015; Simone et al., 2013; Stafford et al., 2010; Wang et al., 2020c; Woolf et al., 2015a, 2015b; Woolf & Scheck, 2015; Xia et al., 2017). The striking feature of the work done to date is that alterations in metabolism have a far-reaching effect on tumor cells, tumors, and the tumor microenvironment, and while the majority of reports are positive, effects on the microenvironment must be taken into account in studies of metabolic alteration as a therapeutic modality (Weiss, 2020).

The use of metabolic alteration for the therapy of brain tumors has been championed by Seyfried and colleagues. They used the VM (Shelton et al., 2010) and CT-2A (Marsh et al., 2008) mouse tumor models to show that a KD, especially when given in restricted amounts, extends survival. D'Agostino and colleagues have added hyperbaric oxygen and exogenous ketone supplementation to demonstrate reduced tumor cell growth and metastatic spread in the VM metastatic tumor model (Poff et al., 2014, 2015). We used the syngeneic intracranial GL261-luc2/albino C57/Bl6 model to demonstrate that CR was not necessary for the antitumor effect of the KD (Stafford et al., 2010), particularly when a 4:1 fat:carbohydrate plus protein formulation is used (Scheck et al., 2012). We used the GL261-luc2 model of malignant glioma (Abdelwahab et al., 2011) to demonstrate that the KD increased blood ketones and inhibited the growth of the tumor when used alone, but most importantly it potentiated radiation and temozolomide therapy (Figure 15.1). Our work and that of others in different systems have shown changes in the formation of ROS and oxidative stress (Allen et al., 2013; Milder & Patel, 2012; Stafford et al., 2010) and reductions in angiogenesis (Puchowicz et al., 2008; Seyfried et al., 2015; Woolf et al., 2015a; Zhou et al., 2007), hypoxia (Maurer et al., 2011; Poff et al., 2015; Woolf et al., 2015a), inflammation and peritumoral edema (Amann & Hellerbrand, 2009; Gluschnaider et al., 2014; Hao et al., 2015; Kim et al., 2012a; Lv et al., 2014; Otto et al., 2008;

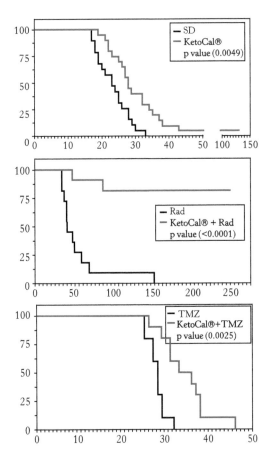

FIGURE 15.1 *Kaplan-Meier Survival Plots*

Animals implanted intracranially with GL261-luc2 malignant glioma cells and (A) maintained on KetoCal® (KC, the 4:1 fat:carbohydrate plus protein formulation of the ketogenic diet) versus standard diet (SD); (B) treated with 2 x 4 Gy radiation versus KC plus radiation, and (C) treated with 50 mg/kg temozolomide (TMZ) versus KC plus TMZ. Animals on KC survived significantly longer when treated with KC alone, when KC was combined with radiation, and when KC was combined with TMZ (Abdelwahab et al., 2012; Scheck et al., 2011).

Poff et al., 2015; Woolf et al., 2015a; Woolf & Scheck, 2015), metastasis and invasion (Amann & Hellerbrand, 2009; Gluschnaider et al., 2014; Hao et al., 2015; Kasumi & Sato, 2019; Lv et al., 2014; Otto et al., 2008; Poff et al., 2015), and the expression of various transcriptional modulators, such as NF-κB (Woolf et al., 2015a) and HIF-1α (Abdelwahab et al., 2012; Scheck et al., 2012; Stafford et al., 2010; Woolf et al., 2015a, 2016). We also demonstrated a decrease in tumor-associated insulinlike growth factor (IGF) expression, and others have demonstrated that ketones and ketogenic diets decrease pERK (Lamichhane et al., 2017) and mTORC1/mTORC2 signaling (Martuscello et al., 2016). Furthermore, we demonstrated that the KD enhanced the antitumor immune response in our syngeneic mouse model (Lussier et al., 2016). These data provide evidence that the KD can alter the expression of major drivers of metabolic remodeling and the consequences of altered metabolism in cancer cells. While many of these effects may be due to the reduction in glucose that results from a KD, we and others have shown that many of these effects can be recapitulated in vitro, even in the absence of glucose reduction. This suggests that the KD may have antitumor effects that go beyond those caused by glucose reduction. The pluripotent antiglioma effects seen with metabolic ketosis suggest that ketones are affecting a fundamental mechanism of gene regulation. Indeed, βHB and alterations in metabolism have been demonstrated to affect epigenetic modifications (Bandera-Merchan et al., 2020; Dąbek et al., 2020; Kinnaird & Michelakis, 2015; Ordway et al., 2020; Zhang & Kutateladze, 2018). βHB alters histone acetylation (Koppel & Swerdlow, 2018; Mehdikhani et al., 2019; Zhao et al., 2017) in part through its activity as a HDAC inhibitor (Shimazu et al., 2013) and it affects DNA methylation (Bandera-Merchan et al., 2020; Boison, 2017; Tadipatri et al., 2020) and the expression of a number of microRNAs (miRNAs; Bishop & Ferguson, 2015; Chan et al., 2015; Irani & Hussain, 2015; Wang et al., 2015a, 2015b, 2015c).

We studied the expression of miRNAs in glioma tissue from mice fed a KD and found a significant global upregulation of miRNAs with tumor suppressor function, which are typically downregulated in gliomas, and downregulation of those having an oncogenic role. Many of these miRNAs modulate genes involved in DNA repair as well as genes involved in all the hallmarks of cancer (Figure 15.2; Pazmandi et al., 2015). miRNA-138 was upregulated by 17-fold,

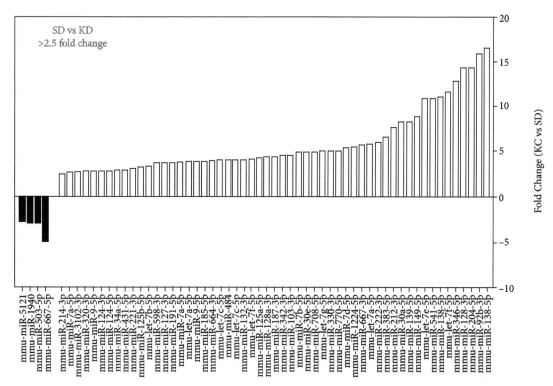

FIGURE 15.2 *Global miRNA Array Expression Analysis of Tumor Tissue from Mice Fed a SD versus a KD* Global array analysis was done to determine the differential expression of miRNAs in four tumors from mice maintained on a SD versus four tumors from mice maintained on a KD. Microarray analysis of miRNA was completed by Primbio, and all significantly differentially expressed miRNAs are shown. Data are expressed as fold change.

and its upregulation has previously been shown to suppress the tumorigenicity of GBM through downregulation of the enhancer of zeste homolog 2 (EZH2). EZH2 is the enzymatic subunit of the polycomb repressive complex 2 (PRC2) responsible for methylating specific residues on histones to promote transcriptional silencing (Qiu et al., 2013). Therapeutic targeting of EZH2 in cancer is an active area of research (Kim & Roberts, 2016). We also observed an increase in the let-7a miRNA, which is involved in the regulation of *MYC*, a gene increasingly recognized as a master regulator of the cancer epigenome and transcriptome (Poole & van Riggelen, 2017). βHB causes a reduction in *MYC* expression in mouse and human malignant glioma cells, as well as *MYC*-amplified medulloblastoma cells (Rossi, 2016). To unravel the potential pathways and gene interactions that could be affected by changes in the expression of these miRNAs, we used various online database tools, including NetworkAnalyst (http://www.network analyst.ca), International Molecular Exchange (IMEx) Interactome, and Reactome. This pooled analysis identified enrichment of pathways

involved in immune regulation. To explore these results further, we proceeded to examine the in vitro effects of βHB on immune cells of the brain, namely microglia. Our studies revealed that βHB is imported and oxidized by microglia in the TCA cycle and promotes their metabolic reprogramming (Benito et al., 2020). In addition to miRNA changes, we examined the effects of the KD on chromatin modifying enzymes. Our results revealed changes in several of these enzymes, but significant changes specifically in the expression of protein methyltransferase 8 (PRMT8) and DNA methyltransferase 3B (DNMT3b), where the former was upregulated and the latter downregulated with KD. The loss of PRMT8 expression and corresponding upregulation of its target genes, such as DHFR and CXCR4, are putative markers in GBM and are thought to contribute to its development (Ehtesham et al., 2006; Gravina et al., 2017; Miyazaki, 2017; Simandi et al., 2015; Stevenson et al., 2008; Walenkamp et al., 2017; Zhao et al., 2019). Indeed, DHFR and CXCR4 inhibitors have been developed and further refined for cancer therapy (Debnath et al., 2013; Raimondi et al.,

2019). DNMT3b is the major de novo DNA methylating enzyme required to establish methylation during development and imprinting (Esteller, 2008), and aberrant expression contributes to hypermethylation in cancer (Rhee et al., 2002). Hence its inhibition can lead to reduced methylation and the reactivation of silenced genes. This is one potential mechanism by which the KD may be exerting its effects in potentiating the effects of radiation in our mouse model (i.e., by upregulating genes involved in radiosensitization). Overall, our findings provide preliminary evidence to suggest that the KD could serve as an adjuvant therapy with existing cancer therapeutics.

KD AS AN ADJUVANT TO CANCER THERAPIES

Although evidence suggests that the KD provides antitumor benefits on its own, perhaps the most effective use of the KD is in combination with standard cancer therapies, such as radiation and chemotherapy (Allen et al., 2014; Icard et al., 2020; Iyikesici, 2020; Klement, 2017; Klement & Pazienza, 2019; O'Flanagan et al., 2017; Panhans et al., 2020; Scheck et al., 2012; Seyfried et al., 2020; Smyl, 2016; Tajan & Vousden, 2020; Vergati et al., 2017; Wang et al., 2020b; Winter et al., 2017). The KD combined with radiation or temozolomide greatly enhanced survival in a mouse model of malignant glioma when compared to either treatment alone (Figure 15.1; Abdelwahab et al., 2012; Scheck et al., 2011). In a bioluminescent, syngeneic intracranial model of malignant glioma, the KD was shown to significantly potentiate the antitumor effect of radiotherapy. In fact, nine of 11 animals maintained on the KD and treated with radiation had complete and sustained remission of their implanted tumors, even after being switched back to a standard rodent diet (Figure 15.1, Abdelwahab et al., 2012). Allen and colleagues (2013) reported similar results when the KD was combined with radiation and chemotherapy in a lung cancer xenograft model. That is, they found decreased tumor growth rate and increased survival. CR and short-term fasting have also been found to potentiate radiation (Klement et al., 2016) and other anticancer therapeutics in both preclinical and clinical studies (Champ et al., 2013, 2014; Kasumi & Sato, 2019; Klement, 2017; Klement et al., 2020a; Klement & Champ, 2014; Klement & Sweeney, 2016a; Lee et al., 2012, 2010; Lin et al., 2019; Poff et al., 2013; Raffaghello et al., 2008, 2010; Safdie et al., 2012; Saleh et al., 2013; Seyfried et al., 2012; Vidali et al., 2015; Weber et al., 2020; Zorn et al., 2020).

Radiation is a mainstay of cancer therapy, and there are ongoing efforts to identify safe radiosensitizers (Chevalier et al., 2020; Reda et al., 2020; Wanigasooriya et al., 2020). The effectiveness of radiation therapy is due to a number of factors, including relative damage done to tumor cells versus normal tissue and the ability of normal cells and tumor cells to repair the damage (Klement & Champ, 2014). The main effect of ketogenic therapies, such as the KD, fasting, or CR, may be not only in altering the amount of radiation-induced damage, but also in modulating the ability of tumor and normal cells to repair radiation-induced damage (Klement & Champ, 2014; Santivasi & Xia, 2014). Studies have shown that CR can enhance DNA repair in normal cells (Heydari et al., 2007); however, this may not be the case in tumor cells, and the differential response of tumor cells and normal cells to genotoxic stress may be mediated in part by reduced IGF1 and glucose in the tumor cells. We and others have shown that IGF is reduced in animals maintained on a ketogenic diet (Freedland et al., 2008; Klement & Champ, 2014; Mavropoulos et al., 2009; Scheck et al., 2012). Furthermore, a number of studies have shown that reduced activation of the PI3K/Akt pathway, activation of the adenosine monophosphate-activated protein kinase (AMPK) signaling pathway, and reduction of receptor tyrosine kinase growth factor pathways can all reduce radioresistance in tumor cells (Choi et al., 2014; Danhier et al., 2013; Gil Del Alcazar et al., 2014; Li et al., 2014; Medova et al., 2013; Munshi & Ramesh, 2013; Sanli et al., 2014; Wang et al., 2013; Wanigasooriya et al., 2020; Zhang et al., 2014). These changes are not found in normal cells. In addition, it should be noted that although many studies demonstrate reductions in growth and therapy resistance by ketogenic therapies, not all studies show beneficial results and some show mixed results in animals fed a KD (Agliano et al., 2017; Bartmann et al., 2018; Khodadadi et al., 2017; Tang et al., 2018; Xia et al., 2017). Furthermore, while it has been suggested that ketolytic enzyme levels may be biomarkers of the efficacy of a KD in the treatment of cancer, this has yet to be verified, and it has not been tested when the KD is used in combination with other therapies (Chang et al., 2013; Zhang & Kutateladze, 2018).

Metabolism is tightly linked to the immune response, so much so that there is now a field called immunometabolism (Banerjee et al., 2020; Cuyàs et al., 2020; Liang et al., 2020; Lio & Huang, 2020; Saravia et al., 2020; Zhao et al., 2020). It is therefore no surprise that ketones and the KD have been shown to affect the immune system, and we have shown that the KD also reverses tumor-mediated immune suppression in a mouse model of malignant glioma. We showed that mice fed a KD had increased innate and adaptive immune responses, along with a significant blockade of the PD1 and CTLA-4 immune checkpoints in glioma (Lussier et al., 2016). As radiation-induced tumor killing is known to expose the immune system to a greater diversity of tumor antigens, it is possible that the KD as an adjuvant works to augment the effect of radiation in part by enhancing immunity against GBM. This also suggests that the KD may be an effective addition to immunotherapies targeting immune checkpoints.

In addition to direct effects of ketogenic therapies (KD, fasting, or CR) on cancer, the KD may have other beneficial effects as an adjuvant therapy—particularly in reducing side effects of therapeutic interventions (O'Flanagan et al., 2017; Zorn et al., 2020). For example, mutations in the phosphatidylinositol-3-kinase (PI3K) pathway are common in tumors, and inhibitors of this pathway showed promising preclinical efficacy; however, the results from clinical trials have been somewhat variable (Paddock et al., 2019). This was shown to be due, at least in part, to resistance to the inhibitor and adverse effects, such as hyperglycemia. Hopkins and colleagues have shown that a ketogenic diet can help mitigate the hyperglycemia that can occur as a side effect of the inhibitors (Hopkins et al., 2018, 2020). In a similar manner, Voss and colleagues (2018) demonstrated that a KD could mitigate the side effects of treatment with the glycolysis inhibitor 2-deoxyglucose and increase the maximum tolerated dose.

A common occurrence in people with advanced cancers is cachexia, or muscle wasting. This causes severe weight loss, loss of appetite, weakness, and fatigue. Although it is less common in patients with glioma, in many cancer patients cachexia severely compromises quality of life and may be exacerbated by cancer therapy. Thus, weight loss in a tumor patient is often viewed as undesirable. The KD has been shown to help prevent muscle loss, improve body condition, and reduce cachexia in several tumor models (Chung & Park, 2017; Fearon et al., 1988; Koutnik et al., 2020; Mitchell et al., 2019; O'Flanagan et al., 2017; Shukla et al., 2014; Yakovenko et al., 2018). This promotes healthy weight loss and reductions in hyperglycemia in patients who are obese. In addition to improvements in quality of life, reductions

in hyperglycemia are associated with improved survival in many tumor types, including gliomas (Adeberg et al., 2016; Chaichana et al., 2010; Derr et al., 2009; Lu et al., 2018; Mayer et al., 2014; McGirt et al., 2008; Tieu et al., 2015).

The pluripotent anticancer effects of ketogenic therapy suggest that it may complement a wide variety of treatment modalities in addition to those mentioned above. Indeed, the KD affects many of molecular alterations currently being investigated as therapeutic targets. While the effects of the KD may not be as robust as those seen with pharmacologic inhibitors, it should be noted that these effects are typically without accompanying side effects. The potential to enhance therapeutic efficacy without increasing toxicity may permit the use of lower doses of therapies, thus reducing adverse effects without reducing the antitumor effect. This may also allow us to "revisit" potentially useful therapies that were not put into general use due to their toxicity, their insufficient efficacy, or the rapid appearance of resistance when they were used alone. While this has not been studied in earnest as yet, combining therapies with similar or intersecting mechanisms of action could be a promising area of research. (Chaul-Barbosa & Marques, 2019; Gravina et al., 2019; Ramezani et al., 2019). For example, the anti-angiogenic drug bevacizumab (Avastin®) is a "second-line" treatment that is often used at tumor recurrence, where it has been shown to reduce treatment toxicity (Dalle Ore et al., 2019; Fleischmann et al., 2019)—possibly due in part to reduced vasogenic edema (Anthony et al., 2019; Villani et al., 2019; Xiao et al., 2018). Bevacizumab increases progression-free survival but not overall survival (Anthony et al., 2019), and tumor recurrence following this treatment is often accompanied by diffuse disease (Hardian et al., 2019). Resistance may involve activation of the PI3K pathway (Gravina et al., 2019; Ramezani et al., 2019). Ketogenic therapy has been shown to inhibit angiogenesis, tumor cell invasion, and tumor cell migration, and it has a negative effect on signaling through the PI3K pathway; thus, it may potentiate the effect of bevacizumab and reduce adverse effects (Poff et al., 2015, 2019; Tajbakhsh et al., 2008; Woolf et al., 2015a, 2016). Ketogenic therapy may also augment the effects of HDAC inhibitors, such as panobinostat and others. HDAC inhibition has been suggested for the treatment of gliomas, particularly in pediatric diffuse intrinsic pontine glioma (DIPG; de Andrade et al., 2016; Lee et al., 2015; Milde et al., 2012; Pont et al., 2015; Qiu et al., 2017; Shi et al.,

2016; Staberg et al., 2017), and HDAC inhibition may even sensitize GBM stemlike cells to radiation and chemotherapy (Reddy et al., 2020). The KD recapitulates many of the therapeutic actions of HDAC inhibitors like panobinostat, including reduction of HIF-1α (Woolf et al., 2015a), a key transcriptional activator involved in regulation of angiogenesis, energy metabolism, tumor cell invasion, and other tumor-associated pathways. Thus, ketogenic therapy may potentiate the activity of HDAC inhibitors without increasing toxicity.

The variety of effects seen when glucose is lowered and/or ketones are increased suggests that this may also potentiate other therapies in addition to the two examples given above, including newer immune and targeted therapies. Concerns that potentiation of the antitumor effect of a particular therapy may also increase its effect on normal brain are valid. However, we and others have shown that the gene expression changes seen in tumor are different from those seen in normal brain (Chang et al., 2013; Maurer et al., 2011; Stafford et al., 2010). Further, the KD is known to have neuroprotective effects (Hartman, 2012; Lund et al., 2009; Maalouf et al., 2009; Puchowicz et al., 2008); thus, it has been postulated that this may actually help to protect the normal brain from the deleterious effects of radiation therapy and chemotherapy. Taken together, the preclinical data provide strong support for the clinical use of the KD or CR as an adjuvant therapy for gliomas and other cancers.

CLINICAL USE OF THE KD FOR TUMORS

Studies of glucose utilization in cancer go back before the 1980s, including studies of metabolism and cancer cachexia (Fearon et al., 1988; Kari et al., 1999; Landau et al., 1958; Magee et al., 1979; Nebeling & Lerner, 1995; Nebeling et al., 1995; Tisdale et al., 1987; Vlashi & Pajonk, 1979; Yamada et al., 1999). These and other studies suggested that a KD consisting of a high percentage of medium-chain triglycerides (MCT) along with various supplements resulted in weight gain and improved nitrogen balance in both animals and humans. In 1995, Nebeling and colleagues published a case report in which they used a similar KD based on MCT oil to treat two female pediatric patients with advanced-stage malignant brain tumors (Nebeling & Lerner, 1995; Nebeling et al., 1995). They demonstrated that diet-induced ketosis decreased the availability of glucose to the tumor without causing a decrease in patient weight or overall nutritional status. Furthermore,

both children had long-term tumor management (Nebeling et al., 1995). Since that time, there have been a number of case reports and reports of small clinical trials using a KD, fasting, metformin, and other metabolic therapies alone or in combination with other therapies (Bauersfeld et al., 2018; Branca et al., 2015; Champ et al., 2014; Cohen et al., 2018, 2020; Cuyàs et al., 2019; de Groot et al., 2015, 2020; Demark-Wahnefried et al., 2016; Dunphy et al., 2018; Erickson et al., 2017; Gresham et al., 2019; Habermann et al., 2015; Hagihara et al., 2020; Iyikesici, 2019, 2020; İyikesici et al., 2017; Katsuya et al., 2015; Kirkham et al., 2018; Klement et al., 2020a, 2020b; Klement & Sweeney, 2016a, 2016b; Laskov et al., 2014; Lende et al., 2019; Li et al., 2015; Murtola et al., 2019; Myers et al., 2018; Parikh et al., 2017; Rieger et al., 2014; Saxton et al., 2014; Smith, 2019; Sturgeon et al., 2018; Vernieri et al., 2019; Voss et al., 2020; Wang et al., 2020b; Wei et al., 2017; Yu et al., 2017; Zahra et al., 2017). Most trials showed efficacy in some patients, but not all. In general, the KD is well tolerated and without severe side effects (Chang et al., 2013; Ludwig, 2020; Mehdikhani et al., 2019; Panhans et al., 2020; Schmidt et al., 2011; Schwartz et al., 2013, 2015, 2018). The number of prospective clinical trials in gliomas and other cancers continues to grow (Lévesque et al., 2019) and the most recent list can be found on the clinicaltrials.gov website.

The results reported to date, along with numerous anecdotal reports, suggest that the KD may be a promising anticancer therapy. However, more work is needed to determine how to best utilize the KD and other metabolic therapies for the treatment of tumors (Ludwig, 2020). Most of the information regarding the most effective way to use the KD comes from the epilepsy literature. A variety of KDs are used for seizure control, and it is not clear if one or more of the different formulations will provide the best results for cancer patients. Indeed, the variability of the diets used and insufficient specification of fasting protocols have made it difficult to directly compare much of the available data (Lubberman et al., 2017; Trimboli et al., 2020). This may be mitigated by the use of blood glucose and ketone levels; however, further research is needed to determine what is optimal for anticancer effects. It has been suggested that a glucose:ketone ratio be calculated for patients (Meidenbauer et al., 2015) to determine if they are in a "therapeutic window." While this may provide additional information for comparing individuals, it will take more data to demonstrate the utility of this measurement. Indeed, it is likely that the efficacy of therapeutic ketosis will depend, to some extent, on the genetic profile of the tumor and perhaps even on the genetic profile of the patient, since this affects the patient's response to nutrients. In addition, while the KD has a long record of safety in the epilepsy community, side effects that occur when KD is used in combination with cancer therapies may differ in type or severity. These data will come from carefully controlled clinical trials that include input from healthcare professionals well versed in the use of the KD. Perhaps the biggest impediment to obtaining high-quality data from the clinical trials is the difficulty encountered in patient enrollment and compliance with the KD. This requires "buy-in" from the medical community and funds for qualified dietitians and nutritionists to support the patients and their caregivers. Physicians must be educated on the therapeutic benefits of metabolic alteration as an adjuvant therapy. Even with the small clinical trials done to date, clinicians trying to use the KD with their patients have repeatedly brought up the same factors (in personal communications) as having the most effect on compliance: (1) prescreening the patients prior to enrollment—only 1 in 4 or 1 in 5 is typically thought to be able to comply with the dietary requirements; (2) physician buy-in and willingness to promote the potential benefits to their patients; and (3) the availability of, and frequent contact with, a dietitian/nutritionist who is well versed in the KD. The patient must also be willing to contact the treatment team if there are any issues that come up, even after the initial period of keto-adaptation. As with any decision regarding therapy, the patient's overall condition, including nutritional status, must be taken into account. As suggested by Klement and Champ (2014), cancer patients should be comprehensively assessed for nutritional needs and tolerability of metabolic interventions.

Concern about patients' quality of life (QOL) is sometimes given as a reason not to employ the KD (Wood & Zabilowicz, 2020). Compliance can be made more difficult by the use of steroids (prescribed for peritumoral edema), which often increase hunger and raise blood glucose levels. To address this, a number of clinical trials now include an analysis of both patient and caregiver QOL. QOL measurements are being added to more clinical trials, as QOL's importance has become recognized at the national level (Boele et al., 2013; Dirven et al., 2014; van den Bent et al., 2011). While some clinicians are concerned that KD compliance will reduce QOL, the patients that do remain on the KD often comment that

it allows them to participate in their own therapy. Parents of children with brain tumors and caregivers report positive feelings about the KD because it allows them to "do something to help their loved one." Despite these caveats, the existing preclinical data suggesting antitumor efficacy and a synergistic effect with standard therapies provide a strong impetus to conduct controlled clinical trials, particularly those that will shed light on the interactions between the KD and other therapies.

CONCLUSION

Improvements in the survival and QOL for patients with malignant brain tumors require the implementation of new therapeutic modalities, especially those that increase the efficacy of current therapies without increasing toxic side effects. While the rapid accumulation of data defining the molecular and genetic aberrations present in these tumors has suggested a host of targets for the development of new treatments, the targeted therapies tried to date have met with limited success. This is at least in part due to the molecular heterogeneity of the tumors, which prevents any one target from being present in all cells. In contrast, metabolic dysregulation is present in virtually all tumor cells, and there is rapidly increasing interest in using metabolic therapies like the KD for the treatment of various cancers, especially brain tumors. Preclinical data have demonstrated that the antitumor effects of the KD and CR are multifaceted, and alterations in energy metabolism can inhibit cancer cell growth and increase the tumor's response to therapy. Furthermore, there are also epigenetic effects beyond those due to changes in energy metabolism. This provides a strong impetus to continue work designed to elucidate the mechanisms through which the KD exerts its anticancer effects, as well as suggesting the need for the design of controlled clinical trials that will shed light on the most effective ways to implement metabolic therapies in combination with standard therapies for the treatment of malignant disease. This is a novel therapeutic paradigm, and we have only begun to scratch the surface in terms of its potential.

REFERENCES
Abdelwahab, M. G., Fenton, K. E., Preul, M. C., Rho, J. M., Lynch, A., Stafford, P., & Scheck, A. C. (2012). The ketogenic diet is an effective adjuvant to radiation therapy for the treatment of malignant glioma. *PLOS ONE, 7,* Article e36197.

Abdelwahab, M. G., Sankar, T., Preul, M. C., & Scheck, A.C. (2011). Intracranial implantation with subsequent in vivo bioluminescent imaging of murine gliomas. *JoVE*, 57, Article e3403.

Adeberg, S., Bernhardt, D., Foerster, R., Bostel, T., Koerber, S. A., Mohr, A., Koelsche, C., Rieken, S., & Debus, J. (2016). The influence of hyperglycemia during radiotherapy on survival in patients with primary glioblastoma. *Acta Oncologica*, 55, 201–207.

Agliano, A., Balarajah, G., Ciobota, D. M., Sidhu, J., Clarke, P. A., Jones, C., Workman, P., Leach, M. O., & Al-Saffar, N. M. S. (2017). Pediatric and adult glioblastoma radiosensitization induced by PI3K/mTOR inhibition causes early metabolic alterations detected by nuclear magnetic resonance spectroscopy. *Oncotarget*, 8, 47969–47983.

Alexandru, O., Horescu, C., Sevastre, A. S., Cioc, C. E., Baloi, C., Oprita, A., & Dricu, A. (2020). Receptor tyrosine kinase targeting in glioblastoma: Performance, limitations and future approaches. *Contemporary Oncology*, 24, 55–66.

Allen, B. G., Bhatia, S. K., Anderson, C. M., Eichenberger-Gilmore, J. M., Sibenaller, Z. A., Mapuskar, K. A., Schoenfeld, J. D., Buatti, J. M., Spitz, D. R., & Fath, M. A. (2014). Ketogenic diets as an adjuvant cancer therapy: History and potential mechanism. *Redox Biology*, 2C, 963–970.

Allen, B. G., Bhatia, S. K., Buatti, J. M., Brandt, K. E., Lindholm, K. E., Button, A. M., Szweda, L. I., Smith, B., Spitz, D. R., & Fath, M.A. (2013). Ketogenic diets enhance oxidative stress and radio-chemo-therapy responses in lung cancer xenografts. *Clinical Cancer Research*, 19, 3905–3913.

Amann, T., & Hellerbrand, C. (2009). GLUT1 as a therapeutic target in hepatocellular carcinoma. *Expert Opinion on Therapeutic Targets*, 13, 1411–1427.

Amberger-Murphy, V. (2009). Hypoxia helps glioma to fight therapy. *Current Cancer Drug Targets*, 9, 381–390.

Anthony, C., Mladkova-Suchy, N., & Adamson, D. C. (2019). The evolving role of antiangiogenic therapies in glioblastoma multiforme: Current clinical significance and future potential. *Expert Opinion on Investigational Drugs*, 28, 787–797.

Augustin, K., Khabbush, A., Williams, S., Eaton, S., Orford, M., Cross, J. H., Heales, S. J. R., Walker, M. C., & Williams, R. S. B. (2018). Mechanisms of action for the medium-chain triglyceride ketogenic diet in neurological and metabolic disorders. *Lancet Neurology*, 17, 84–93.

Azzi, S., Hebda, J. K., & Gavard, J. (2013). Vascular permeability and drug delivery in cancers. *Frontiers in Oncology*, 3, 211.

Bacigalupa, Z. A., & Rathmell, W. K. (2020). Beyond glycolysis: Hypoxia signaling as a master regulator of alternative metabolic pathways and the implications in clear cell renal cell carcinoma. *Cancer Letters*, 489, 19–28.

Bader, J. E., Voss, K., & Rathmell, J. C. (2020). Targeting metabolism to improve the tumor microenvironment for cancer immunotherapy. *Molecular Cell*, 78, 1019–1033.

Badr, C. E., Silver, D. J., Siebzehnrubl, F. A., & Deleyrolle, L. P. (2020). Metabolic heterogeneity and adaptability in brain tumors. *Cellular and Molecular Life Sciences*, 77, 5101–5119.

Baltazar, F., Afonso, J., Costa, M., & Granja, S. (2020). Lactate beyond a waste metabolite: Metabolic affairs and signaling in malignancy. *Frontiers in Oncology*, 10, 231.

Bandera-Merchan, B., Boughanem, H., Crujeiras, A. B., Macias-Gonzalez, M., & Tinahones, F. J. (2020). Ketotherapy as an epigenetic modifier in cancer. *Reviews in Endocrine & Metabolic Disorders*, 21, 509–519.

Banerjee, S., Ghosh, S., Mandal, A., Ghosh, N., & Sil, P. C. (2020). ROS-associated immune response and metabolism: A mechanistic approach with implication of various diseases. *Archives of Toxicology*, 94, 2293–2317.

Baranano, K. W., & Hartman, A. L. (2008). The ketogenic diet: Uses in epilepsy and other neurologic illnesses. *Current Treatment Options in Neurology*, 10, 410–419.

Barker, R. M., Holly, J. M. P., Biernacka, K. M., Allen-Birt, S. J., & Perks, C. M. (2020). Mini review: Opposing pathologies in cancer and Alzheimer's disease; Does the PI3K/Akt pathway provide clues? *Frontiers in Endocrinology*, 11, 403.

Bartmann, C., Janaki Raman, S. R., Flöter, J., Schulze, A., Bahlke, K., Willingstorfer, J., Strunz, M., Wöckel, A., Klement, R. J., Kapp, M., Djuzenova, C. S., Otto, C., & Kämmerer, U. (2018). Beta-hydroxybutyrate (β-OHB) can influence the energetic phenotype of breast cancer cells, but does not impact their proliferation and the response to chemotherapy or radiation. *Cancer & Metabolism*, 6, 8.

Bauersfeld, S. P., Kessler, C. S., Wischnewsky, M., Jaensch, A., Steckhan, N., Stange, R., Kunz, B., Brückner, B., Sehouli, J., & Michalsen, A. (2018). The effects of short-term fasting on quality of life and tolerance to chemotherapy in patients with breast and ovarian cancer: A randomized crossover pilot study. *BMC Cancer*, 18, 476.

Bayley, J. P., & Devilee, P. (2010). Warburg tumours and the mechanisms of mitochondrial tumour suppressor genes: Barking up the right tree? *Current Opinion in Genetics & Development*, 20, 324–329.

Becker, L. M., O'Connell, J. T., Vo, A. P., Cain, M. P., Tampe, D., Bizarro, L., Sugimoto, H., McGow, A. K., Asara, J. M., Lovisa, S. McAndrews, K. M., Zielinski, R., Lorenzi, P. L., Zeisberg, M., Raza, S., LeBleu, V. S., & Kalluri, R. (2020). Epigenetic reprogramming of cancer-associated fibroblasts deregulates glucose metabolism and facilitates progression of breast cancer. *Cell Reports, 31,* Article 107701.

Benito, A., Hajji, N., O'Neill, K., Keun, H. C., & Syed, N. (2020). β-Hydroxybutyrate Oxidation Promotes the Accumulation of Immunometabolites in Activated Microglia Cells. *Metabolites, 10,* 346; doi:10.3390/metabo10090346.

Berrington, A., Schreck, K. C., Barron, B. J., Blair, L., Lin, D. D. M., Hartman, A. L., Kossoff, E., Easter, L., Whitlow, C. T., Jung, Y. Hsu, F. C., Cervenka, M. C., Blakeley, J. O., Barker, P. B., & Strowd, R. E. (2019). Cerebral ketones detected by 3T MR spectroscopy in patients with high-grade glioma on an Atkins-based diet. *American Journal of Neuroradiology, 40,* 1908–1915.

Bi, J., Chowdhry, S., Wu, S., Zhang, W., Masui, K., & Mischel, P. S. (2020). Altered cellular metabolism in gliomas—An emerging landscape of actionable co-dependency targets. *Nature Reviews Cancer, 20,* 57–70.

Bishop, K. S., & Ferguson, L. R. (2015). The interaction between epigenetics, nutrition and the development of cancer. *Nutrients, 7,* 922–947.

Blouin, M. J., Zhao, Y., Zakikhani, M., Algire, C., Piura, E., & Pollak, M. (2010). Loss of function of PTEN alters the relationship between glucose concentration and cell proliferation, increases glycolysis, and sensitizes cells to 2-deoxyglucose. *Cancer Letters, 289,* 246–253.

Boele, F. W., Heimans, J. J., Aaronson, N. K., Taphoorn, M. J., Postma, T. J., Reijneveld, J. C., & Klein, M. (2013). Health-related quality of life of significant others of patients with malignant CNS versus non-CNS tumors: A comparative study. *Journal of Neuro-Oncology, 115,* 87–94.

Boison, D. (2017). New insights into the mechanisms of the ketogenic diet. *Current Opinion in Neurology, 30,* 187–192.

Bordoni, L., & Gabbianelli, R. (2019). Primers on nutrigenetics and nutri(epi)genomics: Origins and development of precision nutrition. *Biochimie, 160,* 156–171.

Bozzetti, F., & Zupec-Kania, B. (2016). Toward a cancer-specific diet. *Clinical Nutrition, 35,* 1188–1195.

Branca, J. J., Pacini, S., & Ruggiero, M. (2015). Effects of pre-surgical vitamin D supplementation and ketogenic diet in a patient with recurrent breast cancer. *Anticancer Research, 35,* 5525–5532.

Branco, A. F., Ferreira, A., Simões, R. F., Magalhães-Novais, S., Zehowski, C., Cope, E., Silva, A. M., Pereira, D., Sardão, V. A., & Cunha-Oliveira, T. (2016). Ketogenic diets: From cancer to mitochondrial diseases and beyond. *European Journal of Clinical Investigation, 46,* 285–298.

Bruzzese, L., Fromonot, J., By, Y., Durand-Gorde, J. M., Condo, J., Kipson, N., Guieu, R., Fenouillet,

E., & Ruf, J. (2014). NF-κB enhances hypoxia-driven T-cell immunosuppression via upregulation of adenosine A$_{2A}$ receptors. *Cellular Signalling, 26,* 1060–1067.

Cahill, G. F., Jr., & Veech, R. L. (2003). Ketoacids? Good medicine? *Transactions of the American Clinical and Climatological Association, 114,* 149–161.

Cahill, K. E., Morshed, R. A., & Yamini, B. (2016). Nuclear factor-κB in glioblastoma: Insights into regulators and targeted therapy. *Neuro-Oncology, 18,* 329–339.

Cantor, J. R., & Sabatini, D. M. (2012). Cancer cell metabolism: One hallmark, many faces. *Cancer Discovery, 2,* 881–898.

Casey, S. C., Amedei, A., Aquilano, K., Azmi, A. S., Benencia, F., Bhakta, D., Bilsland, A. E., Boosani, C. S., Chen, S., Ciriolo, M. R. Crawford, S., Fujii, H., Georgakilas, A. G., Guha, G., Halicka, D., Helferich, W. G., Heneberg, P., Honoki, K., Keith, W. N., . . . Felsher, D. W. (2015). Cancer prevention and therapy through the modulation of the tumor microenvironment. *Seminars in Cancer Biology,* Dec; 35(Suppl): S199–S223.

Caso, J., Masko, E. M., Ii, J. A., Poulton, S. H., Dewhirst, M., Pizzo, S. V., & Freedland, S. J. (2013). The effect of carbohydrate restriction on prostate cancer tumor growth in a castrate mouse xenograft model. *Prostate, 73,* 449–454.

Cassim, S., Vučetić, M., Ždralević, M., & Pouyssegur, J. (2020). Warburg and beyond: The power of mitochondrial metabolism to collaborate or replace fermentative glycolysis in cancer. *Cancers, 12,* 1119–1141.

Chaichana, K. L., McGirt, M. J., Woodworth, G. F., Datoo, G., Tamargo, R. J., Weingart, J., Olivi, A., Brem, H., & Quinones-Hinojosa, A. (2010). Persistent outpatient hyperglycemia is independently associated with survival, recurrence and malignant degeneration following surgery for hemispheric low grade gliomas. *Neurological Research, 32,* 442–448.

Chakraborty, A. A. (2020). Coalescing lessons from oxygen sensing, tumor metabolism, and epigenetics to target VHL loss in kidney cancer. *Seminars in Cancer Biology, 67,* 34–42.

Champ, C. E., Baserga, R., Mishra, M. V., Jin, L., Sotgia, F., Lisanti, M. P., Pestell, R. G., Dicker, A. P., & Simone, N. L. (2013). Nutrient restriction and radiation therapy for cancer treatment: When less is more. *Oncologist, 18,* 97–103.

Champ, C. E., Palmer, J. D., Volek, J. S., Werner-Wasik, M., Andrews, D. W., Evans, J. J., Glass, J., Kim, L., & Shi, W. (2014). Targeting metabolism with a ketogenic diet during the treatment of glioblastoma multiforme. *Journal of Neuro-Oncology, 117,* 125–131.

Chan, B., Manley, J., Lee, J., & Singh, S. R. (2015). The emerging roles of microRNAs in cancer metabolism. *Cancer Letters, 356,* 301–308.

Chan, S. L. (2020). Microbiome and cancer treatment: Are we ready to apply in clinics? *Progress in Molecular Biology and Translational Science, 171*, 301–308.

Chang, H. T., Olson, L. K., & Schwartz, K. A. (2013). Ketolytic and glycolytic enzymatic expression profiles in malignant gliomas: Implication for ketogenic diet therapy. *Nutrition & Metabolism, 10*, 47.

Chaul-Barbosa, C., & Marques, D. F. (2019). How we treat recurrent glioblastoma today and current evidence. *Current Oncology Reports, 21*, 94.

Chen, R., Cohen, A. L., & Colman, H. (2016). Targeted therapeutics in patients with high-grade gliomas: Past, present, and future. *Current Treatment Options in Oncology, 17*, 42.

Chevalier, B., Pasquier, D., Lartigau, E. F., Chargari, C., Schernberg, A., Jannin, A., Mirabel, X., Vantyghem, M. C., & Escande, A. (2020). Metformin: (Future) best friend of the radiation oncologist? *Radiotherapy and Oncology, 151*, 95–105.

Choi, E. J., Cho, B. J., Lee, D. J., Hwang, Y. H., Chun, S. H., Kim, H. H., & Kim, I. A. (2014). Enhanced cytotoxic effect of radiation and temozolomide in malignant glioma cells: Targeting PI3K-AKT-mTOR signaling, HSP90 and histone deacetylases. *BMC Cancer, 14*, 17.

Chung, H. Y., & Park, Y. K. (2017). Rationale, feasibility and acceptability of ketogenic diet for cancer treatment. *Journal of Cancer Prevention, 22*, 127–134.

Ciechomska, I. A., Jayaprakash, C., Maleszewska, M., & Kaminska, B. (2020). Histone modifying enzymes and chromatin modifiers in glioma pathobiology and therapy responses. *Advances in Experimental Medicine and Biology, 1202*, 259–279.

Cohen, C. W., Fontaine, K. R., Arend, R. C., Alvarez, R. D., Leath, C. A., III, Huh, W. K., Bevis, K. S., Kim, K. H., Straughn, J. M., Jr., & Gower, B. A. (2018). A ketogenic diet reduces central obesity and serum insulin in women with ovarian or endometrial cancer. *Journal of Nutrition, 148*, 1253–1260.

Cohen, C. W., Fontaine, K. R., Arend, R. C., & Gower, B. A. (2020). A ketogenic diet is acceptable in women with ovarian and endometrial cancer and has no adverse effects on blood lipids: A randomized, controlled trial. *Nutrition and Cancer, 72*, 584–594.

Coleman, M. F., Cozzo, A. J., Pfeil, A. J., Etigunta, S. K., & Hursting, S. D. (2020). Cell intrinsic and systemic metabolism in tumor immunity and immunotherapy. *Cancers, 12*, 852–882.

Corbet, C., & Feron, O. (2015). Metabolic and mind shifts: From glucose to glutamine and acetate addictions in cancer. *Current Opinion in Clinical Nutrition and Metabolic Care, 18*, 346–353.

Costa, A., Scholer-Dahirel, A., & Mechta-Grigoriou, F. (2014). The role of reactive oxygen species and metabolism on cancer cells and their microenvironment. *Seminars in Cancer Biology, 25*, 23–32.

Courtnay, R., Ngo, D. C., Malik, N., Ververis, K., Tortorella, S. M., & Karagiannis, T. C. (2015). Cancer metabolism and the Warburg effect: The role of HIF-1 and PI3K. *Molecular Biology Reports, 42*, 841–851.

Cross, J. H. (2013). New research with diets and epilepsy. *Journal of Child Neurology, 28*, 970–974.

Cuyàs, E., Fernández-Arroyo, S., Buxó, M., Pernas, S., Dorca, J., Álvarez, I., Martínez, S., Pérez-Garcia, J. M., Batista-López, N., Rodríguez-Sánchez, C. A., Amillano, K., Domínguez, S., Luque, M., Morilla, I., Stradella, A., Viñas, G., Cortés, J., Verdura, S., Brunet, J., López-Bonet, E., . . . Menendez, J. A. (2019). Metformin induces a fasting- and antifolate-mimicking modification of systemic host metabolism in breast cancer patients. *Aging, 11*, 2874–2888.

Cuyàs, E., Verdura, S., Martin-Castillo, B., Alarcón, T., Lupu, R., Bosch-Barrera, J., & Menendez, J. A. (2020). Tumor cell-intrinsic immunometabolism and precision nutrition in cancer immunotherapy. *Cancers, 12*, 1757–1784.

Dąbek, A., Wojtala, M., Pirola, L., & Balcerczyk, A. (2020). Modulation of cellular biochemistry, epigenetics and metabolomics by ketone bodies: Implications of the ketogenic diet in the physiology of the organism and pathological states. *Nutrients, 12*, 788.

Dalle Ore, C. L., Chandra, A., Rick, J., Lau, D., Shahin, M., Nguyen, A. T., McDermott, M., Berger, M. S., & Aghi, M. K. (2019). Presence of histopathological treatment effects at resection of recurrent glioblastoma: Incidence and effect on outcome. *Neurosurgery, 85*, 793–800.

Danhier, P., De Saedeleer, C. J., Karroum, O., De Preter, G., Porporato, P. E., Jordan, B. F., Gallez, B., & Sonveaux, P. (2013). Optimization of tumor radiotherapy with modulators of cell metabolism: Toward clinical applications. *Seminars in Radiation Oncology, 23*, 262–272.

de Andrade, P. V., Andrade, A. F., de Paula Queiroz, R. G., Scrideli, C. A., Tone, L. G., & Valera, E. T. (2016). The histone deacetylase inhibitor PCI-24781 as a putative radiosensitizer in pediatric glioblastoma cell lines. *Cancer Cell International, 16*, 31.

de Groot, S., Lugtenberg, R. T., Cohen, D., Welters, M. J. P., Ehsan, I., Vreeswijk, M. P. G., Smit, V., de Graaf, H., Heijns, J. B., Portielje, J. E. A., van de Wouw, A. J., Imholz, A. L. T., Kessels, L. W., Vrijaldenhoven, S., Baars, A., Kranenbarg, E. M., Carpentier, M. D., Putter, H., van der Hoeven, J. J. M., . . . Kroep, J. R. (2020). Fasting mimicking diet as an adjunct to neoadjuvant chemotherapy for breast cancer in the multicentre randomized phase 2 DIRECT trial. *Nature Communications*, 11, 3083.

de Groot, S., Vreeswijk, M. P., Welters, M. J., Gravesteijn, G., Boei, J. J., Jochems, A., Houtsma, D., Putter, H., van der Hoeven, J. J., Nortier, J. W., Pijl, H., & Kroep, J. R. (2015). The effects of short-term fasting on tolerance to (neo) adjuvant chemotherapy in HER2-negative breast cancer patients: A randomized pilot study. *BMC Cancer*, 15, 652.

Debnath, B., Xu, S., Grande, F., Garofalo, A., & Neamati, N. (2013). Small molecule inhibitors of CXCR4. *Theranostics*, 3, 47–75.

deCampo, D. M., & Kossoff, E. H. (2019). Ketogenic dietary therapies for epilepsy and beyond. *Current Opinion in Clinical Nutrition and Metabolic Care*, 22, 264–268.

Delgado-López, P. D., Saiz-López, P., Gargini, R., Sola-Vendrell, E., & Tejada, S. (2020). A comprehensive overview on the molecular biology of human glioma: What the clinician needs to know. *Clinical & Translational Oncology*, 22, 1909–1922.

Demark-Wahnefried, W., Nix, J. W., Hunter, G. R., Rais-Bahrami, S., Desmond, R. A., Chacko, B., Morrow, C. D., Azrad, M., Frugé, A. D., Tsuruta, Y., Ptacek, T., Tully, S. A., Segal, R., & Grizzle, W. E. (2016). Feasibility outcomes of a presurgical randomized controlled trial exploring the impact of caloric restriction and increased physical activity versus a wait-list control on tumor characteristics and circulating biomarkers in men electing prostatectomy for prostate cancer. *BMC Cancer*, 16, 61.

Derr, R. L., Ye, X., Islas, M. U., Desideri, S., Saudek, C. D., & Grossman, S. A. (2009). Association between hyperglycemia and survival in patients with newly diagnosed glioblastoma. *Journal of Clinical Oncology*, 27, 1082–1086.

Desbats, M. A., Giacomini, I., Prayer-Galetti, T., & Montopoli, M. (2020). Metabolic plasticity in chemotherapy resistance. *Frontiers in Oncology*, 10, 281.

Dewhirst, M. W. (2009). Relationships between cycling hypoxia, HIF-1, angiogenesis and oxidative stress. *Radiation Research*, 172, 653–665.

Dibble, C. C., & Cantley, L. C. (2015). Regulation of mTORC1 by PI3K signaling. *Trends in Cell Biology*, 25, 545–555.

Dirven, L., Taphoorn, M. J., Reijneveld, J. C., Blazeby, J., Jacobs, M., Pusic, A., La, S. E., Stupp, R., Fayers, P., & Efficace, F. (2014). The level of patient-reported outcome reporting in randomised controlled trials of brain tumour patients: A systematic review. *European Journal of Cancer*, 50, 2432–2448.

Dong, Y., Tu, R., Liu, H., & Qing, G. (2020). Regulation of cancer cell metabolism: Oncogenic MYC in the driver's seat. *Signal Transduction and Targeted Therapy*, 5, 124.

Dong, Z., & Cui, H. (2019). Epigenetic modulation of metabolism in glioblastoma. *Seminars in Cancer Biology*, 57, 45–51.

Duchatel, R. J., Jackson, E. R., Alvaro, F., Nixon, B., Hondermarck, H., & Dun, M. D. (2019). Signal transduction in diffuse intrinsic pontine glioma. *Proteomics*, 19, Article e1800479.

Duffy, M. J., & Crown, J. (2020). Drugging "undruggable" genes for cancer treatment: Are we making progress? *International Journal of Cancer*, 148, 8–17.

Dunphy, M. P. S., Harding, J. J., Venneti, S., Zhang, H., Burnazi, E. M., Bromberg, J., Omuro, A. M., Hsieh, J. J., Mellinghoff, I. K., Staton, K., Pressl, C., Beattie, B. J., Zanzonico, P. B., Gerecitano, J. F., Kelsen, D. P., Weber, W., Lyashchenko, S. K., Kung, H. F., & Lewis, J. S. (2018). In vivo PET assay of tumor glutamine flux and metabolism: In-human trial of ^{18}F-(2S,4R)-4-fluoroglutamine. *Radiology*, 287, 667–675.

Ehtesham, M., Winston, J. A., Kabos, P., & Thompson, R. C. (2006). CXCR4 expression mediates glioma cell invasiveness. *Oncogene*, 25, 2801–2806.

Erickson, N., Boscheri, A., Linke, B., & Huebner, J. (2017). Systematic review: Isocaloric ketogenic dietary regimes for cancer patients. *Medical Oncology*, 34, 72.

Esteller, M. (2008). Epigenetics in cancer. *New England Journal of Medicine*, 358, 1148–1159.

Faubert, B., Solmonson, A., & DeBerardinis, R. J. (2020). Metabolic reprogramming and cancer progression. *Science*, 368, 152–162.

Faubert, B., Vincent, E. E., Poffenberger, M. C., & Jones, R. G. (2015). The AMP-activated protein kinase (AMPK) and cancer: Many faces of a metabolic regulator. *Cancer Letters*, 356, 165–170.

Fearon, K. C., Borland, W., Preston, T., Tisdale, M. J., Shenkin, A., & Calman, K. C. (1988). Cancer cachexia: Influence of systemic ketosis on substrate levels and nitrogen metabolism. *American Journal of Clinical Nutrition*, 47, 42–48.

Feinberg, A. P., Ohlsson, R., & Henikoff, S. (2006). The epigenetic progenitor origin of human cancer. *Nature Reviews Genetics*, 7, 21–33.

Fischer, S., Wobben, M., Marti, H. H., Renz, D., & Schaper, W. (2002). Hypoxia-induced hyperpermeability in brain microvessel endothelial cells involves VEGF-mediated changes in the expression of zonula occludens-1. *Microvascular Research*, 63, 70–80.

Fleischmann, D. F., Jenn, J., Corradini, S., Ruf, V., Herms, J., Forbrig, R., Unterrainer, M., Thon, N., Kreth, F.W., Belka, C., & Niyazi, M. (2019). Bevacizumab reduces toxicity of reirradiation in recurrent high-grade glioma. *Radiotherapy and Oncology*, 138, 99–105.

Fredericks, M., & Ramsey, R. B. (1978). 3-Oxo acid coenzyme A transferase activity in brain and tumors of the nervous system. *Journal of Neurochemistry, 31*, 1529–1531.

Freedland, S. J., Mavropoulos, J., Wang, A., Darshan, M., Demark-Wahnefried, W., Aronson, W. J., Cohen, P., Hwang, D., Peterson, B., Fields, T., Pizzo, S. V., & Isaacs, W. B. (2008). Carbohydrate restriction, prostate cancer growth, and the insulin-like growth factor axis. *Prostate, 68*, 11–19.

Fruehauf, J. P., & Meyskens, F. L., Jr. (2007). Reactive oxygen species: A breath of life or death? *Clinical Cancer Research, 13*, 789–794.

Fuchs, Q., Pierrevelcin, M., Messe, M., Lhermitte, B., Blandin, A. F., Papin, C., Coca, A., Dontenwill, M., & Entz-Werlé, N. (2020). Hypoxia inducible factors' signaling in pediatric high-grade gliomas: Role, modelization and innovative targeted approaches. *Cancers, 12*, 979–992.

Fujiwara, S., Nakagawa, K., Harada, H., Nagato, S., Furukawa, K., Teraoka, M., Seno, T., Oka, K., Iwata, S., & Ohnishi, T. (2007). Silencing hypoxia-inducible factor-1α inhibits cell migration and invasion under hypoxic environment in malignant gliomas. *International Journal of Oncology, 30*, 793–802.

Gargini, R., Segura-Collar, B., & Sánchez-Gómez, P. (2020). Cellular plasticity and tumor microenvironment in gliomas: The struggle to hit a moving target. *Cancers, 12*, 1622–1646.

Gasior, M., Rogawski, M. A., & Hartman, A. L. (2006). Neuroprotective and disease-modifying effects of the ketogenic diet. *Behavioural Pharmacology, 17*, 431–439.

Gatenby, R. A., & Gillies, R. J. (2004). Why do cancers have high aerobic glycolysis? *Nature Reviews Cancer, 4*, 891–899.

Gaude, E., & Frezza, C. (2014). Defects in mitochondrial metabolism and cancer. *Cancer Metabolism, 2*, 10–12.

Ghoneum, A., Abdulfattah, A. Y., Warren, B. O., Shu, J., & Said, N. (2020). Redox homeostasis and metabolism in cancer: A complex mechanism and potential targeted therapeutics. *International Journal of Molecular Sciences, 21*, 3100.

Giannone, G., Ghisoni, E., Genta, S., Scotto, G., Tuninetti, V., Turinetto, M., & Valabrega, G. (2020). Immuno-metabolism and microenvironment in cancer: Key players for immunotherapy. *International Journal of Molecular Sciences, 21*, 4414–4436.

Gil Del Alcazar, C. R., Hardebeck, M. C., Mukherjee, B., Tomimatsu, N., Gao, X., Yan, J., Xie, X. J., Bachoo, R., Li, L., Habib, A. A., & Burma, S. (2014). Inhibition of DNA double-strand break repair by the dual PI3K/mTOR inhibitor NVP-BEZ235 as a strategy for radiosensitization of glioblastoma. *Clinical Cancer Research, 20*, 1235–1248.

Gluschnaider, U., Hertz, R., Ohayon, S., Smeir, E., Smets, M., Pikarsky, E., & Bar-Tana, J. (2014). Long-chain fatty acid analogues suppress breast tumorigenesis and progression. *Cancer Research, 74*, 6991–7002.

Golonka, R. M., Xiao, X., Abokor, A. A., Joe, B., & Vijay-Kumar, M. (2020). Altered nutrient status reprograms host inflammation and metabolic health via gut microbiota. *Journal of Nutritional Biochemistry, 80*, 108360.

Gozzelino, L., De Santis, M. C., Gulluni, F., Hirsch, E., & Martini, M. (2020). PI(3,4)P2 signaling in cancer and metabolism. *Frontiers in Oncology, 10*, 360.

Gravina, G. L., Mancini, A., Colapietro, A., Delle Monache, S., Sferra, R., Pompili, S., Vitale, F., Martellucci, S., Marampon, F., Mattei, V., Biordi, L., Sherris, D., & Festuccia, C. (2019). The brain penetrating and dual TORC1/TORC2 inhibitor, RES529, elicits anti-glioma activity and enhances the therapeutic effects of anti-angiogenetic compounds in preclinical murine models. *Cancers, 11*, 1604–1630.

Gravina, G. L., Mancini, A., Marampon, F., Colapietro, A., Delle Monache, S., Sferra, R., Vitale, F., Richardson, P. J., Patient, L., Burbidge, S., & Festuccia, C. (2017). The brain-penetrating CXCR4 antagonist, PRX177561, increases the antitumor effects of bevacizumab and sunitinib in preclinical models of human glioblastoma. *Journal of Hematology & Oncology, 10*, 5.

Gray, A., Dang, B. N., Moore, T. B., Clemens, R., & Pressman, P. (2020). A review of nutrition and dietary interventions in oncology. *SAGE Open Medicine, 8*, Article 2050312120926877.

Gresham, G., Amaral, L., Lockshon, L., Levin, D., Rudnick, J., Provisor, A., Shiao, S., Bhowmick, N., Irwin, S., Freedland, S., & Hu, J. (2019). ACTR-15: Phase 1 trial of a ketogenic diet in patients receiving standard-of-care treatment for recently diagnosed glioblastoma. *Neuro-Oncology, 21*, vi15–vi15.

Guo, D., Bell, E. H., Mischel, P., & Chakravarti, A. (2014). Targeting SREBP-1-driven lipid metabolism to treat cancer. *Current Pharmaceutical Design, 20*, 2619–2626.

Gusyatiner, O., & Hegi, M. E. (2018). Glioma epigenetics: From subclassification to novel treatment options. *Seminars in Cancer Biology, 51*, 50–58.

Gwak, H. S., & Park, H. J. (2017). Developing chemotherapy for diffuse pontine intrinsic gliomas (DIPG). *Critical Reviews in Oncology/Hematology, 120*, 111–119.

Habermann, N., Makar, K. W., Abbenhardt, C., Xiao, L., Wang, C. Y., Utsugi, H. K., Alfano, C. M., Campbell, K. L., Duggan, C., Foster-Schubert, K. E., Mason, C. E., Imayama, I., Blackburn, G. L., Potter, J. D., McTiernan, A., & Ulrich, C. M.

(2015). No effect of caloric restriction or exercise on radiation repair capacity. *Medicine and Science in Sports and Exercise, 47,* 896–904.

Hagihara, K., Kajimoto, K., Osaga, S., Nagai, N., Shimosegawa, E., Nakata, H., Saito, H., Nakano, M., Takeuchi, M., Kanki, H., Kagitani-Shimono, K., & Kijima, T. (2020). Promising effect of a new ketogenic diet regimen in patients with advanced cancer. *Nutrients, 12,* 1473–1485.

Hanahan, D., & Weinberg, R. A. (2011). Hallmarks of cancer: The next generation. *Cell, 144,* 646–674.

Hao, G. W., Chen, Y. S., He, D. M., Wang, H. Y., Wu, G. H., & Zhang, B. (2015). Growth of human colon cancer cells in nude mice is delayed by ketogenic diet with or without omega-3 fatty acids and medium-chain triglycerides. *Asian Pacific Journal of Cancer Prevention, 16,* 2061–2068.

Hardian, R. F., Goto, T., Kuwabara, H., Hanaoka, Y., Kobayashi, S., Kanno, H., Shimojo, H., Horiuchi, T., & Hongo, K. (2019). An autopsy case of widespread brain dissemination of glioblastoma unnoticed by magnetic resonance imaging after treatment with bevacizumab. *Surgical Neurology International, 10,* 137.

Hartman, A. L. (2012). Neuroprotection in metabolism-based therapy. *Epilepsy Research, 100,* 286–294.

Hartman, R. E., & Patel, D. (2020). Dietary approaches to the management of autism spectrum disorders. *Advances in Neurobiology, 24,* 547–571.

Hattingen, E., Jurcoane, A., Bahr, O., Rieger, J., Magerkurth, J., Anti, S., Steinbach, J. P., & Pilatus, U. (2011). Bevacizumab impairs oxidative energy metabolism and shows antitumoral effects in recurrent glioblastomas: A $^{31}P/^1H$ MRSI and quantitative magnetic resonance imaging study. *Neuro-Oncology, 13,* 1349–1363.

Hayashi, Y., Edwards, N. A., Proescholdt, M. A., Oldfield, E. H., & Merrill, M. J. (2007). Regulation and function of aquaporin-1 in glioma cells. *Neoplasia, 9,* 777–787.

Heydari, A. R., Unnikrishnan, A., Lucente, L. V., & Richardson, A. (2007). Caloric restriction and genomic stability. *Nucleic Acids Research, 35,* 7485–7496.

Hopkins, B. D., Goncalves, M. D., & Cantley, L. C. (2020). Insulin-PI3K signalling: An evolutionarily insulated metabolic driver of cancer. *Nature Reviews Endocrinology, 16,* 276–283.

Hopkins, B. D., Pauli, C., Du, X., Wang, D. G., Li, X., Wu, D., Amadiume, S. C., Goncalves, M. D., Hodakoski, C., Lundquist, M. R., Bareja, R., Ma, Y., Harris, E. M., Sboner, A., Beltran, H., Rubin, M. A., Mukherjee, S., & Cantley, L. C. (2018). Suppression of insulin feedback enhances the efficacy of PI3K inhibitors. *Nature, 560,* 499–503.

Horing, E., Harter, P. N., Seznec, J., Schittenhelm, J., Buhring, H. J., Bhattacharyya, S., von, H. E., Zachskorn, C., Mittelbronn, M., & Naumann, U.

(2012). The "go or grow" potential of gliomas is linked to the neuropeptide processing enzyme carboxypeptidase E and mediated by metabolic stress. *Acta Neuropathologica, 124,* 83–97.

Hu, A., Xu, Z., Kim, R. Y., Nguyen, A., Lee, J. W., & Kesari, S. (2011). Seizure control: A secondary benefit of chemotherapeutic temozolomide in brain cancer patients. *Epilepsy Research, 95,* 270–272.

Huang, J., Jiang, Z., Wang, Y., Fan, X., Cai, J., Yao, X., Liu, L., Huang, J., He, J., Xie, C., Wu, Q., Cao, Y., & Leung, E. L. (2020). Modulation of gut microbiota to overcome resistance to immune checkpoint blockade in cancer immunotherapy. *Current Opinion in Pharmacology, 54,* 1–10.

Icard, P., Ollivier, L., Forgez, P., Otz, J., Alifano, M., Fournel, L., Loi, M., & Thariat, J. (2020). Perspective: Do fasting, caloric restriction, and diets increase sensitivity to radiotherapy? A literature review. *Advances in Nutrition, 11,* 1089–1101.

Inamura, K. (2021). Gut microbiota contributes towards immunomodulation against cancer: New frontiers in precision cancer therapeutics. *Seminars in Cancer Biology, 70,* 11–23.

Irani, S., & Hussain, M. M. (2015). Role of microRNA-30c in lipid metabolism, adipogenesis, cardiac remodeling and cancer. *Current Opinion in Lipidology, 26,* 139–146.

Iurlaro, R., Leon-Annicchiarico, C. L., & Munoz-Pinedo, C. (2014). Regulation of cancer metabolism by oncogenes and tumor suppressors. *Methods in Enzymology, 542,* 59–80.

Iyikesici, M. S. (2019). Feasibility study of metabolically supported chemotherapy with weekly carboplatin/paclitaxel combined with ketogenic diet, hyperthermia and hyperbaric oxygen therapy in metastatic non-small cell lung cancer. *International Journal of Hyperthermia, 36,* 446–455.

Iyikesici, M. S. (2020). Survival outcomes of metabolically supported chemotherapy combined with ketogenic diet, hyperthermia, and hyperbaric oxygen therapy in advanced gastric cancer. *Nigerian Journal of Clinical Practice, 23,* 734–740.

İyikesici, M. S., Slocum, A. K., Slocum, A., Berkarda, F. B., Kalamian, M., & Seyfried, T. N. (2017). Efficacy of metabolically supported chemotherapy combined with ketogenic diet, hyperthermia, and hyperbaric oxygen therapy for stage IV triple-negative breast cancer. *Cureus, 9,* Article e1445.

Jagust, P., de Luxán-Delgado, B., Parejo-Alonso, B., & Sancho, P. (2019). Metabolism-based therapeutic strategies targeting cancer stem cells. *Frontiers in Pharmacology, 10,* 203.

Jing, X., Yang, F., Shao, C., Wei, K., Xie, M., Shen, H., & Shu, Y. (2019). Role of hypoxia in cancer therapy by regulating the tumor microenvironment. *Molecular Cancer, 18,* 157.

Jones, R. G., Plas, D. R., Kubek, S., Buzzai, M., Mu, J., Xu, Y., Birnbaum, M.J., & Thompson, C. B. (2005). AMP-activated protein kinase induces a p53-dependent metabolic checkpoint. *Molecular Cell, 18*, 283–293.

Joon, Y. A., Bazar, K. A., & Lee, P. Y. (2004). Tumors may modulate host immunity partly through hypoxia-induced sympathetic bias. *Medical Hypotheses, 63*, 352–356.

Jung, J. G., & Le, A. (2018). Targeting metabolic cross talk between cancer cells and cancer-associated fibroblasts. *Advances in Experimental Medicine and Biology, 1063*, 167–178.

Justus, C. R., Sanderlin, E. J., & Yang, L. V. (2015). Molecular connections between cancer cell metabolism and the tumor microenvironment. *International Journal of Molecular Science, 16*, 11055–11086.

Kanarek, N., Petrova, B., & Sabatini, D. M. (2020). Dietary modifications for enhanced cancer therapy. *Nature, 579*, 507–517.

Kang, J. S. (2020). Dietary restriction of amino acids for cancer therapy. *Nutrition & Metabolism, 17*, 20.

Kari, F. W., Dunn, S. E., French, J. E., & Barrett, J. C. (1999). Roles for insulin-like growth factor-1 in mediating the anti-carcinogenic effects of caloric restriction. *Journal of Nutrition, Health & Aging, 3*, 92–101.

Kasumi, E., & Sato, N. (2019). A ketogenic diet improves the prognosis in a mouse model of peritoneal dissemination without tumor regression. *Journal of Clinical Biochemistry and Nutrition, 64*, 201–208.

Katsuya, Y., Fujiwara, Y., Sunami, K., Utsumi, H., Goto, Y., Kanda, S., Horinouchi, H., Nokihara, H., Yamamoto, N., Takashima, Y., Osawa, S., Ohe, Y., Tamura, T., & Hamada, A. (2015). Comparison of the pharmacokinetics of erlotinib administered in complete fasting and 2 h after a meal in patients with lung cancer. *Cancer Chemotherapy and Pharmacology, 76*, 125–132.

Kaur, B., Khwaja, F. W., Severson, E. A., Matheny, S. L., Brat, D. J., & Van Meir, E. G. (2005). Hypoxia and the hypoxia-inducible-factor pathway in glioma growth and angiogenesis. *Neuro-Oncology, 7*, 134–153.

Ke, W., Saba, J. A., Yao, C. H., Hilzendeger, M. A., Drangowska-Way, A., Joshi, C., Mony, V. K., Benjamin, S. B., Zhang, S., Locasale, J., Patti, G. J., Lewis, N., & O'Rourke, E. J. (2020). Dietary serine–microbiota interaction enhances chemotherapeutic toxicity without altering drug conversion. *Nature Communications, 11*, 2587.

Khan, M. R., Xiang, S., Song, Z., & Wu, M. (2017). The p53-inducible long noncoding RNA TRINGS protects cancer cells from necrosis under glucose starvation. *EMBO Journal, 36*, 3483–3500.

Khodadadi, S., Sobhani, N., Mirshekar, S., Ghiasvand, R., Pourmasoumi, M., Miraghajani, M., & Dehsoukhteh, S. S. (2017). Tumor cells growth and survival time with the ketogenic diet in animal models: A systematic review. *International Journal of Preventive Medicine, 8*, 35.

Kim, D. Y., Hao, J., Liu, R., Turner, G., Shi, F. D., & Rho, J. M. (2012a). Inflammation-mediated memory dysfunction and effects of a ketogenic diet in a murine model of multiple sclerosis. *PLOS ONE, 7*, Article e35476.

Kim, D. Y., & Rho, J. M. (2008). The ketogenic diet and epilepsy. *Current Opinion in Clinical Nutrition and Metabolic Care, 11*, 113–120.

Kim, H. S., Masko, E. M., Poulton, S. L., Kennedy, K. M., Pizzo, S. V., Dewhirst, M. W., & Freedland, S. J. (2012b). Carbohydrate restriction and lactate transporter inhibition in a mouse xenograft model of human prostate cancer. *BJU International, 110*, 1062–1069.

Kim, K. H., & Roberts, C. W. (2016). Targeting EZH2 in cancer. *Nature Medicine, 22*, 128–134.

Kinnaird, A., & Michelakis, E. D. (2015). Metabolic modulation of cancer: A new frontier with great translational potential. *Journal of Molecular Medicine, 93*, 127–142.

Kirkham, A. A., Paterson, D. I., Prado, C. M., Mackey, J. R., Courneya, K. S., Pituskin, E., & Thompson, R. B. (2018). Rationale and design of the Caloric Restriction and Exercise protection from Anthracycline Toxic Effects (CREATE) study: A 3-arm parallel group phase II randomized controlled trial in early breast cancer. *BMC Cancer, 18*, 864.

Klement, R. J. (2013). Calorie or carbohydrate restriction? The ketogenic diet as another option for supportive cancer treatment. *Oncologist, 18*, 1056.

Klement, R. J. (2017). Beneficial effects of ketogenic diets for cancer patients: A realist review with focus on evidence and confirmation. *Medical Oncology, 34*, 132.

Klement, R. J., Brehm, N., & Sweeney, R. A. (2020a). Ketogenic diets in medical oncology: A systematic review with focus on clinical outcomes. *Medical Oncology, 37*, 14.

Klement, R. J., & Champ, C. E. (2014). Calories, carbohydrates, and cancer therapy with radiation: Exploiting the five R's through dietary manipulation. *Cancer Metastasis Review, 33*, 217–229.

Klement, R. J., Champ, C. E., Otto, C., & Kämmerer, U. (2016). Anti-tumor effects of ketogenic diets in mice: A meta-analysis. *PLOS ONE, 11*, Article e0155050.

Klement, R. J., & Pazienza, V. (2019). Impact of different types of diet on gut microbiota profiles and cancer prevention and treatment. *Medicina, 55*, 84–94.

Klement, R. J., Schäfer, G., & Sweeney, R. A. (2020b). A ketogenic diet exerts beneficial effects on body composition of cancer patients during radiotherapy: An interim analysis of the KETOCOMP study. *Journal of Traditional and Complementary Medicine, 10,* 180–187.

Klement, R. J., & Sweeney, R. A. (2016a). Impact of a ketogenic diet intervention during radiotherapy on body composition: I. Initial clinical experience with six prospectively studied patients. *BMC Research Notes, 9,* 143.

Klement, R. J., & Sweeney, R. A. (2016b). Impact of a ketogenic diet intervention during radiotherapy on body composition: II. Protocol of a randomised phase I study (KETOCOMP). *Clinical Nutrition ESPEN, 12,* e1–e6.

Koppel, S. J., & Swerdlow, R. H. (2018). Neuroketotherapeutics: A modern review of a century-old therapy. *Neurochemistry International, 117,* 114–125.

Koutnik, A. P., Poff, A. M., Ward, N. P., DeBlasi, J. M., Soliven, M. A., Romero, M. A., Roberson, P. A., Fox, C. D., Roberts, M. D., & D'Agostino, D. P. (2020). Ketone bodies attenuate wasting in models of atrophy. *Journal of Cachexia, Sarcopenia and Muscle, 11,* 973–996.

Kraeuter, A. K., Phillips, R., & Sarnyai, Z. (2020). Ketogenic therapy in neurodegenerative and psychiatric disorders: From mice to men. *Progress in Neuro-Psychopharmacology & Biological Psychiatry, 101,* 109913.

Kung, C. P., Liu, Q., & Murphy, M. E. (2017). The codon 72 polymorphism of p53 influences cell fate following nutrient deprivation. *Cancer Biology & Therapy, 18,* 484–491.

Labuschagne, C. F., Zani, F., & Vousden, K.H. (2018). Control of metabolism by p53—Cancer and beyond. *Biochimica et Biophysica Acta - Reviews on Cancer, 1870,* 32–42.

Lamichhane, S., Bastola, T., Pariyar, R., Lee, E. S., Lee, H. S., Lee, D. H., & Seo, J. (2017). ROS production and ERK activity are involved in the effects of D-beta-hydroxybutyrate and metformin in a glucose deficient condition. *International Journal of Molecular Sciences, 18,* 674–690.

Landau, B. R., Laszlo, J., Stengle, J., & Burk, D. (1958). Certain metabolic and pharmacologic effects in cancer patients given infusions of 2-deoxy-D-glucose. *Journal of the National Cancer Institute, 21,* 485–494.

Larionova, I., Kazakova, E., Patysheva, M., & Kzhyshkowska, J. (2020). Transcriptional, epigenetic and metabolic programming of tumor-associated macrophages. *Cancers, 12,* 1411–1452.

Läsche, M., Emons, G., & Gründker, C. (2020). Shedding new light on cancer metabolism: A metabolic tightrope between life and death. *Frontiers in Oncology, 10,* 409.

Laskov, I., Drudi, L., Beauchamp, M. C., Yasmeen, A., Ferenczy, A., Pollak, M., & Gotlieb, W. H. (2014). Anti-diabetic doses of metformin decrease proliferation markers in tumors of patients with endometrial cancer. *Gynecologic Oncology, 134,* 607–614.

Le Rhun, E., Preusser, M., Roth, P., Reardon, D. A., van den Bent, M., Wen, P., Reifenberger, G., & Weller, M. (2019). Molecular targeted therapy of glioblastoma. *Cancer Treatment Reviews, 80,* 101896.

Lee, C., Raffaghello, L., Brandhorst, S., Safdie, F. M., Bianchi, G., Martin-Montalvo, A., Pistoia, V., Wei, M., Hwang, S., Merlino, A., Emionite, L., de, Cabo R., & Longo, V. D. (2012). Fasting cycles retard growth of tumors and sensitize a range of cancer cell types to chemotherapy. *Science Translational Medicine, 4,* 124–127.

Lee, C., Safdie, F. M., Raffaghello, L., Wei, M., Madia, F., Parrella, E., Hwang, D., Cohen, P., Bianchi, G., & Longo, V. D. (2010). Reduced levels of IGF-I mediate differential protection of normal and cancer cells in response to fasting and improve chemotherapeutic index. *Cancer Research, 70,* 1564–1572.

Lee, E., Yong, R. L., Paddison, P., & Zhu, J. (2018). Comparison of glioblastoma (GBM) molecular classification methods. *Seminars in Cancer Biology, 53,* 201–211.

Lee, P., Murphy, B., Miller, R., Menon, V., Banik, N. L., Giglio, P., Lindhorst, S. M., Varma, A. K., Vandergrift, W. A., III, Patel, S. J., & Das, A. (2015). Mechanisms and clinical significance of histone deacetylase inhibitors: Epigenetic glioblastoma therapy. *Anticancer Research, 35,* 615–625.

Lee, S. H., & Griffiths, J. R. (2020). How and why are cancers acidic? Carbonic anhydrase IX and the homeostatic control of tumour extracellular pH. *Cancers, 12,* 1616–1641.

Lende, T. H., Austdal, M., Varhaugvik, A. E., Skaland, I., Gudlaugsson, E., Kvaløy, J. T., Akslen, L. A., Søiland, H., Janssen, E. A. M., & Baak, J. P. A. (2019). Influence of pre-operative oral carbohydrate loading vs. standard fasting on tumor proliferation and clinical outcome in breast cancer patients—A randomized trial. *BMC Cancer, 19,* 1076.

Lévesque, S., Pol, J. G., Ferrere, G., Galluzzi, L., Zitvogel, L., & Kroemer, G. (2019). Trial watch: Dietary interventions for cancer therapy. *Oncoimmunology, 8,* 1591878.

Lewis, N. E., & Abdel-Haleem, A. M. (2013). The evolution of genome-scale models of cancer metabolism. *Frontiers in Physiology, 4,* 237.

Lhermitte, B., Blandin, A. F., Coca, A., Guerin, E., Durand, A., & Entz-Werlé, N. (2018). Signaling pathway deregulation and molecular alterations across pediatric medulloblastomas. *Neurochirurgie, 67,* 39–45.

Li, J. H., Han, L., Du, T. P., & Guo, M. J. (2015). The effect of low-nitrogen and low-calorie parenteral nutrition combined with enteral nutrition on inflammatory cytokines and immune functions in patients with gastric cancer: A double blind placebo trial. *European Review for Medical and Pharmacological Sciences, 19,* 1345–1350.

Li, R. J., Liu, Y., Liu, H. Q., & Li, J. (2020). Ketogenic diets and protective mechanisms in epilepsy, metabolic disorders, cancer, neuronal loss, and muscle and nerve degeneration. *Journal of Food Biochemistry, 44,* Article e13140.

Li, W., Guo, F., Wang, P., Hong, S., & Zhang, C. (2014). miR-221/222 confers radioresistance in glioblastoma cells through activating Akt independent of PTEN status. *Current Molecular Medicine, 14,* 185–195.

Li, X., Yu, X., Dai, D., Song, X., & Xu, W. (2016). The altered glucose metabolism in tumor and a tumor acidic microenvironment associated with extracellular matrix metalloproteinase inducer and monocarboxylate transporters. *Oncotarget, 7,* 15.

Liang, S., Ji, L., Kang, L., & Hu, X. (2020). Metabolic regulation of innate immunity. *Advances in Immunology, 145,* 129–157.

Lin, J., Xia, L., Liang, J., Han, Y., Wang, H., Oyang, L., Tan, S., Tian, Y., Rao, S., Chen, X., Tang, Y., Su, M., Luo, X., Wang, Y., Wang, H., Zhou, Y., & Liao, Q. (2019). The roles of glucose metabolic reprogramming in chemo- and radio-resistance. *Journal of Experimental & Clinical Cancer Research, 38,* 218.

Lio, C. J., & Huang, S. C. (2020). Circles of life: Linking metabolic and epigenetic cycles to immunity. *Immunology, 161,* 165–174.

Lorito, N., Bacci, M., Smiriglia, A., Mannelli, M., Parri, M., Comito, G., Ippolito, L., Giannoni, E., Bonechi, M., Benelli, M., Migliaccio, I., Malorni, L., Chiarugi, P., & Morandi, A. (2020). Glucose metabolic reprogramming of ER breast cancer in acquired resistance to the CDK4/6 inhibitor palbociclib. *Cells, 9,* 668–690.

Lu, V. M., Goyal, A., Vaughan, L. S., & McDonald, K. L. (2018). The impact of hyperglycemia on survival in glioblastoma: A systematic review and meta-analysis. *Clinical Neurology and Neurosurgery, 170,* 165–169.

Lubberman, F. J. E., Burger, D., & van Erp, N. P. (2017). Poorly specified fasting conditions in clinical research could lead to treatment failure. *Lancet Oncology, 18,* 571–573.

Ludwig, D. S. (2020). The ketogenic diet: Evidence for optimism but high-quality research needed. *Journal of Nutrition, 150,* 1354–1359.

Lund, T. M., Risa, O., Sonnewald, U., Schousboe, A., & Waagepetersen, H. S. (2009). Availability of neurotransmitter glutamate is diminished when beta-hydroxybutyrate replaces glucose in cultured neurons. *Journal of Neurochemistry, 110,* 80–91.

Lussier, D. M., Woolf, E. C., Johnson, J. L., Brooks, K. S., Blattman, J. N., & Scheck, A. C. (2016).

Enhanced immunity in a mouse model of malignant glioma is mediated by a therapeutic ketogenic diet. *BMC Cancer, 16,* 310.

Lv, M., Zhu, X., Wang, H., Wang, F., & Guan, W. (2014). Roles of caloric restriction, ketogenic diet and intermittent fasting during initiation, progression and metastasis of cancer in animal models: A systematic review and meta-analysis. *PLOS ONE, 9,* Article e115147.

Maalouf, M., Rho, J. M., & Mattson, M. P. (2009). The neuroprotective properties of calorie restriction, the ketogenic diet, and ketone bodies. *Brain Research Reviews, 59,* 293–315.

Magee, B. A., Potezny, N., Rofe, A. M., & Conyers, R. A. (1979). The inhibition of malignant cell growth by ketone bodies. *Australian Journal of Experimental Biology and Medical Science, 57,* 529–539.

Mai, W. X., Gosa, L., Daniels, V. W., Ta, L., Tsang, J. E., Higgins, B., Gilmore, W. B., Bayley, N. A., Harati, M. D., Lee, J. T., Yong, W. H., Kornblum, H. I., Bensinger, S. J., Mischel, P. S., Rao, P. N., Clark, P. M., Cloughesy, T. F., Letai, A., & Nathanson, D. A. (2017). Cytoplasmic p53 couples oncogene-driven glucose metabolism to apoptosis and is a therapeutic target in glioblastoma. *Nature Medicine, 23,* 1342–1351.

Marchiq, I., & Pouyssegur, J. (2016). Hypoxia, cancer metabolism and the therapeutic benefit of targeting lactate/H symporters. *Journal of Molecular Medicine, 94,* 155–171.

Marie, S. K., & Shinjo, S. M. (2011). Metabolism and brain cancer. *Clinics* (Sao Paulo), 66(Suppl. 1), 33–43.

Maroon, J. C., Seyfried, T. N., Donohue, J. P., & Bost, J. (2015). The role of metabolic therapy in treating glioblastoma multiforme. *Surgical Neurology International, 6,* 61. https://doi.org/10.4103/2152-7806.155259

Marsh, J., Mukherjee, P., & Seyfried, T. N. (2008). Drug/diet synergy for managing malignant astrocytoma in mice: 2-Deoxy-D-glucose and the restricted ketogenic diet. *Nutrition & Metabolism, 5,* 33.

Martuscello, R. T., Vedam-Mai, V., McCarthy, D. J., Schmoll, M. E., Jundi, M. A., Louviere, C. D., Griffith, B. G., Skinner, C. L., Suslov, O., Deleyrolle, L. P., & Reynolds, B. A. (2016). A supplemented high-fat low-carbohydrate diet for the treatment of glioblastoma. *Clinical Cancer Research, 22,* 2482–2495.

Masson, N., & Ratcliffe, P. J. (2014). Hypoxia signaling pathways in cancer metabolism: The importance of co-selecting interconnected physiological pathways. *Cancer Metabolism, 2,* 3.

Masui, K., Cavenee, W. K., & Mischel, P. S. (2015). mTORC2 and metabolic reprogramming in GBM: At the interface of genetics and environment. *Brain Pathology, 25,* 755–759.

Masui, K., Cavenee, W. K., & Mischel, P. S. (2016). Cancer metabolism as a central driving force of glioma pathogenesis. *Brain Tumor Pathology*, 33, 161–168.

Masui, K., Harachi, M., Cavenee, W. K., Mischel, P. S., & Shibata, N. (2020). Codependency of metabolism and epigenetics drives cancer progression: A review. *Acta Histochemica et Cytochemica*, 53, 1–10.

Masui, K., Onizuka, H., Cavenee, W. K., Mischel, P. S., & Shibata, N. (2019). Metabolic reprogramming in the pathogenesis of glioma: Update. *Neuropathology*, 39, 3–13.

Maurer, G. D., Brucker, D. P., Bahr, O., Harter, P. N., Hattingen, E., Walenta, S., Mueller-Klieser, W., Steinbach, J. P., & Rieger, J. (2011). Differential utilization of ketone bodies by neurons and glioma cell lines: A rationale for ketogenic diet as experimental glioma therapy. *BMC Cancer*, 11, 315.

Mavropoulos, J. C., Buschemeyer, W. C., III, Tewari, A. K., Rokhfeld, D., Pollak, M., Zhao, Y., Febbo, P. G., Cohen, P., Hwang, D., Devi, G., Demark-Wahnefried, W., Westman, E. C., Peterson, B. L., Pizzo, S. V., & Freedland, S. J. (2009). The effects of varying dietary carbohydrate and fat content on survival in a murine LNCaP prostate cancer xenograft model. *Cancer Prevention Research*, 2, 557–565.

Mayer, A., Vaupel, P., Struss, H. G., Giese, A., Stockinger, M., & Schmidberger, H. (2014). Strong adverse prognostic impact of hyperglycemic episodes during adjuvant chemoradiotherapy of glioblastoma multiforme. *Strahlentherapie und Onkologie*, 190, 933–938.

McGirt, M. J., Chaichana, K. L., Gathinji, M., Attenello, F., Than, K., Ruiz, A. J., Olivi, A., & Quinones-Hinojosa, A. (2008). Persistent outpatient hyperglycemia is independently associated with decreased survival after primary resection of malignant brain astrocytomas. *Neurosurgery*, 63, 286–291.

McLaughlin, M., Patin, E. C., Pedersen, M., Wilkins, A., Dillon, M. T., Melcher, A. A., & Harrington, K. J. (2020). Inflammatory microenvironment remodelling by tumour cells after radiotherapy. *Nature Reviews Cancer*, 20, 203–217.

Medova, M., Aebersold, D. M., & Zimmer, Y. (2013). The molecular crosstalk between the MET receptor tyrosine kinase and the DNA damage response—Biological and clinical aspects. *Cancers*, 6, 1–27.

Mehdikhani, F., Ghahremani, H., Nabati, S., Tahmouri, H., Sirati-Sabet, M., & Salami, S. (2019). Histone butyrylation/acetylation remains unchanged in triple negative breast cancer cells after a long term metabolic reprogramming. *Asian Pacific Journal of Cancer Prevention*, 20, 3597–3601.

Mehrian-Shai, R., Reichardt, J. K. V., Harris, C. C., & Toren, A. (2019). The gut–brain axis, paving the way to brain cancer. *Trends in Cancer, 5,* 200–207.

Meidenbauer, J. J., Mukherjee, P., & Seyfried, T. N. (2015). The glucose ketone index calculator: A simple tool to monitor therapeutic efficacy for metabolic management of brain cancer. *Nutrition & Metabolism*, 12, 12. https://doi.org/10.1186/s12986-015-0009-2

Menyhárt, O., Giangaspero, F., & Győrffy, B. (2019). Molecular markers and potential therapeutic targets in non-WNT/non-SHH (group 3 and group 4) medulloblastomas. *Journal of Hematology & Oncology*, 12, 29.

Metallo, C. M., Gameiro, P. A., Bell, E. L., Mattaini, K. R., Yang, J., Hiller, K., Jewell, C. M., Johnson, Z. R., Irvine, D. J., Guarente, L., Kelleher, J. K., Vander Heiden, M. G., Iliopoulos, O., & Stephanopoulos, G. (2011). Reductive glutamine metabolism by IDH1 mediates lipogenesis under hypoxia. *Nature*, 481, 380–384.

Milde, T., Lodrini, M., Savelyeva, L., Korshunov, A., Kool, M., Brueckner, L. M., Antunes, A. S., Oehme, I., Pekrun, A., Pfister, S. M., Kulozik, A. E., Witt, O., & Deubzer, H. E. (2012). HD-MB03 is a novel Group 3 medulloblastoma model demonstrating sensitivity to histone deacetylase inhibitor treatment. *Journal of Neuro-Oncology*, 110, 335–348.

Milder, J., & Patel, M. (2012). Modulation of oxidative stress and mitochondrial function by the ketogenic diet. *Epilepsy Research*, 100, 295–303.

Miller, D. M., Thomas, S. D., Islam, A., Muench, D., & Sedoris, K. (2012). c-Myc and cancer metabolism. *Clinical Cancer Research*, 18, 5546–5553.

Miller, J. J., & Wen, P. Y. (2016). Emerging targeted therapies for glioma. *Expert Opinion on Emerging Drugs*, 21, 441–452.

Mitchell, T., Clarke, L., Goldberg, A., & Bishop, K. S. (2019). Pancreatic cancer cachexia: The role of nutritional interventions. *Healthcare*, 7, 89–108.

Miyazaki, T., Uemae, Y., & Ishikawa, E. (2017). CXCL12/CXCR4 signaling in glioma stem cells—Prospects for therapeutic intervention. *Translational Cancer Research*, 6, S434–S437.

Moldogazieva, N. T., Mokhosoev, I. M., & Terentiev, A. A. (2020). Metabolic heterogeneity of cancer cells: An interplay between HIF-1, GLUTs, and AMPK. *Cancers*, 12, 862–893.

Molon, B., Cali, B., & Viola, A. (2016). T cells and cancer: How metabolism shapes immunity. *Frontiers in Immunology*, 7, 20.

Mondesir, J., Willekens, C., Touat, M., & de Botton, S. (2016). IDH1 and IDH2 mutations as novel therapeutic targets: Current perspectives. *Journal of Blood Medicine*, 7, 171–180.

Morris, A. A. M. (2005). Cerebral ketone body metabolism. *Journal of Inherited Metabolic Diseases*, 28, 109–121.

Mou, K., Chen, M., Mao, Q., Wang, P., Ni, R., Xia, X., & Liu, Y. (2010). AQP-4 in peritumoral edematous tissue is correlated with the degree of glioma and with expression of VEGF and HIF-1α. *Journal of Neuro-Oncology, 100*, 375–383.

Munksgaard Thorén, M., Vaapil, M., Staaf, J., Planck, M., Johansson, M. E., Mohlin, S., & Påhlman, S. (2017). Myc-induced glutaminolysis bypasses HIF-driven glycolysis in hypoxic small cell lung carcinoma cells. *Oncotarget, 8*, 48983–48995.

Munshi, A., & Ramesh, R. (2013). Mitogen-activated protein kinases and their role in radiation response. *Genes & Cancer, 4*, 401–408.

Murtola, T. J., Sälli, S. M., Talala, K., Taari, K., Tammela, T. L. J., & Auvinen, A. (2019). Blood glucose, glucose balance, and disease-specific survival after prostate cancer diagnosis in the Finnish Randomized Study of Screening for Prostate Cancer. *Prostate Cancer and Prostatic Diseases, 22*, 453–460.

Myers, T. R., Zittel, M., & Goldhamer, A. C. (2018). Follow-up of water-only fasting and an exclusively plant food diet in the management of stage IIIa, low-grade follicular lymphoma. *BMJ Case Reports, 2018*, doi:10.1136/bcr-2018-225520

Nadeem Abbas, M., Kausar, S., Wang, F., Zhao, Y., & Cui, H. (2019). Advances in targeting the epidermal growth factor receptor pathway by synthetic products and its regulation by epigenetic modulators as a therapy for glioblastoma. *Cells, 8*, 350–372.

Nagao, A., Kobayashi, M., Koyasu, S., Chow, C. C. T., & Harada, H. (2019). HIF-1-dependent reprogramming of glucose metabolic pathway of cancer cells and its therapeutic significance. *International Journal of Molecular Sciences, 20*, 238–251.

Nazemi, M., & Rainero, E. (2020). Cross-talk between the tumor microenvironment, extracellular matrix, and cell metabolism in cancer. *Frontiers in Oncology, 10*, 239.

Nebeling, L. C., & Lerner, E. (1995). Implementing a ketogenic diet based on medium-chain triglyceride oil in pediatric patients with cancer. *Journal of the American Dietetic Association, 95*, 693–697.

Nebeling, L. C., Miraldi, F., Shurin, S. B., & Lerner, E. (1995). Effects of a ketogenic diet on tumor metabolism and nutritional status in pediatric oncology patients: Two case reports. *Journal of the American College of Nutrition, 14*, 202–208.

Newman, J. C., & Verdin, E. (2014a). Beta-hydroxybutyrate: Much more than a metabolite. *Diabetes Research and Clinical Practice, 106*, 173–181.

Newman, J. C., & Verdin, E. (2014b). Ketone bodies as signaling metabolites. *Trends in Endocrinology and Metabolism, 25*, 42–52.

Nijsten, M. W., & van Dam, G. M. (2009). Hypothesis: Using the Warburg effect against cancer by reducing glucose and providing lactate. *Medical Hypotheses, 73*, 48–51.

O'Flanagan, C. H., Smith, L. A., McDonell, S. B., & Hursting, S. D. (2017). When less may be more: Calorie restriction and response to cancer therapy. *BMC Medicine, 15*, 106.

Obara-Michlewska, M., & Szeliga, M. (2020). Targeting glutamine addiction in gliomas. *Cancers, 12*, 310.

Obre, E., & Rossignol, R. (2015). Emerging concepts in bioenergetics and cancer research: Metabolic flexibility, coupling, symbiosis, switch, oxidative tumors, metabolic remodeling, signaling and bioenergetic therapy. *International Journal of Biochemistry and Cell Biology, 59C*, 167–181. https://doi.org/10.1016/j.biocel.2014.12.008

Ordway, B., Swietach, P., Gillies, R. J., & Damaghi, M. (2020). Causes and consequences of variable tumor cell metabolism on heritable modifications and tumor evolution. *Frontiers in Oncology, 10*, 373.

Otto, C., Kaemmerer, U., Illert, B., Muehling, B., Pfetzer, N., Wittig, R., Voelker, H. U., Thiede, A., & Coy, J. F. (2008). Growth of human gastric cancer cells in nude mice is delayed by a ketogenic diet supplemented with omega-3 fatty acids and medium-chain triglycerides. *BMC Cancer, 8*, 122.

Ou, Y., Wang, S. J., Jiang, L., Zheng, B., & Gu, W. (2015). p53 protein-mediated regulation of phosphoglycerate dehydrogenase (PHGDH) is crucial for the apoptotic response upon serine starvation. *Journal of Biological Chemistry, 290*, 457–466.

Paddock, M. N., Field, S. J., & Cantley, L. C. (2019). Treating cancer with phosphatidylinositol-3-kinase inhibitors: Increasing efficacy and overcoming resistance. *Journal of Lipid Research, 60*, 747–752.

Panhans, C. M., Gresham, G., Amaral, J. L., & Hu, J. (2020). Exploring the feasibility and effects of a ketogenic diet in patients with CNS malignancies: A retrospective case series. *Frontiers in Neuroscience, 14*, 390.

Parikh, A. B., Kozuch, P., Rohs, N., Becker, D. J., & Levy, B. P. (2017). Metformin as a repurposed therapy in advanced non-small cell lung cancer (NSCLC): Results of a phase II trial. *Investigational New Drugs, 35*, 813–819.

Parrales, A., & Iwakuma, T. (2016). p53 as a regulator of lipid metabolism in cancer. *International Journal of Molecular Sciences, 17*, 2074–2085.

Pavlova, N. N., & Thompson, C. B. (2016). The emerging hallmarks of cancer metabolism. *Cell Metabolism, 23*, 27–47.

Pazmandi, J., O'Neill, K., Scheck, A. C., Szlosarek, P., Woolf, E. C., Brooks, K. S., & Syed, N. (2015). *The ketogenic diet alters the expression of microRNAs that play key roles in tumor development* [Paper presentation]. 106th Annual Meeting of the American Association for Cancer Research (Philadelphia, PA).

Peck, B., & Schulze, A. (2019). Lipid metabolism at the nexus of diet and tumor microenvironment. *Trends in Cancer, 5,* 693–703.

Poff, A., Koutnik, A. P., Egan, K. M., Sahebjam, S., D'Agostino, D., & Kumar, N. B. (2019). Targeting the Warburg effect for cancer treatment: Ketogenic diets for management of glioma. *Seminars in Cancer Biology, 56,* 135–148.

Poff, A. M., Ari, C., Arnold, P., Seyfried, T. N., & D'Agostino, D. P. (2014). Ketone supplementation decreases tumor cell viability and prolongs survival of mice with metastatic cancer. *International Journal of Cancer, 135,* 1711–1720.

Poff, A. M., Ari, C., Seyfried, T. N., & D'Agostino, D. P. (2013). The ketogenic diet and hyperbaric oxygen therapy prolong survival in mice with systemic metastatic cancer. *PLOS ONE, 8,* Article e65522.

Poff, A. M., Ward, N., Seyfried, T. N., Arnold, P., & D'Agostino, D. P. (2015). Non-toxic metabolic management of metastatic cancer in VM mice: Novel combination of ketogenic diet, ketone supplementation, and hyperbaric oxygen therapy. *PLOS ONE, 10,* Article e0127407.

Poli, V., & Camporeale, A. (2015). STAT3-mediated metabolic reprogramming in cellular transformation and implications for drug resistance. *Frontiers in Oncology, 5,* 121.

Pont, L. M., Naipal, K., Kloezeman, J. J., Venkatesan, S., van den Bent, M., van Gent, D. C., Dirven, C. M., Kanaar, R., Lamfers, M. L., & Leenstra, S. (2015). DNA damage response and anti-apoptotic proteins predict radiosensitization efficacy of HDAC inhibitors SAHA and LBH589 in patient-derived glioblastoma cells. *Cancer Letters, 356,* 525–535.

Poole, C. J., & van Riggelen, J. (2017). MYC—Master regulator of the cancer epigenome and transcriptome. *Genes, 8,* 142–170.

Pore, N., Jiang, Z., Shu, H. K., Bernhard, E., Kao, G. D., & Maity, A. (2006). Akt1 activation can augment hypoxia-inducible factor-1alpha expression by increasing protein translation through a mammalian target of rapamycin-independent pathway. *Molecular Cancer Research, 4,* 471–479.

Proescholdt, M. A., Merrill, M. J., Stoerr, E. M., Lohmeier, A., Pohl, F., & Brawanski, A. (2012). Function of carbonic anhydrase IX in glioblastoma multiforme. *Neuro-Oncology, 14,* 1357–1366.

Puchowicz, M. A., Zechel, J. L., Valerio, J., Emancipator, D. S., Xu, K., Pundik, S., LaManna, J. C., & Lust, W. D. (2008). Neuroprotection in diet-induced ketotic rat brain after focal ischemia. *Journal of Cerebral Blood Flow and Metabolism, 28,* 1907–1916.

Puzio-Kuter, A. M. (2011). The role of p53 in metabolic regulation. *Genes & Cancer, 2,* 385–391.

Qiu, S., Huang, D., Yin, D., Li, F., Li, X., Kung, H. F., & Peng, Y. (2013). Suppression of tumorigenicity by microRNA-138 through inhibition of EZH2-CDK4/6-pRb-E2F1 signal loop in glioblastoma multiforme. *Biochimica et Biophysica Acta, 1832,* 1697–1707.

Qiu, X., Xiao, X., Li, N., & Li, Y. (2017). Histone deacetylases inhibitors (HDACIs) as novel therapeutic application in various clinical diseases. *Progress in Neuro-Psychopharmacology & Biological Psychiatry, 72,* 60–72.

Raffaghello, L., Lee, C., Safdie, F. M., Wei, M., Madia, F., Bianchi, G., & Longo, V. D. (2008). Starvation-dependent differential stress resistance protects normal but not cancer cells against high-dose chemotherapy. *Proceedings of the National Academy of Sciences of the United States of America, 105,* 8215–8220.

Raffaghello, L., Safdie, F., Bianchi, G., Dorff, T., Fontana, L., & Longo, V. D. (2010). Fasting and differential chemotherapy protection in patients. *Cell Cycle, 9,* 4474–4476.

Raimondi, M. V., Randazzo, O., La Franca, M., Barone, G., Vignoni, E., Rossi, D., & Collina, S. (2019). DHFR inhibitors: Reading the past for discovering novel anticancer agents. *Molecules, 24,* 1140–1159.

Ramalho, R., Rao, M., Zhang, C., Agrati, C., Ippolito, G., Wang, F. S., Zumla, A., & Maeurer, M. (2020). Immunometabolism: New insights and lessons from antigen-directed cellular immune responses. *Seminars in Immunopathology, 42,* 279–313.

Ramezani, S., Vousooghi, N., Joghataei, M. T., & Chabok, S. Y. (2019). The role of kinase signaling in resistance to bevacizumab therapy for glioblastoma multiforme. *Cancer Biotherapy & Radiopharmaceuticals, 34,* 345–354.

Reda, M., Bagley, A. F., Zaidan, H. Y., & Yantasee, W. (2020). Augmenting the therapeutic window of radiotherapy: A perspective on molecularly targeted therapies and nanomaterials. *Radiotherapy and Oncology, 150,* 225–235.

Reddy, R. G., Bhat, U. A., Chakravarty, S., & Kumar, A. (2020). Advances in histone deacetylase inhibitors in targeting glioblastoma stem cells. *Cancer Chemotherapy and Pharmacology, 86,* 165–179.

Reid, M. A., Wang, W. I., Rosales, K. R., Welliver, M. X., Pan, M., & Kong, M. (2013). The B55α subunit of PP2A drives a p53-dependent metabolic adaptation to glutamine deprivation. *Molecular Cell, 50,* 200–211.

Rhee, I., Bachman, K. E., Park, B. H., Jair, K. W., Yen, R. W., Schuebel, K. E., Cui, H., Feinberg, A. P., Lengauer, C., Kinzler, K. W., Baylin, S. B., & Vogelstein, B. (2002). DNMT1 and DNMT3b cooperate to silence genes in human cancer cells. *Nature*, *416*, 552–556.

Ricci, A., Idzikowski, M. A., Soares, C. N., & Brietzke, E. (2020). Exploring the mechanisms of action of the antidepressant effect of the ketogenic diet. *Reviews in the Neurosciences*, *31*, 637–648.

Rieger, J., Bahr, O., Maurer, G. D., Hattingen, E., Franz, K., Brucker, D., Walenta, S., Kammerer, U., Coy, J. F., Weller, M., & Steinbach, J. P. (2014). ERGO: A pilot study of ketogenic diet in recurrent glioblastoma. *International Journal of Oncology*, *44*, 1843–1852.

Rizzo, D., Ruggiero, A., Amato, M., Maurizi, P., & Riccardi, R. (2016). BRAF and MEK inhibitors in pediatric glioma: New therapeutic strategies, new toxicities. *Expert Opinion on Drug Metabolism & Toxicology*, *12*, 1397–1405.

Roberts, D. J., & Miyamoto, S. (2015). Hexokinase II integrates energy metabolism and cellular protection: Akting on mitochondria and TORCing to autophagy. *Cell Death and Differentiation*, *22*, 248–257.

Robey, R. B., Weisz, J., Kuemmerle, N. B., Salzberg, A. C., Berg, A., Brown, D. G., Kubik, L., Palorini, R., Al-Mulla, F., Al-Temaimi, R., Colacci, A., Mondello, C., Raju, J., Woodrick, J., Scovassi, A. I., Singh, N., Vaccari, M., Roy, R., Forte, S., & Ryan, E. P. (2015). Metabolic reprogramming and dysregulated metabolism: Cause, consequence and/or enabler of environmental carcinogenesis? *Carcinogenesis*, *36*, S203–S231.

Rodrigues, L. M., Uribe-Lewis, S., Madhu, B., Honess, D. J., Stubbs, M., & Griffiths, J. R. (2017). The action of beta-hydroxybutyrate on the growth, metabolism and global histone H3 acetylation of spontaneous mouse mammary tumours: Evidence of a beta-hydroxybutyrate paradox. *Cancer Metabolism*, *5*, 4.

Rodríguez-Hernández, M. A., Cruz-Ojeda, P., López-Grueso, M. J., Navarro-Villarán, E., Requejo-Aguilar, R., Castejón-Vega, B., Negrete, M., Gallego, P., Vega-Ochoa, Á., Victor, V. M., Cordero, M. D., Del Campo, J. A., Bárcena, J. A., Padilla, C. A., & Muntané, J. (2020). Integrated molecular signaling involving mitochondrial dysfunction and alteration of cell metabolism induced by tyrosine kinase inhibitors in cancer. *Redox Biology*, *36*, 101510.

Rossi, A. P., Silva-Nichols, H. B., Woolf, E. C., & Scheck, A. C. (2016). The ketone body β-hydroxybutyrate down regulates c-Myc signaling in a malignant glioma model. In: Proceedings of the 107th Annual Meeting of the American Association for Cancer Research; 2016 Apr 16–20; New Orleans, LA. Philadelphia (PA): AACR; *Cancer Research*, 2016;76 (14 Suppl):Abstract nr 1022.

Ryall, S., Tabori, U., & Hawkins, C. (2020). Pediatric low-grade glioma in the era of molecular diagnostics. *Acta Neuropathologica Communications*, *8*, 30.

Safdie, F., Brandhorst, S., Wei, M., Wang, W., Lee, C., Hwang, S., Conti, P. S., Chen, T. C., & Longo, V. D. (2012). Fasting enhances the response of glioma to chemo- and radiotherapy. *PLOS ONE*, *7*, Article e44603.

Saleh, A. D., Simone, B. A., Palazzo, J., Savage, J. E., Sano, Y., Dan, T., Jin, L., Champ, C. E., Zhao, S., Lim, M., Sotgia, F., Camphausen, K., Pestell, R. G., Mitchell, J. B., Lisanti, M. P., & Simone, N. L. (2013). Caloric restriction augments radiation efficacy in breast cancer. *Cell Cycle*, *12*, 1955–1963.

Sanegre, S., Lucantoni, F., Burgos-Panadero, R., de La Cruz-Merino, L., Noguera, R., & Álvaro Naranjo, T. (2020). Integrating the tumor microenvironment into cancer therapy. *Cancers*, *12*, 1677–1698.

Sanli, T., Steinberg, G. R., Singh, G., & Tsakiridis, T. (2014). AMP-activated protein kinase (AMPK) beyond metabolism: A novel genomic stress sensor participating in the DNA damage response pathway. *Cancer Biology & Therapy*, *15*, 156–169.

Santivasi, W. L., & Xia, F. (2014). Ionizing radiation-induced DNA damage, response, and repair. *Antioxidants & Redox Signaling*, *21*, 251–259.

Saravia, J., Raynor, J. L., Chapman, N. M., Lim, S. A., & Chi, H. (2020). Signaling networks in immunometabolism. *Cell Research*, *30*, 328–342.

Sassone-Corsi, P. (2013). Physiology: When metabolism and epigenetics converge. *Science*, *339*, 148–150.

Saxton, J. M., Scott, E. J., Daley, A. J., Woodroofe, M., Mutrie, N., Crank, H., Powers, H. J., & Coleman, R. E. (2014). Effects of an exercise and hypocaloric healthy eating intervention on indices of psychological health status, hypothalamic-pituitary-adrenal axis regulation and immune function after early-stage breast cancer: A randomised controlled trial. *Breast Cancer Research*, *16*, R39.

Scanlon, S. E., & Glazer, P. M. (2015). Multifaceted control of DNA repair pathways by the hypoxic tumor microenvironment. *DNA Repair*, *32*, 180–189.

Scheck, A. C., Abdelwahab, M. G., Fenton, K., & Stafford, P. (2012). The ketogenic diet for the treatment of glioma: Insights from genetic profiling. *Epilepsy Research*, *100*, 327–337.

Scheck, A. C., Abdelwahab, M. G., Stafford, P., Kim, D. Y., Iwai, S., Preul, M. C., & Rho, J. M. (2011). Mechanistic studies of the ketogenic diet as an adjuvant therapy for malignant gliomas. *Cancer Research*, *70*, Abstract 638.

Schmidt, M., Pfetzer, N., Schwab, M., Strauss, I., & Kammerer, U. (2011). Effects of a ketogenic diet on the quality of life in 16 patients with advanced cancer: A pilot trial. *Nutrition & Metabolism*, *8*, 54.

Schwartz, K., Chang, H., Nikolai, M., Kurniali, P., Olson, K., Pernicine, J., Sweeley, C., & Noel, M. (2013). Treatment of malignant gliomas with an energy restricted ketogenic diet: Case report and literature summary. *Neuro-oncology*, 15(Suppl. 3), Abstract NO–122.

Schwartz, K., Chang, H. T., Nikolai, M., Pernicone, J., Rhee, S., Olson, K., Kurniali, P. C., Hord, N. G., & Noel, M. (2015). Treatment of glioma patients with ketogenic diets: Report of two cases treated with an IRB-approved energy-restricted ketogenic diet protocol and review of the literature. *Cancer Metabolism*, 3, 3–13.

Schwartz, K. A., Noel, M., Nikolai, M., & Chang, H. T. (2018). Investigating the ketogenic diet as treatment for primary aggressive brain cancer: Challenges and lessons learned. *Frontiers in Nutrition*, 5, 11.

Semenza, G. L. (2013). HIF-1 mediates metabolic responses to intratumoral hypoxia and oncogenic mutations. *Journal of Clinical Investigation*, 123, 3664–3671.

Seyfried, B. T., Kiebish, M., Marsh, J., & Mukherjee, P. (2009). Targeting energy metabolism in brain cancer through calorie restriction and the ketogenic diet. *Journal of Cancer Research and Therapeutics*, 5(Suppl. 1), S7–S15.

Seyfried, T. N. (2012). *Cancer as a metabolic disease: On the origin, management and prevention of cancer*. John Wiley & Sons.

Seyfried, T. N., Flores, R., Poff, A. M., D'Agostino, D. P., & Mukherjee, P. (2015). Metabolic therapy: A new paradigm for managing malignant brain cancer. *Cancer Letters*, 356, 289–300.

Seyfried, T. N., Kiebish, M. A., Marsh, J., Shelton, L. M., Huysentruyt, L. C., & Mukherjee, P. (2011). Metabolic management of brain cancer. *Biochimica et Biophysica Acta*, 1807, 577–594.

Seyfried, T. N., Marsh, J., Shelton, L. M., Huysentruyt, L. C., & Mukherjee, P. (2012). Is the restricted ketogenic diet a viable alternative to the standard of care for managing malignant brain cancer? *Epilepsy Research*, 100, 310–326.

Seyfried, T. N., & Mukherjee, P. (2005). Targeting energy metabolism in brain cancer: Review and hypothesis. *Nutrition & Metabolism*, 2, 30–38.

Seyfried, T. N., Mukherjee, P., Iyikesici, M. S., Slocum, A., Kalamian, M., Spinosa, J. P., & Chinopoulos, C. (2020). Consideration of ketogenic metabolic therapy as a complementary or alternative approach for managing breast cancer. *Frontiers in Nutrition*, 7, 21.

Seystahl, K., Wick, W., & Weller, M. (2016). Therapeutic options in recurrent glioblastoma—An update. *Critical Reviews in Oncology/Hematology*, 99, 389–408.

Shahcheraghi, S. H., Tchokonte-Nana, V., Lotfi, M., Lotfi, M., Ghorbani, A., & Sadeghnia, H. R. (2020). Wnt/beta-catenin and PI3K/Akt/mTOR signaling pathways in glioblastoma: Two main targets for drug design; A review. *Current Pharmaceutical Design*, 26, 1729–1741.

Shelton, L. M., Huysentruyt, L. C., Mukherjee, P., & Seyfried, T. N. (2010). Calorie restriction as an anti-invasive therapy for malignant brain cancer in the VM mouse. *ASN NEURO*, 2, Article e00038.

Shen, Y. A., Pan, S. C., Chu, I., Lai, R. Y., & Wei, Y. H. (2020). Targeting cancer stem cells from a metabolic perspective. *Experimental Biology and Medicine*, 245, 465–476.

Shi, W., Palmer, J. D., Werner-Wasik, M., Andrews, D. W., Evans, J. J., Glass, J., Kim, L., Bar-Ad, V., Judy, K., Farrell, C., Simone, N., Liu, H., Dicker, A. P., & Lawrence, Y. R. (2016). Phase I trial of panobinostat and fractionated stereotactic re-irradiation therapy for recurrent high grade gliomas. *Journal of Neuro-Oncology*, 127, 535–539.

Shimazu, T., Hirschey, M. D., Newman, J., He, W., Shirakawa, K., Le Moan, N., Grueter, C. A., Lim, H., Saunders, L. R., Stevens, R. D., Newgard, C. B., Farese, R. V., Jr., de, Cabo R., Ulrich, S., Akassoglou, K., & Verdin, E. (2013). Suppression of oxidative stress by beta-hydroxybutyrate, an endogenous histone deacetylase inhibitor. *Science*, 339, 211–214.

Shingler, E., Perry, R., Mitchell, A., England, C., Perks, C., Herbert, G., Ness, A., & Atkinson, C. (2019). Dietary restriction during the treatment of cancer: Results of a systematic scoping review. *BMC Cancer*, 19, 811.

Shukla, S. K., Gebregiworgis, T., Purohit, V., Chaika, N. V., Gunda, V., Radhakrishnan, P., Mehla, K., Pipinos, I. I., Powers, R., Yu, F., & Singh, P. K. (2014). Metabolic reprogramming induced by ketone bodies diminishes pancreatic cancer cachexia. *Cancer Metabolism*, 2, 18. https://doi.org/10.1186/2049-3002-2-18

Shweiki, D., Neeman, M., Itin, A., & Keshet, E. (1995). Induction of vascular endothelial growth factor expression by hypoxia and by glucose deficiency in multicell spheroids: Implications for tumor angiogenesis. *Proceedings of the National Academy of Sciences of the United States of America*, 92, 768–772.

Simandi, Z., Czipa, E., Horvath, A., Koszeghy, A., Bordas, C., Póliska, S., Juhász, I., Imre, L., Szabó, G., Dezso, B., Barta, E., Sauer, S., Karolyi, K., Kovacs, I., Hutóczki, G., Bognár, L., Klekner, Á., Szucs, P., Bálint, B. L., & Nagy, L. (2015). PRMT1 and PRMT8 regulate retinoic acid-dependent neuronal differentiation with implications to neuropathology. *Stem Cells*, 33, 726–741.

Simone, B. A., Champ, C. E., Rosenberg, A. L., Berger, A. C., Monti, D. A., Dicker, A. P., & Simone, N. L. (2013). Selectively starving cancer cells through dietary manipulation: Methods and clinical implications. *Future Oncology*, 9, 959–976.

Singh, A., Nayak, N., Rathi, P., Verma, D., Sharma, R., Chaudhary, A., Agarwal, A., Tripathi, Y. B., &

Garg, N. (2021). Microbiome and host crosstalk: A new paradigm to cancer therapy. *Seminars in Cancer Biology, 70,* 71–84.

Singh, R. P., Bashir, H., & Kumar, R. (2021). Emerging role of microbiota in immunomodulation and cancer immunotherapy. *Seminars in Cancer Biology, 70,* 37–52.

Skinner, R., Trujillo, A., Ma, X., & Beierle, E. A. (2009). Ketone bodies inhibit the viability of human neuroblastoma cells. *Journal of Pediatric Surgery, 44,* 212–216.

Smith, K. (2019). INNV-01. Ketogenic metabolic therapy significantly improves radiographic and clinical response to salvage temozolomide in patients with recurrent high grade gliomas. *Neuro-Oncology, 21*(Suppl. 6), vi130.

Smyl, C. (2016). Ketogenic diet and cancer—A perspective. *Recent Results in Cancer Research, 207,* 233–240.

Staberg, M., Michaelsen, S. R., Rasmussen, R. D., Villingshoj, M., Poulsen, H. S., & Hamerlik, P. (2017). Inhibition of histone deacetylases sensitizes glioblastoma cells to lomustine. *Cellular Oncology, 40,* 21–32.

Stafford, P., Abdelwahab, M. G., Kim, D. Y., Preul, M. C., Rho, J. M., & Scheck, A. C. (2010). The ketogenic diet reverses gene expression patterns and reduces reactive oxygen species levels when used as an adjuvant therapy for glioma. *Nutrition & Metabolism, 7,* 74.

Stafstrom, C. E., & Rho, J. M. (2012). The ketogenic diet as a treatment paradigm for diverse neurological disorders. *Frontiers in Pharmacology, 3,* 59.

Stegeman, H., Span, P. N., Kaanders, J. H., & Bussink, J. (2014). Improving chemoradiation efficacy by PI3-K/AKT inhibition. *Cancer Treatment Reviews, 40,* 1182–1191.

Stevenson, C. B., Ehtesham, M., McMillan, K. M., Valadez, J. G., Edgeworth, M. L., Price, R. R., Abel, T. W., Mapara, K. Y., & Thompson, R. C. (2008). CXCR4 expression is elevated in glioblastoma multiforme and correlates with an increase in intensity and extent of peritumoral T2-weighted magnetic resonance imaging signal abnormalities. *Neurosurgery, 63,* 560–569; discussion 569–570.

Stine, Z. E., Walton, Z. E., Altman, B. J., Hsieh, A. L., & Dang, C. V. (2015). MYC, metabolism, and cancer. *Cancer Discovery, 5,* 1024–1039.

Sturgeon, K. M., Foo, W., Heroux, M., & Schmitz, K. (2018). Change in inflammatory biomarkers and adipose tissue in BRCA1/2(+) breast cancer survivors following a yearlong lifestyle modification program. *Cancer Prevention Research, 11,* 545–550.

Sun, Y., Bailey, C. P., Sadighi, Z., Zaky, W., & Chandra, J. (2020). Pediatric high-grade glioma: Aberrant epigenetics and kinase signaling define emerging therapeutic opportunities. *Journal of Neuro-Oncology, 150,* 17–26.

Suraya, R., Nagano, T., Kobayashi, K., & Nishimura, Y. (2020). Microbiome as a target for cancer therapy. *Integrative Cancer Therapies, 19,* 1–11.

Syn, N. L., Yong, W. P., Goh, B. C., & Lee, S. C. (2016). Evolving landscape of tumor molecular profiling for personalized cancer therapy: A comprehensive review. *Expert Opinion on Drug Metabolism & Toxicology, 12,* 911–922.

Tadipatri, R., Lyon, K., Azadi, A., & Fonkem, E. (2020). A view of the epidemiologic landscape: How population-based studies can lend novel insights regarding the pathophysiology of glioblastoma. *Chinese Clinical Oncology, 10,* 35. http://dx.doi.org/10.21037/cco.2020.02.07

Tajan, M., & Vousden, K. H. (2020). Dietary approaches to cancer therapy. *Cancer Cell, 37,* 767–785.

Tajbakhsh, M., Houghton, P. J., Morton, C. L., Kolb, E. A., Gorlick, R., Maris, J. M., Keir, S. T., Wu, J., Reynolds, C. P., Smith, M. A., & Lock, R. B. (2008). Initial testing of cisplatin by the pediatric preclinical testing program. *Pediatric Blood & Cancer, 50,* 992–1000.

Tan, C. S., Cho, B. C., & Soo, R. A. (2016). Next-generation epidermal growth factor receptor tyrosine kinase inhibitors in epidermal growth factor receptor-mutant non-small cell lung cancer. *Lung Cancer, 93,* 59–68.

Tanaka, K., Sasayama, T., Irino, Y., Takata, K., Nagashima, H., Satoh, N., Kyotani, K., Mizowaki, T., Imahori, T., Ejima, Y., Masui, K., Gini, B., Yang, H., Hosoda, K., Sasaki, R., Mischel, P. S., & Kohmura, E. (2015). Compensatory glutamine metabolism promotes glioblastoma resistance to mTOR inhibitor treatment. *Journal of Clinical Investigation, 125,* 1591–1602.

Tang, L., Wei, F., Wu, Y., He, Y., Shi, L., Xiong, F., Gong, Z., Guo, C., Li, X., Deng, H., Cao, K., Zhou, M., Xiang, B., Li, X., Li, Y., Li, G., Xiong, W., & Zeng, Z. (2018). Role of metabolism in cancer cell radioresistance and radiosensitization methods. *Journal of Experimental & Clinical Cancer Research, 37,* 87.

Tieu, M. T., Lovblom, L. E., McNamara, M. G., Mason, W., Laperriere, N., Millar, B. A., Ménard, C., Kiehl, T. R., Perkins, B. A., & Chung, C. (2015). Impact of glycemia on survival of glioblastoma patients treated with radiation and temozolomide. *Journal of Neuro-Oncology, 124,* 119–126.

Tisdale, M. J., & Brennan, R. A. (1983). Loss of acetoacetate coenzyme A transferase activity in tumours of peripheral tissues. *British Journal of Cancer, 47,* 293–297.

Tisdale, M. J., Brennan, R. A., & Fearon, K. C. (1987). Reduction of weight loss and tumour size in a cachexia model by a high fat diet. *British Journal of Cancer, 56,* 39–43.

Trimboli, P., Castellana, M., Bellido, D., & Casanueva, F. F. (2020). Confusion in the nomenclature of ketogenic diets blurs evidence. *Reviews in Endocrine & Metabolic Disorders, 21,* 1–3.

Turdo, A., Porcelli, G., D'Accardo, C., Franco, S. D., Verona, F., Forte, S., Giuffrida, D., Memeo, L., Todaro, M., & Stassi, G. (2020). Metabolic escape routes of cancer stem cells and therapeutic opportunities. *Cancers, 12,* 1436–1463.

van den Bent, M. J., Wefel, J. S., Schiff, D., Taphoorn, M. J., Jaeckle, K., Junck, L., Armstrong, T., Choucair, A., Waldman, A. D., Gorlia, T., Chamberlain, M., Baumert, B. G., Vogelbaum, M. A., MacDonald, D. R., Reardon, D. A., Wen, P. Y., Chang, S. M., & Jacobs, A. H. (2011). Response assessment in neuro-oncology (a report of the RANO group): Assessment of outcome in trials of diffuse low-grade gliomas. *Lancet Oncology, 12,* 583–593.

Vander Heiden, M. G., Cantley, L. C., & Thompson, C. B. (2009). Understanding the Warburg effect: The metabolic requirements of cell proliferation. *Science, 324,* 1029–1033.

Vanitallie, T. B., & Nufert, T. H. (2003). Ketones: Metabolism's ugly duckling. *Nutrition Reviews, 61,* 327–341.

Veech, R. L., Chance, B., Kashiwaya, Y., Lardy, H. A., & Cahill, G. F., Jr. (2001). Ketone bodies, potential therapeutic uses. *IUBMB Life, 51,* 241–247.

Venneti, S., & Mischel, P. S. (2015). Metabolic reprogramming in brain cancer: A coordinated effort. *Brain Pathology, 25,* 753–754.

Venneti, S., & Thompson, C. B. (2013). Metabolic modulation of epigenetics in gliomas. *Brain Pathology, 23,* 217–221.

Venneti, S., & Thompson, C. B. (2017). Metabolic reprogramming in brain tumors. *Annual Review of Pathology, 12,* 515–545.

Vergati, M., Krasniqi, E., Monte, G. D., Riondino, S., Vallone, D., Guadagni, F., Ferroni, P., & Roselli, M. (2017). Ketogenic diet and other dietary intervention strategies in the treatment of cancer. *Current Medicinal Chemistry, 24,* 1170–1185.

Vernieri, C., Signorelli, D., Galli, G., Ganzinelli, M., Moro, M., Fabbri, A., Tamborini, E., Marabese, M., Caiola, E., Broggini, M., Hollander, L., Gallucci, R., Vandoni, G., Gavazzi, C., Triulzi, T., Colombo, M. P., Rizzo, A. M., Corsetto, P. A., Pruneri, G., . . . Garassino, M. C. (2019). Exploiting FAsting-mimicking diet and MEtformin to improve the efficacy of platinum-pemetrexed chemotherapy in advanced LKB1-inactivated lung adenocarcinoma: The FAME Trial. *Clinical Lung Cancer, 20,* e413–e417.

Vidali, S., Aminzadeh, S., Lambert, B., Rutherford, T., Sperl, W., Kofler, B., & Feichtinger, R. G. (2015). Mitochondria: The ketogenic diet—A metabolism-based therapy. *International Journal of Biochemistry and Cell Biology, 63,* 55–59.

Villani, V., Fabi, A., Tanzilli, A., Pasqualetti, F., Lombardi, G., Vidiri, A., Gonnelli, A., Molinari, A., Cantarella, M., Bellu, L., Terrenato, I., Carosi, M., Maschio, M., Telera, S. M., Carapella, C. M., Cognetti, F., Paiar, F., Zagonel, V., & Pace, A. (2019). A multicenter real-world study of bevacizumab in heavily pretreated malignant gliomas: Clinical benefit is a plausible end point? *Future Oncology, 15,* 1717–1727.

Vlashi, E., & Pajonk, F. (2015). The metabolic state of cancer stem cells—A valid target for cancer therapy? *Free Radical Biology and Medicine, 79,* 264–268.

Voss, M., Lorenz, N. I., Luger, A. L., Steinbach, J. P., Rieger, J., & Ronellenfitsch, M. W. (2018). Rescue of 2-deoxyglucose side effects by ketogenic diet. *International Journal of Molecular Sciences, 19,* 2462–2474.

Voss, M., Marlies, W., von Mettenheim, N., Harter, P. N., Wenger, K. J., Franz, K., Bojunga, J., Vetter, M., Gerlach, R., Glatzel, M., Paulsen, F., Hattingen, E., Baehr, O., Ronellenfitsch, M. W., Fokas, E., Imhoff, D., Steinbach, J. P., Rödel, C., & Rieger, J. (2020). ERGO2: A prospective randomized trial of calorie restricted ketogenic diet and fasting in addition to re-irradiation for malignant glioma. *International Journal of Radiation Oncology · Biology · Physics, 108,* 987–995.

Walenkamp, A. M. E., Lapa, C., Herrmann, K., & Wester, H. J. (2017). CXCR4 ligands: The next big hit? *Journal of Nuclear Medicine, 58,* 77s–82s.

Wallace, D. C., Fan, W., & Procaccio, V. (2010). Mitochondrial energetics and therapeutics. *Annual Review of Pathology, 5,* 297–348.

Wang, B., Li, K., Wang, H., Shen, X., & Zheng, J. (2020a). Systemic chemotherapy promotes HIF-1α mediated glycolysis and IL-17F pathways in cutaneous T cell lymphoma. *Experimental Dermatology, 29,* 987–992.

Wang, G., Wang, J., Zhao, H., Wang, J., & Tony To, S. S. (2015a). The role of Myc and let-7a in glioblastoma, glucose metabolism and response to therapy. *Archives of Biochemistry and Biophysics, 15*(580), 84–92.

Wang, H., Xu, T., Jiang, Y., Yan, Y., Qin, R., & Chen, J. (2015b). MicroRNAs in human glioblastoma: From bench to beside. *Frontiers in Bioscience, 20,* 105–118.

Wang, T., Wang, G., Hao, D., Liu, X., Wang, D., Ning, N., & Li, X. (2015c). Aberrant regulation of the LIN28A/LIN28B and let-7 loop in human malignant tumors and its effects on the hallmarks of cancer. *Molecular Cancer, 14,* 125.

Wang, Y., Jing, M. X., Jiang, L., Jia, Y. F., Ying, E., Cao, H., Guo, X. Y., & Sun, T. (2020b). Does a ketogenic diet as an adjuvant therapy for drug treatment enhance chemotherapy sensitivity and reduce target lesions in patients with locally recurrent or metastatic Her-2-negative breast cancer? Study protocol for a randomized controlled trial. *Trials*, *21*, 487.

Wang, Y., Yuan, J. L., Zhang, Y. T., Ma, J. J., Xu, P., Shi, C. H., Zhang, W., Li, Y. M., Fu, Q., Zhu, G. F., Xue, W., Lei, Y. H., Gao, J. Y., Wang, J. Y., Shao, C., Yi, C. G., & Wang, H. (2013). Inhibition of both EGFR and IGF1R sensitized prostate cancer cells to radiation by synergistic suppression of DNA homologous recombination repair. *PLOS ONE*, *8*, Article e68784.

Wang, Y. H., Suk, F. M., & Liao, Y. J. (2020c). Loss of HMGCS2 enhances lipogenesis and attenuates the protective effect of the ketogenic diet in liver cancer. *Cancers*, *12*, 1797–1813.

Wanigasooriya, K., Tyler, R., Barros-Silva, J. D., Sinha, Y., Ismail, T., & Beggs, A. D. (2020). Radiosensitising cancer using phosphatidylinositol-3-kinase (PI3K), protein kinase B (AKT) or mammalian target of rapamycin (mTOR) inhibitors. *Cancers*, *12*, 1278–1307.

Warburg, O., Wind, F., & Negelein, E. (1927). The metabolism of tumors in the body. *Journal of General Physiology*, *8*, 519–530.

Ward, P. S., & Thompson, C. B. (2012). Metabolic reprogramming: A cancer hallmark even Warburg did not anticipate. *Cancer Cell*, *21*, 297–308.

Weathers, S. S., & Gilbert, M. R. (2016). Toward personalized targeted therapeutics: An overview. *Neurotherapeutics*, *14*, 256–264.

Weber, D. D., Aminzadeh-Gohari, S., Tulipan, J., Catalano, L., Feichtinger, R. G., & Kofler, B. (2020). Ketogenic diet in the treatment of cancer—Where do we stand? *Molecular Metabolism*, *33*, 102–121.

Wei, J., Wu, A., Kong, L. Y., Wang, Y., Fuller, G., Fokt, I., Melillo, G., Priebe, W., & Heimberger, A. B. (2011). Hypoxia potentiates glioma-mediated immunosuppression. *PLOS ONE*, *6*, Article e16195.

Wei, M., Brandhorst, S., Shelehchi, M., Mirzaei, H., Cheng, C. W., Budniak, J., Groshen, S., Mack, W. J., Guen, E., Di Biase, S., Cohen, P., Morgan, T. E., Dorff, T., Hong, K., Michalsen, A., Laviano, A., & Longo, V. D. (2017). Fasting-mimicking diet and markers/risk factors for aging, diabetes, cancer, and cardiovascular disease. *Science Translational Medicine*, *9*, 1–12.

Wei, W., Shi, Q., Remacle, F., Qin, L., Shackelford, D. B., Shin, Y. S., Mischel, P. S., Levine, R. D., & Heath, J. R. (2013). Hypoxia induces a phase transition within a kinase signaling network in cancer cells. *Proceedings of the National Academy of Sciences of the United States of America*, *110*, E1352–E1360.

Weinberg, F., & Chandel, N. S. (2009). Reactive oxygen species-dependent signaling regulates cancer. *Cellular and Molecular Life Sciences*, *66*, 3663–3673.

Weiss, J. M. (2020). The promise and peril of targeting cell metabolism for cancer therapy. *Cancer Immunology, Immunotherapy*, *69*, 255–261.

Winter, S. F., Loebel, F., & Dietrich, J. (2017). Role of ketogenic metabolic therapy in malignant glioma: A systematic review. *Critical Reviews in Oncology/Hematology*, *112*, 41–58.

Wolf, A., Agnihotri, S., & Guha, A. (2010). Targeting metabolic remodeling in glioblastoma multiforme. *Oncotarget*, *1*, 552–562.

Wood, S., & Zabilowicz, C. (2020). The brain tumour patient experience of ketogenic diet therapy. *Neurodigest*, *5*, 16–20.

Woolf, E. C., Curley, K. L., Liu, Q., Turner, G. H., Charlton, J. A., Preul, M. C., & Scheck, A. C. (2015a). The ketogenic diet alters the hypoxic response and affects expression of proteins associated with angiogenesis, invasive potential and vascular permeability in a mouse glioma model. *PLOS ONE*, *10*, Article e0130357.

Woolf, E. C., Johnson, J. L., Lussier, D. M., Brooks, K. S., Blattman, J. N., & Scheck, A. C. (2015b). The ketogenic diet enhances immunity in a mouse model of malignant glioma. In: Proceedings of the 106th Annual Meeting of the American Association for Cancer Research; 2015 Apr 18-22; Philadelphia, PA. Philadelphia (PA): AACR; *Cancer Res* 2015;75(15 Suppl):Abstract nr 1344. doi:10.1158/1538-7445.AM2015-1344

Woolf, E. C., & Scheck, A. C. (2015). The ketogenic diet for the treatment of malignant glioma. *Journal of Lipid Research*, *56*, 5–10.

Woolf, E. C., Syed, N., & Scheck, A. C. (2016). Tumor metabolism, the ketogenic diet and beta-hydroxybutyrate: Novel approaches to adjuvant brain tumor therapy. *Frontiers in Molecular Neuroscience*, *9*, 122.

Xia, S., Lin, R., Jin, L., Zhao, L., Kang, H. B., Pan, Y., Liu, S., Qian, G., Qian, Z., Konstantakou, E., Zhang, B., Dong, J. T., Chung, Y. R., Abdel-Wahab, O., Merghoub, T., Zhou, L., Kudchadkar, R. R., Lawson, D. H., Khoury, H. J., . . . Chen, J. (2017). Prevention of dietary-fat-fueled ketogenesis attenuates BRAF V600E tumor growth. *Cell Metabolism*, *25*, 358–373.

Xiao, Q., Yang, S., Ding, G., & Luo, M. (2018). Antivascular endothelial growth factor in glioblastoma: A systematic review and meta-analysis. *Neurological Sciences*, *39*, 2021–2031.

Yakovenko, A., Cameron, M., & Trevino, J. G. (2018). Molecular therapeutic strategies targeting pancreatic cancer induced cachexia. *World Journal of Gastrointestinal Surgery*, *10*, 95–106.

Yamada, M., Tomida, A., Yun, J., Cai, B., Yoshikawa, H., Taketani, Y., & Tsuruo, T. (1999). Cellular sensitization to cisplatin and carboplatin with decreased removal of platinum-DNA adduct by glucose-regulated stress. *Cancer Chemotherapy and Pharmacology, 44,* 59–64.

Yang, L., Lin, C., Wang, L., Guo, H., & Wang, X. (2012). Hypoxia and hypoxia-inducible factors in glioblastoma multiforme progression and therapeutic implications. *Experimental Cell Research, 318,* 2417–2426.

Yang, L., Shi, P., Zhao, G., Xu, J., Peng, W., Zhang, J., Zhang, G., Wang, X., Dong, Z., Chen, F., & Cui, H. (2020). Targeting cancer stem cell pathways for cancer therapy. *Signal Transduction and Targeted Therapy, 5,* 8.

Yoshida, G. J. (2020). Beyond the Warburg effect: N-Myc contributes to metabolic reprogramming in cancer cells. *Frontiers in Oncology, 10,* 791.

Yu, G., Li, G. F., Wang, D. X., Wang, J., & Zhou, H. H. (2017). Fasting conditions in clinical oncology trials and drug labelling. *Lancet Oncology, 18,* e506.

Zahra, A., Fath, M. A., Opat, E., Mapuskar, K. A., Bhatia, S. K., Ma, D. C., Rodman, S. N., III, Snyders, T. P., Chenard, C. A., Eichenberger-Gilmore, J. M., Bodeker, K. L., Ahmann, L., Smith, B. J., Vollstedt, S. A., Brown, H. A., Hejleh, T. A., Clamon, G. H., Berg, D. J., Szweda, L. I., . . . Allen, B. G. (2017). Consuming a ketogenic diet while receiving radiation and chemotherapy for locally advanced lung cancer and pancreatic cancer: The University of Iowa experience of two Phase 1 clinical trials. *Radiation Research, 187,* 743–754.

Zam, W., Ahmed, I., & Yousef, H. (2021). Warburg effects on cancer cells survival: The role of sugar starvation in cancer therapy. *Current Clinical Pharmacology, 16,* 30–38.

Zhang, H., Gu, C., Yu, J., Wang, Z., Yuan, X., Yang, L., Wang, J., Jia, Y., Liu, J., & Liu, F. (2014). Radiosensitization of glioma cells by TP53-induced glycolysis and apoptosis regulator knockdown is dependent on thioredoxin-1 nuclear translocation. *Free Radical Biology and Medicine, 69C,* 239–248.

Zhang, Y., & Kutateladze, T. G. (2018). Diet and the epigenome. *Nature Communications, 9,* 3375.

Zhao, H., Raines, L. N., & Huang, S. C. (2020). Carbohydrate and amino acid metabolism as hallmarks for innate immune cell activation and function. *Cells, 9,* 562–584.

Zhao, M., Huang, X., Cheng, X., Lin, X., Zhao, T., Wu, L., Yu, X., Wu, K., Fan, M., & Zhu, L. (2017). Ketogenic diet improves the spatial memory impairment caused by exposure to hypobaric hypoxia through increased acetylation of histones in rats. *PLOS ONE, 12,* Article e0174477.

Zhao, M., Tan, B., Dai, X., Shao, Y., He, Q., Yang, B., Wang, J., & Weng, Q. (2019). DHFR/TYMS are positive regulators of glioma cell growth and modulate chemo-sensitivity to temozolomide. *European Journal of Pharmacology, 863,* 172665.

Zhou, W., Mukherjee, P., Kiebish, M. A., Markis, W. T., Mantis, J. G., & Seyfried, T. N. (2007). The calorically restricted ketogenic diet, an effective alternative therapy for malignant brain cancer. *Nutrition & Metabolism, 4*(5), 5.

Zorn, S., Ehret, J., Schäuble, R., Rautenberg, B., Ihorst, G., Bertz, H., Urbain, P., & Raynor, A. (2020). Impact of modified short-term fasting and its combination with a fasting supportive diet during chemotherapy on the incidence and severity of chemotherapy-induced toxicities in cancer patients—A controlled cross-over pilot study. *BMC Cancer, 20,* 578.

Zou, Z., Tao, T., Li, H., & Zhu, X. (2020). mTOR signaling pathway and mTOR inhibitors in cancer: Progress and challenges. *Cell & Bioscience, 10,* 31.

16

Ketogenic Diet, Social Behavior, and Autism

Insights from Animal Models

NING CHENG, PHD, SUSAN A. MASINO, PHD, AND JONG M. RHO, MD

The ketogenic diet (KD) is a metabolic therapy that has been used clinically for the past century. It is characterized by a high-fat and low-carbohydrate content, and a prospective, controlled study in pediatric patients confirmed its efficacy against medically intractable epilepsy (Neal et al., 2008). Recently, increasing numbers of studies have applied the KD (or its variants) in a much wider array of neurologic diseases and conditions, such as neurodegenerative disorders, sleep disorders, neuroimmune conditions, brain trauma, stroke, pain, and brain cancer (Boison, 2016; Cheng et al., 2017; Gano et al., 2014; Gasior et al., 2006; Lutas & Yellen, 2013; Stafstrom & Rho, 2012; Yudkoff et al., 2007). In addition, although limited in scope and sample size, several studies have demonstrated beneficial effects in patients with autism spectrum disorder (ASD) and related neurodevelopmental syndromes (Bostock et al., 2017; Evangeliou et al., 2003; Herbert & Buckley, 2013; Lee et al., 2018; Liebhaber et al., 2003). Furthermore, this dietary therapy also showed promising results in several rodent models of autism, including reducing deficits in social and repetitive behaviors and rescuing comorbid conditions, such as epileptic seizures (Ahn et al., 2014; Cheng et al., 2017; Kraeuter et al., 2020; Nylen et al., 2008; Ruskin et al., 2013, 2016, 2017; Westmark et al., 2020).

ASD is a prevalent neurodevelopmental condition, characterized by deficits in social function and language development, as well as repetitive and restrictive behaviors. It is one of the most common neurodevelopmental disorders and encompasses a broad spectrum of symptom severity and comorbid medical conditions (Lai et al., 2014). The prevalence of ASD has dramatically increased over the past two decades worldwide, regardless of race, ethnicity, or socioeconomic status. Although ASD prevalence differs from country to country, it is usually around 1% or greater in the general population globally, based on recent estimates (Chiarotti & Venerosi, 2020; Maenner et al., 2020). Consequently, autism not only affects many individuals around the world but also requires a huge amount of resources for support of an affected individual throughout life. It was estimated that the lifetime cost of an individual diagnosed with autism is approximately $1.2 million to $4.7 million (Buescher et al., 2014; Leigh & Du, 2015; Rogge & Janssen, 2019).

Presently there is no effective medical treatment for the core symptoms of ASD. Current therapeutics can address some of the comorbidities, including epileptic seizures, aggression, and irritability, but fail to correct the core deficits. The etiology of ASD is heterogeneous and complex, likely involving both genetic and environmental factors, and the pathophysiologic mechanisms remain largely unknown. Clinical manifestations are similarly diverse. These facts contribute to the difficulty in finding effective treatments for ASD (DiCicco-Bloom et al., 2006; Lai et al., 2014).

Not surprisingly, the molecular and cellular pathways implicated in ASD are also highly complex and include diverse and interconnected processes, such as synaptic function and plasticity of various neurotransmitter systems, transcriptional and chromatin regulation, and protein translation and modification, as well as glial cell function and neuroimmunologic modulation (DiCicco-Bloom et al., 2006; Lai et al., 2014). In addition, ASD has been proposed to involve metabolic dysregulation. As many as 30% of children with ASD experience metabolic abnormalities and changes associated with mitochondrial dysfunction (Cheng et al., 2017;

Rossignol & Frye, 2012). In addition, genes with mutations associated with ASD encode proteins that are known to play a role in energy metabolism, including phosphatase and tensin (PTEN) homolog, branched-chain ketoacid dehydrogenase kinase, ubiquitin-protein ligase E3A, fragile X mental retardation protein (FMRP), and tuberous sclerosis proteins (de la Torre-Ubieta et al., 2016; Rivell & Mattson, 2019). Furthermore, gene expression analyses indicate that altered levels of expression are common in pathways involved in metabolism (Quesnel-Vallières et al., 2019; Wen et al., 2016).

ANIMAL MODELS OF AUTISM

Development of therapeutics for ASD is complicated by the disorder's heterogeneous etiology, which includes genetic, epigenetic, and environmental factors. The majority of ASD cases are idiopathic; that is, the underlying causes are unknown and presumed to be genetic in origin (DiCicco-Bloom et al., 2006; Lai et al., 2014). To investigate the mechanisms and uncover treatments, many animal models have been developed, including ones that model genetic alterations, such as Shank1/2/3, neuroligin-3/4, Tsc2, Fmr1, En2, 15q11-13, and 16p11.2, as well as

ones mimicking environmental risks, including maternal immune activation and exposure to valproic acid during gestation (Ellegood & Crawley, 2015). Most of these models are mouse-based; however, models using other species, such as rat, fruit fly, and zebrafish, have also been developed and studied (Chadman, 2017).

There are also a few models of idiopathic ASD. The BTBR T+tf/J (BTBR) inbred mouse strain has been well characterized using various tests for social interaction and communication (including ultrasonic vocalization), as well as for repetitive behaviors, traits that model the defining symptoms of ASD (Meyza & Blanchard, 2017). In general, BTBR mice display a robust phenotype in these behavioral assays (Figures 16.1 to 16.3). In addition, a relevant anatomical feature of BTBR mice is agenesis of the corpus callosum (Khanbabaei et al., 2019; Meyza & Blanchard 2017), an anomaly that has been observed in human studies (Frazier & Hardan, 2009; Wolff et al., 2015; Paul et al., 2014). Thus, the BTBR mouse has been considered a valuable model of multifactorial idiopathic autism and has been increasingly used to test many potential therapies. Indeed, findings in the BTBR mouse have provided the scientific rationale for a number of clinical trials (Kazdoba et al., 2016).

Experimental setting

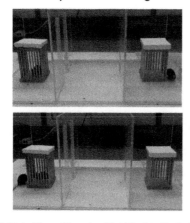

Track visualization

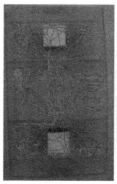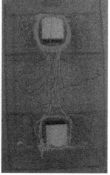

Habituation   **Testing**

FIGURE 16.1 *Three-Chamber Test Used to Probe Sociability*

Left: Experimental setting. The chamber is partitioned into three parts, with doors providing access from the middle chamber to the two side chambers. After the subject is habituated to the whole chamber, an empty wire cage serving as the novel object is introduced to one side chamber, and a wire cage with a stranger mouse inside is introduced to the other side chamber. Typically, the subject mouse will investigate both the novel object (upper image) and the novel mouse (lower image). Right: The location of the subject mouse can be tracked (red traces) by automated software, and the time it spends in each chamber can be used as an indication of its preference for novel object versus novel mouse, a measure of sociability.

Recording

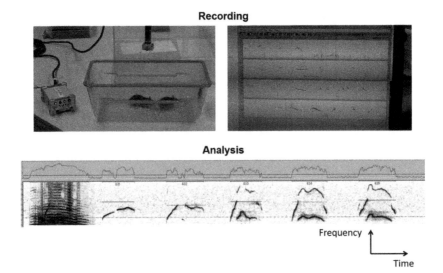

Analysis

Frequency ↑

Time

FIGURE 16.2 *Ultrasonic Vocalization Test for Vocal Communication*

During social interaction, in this case between a male and a female, vocalizations can be recorded by an ultrasound-sensitive microphone and converted to computer-recognizable signal (upper panels). The signal can be analyzed offline by software and methods to quantify both the amount and structure of the vocalizations.

Previous reports have pointed to links between metabolism and behavior in BTBR mice through various pathogenic processes involving neuroinflammation, neurogenesis, transcriptome/proteome, and microbiota, similar to the processes that have been proposed for humans with ASD (Currais et al., 2016; Daimon et al., 2015; Flowers et al., 2007; Golubeva et al., 2017; Stern, 2011).

The EL mouse is also considered a model of idiopathic ASD. In addition, this mouse models the comorbidity of autism and epilepsy (Meidenbauer et al., 2011). The EL mouse has long been studied as a natural model of generalized epilepsy, and it has been reported that these mice also display several atypical behaviors characteristic of ASD, including impaired social

Self-grooming   **Marble-burying**

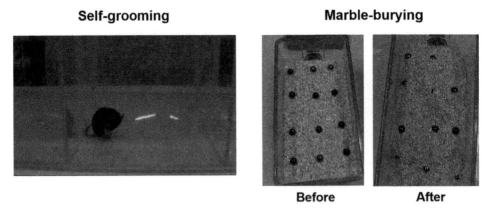

Before   **After**

FIGURE 16.3 *Examples of Assays to Model Repetitive Behaviors in Rodents*

Left: After a habituation period to the chamber, the self-grooming behavior of the subject can be recorded and measured. Right: In the marble-burying assay, the subject is introduced to a cage with an array of marbles laid on top of bedding. After 30 min, the subject is removed from the testing cage and the marbles buried during this period by the subject are counted.

interactions and restricted patterns of behaviors (Meidenbauer et al., 2011; Ruskin et al., 2016).

EFFECTS OF THE KD IN ANIMAL MODELS OF AUTISM

The KD has been utilized in several animal models of ASD. Consistent with clinical studies, reports have been generally positive in both genetic and idiopathic animal models (Table 16.1). In an animal model of succinic semialdehyde dehydrogenase (SSADH) deficiency, wherein the gene encoding SSADH is deleted, it was reported that the KD restored certain electrophysiologic features and reduced seizure susceptibility (Nylen et al., 2008). In a separate study, results showed that either restriction of standard diet or KD improved motor behavior and reduced anxiety in *Mecp2* mutant animals (Mantis et al., 2009), a mouse model of Rett syndrome—a syndrome in which patients often exhibit autistic behaviors during the early stages of the disease (Amir et al., 1999). Mutations in the *En2* gene could lead to neurodevelopmental changes and autism-related behaviors as well (Benayed et al., 2009). A study examined *En2* knockout and wild-type mice fed a KD from weaning to adulthood for about 40 days, after which the KD was discontinued and animals were fed standard chow for 2 days. Results indicated that KD treatment during the juvenile stage led to improved social interactions, reduced repetitive behaviors, and appropriate exploratory behaviors in the knockout mice (Verpeut et al., 2016).

Fragile X syndrome is the leading monogenic cause of ASD and is caused by changes in the *Fmr1* gene that reduce levels of FMRP protein (Abbeduto et al., 2014; Hagerman et al., 2017). Recently, a research group investigated the effects of chronic KD treatment in an *Fmr1* knockout mouse model of fragile X syndrome (Westmark et al., 2020). They found that KD selectively reduced seizures in male, but not female, *Fmr1* knockout mice. In addition, the KD differentially influenced gain in body weight and circadian activity levels depending on genotype, sex, and age of the subject mice.

As mentioned, environmental factors also contribute to the risk of developing ASD. For example, maternal immune activation due to viral or bacterial infection during the first trimester may contribute to an elevated incidence of autism (Boulanger-Bertolus et al., 2018; Lombardo et al., 2018). Ruskin and colleagues found that treatment with a KD partially or completely reversed all behavioral deficits induced by maternal immune activation in male offspring (Ruskin et al., 2017). Interestingly, female offspring were not affected by maternal immune activation and their behavioral phenotype was not influenced by KD treatment. Another exogenous modulator of ASD susceptibility is valproic acid (VPA), a drug that is used primarily for the treatment of epilepsy and migraine. Intriguingly, VPA use during pregnancy is associated with an increased risk of ASD in the offspring (Bromley et al., 2013; Christensen et al., 2013). Using rodent models of VPA exposure (Chomiak et al., 2013; Roullet et al., 2013), it was reported that the KD improved social behavior and mitochondrial respiration (Ahn et al., 2014; Castro et al., 2016).

Most genetic risks associated with ASD are common variations, and the majority of diagnosed cases have unknown genetic underpinnings (Gaugler et al., 2014). Animal models of multifactorial etiology have been characterized that display autistic symptomatology. Using the BTBR mouse model of idiopathic ASD, Ruskin and colleagues reported that the KD increased sociability in the three-chamber test, decreased self-directed repetitive behaviors, and improved social communication in a food preference assay (Ruskin et al., 2013). In addition, studies conducted by Ruskin and colleagues also demonstrated behavioral improvements induced by the KD in the EL mouse, which is a model of comorbid autism-associated behaviors and progressive spontaneous epilepsy (Meidenbauer et al., 2011). The KD improved sociability and reduced repetitive behaviors in the EL mouse. Intriguingly, these effects were more pronounced in females (Ruskin et al., 2016). Specifically, the KD improved several measurements of sociability and decreased repetitive behaviors in female EL mice, but its effects in males were limited. Additionally, the authors observed that a less stringent, more clinically applicable dietary formula was equally effective in female mice in terms of improving social and repetitive behaviors.

Impairment of development and usage of language is a hallmark of ASD (Krishnan et al., 2016; Mayes et al., 2015; Rapin & Dunn 2003; Stefanatos & Baron, 2011); on one extreme of the autism spectrum, about 30% of children either fail to develop functional language or are minimally verbal (Brignell et al., 2018). Social communication is a cornerstone in human society. Not surprisingly, studies have found that difficulties with language are associated with an array of adverse outcomes, such as poorer academic achievement, behavioral difficulties, and overall reduced quality of

TABLE 16.1

■ Deficit and improved
▨ Deficit but not improved
□ No deficit
▨ To be determined

MODEL	sex	Social Behavior				Repetitive Self-Directed Behavior	
		sociability	social novelty	social contact	social communication	Alone	social
Maternal immune activation mouse offspring	M	+	+	+	ND	+	+
	F	ND	ND	+	ND	ND	ND
BTBR mice	M	+	+	+	+	ND	+
	F	0	0	?	?	0	0
EL mice	M	+	ND	0	0	+	ND
	F	+	+	+	ND	+	0
Adenosine A_1R knockout mouse	M	+	ND	+	ND	0	+
Control mice		ND	ND	ND	ND	ND	ND

life. Conversely, functional language usage is associated with improved long-term outcomes in patients with autism (Paul, 2008). Currently, there are no effective treatments for language deficits, as the underlying mechanisms remain mostly unclear. Behavioral therapies thus far are the main available option, but they are highly variable and have led to mixed results (Brignell et al., 2018; Spreckley & Boyd, 2009). In addition, the cost of behavioral therapies is high. With the huge burden associated with ASD (Buescher et al., 2014; Leigh & Du, 2015; Rogge & Janssen, 2019), effective therapies are urgently needed.

Animal models have been used to study vocal communication, including in mice (Fischer & Hammerschmidt, 2011; Konopka & Roberts, 2016; Lahvis et al., 2011). Ultrasonic vocalizations in mice are biologically meaningful signals that are remarkably complex (Arriaga et al., 2012; Lahvis et al., 2011; Portfors & Perkel, 2014). Features in mouse vocalization that could convey communicative value include both the amount and the structure of vocalizations. The latter further encompass acoustic features of individual calls, temporal structures of call organization, and sonographic categories (Castellucci et al., 2018; Holy & Guo, 2005; Panksepp et al., 2007; Takahashi et al., 2015; Wang et al., 2008). Many rodent models of ASD display altered vocalizations (Brunner et al., 2015; Cezar et al., 2018; Jamain et al., 2008; Ju et al., 2014; Kogan et al., 2015; Malkova et al., 2012; Rotschafer et al., 2012; Stoppel et al., 2018; Wohr, 2014; Yang et al., 2015; Young et al., 2010). In addition, several genes involved in human language, such as *Foxp2*, *Foxp1*, and *Catnap2*, are associated with ASD and play a role in rodent vocalization as well (Brunner et al., 2015; Castellucci, et al., 2016; Chabout et al., 2016; Penagarikano et al., 2011; Schaafsma et al., 2017; Usui et al., 2017). However, unlike other core autism-associated traits, such as social approach and repetitive behaviors, which have been shown to respond to diverse therapeutic approaches in many animal models (Kazdoba et al., 2016), only a few studies have reported that vocalization is improved after treatments (Cezar et al., 2018; Rotschafer et al., 2012). In these studies, vocalization amount, but not structure, was affected in the animal models examined and was rescued by drug treatments.

In a recent study, we tested how the KD affected vocalization in BTBR mice, which display robust deficits in this behavior (Scattoni et al., 2011). Adolescent and adult male BTBR mice were fed either standard diet or KD for 11 days. At the end of the treatment, their vocalizations were quantified during male–female interactions. In addition, we investigated C57BL/6J (B6) mice, which exhibit normal levels of social behaviors (Meyza & Blanchard, 2017) and vocalization (Kim et al., 2016; Scattoni et al., 2008, 2011, 2013; Schwartzer et al., 2013; Wohr, 2015). Our results revealed that treatment with the KD robustly improved both the amount and structure of vocalizations in adolescent BTBR mice. Conversely, only subtle changes were observed in the same parameters in B6 mice. In addition, adult BTBR mice were less affected by the dietary treatment (Murari et al., 2021).

The different results from juvenile and adult BTBR mice in this study suggest that early treatment could have more impact. This aligns with studies in patients with ASD, which have shown that early diagnosis and interventions are more likely to lead to long-term positive effects (Sullivan et al., 2014). However, findings in animal models have been more variable. For example, in mouse models of Rett syndrome, studies have shown that impairment could be reversed at any developmental stage, from neonatal to adult animals, by re-expression of the *Mecp2* gene (Gadalla et al., 2013; Garg et al., 2013; Guy et al., 2007). In other animal models of autism, however, results indicate that better outcomes are associated with early treatment. For example, using a mouse model of Angelman syndrome, Silva-Santos and colleagues (2015) have observed that most syndrome-associated phenotypes were rescued if introduction of the *Ube3a* allele was accomplished early in development. However, much more restricted effects were obtained when the same strategy was used later during adolescence. In a separate study, chronic treatment with oxytocin in the Cntnap2 mouse model during early postnatal stage resulted in lasting behavioral recovery (Penagarikano et al., 2011). Furthermore, in a Shank3 mouse model of autism, improvements in social interaction and repetitive behavior, but not in anxiety or motor

coordination deficits, were observed by restoring the expression of *Shank3* gene in adult mice (Mei et al., 2016). Finally, in a recent study using a rat model of fragile X syndrome, sustained correction of deficits in associative learning over several months in adulthood resulted from a brief pharmacologic treatment during the adolescent and young adult stage (Asiminas et al., 2019). Together, these results suggest that critical intervention windows during development may exist for optimal outcomes in ASD.

MECHANISMS OF KD ACTION IN ANIMAL MODELS OF ASD

The KD is a proven therapy for medically intractable epilepsy, especially in children (Neal et al., 2008). It was designed to mimic the metabolic changes in the body in response to fasting or starvation. Historically, it has been observed that these methods have antiseizure effects. The KD induces two key metabolic changes: increased fatty acids and ketone bodies in the blood that are produced by the liver, and decreased blood glucose levels. In addition, results from animal models of distinct diseases have revealed that the KD may regulate energy metabolism and mitochondrial function to induce neuroprotective effects (Gano et al., 2014). However, it could also target additional molecular and cellular pathways (Boison, 2016; Cheng et al., 2017; Gano et al., 2014; Gasior et al., 2006; Lutas & Yellen, 2013; Napoli et al., 2014; Stafstrom & Rho, 2012; Yudkoff et al. 2007). The multitude and diversity of cellular and molecular processes influenced by the diet makes it challenging to identify key mechanisms underlying behavioral changes. In addition, it is quite possible that the KD induces different changes in ASD than in other disease states, such as epilepsy, although epilepsy and ASD are major reciprocal comorbidities.

To investigate whether the KD affords beneficial effects by general neuroprotective mechanisms or by reversing distinct pathologic processes underlying individual diseases, several studies have examined consequences of KD treatment in normal rodents. Huang and colleagues fed adult B6 mice a KD for 3 months and observed that mice fed ketogenic or control diets behaved similarly in tests for motor coordination, anxiety, spatial learning and memory, sociability, and depression. In addition, synaptic transmission and long-term potentiation were also similar between the two groups. However, mice fed the KD had slower weight gain and an increased seizure threshold (Huang et al., 2019). In a separate study, juvenile male rats were fed the KD for 4 weeks, and subsequent behavioral tests revealed that KD-fed rats displayed increased social exploration, with no changes in mobility, anxiety, or working memory. Notably, there were no changes in social behaviors in animals receiving exogenous ketone bodies (β-hydroxybutyrate or acetone; Kasprowska-Liśkiewicz et al., 2017). Another study examined the impact on offspring development of gestational exposure to the KD. Male and female CD-1 mice were exposed to either a standard diet or KD gestationally and then were cross-fostered with dams at birth and remained on standard diet afterward. Behavioral tests revealed that gestational exposure to the KD enhanced sociability and decreased depression-associated behaviors. Oxytocin expression in hypothalamic and limbic areas was not altered by the treatment (Arqoub et al., 2020). Together, these results suggest that the KD may increase social interaction in normal animals under certain circumstances, suggesting that it could influence social behavior through shared mechanisms in normal animals and disease models. This issue needs to be further explored in future studies.

In the study that examined En2 knockout mice, the authors also measured monoamine levels in different regions of the brain. They found norepinephrine levels were increased in hypothalamus of the wild-type mice by the KD, while it did not change regional monoamine levels in the knockout mice. In addition, they observed more c-FOS-positive cells in the cingulate cortex, lateral septal nuclei, and anterior bed nucleus of the stria terminalis in both wild-type and knockout mice fed the KD than in those fed control diet, after the subject mice interacted with a novel mouse (Verpeut et al., 2016).

As mentioned earlier, accumulating evidence indicates that metabolic dysregulation could play an important role in autism; as many as 30% of children with autism experience abnormalities associated with metabolism (Frye, 2015). The KD is designed to mimic the effects of fasting, and thus it is believed to be a metabolism-based approach (Boison, 2016; Cheng et al., 2017; Gano et al., 2014; Gasior et al., 2006; Lutas & Yellen, 2013; Napoli et al., 2014; Stafstrom & Rho, 2012; Yudkoff et al., 2007). Therefore, in a recent study, we examined metabolic profiles of cortical tissue using LC-QTOF-MS-based metabolomics. Our results revealed that multiple metabolites and pathways were altered by the KD in both BTBR

and B6 mice (Mayengbam et al., 2021). A subset of the identified metabolites was also recognized by a previous study, which quantified metabolomics of hippocampus and plasma in KD-fed and/or calorie-restricted rats (Heischmann et al., 2018). The metabolites include ones that are associated with taurine metabolism, steroid hormone biosynthesis, and dopamine metabolism. The results suggest that changes in metabolism resulting from the KD could be partially shared across species and brain regions.

Our study also demonstrated that the KD altered brain metabolic profiles of BTBR and B6 mice through both shared and divergent pathways (Mayengbam et al., 2021). Metabolites associated with bile acid metabolism were highly increased by the KD in both mouse strains. This might result from altered cholesterol metabolism due to the high fat content of the diet. It has been shown that impaired bile acid metabolism is linked to social deficits in BTBR mice (Golubeva et al., 2017). Therefore, upregulation of bile acid metabolites in the brain might be beneficial. Consistent with previous studies (Yudkoff et al., 2007), glutamine levels were increased in the brain of both BTBR and B6 mice. Glutamine is essential for the biosynthesis of GABA, the brain's major inhibitory neurotransmitter. Previous studies suggest that this pathway is one of the mechanisms of the anti-seizure effect of the KD, and it needs to be further investigated in the context of ASD. One-carbon and folate metabolism were also affected by the diet in both mouse strains, in that it upregulated folate in B6 mice and increased dihydrofolate in BTBR mice. Notably, previous studies have suggested that low levels of circulating folate may be associated with ASD (Al-Farsi et al., 2013; Altun et al., 2018). In support of this hypothesis, it has been reported that use of one-carbon-linked B vitamins and folate as supplements improved the clinical evaluations in patients with ASD (Adams & Holloway, 2004). Last, our results revealed that the levels of cortical pantothenate in both B6 and BTBR mice were increased by the KD. Pantothenate is obligatory in the biosynthesis of CoA, which plays central roles in many cellular processes. It has been shown from previous studies that patients with ASD have decreased levels of pantothenate biosynthesis (Gevi et al., 2016; Stewart et al., 2015), thus suggesting that increased pantothenate levels with the KD might be protective.

In contrast to the above, distinct pathways impacted by the KD were identified in either mouse strain. For example, glutathione levels were increased only in BTBR mice. Glutathione plays a critical role in quenching the formation of reactive oxygen species and in protecting proteins from oxidative damage by introducing covalent modifications (Mailloux et al., 2013). Oxidative damage is believed to be an important factor in the pathophysiology of autism (Rossignol & Frye, 2014). Therefore, another possible mechanism underlying the beneficial effects of the KD is to enhance antioxidant functions that could lead to neuroprotection. Our metabolic results also showed that purine and pyrimidine metabolism pathways were altered, and inosine levels were decreased by the KD, but only in BTBR cortical tissue. Existing evidence suggests these pathways are dysregulated in patients with ASD (Fumagalli et al., 2017; Gevi et al., 2016), and studies in animal models, including models of maternal immune activation and fragile X syndrome, demonstrated that treatment with a nonselective purinergic antagonist (suramin) reversed autism-like phenotypes in these two models (J. C. Naviaux et al., 2014, 2015; R. K. Naviaux et al., 2013).

Together, these results suggest that the KD may reverse the changes observed in ASD through regulation of several metabolic pathways. In our previous studies, we found that BTBR mice display several changes during early postnatal neurodevelopment (Cheng et al., 2016, 2017; Khanbabaei et al., 2019). Whether these changes are associated with metabolism in the brain, and whether they could be reversed by the KD, are questions that could be addressed in future studies.

In addition to metabolic profiling, we also examined cortical electroencephalography (EEG) in BTBR and B6 mice fed either the KD or a control diet. It has been proposed that EEG could be used as a potential translational biomarker, to facilitate diagnosis and treatment monitoring in autism (Ewen et al., 2019; Gurau et al., 2017; Sahin et al., 2018). Accumulating evidence has shown that there are robust differences in EEG signal between autistic and neurotypical subjects. Specifically, results from some studies suggest that a U-shaped profile of EEG power is associated with a subset of people with autism, who display greater power in low- and high-frequency bands when compared with control subjects (Gurau et al., 2017; O'Reilly et al., 2017; Wang et al., 2013). However, as is typical of most measurements in the autistic population, highly variable findings have been reported. The possible reasons include the intrinsic heterogeneity of autism as a spectrum

disorder (indeed, as explicitly stated by the name), nonuniform methods used in different studies, and generally limited sample sizes. In our study, we observed that EEG power was greater in theta, beta, and gamma bands, but similar in delta and alpha bands, in BTBR mice when compared with B6 mice. This is reminiscent of the U-shaped profile observed in some people with autism, as mentioned above. Yet following treatment with a KD, the pattern of cortical EEG power was not altered, indicating a dissociation from the impaired social interaction/communication and repetitive behaviors in BTBR mice that were robustly improved by the diet. Together, these findings suggest that while it is plausible that EEG patterns could be a potential diagnostic biomarker for ASD, EEG may not be a reliable method in all cases for monitoring responses to treatment.

LIMITATIONS AND FUTURE DIRECTIONS

Although extremely powerful and indispensable, animal models of human conditions do have limitations. Studies need to focus on the conserved aspects of biology between human and animal models, but consideration should always be given to areas of divergence. For example, although sharing certain features and genetic/anatomical pathways, mouse vocalization is unlikely to model every aspect of human language development or dysfunction. Currently, evidence suggests that vocalization in mice is a largely innate function, while human language requires the ability to imitate novel sounds (Arriaga & Jarvis, 2013). Thus, results obtained using animal models need to be considered within this general context and carefully interpreted.

Only a few studies using animal models thus far have investigated sex differences with respect to KD effects (Arqoub et al., 2020; Ruskin et al., 2017; Westmark et al., 2020); the majority of studies have employed only male mice. It is important to investigate the effects of the KD in female mouse models of ASD as well, not only due to the numerous differences in physiology and responses between males and females, but also because of the fact that, in humans, both males and females are diagnosed with ASD (Ratto et al., 2018). Although the prevalence of ASD is higher in human males than in females (Loomes et al., 2017), it cannot be assumed that findings from males are also applicable to females.

In addition, several issues also need to be considered regarding the administration of the KD.

Due to the stringent high-fat and low-carbohydrate requirements, the KD is highly restrictive and can be difficult to follow over an extended time. This is especially true for many people with ASD, who already have meal-related challenges and/or narrow food preferences, or who experience very common gastrointestinal problems. In addition, side effects should also be considered. Although most of them are reported to be transient and manageable with relative ease, they need to be carefully monitored (Duchowny, 2005). Furthermore, the potential influence on development needs to be considered. As mentioned above, based on results from animal models, the KD might be more effective when given to infants rather than adolescents and adults. In humans, studies have shown the KD's beneficial influences on cognition and behavior during development (Hallbook et al., 2012; Pulsifer et al., 2001). However, its impact on development, especially neurodevelopment, is in need of further investigation (Bostock et al., 2017; Mayengbam et al., 2021; Scichilone et al., 2016).

Due to these limitations, future investigations are urgently needed to unravel the molecular mechanisms accounting for the clinical activity of the KD, such as the specific metabolic pathways identified in previous studies. Knowledge gathered from additional investigations will hopefully reveal novel interventional targets, which could then be selectively exploited with more specific and potentially personalized approaches.

Other dietary interventions have also been shown to regulate social behavior. For example, an interesting study fed diets with different glycemic indices to BTBR mice. The glycemic index measures the degree of blood glucose levels affected by the carbohydrate content in a diet. The authors found that behavioral and biochemical phenotypes in the BTBR mice were significantly impacted by dietary glycemic index (Currais et al., 2016). Together with the studies mentioned earlier using the KD, these findings provide support for the hypothesis that in the context of genetic predisposition to ASD, metabolism-based dietary interventions could potentially modify symptoms of the disease, including core symptoms. As mentioned, there is no effective medical treatment or cure for the core symptoms of ASD. Future studies could further validate the effects of the KD in both humans and animal models and continue to unravel the underlying mechanisms using multiple complementary approaches.

REFERENCES

Abbeduto, L., McDuffie, A., & Thurman, A. J. (2014). The fragile X syndrome-autism comorbidity: What do we really know? *Frontiers in Genetics, 5*, 355.

Adams, J. B., & Holloway, C. (2004). Pilot study of a moderate dose multivitamin/mineral supplement for children with autistic spectrum disorder. *Journal of Alternative and Complementary Medicine, 10*(6), 1033–1039.

Ahn, Y., Narous, M., Tobias, R., Rho, J. M., & Mychasiuk, R. (2014). The ketogenic diet modifies social and metabolic alterations identified in the prenatal valproic acid model of autism spectrum disorder. *Developmental Neuroscience, 36*(5), 371–380.

Al-Farsi, Y. M., Waly, M. I., Deth, R. C., Al-Sharbati, M. M., Al-Shafaee, M., Al-Farsi, O., Al-Khaduri, M. M., et al. (2013). Low folate and vitamin B12 nourishment is common in Omani children with newly diagnosed autism. *Nutrition, 29*(3), 537–541.

Altun, H., Kurutas, E. B., Sahin, N., Gungor, O., & Findikli, E. (2018). The levels of vitamin D, vitamin D receptor, homocysteine and complex B vitamin in children with autism spectrum disorders. *Clinical Psychopharmacology and Neuroscience, 16*(4), 383–390.

Amir, R. E., Van den Veyver, I. B., Wan, M., Tran, C. Q., Francke, U., & Zoghbi, H. Y. (1999). Rett syndrome is caused by mutations in X-linked MECP2, encoding methyl-CpG-binding protein 2. *Nature Genetics, 23*(2), 185–188.

Arqoub, A. M. S., Flynn, K. G., & Martinez, L. A. (2020). Gestational exposure to a ketogenic diet increases sociability in CD-1 mice. *Behavioral Neuroscience.* https://doi.org/10.1037/bne0000368

Arriaga, G., & Jarvis, E. D. (2013). Mouse vocal communication system: Are ultrasounds learned or innate? *Brain and Language, 124*(1), 96–116.

Arriaga, G., Zhou, E. P., & Jarvis, E. D. (2012). Of mice, birds, and men: The mouse ultrasonic song system has some features similar to humans and song-learning birds. *PLOS ONE, 7*(10), Article e46610.

Asiminas, A., Jackson, A. D., Louros, S. R., Till, S. M., Spano, T., Dando, O., Bear, M. F., et al. (2019). Sustained correction of associative learning deficits after brief, early treatment in a rat model of fragile X syndrome. *Science Translational Medicine, 11*(494). https://doi.org/10.1126/scitranslmed.aao0498

Benayed, R., Choi, J., Matteson, P. G., Gharani, N., Kamdar, S., Brzustowicz, L. M., & Millonig, J. H. (2009). Autism-associated haplotype affects the regulation of the homeobox gene, *ENGRAILED 2. Biological Psychiatry, 66*(10), 911–917.

Boison, D. (2016). The biochemistry and epigenetics of epilepsy: Focus on adenosine and glycine. *Frontiers in Molecular Neuroscience, 9*, 26.

Bostock, E. C., Kirkby, K. C., & Taylor, B. V. (2017). The current status of the ketogenic diet in psychiatry. *Frontiers in Psychiatry, 8*, 43.

Boulanger-Bertolus, J., Pancaro, C., & Mashour, G. A. (2018). Increasing role of maternal immune activation in neurodevelopmental disorders. *Frontiers in Behavioral Neuroscience, 12*(October), 230.

Brignell, A., Chenausky, K. V., Song, H., Zhu, J., Suo, C., & Morgan, A. T. (2018). Communication interventions for autism spectrum disorder in minimally verbal children. *Cochrane Database of Systematic Reviews, 11*, CD012324.

Bromley, R. L., Mawer, G. E., Briggs, M., Cheyne, C., Clayton-Smith, J., Garcia-Finana, M., Kneen, R., et al. (2013). The prevalence of neurodevelopmental disorders in children prenatally exposed to antiepileptic drugs. *Journal of Neurology, Neurosurgery, and Psychiatry, 84*(6), 637–643.

Brunner, D., Kabitzke, P., He, D., Cox, K., Thiede, L., Hanania, T., Sabath, E., et al. (2015). Comprehensive analysis of the 16p11.2 deletion and null Cntnap2 mouse models of autism spectrum disorder. *PLOS ONE, 10*(8), Article e0134572.

Buescher, A. V., Cidav, Z., Knapp, M., & Mandell, D. S. (2014). Costs of autism spectrum disorders in the United Kingdom and the United States. *JAMA Pediatrics, 168*(8), 721–728.

Castellucci, G. A., Calbick, D., & McCormick, D. (2018). The temporal organization of mouse ultrasonic vocalizations. *PLOS ONE, 13*(10), Article e0199929.

Castellucci, G. A., McGinley, M. J., & McCormick, D. A. (2016). Knockout of Foxp2 disrupts vocal development in mice. *Scientific Reports, 6*, 23305.

Castro, K., Baronio, D., Perry, I. S., Riesgo, R. D., & Gottfried, C. (2016). The effect of ketogenic diet in an animal model of autism induced by prenatal exposure to valproic acid. *Nutritional Neuroscience.* https://doi.org/10.1080/1028415X.2015.1133029

Cezar, L. C., Kirsten, T. B., da Fonseca, C. C. N., de Lima, A. P. N., Bernardi, M. M., & Felicio, L. F. (2018). Zinc as a therapy in a rat model of autism prenatally induced by valproic acid. *Progress in Neuro-Psychopharmacology & Biological Psychiatry, 84*(Part A), 173–180.

Chabout, J., Sarkar, A., Patel, S. R., Radden, T., Dunson, D. B., Fisher, S. E., & Jarvis, E. D. (2016). A *Foxp2* mutation implicated in human speech deficits alters sequencing of ultrasonic vocalizations in adult male mice. *Frontiers in Behavioral Neuroscience, 10*, 197.

Chadman, K. K. (2017). Animal models for autism in 2017 and the consequential implications to drug discovery. *Expert Opinion on Drug Discovery, 12*(12), 1187–1194.

Cheng, N., Alshammari, F., Hughes, E., Khanbabaei, M., & Rho, J. M. (2017). Dendritic overgrowth and elevated ERK signaling during neonatal development in a mouse model of autism. *PLOS ONE, 12*(6), Article e0179409.

Cheng, N., Khanbabaei, M., Murari, K, & Rho, J. M. (2016) . Disruption of visual circuit formation and refinement in a mouse model of autism. *Autism Research*, https://doi.org/10.1002/aur.1687

Cheng, N., Rho, J. M., & Masino, S. A. (2017). Metabolic dysfunction underlying autism spectrum disorder and potential treatment approaches. *Frontiers in Molecular Neuroscience, 10*, 34.

Chiarotti, F., & Venerosi, A. (2020). Epidemiology of autism spectrum disorders: A review of worldwide prevalence estimates since 2014. *Brain Sciences, 10*(5). https://doi.org/10.3390/brainsci10050274

Chomiak, T., Turner, N., & Hu, B. (2013). What we have learned about autism spectrum disorder from valproic acid. *Pathology Research International, 2013*, 712758.

Christensen, J., Gronborg, T. K., Sorensen, M. J., Schendel, D., Parner, E. T., Pedersen, L. H., & Vestergaard, M. (2013). Prenatal valproate exposure and risk of autism spectrum disorders and childhood autism. *JAMA, 309*(16), 1696–1703.

Currais, A., Farrokhi, C., Dargusch, R., Goujon-Svrzic, M., & Maher, P. (2016). Dietary glycemic index modulates the behavioral and biochemical abnormalities associated with autism spectrum disorder. *Molecular Psychiatry, 21*(3), 426–436.

Daimon, C. M., Jasien, J. M., Wood, W. H., III, Zhang, Y., Becker, K. G., Silverman, J. L., Crawley, J. N., Martin, B., & Maudsley, S. (2015). Hippocampal transcriptomic and proteomic alterations in the BTBR mouse model of autism spectrum disorder. *Frontiers in Physiology, 6*, 324.

de la Torre-Ubieta, L., Won, H., Stein, J. L., & Geschwind, D. H. (2016). Advancing the understanding of autism disease mechanisms through genetics. *Nature Medicine, 22*(4), 345–361.

DiCicco-Bloom, E., Lord, C., Zwaigenbaum, L., Courchesne, E., Dager, S. R., Schmitz, C., Schultz, R. T., Crawley, J., & Young, L. J. (2006). The developmental neurobiology of autism spectrum disorder. *Journal of Neuroscience, 26*(26), 6897–6906.

Duchowny, M. S. (2005). Food for thought: The ketogenic diet and adverse effects in children. *Epilepsy Currents, 5*(4), 152–154.

Ellegood, J., & Crawley, J. N. (2015). Behavioral and neuroanatomical phenotypes in mouse models of autism. *Neurotherapeutics, 12*(3), 521–533.

Evangeliou, A., Vlachonikolis, I., Mihailidou, H., Spilioti, M., Skarpalezou, A., Makaronas, N., Prokopiou, A., et al. (2003). Application of a ketogenic diet in children with autistic behavior: Pilot study. *Journal of Child Neurology, 18*(2), 113–118.

Ewen, J. B., Sweeney, J. A., & Potter, W. Z. (2019). Conceptual, regulatory and strategic imperatives in the early days of EEG-based biomarker validation for neurodevelopmental disabilities. *Frontiers in Integrative Neuroscience, 13*, 45.

Fischer, J., & Hammerschmidt, K. (2011). Ultrasonic vocalizations in mouse models for speech and socio-cognitive disorders: Insights into the evolution of vocal communication. *Genes, Brain, and Behavior, 10*(1), 17–27.

Flowers, J. B., Oler, A. T., Nadler, S. T., Choi, Y., Schueler, K. L., Yandell, B. S., Kendziorski, C. M., & Attie, A. D. (2007). Abdominal obesity in BTBR male mice is associated with peripheral but not hepatic insulin resistance. *American Journal of Physiology. Endocrinology and Metabolism, 292*(3), E936–E945.

Frazier, T. W., & Hardan, A. Y. (2009). A meta-analysis of the corpus callosum in autism. *Biological Psychiatry, 66*(10), 935–941.

Frye, R. E. (2015). Metabolic and mitochondrial disorders associated with epilepsy in children with autism spectrum disorder. *Epilepsy & Behavior, 47*(June), 147–157.

Fumagalli, M., Lecca, D., Abbracchio, M. P., & Ceruti, S. (2017). Pathophysiological role of purines and pyrimidines in neurodevelopment: Unveiling new pharmacological approaches to congenital brain diseases. *Frontiers in Pharmacology, 8*, 941.

Gadalla, K. K., Bailey, M. E., Spike, R. C., Ross, P. D., Woodard, K. T., Kalburgi, S. N., Bachaboina, L., et al. (2013). Improved survival and reduced phenotypic severity following *AAV9/MECP2* gene transfer to neonatal and juvenile male *Mecp2* knockout mice. *Molecular Therapy, 21*(1), 18–30.

Gano, L. B., Patel, M., & Rho, J. M. (2014). Ketogenic diets, mitochondria, and neurological diseases. *Journal of Lipid Research, 55*(11), 2211–2228.

Garg, S. K., Lioy, D. T., Cheval, H., McGann, J. C., Bissonnette, J. M., Murtha, M. J., Foust, K. D., Kaspar, B. K., Bird, A., & Mandel, G. (2013). Systemic delivery of MeCP2 rescues behavioral and cellular deficits in female mouse models of Rett syndrome. *Journal of Neuroscience, 33*(34), 13612–13620.

Gasior, M., Rogawski, M. A., & Hartman, A. L. (2006). Neuroprotective and disease-modifying effects of the ketogenic diet. *Behavioural Pharmacology, 17*(5–6), 431–439.

Gaugler, T., Klei, L., Sanders, S. J., Bodea, C. A., Goldberg, A. P., Lee, A. B., Mahajan, M., et al. (2014). Most genetic risk for autism resides with common variation. *Nature Genetics, 46*(8), 881–885.

Gevi, F., Zolla, L., Gabriele, S., & Persico, A. M. (2016). Urinary metabolomics of young Italian autistic children supports abnormal tryptophan and purine metabolism. *Molecular Autism, 7*, 47.

Golubeva, A. V., Joyce, S. A., Moloney, G., Burokas, A., Sherwin, E., Arboleya, S., Flynn, I., et al. (2017). Microbiota-related changes in bile acid & tryptophan metabolism are associated with gastrointestinal dysfunction in a mouse model of autism. *EBioMedicine, 24*(October), 166–178.

Gurau, O., Bosl, W. J., & Newton, C. R. (2017). How useful is electroencephalography in the diagnosis of autism spectrum disorders and the delineation of subtypes: A systematic review. *Frontiers in Psychiatry, 8*, 121.

Guy, J., Gan, J., Selfridge, J., Cobb, S., & Bird, A. (2007). Reversal of neurological defects in a mouse model of Rett syndrome. *Science, 315*(5815), 1143–1147.

Hagerman, R. J., Berry-Kravis, E., Hazlett, H. C., Bailey, D. B., Jr., Moine, H., Kooy, R. F., Tassone, F., et al. (2017). Fragile X syndrome. *Nature Reviews Disease Primers, 3*(September), 17065.

Hallbook, T., Ji, S., Maudsley, S., & Martin, B. (2012). The effects of the ketogenic diet on behavior and cognition. *Epilepsy Research, 100*(3), 304–309.

Heischmann, S., Gano, L. B., Quinn, K., Liang, L. P., Klepacki, J., Christians, U., Reisdorph, N., & Patel, M. (2018). Regulation of kynurenine metabolism by a ketogenic diet. *Journal of Lipid Research, 59*(6), 958–966.

Herbert, M. R., & Buckley, J. A. (2013). Autism and dietary therapy: Case report and review of the literature. *Journal of Child Neurology, 28*(8), 975–982.

Holy, T. E., & Guo, Z. (2005). Ultrasonic songs of male mice. *PLOS Biology, 3*(12), Article e386.

Huang, J., Li, Y.-Q., Wu, C.-H., Zhang, Y.-L., Zhao, S.-T., Chen, Y.-J., Deng, Y.-H., Xuan, A., & Sun, X.-D. (2019). The effect of ketogenic diet on behaviors and synaptic functions of naive mice. *Brain and Behavior, 9*(4), e01246.

Jamain, S., Radyushkin, K., Hammerschmidt, K., Granon, S., Boretius, S., Varoqueaux, F., Ramanantsoa, N., et al. (2008). Reduced social interaction and ultrasonic communication in a mouse model of monogenic heritable autism. *Proceedings of the National Academy of Sciences of the United States of America, 105*(5), 1710–1715.

Ju, A., Hammerschmidt, K., Tantra, M., Krueger, D., Brose, N., & Ehrenreich, H. (2014). Juvenile manifestation of ultrasound communication deficits in the neuroligin-4 null mutant mouse model of autism. *Behavioural Brain Research, 270*, 159–164.

Kasprowska-Liśkiewicz, D., Liśkiewicz, A. D., Nowacka-Chmielewska, M. M., Nowicka, J., Małecki, A., & Barski, J. J. (2017). The ketogenic diet affects the social behavior of young male rats. *Physiology & Behavior, 179*(October), 168–177.

Kazdoba, T. M., Leach, P. T., Yang, M., Silverman, J. L., Solomon, M., & Crawley, J. N. (2016). Translational mouse models of autism: Advancing toward pharmacological therapeutics. *Current Topics in Behavioral Neurosciences, 28*, 1–52.

Khanbabaei, M., Hughes, E., Ellegood, J., Qiu, L. R., Yip, R., Dobry, J., Murari, K., Lerch, J. P., Rho, J. M., & Cheng, N. (2019). Precocious myelination in a mouse model of autism. *Translational Psychiatry, 9*(1), 251.

Kim, H., Son, J., Yoo, H., Kim, H., Oh, J., Han, D., Hwang, Y., & Kaang, B. K. (2016) . Effects of the female estrous cycle on the sexual behaviors and ultrasonic vocalizations of male C57BL/ 6 and autistic BTBR T+tf/J mice. *Experimental Neurobiology, 25*(4), 156–162.

Kogan, J. H., Gross, A. K., Featherstone, R. E., Shin, R., Chen, Q., Heusner, C. L., Adachi, M., et al. (2015). Mouse model of chromosome 15q13.3 microdeletion syndrome demonstrates features related to autism spectrum disorder. *Journal of Neuroscience, 35*(49), 16282–16294.

Konopka, G., & Roberts, T. F. (2016). Animal models of speech and vocal communication deficits associated with psychiatric disorders. *Biological Psychiatry, 79*(1), 53–61.

Kraeuter, A.-K., Phillips, R., & Sarnyai, Z. (2020). Ketogenic therapy in neurodegenerative and psychiatric disorders: From mice to men. *Progress in Neuro-Psychopharmacology & Biological Psychiatry, 101*(July), 109913.

Krishnan, S., Watkins, K. E., & Bishop, D. V. M. (2016). Neurobiological basis of language learning difficulties. *Trends in Cognitive Sciences, 20*(9), 701–714.

Lahvis, G. P., Alleva, E., & Scattoni, M. L. (2011). Translating mouse vocalizations: Prosody and frequency modulation. *Genes, Brain, and Behavior, 10*(1), 4–16.

Lai, M. C., Lombardo, M. V., & Baron-Cohen, S. (2014). Autism. *Lancet, 383*(9920), 896–910.

Lee, R. W. Y., Corley, M. J., Pang, A., Arakaki, G., Abbott, L., Nishimoto, M., Miyamoto, R., et al. (2018). A modified ketogenic gluten-free diet with MCT improves behavior in children with autism spectrum disorder. *Physiology & Behavior, 188,* 205–211.

Leigh, J. P., & Du, J. (2015). Brief report: Forecasting the economic burden of autism in 2015 and 2025 in the United States. *Journal of Autism and Developmental Disorders, 45*(12), 4135–4139.

Liebhaber, G. M., Riemann, E., & Baumeister, F. A. (2003). Ketogenic diet in Rett syndrome. *Journal of Child Neurology, 18*(1), 74–75.

Lombardo, M. V., Courchesne, E., Lewis, N. E., & Pramparo, T. (2017) . Hierarchical cortical transcriptome disorganization in autism. *Molecular Autism, 8*(June), 29.

Lombardo, M. V., Moon, H. M., Su, J., Palmer, T. D., Courchesne, E., & Pramparo, T. (2018). Maternal immune activation dysregulation of the fetal brain transcriptome and relevance to the pathophysiology of autism spectrum disorder. *Molecular Psychiatry, 23*(4), 1001–1013.

Loomes, R., Hull, L., & Mandy, W. P. L. (2017). What is the male-to-female ratio in autism spectrum disorder? A systematic review and meta-analysis. *Journal of the American Academy of Child and Adolescent Psychiatry, 56*(6), 466–474.

Lutas, A., & Yellen, G. (2013). The ketogenic diet: Metabolic influences on brain excitability and epilepsy. *Trends in Neurosciences, 36*(1), 32–40.

Maenner, M. J., Shaw, K. A., Baio, J., EdS1, Washington, A., Patrick, M., DiRienzo, M., et al. (2020). Prevalence of autism spectrum disorder among children aged 8 years—Autism and Developmental Disabilities Monitoring Network, 11 Sites, United States, 2016. *Morbidity and Mortality Weekly Report Surveillance Summaries, 69*(4), 1–12.

Mailloux, R. J., McBride, S. L., & Harper, M. E. (2013). Unearthing the secrets of mitochondrial ROS and glutathione in bioenergetics. *Trends in Biochemical Sciences, 38*(12), 592–602.

Malkova, N. V., Yu, C. Z., Hsiao, E. Y., Moore, M. J., & Patterson, P. H. (2012). Maternal immune activation yields offspring displaying mouse versions of the three core symptoms of autism. *Brain, Behavior, and Immunity, 26*(4), 607–616.

Mantis, J. G., Fritz, C. L., Marsh, J., Heinrichs, S. C., & Seyfried, T. N. (2009). Improvement in motor and exploratory behavior in Rett syndrome mice with restricted ketogenic and standard diets. *Epilepsy & Behavior, 15*(2), 133–141.

Mayengbam, S. S., Ellegood, J., Kesler, M., Reimer, R. A., Shearer, J., Murari, K., Rho, J. M., Lerch, J. P. & Cheng, N. "A ketogenic diet affects brain volume and metabolomics in juvenile mice". *Under review by NeuroImage.*

Mayes, A. K., Reilly, S., & Morgan, A. T. (2015). Neural correlates of childhood language disorder: A systematic review. *Developmental Medicine and Child Neurology, 57*(8), 706–717.

Meidenbauer, J. J., Mantis, J. G., & Seyfried, T. N. (2011). The EL mouse: A natural model of autism and epilepsy. *Epilepsia, 52*(2), 347–357.

Mei, Y., Monteiro, P., Zhou, Y., Kim, J. A., Gao, X., Fu, Z., & Feng, G. (2016). Adult restoration of Shank3 expression rescues selective autistic-like phenotypes. *Nature, 530*(7591), 481–484.

Meyza, K. Z., & Blanchard, D. C. (2017). The BTBR mouse model of idiopathic autism—Current view on mechanisms. *Neuroscience and Biobehavioral Reviews, 76*(Part A), 99–110.

Mierau, S. B., & Neumeyer, A. M. (2019) . Metabolic interventions in autism spectrum disorder. *Neurobiology of Disease, 132*(December), 104544.

Murari, K., Rho, J. M., & Cheng, N. (2020). Improving vocal communication with a ketogenic diet in a mouse model of autism. *In preparation.*

Napoli, E., Duenas, N., & Giulivi, C. (2014). Potential therapeutic use of the ketogenic diet in autism spectrum disorders. *Frontiers in Pediatrics, 2,* 69.

Naviaux, J. C., Schuchbauer, M. A., Li, K., Wang, L., Risbrough, V. B., Powell, S. B., & Naviaux, R. K. (2014). Reversal of autism-like behaviors and metabolism in adult mice with single-dose antipurinergic therapy. *Translational Psychiatry*, 4, e400.

Naviaux, J. C., Wang, L., Li, K., Bright, A. T., Alaynick, W. A., Williams, K. R., Powell, S. B., & Naviaux, R. K. (2015). Antipurinergic therapy corrects the autism-like features in the fragile X (*Fmr1* knock-out) mouse model. *Molecular Autism*, 6, 1.

Naviaux, R. K., Zolkipli, Z., Wang, L., Nakayama, T., Naviaux, J. C., Le, T. P., Schuchbauer, M. A., et al. (2013). Antipurinergic therapy corrects the autism-like features in the poly(IC) mouse model. *PLOS ONE*, 8(3), Article e57380.

Neal, E. G., Chaffe, H., Schwartz, R. H., Lawson, M. S., Edwards, N., Fitzsimmons, G., Whitney, A., & Cross, J. H. (2008). The ketogenic diet for the treatment of childhood epilepsy: A randomised controlled trial. *Lancet Neurology*, 7(6), 500–506.

Nylen, K., Velazquez, J. L., Likhodii, S. S., Cortez, M. A., Shen, L., Leshchenko, Y., Adeli, K., Gibson, K. M., Burnham, W. M., & Snead, O. C., III. (2008). A ketogenic diet rescues the murine succinic semialdehyde dehydrogenase deficient phenotype. *Experimental Neurology*, 210(2), 449–457.

O'Reilly, C., Lewis, J. D., & Elsabbagh, M. (2017). Is functional brain connectivity atypical in autism? A systematic review of EEG and MEG studies. *PLOS ONE*, 12(5), Article e0175870.

Panksepp, J. B., Jochman, K. A., Kim, J. U., Koy, J. J., Wilson, E. D., Chen, Q., Wilson, C. R., & Lahvis, G. P. (2007). Affiliative behavior, ultrasonic communication and social reward are influenced by genetic variation in adolescent mice. *PLOS ONE*, 2(4), Article e351.

Paul, L. K., Corsello, C., Kennedy, D. P., & Adolphs, R. (2014). Agenesis of the corpus callosum and autism: A comprehensive comparison. *Brain*, 137(Part 6), 1813–1829.

Paul, R. (2008). Interventions to improve communication in autism. *Child and Adolescent Psychiatric Clinics of North America*, 17(4), 835–856.

Penagarikano, O., Abrahams, B. S., Herman, E. I., Winden, K. D., Gdalyahu, A., Dong, H., Sonnenblick, L. I., et al. (2011). Absence of CNTNAP2 leads to epilepsy, neuronal migration abnormalities, and core autism-related deficits. *Cell*, 147(1), 235–246.

Portfors, C. V., & Perkel, D. J. (2014). The role of ultrasonic vocalizations in mouse communication. *Current Opinion in Neurobiology*, 28(October), 115–120.

Pulsifer, M. B., Gordon, J. M., Brandt, J., Vining, E. P., & Freeman, J. M. (2001). Effects of ketogenic diet on development and behavior: Preliminary report of a prospective study. *Developmental Medicine and Child Neurology*, 43(5), 301–306.

Quesnel-Vallières, M., Weatheritt, R. J., Cordes, S. P., & Blencowe, B. J. (2019). Autism spectrum disorder: Insights into convergent mechanisms from transcriptomics. *Nature Reviews Genetics*, 20(1), 51–63.

Rapin, I., & Dunn, M. (2003). Update on the language disorders of individuals on the autistic spectrum. *Brain & Development*, 25(3), 166–172.

Ratto, A. B., Kenworthy, L., Yerys, B. E., Bascom, J., Wieckowski, A. T., White, S. W., Wallace, G. L., et al. (2018). What about the girls? Sex-based differences in autistic traits and adaptive skills. *Journal of Autism and Developmental Disorders*, 48(5), 1698–1711.

Rivell, A., & Mattson, M. P. (2019). Intergenerational metabolic syndrome and neuronal network hyperexcitability in autism. *Trends in Neurosciences*, 42(10), 709–726.

Rogge, N., & Janssen, J. (2019). The economic costs of autism spectrum disorder: A literature review. *Journal of Autism and Developmental Disorders*, 49(7), 2873–2900.

Rossignol, D. A., & Frye, R. E. (2012). Mitochondrial dysfunction in autism spectrum disorders: A systematic review and meta-analysis. *Molecular Psychiatry*, 17(3), 290–314.

Rossignol, D. A., & Frye, R. E. (2014). Evidence linking oxidative stress, mitochondrial dysfunction, and inflammation in the brain of individuals with autism. *Frontiers in Physiology*, 5, 150.

Rotschafer, S. E., Trujillo, M. S., Dansie, L. E., Ethell, I. M., & Razak, K. A. (2012). Minocycline treatment reverses ultrasonic vocalization production deficit in a mouse model of fragile X syndrome. *Brain Research*, 1439, 7–14.

Roullet, F. I., Lai, J. K., & Foster, J. A. (2013). In utero exposure to valproic acid and autism—A current review of clinical and animal studies. *Neurotoxicology and Teratology*, 36, 47–56.

Ruskin, D. N., Fortin, J. A., Bisnauth, S. N., & Masino, S. A. (2016). Ketogenic diets improve behaviors associated with autism spectrum disorder in a sex-specific manner in the EL mouse. *Physiology & Behavior*, 168, 138–145.

Ruskin, D. N., Murphy, M. I., Slade, S. L., & Masino, S. A. (2017). Ketogenic diet improves behaviors in a maternal immune activation model of autism spectrum disorder. *PLOS ONE*, 12(2), Article e0171643.

Ruskin, D. N., Svedova, J., Cote, J. L., Sandau, U., Rho, J. M., Kawamura, M., Jr., Boison, D., & Masino, S. A. (2013). Ketogenic diet improves core symptoms of autism in BTBR mice. *PLOS ONE*, 8(6), Article e65021.

Sahin, M., Jones, S. R., Sweeney, J. A., Berry-Kravis, E., Connors, B. W., Ewen, J. B., Hartman, A. L., Levin, A. R., Potter, W. Z., & Mamounas, L. A. (2018) . Discovering translational biomarkers in neurodevelopmental disorders. *Nature Reviews Drug Discovery*. https://doi.org/10.1038/d41573-018-00010-7

Scattoni, M. L., Gandhy, S. U., Ricceri, L., & Crawley, J. N. (2008). Unusual repertoire of vocalizations in the BTBR T+tf/J mouse model of autism. *PLOS ONE*, 3(8), Article e3067.

Scattoni, M. L., Martire, A., Cartocci, G., Ferrante, A., & Ricceri, L. (2013) . Reduced social interaction, behavioural flexibility and BDNF signalling in the BTBR T+tf/J strain, a mouse model of autism. *Behavioural Brain Research*, 251, 35–40.

Scattoni, M. L., Ricceri, L., & Crawley, J. N. (2011). Unusual repertoire of vocalizations in adult BTBR T+tf/J mice during three types of social encounters. *Genes, Brain, and Behavior*, 10(1), 44–56.

Schaafsma, S. M., Gagnidze, K., Reyes, A., Norstedt, N., Mansson, K., Francis, K., & Pfaff, D. W. (2017). Sex-specific gene–environment interactions underlying ASD-like behaviors. *Proceedings of the National Academy of Sciences of the United States of America*, 114(6), 1383–1388.

Schwartzer, J. J., Careaga, M., Onore, C. E., Rushakoff, J. A., Berman, R. F., & Ashwood, P. (2013). Maternal immune activation and strain specific interactions in the development of autism-like behaviors in mice. *Translational Psychiatry*, 3, e240.

Scichilone, J. M., Yarraguntla, K., Charalambides, A., Harney, J. P., & Butler, D. (2016). Environmental enrichment mitigates detrimental cognitive effects of ketogenic diet in weanling rats. *Journal of Molecular Neuroscience*, 60(1), 1–9.

Silva-Santos, S., van Woerden, G. M., Bruinsma, C. F., Mientjes, E., Jolfaei, M. A., Distel, B., Kushner, S. A., & Elgersma, Y. (2015). Ube3a reinstatement identifies distinct developmental windows in a murine Angelman syndrome model. *Journal of Clinical Investigation*, 125(5), 2069–2076.

Spreckley, M., & Boyd, R. (2009). Efficacy of applied behavioral intervention in preschool children with autism for improving cognitive, language, and adaptive behavior: A systematic review and meta-analysis. *Journal of Pediatrics*, 154(3), 338–344.

Stafstrom, C. E., & Rho, J. M. (2012). The ketogenic diet as a treatment paradigm for diverse neurological disorders. *Frontiers in Pharmacology*, 3, 59.

Stefanatos, G. A., & Baron, I. S. (2011). The ontogenesis of language impairment in autism: A neuropsychological perspective. *Neuropsychology Review*, 21(3), 252–270.

Stern, M. (2011). Insulin signaling and autism. *Frontiers in Endocrinology*, 2, 54.

Stewart, P. A., Hyman, S. L., Schmidt, B. L., Macklin, E. A., Reynolds, A., Johnson, C. R., James, S. J., & Manning-Courtney, P. (2015). Dietary supplementation in children with autism spectrum disorders: Common, insufficient, and excessive.

Journal of the Academy of Nutrition and Dietetics, 115(8), 1237–1248.

Stoppel, L. J., Kazdoba, T. M., Schaffler, M. D., Preza, A. R., Heynen, A., Crawley, J. N., & Bear, M. F. (2018). R-baclofen reverses cognitive deficits and improves social interactions in two lines of 16p11.2 deletion mice. *Neuropsychopharmacology*, 43(3), 513–524.

Sullivan, K., Stone, W. L., & Dawson, G. (2014). Potential neural mechanisms underlying the effectiveness of early intervention for children with autism spectrum disorder. *Research in Developmental Disabilities*, 35(11), 2921–2932.

Takahashi, T., Okabe, S., Broin, P. O., Nishi, A., Ye, K., Beckert, M. V., Izumi, T., et al. (2015). Structure and function of neonatal social communication in a genetic mouse model of autism. *Molecular Psychiatry*. https://doi.org/10.1038/mp.2015.190

Usui, N., Araujo, D. J., Kulkarni, A., Co, M., Ellegood, J., Harper, M., Toriumi, K., Lerch, J. P., & Konopka, G. (2017). Foxp1 regulation of neonatal vocalizations via cortical development. *Genes & Development*, 31(20), 2039–2055.

Verpeut, J. L., DiCicco-Bloom, E., & Bello, N. T. (2016). Ketogenic diet exposure during the juvenile period increases social behaviors and forebrain neural activation in adult *Engrailed 2* null mice. *Physiology & Behavior*, 161(July), 90–98.

Wang, H., Liang, S., Burgdorf, J., Wess, J., & Yeomans, J. (2008). Ultrasonic vocalizations induced by sex and amphetamine in M2, M4, M5 muscarinic and D2 dopamine receptor knockout mice. *PLOS ONE*, 3(4), Article e1893.

Wang, J., Barstein, J., Ethridge, L. E., Mosconi, M. W., Takarae, Y., & Sweeney, J. A. (2013). Resting state EEG abnormalities in autism spectrum disorders. *Journal of Neurodevelopmental Disorders*, 5(1), 24.

Wen, Y., Alshikho, M. J., & Herbert, M. R. (2016). Pathway network analyses for autism reveal multisystem involvement, major overlaps with other diseases and convergence upon MAPK and calcium signaling. *PLOS ONE*, 11(4), Article e0153329.

Westmark, P. R., Gutierrez, A., Gholston, A. K., Wilmer, T. M., & Westmark, C. J. (2020). Preclinical testing of the ketogenic diet in fragile X mice. *Neurochemistry International*, 134(March), 104687.

Wohr, M. (2014). Ultrasonic vocalizations in shank mouse models for autism spectrum disorders: Detailed spectrographic analyses and developmental profiles. *Neuroscience and Biobehavioral Reviews*, 43(June), 199–212.

Wohr, M. (2015). Effect of social odor context on the emission of isolation-induced ultrasonic vocalizations in the BTBR T+tf/J mouse model for autism. *Frontiers in Neuroscience*, 9, 73.

Wolff, J. J., Gerig, G., Lewis, J. D., Soda, T., Styner, M. A., Vachet, C., Botteron, K. N., et al. (2015). Altered corpus callosum morphology associated with autism over the first 2 years of life. *Brain,* *138*(Part 7), 2046–2058.

Yang, M., Mahrt, E. J., Lewis, F., Foley, G., Portmann, T., Dolmetsch, R. E., Portfors, C. V., & Crawley, J. N. (2015). 16p11.2 deletion syndrome mice display sensory and ultrasonic vocalization deficits during social interactions. *Autism Research, 8*(5), 507–521.

Young, D. M., Schenk, A. K., Yang, S. B., Jan, Y. N., & Jan, L. Y. (2010). Altered ultrasonic vocalizations in a tuberous sclerosis mouse model of autism. *Proceedings of the National Academy of Sciences of the United States of America, 107*(24), 11074–11079.

Yudkoff, M., Daikhin, Y., Melo, T. M., Nissim, I., Sonnewald, U., & Nissim, I. (2007). The ketogenic diet and brain metabolism of amino acids: Relationship to the anticonvulsant effect. *Annual Review of Nutrition, 27,* 415–430.

Ketotherapeutics to Rescue Brain Energy Deficits

An Emerging Strategy to Delay Cognitive Decline in Alzheimer's Disease

ÉTIENNE MYETTE-CÔTÉ, PHD, CHRISTIAN-ALEXANDRE CASTELLANO, PHD, MÉLANIE FORTIER, MSC, VALÉRIE ST-PIERRE, MSC, AND STEPHEN C. CUNNANE, PHD

INTRODUCTION

With the global average life expectancy continuously rising, the impact of deteriorating cognitive function in older age has become a major challenge for healthcare systems worldwide. Alzheimer's disease (AD), the most common neurologic disease of aging involving cognitive decline, is debilitating and dehumanizing and is expensive to manage. To make matters worse, the numerous clinical trials with anti-amyloid drugs conducted over the past few decades have consistently failed to yield positive results, leaving little hope for those impacted by the disease. Some major risk factors for AD have long been recognized and include hypertension, high cholesterol, physical inactivity, and insulin-resistant states, such as type 2 diabetes (T2D). Whether intake of certain nutrients, such as omega-3 fatty acids, B vitamins, or polyphenols, can be beneficial in AD is receiving considerable attention but remains unclear and controversial (Choi et al., 2012; Dangour et al., 2010; Mazereeuw et al., 2012). The potential of diabetes treatments and intranasal insulin have been the focus of some promising investigations, but definitive results in AD are still awaited (Claxton et al., 2015; Gejl et al., 2016; Koenig et al., 2017). Preventive strategies using multidomain intervention with exercise have been shown in clinical trials to be beneficial in reducing the progression of lifestyle-related cognitive decline as well as chronic diseases (Marengoni et al., 2018; Ngandu et al., 2015). We speculate that effective strategies to delay the progression of AD probably have at least one feature in common—that of improving brain energy metabolism in older people.

The brain requires a disproportionately large amount of energy; whereas the adult brain represents about 2% of adult body weight, it consumes about 21% of whole-body energy requirements. Within the brain, neural signaling and nonsignaling activities account for about 70% and 30% of ATP consumption, respectively. Given the limited glycogen stores located in astrocytes, continuous supply of glucose and oxygen from the circulation is critical for normal neurologic function. Excitatory neurons are responsible for the majority of energy expenditure (80%–85%), while inhibitory neurons and glial cells account for the remaining 15% to 20% (Yu et al., 2018). Under normal circumstances, glucose is the brain's predominant fuel, but when ketones are elevated in circulation (i.e., during fasting, starvation, ketogenic interventions, or strenuous exercise), they are readily utilized by the brain as an additional fuel. Unlike in other organs, which use free fatty acids directly to compensate for low intracellular glucose availability, in the brain, ketones (and lactate from muscle under exercise-induced hyperlactatemia) are the only significant alternative fuels to glucose. The two ketones that are taken up by the brain are acetoacetate (AcAc) and its reduced form β-hydroxybutyrate (βHB). As the decarboxylation product of AcAc, acetone is mainly excreted via breath.

For over 30 years, it has become increasingly well established that brain glucose uptake and metabolism are defective in AD, a problem that is particularly evident in the parietal and temporal cortex (reviewed in Cunnane et al., 2020). Low brain glucose uptake in AD has generally been interpreted to be a *consequence* of the neuronal failure and death that lead to significant brain atrophy in AD (Li et al., 2016). While fewer functioning neurons would indeed diminish the need for glucose, this perspective does not account for multiple conditions in which regional brain glucose hypometabolism is present presymptomatically in individuals at elevated risk of AD, i.e. before the clinical (cognitive) onset of the disease. The emerging literature discussed here provides several clear examples that: individuals at genetic or lifestyle risk of AD but still presymptomatic already have disrupted brain glucose metabolism; individuals with AD or mild cognitive impairment (MCI) have ketone utilization similar to that in age-matched cognitively healthy controls; and providing additional ketones to the brain can ameliorate cognitive function in MCI and AD. Given that brain function is acutely dependent on a constant supply of glucose and oxygen, it is crucial to know whether latent presymptomatic deterioration in brain glucose uptake and/or utilization could be contributing to AD risk or development. If such is the case, future investigations could focus on prevention and treatment strategies that would bypass or correct it.

We have developed a positron emission tomography (PET) research program using the ketone tracer [¹¹C]acetoacetate to better understand the relation between brain fuel uptake and brain function in people with, or at risk for, AD. In each individual studied, a dual-tracer PET protocol is used to compare the brain uptake of [¹¹C]acetoacetate to that of the glucose tracer [¹⁸F]fluorodeoxyglucose (FDG; Croteau et al., 2018b). We quantify the magnitude of glucose and ketone uptake regionally throughout the brain. To date, we have completed several clinical studies, while other studies using the dual-tracer PET methods are currently underway to test the potential therapeutic utility of ketogenic interventions, such as medium-chain triglycerides (MCT), ketogenic diet (KD), and ketone supplements. Here, the focus is on providing supporting evidence for an emerging "brain energy rescue" strategy that implicates maintenance of brain fuel supply by overcoming the glucose deficit using "keto-neurotherapeutic" approaches to delay the onset of, or to treat, AD.

BRAIN GLUCOSE HYPOMETABOLISM IN COGNITIVELY IMPAIRED POPULATIONS

From Kety's arteriovenous difference (AVD) in vivo studies to Sokoloff's measurement of cerebral metabolic rate (i.e., the amount of a given substrate metabolized by brain cells) by an autoradiographic technique (reviewed in Sokoloff, 1977), there is broad agreement that glucose is the major oxidative energy fuel for the human brain. Whereas the AVD method has provided good information about the global net influx/efflux of glucose and other substrates between blood and brain, FDG-PET is less invasive and permits regional quantification of brain energy metabolism. This method is now the cornerstone of studies on brain energy metabolism in aging and AD (Cunnane et al., 2020).

A report published in 1963 first suggested that brain glucose and oxygen utilization reductions of 22% and 18%, respectively, were present in patients with dementia as compared to healthy older adults (Dastur et al., 1963). This report was subsequently confirmed by further AVD studies in moderate-advanced AD, where global brain glucose uptake was reduced between 25% and 55% (Hoyer, 1992; Hoyer et al., 1988; Lying-Tunell et al., 1981; Ogawa et al., 1996). However, the studies also suggested that cerebral blood flow and oxygen metabolism were normal in early stages of AD (Hoyer et al., 1988) or much less disrupted than brain glucose uptake (Ogawa et al., 1996). The problem with brain energy metabolism in AD seemed to be focused on impaired brain glucose utilization and was interpreted to probably involve impaired glycolysis (Hoyer et al., 1988). These studies were the first to propose that lower brain glucose utilization was an early and possibly presymptomatic problem in AD.

Among the functional neuroimaging techniques, PET coupled with FDG, an analog tracer of glucose, offers the unique capability to both visualize and quantify glucose metabolism in the brain. The gold standard is the calculation of the cerebral metabolic rate of glucose (CMRglc, μmol/100 g/min) based on kinetic modeling of FDG simultaneously in the brain and in the blood (Berti et al., 2013). FDG-PET studies in the 1980s confirmed the global diminution of the glucose utilization rate observed with the AVD method and advanced the field by quantifying for the first time a regional reduction across the brain in individuals with AD (Benson et al., 1983; Chawluk et al., 1987; Cutler et al., 1985; de Leon et al., 1983). These observations have been confirmed, by more recent studies showing that CMRglc for global gray matter was 9% to 13% lower in early AD, with global deficit primarily confined to the parietal cortex and posterior cingulate (Castellano et al., 2015b; Croteau et al., 2018b). An overview of the literature on FDG-PET shows that, depending on the disease stage, *global* CMRglc in AD is 10% to 15% lower, while in specific regions it can be anywhere between 10% and 50% lower than in cognitively healthy older adults, even after adjustment for brain atrophy (Table 17.1). The earliest regional gray matter deficit in CMRglc in AD seems to be in the medial temporal lobe, which includes the hippocampus and entorhinal cortex, followed by the parietotemporal and posterior cingulate cortices. Hypometabolism extends to the frontal lobe in more advanced stages of the disease, whereas in the primary sensorimotor cortex, visual area, and cerebellum, metabolism is relatively preserved (Brown et al., 2014; Mosconi, 2005; Mosconi et al, 2008c).

MCI is the prodromal state of AD, since it is associated with a conversion rate of up 15% per year (Petersen et al., 2009). To emphasize this transitional state between normal and pathologic aging, Albert et al. (2011) introduced the concept of "MCI due to AD," which

TABLE 17.1 DECLINING CEREBRAL METABOLIC RATE OF GLUCOSE SEEN ON FDG-PET IN ALZHEIMER'S DISEASE AND MILD COGNITIVE IMPAIRMENT

Population (*N*)	CMRglc (versus CTL)	Reference
CTL (22), AD (24)	–17% to –24% in frontal, parietal, temporal, caudate, and thalamus	de Leon et al., 1983
CTL (16), AD (8)	–36% to –53% in frontal, parietotemporal, frontoparietal, visual cortex, caudate, and thalamus	Benson et al., 1983
CTL (25), AD (7)	–25% to –50% in frontal, parietal, temporal lobes	Cutler et al., 1985
CTL (17), AD (24)	–12% in whole brain	Chawluk et al., 1987
CTL (17), AD (20)	–13% in whole brain	Alavi et al., 1993
CTL (10), AD (8)	–17% in whole brain; –13% to –41% in the frontal, temporal, occipital, and parietal cortex	Piert et al., 1996
CTL (22), AD (8)	–21% in posterior cingulate and cinguloparietal transitional area.	Minoshima et al., 1997
CTL (29), AD (10)	–13% in global cortex; –16% to –33% in the superior, middle, and inferior temporal regions, supramarginal gyrus, precuneus, angular gyrus, cuneus, posterior cingulate, and thalamus	Castellano et al., 2015b
CTL (11), MCI (15), AD (12)	AD: –17 to –25% in hippocampus, parahippocampal gyrus, fusiform gyrus, middle/inferior temporal gyrus, superior temporal gyrus MCI: –10% in hippocampus; –17% anterior parahippocampal gyrus	De Santi et al., 2001
CTL (15), MCI (10), AD (10)	AD: –15% to –30% in hippocampal complex, thalamus, posterior cingulate, amygdala MCI: –7% to –20% in hippocampal complex, thalamus, posterior cingulate, amygdala	Nestor et al., 2003
CTL (20), MCI (16), AD (12)	AD: –27% in hippocampus MCI: –18% in hippocampus	Mosconi et al., 2005
CTL (7), MCI (13), AD (17)	AD: –11% in gray matter; –13% to –43% in hippocampus, inferior parietal lobe, middle frontal gyrus, posterior cingulate MCI: –16% in hippocampus and –13% in inferior parietal lobe	Li et al., 2008
CTL (24), MCI (20), AD (19)	AD: –9% to –12% in the frontal, parietal, temporal lobes, cingulate gyrus, and whole brain MCI: –7% in the cingulate gyrus	Croteau et al., 2018b

Note. AD = Alzheimer's disease, CMRglc = cerebral metabolic rate of glucose, CTL = control, MCI = mild cognitive impairment, *N* = sample size, PET-FDG = positron emission tomography with [^{18}F]fluorodeoxyglucose.

is a syndrome defined by the following criteria: i) concern about a change in cognition, ii)
evidence of lower performance in one or more
cognitive domains, and iii) preservation of
independence in functional abilities in daily
life (Albert et al., 2011). A number of FDG-
PET studies in MCI showed that brain glucose
hypometabolism could be observed in AD-
sensitive regions, including posterior cingulate
cortex and parietotemporal areas (Croteau et
al., 2018b; Del Sole et al., 2008; Drzezga et al.,
2003; Langbaum et al., 2009; Mosconi et al.,
2005). MCI seems to represent an intermediary state of metabolic decline in which cerebral
glucose metabolism impairments are significant
in comparison to glucose metabolism in healthy
older adults but are of lower magnitude than the
impairments in AD (Table 17.1).

LATENT BRAIN GLUCOSE HYPOMETABOLISM IN POPULATIONS AT RISK FOR AD

Over the last 60 years, it has become clear that
cerebral glucose hypometabolism is a defining
feature of AD. It is also increasingly certain that
brain glucose impairment is present well before
any measurable cognitive AD-specific impairment (Cunnane et al., 2020; Mosconi et al.,
2008b). The early presymptomatic brain metabolic signature of AD development raises the
question of cause versus consequence: Is brain
glucose hypometabolism a consequence of AD, or
part of the cause, or both? This question can be
addressed by measuring brain energy metabolism
in populations at elevated risk of the disease but
in whom cognition is still normal (Table 17.2).

TABLE 17.2 LATENT PRESYMPTOMATIC BRAIN GLUCOSE HYPOMETABOLISM IN INDIVIDUALS AT RISK OF ALZHEIMER'S DISEASE

Population (N)	Mean age (years)	Brain regions affected	Brain glucose hypometabolism (Δ from control)	Reference
Young adult carriers of apolipoprotein-E4 (12)	31	Parietal cortex Temporal cortex Posterior cingulate Prefrontal cortex	–9% to –11%	Reiman et al., 2004
Maternal family history of Alzheimer's disease (24)	43	Parietal cortex Temporal cortex Hippocampus Entorhinal cortex Posterior cingulate	–12 to –21%	Mosconi et al., 2007
Subjective memory complaint (14)	59	Inferior parietal cortex Middle temporal cortex Inferior frontal cortex Parahippocampal gyrus	Up to –18%	Mosconi et al., 2008a
Young adult carriers of presenilin-1 (2)	30	Posterior cingulate Parietal cortex Temporal cortex	–14% to –25%	Schöll et al., 2011
Prediabetes and early type 2 diabetes (23)	74	Temporal cortex Parietal cortex Posterior cingulate Precuneus Prefrontal cortex	Lower % N/A	Baker et al., 2011
Cognitively healthy older adults (24)	72	Frontal cortex Temporal cortex Anterior cingulate	–10% to –18%	Nugent et al., 2014b
Young women with PCOS and insulin resistance (7)	25	Frontal cortex Middle temporal cortex	–9% to –14%	Castellano et al., 2015a

Note. N/A = not available, PCOS = polycystic ovary syndrome, Δ = difference.

Carriers of autosomal dominant mutations, including in the amyloid precursor protein, presenilin-1, or presenilin-2, are at very high risk of developing early-onset AD (Ryman et al., 2014). Carriers of the apolipoprotein E4 allele (Slooter et al., 1998) and persons with a family history of AD (Mosconi et al., 2010) are at 1.7- to 10-fold greater risk of AD. In these at-risk populations, FDG-PET clearly shows that regional brain glucose hypometabolism is present before the onset of cognitive deficit (Bu, 2009; Fox et al., 1997; Kennedy et al., 1995; Mosconi et al., 2006; Reiman et al., 2004; Schöll et al., 2011).

Aging is the most common risk factor for late-onset AD. Population-based studies show that AD incidence increases significantly after age 65 (Kawas et al., 2000; Lobo et al., 2000). Lower brain glucose metabolism has been reported on several previous occasions and appears to be located mostly in the frontal cortex in older people with normal cognition (De Santi et al., 1995; Kalpouzos et al., 2009; Nugent et al., 2014a). Thus, frontal glucose hypometabolism during normal aging seems to differ from (but might be related to) the parietotemporal AD pattern. In fact, both temporal and parietal hypometabolism are considered sensitive predictors of clinical progression to AD (Ewers et al., 2014; Mosconi et al., 2009).

After aging, T2D is the most important non-genetic risk factor for AD (Vagelatos & Eslick, 2013). Although the exact link between the two conditions remains unclear, the development of brain insulin resistance and alteration in insulin action on synaptic activity, metabolism, and neuroinflammation during aging might contribute to the increased risk (Arnold et al., 2018; Talbot et al., 2012). Although glucose transport into the brain is mostly independent of insulin, insulin remains critical for optimal systemic metabolism and brain health (Arnold et al., 2018). Accordingly, T2D and poor glucose control are associated with cerebral glucose hypometabolism in several AD-related brain areas, including the posterior cingulate and parietotemporal regions (Baker et al., 2011; Roberts et al., 2014; Willette et al., 2015). Our group has also shown that young normal-weight women with polycystic ovary syndrome displaying mild to moderate insulin resistance had a 14% reduction in glucose uptake in the frontal cortex (Castellano et al., 2015a). The mild insulin resistance in this population was significantly inversely correlated with CMRglc in several brain regions.

Finally, subjective memory complaints occur in individuals with self-perceived cognitive decline but without any measurable impairment on objective memory performance (Abdulrab & Heun, 2008). Here again, glucose hypometabolism is already present in several brain regions, including the parahippocampal gyrus, the middle temporal gyri, the inferior parietal lobe, the inferior frontal gyrus, the fusiform gyrus, the thalamus, and the putamen (Mosconi et al., 2008a).

Taken together, these examples are a good basis for concluding that brain glucose hypometabolism can commonly be present in those at risk of AD but before any signs of cognitive decline; therefore, presymptomatic brain glucose hypometabolism could be *contributing* to the development of AD. This interpretation does not exclude brain glucose hypometabolism's being a consequence of synaptic dysfunction and neuronal loss, but it suggests that a vicious cycle can develop in which latent presymptomatic brain glucose hypometabolism leads to chronic brain energy deficit, deteriorating neuronal function, further decline in demand for glucose, and further cognitive decline (Figure 17.1; Cunnane et al., 2020). Brain glucose deficit is not necessarily the cause of AD, or even the first abnormality detectable in those at risk of AD. However, because of the high and continuous energy requirements of the brain, the presymptomatic onset of brain glucose hypometabolism in various at-risk populations shows that it is a relatively early problem that would clearly contribute to declining neuronal function.

BRAIN GLUCOSE UPTAKE, METABOLISM, OR BOTH?

AVD studies show the magnitude of the lower glucose "disappearance" in the brain in AD, but they do not establish whether the problem is with brain glucose uptake—i.e., its transport into the brain across the blood–brain barrier (BBB) and/or brain cell membranes—or with metabolism within the brain—i.e., glycolysis, citric acid cycle (CAC), and/or oxidative phosphorylation. Under normal conditions, brain glucose delivery exceeds demand, with glucose influx being 1.6-fold higher than phosphorylation, a situation that largely avoids local energy shortage (Dienel, 2019). However, several studies have shown that there is a problem in AD at the level of cerebral blood flow (Leijenaar et al., 2017), microvasculature (Brown & Thore, 2011), and glucose transport (Piert et al., 1996). Accordingly, individuals with AD display reduced protein levels of the main brain glucose transporters GLUT-1 (in astrocytes, capillary endothelium, BBB) and GLUT-3 (in neuronal membranes; Simpson et al., 1994),

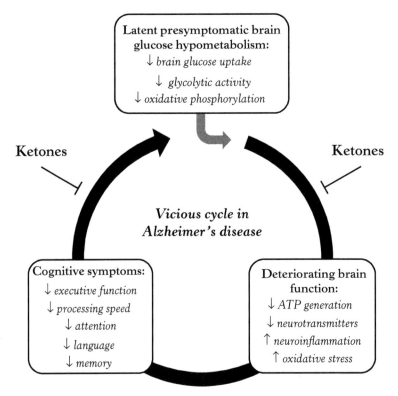

FIGURE 17.1 *Vicious Cycle in Alzheimer's Disease*

Schematic representation of latent brain glucose hypometabolism leading to a vicious cycle of accelerating metabolic deterioration and neuronal dysfunction that increases the risk of developing Alzheimer's disease. Adapted from Cunnane et al. (2020).

but not the insulin-dependent GLUT-4 (Liu et al., 2008). However, these observations provide no information about whether, in addition to defective glucose transport, the metabolic pathways of glucose are also altered.

In vitro studies (Sorbi et al., 1990), in vivo PET (Piert et al., 1996), and postmortem analyses (An et al., 2018) in AD have all reported significant dysregulations along the glycolytic pathway, including at the level of hexokinase, phosphofructokinase, glyceraldehyde-3-phosphate dehydrogenase, and pyruvate kinase. Moreover, the higher brain tissue glucose concentration and lower glycolytic flux among AD, asymptomatic AD, and age-matched controls, suggests a link between brain glucose impairments and the severity of AD pathology (An et al., 2018). In contrast, glucose-6-phosphate dehydrogenase, the rate-limiting enzyme in the pentose phosphate pathway, is upregulated in AD, probably for antioxidant defense against high oxidative stress, which inhibits glycolytic flux (Dong & Brewer, 2019; Russell et al., 1999). Along with glycolysis, mitochondrial multienzyme complexes, including pyruvate

dehydrogenase (Perry et al., 1980; Sorbi et al., 1983), 2-oxoglutarate dehydrogenase in the CAC (Gibson et al., 2010), and cytochrome c oxidase in the electron transport chain (Maurer et al., 2000; Parker et al., 1994), have also been reported to be altered in AD. While the exact mechanism is not fully understood, these impairments in enzymatic functions are probably due, at least in part, to oxidative damage that limits ATP production (Butterfield & Halliwell, 2019). Because brain glucose transport is dependent on brain cell activity, any defects in substrate or oxidative phosphorylation should reduce neural viability and decrease glucose transport into the brain (Cunnane et al., 2020). Taken together, defects in both brain glucose transport and metabolism are present in AD, but their respective contributions to development of AD pathologies remains to be elucidated.

KETONES—THE BRAIN'S PHYSIOLOGIC ALTERNATIVE FUEL

During glucose scarcity, blood insulin decreases, which releases the inhibition on adipose tissue lipolysis, thereby increasing free fatty acid flux in different tissues. In hepatic mitochondria, the increased supply of fatty acid-derived acetyl-CoA, combined with insufficient levels of oxaloacetate to form citrate, leads to ketogenesis by condensation of two acetyl-CoAs. Whereas cerebral ketone supply originates mainly from the liver, astrocytes also possess the capacity to synthesize ketones in the brain, although determination of their net contribution to cerebral ketone metabolism requires further study (Guzmán & Blázquez, 2004).

In adults, ketogenesis occurs primarily from long-chain fatty acids stored in adipose tissue, the release of which is regulated by the glucagon:insulin ratio. Some amino acids, including isoleucine, leucine, and lysine, are also ketogenic (Noda & Ichihara, 1976). In addition to providing an alternative fuel to tissues like the brain and participating in biosynthetic processes, ketones help reduce loss of lean tissue protein needed for gluconeogenesis, a process that becomes pathologic in untreated diabetic ketoacidosis (Flatt, 1972). The human liver can produce ketones at a rate of 100 to 150 g/day (Flatt, 1972; Reichard et al., 1974) or even more in diabetic ketosis (Bondy et al., 1949), which is more than sufficient to account for whole-body ketone utilization, even during prolonged starvation. The energy cost to the liver of gluconeogenesis and ketogenesis during starvation is mostly supplied by hepatic free fatty acid oxidation.

During extended fasting, free fatty acids compete with ketones and become the main fuel to most tissues, including skeletal muscle, with the notable exception of the brain, which has low enzymatic capacity for fatty acid uptake and β-oxidation (Drenick et al., 1972; Owen & Reichard, 1971). The classic studies by Owen et al. (1967) and Drenick et al. (1972) demonstrated for the first time that ketones are the main reserve fuel for the brain, where they can account for well over 50% of total energy when glucose supply is compromised by several weeks of starvation (Drenick et al., 1972; Owen & Reichard, 1971). Gottstein et al. (1971) confirmed under the more physiologic condition of a 12- to 16-hr overnight fast that the brain consumed more ketones. As far as is known, cerebral ketone metabolism is regulated principally by ketone concentration in the blood, transport across the BBB and into the cells, and the activity of the metabolizing enzymes (Morris, 2005).

KETONES AND EARLY BRAIN DEVELOPMENT

Although it is not the subject of this chapter, it has become clear over the past three to four decades that ketones are even more important to the developing brain than to the adult brain. Unlike in adults, in infants, ketones are an *essential* fuel and brain lipid substrate because there is insufficient glucose available for glucose alone to meet brain energy (Patel et al., 1975). At birth, umbilical cord blood and placental tissue fluid have been recorded with βHB levels of 0.8 mM and 2.2 mM, respectively, demonstrating the magnitude of ketone delivery to the fetus during developmental stages (Muneta et al., 2016). In infants, sustained ketosis is common (0.3–1.3 mM βHB + AcAc) for several months after birth (Bougneres et al., 1986; Melichar et al., 1965; Settergren et al., 1976). Ketosis and the brain's dependence on ketones are ensured by the continuous delivery of MCT (i.e., 6–12 carbons; 8%–10% MCFAs) through breast milk (Sarda et al., 1987; Silva et al., 2005), along with ample long-chain fatty acid stores for ketogenesis when fasting. In animal models, while brain ketolytic enzyme (βHB dehydrogenase, succinyl-Coa:3-ketoacid CoA-transferase, and acetyl-CoA C-acetyltransferase) and ketone transporter expression increase during suckling, their concentrations progressively diminish after weaning (Gerhart et al., 1997; Page et al., 1971; Williamson et al., 1971), but this remains to be determined in humans. Still, in children up to 8 years old, hyperketonemia following fasting (4 to 48 hr) is 2- to 5-fold greater than in adults (Cahill, 2006; Elia et al., 1999). The potential utility of ketogenic supplements to the aging brain is perhaps analogous to their important role in the developing brain (Cunnane & Crawford, 2015).

KETONE TRANSPORT AND KINETICS

With the exception of hepatocytes, most cells, including neurons, oligodendrocytes, and astrocytes, can transport ketones into the cell and catabolize them (Edmond et al., 1987). Monocarboxylic acid transporters (MCT) are responsible for active ketone transport, but ketones can also enter tissues through simple diffusion (Tildon & Roeder, 1988). MCT1, MCT2, and sodium-dependent MCT1 carry ketones into and out of the brain, while MCT7 seems to be the key transporter for ketone export out of the liver (Hugo et al., 2012). In the brain, various isoforms of MCT are

TABLE 17.3 MAIN BRAIN KETONE AND GLUCOSE TRANSPORTERS AND THEIR AFFINITIES TO DIFFERENT SUBSTRATES

Transporters	Locations	Substrates K_m (mM)			Reference
Monocarboxylic acid transporters		**Acetoacetate**	**DL-βHB**	**D-βHB**	
MCAT1 (SLC16A1)	BBB, Astrocytes	5.5 ± 0.6	12.5 ± 0.3	10.1 ± 0.5	Carpenter & Halestrap, 1994
MCAT2 (SLC16A7)	Neurons	0.8 ± 0.1	1.2 ± 0.2	1.2 ± 0.2	Broer et al., 1999
SMCAT1 (SLC5A8)	Neurons	0.2 ± 0.0	*2.3 ± 0.2	1.4 ± 0.1	Martin et al., 2006
Glucose transporters		**Glucose**	**Type**		
GLUT1 (SLC2A1)	BBB, Astrocytes	3–7	Insulin-independent		Augustin, 2010 Burant & Bell, 1992
GLUT3 (SLC2A3)	Neurons	1–3	Insulin-independent		Augustin, 2010 Maher et al., 1996
GLUT4 (SLC2A4)	Neurons	4–5	Insulin-dependent		Augustin, 2010 Burant & Bell, 1992

Note. Data are presented as mean ± standard deviation for ketones and as range for glucose. BBB = blood–brain barrier endothelium, βHB = beta-hydroxybutyrate, GLUT = glucose transporter, K_m = Michaelis constant, MCAT = monocarboxylic acid transporters, SLC = solute carrier, SMCAT = sodium-dependent monocarboxylic acid transporters. *Value is for L-βHB.

expressed in the blood, BBB endothelium, and neurons, and at lower levels in astrocytes, where their higher affinities for AcAc favor its uptake over βHB (Table 17.3). In humans, brain uptake responds rapidly to hyperketonemia (Pan et al., 2000, 2001), so, under normal conditions, ketone utilization is directly proportional to the plasma concentration over at least a 165-fold range of βHB (0.04–6.7 mM; Figure 17.2). Within this range, with each 0.1-mM increase in plasma βHB values,

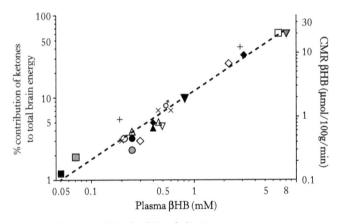

FIGURE 17.2 *Ketones, Brain Energy, and Cerebral Metabolic Rate*

Direct linear relation between plasma β-hydroxybutyrate (βHB) and percentage contribution of ketones (βHB + AcAc) to total brain energy requirement (left-side y axis, r = 0.99, y = 10.19x + 1.532, p < 0.0001) and cerebral metabolic rate of βHB (right-side axis). Data have been combined from several sources: ■ Here healthy older adults (HOA); N = 7, ▨ Here Alzheimer's disease (AD); N = 7 (Ogawa et al., 1996), ● Here HOA; N = 24, ● Here mild cognitive impairment (MCI); N = 20, ○ Here AD; N = 19 (Croteau et al., 2018b), × AD with medium-chain triglycerides (MCT) at three levels of ketonemia; N = 6–11 (Croteau et al., 2018a), ◇ Here healthy young adults (HYA) before and after ketone infusion; N = 8 (Hasselbalch et al., 1996), △ Here HYA; N = 5, ▲ Here HOA; N = 5, ▲ Here AD; N = 12 (Lying-Tunell et al., 1980, 1981), + HYA before and after 3.5 days of starvation; N = 9 (Hasselbalch et al., 1994), ◆ Here HYA before and after a ketogenic diet; N = 10 (Courchesne-Loyer et al., 2017a), ▽ Here HYA; N = 16, ▼ Here clinical patients; N = 8, after a 12- to 16-hr fast (Gottstein et al., 1971), ♂ MCI with MCT; N = 39 (Fortier et al., 2019), ▢ Here adults with obesity after 40 days of starvation; N = 3 (Owen et al., 1967), ▼ Here 60 days of starvation in adults with obesity; N = 5 (Drenick et al., 1972). Some of the data in Drenick et al. (1972) were recalculated. The AcAc contribution was extrapolated using the Owen et al. (1967) study.

ketones contribute an additional 1.0% to 1.2% to total brain energy metabolism. During extreme physiologic ketosis (6.7 mM of βHB), ketones appear to provide up to approximately two thirds of total brain energy (Owen et al., 1967). This two-thirds value is unlikely to be exceeded, as shown by studies in both humans (Drenick et al., 1972) and rats (Chowdhury et al., 2014) where βHB concentration was increased to 8 mM and 17 mM, respectively. One possible exception in which the ketone contribution exceeded this value is when insulin was infused following ≥ 60 days of starvation in obesity (Drenick et al., 1972).

Similar to brain glucose uptake, the transport of ketones into the brain per se may not be the limiting variable in their uptake. Rather, ketones are "pushed" into the brain in proportion to their plasma ketone concentration, which usually only increases when plasma glucose decreases (Cunnane et al., 2016). This contrasts with glucose, which is "pulled" into the brain with an extraction fraction of 10% to 12% (Madsen et al., 1999) down its concentration gradient (blood 5 mM vs. brain 1–2 mM; McNay & Gold, 1999) in proportion to its utilization. Hence, the push–pull strategy ensures that under conditions in which glucose availability decreases, ketone synthesis would normally be stimulated, and the brain's energy supply would be maintained (Figure 17.3).

Elegant kinetic studies show that ketone utilization essentially matches synthesis in healthy adults fasted overnight (Elia et al., 1990; Hall et al., 1984). The rapid utilization of ketones as they are produced during 12 to 15 hr of fasting generally keeps plasma ketones at ≤ 0.3 mM, except in untreated insulin-dependent diabetes, where plasma ketones increase to 1.0 to 2.5 mM because the regulation of ketogenesis by insulin is lacking (Hall et al., 1984; Wahren et al., 1984). After 3 days of fasting, the rates of ketone synthesis and utilization generally increase ketone concentrations to the range of 1.5 to 3.0 mM (Garber et al., 1974a; Owen & Reichard, 1971; Owen et al., 1969). Peak physiologic ketone levels observed after several weeks of starvation (5–10 mM; Drenick et al., 1972; Hall et al., 1984; Owen et al., 1967) arise by a progressive reduction in metabolic clearance by peripheral tissues (mainly βHB) and an increase in renal ketone reabsorption that amplifies their increased production (Féry & Balasse, 1985; Sapir & Owen, 1975).

During mild ketosis, muscle ketone extraction from the blood is about 50% at 0.1 mM and 20% at 1 mM, while brain ketone extraction is considerably lower, at 10%. With increased ketonemia (1–8 mmol/L), muscle ketone extraction progressively falls from 20% to 5% while brain extraction remains stable at 10% (Balasse & Féry,

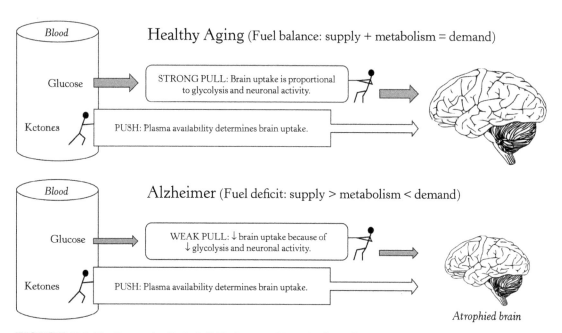

FIGURE 17.3 *The Contrasting Push–Pull Mechanism of Brain Fuel Supply*

Glucose is pulled from the blood into the brain as a function of the metabolic demand by brain cell activation. Under normal conditions, ketones are pushed from the blood into the brain in direct proportion to their plasma concentration. Adapted from Cunnane et al. (2020).

1989). This ketone uptake redistribution from muscle to the brain ensures that ketones are available to complement the lower availability of glucose in meeting the energy needs of the brain. While at rest, muscle ketone uptake reaches saturation between 1.5 and 2.0 mM of βHB during ketone infusion (Mikkelsen et al., 2015), the exact concentration at which brain ketone uptake fully saturates in humans has not yet been determined. Nevertheless, a comparison of results among the studies included in Figure 17.2 suggests that the saturation point in the brain is much higher than the average βHB levels achieved during most types of ketogenic interventions. The progressive accumulation of up to 1 mM βHB in the brain during physiologic ketosis (Novotny, 1996; Pan et al., 2000, 2001) suggests that the oxidation, more than the transport rate, could be limiting cerebral ketone utilization in humans. Accordingly, a recent animal study showed that after maximal βHB oxidation capacity is achieved, βHB within the brain continues to accumulate with further infusion (Chowdhury et al., 2014).

Generally, in fasted and starved adults, exercise at low-to-moderate intensity for 30 min significantly reduces circulating ketones, which rebound to pre-exercise levels or even higher when exercise is prolonged to 60 or 120 min or terminated (Fery & Balasse, 1983, 1986, 1988). However, several studies have demonstrated that basal ketone levels and the means by which hyperketonemia is induced (diabetes, infusion, starvation, KD) can affect ketone kinetic parameters at rest and during exercise (Fery & Balasse, 1983, 1986, 1988; Nosadini et al., 1985). Indeed, evidence in both rats and humans suggests that as compared to states with no or little adaptations (fed state, overnight fast) at similar degree of ketonemia, 3 to 5 days of fasting significantly upregulates ketone transport parameters (Gjedde & Crone, 1975; Pan et al., 2000, 2001).

KETONE METABOLISM AND METABOLIC IMPAIRMENTS

Insulin controls the ebb and flow of plasma glucose, free fatty acids, and ketones, making the body's metabolic response to this hormone crucial for optimal energy metabolism. Indeed, conditions involving decreased insulin responsiveness (e.g., obesity, prediabetes, T2D) are associated with impaired tissue glucose uptake and a vicious cycle of hyperglycemia, hyperinsulinemia, and insulin resistance. These conditions all have in common that they are important risk factors for the development of AD and are associated with brain glucose hypometabolism (Baker et al., 2011; Craft, 2009; Profenno et al., 2010).

The relationship between ketones and insulin sensitivity is controversial, as both insulin resistance (Avogaro et al., 1992) and sensitivity (Mahendran et al., 2013) have been associated with elevated ketone levels. This could potentially be explained in part by the fact that impaired insulin secretion and not insulin resistance per se predicts ketone levels (Mahendran et al., 2013). In T2D, ketone levels are usually high (Avogaro et al., 1996; Mahendran et al., 2013) but numerous studies that evaluated the effects of obesity and insulin resistance on ketone metabolism in humans reported lower ketone synthesis, oxidation, or concentrations in the obese or insulin-resistant subjects as compared to their lean or insulin-sensitive counterparts (Bergman et al., 2007; Bickerton et al., 2008; Elia et al., 1999; Göschke, 1977; Mey et al., 2020; Nosadini et al., 1985; Vega et al., 2009; Vice et al., 2005). Also, while insulin-mediated suppression of ketogenesis showed some degree of insulin resistance in nonobese individuals with T2D (Singh et al., 1993), this same pathway seems normal in individuals with obesity displaying some degree of insulin resistance (Bergman et al., 2007; Soeters et al., 2009). In these populations, defects in adipocyte lipolysis (Reynisdottir et al., 1994; Tan et al., 2015) and mitochondrial dysfunction are often present (Bournat & Brown, 2010; Kim et al., 2008) and could potentially limit ketone synthesis and oxidation regardless of the circulating ketone levels. If ketone metabolism is indeed impaired, it would put the brain of individuals living with these conditions in double jeopardy because the brain is not only getting insufficient glucose but also is getting less of the main alternative fuel, ketones (Cunnane et al., 2020; Mamelak, 2012).

KETOGENESIS FROM MCT

Fasting and KD induce ketosis because long-chain fatty acids from adipose tissue and dietary fats are β-oxidized by the liver to acetyl CoA. Long-chain fatty acids are of 14 to 22 carbons in length and are essentially the only endogenous fatty acids available for energy metabolism, because medium-chain fatty acids are not normally esterified into adipose tissue. Medium-chain fatty acids (6 to 12 carbons) are mostly absorbed through the portal vein, hence gaining direct and more rapid access to the liver than long-chain fatty acids, which are absorbed into the peripheral circulation via the lymph. Medium-chain fatty acids are also transported across the inner mitochondrial membrane without the need to be activated by carnitine. The net result is rapid β-oxidation and ketogenesis. With rare exception, there is normally no further opportunity after breastfeeding to consume medium-chain fatty acids from the diet once breastfeeding is terminated. The exceptions are dietary coconut oil and palm kernel oil, in which medium-chain fatty acids make up about 65%—dodecanoic acid 50%, octanoic acid (C8) and decanoic acid (C10) 15%—and 60%—dodecanoic acid 50%, C8–10 10%—of the fatty acids, respectively. The C8 and C10 fractions of these oils can be concentrated, resulting in a generic medium-chain triglyceride (MCT) product containing mostly C8 and C10 fatty acids, but their content and ratio can vary widely from one MCT product to another. C8 alone or in combination with C10 is more ketogenic than MCT products containing dodecanoic acid or longer chain fatty acids (St-Pierre et al., 2019; Vandenberghe et al., 2017). Notwithstanding the generic nature of the different MCT products used and different study designs to assess their metabolism, a cross-sectional "pseudo-dose-response" analysis showed

a good correlation between the maximal plasma ketone level achieved on oral doses of MCT from 10 to 70 g (Figure 17.4). Moreover, adults consuming a mixture of C8-C10 twice daily for up to 6 months do not show any habituation with respect to the plasma ketone response (Fortier et al., 2020). The addition of MCT to a KD (Harvey et al., 2018) or aerobic exercise (Vandenberghe et al., 2019) can potentiate βHB concentrations (+ 0.2–0.8 mM), which in turn could allow some patients a more permissive form of KD, adherence being the main predictor of long-term diet effectiveness.

Healthy people over 50 years old have a similar or higher plasma ketone response to an acute MCT supplement as adults in their twenties to thirties (Vandenberghe et al., 2020) or during short-term fasting (London et al., 1986). These results confirm the findings of Freemantle et al. (2009), which, in addition to similar ketone concentrations, also observed that the rate of [^{13}C] ketone oxidation to [^{13}C]CO$_2$ after a standard high-fat ketogenic breakfast containing 71 g of MCT was the same among healthy older, middle-aged, or young adults (76 years old versus 50 or 23 years old; Freemantle et al., 2009). Hence, the capacity to produce and utilize ketones does not appear to be reduced during healthy aging. While this study did not distinguish between ketone

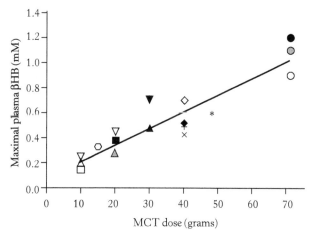

FIGURE 17.4 Direct relationship dose of medium-chain triglycerides (MCT) and maximal observed plasma β-hydroxybutyrate ($R^2 = 0.93$; $y = 0.01219x + 0.08354$, $p < 0.0001$) in young adults unless otherwise specified. MCT were given as a single dose or multiple doses*: (□ 10 g MCT; Alzheimer (AD), $N = 77$, ■ 20 g MCT*; AD, $N = 77$ (Henderson et al., 2009), (▽ 10 g MCT emulsion; $N = 10$, ▼ 20 g MCT emulsion, $N = 10$, ▼ 30 g MCT emulsion; $N = 10$; △ 10 g neat MCT; $N = 10$, ▲ 20 g neat MCT; $N = 10$, ▲ 30 g neat MCT; $N = 10$ (Courchesne-Loyer et al., 2017b), ○ 15 g MCT*; $N = 8$ (Courchesne-Loyer et al., 2013), + 40 g MCT; mild cognitive impairment, AD, $N = 10$ (Reger et al., 2004), × 40 g MCT; type 1 diabetes, $N = 11$ (Page et al., 2009), ◇ 40 g MCT C8*; $N = 9$, ◆ 40 g MCT C8C10*; $N = 9$ (St-Pierre et al., 2019), * 48 g MCT; $N = 7$ (Seaton et al., 1986), ○ 71 g MCT; young adults $N = 11$, ◉ 71 g MCT; middle-age adults, $N = 12$, ● 71 g MCT; older adults, $N = 9$ (Freemantle et al., 2009).

utilization by the brain versus other organs, our brain ketone PET results confirm that the brain has similar ketone uptake and utilization in healthy older and younger persons (Nugent et al., 2014b) and in individuals with mild cognitive impairment and early AD (Croteau et al., 2018b).

BRAIN KETONE UTILIZATION IN AD

Several ground-breaking reports based on AVD methods established the foundation for our current understanding that ketones help meet daily brain energy requirements (Drenick et al., 1972; Owen et al., 1967). Using PET with ^{11}C-βHB tracer, Blomqvist et al. (2002) showed that the uptake was directly proportional to plasma βHB even at very low plasma ketone concentrations (< 0.1 mM; Blomqvist et al., 1995). Despite impaired brain glucose uptake and lower CMRglc in MCI and AD, brain ketone uptake and cerebral metabolic rate of acetoacetate (CMR_{AcAc}) were not significantly different from those in cognitively healthy, age-matched controls (Table 17.4). Importantly, the direct positive relationship between plasma ketone concentration and brain ketone uptake had a similar slope in all groups, which implies that brain ketone utilization during mild ketonemia in these populations was also still normal (Figure 17.5). Brain energetic alteration during aging therefore seems to be a problem specific to glucose metabolism, as shown by a nonsignificant but progressive CMRglc reduction of 6% to 12% over a 4-year follow-up in cognitively healthy older adults, while here again, ketone utilization was unaffected (Castellano et al., 2019).

With the focus on glucose as the predominant brain fuel, until recently, the possibility that brain ketone uptake could be less affected or even remain intact in AD has largely been overlooked. The above findings provide a rationale for the concept that if afforded more ketones, the brain of AD patients would be able to use them, which, in turn, might help it overcome its energetic deficit and hopefully improve cognitive function.

CLINICAL STUDIES OF HYPERKETONEMIA IN CONDITIONS OF COGNITIVE DEFICIT

KDs inducing pronounced ketosis (4–5 mM) have been reported to increase brain ketone utilization while concomitantly reducing brain glucose utilization in healthy rats (LaManna et al., 2009) and humans (Courchesne-Loyer et al., 2017a), resulting in unchanged net whole brain energy utilization. However, the ketone-induced reduction in brain glucose utilization (glucose sparing) does not occur in individuals with cognitive deficits in mild ketosis (0.5–1.0 mM) because the additional supply of ketones partially compensates for the preexisting deficit in glucose metabolism (Croteau et al., 2018a; Fortier et al., 2019; Neth et al., 2020). Thus, in both AD and MCI, a drink containing 15 g of MCT taken twice a day for 1 and 6 months, respectively, did not alter glucose utilization but more than doubled brain CMR of ketones (+ 142% and + 230%), leading to a ~ 4% increase in net global brain energy uptake during the post-MCT period (Croteau et al., 2018a; Fortier et al., 2019; Figure 17.6), an improved situation but one that still left a brain energy gap.

As early as 1972, studies showed that autonomic and neurologic symptoms of acute, severe

TABLE 17.4 DIFFERENCES BETWEEN CEREBRAL METABOLIC RATE OF GLUCOSE AND OF ACETOACETATE IN OLDER ADULTS AND ALZHEIMER'S DISEASE

Method	CMR glucose (µmol/100 g/min)		CMR acetoacetate (µmol/100 g/min)		Reference
	CTL	AD	CTL	AD	
AVD	24.8 (18.8–32.1)	18.7* (11.9–30.3)	0.44 (−0.63+1.7)	0.39 (0.03–2.5)	Lying-Tunell et al., 1981†
AVD	24.9 ± 7.2	11.6** ± 4.0	0.18 ± 0.13	0.09 ± 0.04	Ogawa et al., 1996†
PET	38.3 ± 4.9	34.2* ± 5.0	0.35 ± 0.16	0.31 ± 0.24	Castellano et al., 2015b‡
PET	29.7 ± 2.5	27.0* ± 3.3	0.28 ± 0.19	0.30 ± 0.20	Croteau et al., 2018b‡

Note. Data are presented as mean ± standard deviation, except for Lying-Tunell et al. (1981), where they are presented as median (range). Significantly lower than cognitively healthy older adults (CTL) * $p < 0.05$, ** $p < 0.005$. AD = Alzheimer's disease, AVD = arteriovenous difference, CMR = cerebral metabolic rate, PET = positron emission tomography. † Advanced AD, ‡ mild–moderate AD.

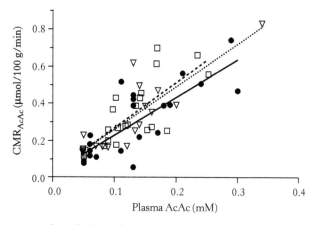

FIGURE 17.5 *Acetoacetate and Cerebral Metabolic Rate*

The direct, linear relationship between cerebral metabolic rate of acetoacetate (CMR_{AcAc}) and plasma AcAc concentration is not altered in mild cognitive impairment (☐ top dotted line, $N = 20$, $r = 0.72$; $y = 2.412x + 0.03178$, $p < 0.0004$) or Alzheimer's disease (▽ middle dotted line, $N = 19$, $r = 0.87$; $y = 2.305x + 0.02826$, $p < 0.0001$) compared to healthy older adults (● bottom solid line, $N = 24$, $r = 0.81$; $y = 2.014x + 0.02954$, $p < 0.0001$). Comparison groups $p = 0.729$. Adapted from Croteau et al. (2018b). The energetic contributions provided here assume no significant provision to the brain from other monocarboxylates, such as lactate, pyruvate, or short-chain fatty acids.

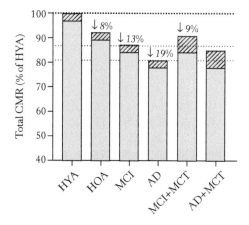

FIGURE 17.6 *Total Brain Energy Metabolism in Different Populations*

Total brain energy metabolism—cerebral metabolic rate (CMR) of ketones + glucose—of healthy young adults (HYA), healthy older adults (HOA), patients with mild cognitive impairment (MCI), and patients with Alzheimer's disease (AD). Percentages above columns represent the average energy deficit as compared to HYA based on reported whole-brain or gray matter CMR percent differences between groups (Castellano et al., 2015b; Croteau et al., 2018b; Li et al., 2008; Nugent et al., 2014b). In each group, the basal daily contribution of ketones to brain energy metabolism is ~ 3%. With provision of 15 g of MCT (carbon 8–10) in MCI (MCI + MCT; Fortier et al., 2019) and in AD (AD + MCT; Croteau et al., 2018a), the additional supply of ketones can reduce the brain energy deficit by ~ 4%.

experimental hypoglycemia could be prevented by providing ketones (Table 17.5). Since then, several reports in MCI and AD have shown that KD and MCT supplementation had beneficial effects on brain energetics and cognitive outcomes after a single dose (Reger et al., 2004) or with regular consumption over several weeks to months (Table 17.6). A systematic review and meta-analysis on the topic concluded that, as compared to placebo, MCT significantly increased blood βHB levels (weighted mean differences = + 0.355) and improved cognitive performance (combined scores of Alzheimer Disease Assessment Scale-Cognitive Subscale and Mini-Mental State Examination; weighted mean differences = − 0.289) in MCI and AD (Avgerinos et al., 2020). While these two common neurocognitive tests are not suitable to assess cognitive changes in MCI, we recently reported significant improvements in this population in several cognitive tests, including episodic memory, language, executive function, and processing speed following 6 months of MCT supplementation (Fortier et al., 2019). In this study, the improvements in cognitive tests were accompanied and positively related to circulating βHB (Figure 17.7).

The cardiometabolic safety of MCT has often been questioned because they are saturated fats. In doses up to 1 g/kg/day provided acutely or daily over several months, they have a robust

TABLE 17.5 STUDIES USING KETONES TO PREVENT BRAIN DYSFUNCTION DUE TO INSULIN-INDUCED HYPOGLYCEMIA

Population (N)	Treatment	Outcomes	Reference
Adults with obesity (9)	2 months fast + acute insulin bolus infusion Peak βHB levels 8.0 mM	↓ hypoglycemic (as low as 0.5 mM) reactions, including mental confusion, anxiety, sweating, tachycardia, blood pressure, catecholamine excretion	Drenick et al., 1972
Healthy adults (8)	72-hr fast + 1-hr hypoglycemic insulin clamp Peak βHB levels N/A	Prevented ↓ mental alertness during hypoglycemia	Fourest-Fontecave et al., 1987
Healthy adults (6)	4-hr hypoglycemic insulin clamp + βHB infusion Peak βHB levels 0.6 mM	↓ hormonal response (adrenaline, noradrenaline, cortisol, growth hormones) to hypoglycemia	Amiel et al., 1991
Healthy adults (13)	6-hr hypoglycemic insulin clamp + 4.5-hr βHB infusion Peak βHB levels 1.9 mM	↓ counterregulatory hormone responses and cognitive dysfunction during hypoglycemia	Veneman et al., 1994
Type 1 diabetes (11)	3-hr euglycemic-hypoglycemic insulin clamp + MCT drink (40 g) Peak βHB levels 0.4 mM	↓ cognitive dysfunction but had no effect on hormonal response to hypoglycemia	Page et al., 2009

Note. βHB = beta-hydroxybutyrate, N/A = not available.

safety record (Traul et al., 2000) and generally induce few if any significant adverse changes in terms of metabolites, hormonal profiles, or body weight in humans (Avgerinos et al., 2020). Secondary side effects of MCT involving gastrointestinal distress have been reported, but they can usually be mitigated by gradual dose titration, emulsification, or splitting up the total daily intake into multiple small doses (Avgerinos et al., 2020; Courchesne-Loyer et al., 2017b). Aside from MCT, AcAc and βHB can also be directly administered orally as salts or esters, but results of randomized controlled trials in AD or MCI are still awaited. With respect to long-term therapeutic use, ketone salts are effective are inducing mild ketosis (1.0 mM) but, theoretically, could potentially lead to sodium overload. The alternative βHB monoester sharply increases the D-isomer of βHB (up to 5 mM) but is poor-tasting and currently very costly. Nevertheless, the safety of βHB monoester in humans (Clarke et al., 2012) and its anecdotal utility in improving some aspects of cognitive function in an advanced case of early-onset Alzheimer's disease have recently been reported (Newport et al., 2015).

ANAPLEROTIC AND CATAPLEROTIC REACTIONS DURING KETOSIS

Even under prolonged starvation, when ketones become the main fuel for the brain, glucose remains essential to replenish CAC intermediates and to synthesize compounds necessary for normal brain function and structure (e.g., the neurotransmitters γ-aminobutyric acid [GABA] and acetylcholine, but also myelin lipids). For example, during ketosis, gluconeogenesis is directly proportional to ketogenesis, possibly because endogenous glucose synthesis stimulates local free fatty acid flux and oxidation, which in turn promote ketogenesis by providing ketogenic substrates and ATP (Garber et al., 1974b). Part of the resulting glucose production is used to sustain anaplerosis, including in the brain (Owen et al., 1967). Hence, glucose not only is a major fuel but also controls the balance between anaplerosis and cataplerosis (Owen et al., 2002), without which the CAC would be rapidly depleted.

Glucose is a CAC substrate that contributes to both cataplerosis and anaplerosis reactions

TABLE 17.6 EXPERIMENTAL STUDIES USING KETOGENIC INTERVENTIONS OF ≥ 3 WEEKS' DURATION AND COGNITIVE OUTCOMES IN MCI AND AD PATIENTS

Intervention	Treatments	Design	Populations (N)	Outcomes	Reference
Diet	Ketogenic (n = 12) or high-carbohydrate (n = 11) diets, 6 weeks	RCT	MCI (23)	↑ Verbal memory performance; Ketone levels positively correlated with memory performance	Krikorian et al., 2012
	Ketogenic (n = 9) or HCLF (n = 5) diets, 12 weeks	RCT	AD, MCI (14)	↑ Memory composite score at week 6	Brandt et al., 2019
	Ketogenic or HCLF diets, 6 weeks	RCT - crossover	SMC, MCI (20)	↑ Memory performance in both diets; ↑ CSF Ab42, ↓ Tau, ↑ cerebral perfusion and ketone uptake	Neth et al., 2020
Supplement	C8 20 g/day (n = 77) or placebo (n = 63), 12 weeks	RCT	AD (140)	Improved ADAS-Cog (−3.4 points versus placebo) in ApoE4(-)	Henderson et al., 2009
	CCO 40 ml/day (n = 22) or placebo (n = 22), 3 weeks	RCT	AD (44)	Cognitive improvement MEC-WOLF test	Hu Yang et al., 2015
	MCT 56 g/day (n = 2) or placebo (n = 2) 24 weeks	RCT	MCI (4)	↑ Memory score in MCT but not in placebo.	Rebello et al., 2015
	C8 20 g/day, 12 weeks	One-arm trial	AD (22)	No cognitive improvements	Ohnuma et al., 2016
	CCO, 60 ml/day (n = 8) or placebo (n = 14), 6 months	RCT	AD (22)	No cognitive improvements	Chan et al., 2017
	C8C10, 30 g/day (n = 19) or placebo (n = 20), 6 months	RCT	MCI (39)	↑ episodic memory, language, executive function, and processing speed associated with ↑ brain ketone uptake	Fortier et al., 2019
	C8C10, 17 g/day or placebo, 4 weeks.	RCT – crossover	AD (APOE4 -/-) (46)	Improved ADAS-Cog (−5.2 points versus placebo)	Xu et al., 2019
	C8C10, 20 g/day, 12 weeks.	One-arm trial	AD (16)	↑ Verbal memory and processing speed	Ota et al., 2019
Diet + Supplement	Ketogenic diet + MCT 21–42 g/day, 12 weeks.	One arm trial	AD (10)	Improved ADAS-Cog (−4.1 points versus baseline)	Taylor et al., 2018
	Mediterranean diet + CCO 40 ml/day or placebo, 3 weeks.	RCT	AD (44)	Improved episodic, temporal orientation and sematic memory.	de la Rubia Ortí et al., 2018

Note. AD = Alzheimer's disease, ADAS-cog = Alzheimer's Disease Assessment Scale cognitive subscale, C8 = eight-carbon chain fatty acids, C10 = ten-carbon chain fatty acids, CCO = coconut oil, CSF Ab42 = cerebrospinal fluid amyloid-β 42, g/day = grams per day, HCLF = high-carbohydrate low-fat, MCI = mild cognitive impairment, ml/day = milliliters per day, RCT = randomized controlled trial, SMC = subjective memory complaints. The population includes only participants who completed the interventions.

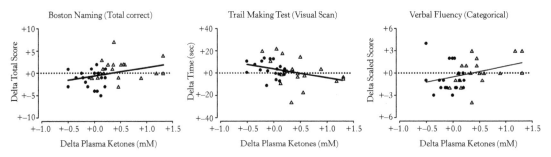

FIGURE 17.7 *Plasma Ketones and Cognition*

Scatter plots of the change in plasma ketones (acetoacetate + beta-hydroxybutyrate; mM) and change in the score for the Boston Naming (r = +0.331, p = 0.042) tests, Trail Making (Visual Scan: r = −0.351, p = 0.031), and the Verbal Fluency (categorical: r = +0.330, p = 0.043).

● placebo (N = 19) and △ medium-chain triglycerides (N = 19). Linear regression (p < 0.05). Adapted from Fortier et al. (2019).

(Brunengraber & Roe, 2006). In contrast, ketones are cataplerotic because they increase CAC activity but do not contribute to anaplerosis (Roy et al., 2015). In isolated rat hearts, perfusing with ketones was reported to reduce CAC intermediates and to lead to cardiac dysfunction when ketones were provided as a sole substrate (Taegtmeyer et al., 1980), but the addition of anaplerotic substrates, such as glucose and pyruvate, reversed these conditions (Russell & Taegtmeyer, 1991a, 1991b; Taegtmeyer, 1983; Taegtmeyer et al., 1980). Alternatively, the addition of ketones to glucose was shown to improved cardiac function and efficiency as compared to glucose alone in some (Sato et al., 1995), but not all, studies (Taegtmeyer et al., 1980). A more recent study showed that adding 21.5% of total calories as dietary ketone ester to a diet moderately high in carbohydrates led to significant increases in hippocampal glycolytic and CAC intermediates in a mouse model of AD (Pawlosky et al., 2017). Taken together, these findings highlight the importance of ensuring sufficient anaplerotic substrates during hyperketonemia and suggest that a combination of both substrates might confer benefits for mitochondrial health and function.

In conditions in which the glucose supply to the brain is more severely limited, such as in inherited GLUT-1 deficiency (Brunengraber & Roe, 2006; Mochel et al., 2005; Roe & Mochel, 2006), there is insufficient glucose to maintain anaplerosis and energy production in the brain. While traditional ketogenic interventions can be beneficial in this population, they may exhaust the CAC over time (Brunengraber & Roe, 2006; Mochel et al., 2005; Roe & Mochel, 2006). Utilization of the 7-carbon MCT triheptanoin was effective at reducing symptoms in this

population and other metabolic diseases (Mochel et al., 2005, 2010; Pascual et al., 2014), possibly because triheptanoin metabolism generates both oxidative and anaplerotic precursors.

Whether the situation is analogous in AD remains to be seen. However, it is clear that, as AD becomes more severe, brain glucose utilization continues to deteriorate, thereby further compromising ATP production and presumably anaplerosis, with the potential to impair ketone oxidation through lower CAC activity. There is most likely a trade-off between supplying more ketones to compensate for the glucose deficit and oversupplying them, thereby further depleting glucose and risking burning out the CAC.

POTENTIAL MECHANISMS OF ACTIONS OF KETONES IN AD

The broadly similar neurologic/cognitive benefit among the different ketogenic interventions implies that the improvement is related to a common denominator of raised plasma ketones and improved brain energy metabolism, although other overlapping effects do exist (reviewed in Maalouf et al., 2009). This is still speculative, as no study has yet provided solid proof as to how ketogenic interventions improve cognitive outcomes. During functional activation, glycolysis is transiently upregulated over oxidative metabolism to sustain brain function, which suggests that an impairment in glycolysis would disrupt the ability of brain cells to increase energy consumption when needed during neurotransmission (Dienel, 2019). Providing ketones would increase ATP availability in the affected brain area with a more efficient fuel than glucose and bypass the chronically impaired steps that limit the supply of acetyl-CoA (i.e., glucose uptake, glycolysis, and pyruvate oxidation; Bubber et al., 2005). Contrary to glucose, which can produce ATP via both glycolysis and oxidative phosphorylation, ketones produce ATP only via the latter. On top of not entering the glycolytic pathway, βHB has previously been shown to inhibit glycolysis through phosphofructokinase (Newsholme et al., 1962) and to convert pyruvate dehydrogenase to its inactive form (Wieland et al., 1971). The observations that ketones are readily utilized in AD and that certain but not all populations with established mitochondrial defects improve their conditions on KD (Kossoff et al., 2009) suggest that mitochondrial capacity must remain at least partially functional and that the specificity of mitochondrial defects might regulate ketogenic treatments' effectiveness.

Brain mitochondria both produce, and are the target of, reactive oxygen species (ROS) that affect their dynamics (fission/fusion) and contribute to the pathogenesis of AD (Wang et al., 2014). Neural protection by ketones could be related to improved mitochondrial function through reduced mitochondrial production of ROS and increased protection against oxidative damage (Kim et al., 2007) and mitochondrial biogenesis (Hasan-Olive et al., 2019). Alternatively, several other potential beneficial effects of ketones on brain cells have been proposed to confer neuroprotection, including reduced apoptosis (Maalouf et al., 2009), more balanced neurotransmitter metabolism (glutamate and GABA; Daikhin & Yudkoff, 1998), increased nicotinamide adenine dinucleotide (NAD^+:NADH) redox state (Xin et al., 2018), and brain-derived neurotrophic factor expression (Hu et al., 2018).

In AD, chronic oxidative stress is associated with glia-induced neuroinflammation, contributing to neurodegeneration (Yin et al., 2016a). Moreover, proinflammatory signaling impairs ketone production (Pailla et al., 2001) and mediates peripheral and neuronal insulin resistance (Olefsky & Glass, 2010). Inflammation and defective insulin signaling within the brain are present in AD and can impair synaptic transmission and neuronal survival, which might exacerbate brain glucose hypometabolism and cognitive dysfunctions (De Felice & Ferreira, 2014). Although βHB and KD possess anti-inflammatory properties (Forsythe et al., 2008; Rahman et al., 2014), the failure of recent trials using anti-inflammatory drugs in AD (Gupta et al., 2015) suggests that it is most likely not the central mechanism by which ketones improve cognition.

Beta-amyloid accumulation in AD could arise as a result of (Velliquette et al., 2005), or contribute to, brain glycolytic (Meier-Ruge & Bertoni-Freddari, 1997) and mitochondrial dysfunction (Wang et al., 2008). While several studies in rodents have highlighted the potential of ketogenic interventions to reduce amyloid and tau accumulation and toxicity, with corresponding improvement in cognitive behaviors (Kashiwaya et al., 2000, 2013; Yin et al., 2016b), further studies in humans (Neth et al., 2020) are required to confirm these findings. Cognitive improvements with ketogenic interventions are observed within hours or days, suggesting that if a reduction in beta-amyloid really occurs, it would be subsequent to brain energy rescue.

PERSPECTIVES

The emerging concept is that brain glucose hypometabolism is already present years before the onset of noticeable cognitive decline associated with AD. The presence of such metabolic dysfunction in presymptomatic individuals strongly suggests that chronic, progressive brain glucose hypometabolism is not simply a consequence of decreased neuronal activity but rather exacerbates (if not causes) AD neuropathology and cognitive decline by preventing sufficient brain fuel supply. In support of the concept of "brain energy rescue" (Cunnane et al., 2020), numerous studies found that interventions elevating ketones were beneficial to both brain energy metabolism and cognitive functions in AD. Importantly, some studies suggested that ketogenic interventions might be less effective in individuals carrying the *APOE4* gene (Henderson et al., 2009; Reger et al., 2004; Torosyan et al., 2018), which has recently been shown to accelerate BBB degeneration (Montagne et al., 2020). Future studies should also investigate if similar differences can be observed between genders, which did not seem to be the case based on exploratory analyses conducted as part of our study (Fortier et al., 2020).

Whether trying to directly correct the problem of impaired glucose uptake-metabolism and deteriorating mitochondrial function should be undertaken concurrently with providing a ketogenic supplement remains to be assessed. Along these lines, exercise can be an important adjunctive treatment for metabolic diseases and has been shown to be moderately beneficial in improving cognitive functions in MCI and AD (Öhman et al., 2014). A pilot study conducted by our group found that 3 months of aerobic exercise significantly increases CMR_{AcAc} by threefold (0.6 ± 0.4

versus 0.2 ± 0.1 mol/100 g/min) even if no keto-genic interventions were provided (Castellano et al., 2017). Given the important effect exercise has on insulin sensitivity, mitochondrial function, and brain substrate delivery, future studies should test the combination of ketogenic interventions and exercise on cognition and progression of MCI to AD.

At plasma βHB concentrations of 0.3 to 0.5 mM, ketones contribute 3% to 6% of total brain energy (see Figure 17.2), which is line with our results showing that a drink containing 15 g of MCT and raising ketones by 0.3 to 0.4 mM reduces the brain energy deficit by ~ 4% (Croteau et al., 2018a; Fortier et al., 2019). Thus, it is likely that the energetic and cognitive benefits of MCT supplementation could be augmented by using an intervention that could elevate blood ketones more than MCT. Accordingly, our team launched a trial assessing the potential of a βHB salt to improve cognitive function in MCI, which should shed further light on the potential utility of keto-neurotherapeutics. Cognitively healthy older adults and MCI populations offer a window of opportunity where potential disease-modifying treatments could slow down, or possibly even prevent, progression to AD. Indeed, with the failure of amyloid-based treatments and the fact that some clinical symptoms begin decades before the onset of AD, much more effort should be invested in prevention and alternative therapeutic targets. Collectively, the literature presented in this chapter highlights the potential benefit of overcoming deteriorating brain glucose metabolism using ketogenic interventions, an approach that should be pursued as a safe and effective tool to prevent and manage cognitive decline associated with AD.

ACKNOWLEDGMENTS

Mélanie Fortier, Valérie St-Pierre, Camille Vandenberghe, Marie-Christine Morin, Maggie Roy, and Étienne Croteau are thanked for their technical assistance. Financial support was provided by a Canada Research Chair and University Research Chair (SCC), CFI, CIHR, NSERC, FRQS, FQRNT, Sojecci II, The Alzheimer Association (USA), The Alzheimer Society of Canada (ASRP), and the Université de Sherbrooke. Some MCT products used in our studies were provided as gifts by Abitec and Nestlé Health Science. Dr. Étienne Myette-Côté is supported by a Postdoctoral Fellowship from the Alzheimer Society Research Program—Alzheimer Society Canada and the Fonds de Recherche en Santé du Québec (FRQS).

CONFLICTS OF INTEREST

S.C.C. declares that he has consulted for and has received honoraria, test products, and/or research funding from Abitec, Accera, Bulletproof, Nestlé, and Servier, is the founder of Senotec, and is co-inventor on a patent for an MCT formulation.

REFERENCES

Abdulrab, K., & Heun, R. (2008). Subjective memory impairment: A review of its definitions indicates the need for a comprehensive set of standardised and validated criteria. *European Psychiatry, 23,* 321–330.

Alavi, A., Newberg, A. B., Souder, E., & Berlin, J. A. (1993). Quantitative analysis of PET and MRI data in normal aging and Alzheimer's disease: Atrophy weighted total brain metabolism and absolute whole brain metabolism as reliable discriminators. *Journal of Nuclear Medicine, 34,* 1681–1687.

Albert, M. S., DeKosky, S. T., Dickson, D., Dubois, B., Feldman, H. H., Fox, N. C., Gamst, A., Holtzman, D. M., Jagust, W. J., & Petersen, R. C. (2011). The diagnosis of mild cognitive impairment due to Alzheimer's disease: Recommendations from the National Institute on Aging-Alzheimer's Association workgroups on diagnostic guidelines for Alzheimer's disease. *Alzheimer's & Dementia, 7,* 270–279.

Amiel, S. A., Archibald, H. R., Chusney, G., Williams, A. J., & Gale, E. A. (1991). Ketone infusion lowers hormonal responses to hypoglycaemia: Evidence for acute cerebral utilization of a non-glucose fuel. *Clinical Science, 81,* 189–194.

An, Y., Varma, V. R., Varma, S., Casanova, R., Dammer, E., Pletnikova, O., Chia, C. W., Egan, J. M., Ferrucci, L., & Troncoso, J. (2018). Evidence for brain glucose dysregulation in Alzheimer's disease. *Alzheimer's & Dementia, 14,* 318–329.

Arnold, S. E., Arvanitakis, Z., Macauley-Rambach, S. L., Koenig, A. M., Wang, H.-Y., Ahima, R. S., Craft, S., Gandy, S., Buettner, C., & Stoeckel, L. E. (2018). Brain insulin resistance in type 2 diabetes and Alzheimer disease: Concepts and conundrums. *Nature Reviews Neurology, 14,* 168.

Augustin, R. (2010). The protein family of glucose transport facilitators: It's not only about glucose after all. *International Union of Biochemistry and Molecular Biology, 62,* 315–333.

Avgerinos, K. I., Egan, J. M., Mattson, M. P., & Kapogiannis, D. (2020). Medium chain triglycerides induce mild ketosis and may improve cognition in Alzheimer's disease: A systematic review and meta-analysis of human studies. *Ageing Research Reviews,* 101001. doi:10.1016/j.arr.2019.101001. Epub 2019 Dec 20. PMID: 31870908; PMCID: PMC7050425.

Avogaro, A., Crepaldi, C., Miola, M., Maran, A., Pengo, V., Tiengo, A., & Del Prato, S. (1996). High blood ketone body concentration in type 2 non-insulin dependent diabetic patients. *Journal of Endocrinological Investigation, 19,* 99–105.

Avogaro, A., Valerio, A., Gnudi, L., Maran, A., Zolli, M., Duner, E., Riccio, A., Del Prato, S., Tiengo, A., & Nosadini, R. (1992). Ketone body metabolism in NIDDM: Effect of sulfonylurea treatment. *Diabetes, 41,* 968–974.

Baker, L. D., Cross, D. J., Minoshima, S., Belongia, D., Watson, G. S., & Craft, S. (2011). Insulin resistance and Alzheimer-like reductions in regional cerebral glucose metabolism for cognitively normal adults with prediabetes or early type 2 diabetes. *Archives of Neurology, 68,* 51–57.

Balasse, E. O., & Féry, F. (1989). Ketone body production and disposal: Effects of fasting, diabetes, and exercise. *Diabetes & Metabolism Reviews, 5,* 247–270.

Benson, D. F., Kuhl, D. E., Hawkins, R. A., Phelps, M. E., Cummings, J. L., & Tsai, S. (1983). The fluorodeoxyglucose 18F scan in Alzheimer's disease and multi-infarct dementia. *Archives of Neurology, 40,* 711–714.

Bergman, B. C., Cornier, M.-A., Horton, T. J., & Bessesen, D. H. (2007). Effects of fasting on insulin action and glucose kinetics in lean and obese men and women. *American Journal of Physiology-Endocrinology and Metabolism, 293,* E1103–E1111.

Berti, V., Vanzi, E., Polito, C., & Pupi, A. (2013). Back to the future: the absolute quantification of cerebral metabolic rate of glucose. *Clinical and Translational Imaging, 1,* 289–296.

Bickerton, A., Roberts, R., Fielding, B., Tornqvist, H., Blaak, E., Wagenmakers, A., Gilbert, M., Humphreys, S., Karpe, F., & Frayn, K. (2008). Adipose tissue fatty acid metabolism in insulin-resistant men. *Diabetologia, 51,* 1466.

Blomqvist, G., Alvarsson, M., Grill, V., Von Heijne, G., Ingvar, M., Thorell, J.-O., Stone-Elander, S., Widen, L., & Ekberg, K. (2002). Effect of acute hyperketonemia on the cerebral uptake of ketone bodies in nondiabetic subjects and IDDM patients. *American Journal of Physiology-Endocrinology and Metabolism, 283,* E20–E28.

Blomqvist, G., Thorell, J., Ingvar, M., Grill, V., Widen, L., & Stone-Elander, S. (1995). Use of R-beta-[1-^{11}C] hydroxybutyrate in PET studies of regional cerebral uptake of ketone bodies in humans. *American Journal of Physiology-Endocrinology and Metabolism, 269,* E948–E959.

Bondy, P. K., Bloom, W. L., Whitner, V. S., & Farrar, B. W. (1949). Studies of the role of the liver in human carbohydrate metabolism by the venous catheter technic. II. Patients with diabetic ketosis, before and after the administration of insulin. *Journal of Clinical Investigation, 28,* 1126–1133.

Bougneres, P., Lemmel, C., Ferre, P., & Bier, D. (1986). Ketone body transport in the human neonate and infant. *Journal of Clinical Investigation, 77,* 42–48.

Bournat, J. C., & Brown, C. W. (2010). Mitochondrial dysfunction in obesity. *Current Opinion in Endocrinology, Diabetes, and Obesity, 17,* 446.

Brandt, J., Buchholz, A., Henry-Barron, B., Vizthum, D., Avramopoulos, D., & Cervenka, M. C. (2019). Preliminary report on the feasibility and efficacy of the modified Atkins diet for treatment of mild cognitive impairment and early Alzheimer's disease. *Journal of Alzheimer's Disease, 68,* 969–981.

Broer, S., Broer, A., Schneider, H. P., Stegen, C., Halestrap, A. P., & Deitmer, J. W. (1999). Characterization of the high-affinity monocarboxylate transporter MCT2 in *Xenopus laevis* oocytes. *Biochemical Journal, 341*(Part 3), 529–535.

Brown, R. K., Bohnen, N. I., Wong, K. K., Minoshima, S., & Frey, K. A. (2014). Brain PET in suspected dementia: Patterns of altered FDG metabolism. *Radiographics, 34,* 684–701.

Brown, W. R., & Thore, C. R. (2011). Cerebral microvascular pathology in ageing and neurodegeneration. *Neuropathology and Applied Neurobiology, 37,* 56–74.

Brunengraber, H., & Roe, C. R. (2006). Anaplerotic molecules: Current and future. *Journal of Inherited Metabolic Disease, 29,* 327–331.

Bu, G. (2009). Apolipoprotein E and its receptors in Alzheimer's disease: Pathways, pathogenesis and therapy. *Nature Reviews Neuroscience, 10,* 333–344.

Bubber, P., Haroutunian, V., Fisch, G., Blass, J. P., & Gibson, G. E. (2005). Mitochondrial abnormalities in Alzheimer brain: Mechanistic implications. *Annals of Neurology, 57,* 695–703.

Burant, C. F., & Bell, G. I. (1992). Mammalian facilitative glucose transporters: Evidence for similar substrate recognition sites in functionally monomeric proteins. *Biochemistry, 31,* 10414–10420.

Butterfield, D. A., & Halliwell, B. (2019). Oxidative stress, dysfunctional glucose metabolism and Alzheimer disease. *Nature Reviews Neuroscience, 20,* 148–160.

Cahill, G. F., Jr. (2006). Fuel metabolism in starvation. *Annual Review of Nutrition, 26,* 1–22.

Carpenter, L., & Halestrap, A. P. (1994). The kinetics, substrate and inhibitor specificity of the lactate transporter of Ehrlich-Lettre tumour cells studied with the intracellular pH indicator BCECF. *Biochemical Journal, 304,* 751–760.

Castellano, C.-A., Baillargeon, J.-P., Nugent, S., Tremblay, S., Fortier, M., Imbeault, H., Duval, J., & Cunnane, S. C. (2015a). Regional brain glucose hypometabolism in young women with polycystic ovary syndrome: Possible link to mild insulin resistance. *PLOS ONE, 10*(12), e0144116.

Castellano, C.-A., Paquet, N., Dionne, I. J., Imbeault, H., Langlois, F., Croteau, E., Tremblay, S., Fortier, M., Matte, J. J., & Lacombe, G. (2017). A 3-month aerobic training program improves brain energy metabolism in mild Alzheimer's disease: Preliminary results from a neuroimaging study. *Journal of Alzheimer's Disease, 56,* 1459–1468.

Castellano, C. A., Hudon, C., Croteau, E., Fortier, M., St-Pierre, V., Vandenberghe, C., Nugent, S., Tremblay, S., Paquet, N., Lepage, M., et al. (2019). Links between metabolic and structural changes in the brain of cognitively normal older adults: A 4-year longitudinal follow-up. *Frontiers in Aging Neuroscience, 11,* 15.

Castellano, C. A., Nugent, S., Paquet, N., Tremblay, S., Bocti, C., Lacombe, G., Imbeault, H., Turcotte, E., Fulop, T., & Cunnane, S. C. (2015b). Lower brain ¹⁸F-fluorodeoxyglucose uptake but normal ¹¹C-acetoacetate metabolism in mild Alzheimer's disease dementia. *Journal of Alzheimer's Disease, 43,* 1343–1353.

Chan, S. C., Esther, G. E., Yip, H. L., Sugathan, S., & Chin, P. S. (2017). Effect of cold pressed coconut oil on cognition and behavior among patients with Alzheimer's disease—A pilot intervention study. *National Journal of Physiology, Pharmacy and Pharmacology, 7,* 1432–1435.

Chawluk, J. B., Alavi, A., Dann, R., Hurtig, H. I., Bais, S., Kushner, M. J., Zimmerman, R. A., & Reivich, M. (1987). Positron emission tomography in aging and dementia: Effect of cerebral atrophy. *Age, 65,* 9.

Choi, D.-Y., Lee, Y.-J., Hong, J. T., & Lee, H.-J. (2012). Antioxidant properties of natural polyphenols and their therapeutic potentials for Alzheimer's disease. *Brain Research Bulletin, 87,* 144–153.

Chowdhury, G. M., Jiang, L., Rothman, D. L., & Behar, K. L. (2014). The contribution of ketone bodies to basal and activity-dependent neuronal oxidation in vivo. *Journal of Cerebral Blood Flow & Metabolism, 34,* 1233–1242.

Clarke, K., Tchabanenko, K., Pawlosky, R., Carter, E., Todd King, M., Musa-Veloso, K., Ho, M., Roberts, A., Robertson, J., Vanitallie, T. B., et al. (2012). Kinetics, safety and tolerability of (R)-3-hydroxybutyl (R)-3-hydroxybutyrate in healthy adult subjects. *Regulatory Toxicology and Pharmacology, 63,* 401–408.

Claxton, A., Baker, L. D., Hanson, A., Trittschuh, E. H., Cholerton, B., Morgan, A., Callaghan, M., Arbuckle, M., Behl, C., & Craft, S. (2015). Long-acting intranasal insulin detemir improves cognition for adults with mild cognitive impairment or early-stage Alzheimer's disease dementia. *Journal of Alzheimer's Disease, 44,* 897–906.

Courchesne-Loyer, A., Croteau, E., Castellano, C.-A., St-Pierre, V., Hennebelle, M., & Cunnane, S.C. (2017a). Inverse relationship between brain glucose and ketone metabolism in adults during short-term moderate dietary ketosis: A dual tracer quantitative positron emission tomography study. *Journal of Cerebral Blood Flow & Metabolism, 37,* 2485–2493.

Courchesne-Loyer, A., Fortier, M., Tremblay-Mercier, J., Chouinard-Watkins, R., Roy, M., Nugent, S., Castellano, C.-A., & Cunnane, S. C. (2013). Stimulation of mild, sustained ketonemia by medium-chain triacylglycerols in healthy humans: Estimated potential contribution to brain energy metabolism. *Nutrition, 29,* 635–640.

Courchesne-Loyer, A., Lowry, C.-M., St-Pierre, V., Vandenberghe, C., Fortier, M., Castellano, C.-A., Wagner, J. R., & Cunnane, S. C. (2017b). Emulsification increases the acute ketogenic effect and bioavailability of medium-chain triglycerides in humans: Protein, carbohydrate, and fat metabolism. *Current Developments in Nutrition, 1,* Article e000851.

Craft, S. (2009). The role of metabolic disorders in Alzheimer disease and vascular dementia: Two roads converged. *Archives of Neurology, 66,* 300–305.

Croteau, E., Castellano, C.-A., Richard, M. A., Fortier, M., Nugent, S., Lepage, M., Duchesne, S., Whittingstall, K., Turcotte, É. E., & Bocti, C. (2018a). Ketogenic medium chain triglycerides increase brain energy metabolism in Alzheimer's disease. *Journal of Alzheimer's Disease, 64,* 551–561.

Croteau, E., Castellano, C., Fortier, M., Bocti, C., Fulop, T., Paquet, N., & Cunnane, S. (2018b). A cross-sectional comparison of brain glucose and ketone metabolism in cognitively healthy older adults, mild cognitive impairment and early Alzheimer's disease. *Experimental Gerontology, 107,* 18–26.

Cunnane, S., Trushina, E., Morland, C., & Prigione, A. (2020). Brain energy rescue: An emerging therapeutic concept for neurodegenerative disorders of ageing. *Nature Reviews Drug Discovery, 19,* 609–633.

Cunnane, S. C., Courchesne-Loyer, A., St-Pierre, V., Vandenberghe, C., Pierotti, T., Fortier, M., Croteau, E., & Castellano, C. A. (2016). Can ketones compensate for deteriorating brain glucose uptake during aging? Implications for the risk and treatment of Alzheimer's disease. *Annals of the New York Academy of Sciences, 1367,* 12–20.

Cutler, N. R., Haxby, J. V., Duara, R., Grady, C. L., Kay, A. D., Kessler, R. M., Sundaram, M., & Rapoport, S. I. (1985). Clinical history, brain metabolism, and neuropsychological function in Alzheimer's disease. *Annals of Neurology, 18,* 298–309.

Daikhin, Y., & Yudkoff, M. (1998). Ketone bodies and brain glutamate and GABA metabolism. *Developmental Neuroscience, 20,* 358–364.

Dangour, A. D., Whitehouse, P. J., Rafferty, K., Mitchell, S. A., Smith, L., Hawkesworth, S., & Vellas, B. (2010). B-vitamins and fatty acids in the prevention and treatment of Alzheimer's disease and dementia: A systematic review. *Journal of Alzheimer's Disease, 22,* 205–224.

Dastur, D. K., Lane, M. H., Hansen, D. B., Kety, S. S., Butler, R. N., Perlin, S., & Sokoloff, L. (1963). Effects of aging on cerebral circulation and metabolism in man. *Human Aging: A Biological and Behavioral Study*, 1, 57–76.

De Felice, F. G., & Ferreira, S. T. (2014). Inflammation, defective insulin signaling, and mitochondrial dysfunction as common molecular denominators connecting type 2 diabetes to Alzheimer disease. *Diabetes*, 63, 2262–2272.

de la Rubia Ortí, J. E., García-Pardo, M. P., Drehmer, E., Sancho Cantus, D., Julián Rochina, M., Aguilar, M. A., & Hu Yang, I. (2018). Improvement of main cognitive functions in patients with Alzheimer's disease after treatment with coconut oil enriched Mediterranean diet: A pilot study. *Journal of Alzheimer's Disease*, 65, 577–587.

de Leon, M. J., Ferris, S. H., George, A. E., Christman, D. R., Fowler, J. S., Gentes, C., Reisberg, B., Gee, B., Emmerich, M., & Yonekura, Y. (1983). Positron emission tomographic studies of aging and Alzheimer disease. *American Journal of Neuroradiology*, 4, 568–571.

De Santi, S., de Leon, M. J., Convit, A., Tarshish, C., Rusinek, H., Tsui, W. H., Sinaiko, E., Wang, G.-J., Bartlet, E., & Volkow, N. (1995). Age-related changes in brain: II. Positron emission tomography of frontal and temporal lobe glucose metabolism in normal subjects. *Psychiatric Quarterly*, 66, 357–370.

De Santi, S., de Leon, M. J., Rusinek, H., Convit, A., Tarshish, C. Y., Roche, A., Tsui, W. H., Kandil, E., Boppana, M., & Daisley, K. (2001). Hippocampal formation glucose metabolism and volume losses in MCI and AD. *Neurobiology of Aging*, 22, 529–539.

Del Sole, A., Clerici, F., Chiti, A., Lecchi, M., Mariani, C., Maggiore, L., Mosconi, L., & Lucignani, G. (2008). Individual cerebral metabolic deficits in Alzheimer's disease and amnestic mild cognitive impairment: An FDG PET study. *European Journal of Nuclear Medicine and Molecular Imaging*, 35, 1357.

Dienel, G. A. (2019). Brain glucose metabolism: Integration of energetics with function. *Physiological Reviews*, 99, 949–1045.

Dong, Y., & Brewer, G. J. (2019). Global metabolic shifts in age and Alzheimer's disease mouse brains pivot at NAD+/NADH redox sites. *Journal of Alzheimer's Disease*, 71, 119–140.

Drenick, E. J., Alvarez, L. C., Tamasi, G. C., & Brickman, A. S. (1972). Resistance to symptomatic insulin reactions after fasting. *Journal of Clinical Investigation*, 51, 2757–2762.

Drzezga, A., Lautenschlager, N., Siebner, H., Riemenschneider, M., Willoch, F., Minoshima, S., Schwaiger, M., & Kurz, A. (2003). Cerebral metabolic changes accompanying conversion of mild cognitive impairment into Alzheimer's disease: A PET follow-up study. *European Journal of Nuclear Medicine and Molecular Imaging*, 30, 1104–1113.

Edmond, J., Robbins, R., Bergstrom, J., Cole, R., & De Vellis, J. (1987). Capacity for substrate utilization in oxidative metabolism by neurons, astrocytes, and oligodendrocytes from developing brain in primary culture. *Journal of Neuroscience Research*, 18, 551–561.

Elia, M., Stubbs, R., & Henry, C. (1999). Differences in fat, carbohydrate, and protein metabolism between lean and obese subjects undergoing total starvation. *Obesity Research*, 7, 597–604.

Elia, M., Wood, S., Khan, K., & Pullicino, E. (1990). Ketone body metabolism in lean male adults during short-term starvation, with particular reference to forearm muscle metabolism. *Clinical Science*, 78, 579–584.

Ewers, M., Brendel, M., Rizk-Jackson, A., Rominger, A., Bartenstein, P., Schuff, N., Weiner, M. W., & Initiative, A.s.D.N. (2014). Reduced FDG-PET brain metabolism and executive function predict clinical progression in elderly healthy subjects. *NeuroImage: Clinical*, 4, 45–52.

Fery, F., & Balasse, E. (1986). Response of ketone body metabolism to exercise during transition from postabsorptive to fasted state. *American Journal of Physiology-Endocrinology and Metabolism*, 250, E495–E501.

Fery, F., & Balasse, E. (1988). Effect of exercise on the disposal of infused ketone bodies in humans. *Journal of Clinical Endocrinology & Metabolism*, 67, 245–250.

Fery, F., & Balasse, E. O. (1983). Ketone body turnover during and after exercise in overnight-fasted and starved humans. *American Journal of Physiology-Endocrinology and Metabolism*, 245, E318–E325.

Féry, F., & Balasse, E. O. (1985). Ketone body production and disposal in diabetic ketosis: A comparison with fasting ketosis. *Diabetes*, 34, 326–332.

Flatt, J. (1972). On the maximal possible rate of ketogenesis. *Diabetes*, 21, 50–53.

Forsythe, C. E., Phinney, S. D., Fernandez, M. L., Quann, E. E., Wood, R. J., Bibus, D. M., Kraemer, W. J., Feinman, R. D., & Volek, J. S. (2008). Comparison of low fat and low carbohydrate diets on circulating fatty acid composition and markers of inflammation. *Lipids*, 43, 65–77.

Fortier, M., Castellano, C.-A., Croteau, E., Langlois, F., Bocti, C., St-Pierre, V., Vandenberghe, C., Bernier, M., Roy, M., & Descoteaux, M. (2019). A ketogenic drink improves brain energy and some measures of cognition in mild cognitive impairment. *Alzheimer's & Dementia*, 15, 625–634.

Fourest-Fontecave, S., Adamson, U., Lins, P., Ekblom, B., Sandahl, C., & Strand, L. (1987). Mental alertness in response to hypoglycaemia in normal man: The effect of 12 hours and 72 hours of fasting. *Diabetes & Metabolism*, 13, 405–410.

Fox, N., Kennedy, A., Harvey, R. J., Lantos, P., Roques, P., Collinge, J., Hardy, J., Hutton, M., Stevens, J., & Warrington, E. (1997). Clinicopathological features of familial Alzheimer's disease associated with the M139V mutation in the presenilin 1 gene: Pedigree but not mutation specific age at onset provides evidence for a further genetic factor. *Brain*, *120*, 491–501.

Freemantle, E., Vandal, M., Tremblay Mercier, J., Plourde, M., Poirier, J., & Cunnane, S. C. (2009). Metabolic response to a ketogenic breakfast in the healthy elderly. *Journal of Nutrition, Health & Aging*, *13*, 293–298.

Garber, A., Menzel, P., Boden, G., & Owen, O. (1974a). Hepatic ketogenesis and gluconeogenesis in humans. *Journal of Clinical Investigation*, *54*, 981–989.

Garber, A. J., Menzel, P. H., Boden, G., & Owen, O. E. (1974b). Hepatic ketogenesis and gluconeogenesis in humans. *Journal of Clinical Investigation*, *54*, 981–989.

Gejl, M., Gjedde, A., Egefjord, L., Møller, A., Hansen, S. B., Vang, K., Rodell, A., Brændgaard, H., Gottrup, H., & Schacht, A. (2016). In Alzheimer's disease, 6-month treatment with GLP-1 analog prevents decline of brain glucose metabolism: Randomized, placebo-controlled, double-blind clinical trial. *Frontiers in Aging Neuroscience*, *8*, 108.

Gerhart, D. Z., Enerson, B. E., Zhdankina, O. Y., Leino, R. L., & Drewes, L. R. (1997). Expression of monocarboxylate transporter MCT1 by brain endothelium and glia in adult and suckling rats. *American Journal of Physiology-Endocrinology and Metabolism*, *273*, E207–E213.

Gibson, G. E., Starkov, A., Blass, J. P., Ratan, R. R., & Beal, M. F. (2010). Cause and consequence: Mitochondrial dysfunction initiates and propagates neuronal dysfunction, neuronal death and behavioral abnormalities in age-associated neurodegenerative diseases. *Biochimica et Biophysica Acta-Molecular Basis of Disease*, *1802*, 122–134.

Gjedde, A., & Crone, C. (1975). Induction processes in blood-brain transfer of ketone bodies during starvation. *American Journal of Physiology-Legacy Content*, *229*, 1165–1169.

Göschke, H. (1977). Mechanism of glucose intolerance during fasting: Differences between lean and obese subjects. *Metabolism*, *26*, 1147–1153.

Gottstein, U., Mueller, W., Berghoff, W., Gaertner, H., & Held, K. (1971). Utilization of non-esterified fatty acids and ketone nbodies in human brain. *Klinische Wochenschrift*, *49*(7), 406–411.

Gupta, P. P., Pandey, R. D., Jha, D., Shrivastav, V., & Kumar, S. (2015). Role of traditional nonsteroidal anti-inflammatory drugs in Alzheimer's disease: A meta-analysis of randomized clinical trials. *American Journal of Alzheimer's Disease & Other Dementias*, *30*, 178–182.

Guzmán, M., & Blázquez, C. (2004). Ketone body synthesis in the brain: Possible neuroprotective effects. *Prostaglandins, Leukotrienes and Essential Fatty Acids*, *70*, 287–292.

Hall, S., Wastney, M., Bolton, T., Braaten, J., & Berman, M. (1984). Ketone body kinetics in humans: The effects of insulin-dependent diabetes, obesity, and starvation. *Journal of Lipid Research*, *25*, 1184–1194.

Harvey, C., Richard, J., Cliff, J., Schofield, G. M., Williden, M., & McQuillan, J. A. (2018). The effect of medium chain triglycerides on time to nutritional ketosis and symptoms of keto-induction in healthy adults: A randomised controlled clinical trial. *Journal of Nutrition and Metabolism*, 2630565. doi:10.1155/2018/2630565. PMID: 29951312; PMCID: PMC5987302.

Hasan-Olive, M. M., Lauritzen, K. H., Ali, M., Rasmussen, L. J., Storm-Mathisen, J., & Bergersen, L. H. (2019). A ketogenic diet improves mitochondrial biogenesis and bioenergetics via the PGC1α-SIRT3-UCP2 axis. *Neurochemical Research*, *44*, 22–37.

Hasselbalch, S. G., Knudsen, G. M., Jakobsen, J., Hageman, L. P., Holm, S., & Paulson, O. B. (1994). Brain metabolism during short-term starvation in humans. *Journal of Cerebral Blood Flow & Metabolism*, *14*, 125–131.

Hasselbalch, S. G., Madsen, P. L., Hageman, L. P., Olsen, K. S., Justesen, N., Holm, S., & Paulson, O. B. (1996). Changes in cerebral blood flow and carbohydrate metabolism during acute hyperketonemia. *American Journal of Physiology-Endocrinology And Metabolism*, *270*, E746–E751.

Henderson, S. T., Vogel, J. L., Barr, L. J., Garvin, F., Jones, J. J., & Costantini, L. C. (2009). Study of the ketogenic agent AC-1202 in mild to moderate Alzheimer's disease: A randomized, double-blind, placebo-controlled, multicenter trial. *Nutrition & Metabolism*, *6*, 31.

Hoyer, S. (1992). Oxidative energy metabolism in Alzheimer brain. *Molecular and Chemical Neuropathology*, *16*, 207–224.

Hoyer, S., Oesterreich, K., & Wagner, O. (1988). Glucose metabolism as the site of the primary abnormality in early-onset dementia of Alzheimer type? *Journal of Neurology*, *235*, 143–148.

Hu, E., Du, H., Zhu, X., Wang, L., Shang, S., Wu, X., Lu, H., & Lu, X. (2018). Beta-hydroxybutyrate promotes the expression of BDNF in hippocampal neurons under adequate glucose supply. *Neuroscience*, *386*, 315–325.

Hu Yang, I., Ortí, R., Selvi Sabater, P., Sancho Castillo, S., Rochina, M. J., Manresa Ramón, N., & Montoya-Castilla, I. (2015). Aceite de coco: Tratamiento alternativo no farmacológico frente a la enfermedad de Alzheimer. *Nutrición Hospitalaria*, *32*, 2822–2827.

Hugo, S. E., Cruz-Garcia, L., Karanth, S., Anderson, R. M., Stainier, D. Y., & Schlegel, A. (2012). A monocarboxylate transporter required for hepatocyte secretion of ketone bodies during fasting. *Genes & Development, 26*, 282–293.

Kalpouzos, G., Chételat, G., Baron, J.-C., Landeau, B., Mevel, K., Godeau, C., Barré, L., Constans, J.-M., Viader, F., & Eustache, F. (2009). Voxel-based mapping of brain gray matter volume and glucose metabolism profiles in normal aging. *Neurobiology of Aging, 30*, 112–124.

Kashiwaya, Y., Bergman, C., Lee, J.-H., Wan, R., King, M. T., Mughal, M. R., Okun, E., Clarke, K., Mattson, M. P., & Veech, R. L. (2013). A ketone ester diet exhibits anxiolytic and cognition-sparing properties, and lessens amyloid and tau pathologies in a mouse model of Alzheimer's disease. *Neurobiology of Aging, 34*, 1530–1539.

Kashiwaya, Y., Takeshima, T., Mori, N., Nakashima, K., Clarke, K., & Veech, R. L. (2000). D-β-Hydroxybutyrate protects neurons in models of Alzheimer's and Parkinson's disease. *Proceedings of the National Academy of Sciences of the United States of America, 97*, 5440–5444.

Kawas, C., Gray, S., Brookmeyer, R., Fozard, J., & Zonderman, A. (2000). Age-specific incidence rates of Alzheimer's disease: The Baltimore Longitudinal Study of Aging. *Neurology, 54*, 2072–2077.

Kennedy, A. M., Frackowiak, R. S., Newman, S. K., Bloomfield, P. M., Seaward, J., Roques, P., Lewington, G., Cunningham, V. J., & Rossor, M. N. (1995). Deficits in cerebral glucose metabolism demonstrated by positron emission tomography in individuals at risk of familial Alzheimer's disease. *Neuroscience Letters, 186*, 17–20.

Kim, D. Y., Davis, L. M., Sullivan, P. G., Maalouf, M., Simeone, T. A., Brederode, J. V., & Rho, J. M. (2007). Ketone bodies are protective against oxidative stress in neocortical neurons. *Journal of Neurochemistry, 101*, 1316–1326.

Kim, J.-A., Wei, Y., & Sowers, J. R. (2008). Role of mitochondrial dysfunction in insulin resistance. *Circulation Research, 102*, 401–414.

Koenig, A. M., Mechanic-Hamilton, D., Xie, S. X., Combs, M. F., Cappola, A. R., Xie, L., Detre, J. A., Wolk, D. A., & Arnold, S. E. (2017). Effects of the insulin sensitizer metformin in Alzheimer's disease: Pilot data from a randomized placebo-controlled crossover study. *Alzheimer Disease and Associated Disorders, 31*, 107.

Kossoff, E. H., Zupec-Kania, B. A., Amark, P. E., Ballaban-Gil, K. R., Christina Bergqvist, A., Blackford, R., Buchhalter, J. R., Caraballo, R. H., Helen Cross, J., & Dahlin, M. G. (2009). Optimal clinical management of children receiving the ketogenic diet: Recommendations of the International Ketogenic Diet Study Group. *Epilepsia, 50*, 304–317.

Krikorian, R., Shidler, M. D., Dangelo, K., Couch, S. C., Benoit, S. C., & Clegg, D. J. (2012). Dietary ketosis enhances memory in mild cognitive impairment. *Neurobiology of Aging, 33*, e419–e427.

LaManna, J. C., Salem, N., Puchowicz, M., Erokwu, B., Koppaka, S., Flask, C., & Lee, Z. (2009). Ketones suppress brain glucose consumption. In Liss P., Hansell P., Bruley D. F., Harrison D. K. (eds.), *Oxygen Transport to Tissue XXX. Advances in Experimental Medicine and Biology, 645*, pp. 301–306. Springer, Boston, MA. https://doi.org/10.1007/978-0-387-85998-9_45

Langbaum, J. B., Chen, K., Lee, W., Reschke, C., Bandy, D., Fleisher, A. S., Alexander, G. E., Foster, N. L., Weiner, M. W., & Koeppe, R. A. (2009). Categorical and correlational analyses of baseline fluorodeoxyglucose positron emission tomography images from the Alzheimer's Disease Neuroimaging Initiative (ADNI). *Neuroimage, 45*, 1107–1116.

Leijenaar, J. F., van Maurik, I. S., Kuijer, J. P., van der Flier, W. M., Scheltens, P., Barkhof, F., & Prins, N. D. (2017). Lower cerebral blood flow in subjects with Alzheimer's dementia, mild cognitive impairment, and subjective cognitive decline using two-dimensional phase-contrast magnetic resonance imaging. *Alzheimer's & Dementia: Diagnosis, Assessment & Disease Monitoring, 9*, 76–83.

Li, W., Risacher, S. L., Huang, E., Saykin, A. J., & Alzheimer's Disease Neuroimaging Initiative. (2016). Type 2 diabetes mellitus is associated with brain atrophy and hypometabolism in the ADNI cohort. *Neurology, 87*, 595–600.

Li, Y., Rinne, J. O., Mosconi, L., Pirraglia, E., Rusinek, H., DeSanti, S., Kemppainen, N., Någren, K., Kim, B.-C., & Tsui, W. (2008). Regional analysis of FDG and PIB-PET images in normal aging, mild cognitive impairment, and Alzheimer's disease. *European Journal of Nuclear Medicine and Molecular Imaging, 35*, 2169–2181.

Liu, Y., Liu, F., Iqbal, K., Grundke-Iqbal, I., & Gong, C.-X. (2008). Decreased glucose transporters correlate to abnormal hyperphosphorylation of tau in Alzheimer disease. *FEBS Letters, 582*, 359–364.

Lobo, A., Launer, L., Fratiglioni, L., Andersen, K., Di Carlo, A., Breteler, M., Copeland, J., Dartigues, J., Jagger, C., & Martinez-Lage, J. (2000). Prevalence of dementia and major subtypes in Europe: A collaborative study of population-based cohorts. *Neurology, 54*, S4.

London, E. D., Margolin, R. A., Duara, R., Holloway, H. W., Robertson-tchabo, E. A., Cutler, N. R., & Rapoport, S. I. (1986). Effects of fasting on ketone body concentrations in healthy men of different ages. *Journal of Gerontology, 41*, 599–604.

Lying-Tunell, U., Lindblad, B., Malmlund, H., & Persson, B. (1980). Cerebral blood flow and metabolic rate of oxygen, glucose, lactate, pyruvate, ketone bodies and amino acids: I. Young and old normal subjects. *Acta Neurologica Scandinavica* 62, 265–275.

Lying-Tunell, U., Lindblad, B., Malmlund, H., & Persson, B. (1981). Cerebral blood flow and metabolic rate of oxygen, glucose, lactate, pyruvate, ketone bodies and amino acids: II. Presinile dementia and normal-pressure hydrocephalus. *Acta Neurologica Scandinavica*, 63, 337–350.

Maalouf, M., Rho, J. M., & Mattson, M. P. (2009). The neuroprotective properties of calorie restriction, the ketogenic diet, and ketone bodies. *Brain Research Reviews*, 59, 293–315.

Madsen, P. L., Cruz, N. F., Sokoloff, L., & Dienel, G. A. (1999). Cerebral oxygen/glucose ratio is low during sensory stimulation and rises above normal during recovery: Excess glucose consumption during stimulation is not accounted for by lactate efflux from or accumulation in brain tissue. *Journal of Cerebral Blood Flow & Metabolism*, 19, 393–400.

Mahendran, Y., Vangipurapu, J., Cederberg, H., Stančáková, A., Pihlajamäki, J., Soininen, P., Kangas, A. J., Paananen, J., Civelek, M., & Saleem, N. K. (2013). Association of ketone body levels with hyperglycemia and type 2 diabetes in 9,398 Finnish men. *Diabetes*, 62, 3618–3626.

Maher, F., Davies-Hill, T. M., & Simpson, I. A. (1996). Substrate specificity and kinetic parameters of GLUT3 in rat cerebellar granule neurons. *Biochemical Journal*, 315, 827–831.

Mamelak, M. (2012). Sporadic Alzheimer's disease: The starving brain. *Journal of Alzheimer's Disease*, 31, 459–474.

Marengoni, A., Rizzuto, D., Fratiglioni, L., Antikainen, R., Laatikainen, T., Lehtisalo, J., Peltonen, M., Soininen, H., Strandberg, T., & Tuomilehto, J. (2018). The effect of a 2-year intervention consisting of diet, physical exercise, cognitive training, and monitoring of vascular risk on chronic morbidity—The FINGER randomized controlled trial. *JAMA*, 19, 355–360.

Martin, P. M., Gopal, E., Ananth, S., Zhuang, L., Itagaki, S., Prasad, B. M., Smith, S. B., Prasad, P. D., & Ganapathy, V. (2006). Identity of SMCT1 (SLC5A8) as a neuron-specific Na+-coupled transporter for active uptake of L-lactate and ketone bodies in the brain. *Journal of Neurochemistry*, 98, 279–288.

Maurer, I., Zierz, S., & Möller, H. J. (2000). A selective defect of cytochrome c oxidase is present in brain of Alzheimer disease patients. *Neurobiology of Aging*, 21, 455–462.

Mazereeuw, G., Lanctot, K. L., Chau, S. A., Swardfager, W., & Herrmann, N. (2012). Effects of omega-3 fatty acids on cognitive performance: A meta-analysis. *Neurobiology of Aging*, 33, e1417–e1428.

McNay, E. C., & Gold, P. E. (1999). Extracellular glucose concentrations in the rat hippocampus measured by zero-net-flux: Effects of microdialysis flow rate, strain, and age. *Journal of Neurochemistry*, 72, 785–790.

Meier-Ruge, W., & Bertoni-Freddari, C. (1997). Pathogenesis of decreased glucose turnover and oxidative phosphorylation in ischemic and trauma-induced dementia of the Alzheimer type. *Annals of the New York Academy of Sciences*, 826, 229–241.

Melichar, V., Drahota, Z., & Hahn, P. (1965). Changes in the blood levels of acetoacetate and ketone bodies in newborn infants. *Biology of the Neonate*, 8, 348–352.

Mey, J. T., Erickson, M. L., Axelrod, C. L., King, W. T., Flask, C. A., McCullough, A. J., & Kirwan, J. P. (2020). ß-Hydroxybutyrate is reduced in humans with obesity-related NAFLD and displays a dose-dependent effect on skeletal muscle mitochondrial respiration in vitro. *American Journal of Physiology-Endocrinology and Metabolism*, 319, E187–E195.

Mikkelsen, K. H., Seifert, T., Secher, N. H., Grøndal, T., & van Hall, G. (2015). Systemic, cerebral and skeletal muscle ketone body and energy metabolism during acute hyper-D-β-hydroxybutyratemia in post-absorptive healthy males. *Journal of Clinical Endocrinology & Metabolism*, 100, 636–643.

Minoshima, S., Giordani, B., Berent, S., Frey, K. A., Foster, N. L., & Kuhl, D. E. (1997). Metabolic reduction in the posterior cingulate cortex in very early Alzheimer's disease. *Annals of Neurology*, 42, 85–94.

Mochel, F., DeLonlay, P., Touati, G., Brunengraber, H., Kinman, R. P., Rabier, D., Roe, C. R., & Saudubray, J. M. (2005). Pyruvate carboxylase deficiency: Clinical and biochemical response to anaplerotic diet therapy. *Molecular Genetics and Metabolism*, 84, 305–312.

Mochel, F., Duteil, S., Marelli, C., Jauffret, C., Barles, A., Holm, J., Sweetman, L., Benoist, J.-F., Rabier, D., & Carlier, P. G. (2010). Dietary anaplerotic therapy improves peripheral tissue energy metabolism in patients with Huntington's disease. *European Journal of Human Genetics*, 18, 1057–1060.

Montagne, A., Nation, D. A., Sagare, A. P., Barisano, G., Sweeney, M. D., Chakhoyan, A., Pachicano, M., Joe, E., Nelson, A. R., & D'Orazio, L. M. (2020). APOE4 leads to blood–brain barrier dysfunction predicting cognitive decline. *Nature*, 581, 71–76.

Morris, A. (2005). Cerebral ketone body metabolism. *Journal of Inherited Metabolic Disease*, 28, 109–121.

Mosconi, L. (2005). Brain glucose metabolism in the early and specific diagnosis of Alzheimer's disease. *European Journal of Nuclear Medicine and Molecular Imaging*, 32, 486–510.

Mosconi, L., Berti, V., Swerdlow, R. H., Pupi, A., Duara, R., & de Leon, M. (2010). Maternal transmission of Alzheimer's disease: Prodromal metabolic phenotype and the search for genes. *Human Genomics, 4,* 170.

Mosconi, L., Brys, M., Switalski, R., Mistur, R., Glodzik, L., Pirraglia, E., Tsui, W., De Santi, S., & de Leon, M. J. (2007). Maternal family history of Alzheimer's disease predisposes to reduced brain glucose metabolism. *Proceedings of the National Academy of Sciences of the United States of America, 104,* 19067–19072.

Mosconi, L., De Santi, S., Brys, M., Tsui, W. H., Pirraglia, E., Glodzik-Sobanska, L., Rich, K. E., Switalski, R., Mehta, P. D., & Pratico, D. (2008a). Hypometabolism and altered cerebrospinal fluid markers in normal apolipoprotein E E4 carriers with subjective memory complaints. *Biological Psychiatry, 63,* 609–618.

Mosconi, L., Mistur, R., Switalski, R., Tsui, W. H., Glodzik, L., Li, Y., Pirraglia, E., De Santi, S., Reisberg, B., & Wisniewski, T. (2009). FDG-PET changes in brain glucose metabolism from normal cognition to pathologically verified Alzheimer's disease. *European Journal of Nuclear Medicine and Molecular Imaging, 36,* 811–822.

Mosconi, L., Pupi, A., & De Leon, M. J. (2008b). Brain glucose hypometabolism and oxidative stress in preclinical Alzheimer's disease. *Annals of the New York Academy of Sciences, 1147,* 180.

Mosconi, L., Sorbi, S., De Leon, M. J., Li, Y., Nacmias, B., Myoung, P. S., Tsui, W., Ginestroni, A., Bessi, V., & Fayyazz, M. (2006). Hypometabolism exceeds atrophy in presymptomatic early-onset familial Alzheimer's disease. *Journal of Nuclear Medicine, 47,* 1778–1786.

Mosconi, L., Tsui, W.-H., De Santi, S., Li, J., Rusinek, H., Convit, A., Li, Y., Boppana, M., & De Leon, M. (2005). Reduced hippocampal metabolism in MCI and AD: Automated FDG-PET image analysis. *Neurology, 64,* 1860–1867.

Mosconi, L., Tsui, W. H., Herholz, K., Pupi, A., Drzezga, A., Lucignani, G., Reiman, E. M., Holthoff, V., Kalbe, E., & Sorbi, S. (2008c). Multicenter standardized ^{18}F-FDG PET diagnosis of mild cognitive impairment, Alzheimer's disease, and other dementias. *Journal of Nuclear Medicine, 49,* 390–398.

Muneta, T., Kawaguchi, E., Nagai, Y., Matsumoto, M., Ebe, K., Watanabe, H., & Bando, H. (2016). Ketone body elevation in placenta, umbilical cord, newborn and mother in normal delivery. *Glycative Stress Research, 3,* 133–140.

Nestor, P. J., Fryer, T. D., Smielewski, P., & Hodges, J. R. (2003). Limbic hypometabolism in Alzheimer's disease and mild cognitive impairment. *Annals of Neurology, 54,* 343–351.

Neth, B. J., Mintz, A., Whitlow, C., Jung, Y., Sai, K. S., Register, T. C., Kellar, D., Lockhart, S. N.,

Hoscheidt, S., & Maldjian, J. (2020). Modified ketogenic diet is associated with improved cerebrospinal fluid biomarker profile, cerebral perfusion, and cerebral ketone body uptake in older adults at risk for Alzheimer's disease: A pilot study. *Neurobiology of Aging, 86,* 54–63.

Newport, M. T., Van Itallie, T. B., Kashiwaya, Y., King, M. T., & Veech, R. L. (2015). A new way to produce hyperketonemia: Use of ketone ester in a case of Alzheimer's disease. *Alzheimers Dementia, 11,* 99–103.

Newsholme, E., Randle, P., & Manchester, K. (1962). Inhibition of the phosphofructokinase reaction in perfused rat heart by respiration of ketone bodies, fatty acids and pyruvate. *Nature, 193,* 270–271.

Ngandu, T., Lehtisalo, J., Solomon, A., Levälahti, E., Ahtiluoto, S., Antikainen, R., Bäckman, L., Hänninen, T., Jula, A., and Laatikainen, T. (2015). A 2 year multidomain intervention of diet, exercise, cognitive training, and vascular risk monitoring versus control to prevent cognitive decline in at-risk elderly people (FINGER): A randomised controlled trial. *Lancet, 385,* 2255–2263.

Noda, C., & Ichihara, A. (1976). Control of ketogenesis from amino acids. *Journal of Biochemistry, 80*(5), 1159–1164.

Nosadini, R., Avogaro, A., Trevisan, R., Duner, E., Marescotti, C., Iori, E., Cobelli, C., & Toffolo, G. (1985). Acetoacetate and 3-hydroxybutyrate kinetics in obese and insulin-dependent diabetic humans. *American Journal of Physiology-Regulatory, Integrative and Comparative Physiology, 248,* R611–R620.

Novotny, E. (1996). Observation of cerebral ketone bodies by ^{1}H NMR spectroscopy. *Annals of Neurology, 40,* 385.

Nugent, S., Castellano, C. A., Goffaux, P., Whittingstall, K., Lepage, M., Paquet, N., Bocti, C., Fulop, T., & Cunnane, S. C. (2014a). Glucose hypometabolism is highly localized, but lower cortical thickness and brain atrophy are widespread in cognitively normal older adults. *American Journal of Physiology-Endocrinology and Metabolism, 306*(11), E1315–E1321.

Nugent, S., Tremblay, S., Chen, K. W., Ayutyanont, N., Roontiva, A., Castellano, C.-A., Fortier, M., Roy, M., Courchesne-Loyer, A., & Bocti, C. (2014b). Brain glucose and acetoacetate metabolism: A comparison of young and older adults. *Neurobiology of Aging, 35,* 1386–1395.

Ogawa, M., Fukuyama, H., Ouchi, Y., Yamauchi, H., & Kimura, J. (1996). Altered energy metabolism in Alzheimer's disease. *Journal of the Neurological Sciences, 139,* 78–82.

Öhman, H., Savikko, N., Strandberg, T. E., & Pitkälä, K. H. (2014). Effect of physical exercise on cognitive performance in older adults with mild cognitive impairment or dementia: A systematic review. *Dementia and Geriatric Cognitive Disorders*, 38, 347–365.

Ohnuma, T., Toda, A., Kimoto, A., Takebayashi, Y., Higashiyama, R., Tagata, Y., Ito, M., Ota, T., Shibata, N., & Arai, H. (2016). Benefits of use, and tolerance of, medium-chain triglyceride medical food in the management of Japanese patients with Alzheimer's disease: A prospective, open-label pilot study. *Clinical Interventions in Aging*, 11, 29.

Olefsky, J. M., & Glass, C. K. (2010). Macrophages, inflammation, and insulin resistance. *Annual Review of Physiology*, 72, 219–246.

Ota, M., Matsuo, J., Ishida, I., Takano, H., Yokoi, Y., Hori, H., Yoshida, S., Ashida, K., Nakamura, K., & Takahashi, T. (2019). Effects of a medium-chain triglyceride-based ketogenic formula on cognitive function in patients with mild-to-moderate Alzheimer's disease. *Neuroscience Letters*, 690, 232–236.

Owen, O., & Reichard, G. A. (1971). Human forearm metabolism during progressive starvation. *Journal of Clinical Investigation*, 50, 1536–1545.

Owen, O. E., Felig, P., Morgan, A. P., Wahren, J., & Cahill, G. F. (1969). Liver and kidney metabolism during prolonged starvation. *Journal of Clinical Investigation*, 48, 574–583.

Owen, O. E., Kalhan, S. C., & Hanson, R. W. (2002). The key role of anaplerosis and cataplerosis for citric acid cycle function. *Journal of Biological Chemistry*, 277, 30409–30412.

Owen, O. E., Morgan, A. P., Kemp, H. G., Sullivan, J. M., Herrera, M. G., & Cahill, G. F., Jr. (1967). Brain metabolism during fasting. *Journal of Clinical Investigation*, 46, 1589–1595.

Page, K. A., Williamson, A., Yu, N., McNay, E. C., Dzuira, J., McCrimmon, R. J., & Sherwin, R. S. (2009). Medium-chain fatty acids improve cognitive function in intensively treated type 1 diabetic patients and support in vitro synaptic transmission during acute hypoglycemia. *Diabetes*, 58, 1237–1244.

Page, M. A., Krebs, H., & Williamson, D. (1971). Activities of enzymes of ketone-body utilization in brain and other tissues of suckling rats. *Biochemical Journal*, 121, 49–53.

Pan, J. W., Rothman, D. L., Behar, K. L., Stein, D. T., & Hetherington, H. P. (2000). Human brain β-hydroxybutyrate and lactate increase in fasting-induced ketosis. *Journal of Cerebral Blood Flow & Metabolism*, 20, 1502–1507.

Pan, J. W., Telang, F. W., Lee, J. H., de Graaf, R. A., Rothman, D. L., Stein, D. T., & Hetherington, H. P. (2001). Measurement of beta-hydroxybutyrate in acute hyperketonemia in human brain. *Journal of Neurochemistry*, 79, 539–544.

Parker, W. D., Parks, J., Filley, C. M., & Kleinschmidt-DeMasters, B. (1994). Electron transport chain defects in Alzheimer's disease brain. *Neurology*, 44, 1090–1090.

Pascual, J. M., Liu, P., Mao, D., Kelly, D. I., Hernandez, A., Sheng, M., Good, L. B., Ma, Q., Marin-Valencia, I., & Zhang, X. (2014). Triheptanoin for glucose transporter type I deficiency (G1D): Modulation of human ictogenesis, cerebral metabolic rate, and cognitive indices by a food supplement. *JAMA Neurology*, 71, 1255–1265.

Patel, M., Johnson, C., Rajan, R., & Owen, O. (1975). The metabolism of ketone bodies in developing human brain: Development of ketone-body-utilizing enzymes and ketone bodies as precursors for lipid synthesis. *Journal of Neurochemistry*, 25, 905–908.

Pawlosky, R. J., Kemper, M. F., Kashiwaya, Y., King, M. T., Mattson, M. P., & Veech, R. L. (2017). Effects of a dietary ketone ester on hippocampal glycolytic and tricarboxylic acid cycle intermediates and amino acids in a 3xTg AD mouse model of Alzheimer's disease. *Journal of Neurochemistry*, 141, 195–207.

Perry, E. K., Perry, R. H., Tomlinson, B. E., Blessed, G., & Gibson, P. H. (1980). Coenzyme A-acetylating enzymes in Alzheimer's disease: Possible cholinergic 'compartment' of pyruvate dehydrogenase. *Neuroscience Letters*, 18, 105–110.

Petersen, R. C., Roberts, R. O., Knopman, D. S., Boeve, B. F., Geda, Y. E., Ivnik, R. J., Smith, G. E., & Jack, C. R. (2009). Mild cognitive impairment: Ten years later. *Archives of Neurology*, 66, 1447–1455.

Piert, M., Koeppe, R. A., Giordani, B., Berent, S., & Kuhl, D. E. (1996). Diminished glucose transport and phosphorylation in Alzheimer's disease determined by dynamic FDG-PET. *Journal of Nuclear Medicine*, 37, 201–208.

Profenno, L. A., Porsteinsson, A. P., & Faraone, S. V. (2010). Meta-analysis of Alzheimer's disease risk with obesity, diabetes, and related disorders. *Biological Psychiatry*, 67, 505–512.

Rahman, M., Muhammad, S., Khan, M. A., Chen, H., Ridder, D. A., Müller-Fielitz, H., Pokorná, B., Vollbrandt, T., Stölting, I., & Nadrowitz, R. (2014). The β-hydroxybutyrate receptor HCA 2 activates a neuroprotective subset of macrophages. *Nature Communications*, 5, 1–11.

Rebello, C. J., Keller, J. N., Liu, A. G., Johnson, W. D., & Greenway, F. L. (2015). Pilot feasibility and safety study examining the effect of medium chain triglyceride supplementation in subjects with mild cognitive impairment: A randomized controlled trial. *BBA Clinical*, 3, 123–125.

Reger, M. A., Henderson, S. T., Hale, C., Cholerton, B., Baker, L. D., Watson, G. S., Hyde, K., Chapman, D., & Craft, S. (2004). Effects of beta-hydroxybutyrate on cognition in memory-impaired adults. *Neurobiology of Aging*, 25, 311–314.

Reichard, G., Owen, O., Haff, A., Paul, P., & Bortz, W. (1974). Ketone-body production and oxidation in fasting obese humans. *Journal of Clinical Investigation*, 53, 508–515.

Reiman, E. M., Chen, K., Alexander, G. E., Caselli, R. J., Bandy, D., Osborne, D., Saunders, A. M., & Hardy, J. (2004). Functional brain abnormalities in young adults at genetic risk for late-onset Alzheimer's dementia. *Proceedings of the National Academy of Sciences of the United States of America*, 101, 284–289.

Reynisdottir, S., Ellerfeldt, K., Wahrenberg, H., Lithell, H., & Arner, P. (1994). Multiple lipolysis defects in the insulin resistance (metabolic) syndrome. *Journal of Clinical Investigation* 93, 2590–2599.

Roberts, R. O., Knopman, D. S., Cha, R. H., Mielke, M. M., Pankratz, V. S., Boeve, B. F., Kantarci, K., Geda, Y. E., Jack, C. R., & Petersen, R. C. (2014). Diabetes and elevated hemoglobin A1c levels are associated with brain hypometabolism but not amyloid accumulation. *Journal of Nuclear Medicine*, 55, 759–764.

Roe, C. R., & Mochel, F. (2006). Anaplerotic diet therapy in inherited metabolic disease: Therapeutic potential. *Journal of Inherited Metabolic Disease*, 29, 332–340.

Roy, M., Beauvieux, M. C., Naulin, J., El Hamrani, D., Gallis, J. L., Cunnane, S. C., & Bouzier-Sore, A. K. (2015). Rapid adaptation of rat brain and liver metabolism to a ketogenic diet: An integrated study using ¹H- and ¹³C-NMR spectroscopy. *Journal of Cerebral Blood Flow & Metababolism*, 35, 1154–1162.

Russell, R., & Taegtmeyer, H. (1991a). Changes in citric acid cycle flux and anaplerosis antedate the functional decline in isolated rat hearts utilizing acetoacetate. *Journal of Clinical Investigation*, 87, 384–390.

Russell, R., and Taegtmeyer, H. (1991b). Pyruvate carboxylation prevents the decline in contractile function of rat hearts oxidizing acetoacetate. *American Journal of Physiology-Heart and Circulatory Physiology*, 261, H1756–H1762.

Russell, R. L., Siedlak, S. L., Raina, A. K., Bautista, J. M., Smith, M. A., & Perry, G. (1999). Increased neuronal glucose-6-phosphate dehydrogenase and sulfhydryl levels indicate reductive compensation to oxidative stress in Alzheimer disease. *Archives of Biochemistry and Biophysics*, 370, 236–239.

Ryman, D. C., Acosta-Baena, N., Aisen, P. S., Bird, T., Danek, A., Fox, N. C., Goate, A., Frommelt, P., Ghetti, B., & Langbaum, J. B. (2014). Symptom onset in autosomal dominant Alzheimer disease: A systematic review and meta-analysis. *Neurology*, 83, 253–260.

Sapir, D., & Owen, O. (1975). Renal conservation of ketone bodies during starvation. *Metabolism*, 24, 23–33.

Sarda, P., Lepage, G., Roy, C. C., & Chessex, P. (1987). Storage of medium-chain triglycerides in adipose tissue of orally fed infants. *American Journal of Clinical Nutrition*, 45, 399–405.

Sato, K., Kashiwaya, Y., Keon, C., Tsuchiya, N., King, M., Radda, G., Chance, B., Clarke, K., & Veech, R. (1995). Insulin, ketone bodies, and mitochondrial energy transduction. *The Federation of American Societies for Experimental Biology Journal*, 9, 651–658.

Schöll, M., Almkvist, O., Bogdanovic, N., Wall, A., Långström, B., Viitanen, M., & Nordberg, A. (2011). Time course of glucose metabolism in relation to cognitive performance and postmortem neuropathology in Met146Val PSEN1 mutation carriers. *Journal of Alzheimer's Disease*, 24, 495–506.

Seaton, T. B., Welle, S. L., Warenko, M. K., & Campbell, R. G. (1986). Thermic effect of medium-chain and long-chain triglycerides in man. *American Journal of Clinical Nutrition*, 44, 630–634.

Settergren, G., Lindblad, B., & Persson, B. (1976). Cerebral blood flow and exchange of oxygen, glucose, ketone bodies, lactate, pyruvate and amino acids in infants. *Acta Pædiatrica*, 65, 343–353.

Silva, M. H. L., Silva, M. T. C., Brandão, S. C. C., Gomes, J. C., Peternelli, L. A., & Franceschini, S. do C. C. (2005). Fatty acid composition of mature breast milk in Brazilian women. *Food Chemistry*, 93, 297–303.

Simpson, I. A., Chundu, K. R., Davies-Hill, T., Honer, W. G., & Davies, P. (1994). Decreased concentrations of GLUT1 and GLUT3 glucose transporters in the brains of patients with Alzheimer's disease. *Annals of Neurology*, 35, 546–551.

Singh, B., Krentz, A., & Nattrass, M. (1993). Insulin resistance in the regulation of lipolysis and ketone body metabolism in non-insulin dependent diabetes is apparent at very low insulin concentrations. *Diabetes Research and Clinical Practice*, 20, 55 62.

Slooter, A. J., Cruts, M., Kalmijn, S., Hofman, A., Breteler, M. M., Van Broeckhoven, C., & van Duijn, C. M. (1998). Risk estimates of dementia by apolipoprotein E genotypes from a population-based incidence study: The Rotterdam Study. *Archives of Neurology*, 55, 964–968.

Soeters, M. R., Sauerwein, H. P., Faas, L., Smeenge, M., Duran, M., Wanders, R. J., Ruiter, A. F., Ackermans, M. T., Fliers, E., & Houten, S. M. (2009). Effects of insulin on ketogenesis following fasting in lean and obese men. *Obesity*, 17, 1326–1331.

Sokoloff, L. (1977). Relation between physiological function and energy metabolism in the central nervous system. *Journal of Neurochemistry*, 29, 13–26.

Sorbi, S., Bird, E. D., & Blass, J. P. (1983). Decreased pyruvate dehydrogenase complex activity in

Huntington and Alzheimer brain. *Annals of Neurology, 13*, 72–78.

Sorbi, S., Mortilla, M., Piacentini, S., Tonini, S., & Amaducci, L. (1990). Altered hexokinase activity in skin cultured fibroblasts and leukocytes from Alzheimer's disease patients. *Neuroscience Letters, 117*, 165–168.

St-Pierre, V., Vandenberghe, C., Lowry, C.-M., Fortier, M., Castellano, C.-A., Wagner, R., & Cunnane, S. C. (2019). Plasma ketone and medium chain fatty acid response in humans consuming different medium chain triglycerides during a metabolic study day. *Frontiers in Nutrition, 6*, 46.

Taegtmeyer, H. (1983). On the inability of ketone bodies to serve as the only energy providing substrate for rat heart at physiological work load. *Basic Research in Cardiology, 78*, 435–450.

Taegtmeyer, H., Hems, R., & Krebs, H. A. (1980). Utilization of energy-providing substrates in the isolated working rat heart. *Biochemical Journal, 186*, 701–711.

Talbot, K., Wang, H.-Y., Kazi, H., Han, L.-Y., Bakshi, K. P., Stucky, A., Fuino, R. L., Kawaguchi, K. R., Samoyedny, A. J., & Wilson, R. S. (2012). Demonstrated brain insulin resistance in Alzheimer's disease patients is associated with IGF-1 resistance, IRS-1 dysregulation, and cognitive decline. *Journal of Clinical Investigation, 122*, 1316–1338.

Tan, S.-X., Fisher-Wellman, K. H., Fazakerley, D. J., Ng, Y., Pant, H., Li, J., Meoli, C. C., Coster, A. C., Stöckli, J., & James, D. E. (2015). Selective insulin resistance in adipocytes. *Journal of Biological Chemistry, 290*, 11337–11348.

Taylor, M. K., Sullivan, D. K., Mahnken, J. D., Burns, J. M., & Swerdlow, R. H. (2018). Feasibility and efficacy data from a ketogenic diet intervention in Alzheimer's disease. *Alzheimer's & Dementia: Translational Research & Clinical Interventions, 4*, 28–36.

Tildon, J. T., & Roeder, L. M. (1988). Transport of 3-hydroxy [3-14C] butyrate by dissociated cells from rat brain. *American Journal of Physiology-Cell Physiology, 255*, C133–C139.

Torosyan, N., Sethanandha, C., Grill, J. D., Dilley, M. L., Lee, J., Cummings, J. L., Ossinalde, C., & Silverman, D. H. (2018). Changes in regional cerebral blood flow associated with a 45 day course of the ketogenic agent, caprylidene, in patients with mild to moderate Alzheimer's disease: Results of a randomized, double-blinded, pilot study. *Experimental Gerontology, 111*, 118–121.

Traul, K. A., Driedger, A., Ingle, D. L., & Nakhasi, D. (2000). Review of the toxicologic properties of medium-chain triglycerides. *Food & Chemical Toxicology, 38*, 79–98.

Vagelatos, N. T., & Eslick, G. D. (2013). Type 2 diabetes as a risk factor for Alzheimer's disease: The confounders, interactions, and neuropathology associated with this relationship. *Epidemiologic Reviews, 35*, 152–160.

Vandenberghe, C., Castellano, C.-A., Maltais, M., Fortier, M., St-Pierre, V., Dionne, I. J., & Cunnane, S. C. (2019). A short-term intervention combining aerobic exercise with medium-chain triglycerides (MCT) is more ketogenic than either MCT or aerobic exercise alone: A comparison of normoglycemic and prediabetic older women. *Applied Physiology, Nutrition, and Metabolism, 44*, 66–73.

Vandenberghe, C., St-Pierre, V., Fortier, M., Castellano, C.-A., Cuenoud, B., & Cunnane, S. C. (2020). Medium chain triglycerides modulate the ketogenic effect of a metabolic switch. *Frontiers in Nutrition, 7*, 3.

Vandenberghe, C., St-Pierre, V., Pierotti, T., Fortier, M., Castellano, C.-A., & Cunnane, S. C. (2017). Tricaprylin alone increases plasma ketone response more than coconut oil or other medium-chain triglycerides: An acute crossover study in healthy adults. *Current Developments in Nutrition, 1*, e000257.

Vega, G. L., Dunn, F. L., & Grundy, S. M. (2009). Impaired hepatic ketogenesis in moderately obese men with hypertriglyceridemia. *Journal of Investigative Medicine, 57*, 590–594.

Velliquette, R. A., O'Connor, T., & Vassar, R. (2005). Energy inhibition elevates β-secretase levels and activity and is potentially amyloidogenic in APP transgenic mice: Possible early events in Alzheimer's disease pathogenesis. *Journal of Neuroscience, 25*, 10874–10883.

Veneman, T., Mitrakou, A., Mokan, M., Cryer, P., & Gerich, J. (1994). Effect of hyperketonemia and hyperlacticacidemia on symptoms, cognitive dysfunction, and counterregulatory hormone responses during hypoglycemia in normal humans. *Diabetes, 43*, 1311–1317.

Vice, E., Privette, J. D., Hickner, R. C., & Barakat, H. A. (2005). Ketone body metabolism in lean and obese women. *Metabolism, 54*, 1542–1545.

Wahren, J., Sato, Y., Ostman, J., Hagenfeldt, L., & Felig, P. (1984). Turnover and splanchnic metabolism of free fatty acids and ketones in insulin-dependent diabetics at rest and in response to exercise. *Journal of Clinical Investigation, 73*, 1367–1376.

Wang, X., Su, B., Siedlak, S. L., Moreira, P. I., Fujioka, H., Wang, Y., Casadesus, G., & Zhu, X. (2008). Amyloid-β overproduction causes abnormal mitochondrial dynamics via differential modulation of mitochondrial fission/fusion proteins. *Proceedings of the National Academy of Sciences of the United States of America, 105*, 19318–19323.

Wang, X., Wang, W., Li, L., Perry, G., Lee, H.-G., & Zhu, X. (2014). Oxidative stress and mitochondrial dysfunction in Alzheimer's disease. *Biochimica et Biophysica Acta Molecular Basis of Disease, 1842*, 1240–1247.

Wieland, O., Funcke, H., & Löffler, G. (1971). Interconversion of pyruvate dehydrogenase in rat heart muscle upon perfusion with fatty acids or ketone bodies. *FEBS Letters, 15*, 295–298.

Willette, A. A., Bendlin, B. B., Starks, E. J., Birdsill, A. C., Johnson, S. C., Christian, B. T., Okonkwo, O. C., La Rue, A., Hermann, B. P., & Koscik, R. L. (2015). Association of insulin resistance with cerebral glucose uptake in late middle-aged adults at risk for Alzheimer disease. *JAMA Neurology, 72*, 1013–1020.

Williamson, D., Bates, M. W., Page, M. A., & Krebs, H. (1971). Activities of enzymes involved in acetoacetate utilization in adult mammalian tissues. *Biochemical Journal, 121*, 41–47.

Xin, L., Ipek, Ö., Beaumont, M., Shevlyakova, M., Christinat, N., Masoodi, M., Greenberg, N., Gruetter, R., & Cuenoud, B. (2018). Nutritional ketosis increases NAD$^+$/NADH ratio in healthy human brain: An in vivo study by ^{31}P-MRS. *Frontiers in Nutrition, 5*, 62.

Xu, Q., Zhang, Y., Zhang, X., Liu, L., Zhou, B., Mo, R., Li, Y., Li, H., Li, F., & Tao, Y. (2019). Medium-chain triglycerides improved cognition and lipid metabolomics in mild to moderate Alzheimer's disease patients with APOE4$^{-/-}$: A double-blind, randomized, placebo-controlled crossover trial. *Clinical Nutrition, 39*, 2092–2105.

Yin, F., Sancheti, H., Patil, I., & Cadenas, E. (2016a). Energy metabolism and inflammation in brain aging and Alzheimer's disease. *Free Radical Biology and Medicine, 100*, 108–122.

Yin, J. X., Maalouf, M., Han, P., Zhao, M., Gao, M., Dharshaun, T., Ryan, C., Whitelegge, J., Wu, J., & Eisenberg, D. (2016b). Ketones block amyloid entry and improve cognition in an Alzheimer's model. *Neurobiology of Aging, 39*, 25–37.

Yu, Y., Herman, P., Rothman, D. L., Agarwal, D., & Hyder, F. (2018). Evaluating the gray and white matter energy budgets of human brain function. *Journal of Cerebral Blood Flow & Metabolism, 38*, 1339–1353.

18

Ketogenic Diet and Ketones for Improving Neurologic Outcomes after Acute Neurotrauma

OSCAR SEIRA, PHD, KATHLEEN L. KOLEHMAINEN, PHD,
WARD T. PLUNET, PHD, CEREN YARAR-FISHER, PHD,
AND WOLFRAM TETZLAFF, MD, PHD

INTRODUCTION

In the United States alone, approximately 17,810 people sustain a traumatic spinal cord injury (SCI) every year and several hundred thousand are estimated to live with SCI (National Spinal Cord Injury Statistical Centre, https://www.nscisc.uab.edu/). The global incidence and prevalence of SCI are estimated to be around 1 million and 27 million, respectively (Global-Collaborators, 2019). The global incidence of traumatic brain injury (TBI) is about 30 times higher (27 million) and the prevalence is 55 million (Global-Collaborators, 2019). SCI has a devastating impact on the quality of life that goes beyond the obvious paralysis, including pain, spasticity, sexual dysfunction, respiratory problems, bowel and bladder disorders, skin ulcers, autonomic blood pressure dysregulation, cardiovascular disease, and metabolic disease, leading to a greatly reduced life expectancy. The economic burden of traumatic SCI is enormous, and the estimated lifetime costs range from $1.2 million for a person with incomplete paraplegia at age 50, to over $5 million for a person with complete tetraplegia at age 25 (NSCISC, 2020). This number does not include the loss of income and personal opportunities. In addition, the greatly reduced life expectancy—by up to 25 years—is often overlooked (NSCISC, 2020).

The acute management of SCI is mainly focused on surgical stabilization of the spinal column and decompression of the spinal cord to relieve extrinsic pressure from bone fragments (Hachem et al., 2017), and more recently the management of SCI has focused on tight blood pressure control (Squair et al., 2017). There are currently no neuroprotective or neurorestorative therapies available for SCI patients. Methylprednisolone, the only drug approved by the U.S. Food and Drug Administration (FDA),

showed only marginal neuroprotective effects when administered within 8 hr after injury (Bracken et al., 1998). Methylprednisolone has become the subject of lively debates over the past decades and is presently merely optional. The reality is that the only effective treatments for people with SCI to date are rehabilitation programs, together with medical care for the wide range of secondary complications listed above (scireproject.com). Rehabilitation interventions have led to significant improvements in the neurologic outcome after motor incomplete SCI, and promising unexpected strides were made in a few individuals with functionally complete SCI (Harkema et al., 2012). More recently, epidural stimulation protocols yielded remarkable improvements of locomotor (Angeli et al., 2018) and autonomic functions (West et al., 2018) in people with SCI that had been classified as functionally complete but evidently had some anatomical sparing.

However, there is still a large unmet clinical need for treatments to protect the damaged spinal cord from secondary damage in the wake of a primary injury. While little can be done for the immediate necrosis of the tissue due to mechanical destruction by the primary impact, the injury triggers a cascade of secondary damage due to vascular disruption, hemorrhage, edema, and ischemia, leading to energy depletion and ion pump failures, membrane depolarization, excitotoxicity, calcium overload, activation of proteases, free oxygen radical formation, cell membrane compromise, lipid peroxidation, protein nitrosylation, inflammation, and cell death through various mechanisms. Such secondary damage results in oligodendrocyte death with demyelination, axonal and neuronal losses, and permanent functional impairments (for reviews, see (Bareyre and Schwab, 2003; Hilton et al., 2017; Oyinbo, 2011).

The quest for treatments to mitigate secondary injury after neurotrauma has led to the preclinical discovery of numerous "neuroprotective" drug candidates (Kwon et al., 2011) as well as metabolic and dietary treatments/supplements. The latter include a number of health supplements and dietary regimes that are neuroprotective after acute SCI in rodents, including acetyl-L-carnitine (Patel et al., 2012), N-acetylcysteine (Patel et al., 2014), creatine (Rabchevsky et al., 2003), melatonin (Yang et al., 2016a), natural polyphenols from green tea, olive oil, resveratrol, and turmeric (for review, see (Khalatbary, 2014; Khalatbary and Khademi, 2020), inosine (Kim et al., 2013), and omega-3 enriched fish oils (Michael-Titus, 2007; Michael-Titus and Priestley, 2014) containing DHA (docosahexaenoic acid) and EPA (eicosapentaenoic acid) (Thau-Zuchman et al., 2020). Many of these approaches with "naturally occurring" nutrients and over-the-counter health supplements appear to have anti-inflammatory, anti-apoptotic, and antioxidant properties by mechanisms that are only partially understood, while some also enhance synaptic plasticity in the injured spinal cord of rodents (Kim et al., 2013). However, these treatment candidates have yet to be validated in clinical trials before becoming standard of care. Surprisingly, the nutritional guidelines for acute SCI are based on expert opinions and a few very small cohort studies (Class III/IV evidence;(Consortium_for_Spinal_Cord_Medicine, 2008; Rodriguez et al., 1997; Thibault-Halman et al., 2011). Nutrition is generally recommended within 24 hours after injury using a "balanced" enteral formula composed of carbohydrates, fat, and protein (Consortium_for_Spinal_Cord_Medicine, 2008; Thibault-Halman et al., 2011).

In contrast to the clinical guidelines, our laboratory discovered in rats that a form of caloric restriction known as intermittent fasting (every other day fasting—EODF) improved outcomes in acute cervical and thoracic SCI by promoting neuroprotection and neuroplasticity (Jeong et al., 2011; Plunet et al., 2010; Plunet et al., 2008). These results raise new and interesting questions, especially given the widely appreciated notion that intermittent fasting can have a positive impact on multiple chronic diseases in animal models and on parameters of metabolic, cardiovascular, and inflammatory diseases in humans (Longo and Mattson, 2014; Maalouf et al., 2009; Mattson et al., 2017). Despite the growing enthusiasm

for fasting in the research field in recent years, introducing such a regimen to acutely injured patients is met with little enthusiasm from clinicians, despite the fact that the caloric basal metabolic rate and energy expenditure requirements are drastically reduced after SCI due to paralysis (Cook et al., 2008; Magnuson et al., 2011), unlike in traumatic brain injury (TBI), where they may be increased (Cook et al., 2008). Fasting affects multiple pathways, including the generation of ketone bodies, most prominently D-β-hydroxybutyrate (βHB) and acetoacetate (AcAc), which have become increasingly known to be "neuroprotective" through their intensely studied role in ketogenic diets (KDs) for epilepsy (for reviews, see (Gano et al., 2014; Rho, 2015) and other chapters in this book). KDs are high in fat (typically 65% to 80%), adequate in protein (typically under 25%), and very low in carbohydrates (typically under 5%) and induce a fasting-like state without effectively fasting. The KDs or ketone supplementations have been shown to be beneficial in many neurologic disorders and models. About one third of the 226 hits in a search on the term *ketogenic diet* in the clinical trials.gov registry are trials for disorders of the nervous system (www.clinicaltrials.gov, July 2020).

This chapter reviews the neuroprotective effects of KDs and ketones as they relate to SCI and TBI, places them in context with data from using KDs in rodents with acute SCI, and discusses the KD's potential mechanisms. Due to the overlapping pathophysiology of SCI and TBI, the possible benefits of KD for both conditions are discussed.

KD IMPROVES FUNCTIONAL OUTCOME IN RODENT MODELS OF SCI

In addition to previously shown neuroprotective effects of KD/ketone administration, rats treated with intermittent fasting after SCI showed ketosis every second day. This evidence supported the rationale for performing a battery of tests to assess whether KD after rodent SCI could promote neuroprotection and neurorecovery (Streijger et al., 2013). A unilateral hemicontusion model of the cervical spinal cord was developed and applied in adult rats (Lee et al., 2012). At 4 hr after injury, access to ad lib KD consisting of a fat: protein + carbohydrate ratio of 3:1 was given and maintained for 12 weeks. Ketone levels reached 0.7 mmol/L at 24 hr and peaked around 1.8 mmol/L at 7 days after injury. While spinal cord injured rats showed a lower food intake on the first 2 days and lost more weight acutely after SCI, their weights returned to normal values within approximately 2 weeks, and both standard diet (SD) and KD rats gained weight above preinjury levels thereafter. We ruled out the possibility that the instinctive rejection of the novel food (KD) in the first days after injury was de facto fasting the rats and hence responsible for the improved recoveries seen with KD. The KD-fed rats used the forelimb on their injured side more frequently than carbohydrate-based SD-fed controls during vertical exploration of their environment in a cylinder. Importantly, this improvement was maintained beyond Week 12, when the KD was replaced by a SD. The KD-fed rats also displayed a greater active range of forelimb movement during grooming.

Given that hand function is the most coveted function in people with cervical SCI (Anderson, 2004), the rats were given two different reaching tests, and on both tasks the KD-fed rats showed an improved ability to reach forward and grasp a small pellet compared to SD-fed animals. Because reaching success indicates little about the strategy the animal uses to obtain the pellet, reaching can be broken down into discrete components of motion in time-lapse video analysis (Whishaw and Gorny, 1994). In our experiments, KD improved the pellet grasp and the subsequent supination that directs the pellet toward the mouth. Histologic analysis revealed that KD treatment resulted in smaller gray matter damage and greater protection of neuronal survival in the vicinity of the lesion, as well as less infiltration by inflammatory cells, when compared to the SD.

More recently, we added exogenous ketone (sodium salt) supplementation to a KD on the first 4 days after a similar cervical hemicontusion injury to provide a faster increase in ketone levels (Tan et al., 2020). This provided only a transient acceleration in the increase in β-hydroxybutyrate (βHB) levels during the hour after gavage, but otherwise the βHB levels were comparable to what were observed in our earlier study discussed above. Similarly, the behavioral improvements were comparable to the ones observed previously (Streijger et al., 2013) and included improved performance when reaching for food pellets and improved usage of the forepaw during vertical exploration. While the neuroprotective effects were not apparent with standard white matter staining using Eriochrome cyanine, there was significant sparing of corticospinal axons, which could be a plausible explanation for the improved distal limb function (Tan et al., 2020). These behavioral benefits of KD initiated 4 hr

after injury in rats were confirmed by Lu and coworkers, who visited our laboratories to adopt our cervical hemicontusion model and later independently reported increased limb usage in a cylinder test and an increased success rate of pellets reached in rats on KD (Lu et al., 2018). These authors also followed up on possible anti-oxidant and anti-inflammatory mechanisms of KD (which are discussed below). In a finding that is interesting from a mechanistic standpoint, Qian and colleagues (Qian et al., 2017) found that application of βHB (1.6 mmol/kg/day subcutaneously via osmotic pump) at 6 hr after T9 thoracic contusion injury improved open-field locomotor scores and raised pain thresholds. These authors also reported increased numbers of neurons and decreased GFAP and Iba1 immunoreactivity, markers for astroglial and microglial/macrophage activation, respectively. Unfortunately, their data where not corroborated by strict stereologic morphologic assessments.

Taken together, manipulating the composition and timing of macronutrient intake can have significant effects on neurologic outcomes early after SCI in rodents, which challenges the current clinical nutritional guidelines for SCI, which have insufficient evidence. How KD and ketone bodies enhance behavioral recovery after neurotrauma is partially understood and is further discussed in the sections following the next section.

KD IMPROVES OUTCOME IN RODENT MODELS OF TBI

Several studies reported that a KD fed prior to traumatic brain injury (TBI) or started after injury may improve recovery from TBI (for review, see (McDougall et al., 2018). Using a controlled cortical impact (CCI) model that is delivered with an electromagnetic device onto the dura through a drill hole in the skull (craniotomy), Prins and Hovda were the first to show that a 7-day KD regimen (containing as little as 0.8% carbohydrates), started immediately after TBI in adolescent rats (35–45 days old), reduced cortical lesion size and improved cognition in a water maze as well as motor performance in walking on a narrow beam. However, no improvements have been shown in young adult rats (65–75 days old; (Appelberg et al., 2009; Prins et al., 2005). Another group also found histologic evidence for neuroprotection, with reduced edema, lesion volumes, and cell death in the cortex of adolescent rats, using a somewhat similar weight drop TBI model and initiating a KD after injury (4:1 with 0% carbohydrates; (Hu et al., 2009a; Hu et al., 2009b). The well-known antiepileptogenic effects of the KD were assessed following fluid percussion injury (FPI) of the brain, which is another widely used open-skull model of TBI that sends a sudden fluid pressure wave through a small craniotomy (Schwartzkroin et al., 2010). However, in this latter study, the KD was only effective when given before, but not when started after, injury. With the recognition of chronic traumatic encephalitis (CTE) as a result of mild repetitive brain injuries, several animal models of repeated mild TBI have been developed to mimic a series of concussions, as they often occur in sports (Bolton-Hall et al., 2019; VanItallie, 2019). While a single mild TBI does not usually trigger overt brain damage in rodents, repeated injuries may cause distinct histopathology. A KD, started after the first of three repeated mild FPIs (one every 24 hr), improved motor recovery (beam balance) by 7 days after injury, along with reduced brain edema revealed by T2-rated MRI in 35-day-old male rats (Zhang et al., 2018). Another group extended the age range to 47-day-old rats of both sexes and administered a KD (6:1 with 3.2% carbohydrates) either 17 days before, or immediately after, a single lateral impact mild TBI applied by propelling a 50-g weight against the rat's head, which is protected against fracture by a "helmet" (Salberg et al., 2019). The KD pretreatment led to improved behavioral outcomes on the beam walk, increased exploration in the open-field test, and improved neuroprotection, as measured by brain weight:body weight ratio. The post-injury KD treatment reduced a measurement of depressive behavior (amount of time spent immobile in the swim test) and was also neuroprotective. Collectively, these studies indicate that the KD can be an effective therapy to improve pathologic and cognitive outcomes after various models of TBI.

In TBI treatment, a possible alternative to a dietary increase of ketones by carbohydrate restriction could be the direct intake of ketones, which contributes to our mechanistic understanding by dissociating the effects of carbohydrate starvation from the actions of ketones. Infusion of βHB (30 mg/kg/hr for 6 hr) via the femoral vein after a lateral fluid percussion TBI (Orhan et al., 2016) reduced the increase of the blood–brain barrier permeability (HRP extravasation) after TBI in the cortex and hippocampus. Somewhat concerning, though, was an increase in the blood–brain barrier permeability in uninjured animals given βHB. However, the dose used was about 4.5 times higher than in the SCI study by Qian et al. (Qian et al., 2017), indicating the need to establish toxicity data on this alternative route for increasing ketone levels.

POSSIBLE MECHANISMS OF ACTION OF KDS AND KETONES IN SCI AND TBI

Ketones as an Alternative Source of Energy

It is well known that a physiologically low intake of carbohydrates during consumption of KD or fasting typically causes hepatic ketogenesis fueled by the β-oxidation of fatty acids, resulting in increased blood levels of the ketone bodies βHB, AcAc, and acetone (Cahill, 2006). The ketone bodies cross the blood–brain/spinal cord barrier and enter neuronal and glial cells via monocarboxylate transporters (MCTs; (Nijland et al., 2014; Pierre and Pellerin, 2005). In the cells, ketone bodies are converted into acetoacetyl-CoA by the enzyme succinyl-CoA:3CoA transferase (SCOT) and are broken down into two molecules of acetyl-CoA that are subsequently used in the Krebs cycle (see (Fukao et al., 2014; Kim and Rho, 2008). Interestingly, brain astrocytes are an additional site for ketogenesis (Auestad et al., 1991; Guzman and Blazquez, 2001). Taken together, KDs provide an effective source of energy without the need for glycolysis or mitochondrial complex I and the associated free oxygen radical byproducts. The human brain can utilize ketones for up to 60% of its energy demands (Owen et al., 1967). This can provide an important alternative source of energy when the activity of pyruvate dehydrogenase is low, as is true after both SCI and TBI (McEwen et al., 2011; Sharma et al., 2009). Pyruvate dehydrogenase converts pyruvate to acetyl-CoA, which is used for mitochondrial ATP production. Low activity of the enzyme may trigger an energy crisis. Hence, some of the benefits of the KD observed after SCI as well as TBI (Prins and Matsumoto, 2014) could be due to metabolic rescue by ketones.

A TBI triggers a transient increase and subsequent depression in glucose uptake, accompanied by decreased glycolysis (Prins and Matsumoto, 2014). Oxidative damage-driven activation of the DNA repair enzyme poly (ADP-ribose) polymerase (PARP) may lead to depletion of NAD^+ (Besson et al., 2003; LaPlaca et al., 1999), which would cause a decrease in glyceraldehyde phosphate dehydrogenase activity. Together with an oxidative damage-driven decrease in pyruvate dehydrogenase activity, less glucose is available to be utilized for ATP generation in the TCA cycle, and energy failure ensues (Lee et al.,

1999; Sharma et al., 2009; Singh et al., 2006). Exogenously applied βHB is readily taken up by the injured brain after a TBI by CCI and is used to restore the depleted ATP stores (Prins et al., 2004). Such uptake is not seen in the uninjured brain, where energy supplies are largely glucose-derived (Prins et al., 2004). Interestingly, the brains of P70 rats started to experience a reduction in energy metabolites within 6 hr after TBI (on a standard diet), while in contrast, P35 animals did not begin to experience these changes until 24 hr after injury (Prins et al., 2005) This time difference might be critical, since injury triggers an immediate secondary cascade, and the rescue of neuronal tissue after injury is time sensitive; the age-specific differences in neuroprotection seen with KD treatment after TBI are likely related. Moreover, blood ketones of animals on a KD indicated that P35 rats had 43% higher levels of blood ketone measurements compared to P70 rats (Deng-Bryant et al., 2011). Administration of βHB results in a more pronounced increase in βHB levels in the brains of younger rats and restores their energy stores more effectively than in older rats. This could be explained by the fact that young rats express higher level of MCTs for the uptake of ketone bodies into the brain than older rats express (Prins and Giza, 2006). An important consideration for clinical translation is that adult humans are in general more responsive to a KD than rodents; therefore, adult humans' response to a KD might be more like that of adolescent rats than that of adult rats (Cahill, 2006; Prins, 2012). For example, the brain of an adult rat can at most utilize ketones for 25% of its energy needs, while the brain of an adult human can use ketones to fuel up to 60% of its metabolic requirements (Cahill, 2006; Owen et al., 1967). There are similar differences for the level of brain ketone-uptake measurements, with adult humans having the ability to increase their levels 13-fold, while adult rats are only able to manage around a 5-fold increase (Hasselbalch et al., 1995; Owen et al., 1967; Prins, 2008). Therefore, the differences in outcomes in TBI models between adolescent and adult rats on the KD might not be observed in human studies trialing a KD to treat various CNS traumatic injuries.

Ketones as Signaling Metabolites in the Context of Traumatic Injuries

It has become increasingly clear that ketone bodies have direct nonmetabolic actions as ligands for various receptors, transporters, and regulators of enzymes. These actions likely contribute to the beneficial effects of KDs in a wide range of neurologic disorders (which are covered in other chapters of this book). Of particular interest in the context of SCI and TBI are the rescue of mitochondrial bioenergetics and the antioxidant and the anti-inflammatory actions. A combination of multiple mechanisms may lead to the beneficial effects of KDs and ketones after neurotrauma; these mechanisms are illustrated in Figure 18.1 and are discussed in turn below.

Ketones Rescue Mitochondrial Bioenergetics

Ketone bodies provide an alternative energy source that improves mitochondrial efficiency under physiologic conditions and in models of various neurologic diseases, such as Parkinson's disease, Alzheimer's disease, amyotrophic lateral sclerosis, epilepsy, and neurotrauma (Fortier et al., 2019; Hasan-Olive et al., 2019; Kephart et al., 2017; Norwitz et al., 2019; Pandya et al., 2019; Prins and Matsumoto, 2014; Sullivan et al., 2004; Veyrat-Durebex et al., 2018; Zhao et al., 2006). Indeed, a growing number of publications support the idea that a shift in energy metabolism toward ketogenesis and fatty acid oxidation may play a key role in controlling mitochondrial function and mitohormesis (Miller et al., 2018). For example, Greco et al. showed that 24 hr after TBI by CCI in rats, ketones decreased oxidative stress and improved mitochondrial bioenergetics by: (1) increasing the expression of the antioxidant enzymes NAD(P)H dehydrogenase quinone 1 (NQO1) and superoxide dismutase (SOD1/2) and decreasing the protein oxidation markers 4-hydroxynonenal (4-HNE) and 3-nitrotyrosine (3-NT); and (2) by inducing an amelioration in mitochondrial Complex II + III activity (Greco et al., 2016). Furthermore, as already mentioned, in vitro work in neurons suggests that ketones reduce production of reactive oxygen species (ROS) by increasing NADH oxidation (Maalouf et al., 2007), which is complemented further by fatty acid-induced activation of mitochondrial uncoupling proteins (UCPs; (Sullivan et al., 2004). Moreover, βHB administration rescues H_2O_2-mediated deficits in coupled mitochondrial respiration in rat hippocampal neurons both in vitro and in vivo (Hasan-Olive et al., 2019).

Data from our laboratory, in which we assessed the therapeutic effect of KD administration initiated acutely after a cervical SCI on the

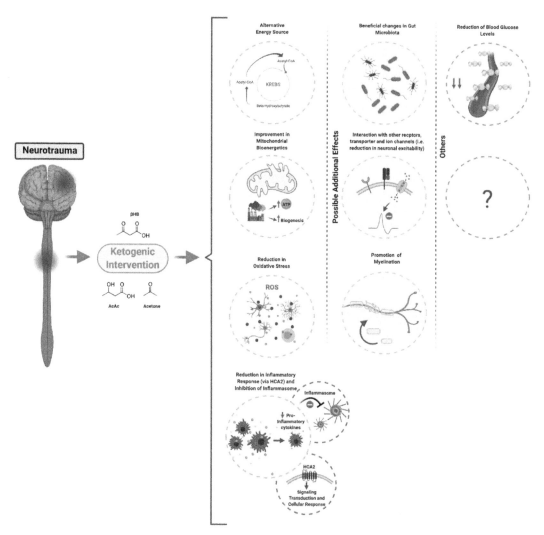

FIGURE 18.1 *Possible Beneficial Mechanisms and Effects of a Ketogenic Intervention after Neurotrauma*
There are multiple strongly supported mechanisms behind the beneficial effects of ketones after central neurotrauma. As an alternative to glucose as an energy source, ketones may help overcome the energy deficit seen during trauma. Ketones may improve mitochondrial function and increase mitochondrial volume. Ketones can reduce free radical production and oxidative stress. Ketones have been shown to reduce the inflammatory response by inhibiting the inflammasome complex and reducing infiltrating macrophages (via the niacin receptor HCA2), which consequently may contribute to decreased pro-inflammatory cytokine production. Additionally, growing evidence suggests that the KD may help to restore health by regulating the gut microbiota in order to overcome the dysbiosis that occurs after trauma. The newly discovered interactions of ketones with other receptors and ion channels may lead to a reduction in neuronal excitability after trauma. New evidence suggests that ketones can also promote myelin production. Finally, ketones reduce blood glucose levels. Other beneficial effects or mechanisms of action of ketone bodies still need to be unraveled. Created with BioRender.com.

restoration of mitochondrial bioenergetics, shed some light in the mechanism behind the KD's beneficial effects. Our research demonstrated how the KD modulates the expression and activity of some key kinases and transcription factors involved in the control of the transcriptional and translational machineries (both mitochondrial and nuclear) that might be associated with the rescue of mitochondrial bioenergetics by a KD (Seira et al., 2021). In the injured spinal cord, this is accompanied by mitochondrial biogenesis (Seira et al., 2021), and similar observations have been made by others in different systems (e.g., in rat hippocampi after several weeks of KD treatment; (Bough and Rho, 2007).

KD and βHB Increase Antioxidant Proteins

Oxidative stress and damage occur extensively after SCI and TBI (for review, see (Bains and Hall, 2012). In both TBI and SCI, the byproducts of oxidative damage can be measured within minutes of injury, and both 3-NT and 4-HNE peak between 1 and 3 days. ROS cause perturbation of many cellular processes, including Ca^{2+} and Na^+/K^+ pumps. These failures lead to Ca^{2+} overload, mitochondrial damage, and further ROS production. This implies some urgency when attempting to prevent secondary injury with an antioxidant treatment. Indeed, in laboratory animals, most neuroprotective treatments are effective if given prior to, or at the time of, injury, but they lose efficacy when administered with a delay of several hours after SCI (Kwon et al., 2011). This implies that any diet-induced benefit provided by the initiation of KD in the acute stage of injury would likely miss some of the oxidative damage during the first day of injury, since it takes 16 to 20 hr for the endogenous ketone levels to significantly rise. To solve this, the use of external oral ketone esters as an initial and acute way to increase the circulatory ketone levels would be a rational approach.

The antioxidant effects of KDs have been extensively reviewed (Gano et al., 2014; Rojas-Morales et al., 2020; Yang et al., 2019). The KD upregulates mitochondrial glutathione (GSH) biosynthesis in the brain (Jarrett et al., 2008), enhances mitochondrial antioxidant status, and reduces ROS production (Maalouf et al., 2007), protecting mtDNA from oxidant-induced damage. The exact mechanism of the GSH increase is unknown. The GSH is synthetized by glutamate cysteine ligase (GCL) forming gamma-glutamylcysteine, to which glycine is added by glutathione synthase. The activity of GCL, which is rate limiting, is increased by the KD (Jarrett et al., 2008) and could be mediated by the transcription factor Nrf2 that is found in nuclear fractions of KD-fed rats (Milder et al., 2010). In response to stimuli, Nrf2 detaches from Keap1 in the cytosol and translocates into the nucleus, where it binds to antioxidant response elements (ARE), leading to the expression of antioxidant response genes (Nguyen et al., 2000), including GCL (Milder and Patel, 2012). This complex functions as a redox sensor, releasing Nrf2 in situations of stress and high ROS levels. Interestingly, there is an increase in Nrf2-ARE-regulated antioxidant genes after TBI, but it does not occur until 24 to 48 hr after injury (Miller et al., 2014), which may be too late to prevent much secondary damage. Acceleration of Nrf2-ARE activation with carnosic acid provides effective protection when carnosic acid is given within 15 min of injury, and some benefits, such as reduced cytoskeletal breakdown, are observed with its application at 8 hr after TBI (Miller et al., 2015). Furthermore, data from Lu et al., together with data from our laboratory, indicate that KD treatment activates the Nrf2-dependent antioxidant pathway after SCI in vivo (Lu et al., 2018); (Seira et al., 2021). Interestingly, our microarray data indicate that KD regulates genes like *Nrf1* and *Gsta5*, which are also associated with cell defense mechanisms (Seira et al., 2021). Nrf2 also has a role in regulating mitochondrial function through modulating the availability of substrates for mitochondrial respiration (NADH and $FADH_2$), which are important for the function of antioxidant enzymes (Holmstrom et al., 2013). Despite all these correlative data, it remains to be shown whether the KD or administration of ketone bodies will be able to elicit such a protective response via the Nrf2-ARE pathway in the time-sensitive setting of acute neurotrauma.

A recognized indirect antioxidant effect of βHB is mediated through its action as an endogenous inhibitor of class I histone deacetylases (HDACs) at concentrations that occur with KD administration (EC_{50} between 2.5 and 5 mM; Shimazu et al., 2013). Kidneys of mice fasted for 24 hr showed increased acetylation at the *Foxo3a* and *Mt2* (metallothionin 2) promoters due to HDAC1 inhibition by βHB. Both genes protect against oxidative stress, whereby *Foxo3a* increases the expression of mitochondrial antioxidant manganese superoxide dismutase (MnSOD) and catalase (Newman & Verdin, 2017; Shimazu et al., 2013). In fact, recent work demonstrated that a similar inhibition of class I HDACs by βHB (or a KD) occurs in the spinal cord after injury (Kong et al., 2017; Wang et al., 2017). This inhibition would lead to the regulation of genes associated with the antioxidant effects of ketogenic metabolism, such as *Sod*, *Foxo3a*, *catalase*, *Mt2*, *Nox2*, and *Nox4* (Kong et al., 2017; Wang et al., 2017). Overall, these may contribute to the reduction of the oxidative damage in the spinal cord tissue after injury, although a causal link has not been firmly established.

Anti-Inflammatory Effects of Ketones

The KD has been shown to reduce inflammation in several disorders, including models of multiple sclerosis (Kim et al., 2012), stroke (Rahman et al., 2014), pain (Ruskin et al., 2009), glaucoma (Harun-Or-Rashid and Inman, 2018), and SCI (Lu et al., 2018). Following SCI, spinal cord-resident microglia and astrocytes are the first to be activated, releasing pro-inflammatory cytokines and recruiting additional immune cells. Neutrophils then rapidly infiltrate the injury site, followed by macrophages, T cells, and finally B cells (Orr and Gensel, 2017). These cells have been shown to fulfill both pro-inflammatory and anti-inflammatory roles. For example, macrophages can be inflammatory or reparative; they are often referred to as M1 and M2 macrophages, respectively. Inflammation is a particularly deleterious component of the secondary injury cascade following SCI. The inflammatory response following SCI contributes to axonal regeneration failure through the lesion site (Evans et al., 2014) and persists chronically. Multiple studies have indicated that dampening the inflammatory response can improve recovery from SCI (for a review, see (Orr and Gensel, 2018). This can be accomplished in a number of ways: diminishing recruitment of immune cells to the injury site, shifting cells to an anti-inflammatory subtype, or inhibiting specific inflammatory pathways. Established targets for the inflammatory response after SCI include TNF-α, NF-κB, iNOS, IL-1β, IL-18, and FasL (Jorge et al., 2019). Importantly, some of these targets, particularly NF-κB, are upstream or downstream of NLRP3 inflammasome activation. Inhibition of the NF-κB pathway by the KD has been reported after SCI in rats (Lu et al., 2018), and other treatments that target NF-κB either directly or indirectly have also been shown to reduce inflammation and improve recovery from SCI (Brambilla et al., 2005; Huang et al., 2019; Liu et al., 2017).

βHB Inhibits the NLRP3 Inflammasome at Concentrations Reached by the KD

The NLRP3 inflammasome is a multiprotein complex including oligomers of pyrin domain-containing protein 3 (NLRP3), apoptosis-associated speck-like protein containing a caspase-recruitment domain (ASC), and procaspase-1. By bringing procaspase-1 into close proximity, NLRP3 allows ASC to activate caspase-1 via proteolytic cleavage; activated caspase-1 subsequently cleaves pro-IL-1β and pro-IL-18 to their mature forms

(for review, see Kelley et al., 2019; Swanson et al., 2019). Importantly, at concentrations reached by the KD, the ketone βHB directly inhibits caspase-1 cleavage by the NLRP3 inflammasome, which ultimately dampens the increases in IL-1β and IL-18 that are seen in many inflammatory states and contributes to the anti-inflammatory actions of ketones (Youm et al., 2015). The authors tested a battery of NLRP3 activators, including the fatty acids palmitate, ceramide, and sphingosine, in vitro and consistently showed inhibition by βHB (see also the chapter by Youm in this book). Priming macrophages with Toll-like agonists revealed a potent inhibition of Pro-IL1β cleavage by βHB treatment at similar concentrations. These βHB effects were specific to the NLRP3 inflammasome. In vivo, βHB reduced peritoneal infiltration by neutrophils and IL-1β-secreting macrophages following intraperitoneal injection of uric acid crystals in mice. Mice carrying a *Nlrp3* mutation that leads to NLRP3 inflammasome activation showed severe peritoneal neutrophilia, which was greatly reduced by feeding of oral ketone esters. Thus, in vivo, even with levels on the order of 1 mM, which can easily by achieved by a KD, βHB is an effective and specific inhibitor of the NLRP3 inflammasome (Youm et al., 2015). Importantly, these actions are independent of the presence of GPR109A, also known as hydroxyl-carboxylic acid (HCA2) receptor, the mitochondrial UCP2, and the metabolic function of βHB in the TCA cycle.

Activation of the NLRP3 inflammasome following SCI and TBI has been repeatedly observed in multiple studies that have been well summed up in recent publications (Irrera et al., 2020; Mortezaee et al., 2018). A correlation of reduced NLRP3 activation and improved outcome from SCI has been reported using a wide variety of NLPR3-inhibiting compounds, including miR-223 (Zhang et al., 2020) and the NLRP3 inhibitors MCC950 (Jiao et al., 2020; Zhang et al., 2020) and BAY 11-7082 (Jiang et al., 2017), as well as melatonin (Xu et al., 2019) and 17β-estradiol (Slowik et al., 2018; Zendedel et al., 2018). While the specificity of these compounds varies and may include other targets, mice with gene deletion of ASC, a critical part of the NLRP3 inflammasome complex, showed improved motor outcomes after SCI (Shiraishi et al., 2020), a finding further supporting the concept that the NLRP3 complex plays a significant role in the secondary inflammatory damage cascades after SCI. The multiple triggers activating NLRP3 and their cell-specific involvement remain incompletely understood (Kelley et al., 2019; Swanson et al., 2019). Administration of βHB to mice via subcutaneous osmotic minipumps (1.6 mmol/kg/day for 7 days) improved open-field locomotion and sensory thresholds after moderate thoracic spinal cord contusion injury (Qian et al., 2017). The biochemical effects included, but were not limited to, reduced NLRP3 protein expression, with reduction of both IL-1β and IL-18 proteins. Other beneficial effects reported were an inhibition of HDACs, with increased AcH3K9 epitopes on histone 3, leading to rescue of antioxidant proteins. These βHB-induced effects may contribute to the observed neuroprotection after SCI and include a mitigated astrocytic and microglial reaction and increased neuronal survival. Surprisingly, whether a similar inhibition of the NLRP3 inflammasome after SCI can occur with KD treatment has yet to be determined, although serum concentrations around 1 mM βHB are quite achievable with the KD.

The role of the NLRP3 inflammasome in the secondary cascades after TBI has been supported by over a dozen experimental studies using NLRP3 inhibitors—mostly in CCI models (Irrera et al., 2017; Irrera et al., 2020; Ismael et al., 2021) as well as in a NLRP$^{-/-}$ knockout mouse using a closed skull model (Irrera et al., 2017). Importantly, in humans the levels of NLRP3 in the cerebrospinal fluid (CSF) become detectable after TBI, and high levels correlate with poor outcomes (Wallisch et al., 2017). This could make CSF NLRP3 a candidate biomarker and surrogate target for monitoring therapeutic interventions after TBI (O'Brien et al., 2020). Despite the linkage of KD/βHB to NLRP3 inhibition and the established role of NLPR3 in secondary inflammation, we could not find reports showing that the benefits of KD administration after TBI in animals are at least in part due to NLPR3 inhibition.

βHB Dampens Inflammation via Activation of the HCA2 Receptor

An additional way to directly modify inflammation by ketones is through activation of the HCA2 receptor (also known as GPR109A, PUMA-G, or niacin receptor). Endogenous levels of niacin are too low to activate this receptor and βHB is the main known endogenous ligand of the HCA2 receptor at concentrations that are easily reached by fasting or KD treatment (EC$_{50}$ 0.7 mM; (Taggart et al., 2005). This receptor has received much attention due to its favorable role in dyslipidemia and the anti-inflammatory actions responsible for the cardiovascular benefits of niacin at high doses (10–25 mg/kg; (Gille et al., 2008; Lukasova et al., 2011). While the HCA2 receptor is widely expressed in adipose tissue, where it regulates lipolysis (Taggart et al., 2005), it is also found on immune cells, such as neutrophils, macrophages, and microglia, but not on astrocytes or neurons (Kostylina et al., 2008; Rahman et al., 2014). HCA2 receptor activation promotes neutrophil apoptosis (Kostylina et al., 2008), and on macrophages/monocytes it activates/attracts a neuroprotective Ly-6^{Lo} subset (Rahman et al., 2014). Mice fed the KD after ischemic stroke showed reduced infarct volume and improved behavioral recovery (Rahman et al., 2014). Importantly, this protection by the KD was not seen in HCA2$^{-/-}$ mice. Transplantation of bone marrow from HCA2$^{+/+}$ wild-type mice into HCA2$^{-/-}$ mice restored the protective effect of the KD, demonstrating that monocyte/macrophage HCA2 expression is required. Apart from βHB, HCA2 can also be activated by exogenous dosing of niacin, a widely used cholesterol-lowering drug (Gille et al., 2008; Lukasova et al., 2011), monomethylfumarate used for psoriasis and multiple sclerosis (Tang et al., 2008), and butyrate produced by some gut bacteria (Thangaraju et al., 2009). Studies of HCA2 activation through these molecules have also shown anti-inflammatory effects. For example, activation of HCA2 by niacin in LPS-primed bone marrow-derived macrophages was able to reduce production of multiple pro-inflammatory cytokines, including TNFα, IL-6, and IL-1β, to reduce NF-κB phosphorylation, and to inhibit the recruitment of macrophages elicited by the chemokine MCP-1 (Zandi-Nejad et al., 2013). These effects were all lost in macrophages derived from bone marrow of HCA2$^{-/-}$ mice, indicating that activation of HCA2 is required for the anti-inflammatory effects of niacin (Zandi-Nejad et al., 2013). Interestingly, mice given a 50-kdyne T9 contusive SCI and treated with niacin (100 mg/kg by oral gavage once daily) showed reduced production of pro-inflammatory cytokines, increased anti-inflammatory cytokine production, and reduced levels of pro-inflammatory M1 macrophages, while anti-inflammatory M2 macrophages were increased (Yang et al., 2016b) Phosphorylated NF-κB was also reduced with niacin treatment in the injured spinal cord, a finding consistent with activation of the HCA2 receptor. Interestingly, in vitro, this effect of niacin was only seen in M1, but not M2, primed macrophages; the HCA2 receptor was expressed on the cell surface of M1 macrophages but was largely cytosolic in M2 macrophages. Membrane-localized HCA2 underwent endocytosis in response to niacin treatment, and niacin itself could reduce M1 markers while significantly increasing M2 markers (Yang et al., 2016b). Together, these data support the concept that niacin induces a phenotypic switch in macrophages through the HCA2 receptor. It will be very interesting to see if βHB or KD can similarly alter macrophage phenotype in the injured spinal cord or brain through HCA2 activation. In our own laboratory, we see differences in the cytokine and inflammatory cell profiles in the injured spinal cord of HCA2$^{-/-}$ mice fed a KD compared to their wild-type littermates (Kolehmainen et al., in preparation; for further general discussion of the anti-inflammatory roles of HCA2, see (Graff et al., 2016; Offermanns and Schwaninger, 2015; Wannick et al., 2018). Many questions still need to be addressed. What exactly is the role of HCA2, and is it required for the beneficial effects of the KD and βHB after SCI? What cell types are being targeted, and can βHB differentially affect resident CNS versus infiltrating immune cells? Is βHB able to induce a phenotypic switch to anti-inflammatory macrophages, as seen with niacin activation of HCA2? And, finally, is a restrictive KD required or can ketone esters, which provide exogenous βHB, be used instead to reduce inflammation after SCI? Clearly, additional research is warranted. Notwithstanding their limitations, these studies provide promising support for the ability of KD to reduce inflammation after SCI.

Additional Possible Effects of KD Relevant in Neurotrauma

In summary, it is becoming increasingly clear that ketone bodies have metabolic as well as nonmetabolic actions as ligands for various receptors, transporters, and regulators of enzymes that may contribute to the beneficial effects of KDs for a wide range of neurologic disorders. In addition to the bioenergetic, antioxidant, and anti-inflammatory actions of ketone bodies themselves, there are possible neuroprotective effects of KD through dampened neuronal excitability (Achanta and Rae, 2017; Juge et al., 2010; Martinez-Francois et al., 2018), changes in circulating polyunsaturated fatty acids (Michael-Titus and Priestley, 2014; Taha et al., 2010), and changes in gut microbiome composition. The KD induces changes in the microbiome that have recently been causally linked to antiepileptic effects mediated by enteral bacteria of *Akkermansia* and *Parabacteroides* species (Olson et al., 2018). Possible links of the KD-induced microbiome changes to the beneficial effects seen in SCI and TBI remain to be explored.

Of interest in the context of neurotrauma is the beneficial effect of the KD for remyelination in the aftermath of injury, when lipids and metabolic energy are in high demand. Demyelination is regularly seen after SCI in parallel with apoptosis of oligodendrocytes (Crowe et al., 1997). Remyelination is notoriously sluggish in the CNS (Franklin and Ffrench-Constant, 2008), and demyelinated axons have an increased energy demand that leaves them vulnerable to degeneration. The Nave group recently found that an extreme KD (94% of calories from fat, 5% from protein, 1% from carbohydrates) ameliorates axonal defects and promotes myelination in Pelizaeus-Merzbacher disease as well as in the cuprizone-induced model of demyelination and remyelination (Stumpf et al., 2019). This report contributes further to the mechanisms of the KD as a potential therapy for multiple sclerosis, which is currently being clinically trialed (Bahr et al., 2020)

HUMAN TRIALS

In the light of this emerging body of preclinical data, it is timely that the KD or ketogenic therapeutic approaches have been taken to clinical trials. An open-label clinical trial of a KD in 10 patients with acute SCI evaluated its safety and feasibility (Guo et al., 2014). All patients developed ketone levels above 2 mM (typically ~ 3 mmol/L) while maintaining normal glucose levels (9 out of 10). Routine blood tests for electrolytes and for liver and kidney function showed no changes. This demonstrates that diet-induced ketosis in patients with SCI is feasible and that the KD seems safe when initiated after SCI in the hospital setting. Yet, there were some transient gastrointestinal side effects (i.e., diarrhea, nausea, poor appetite, gastric pain, and abdominal distension) in five patients and a low enthusiasm for the Chinese KD formulation. This underscores the translatability of this dietary approach but provides motivation to improve the treatment in order to minimize unpleasant side effects and thereby to increase compliance.

A recent randomized clinical trial at the University of Birmingham (Alabama) initiated the KD in humans within 72 hr of acute SCI (Yarar-Fisher et al., 2018). While the numbers of four KD-fed patients and three control patients are too small for any firm conclusions, this study also showed that it is logistically feasible to start

KD via enteral tube feeding followed by a solid KD with about 65% of the total energy as fat, 27% as protein, and 8% as carbohydrate and fiber. Higher levels of lysoPC 16:0, an anti-inflammatory lysophospholipid, were found in the KD group compared with the control diet group, and, interestingly, fibrinogen—a known proinflammatory protein (Davalos and Akassoglou, 2012)—was lower in all four KD-treated patients. Whether the improved upper extremity motor scores in the KD group will be robust with the enrollment of more patients remains unknown. Altogether, KD appears feasible in the acute SCI setting, and the preliminary data show promise.

A prospective interventional phase II trial enrolled 20 ventilated critically ill patients with a recent TBI (15) or stroke or hemorrhage and administered an enteral ketogenic formulation (KetoCal[R]; (White et al., 2020). Blood ketone levels were increased in proportion to the KetoCal[R] intake. There was no correlation between ketone levels and cerebral hypertension or hypoperfusion in this study. The ketogenic formulation was well tolerated and could be safely administered.

Overall, clinical translation of a ketogenic regimen is feasible and safe in the acute setting of neurotrauma, and larger studies are eagerly awaited. Many questions remain to be answered regarding the therapeutic window of diet onset, the need to initiate with an enteral formula, the optimal duration of the treatment in the acute setting, the degree of strictness/relaxation of the ketogenic regimen, and the optimal level of ketones in the blood required for protection.

FUTURE DIRECTIONS

Aside from the obvious motor, sensory, and autonomic impairments, in the chronic stage of SCI, metabolic syndrome, systemic inflammation, obesity, heightened risk for cardiovascular disease, and cognitive decline contribute to morbidity and reduced life expectancy. Many aspects of this chronic stage may benefit from a metabolic treatment with ketogenic effects that target inflammation and oxidative stress. However, long-term treatment with the KD seems less than ideal, due to the inherent challenge of having patients adhere to a strict dietary regimen for lengthy periods of time. Poor compliance with the restricted protein and carbohydrate intake of a KD may suppress ketosis and thereby bring a person closer to the unhealthy effects of a high-fat diet without ketosis. The use of high amounts of animal fats and meat in the classic KDs should be revisited in the light of the long-term population studies that link these food sources to cardiovascular complications, increased cancer risk, and greater mortality (Levine et al., 2014; Seidelmann et al., 2018). The reported superiority of vegetarian or vegan approaches in these large population studies begs the question whether a vegetarian or a modified Mediterranean KD could bring together the best of both worlds for people with chronic SCI. The Internet is full of KD recipes, and some are vegetarian or are inspired by the Mediterranean diet and could be suitable for the implementation of a healthy ketogenic lifestyle. Other alternatives and more liberal KDs are discussed in this book and the authors refer to those chapters.

An alternative to a KD for the treatment of TBI, Parkinson's disease, and Alzheimer's disease has been envisioned by Richard Veech and colleagues, specifically the use of oral ketone-ester supplementation accompanying a regular diet (Norwitz et al., 2020); (Soto-Mota et al., 2020; Veech et al., 2012). In vivo oral administration of ketone esters readily increases βHB levels to the desired range of 3 to 4 mmol/L and has been shown to improve cognition and histopathology in 3xTgAD mice, which are a model for Alzheimer's disease (Kashiwaya et al., 2013). A clinical study in patients with Parkinson's disease is currently under way (clinicaltrials.gov NCT04477161). Whether or not supplementation with oral ketone esters after acute TBI and SCI is as effective as KD, thus representing a "diet in a bottle," is currently under investigation in our laboratories.

ACKNOWLEDGMENTS

Research in W. T.'s laboratory is supported by the Craig H. Neilsen Foundation, the Canadian Institutes for Health Research (CIHR), the National Science and Engineering Research Council, Wings for Life, the Canadian Stem Cell Network, and the Rick Hansen Foundation. W.T. holds the John and Penny Ryan Chair in Spinal Cord Injury Research.

Research in the laboratory of C. Yarar-Fisher is supported by grants from the UAB Center for Clinical and Translational Science (UL1-TR-001417- KL2TR001419-01), the National Institute of Health (NIH)/National Institute of Nursing (NINR-1R01NR016443), and the NIH/National Institute of Child Health and Human Development (NICHD-1K01HD087463).

REFERENCES

Achanta, L. B., & Rae, C. D. (2017). β-Hydroxybutyrate in the brain: One molecule, multiple mechanisms. *Neurochemical Research. 42*, 35–49.

Ahuja, C. S., Wilson, J. R., Nori, S., Kotter, M. R. N., Druschel, C., Curt, A., & Fehlings, M. G. (2017). Traumatic spinal cord injury. *Nature Reviews Disease Primers. 3*, 17018.

Anderson, K. D. (2004). Targeting recovery: Priorities of the spinal cord-injured population. *Journal of Neurotrauma, 21*, 1371–1383.

Angeli, C. A., Boakye, M., Morton, R. A., Vogt, J., Benton, K., Chen, Y., Ferreira, C. K., & Harkema, S. J. (2018). Recovery of over-ground walking after chronic motor complete spinal cord injury. *New England Journal of Medicine, 379*, 1244–1250.

Appelberg, K. S., Hovda, D. A., & Prins, M. L. (2009). The effects of a ketogenic diet on behavioral outcome after controlled cortical impact injury in the juvenile and adult rat. *Journal of Neurotrauma, 26*, 497–506.

Auestad, N., Korsak, R. A., Morrow, J. W., & Edmond, J. (1991). Fatty acid oxidation and ketogenesis by astrocytes in primary culture. *Journal of Neurochemistry, 56*, 1376–1386.

Bahr, L. S., Bock, M., Liebscher, D., Bellmann-Strobl, J., Franz, L., Pruss, A., Schumann, D., Piper, S. K., Kessler, C. S., Steckhan, N., Michalsen, A., Paul, F., & Mahler, A. (2020). Ketogenic diet and fasting diet as nutritional approaches in multiple sclerosis (NAMS): Protocol of a randomized controlled study. *Trials, 21*, 3.

Bains, M., & Hall, E. D. (2012). Antioxidant therapies in traumatic brain and spinal cord injury. *Biochimica et Biophysica Acta, 1822*, 675–684.

Bareyre, F. M., & Schwab, M. E. (2003). Inflammation, degeneration and regeneration in the injured spinal cord: Insights from DNA microarrays. *Trends in Neuroscience, 26*, 555–563.

Besson, V. C., Croci, N., Boulu, R. G. Plotkine, M., & Marchand-Verrecchia, C. (2003). Deleterious poly(ADP ribose)polymerase-1 pathway activation in traumatic brain injury in rat. *Brain Research, 989*, 58–66.

Bolton-Hall, A. N., Hubbard, W. B., & Saatman, K. E. (2019). Experimental designs for repeated mild traumatic brain injury: Challenges and considerations. *Journal of Neurotrauma, 36*, 1203–1221.

Bough, K. J., & Rho, J. M. (2007). Anticonvulsant mechanisms of the ketogenic diet. *Epilepsia, 48*, 43–58.

Bracken, M. B., Shepard, M. J., Holford, T. R., Leo-Summers, L., Aldrich, E. F., Fazl, M., Fehlings, M. G., Herr, D. L., Hitchon, P. W., Marshall, L. F., Nockels, R. P., Pascale, V., Perot, P. L., Jr., Piepmeier, J., Sonntag, V. K., Wagner, F., Wilberger, J. E., Winn, H. R., & Young, W. (1998). Methylprednisolone or tirilazad mesylate administration after acute spinal cord injury: 1-year follow up. Results of the third national acute spinal cord injury randomized controlled trial. *Journal of Neurosurgery, 89*, 699–706.

Brambilla, R., Bracchi-Ricard, V., Hu, W. H., Frydel, B., Bramwell, A., Karmally, S., Green, E. J., & Bethea, J. R. (2005). Inhibition of astroglial nuclear factor κB reduces inflammation and improves functional recovery after spinal cord injury. *Journal of Experimental Medicine, 202*, 145–156.

Cahill, G. F., Jr. (2006). Fuel metabolism in starvation. *Annual Review of Nutrition, 26*, 1–22.

Consortium_for_Spinal_Cord_Medicine. (2008). *Early acute management in adults with spinal cord injury*. http://www.nxtbook.com/nxtbooks/pva/earlyacutemanagement/index.php

Cook, A. M., Peppard, A., & Magnuson, B. (2008). Nutrition considerations in traumatic brain injury. *Nutrition in Clinical Practice, 23*, 608–620.

Crowe, M. J., Bresnahan, J. C., Shuman, S. L., Masters, J. N., & Beattie, M. S. (1997). Apoptosis and delayed degeneration after spinal cord injury in rats and monkeys. *Nature Medicine, 3*, 73–76.

Davalos, D., & Akassoglou, K. (2012). Fibrinogen as a key regulator of inflammation in disease. *Seminars in Immunopathology. 34*, 43–62.

Deng-Bryant, Y., Prins, M. L., Hovda, D. A., & Harris, N. G. (2011). Ketogenic diet prevents alterations in brain metabolism in young but not adult rats after traumatic brain injury. *Journal of Neurotrauma, 28*, 1813–1825.

Evans, T. A., Barkauskas, D. S., Myers, J. T., Hare, E. G., You, J. Q., Ransohoff, R. M., Huang, A. Y., & Silver, J. (2014). High-resolution intravital imaging reveals that blood-derived macrophages but not resident microglia facilitate secondary axonal dieback in traumatic spinal cord injury. *Experimental Neurology, 254*, 109–120.

Fehlings, M. G., Wilson, J. R., Tetreault, L. A., Aarabi, B., Anderson, P., Arnold, P. M., Brodke, D. S., Burns, A. S., Chiba, K., Dettori, J. R., Furlan, J. C., Hawryluk, G., Holly, L. T., Howley, S., Jeji, T., Kalsi-Ryan, S., Kotter, M., Kurpad, S., Kwon, B. K., . . . Harrop, J. S. (2017). A clinical practice guideline for the management of patients with acute spinal cord injury: Recommendations on the use of methylprednisolone sodium succinate. *Global Spine Journal, 7*, 203S–211S.

Fortier, M., Castellano, C. A., Croteau, E., Langlois, F., Bocti, C., St-Pierre, V., Vandenberghe, C., Bernier, M., Roy, M., Descoteaux, M., Whittingstall, K., Lepage, M., Turcotte, E. E., Fulop, T., & Cunnane, S. C. (2019). A ketogenic drink improves brain energy and some measures of cognition in mild cognitive impairment. *Alzheimer's & Dementia, 15*, 625–634.

Franklin, R. J., & Ffrench-Constant, C. (2008). Remyelination in the CNS: From biology to therapy. *Nauret Reviews Neuroscience, 9,* 839–855.

Fukao, T., Mitchell, G., Sass, J. O., Hori, T., Orii, K., & Aoyama, Y. (2014). Ketone body metabolism and its defects. *Journal of Inherited Metabolic Disease, 37,* 541–551.

Gano, L. B., Patel, M., & Rho, J. M. (2014). Ketogenic diets, mitochondria, and neurological diseases. *Journal of Lipid Research, 55,* 2211–2228.

Gille, A., Bodor, E. T., Ahmed, K., & Offermanns, S. (2008). Nicotinic acid: Pharmacological effects and mechanisms of action. *Annual Review of Pharmacology and Toxicology, 48,* 79–106.

Global-Collaborators. (2019). Global, regional, and national burden of traumatic brain injury and spinal cord injury, 1990-2016: a systematic analysis for the Global Burden of Disease Study 2016. *Lancet Neurology, 18,* 56–87.

Graff, E. C., Fang, H., Wanders, D., & Judd, R. L. (2016). Anti-inflammatory effects of the hydroxy-carboxylic acid receptor 2. *Metabolism, 65,* 102–113.

Greco, T., Glenn, T. C., Hovda, D. A., & Prins, M. L. (2016). Ketogenic diet decreases oxidative stress and improves mitochondrial respiratory complex activity. *Journal of Cerebral Blood Flow & Metabolism, 36,* 1603–1613.

Guzman, M., & Blazquez, C. (2001). Is there an astrocyte-neuron ketone body shuttle? *Trends in Endocrinology Metabolism, 12,* 169–173.

Hachem, L. D., Ahuja, C. S., & Fehlings, M. G. (2017). Assessment and management of acute spinal cord injury: From point of injury to rehabilitation. *Journal of Spinal Cord Medicine, 40,* 665–675.

Harkema, S. J., Hillyer, J., Schmidt-Read, M., Ardolino, E., Sisto, S. A., & Behrman, A. L. (2012). Locomotor training: As a treatment of spinal cord injury and in the progression of neurologic rehabilitation. *Archives of Physical Medicine and Rehabilitation, 93,* 1588–1597.

Harun-Or-Rashid, M., & Inman, D. M. (2018). Reduced AMPK activation and increased HCAR activation drive anti-inflammatory response and neuroprotection in glaucoma. *Journal of Neuroinflammation, 15,* 313.

Hasan-Olive, M. M., Lauritzen, K. H., Ali, M., Rasmussen, L. J., Storm-Mathisen, J., & Bergersen, L. H. (2019). A ketogenic diet improves mitochondrial biogenesis and bioenergetics via the PGC1alpha-SIRT3-UCP2 axis. *Neurochemical Research, 44,* 22–37.

Hasselbalch, S. G., Knudsen, G. M., Jakobsen, J., Hageman, L. P., Holm, S., & Paulson, O. B. (1995). Blood-brain barrier permeability of glucose and ketone bodies during short-term starvation in humans. *American Journal of Physiology, 268,* E1161–E1166.

Hilton, B. J., Moulson, A. J., & Tetzlaff, W. (2017). Neuroprotection and secondary damage following spinal cord injury: Concepts and methods. *Neuroscience Letters, 652,* 3–10.

Holmstrom, K. M., Baird, L., Zhang, Y., Hargreaves, I., Chalasani, A., Land, J. M., Stanyer, L., Yamamoto, M., Dinkova-Kostova, A. T., & Abramov, A. Y. (2013). Nrf2 impacts cellular bio-energetics by controlling substrate availability for mitochondrial respiration. *Biology Open, 2,* 761–770.

Hu, Z. G., Wang, H. D., Jin, W., & Yin, H. X. (2009a). Ketogenic diet reduces cytochrome c release and cellular apoptosis following traumatic brain injury in juvenile rats. *Annals of Clinical & Laboratory Science, 39,* 76–83.

Hu, Z. G., Wang, H. D., Qiao, L., Yan, W., Tan, Q. F., & Yin, H. X. (2009b). The protective effect of the ketogenic diet on traumatic brain injury-induced cell death in juvenile rats. *Brain Injury, 23,* 459–465.

Huang, Y., Zhu, N., Chen, T., Chen, W., Kong, J., Zheng, W., & Ruan, J. (2019). Triptolide suppressed the microglia activation to improve spinal cord injury through miR-96/IKKβ/NF-κB pathway. *Spine, 44,* E707–E714.

Irrera, N., Pizzino, G., Calo, M., Pallio, G., Mannino, F., Fama, F., Arcoraci, V., Fodale, V., David, A., Francesca, C., Minutoli, L., Mazzon, E., Bramanti, P., Squadrito, F., Altavilla, D., & Bitto, A. (2017). Lack of the Nlrp3 inflammasome improves mice recovery following traumatic brain injury. *Frontiers in Pharmacology, 8,* 459.

Irrera, N., Russo, M., Pallio, G., Bitto, A., Mannino, F., Minutoli, L., Altavilla, D., & Squadrito, F. (2020). The role of NLRP3 inflammasome in the pathogenesis of traumatic brain injury. *International Journal of Molecular Sciences, 21.*

Ismael, S., Ahmed, H. A., Adris, T., Parveen, K., Thakor, P., & Ishrat, T. (2021). The NLRP3 inflammasome: A potential therapeutic target for traumatic brain injury. *Neural Regeneration Research, 16,* 49–57.

Jarrett, S. G., Milder, J. B., Liang, L. P., & Patel, M. (2008). The ketogenic diet increases mitochondrial glutathione levels. *Journal of Neurochemistry, 106,* 1044–1051.

Jeong, M. A., Plunet, W., Streijger, F., Lee, J. H., Plemel, J. R., Park, S., Lam, C. K., Liu, J., & Tetzlaff, W. (2011). Intermittent fasting improves functional recovery after rat thoracic contusion spinal cord injury. *Journal of Neurotrauma, 28,* 479–492.

Jiang, W., Li, M., He, F., Zhou, S., & Zhu, L. (2017). Targeting the NLRP3 inflammasome to attenuate spinal cord injury in mice. *Journal of Neuroinflammation, 14,* 207.

Jiao, J., Zhao, G., Wang, Y., Ren, P., & Wu, M. (2020). MCC950, a selective inhibitor of NLRP3 inflammasome, reduces the inflammatory response and improves neurological outcomes in mice model of spinal cord injury. *Frontiers in Molecular Bioscience, 7*, 37.

Jorge, A., Taylor, T., Agarwal, N., & Hamilton, D. K. (2019). Current agents and related therapeutic targets for inflammation after acute traumatic spinal cord injury. *World Neurosurgery, 132*, 138–147.

Juge, N., Gray, J. A., Omote, H., Miyaji, T., Inoue, T., Hara, C., Uneyama, H., Edwards, R. H., Nicoll, R. A., & Moriyama, Y. (2010). Metabolic control of vesicular glutamate transport and release. *Neuron, 68*, 99–112.

Kashiwaya, Y., Bergman, C., Lee, J. H., Wan, R., King, M. T., Mughal, M. R., Okun, E., Clarke, K., Mattson, M. P., & Veech, R. L. (2013). A ketone ester diet exhibits anxiolytic and cognition-sparing properties, and lessens amyloid and tau pathologies in a mouse model of Alzheimer's disease. *Neurobiology of Aging, 34*, 1530–1539.

Kelley, N., Jeltema, D., Duan, Y., & He, Y. (2019). The NLRP3 inflammasome: An overview of mechanisms of activation and regulation. *International Journal of Molecular Sciences, 20*.

Kephart, W. C., Mumford, P. W., Mao, X., Romero, M. A., Hyatt, H. W., Zhang, Y., Mobley, C. B., Quindry, J. C., Young, K. C., Beck, D. T., Martin, J. S., McCullough, D. J., D'Agostino, D. P., Lowery, R. P., Wilson, J. M., Kavazis, A. N., & Roberts, M. D. (2017). The 1-week and 8-month effects of a ketogenic diet or ketone salt supplementation on multi-organ markers of oxidative stress and mitochondrial function in rats. *Nutrients, 9*.

Khalatbary, A. R. (2014). Natural polyphenols and spinal cord injury. *Iranian Biomedical Journal, 18*, 120–129.

Khalatbary, A. R., & Khademi, E. (2020). The green tea polyphenolic catechin epigallocatechin gallate and neuroprotection. *Nutritional Neuroscience. 23*, 281–294.

Kim, D., Zai, L., Liang, P., Schaffling, C., Ahlborn, D., & Benowitz, L. I. (2013). Inosine enhances axon sprouting and motor recovery after spinal cord injury. *PLOS ONE, 8*, Article e81948.

Kim, D. Y., Hao, J., Liu, R., Turner, G., Shi, F. D., & Rho, J. M. (2012). Inflammation-mediated memory dysfunction and effects of a ketogenic diet in a murine model of multiple sclerosis. *PLOS ONE, 7*, Article e35476.

Kim, D. Y., & Rho, J. M. (2008). The ketogenic diet and epilepsy. *Current Opinion in Clinical Nutrition and Metabolic Care, 11*, 113–120.

Kong, G., Huang, Z., Ji, W., Wang, X., Liu, J., Wu, X., Huang, Z., Li, R., & Zhu, Q. (2017). The ketone metabolite β-hydroxybutyrate attenuates oxidative stress in spinal cord injury by suppression of class I histone deacetylases. *Journal of Neurotrauma, 34*, 2645–2655.

Kostylina, G., Simon, D., Fey, M. F., Yousefi, S., & Simon, H. U. (2008). Neutrophil apoptosis mediated by nicotinic acid receptors (GPR109A). *Cell Death and Differentiation, 15*, 134–142.

Kwon, B. K., Okon, E., Hillyer, J., Mann, C., Baptiste, D., Weaver, L. C., Fehlings, M. G., & Tetzlaff, W. (2011). A systematic review of non-invasive pharmacologic neuroprotective treatments for acute spinal cord injury. *Journal of Neurotrauma, 28*, 1545–1588.

LaPlaca, M. C., Raghupathi, R., Verma, A., Pieper, A. A., Saatman, K. E., Snyder, S. H., & McIntosh, T. K. (1999). Temporal patterns of poly(ADP-ribose) polymerase activation in the cortex following experimental brain injury in the rat. *Journal of Neurochemistry, 73*, 205–213.

Lee, J. H., Streijger, F., Tigchelaar, S., Maloon, M., Liu, J., Tetzlaff, W., & Kwon, B. K. (2012). A contusive model of unilateral cervical spinal cord injury using the infinite horizon impactor. *Journal of Visual Experiments, 65*, 3313.

Lee, S. M., Wong, M. D., Samii, A., & Hovda, D. A. (1999). Evidence for energy failure following irreversible traumatic brain injury. *Annales of the New York Academy of Science, 893*, 337–340.

Levine, M. E., Suarez, J. A., Brandhorst, S., Balasubramanian, P., Cheng, C. W., Madia, F., Fontana, L., Mirisola, M. G., Guevara-Aguirre, J., Wan, J., Passarino, G., Kennedy, B. K., Wei, M., Cohen, P., Crimmins, E. M., & Longo, V. D. (2014). Low protein intake is associated with a major reduction in IGF-1, cancer, and overall mortality in the 65 and younger but not older population. *Cell Metabolism, 19*, 407–417.

Liu, G., Fan, G., Guo, G., Kang, W., Wang, D., Xu, B., & Zhao, J. (2017). FK506 attenuates the inflammation in rat spinal cord injury by inhibiting activation of NF-κB in microglia cells. *Cellular and Molecular Neurobiology, 37*, 843–855.

Longo, V. D., & Mattson, M. P. (2014). Fasting: Molecular mechanisms and clinical applications. *Cell Metabolism, 19*, 181–192.

Lu, Y., Yang, Y. Y., Zhou, M. W., Liu, N., Xing, H. Y., Liu, X. X., & Li, F. (2018). Ketogenic diet attenuates oxidative stress and inflammation after spinal cord injury by activating Nrf2 and suppressing the NF-κB signaling pathways. *Neuroscience Letters, 683*, 13–18.

Lukasova, M., Hanson, J., Tunaru, S., & Offermanns, S. (2011). Nicotinic acid (niacin): New lipid-independent mechanisms of action and therapeutic potentials. *Trends in Pharmacological Sciences, 32*, 700–707.

Maalouf, M., Rho, J. M., & Mattson, M. P. (2009). The neuroprotective properties of calorie restriction, the ketogenic diet, and ketone bodies. *Brain Research Reviews, 59*, 293–315.

Maalouf, M., Sullivan, P. G., Davis, L., Kim, D. Y., & Rho, J. M. (2007). Ketones inhibit mitochondrial production of reactive oxygen species production following glutamate excitotoxicity by increasing NADH oxidation. *Neuroscience, 145*, 256–264.

Magnuson, B., Peppard, A., & Auer Flomenhoft, D. (2011). Hypocaloric considerations in patients with potentially hypometabolic disease States. *Nutrition in Clinical Practice, 26*, 253–260.

Martinez-Francois, J. R., Fernandez-Aguera, M. C., Nathwani, N., Lahmann, C., Burnham, V. L., Danial, N. N., & Yellen, G. (2018). BAD and KATP channels regulate neuron excitability and epileptiform activity. *Elife, 7*.

Mattson, M. P., V.D. Longo, & M. Harvie. (2017). Impact of intermittent fasting on health and disease processes. *Ageing Research Reviews, 39*, 46–58.

McDougall, A., Bayley, M., & Munce, S. E. (2018). The ketogenic diet as a treatment for traumatic brain injury: A scoping review. *Brain Injury, 32*, 416–422.

McEwen, M. L., Sullivan, P. G., Rabchevsky, A. G., & Springer, J. E. (2011). Targeting mitochondrial function for the treatment of acute spinal cord injury. *Neurotherapeutics, 8*, 168–179.

Michael-Titus, A. T. (2007). Omega-3 fatty acids and neurological injury. *Prostaglandins, Leukotrienes and Essential Fatty Acids, 77*, 295–300.

Michael-Titus, A. T., & Priestley, J. V. (2014). Omega-3 fatty acids and traumatic neurological injury: From neuroprotection to neuroplasticity? *Trends in Neuroscience, 37*, 30–38.

Milder, J., & Patel, M. (2012). Modulation of oxidative stress and mitochondrial function by the ketogenic diet. *Epilepsy Research, 100*, 295–303.

Milder, J. B., Liang, L. P., & Patel, M. (2010). Acute oxidative stress and systemic Nrf2 activation by the ketogenic diet. *Neurobiology of Disease, 40*, 238–244.

Miller, D. M., Singh, I. N., Wang, J. A., & Hall, E. D. (2015). Nrf2-ARE activator carnosic acid decreases mitochondrial dysfunction, oxidative damage and neuronal cytoskeletal degradation following traumatic brain injury in mice. *Experimetal Neurology, 264*, 103–110.

Miller, D. M., Wang, J. A., Buchanan, A. K., & Hall, E. D. (2014). Temporal and spatial dynamics of nrf2-antioxidant response elements mediated gene targets in cortex and hippocampus after controlled cortical impact traumatic brain injury in mice. *Journal of Neurotrauma, 31*, 1194–1201.

Miller, V. J., Villamena, F. A., & Volek, J. S. (2018). Nutritional ketosis and mitohormesis: Potential implications for mitochondrial function and human health. *Journal or Nutrition and Metabolism, 2018*, 5157645.

Mortezaee, K., Khanlarkhani, N., Beyer, C., & Zendedel, A. (2018). Inflammasome: Its role in traumatic brain and spinal cord injury. *Journal of Cellular Physiology, 233*, 5160–5169.

Newman, J. C., & Verdin, E. (2017). β-Hydroxybutyrate: A signaling metabolite. *Annual Review of Nutrition, 37*, 51–76.

Nguyen, T., Huang, H. C., & Pickett, C. B. (2000). Transcriptional regulation of the antioxidant response element: Activation by Nrf2 and repression by MafK. *Journal of Biologica Chemistry, 275*, 15466–15473.

Nijland, P. G., Michailidou, I., Witte, M. E., Mizee, M. R., van der Pol, S. M., van Het Hof, B., Reijerkerk, A., Pellerin, L., van der Valk, P., de Vries, H. E., & van Horssen, J. (2014). Cellular distribution of glucose and monocarboxylate transporters in human brain white matter and multiple sclerosis lesions. *Glia, 62*, 1125–1141.

Norwitz, N. G., Hu, M. T., & Clarke, K. (2019). The mechanisms by which the ketone body D-β-hydroxybutyrate may improve the multiple cellular pathologies of Parkinson's disease. *Frontiers in Nutrition, 6*, 63.

Norwitz, N. G., Jaramillo, J. G., Clarke, K., & Soto, A. (2020). Ketotherapeutics for neurodegenerative diseases. *International Review of Neurobiology, 155*, 141–168.

National Spinal Cord Injury Statistical Center (NSCISC). (2020). *National Spinal Cord Injury Statistical Center: Facts and figures at a glance.* https://msktc.org/sites/default/files/Facts-Figures-2020-508.pdf

O'Brien, W. T., Pham, L., Symons, G. F., Monif, M., Shultz, S. R., & McDonald, S. J. (2020). The NLRP3 inflammasome in traumatic brain injury: Potential as a biomarker and therapeutic target. *Journal of Neuroinflammation, 17*, 104.

Offermanns, S., & Schwaninger, M. (2015). Nutritional or pharmacological activation of HCA(2) ameliorates neuroinflammation. *Trends in Molecular Medicine, 21*, 245–255.

Olson, C. A., Vuong, H. E., Yano, J. M., Liang, Q. Y., Nusbaum, D. J., & Hsiao, E. Y. (2018). The gut microbiota mediates the anti-seizure effects of the ketogenic diet. *Cell, 173*, 1728–1741.

Orhan, N., Ugur Yilmaz, C., Ekizoglu, O., Ahishali, B., Kucuk, M., Arican, N., Elmas, I., Gurses, C., & Kaya, M. (2016). Effects of beta-hydroxybutyrate on brain vascular permeability in rats with traumatic brain injury. *Brain Research, 1631*, 113–126.

Orr, M. B., & Gensel, J. C. (2017). Interactions of primary insult biomechanics and secondary cascades in spinal cord injury: Implications for therapy. *Neural Regeneration Research, 12*, 1618–1619.

Orr, M. B., & Gensel, J. C. (2018). Spinal cord injury scarring and inflammation: Therapies targeting glial and inflammatory responses. *Neurotherapeutics, 15*, 541–553.

Owen, O. E., Morgan, A. P., Kemp, H. G., Sullivan, J. M., Herrera, M. G., & Cahill, G. F., Jr. (1967). Brain metabolism during fasting. *Journal of Clinical Investigation, 46*, 1589–1595.

Oyinbo, C. A. (2011). Secondary injury mechanisms in traumatic spinal cord injury: A nugget of this multiply cascade. *Acta Neurobiologiae Experimentalis, 71*, 281–299.

Pandya, J. D., Leung, L. Y., Yang, X., Flerlage, W. J., Gilsdorf, J. S., Deng-Bryant, Y., & Shear, D. A. (2019). Comprehensive profile of acute mitochondrial dysfunction in a preclinical model of severe penetrating TBI. *Frontiers in Neurology, 10*, 605.

Patel, S. P., Sullivan, P. G., Lyttle, T. S., Magnuson, D. S., & Rabchevsky, A. G. (2012). Acetyl-L-carnitine treatment following spinal cord injury improves mitochondrial function correlated with remarkable tissue sparing and functional recovery. *Neuroscience, 210*, 296–307.

Patel, S. P., Sullivan, P. G., Pandya, J. D., Goldstein, G. A., VanRooyen, J. L., Yonutas, H. M., Eldahan, K. C., Morehouse, J., Magnuson, D. S., & Rabchevsky, A. G. (2014). N-Acetylcysteine amide preserves mitochondrial bioenergetics and improves functional recovery following spinal trauma. *Experimental Neurology, 257*, 95–105.

Pierre, K., & Pellerin, L. (2005). Monocarboxylate transporters in the central nervous system: Distribution, regulation and function. *Journal of Neurochemistry, 94*, 1–14.

Plunet, W. T., Lam, C. K., Lee, J. H., Liu, J., & Tetzlaff, W. (2010). Prophylactic dietary restriction may promote functional recovery and increase lifespan after spinal cord injury. *Annals of the New York Academy of Sciences, 1198*(Suppl. 1), E1–E11.

Plunet, W. T., Streijger, F., Lam, C. K., Lee, J. H., Liu, J., & Tetzlaff, W. (2008). Dietary restriction started after spinal cord injury improves functional recovery. *Experimental Neurology, 213*, 28–35.

Prins, M. L. (2008). Cerebral metabolic adaptation and ketone metabolism after brain injury. *Journal of Cerebral Blood Flow and Metabolism, 28*, 1–16.

Prins, M. L. (2012). Cerebral ketone metabolism during development and injury. *Epilepsy Research, 100*, 218–223.

Prins, M. L., Fujima, L. S., & Hovda, D. A. (2005). Age-dependent reduction of cortical contusion volume by ketones after traumatic brain injury. *Journal of Neuroscience Research, 82*, 413–420.

Prins, M. L., & Giza, C. C. (2006). Induction of monocarboxylate transporter 2 expression and ketone transport following traumatic brain injury in juvenile and adult rats. *Developmental Neuroscience, 28*, 447–456.

Prins, M. L., Lee, S. M., Fujima, L. S., & Hovda, D. A. (2004). Increased cerebral uptake and oxidation of exogenous βHB improves ATP following traumatic brain injury in adult rats. *Journal of Neurochemistry, 90*, 666–672.

Prins, M. L., & Matsumoto, J. H. (2014). The collective therapeutic potential of cerebral ketone metabolism in traumatic brain injury. *Journal of Lipid Research, 55*, 2450–2457.

Qian, J., Zhu, W., Lu, M., Ni, B., & Yang, J. (2017). D-β-Hydroxybutyrate promotes functional recovery and relieves pain hypersensitivity in mice with spinal cord injury. *British Journal of Pharmacology, 174*, 1961–1971.

Rabchevsky, A. G., Sullivan, P. G., Fugaccia, I., & Scheff, S. W. (2003). Creatine diet supplement for spinal cord injury: Influences on functional recovery and tissue sparing in rats. *Journal of Neurotrauma, 20*, 659–669.

Rahman, M., Muhammad, S., Khan, M. A., Chen, H., Ridder, D. A., Muller-Fielitz, H., Pokorna, B., Vollbrandt, T., Stolting, I., Nadrowitz, R., Okun, J. G., Offermanns, S., & Schwaninger, M. (2014). The β-hydroxybutyrate receptor HCA2 activates a neuroprotective subset of macrophages. *Nature Communication, 5*, 3944.

Rho, J. M. (2015). How does the ketogenic diet induce anti-seizure effects? *Neuroscience Letters,*

Rodriguez, D. J., Benzel, E. C., & Clevenger, F. W. (1997). The metabolic response to spinal cord injury. *Spinal Cord, 35*, 599–604.

Rojas-Morales, P., Pedraza-Chaverri, J., & Tapia, E. (2020). Ketone bodies, stress response, and redox homeostasis. *Redox Biology, 29*, 101395.

Ruskin, D. N., Kawamura, M., & Masino, S. A. (2009). Reduced pain and inflammation in juvenile and adult rats fed a ketogenic diet. *PLOS ONE, 4*, Article e8349.

Salberg, S., Weerwardhena, H., Collins, R., Reimer, R. A., & Mychasiuk, R. (2019). The behavioural and pathophysiological effects of the ketogenic diet on mild traumatic brain injury in adolescent rats. *Behavioral Brain Research, 376*, 112225.

Schwartzkroin, P. A., Wenzel, H. J., Lyeth, B. G., Poon, C. C., Delance, A., Van, K. C., Campos, L., & Nguyen, D. V. (2010). Does ketogenic diet alter seizure sensitivity and cell loss following fluid percussion injury? *Epilepsy Research, 92*, 74–84.

Seidelmann, S. B., Claggett, B., Cheng, S., Henglin, M., Shah, A., Steffen, L. M., Folsom, A. R., Rimm, E. B., Willett, W. C., & Solomon, S. D. (2018). Dietary carbohydrate intake and mortality: a prospective cohort study and meta-analysis. *Lancet Public Health, 3*, e419–e428.

Seira, O., Kolehmainen, K., Liu, J., Streijger, F., Haegert, A., Lebihan, S., Boushel, R., & Tetzlaff, W. (2021). Ketogenesis controls mitochondrial gene expression and rescues mitochondrial bioenergetics after cervical spinal cord injury in rats. *Scientific Reports, 11*, 16359.

Sharma, P., Benford, B., Li, Z. Z., & Ling, G. S. (2009). Role of pyruvate dehydrogenase complex in traumatic brain injury and measurement of pyruvate dehydrogenase enzyme by dipstick test. *Journal of Emergencies Trauma and Shock. 2*, 67–72.

Shimazu, T., Hirschey, M. D., Newman, J., He, W., Shirakawa, K., Le Moan, N., Grueter, C. A., Lim, H., Saunders, L. R., Stevens, D. R., Newgard,

C. B., Farese, R. V., Jr., de Cabo, R., Ulrich, S., Akassoglou, K., & Verdin, E. (2013). Suppression of oxidative stress by beta-hydroxybutyrate, an endogenous histone deacetylase inhibitor. *Science, 339,* 211–214.

Shiraishi, Y., Kimura, A., Kimura, H., Ohmori, T., Takahashi, M., & Takeshita, K. (2020). Deletion of inflammasome adaptor protein ASC enhances functional recovery after spinal cord injury in mice. *Journal of Orthopaedic Science.*

Singh, I. N., Sullivan, P. G., Deng, Y., Mbye, L. H., & Hall, E. D. (2006). Time course of post-traumatic mitochondrial oxidative damage and dysfunction in a mouse model of focal traumatic brain injury: Implications for neuroprotective therapy. *Journal of Cerebral Blood Flow and Metabolism, 26,* 1407–1418.

Slowik, A., Lammerding, L., Zendedel, A., Habib, P., & Beyer, C. (2018). Impact of steroid hormones E2 and P on the NLRP3/ASC/Casp1 axis in primary mouse astroglia and BV-2 cells after in vitro hypoxia. *Journal of Steroid Biochemistry and Molecular Biology, 183,* 18–26.

Soto-Mota, A., Norwitz, N. G., & Clarke, K. (2020). Why a D-β-hydroxybutyrate monoester? *Biochemistry Society Transactions, 48,* 51–59.

Squair, J. W., Belanger, L. M., Tsang, A., Ritchie, L., Mac-Thiong, J. M., Parent, S., Christie, S., Bailey, C., Dhall, S., Street, J., Ailon, T., Paquette, S., Dea, N., Fisher, C. G., Dvorak, M. F., West, C. R., & Kwon, B. K. (2017). Spinal cord perfusion pressure predicts neurologic recovery in acute spinal cord injury. *Neurology, 89,* 1660–1667.

Streijger, F., Plunet, W. T., Lee, J. H., Liu, J., Lam, C. K., Park, S., Hilton, B. J., Fransen, B. L., Matheson, K. A., Assinck, P., Kwon, B. K., & Tetzlaff, W. (2013). Ketogenic diet improves forelimb motor function after spinal cord injury in rodents. *PLOS ONE, 8,* Article e78765.

Stumpf, S. K., Berghoff, S. A., Trevisiol, A., Spieth, L., Duking, T., Schneider, L. V., Schlaphoff, L., Dreha-Kulaczewski, S., Bley, A., Burfeind, D., Kusch, K., Mitkovski, M., Ruhwedel, T., Guder, P., Rohse, H., Denecke, J., Gartner, J., Mobius, W., Nave, K. A., & Saher, G. (2019). Ketogenic diet ameliorates axonal defects and promotes myelination in Pelizaeus-Merzbacher disease. *Acta Neuropathologica, 138,* 147–161.

Sullivan, P. G., Rippy, N. A., Dorenbos, K., Concepcion, R. C., Agarwal, A. K., & Rho, J. M. (2004). The ketogenic diet increases mitochondrial uncoupling protein levels and activity. *Annals of Neurology, 55,* 576–580.

Swanson, K. V., Deng, M., & Ting, J. P. (2019). The NLRP3 inflammasome: Molecular activation and regulation to therapeutics. *Nature Reviews Immunology, 19,* 477–489.

Taggart, A. K., Kero, J., Gan, X., Cai, T. Q., Cheng, K., Ippolito, M., Ren, N., Kaplan, R., Wu, K., Wu, T. J.,

Jin, L., Liaw, C., Chen, R., Richman, J., Connolly, D., Offermanns, S., Wright, S. D., & Waters, M. G. (2005). (D)-β-Hydroxybutyrate inhibits adipocyte lipolysis via the nicotinic acid receptor PUMA-G. *Journal of Biological Chemistry, 280,* 26649–26652.

Taha, A. Y., Burnham, W. M., & Auvin, S. (2010). Polyunsaturated fatty acids and epilepsy. *Epilepsia, 51,* 1348–1358.

Tan, B. T., Jiang, H., Moulson, A. J., Wu, X. L., Wang, W. C., Liu, J., Plunet, W. T., & Tetzlaff, W. (2020). Neuroprotective effects of a ketogenic diet in combination with exogenous ketone salts following acute spinal cord injury. *Neural Regeneration Research, 15,* 1912–1919.

Tang, H., Lu, J. Y., Zheng, X., Yang, Y., & Reagan, J. D. (2008). The psoriasis drug monomethylfumarate is a potent nicotinic acid receptor agonist. *Biochemical and Biophysical Research Communications, 375,* 562–565.

Thangaraju, M., Cresci, G. A., Liu, K., Ananth, S., Gnanaprakasam, J. P., Browning, D. D., Mellinger, J. D., Smith, S. B., Digby, G. J., Lambert, N. A., Prasad, P. D., & Ganapathy, V. (2009). GPR109A is a G-protein-coupled receptor for the bacterial fermentation product butyrate and functions as a tumor suppressor in colon. *Cancer Research, 69,* 2826–2832.

Thau-Zuchman, O., Ingram, R., Harvey, G. G., Cooke, T., Palmas, F., Pallier, P. N., Brook, J., Priestley, J. V., Dalli, J., Tremoleda, J. L., & Michael-Titus, A. T. (2020). A single injection of docosahexaenoic acid induces a pro-resolving lipid mediator profile in the injured tissue and a long-lasting reduction in neurological deficit after traumatic brain injury in mice. *Journal of Neurotrauma, 37,* 66–79.

Thibault-Halman, G., Casha, S., Singer, S., & Christie, S. (2011). Acute management of nutritional demands after spinal cord injury. *Journal of Neurotrauma, 28,* 1497–1507.

VanItallie, T. B. (2019). Traumatic brain injury (TBI) in collision sports: Possible mechanisms of transformation into chronic traumatic encephalopathy (CTE). *Metabolism, 100S,* 153943.

Veech, R. L., Valeri, C. R., & VanItallie, T. B. (2012). The mitochondrial permeability transition pore provides a key to the diagnosis and treatment of traumatic brain injury. *IUBMB Life, 64,* 203–207.

Veyrat-Durebex, C., Reynier, P., Procaccio, V., Hergesheimer, R., Corcia, P., Andres, C. R., & Blasco, H. (2018). How can a ketogenic diet improve motor function? *Frontiers in Molecular Neuroscience, 11,* 15.

Wallisch, J. S., Simon, D. W., Bayir, H., Bell, M. J., Kochanek, P. M., & Clark, R. S. B. (2017). Cerebrospinal fluid NLRP3 is increased after severe traumatic brain injury in infants and children. *Neurocritical Care, 27,* 44–50.

Wang, X., Wu, X., Liu, Q., Kong, G., Zhou, J., Jiang, J., Wu, X., Huang, Z., Su, W., & Zhu, Q. (2017). Ketogenic metabolism inhibits histone deacetylase (HDAC) and reduces oxidative stress after spinal cord injury in rats. *Neuroscience, 366,* 36–43.

Wannick, M., Assmann, J. C., Vielhauer, J. F., Offermanns, S., Zillikens, D., Sadik, C. D., & Schwaninger, M. (2018). The immunometabolomic interface receptor hydroxycarboxylic acid receptor 2 mediates the therapeutic effects of dimethyl fumarate in autoantibody-induced skin inflammation. *Frontiers in Immunology, 9,* 1890.

West, C. R., Phillips, A. A., Squair, J. W., Williams, A. M., Walter, M., Lam, T., & Krassioukov, A. V. (2018). Association of epidural stimulation with cardiovascular function in an individual with spinal cord injury. *JAMA Neurology, 75,* 630–632.

Whishaw, I. Q., & Gorny, B. (1994). Arpeggio and fractionated digit movements used in prehension by rats. *Behavioral Brain Research, 60,* 15–24.

White, H., Venkatesh, B., Jones, M., Kruger, P. S., Walsham, J., & Fuentes, H. (2020). Inducing ketogenesis via an enteral formulation in patients with acute brain injury: A phase II study. *Neurological Research, 42,* 275–285.

Xu, G., Shi, D., Zhi, Z., Ao, R., & Yu, B. (2019). Melatonin ameliorates spinal cord injury by suppressing the activation of inflammasomes in rats. *Journal of Cellular Biochemistry, 120,* 5183–5192.

Yang, H., Shan, W., Zhu, F., Wu, J., & Wang, Q. (2019). Ketone bodies in neurological diseases: Focus on neuroprotection and underlying mechanisms. *Frontiers in Neurology, 10,* 585.

Yang, L., Yao, M., Lan, Y., Mo, W., Sun, Y. L., Wang, J., Wang, Y. J., & Cui, X. J. (2016a). Melatonin for spinal cord injury in animal models: A systematic review and network meta-analysis. *Journal of Neurotrauma, 33,* 290–300.

Yang, R., He, J., & Wang, Y. (2016b). Activation of the niacin receptor HCA2 reduces demyelination and neurofilament loss, and promotes functional recovery after spinal cord injury in mice. *European Journal of Pharmacology, 791,* 124–136.

Yarar-Fisher, C., Kulkarni, A., Li, J., Farley, P., Renfro, C., Aslam, H., Bosarge, P., Wilson, L., & Barnes, S. (2018). Evaluation of a ketogenic diet for improvement of neurological recovery in individuals with acute spinal cord injury: A pilot, randomized safety and feasibility trial. *Spinal Cord Series and Cases, 4,* 88.

Youm, Y. H., Nguyen, K. Y., Grant, R. W., Goldberg, E. L., Bodogai, M., Kim, D., D'Agostino, D., Planavsky, N., Lupfer, C., Kanneganti, T. D., Kang, S., Horvath, T. L., Fahmy, T. M., Crawford, P. A., Biragyn, A., Alnemri, E., & Dixit, V. D. (2015). The ketone metabolite beta-hydroxybutyrate blocks NLRP3 inflammasome-mediated inflammatory disease. *Nature Medicine, 21,* 263–269.

Zandi-Nejad, K., Takakura, A., Jurewicz, M., Chandraker, A. K., Offermanns, S., Mount, D., & Abdi, R. (2013). The role of HCA2 (GPR109A) in regulating macrophage function. *FASEB Journal, 27,* 4366–4374.

Zendedel, A., Monnink, F., Hassanzadeh, G., Zaminy, A., Ansar, M. M., Habib, P., Slowik, A., Kipp, M., & Beyer, C. (2018). Estrogen attenuates local inflammasome expression and activation after spinal cord injury. *Molecular Neurobiology, 55,* 1364–1375.

Zhang, F., Wu, H., Jin, Y., & Zhang, X. (2018). Proton magnetic resonance spectroscopy (H1-MRS) study of the ketogenic diet on repetitive mild traumatic brain injury in adolescent rats and its effect on neurodegeneration. *World Neurosurgery, 120,* e1193–e1202.

Zhang, M., Wang, L., Huang, S., & He, X. (2020). MicroRNA-223 targets NLRP3 to relieve inflammation and alleviate spinal cord injury. *Life Sciences, 254,* 117796.

Zhao, Z., Lange, D. J., Voustianiouk, A., MacGrogan, D., Ho, L., Suh, J., Humala, N., Thiyagarajan, M., Wang, J., & Pasinetti, G. M. (2006). A ketogenic diet as a potential novel therapeutic intervention in amyotrophic lateral sclerosis. *BMC Neuroscience, 7,* 29.

19

Ketogenic Diets and Neuroinflammation

DAVID RUSKIN, PHD, NINA DUPUIS, PHD, AND
STÉPHANE AUVIN, MD, PHD

INTRODUCTION

The ketogenic diet (KD) is a high-fat, low-carbohydrate diet that results in ketosis, modulation of glycemia, relative caloric restriction, and elevations in the levels of certain fatty acids. In clinical practice, the KD is an established treatment for pharmacoresistant epilepsy, and it is increasingly being explored for some inflammation-induced epileptic encephalopathies, such as febrile infection-related epilepsy syndrome (FIRES; Nabbout et al., 2011). FIRES begins with severe seizures evolving into status epilepticus, and it is preceded by fever or a common viral infection but without an identifiable cause (Dupuis & Auvin, 2015). Whether fever itself or some other factor is the trigger remains to be determined. The outcome is very severe, with adverse motor and cognitive consequences as well as medically refractory epilepsy (Kramer et al., 2011). It is hypothesized that the synergy between inflammation and status epilepticus, the latter resulting partly from inflammation itself and contributing to the induction of inflammation, generates a vicious cycle that leads to major neurologic consequences (Nabbout et al., 2011). Indeed, FIRES has become the hallmark disorder underscoring the clinical anti-inflammatory effects of the KD.

While the antiseizure mechanisms of the KD remain unclear, new uses for this metabolic therapy are increasingly suggested, given its broad efficacy in various experimental models, including animal models exhibiting prominent inflammatory changes. This chapter reviews the data supporting the anti-inflammatory profile of the KD and links improvements in various animal models of neurologic disease with KD-induced modulation of inflammation. Finally, the possible mechanisms underlying the anti-inflammatory properties of the KD are discussed.

KD EXHIBITS ANTI-INFLAMMATORY PROPERTIES

The use of the KD in a pain model first led to the idea that this dietary treatment might induce anti-inflammatory activity. In this study, the KD attenuated thermal nociception and decreased peripheral edema (Ruskin et al., 2009). Later, the anti-inflammatory effects of the KD were demonstrated in a rat model of induced fever (Dupuis et al., 2015). In Wistar rats, 2 weeks of KD treatment before lipopolysaccharide (LPS) intraperitoneal injection reduced the fever response as well as pro-inflammatory cytokine levels. In this fever model, the body temperature did not rise in KD-treated animals the way it did in the controls. Body temperature was actually significantly lower in the KD group (around 37.6°C, versus 38.5°C in controls) from 1.5 hr to 4 hr after LPS administration (Dupuis et al., 2015). The fever profile correlated with plasma interleukin 1β (IL-1β) levels: 1 hr after injection, it was 130.8 ± 36.3 pg/ml in controls versus 51.4 ± 9.1 pg/ml in KD-treated rats ($p < 0.05$); 2 hr after injection, it was 203.3 ± 65.8 pg/ml in controls, versus 171.9 ± 38.8 pg/ml in the KD-treated group ($p < 0.05$). Four hours after LPS injection, plasma levels of tumor necrosis factor α (TNF-α) were significantly lower in the KD group than in the control group, although no difference was observed before LPS injection. In contrast, 4 hr after LPS injection, prostaglandin E_2 (PGE$_2$) plasma levels were not different between the two groups. Interestingly, 4 hr after LPS injection, the KD group also showed lower IL-1β mRNA levels in the hippocampus compared with controls. As expected, total fatty acid levels were increased after 14 days of KD treatment compared with a standard diet. The levels of the long-chain omega-3 (n-3) polyunsaturated fatty acids (PUFAs) eicosapentaenoic acid (EPA; C20:5 n-3) and docosahexaenoic acid

(DHA; C22:6 n-3), which are precursors of some anti-inflammatory agents, were decreased in the KD group. In contrast, arachidonic acid (AA; C20:4 n-6), an n-6 PUFA that is a precursor for the synthesis of some pro-inflammatory eicosanoids, was also reduced by the KD (Dupuis et al., 2015).

The KD further modulated fever by decreasing peripheral inflammation and brain IL-1β expression. Although we cannot exclude an effect of ketone bodies and/or caloric restriction in our study, we propose that the decrease of AA may be a key factor in the anti-inflammatory properties of the KD. This suggestion is underscored by our previous report of a decrease in AA levels in patients responding to KD (Porta et al., 2009).

Another recent study evaluated the effect of a KD on inflammation and the cell signaling protein fibroblast growth factor 21 (FGF21; Asrih et al., 2015). The authors first established that the KD promoted weight loss through increased energy expenditure and reduced food intake. The mice treated with a KD had increased plasma levels of FGF21; FGF21 gene expression was also increased in the liver but was decreased in white adipose tissue. FGF21 is produced principally in the liver and mainly acts on adipocytes. It has been shown that by targeting adipose tissue, FGF21 promotes adiponectin production and secretion; adiponectin subsequently mediates the systemic effects of FGF21 (Holland et al., 2013; Lin et al., 2013). The authors reported an increase in the expression of pro-inflammatory cytokines and macrophage accumulation. In addition, a key mediator of the inflammasome NOD-, LRR-, and pyrin domain-containing 3 (NLRP3) was significantly increased in the liver of mice treated with a KD. Interestingly, these inflammatory markers were decreased in adipose tissue of KD-fed mice (Asrih et al., 2015).

KD IMPROVES THE OUTCOME OF NEUROLOGIC DISEASE IN ANIMAL MODELS WITH INVOLVEMENT OF INFLAMMATION

The KD has been widely studied in experimental models of seizure and epilepsy, but it has also been explored in other models of neurologic diseases, such as pain, multiple sclerosis, and Parkinson's disease. In these latter conditions, the KD appears to render broad neuroprotective effects.

Pain

Our animal studies showed that KDs have a clear antinociceptive effect in acute thermal pain. This effect was present in both male and female adolescent rats (Figure 19.1) and was found using a KD comprising a ~ 6:1 fat:(carbohydrate + protein) ratio, as well as a more clinical strength ratio of 3:1 (Ruskin et al., 2013). There was also a significant effect in adult rats, although of smaller magnitude (Ruskin et al., 2009). Notably, the progressive effect had a slower onset than ketosis and lowered blood glucose (Figure 19.2), both of which were already significant at 2 days of KD feeding (Ruskin et al., 2013), a finding suggesting that these biochemical changes are not directly involved.

Chronic pain persists or progresses over a long period of time. It seems that some chronic pain patients suffer from long-term immune-system activation, resulting in continuous release of pro-inflammatory cytokines. In contrast, there is evidence that levels of anti-inflammatory cytokines are decreased in patients with widespread pain (Uceyler et al., 2006) and neuropathic pain (Uceyler et al., 2007). This explains why chronic pain may arise through an increase in pro-inflammatory cytokines and the resulting inhibition of anti-inflammatory cytokines.

KD feeding significantly reduced the inflammatory swelling produced by intraplantar injection of complete Freund's adjuvant (CFA), at least in part by reducing the amount of plasma extravasation (Ruskin et al., 2009). Notably, regarding sensory effects, KD pretreatment promotes reversal of plantar tactile allodynia in the days after a CFA injection (Figure 19.3). KD feeding was shown also to reverse the tactile allodynia produced in a mouse model of metabolic syndrome (Cooper et al., 2018). Strikingly, KD restored nerve fiber density in footpads and increased neurite growth from dorsal root ganglia in vitro. Allodynia in metabolic syndrome relates to inflammation in the peripheral nervous system (Cooper et al., 2017), and because diabetic neuropathy is thought to involve inflammation in the spinal cord (Wang et al., 2014), beneficial effects of the KD against pain syndromes involving inflammation could be peripheral, central, or both.

Clinically, the KD was used very early as a treatment for pain (Maggioni et al., 2011). For instance, in one study, KD feeding improved or completely controlled migraine, a syndrome involving neurogenic inflammation, in 39 of 50

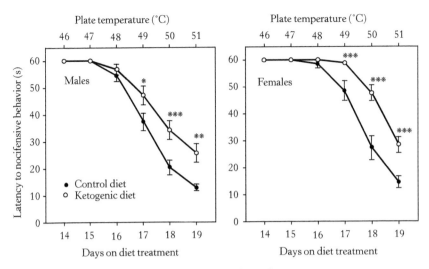

FIGURE 19.1 *The Antinociceptive Effect of the KD in Acute Thermal Pain*

Sprague-Dawley rats on a control diet or a ~ 6:1 KD were challenged with a temperature-response curve for nocifensive behavior. One temperature was tested per day. Top and bottom x-axes illustrate hotplate temperature and days on diet, respectively. Three-week dietary treatment began at 3 to 3½ weeks of age. The y-axis indicates latency to avoidance behavior (e.g., paw lifting, licking, or fluttering). All tests had a 60-s ceiling. At left, KD treatment in adolescent male rats caused heat hypoalgesia at moderate 49°C, 50°C, and 51°C temperatures. Diet $F = 5.7$, $p = 0.19$; Temperature $F = 158.4$, $p < 0.001$; Diet × Temperature interaction $F = 4.0$, $p < 0.001$; $N = 18-20$. Neuman-Keuls comparisons at each temperature: *$p < 0.05$, **$p < 0.01$, ***$p < 0.001$ compared to control. At right, KD treatment in adolescent female rats also caused heat hypoalgesia at the same temperatures. Diet $F = 28.2$, $p < 0.001$; Temperature $F = 134.2$, $p < 0.001$; Diet × Temperature interaction $F = 9.6$, $p < 0.001$; $N = 12-16$. All points are mean ± standard error. Neuman-Keuls comparisons at each temperature: ***$p < 0.001$. From S. A. Masino (Ed.), *Ketogenic Diet and Metabolic Therapies: Expanded Roles in Health and Disease*, 2017; left panel originally adapted from Ruskin et al. (2013).

patients (Baborka, 1930). More recent results support its antimigraine efficacy (Di Lorenzo et al., 2019). KD treatment was effective in treating inflammatory bowel syndrome, including its pain symptoms (Austin et al., 2009).

Some antinociceptive effects of the KD might relate directly to its high fat content. The G-protein-coupled receptor 40 (GPR40) binds and is activated by free medium- and long-chain fatty acids, and thus is sometimes called free fatty acid receptor 1 (Covington et al., 2006). This nutrient sensor is expressed in the central nervous system (CNS). In animal testing, synthetic GPR40 agonists and natural ligands injected intrathecally or intracerebroventricularly reduce inflammatory (and neuropathic) pain in numerous models (Harada et al., 2014; Karki et al., 2015; Nakamoto et al., 2013, 2015). There are electrophysiologic correlates of these behavioral effects (Karki et al., 2015).

Multiple Sclerosis

Multiple sclerosis (MS) is an autoimmune inflammatory disorder of the CNS affecting the white matter. This demyelinating disorder results in a wide range of symptoms, including motor, cognitive, and sometimes psychiatric problems. MS can be modeled in mice by inducing autoimmune encephalomyelitis or by chronic administration of cuprizone. These models are characterized by CNS neurodegeneration and synaptic loss, particularly in the hippocampus, with resulting spatial learning and memory deficits and motor impairment. Studies have shown that pretreatment with KD improves overall clinical score, exploration, motor coordination, and swim speed (Choi et al., 2016; Kim et al., 2012; Liu et al., 2020). Cognitively, impairments in a spatial reference learning and memory task are prevented by a KD (Kim et al., 2012; Liu et al., 2020), as are deficits in hippocampal long-term synaptic potentiation (Kim et al., 2012). A KD reduced the size of periventricular lesions, prevented the reduction in hippocampal volume (Kim et al., 2012), and increased hippocampal expression of mature oligodendrocytes, while inhibiting the activation of microglia and reactive astrocytes (Liu et al., 2020). In these models, the KD reduced many inflammatory mediators in brain, lymph nodes, and blood (Kim et al., 2012; Liu et al., 2020); the KD reduced by over

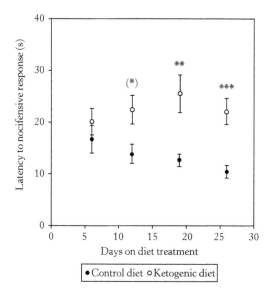

FIGURE 19.2 *The Development of the Antinociceptive Effects of the KD Over Time*

Male Sprague-Dawley rats were placed on a control diet or a 6:1 KD at 3 to 3½ weeks of age. Temperature-response curves are as in Figure 19.1; for clarity of the progressive effect, data from only the highest (51°C) tested temperature are shown. Each point represents a different squad of rats. Several days of treatment are necessary for the KD-related heat hypoalgesia to emerge. At each length of treatment, *t*-tests were protected for multiple comparisons. * $p = 0.056$, **$p < 0.01$, ***$p < 0.001$; $N = 12$–20. From S. A. Masino (Ed.), *Ketogenic Diet and Metabolic Therapies: Expanded Roles in Health and Disease*, 2017; originally adapted from Ruskin et al. (2009, 2013).

twofold the number of CD4[+] T cells and CD11b/CD45[+] macrophages/microglia (Kim et al., 2012), increased glial expression of the neuroprotective protein sirtuin-1 (Liu et al., 2020), and improved oxidative stress in brain by reducing reactive oxygen species (ROS) and malondialdehyde content and increasing glutathione (Kim et al., 2012; Liu et al., 2020).

Clinical work to date has mostly involved the relapsing-remitting form of MS. The KD is tolerated well in MS patients, with high compliance, and has had positive effects on health-related quality of life and disability status (Choi et al., 2016). KD treatment decreased leukocyte expression of enzymes that produce pro-inflammatory cytokines, such as lipoxygenase (ALOX) 2 and cyclooxygenase (COX) 1 and 2, and quality of life inversely correlated with ALOX2 and COX1 expression (Bock et al., 2018). Also, a low-sugar diet supplemented with medium-chain triglycerides led to increased percent lean body mass, decreased hunger, and increased blood paraoxonase 1 (a marker associated with low levels of oxidative stress and inflammation; Benlloch et al., 2019).

Parkinson's Disease

Parkinson's disease (PD) is a progressive neurodegenerative disorder characterized by abnormal shaking, rigidity, and slowness. The symptoms arise from the death of dopaminergic neurons in

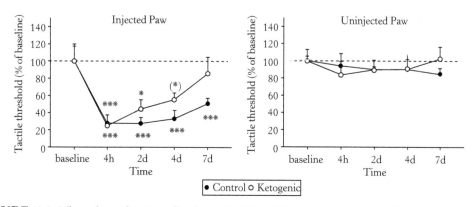

FIGURE 19.3 *Effects of Complete Freund's Adjuvant (CFA) and KD Treatment on Tactile Allodynia in Mice*

Mice were assessed by electronic von Frey probe. Male C57Bl/6 mice were placed on a control diet or a 6:1 KD for 4 weeks at 6 to 8 weeks of age. Responses are presented as percent of baseline. Injected paws became strongly hypersensitive after CFA injection in both diet groups, but the rate of recovery differed in the groups. Control diet-fed mice were still strongly hypersensitive at the last examined time, whereas a gradual and complete recovery occurred in KD-fed mice. There were no effects in the uninjected paw. Control diet $n = 6$, KD $n = 8$. *$p = 0.071$, **$p < 0.05$, ***$p < 0.001$ compared to baseline. Used with permission from Ruskin et al. (2020), *Scientific Reports*, doi.org/10.1038/s41598-020-80727-x the substantia nigra. Despite abundant clinical information about PD, the mechanisms of neurodegeneration in the substantia nigra remain unclear. Nevertheless, there is some evidence for the role of inflammation in PD, since activated microglia have been implicated in the pathogenesis and progression of PD (Hirsch & Hunot, 2009).

The murine 1-methyl-4-phenyl-1,2,3,6-tetrahydropyridine (MPTP) and rat 6-hydroxydopamine (6-OHDA) models of PD recapitulate the motor dysfunction and neurochemical changes observed in humans diagnosed with this disorder. Like patients with PD, treated rodents are characterized by selective progressive loss of dopaminergic neurons in the substantia nigra and their projections to the striatum. KD pretreatment provided neuroprotective effects in both MPTP and 6-OHDA models: nigral cell loss was significantly alleviated, as measured by tyrosine hydroxylase-positive neurons or neuron density per se, as was the loss of dopamine and its metabolites in the striatum (Cheng et al., 2009; Yang & Cheng, 2010). This effect was associated with moderate improvements in motor function in both models (Shaafi et al., 2016; Yang & Cheng, 2010). In the mouse MPTP model, KD feeding was shown to reduce inflammation—there were moderate reductions in nigral pro-inflammatory cytokines and activated microglia (Yang & Cheng, 2010). In the rat 6-OHDA model, KD feeding was found to significantly reverse the toxin-related decrease in nigral and striatal glutathione, suggesting improvements in oxidative status may also be involved in the KD's neuroprotective effects (Cheng et al., 2009).

Other ketogenic strategies have been tested. In the mouse MPTP model, octanoic acid (caprylic acid) was administered: like other medium-chain fatty acids, this compound is easily metabolized to ketone bodies. The caprylic acid treatment moderately reversed dopamine decreases and completely reversed dopamine metabolite decreases in striatum (Joniec-Maciejak et al., 2018). Octanoic acid was also found to increase striatal peroxisome proliferator-activated receptor γ (PPARγ) coactivator 1-α, impairment of which is implicated in PD pathogenesis (Choong & Mochizuki, 2017). However, this effect was not investigated in the MPTP-treated state. In addition, ketosis was not confirmed. Also in the mouse MPTP model, the ketone body β-hydroxybutyrate (βHB) was administered by subcutaneous minipump, which moderately ameliorated substantia nigra neuron loss and tyrosine-positive innervation loss in striatum, as well as loss of tissue dopamine and its

metabolites in both structures (Tieu et al., 2003). The impairment of motor coordination was completely prevented. Detailed study of brain respiration suggested that this effect is mediated by support of oxidative phosphorylation.

Clinically, the KD is tolerated well in PD patients and was associated with improvements in all four sections of the Movement Disorder Society Unified Parkinson's Disease Rating Scale, with the largest improvement in the "nonmotor daily living experiences," including pain, fatigue, and cognitive impairment (Phillips et al., 2018). Specifically in PD patients with speech problems, KD treatment significantly improved all parameters in the Voice Handicap Index-10 (Koyuncu et al., 2020).

POSSIBLE MECHANISMS OF THE ANTI-INFLAMMATORY EFFECT OF THE KD

Although the clinical efficacy of the KD against forms of pharmacoresistant epilepsy is well established, the underlying mechanisms are incompletely understood. Some intriguing hypotheses have been advanced to explain the KD's action (Lutas & Yellen, 2013; Masino & Rho, 2012). However, it is unlikely that a single mechanism can explain all the clinical effects of the KD. In the context of the present chapter, there are also probably multiple mechanisms involved in the anti-inflammatory effect of the KD (Figure 19.4).

Ketone Bodies

The ketone bodies βHB and acetoacetate (AcAc) are the products of fatty acid oxidation in hepatic mitochondria. Several lines of research have supported a direct role for βHB as an anti-inflammatory mediator (Rahman et al., 2014; Youm et al., 2015). βHB has been shown to directly inhibit the NLRP3 inflammasome assembly, which is responsible for caspase-1 activation and the release of the pro-inflammatory cytokines IL-1β and IL-18. The NLRP3 functions primarily in cells of the myeloid lineage. In mouse bone-marrow-derived macrophages and human monocytes, βHB inhibited ATP-induced cleavage of caspase-1 and the processing of the active form of IL-1β in LPS-primed cells (Youm et al., 2015). This effect was independent of fasting-regulated mechanisms, such as ROS production and inhibition of glycolysis and autophagy, both of which are known to regulate the NLRP3 inflammasome. The inhibitory effect of βHB appears specific to NLRP3, because βHB does not inhibit caspase-1 activation in response

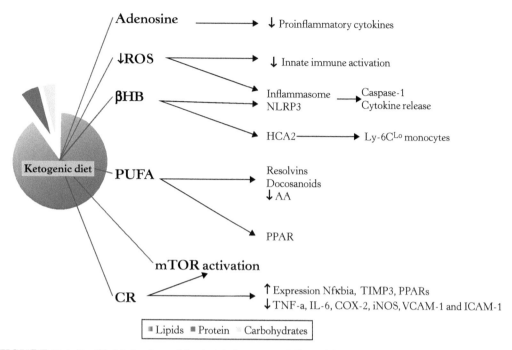

FIGURE 19.4 *Possible Mechanisms of the Anti-inflammatory Effects of the KD*

AA = arachidonic acid; βHB = β-hydroxybutyrate; CR = caloric restriction; HCA2 = hydroxyl-carboxylic acid receptor 2; NFκBiα = NF-κB inhibitor alpha; NLRP3 = NOD-, LRR- and pyrin domain-containing 3; mTOR = mammalian target of rapamycin; PPARs = peroxisome proliferator-activated receptors; PUFA = polyunsaturated fatty acids; TIMP3 = tissue inhibitor of metalloproteinases-3. From S. A. Masino (Ed.), *Ketogenic Diet and Metabolic Therapies: Expanded Roles in Health and Disease*, 2017.

to pathogens activating other inflammasomes— namely, NLR family CARD domain containing 4 (NLRC4) and absent in melanoma 2 (AIM2; Youm et al., 2015). Additionally, βHB was shown to inhibit caspase-1 activation and IL-1β secretion in mouse models of Muckle-Wells syndrome, a condition associated with a mutation in NLRP3. Finally, the KD and the associated elevation in βHB levels protected mice bearing the missense NLRP3 mutation that leads to familial cold auto-inflammatory syndrome (Youm et al., 2015).

βHB has also been shown to be a potent modulator of the HCA2 (hydroxyl-carboxylic acid 2) receptor (HCA2R), and through this target it exerts neuroprotective effects in a rodent model of stroke (Rahman et al., 2014). HCA2R activation by βHB induces Ly-6CLo monocytes and/or macrophages to deliver a neuroprotective signal to the brain (Rahman et al., 2014).

Caloric Restriction

The KD is frequently associated with a reduced calorie intake, and it has been shown that the KD promotes weight loss through increased energy expenditure and reduced food intake (Asrih et

al., 2015). Caloric restriction (CR) is a pragmatic strategy for handling excess energy stored in adipose tissues, which might contribute to systemic inflammation (Ye & Keller, 2010). CR can increase gene expression of anti-inflammatory mediators like NF-κB inhibitor alpha (NFκBiα), tissue inhibitor of metalloproteinases-3 (TIMP3), and PPARs (Sung et al., 2004; Swindell, 2009), and conversely it can inhibit pro-inflammatory genes, such as those producing TNF-α, IL-6, COX-2, inducible nitric oxide synthase, vascular cell adhesion molecule 1, and intercellular adhesion molecule 1 (Higami et al., 2006; Jung et al., 2009).

Despite these data, evidence for the potential anti-inflammatory mechanisms of CR in humans is more limited, and most of the studies addressing this topic have been developed in obese patients. In this context, CR appears to reduce pro-inflammatory molecules (Lee et al., 2010; Salas-Salvado et al., 2006), but the data reflect more the correction of an abnormal state to the nonpathologic state than the changes induced by CR under healthy conditions.

There is abundant experimental evidence for antinociceptive effects of CR in inflammatory pain (Hargraves & Hentall, 2005) and in heat hyperalgesia in arthritis models (Jurcovicova et al., 2001). Clinically, CR (applied for 12 weeks to 1 year, and typically combined with exercise) in overweight patients reduced back, knee, and overall body pain, all of which are thought to involve inflammation (Landaeta-Diaz et al., 2013; Roffey et al., 2011; White et al., 2015). Fasting (either every other day or for multiple-day periods) may be considered the ultimate CR. Seven days of fasting significantly alleviated joint pain and stiffness in rheumatoid arthritis sufferers (Kroker et al., 1984; Michalsen et al., 2005; Sköldstam et al., 1979), apparently through anti-inflammatory actions, including modified neutrophil function (Hafström et al., 1988; Udén et al., 1983). A 24-hr clinical fast is sufficient to limit activation of the NLRP3 inflammasome (Traba et al., 2015), which is associated with hyperalgesia (Bullón et al., 2016); therefore, fasting every other day might be beneficial in rheumatoid arthritis.

Overall, the underlying mechanisms explaining the anti-inflammatory effects of CR are not well understood. However, since many nutrients and growth factors can activate mammalian target of rapamycin (mTOR), the anti-inflammatory effect of CR may be in part the result of stimulating this pathway. Laboratory studies have already demonstrated that the KD inhibits mTOR signaling in the brain and liver of normal rats (McDaniel et al., 2011). This inhibition is thought to be related to a decrease in Akt signaling in the brain and the liver. McDaniel and colleagues also showed that the KD prevented mTOR hyperactivation after kainate-induced status epilepticus (McDaniel et al., 2011). However, their study did not correlate the modulation of the mTOR by the KD with any status epilepticus-induced pro-inflammatory changes.

PUFAs

PUFAs are dietary lipids that contain more than one double bond. There are two groups of PUFAs: the omega-3 (n-3) and the omega-6 (n-6) PUFAs. This nomenclature refers to the position of the double bond relative to the methyl terminal of the molecule (Taha et al., 2010). Diet is an important source of PUFAs. Dietary n-3 PUFAs are found in flaxseed, in some nuts, in marine fish, and in marine mammals, such as seals. In contrast, n-6 PUFAs are found in a variety of animal products and in vegetable oils, such as canola and corn oil, and they make up

the majority of PUFAs in the modern Western diet (Taha et al., 2010).

With normal dietary intake, n-3 PUFAs can decrease the production of inflammatory eicosanoids, cytokines, and ROS as well as the expression of adhesion molecules. Toward these ends, n-3 PUFAs act both directly (by replacing AA as an eicosanoid substrate and inhibiting AA metabolism) and indirectly (by altering the expression of inflammatory genes through effects on transcription factor activation). The n-3 PUFAs, particularly EPA and DHA, also have anti-inflammatory actions, mediated primarily by their hydroxylated metabolites, which include resolvins and docosanoids (Hong et al., 2003). For instance, EPA and DHA have been reported to incorporate into human neutrophil cells and to decrease the production of pro-inflammatory PGE_2 in a dose-dependent manner (Rees et al., 2006).

KD treatment not only increases fatty acid levels in the blood but also increases levels of specific PUFAs that can bind to and activate PPARs. The PPARs have been considered potential drug targets for seizure control (Sampath & Ntambi, 2005). Both PPARα and PPARγ are activated by PUFAs and their eicosanoid derivatives, as well as by synthetic ligands, such as the fibrates (Kersten et al., 2000). Activation of PPARs stimulates the transcription of the genes involved in fatty acid oxidation via the formation of heterodimeric transcription-factor complexes with the retinoid X receptor (Smith, 2002). Three types of PPARs have been identified—α, β, and γ: PPARα is expressed mainly in liver, kidney, and heart muscle; PPARβ is expressed in several tissues, such as brain, adipose tissue, and skin; PPARγ is also expressed in the brain. Both linolenic and linoleic fatty acids have a greater binding affinity for PPARα than EPA or DHA (Lin et al., 1999). Synthetic PPAR agonists reduce experimentally induced inflammation (Cuzzocrea et al., 2003, 2004; LoVerme et al., 2005). This effect is the result of the inhibition of pro-inflammatory pathways involving NF-κB, signal transduction and transcription-1, and nuclear factor of activated T cells (Blanquart et al., 2003). Activation of the PPARγ subtype alleviated inflammatory and neuropathic pain in animal models (Morgenweck et al., 2010, 2013), and PPARα agonists given to patients reduced pain in a number of inflammatory (and neuropathic) conditions (Freitag & Miller, 2014). In addition, PUFAs activate the nutrient receptor

GPR120 (also known as free fatty acid receptor 4), which is known to be anti-inflammatory (Cintra et al., 2012). Certain PUFAs also block pain due to activation of the heat-sensing transient receptor potential vanilloid-1 (TRPV1; the "capsaicin receptor"), an inflammation-related receptor expressed by peripheral nociceptive neurons (Matta et al., 2007). Regardless of mechanism, specific PUFAs appear effective against inflammatory pain (Goldberg & Katz, 2007; Lee et al., 2012).

Adenosine Modulation

The KD has been shown to modulate adenosine levels. Astrocytic adenosine kinase (ADK) is an enzyme responsible for adenosine phosphorylation and clearance of adenosine from the extracellular space. Expression of ADK is reduced by the KD, thereby increasing extracellular levels of adenosine and the activation of inhibitory adenosine A_1 receptor (A_1R; Masino et al., 2011). Importantly, the effect of the KD on adenosine has been linked to a decrease in electrographic seizure activity (Masino et al., 2011). The anti-inflammatory effects of the KD may be explained in part by adenosine, as this metabolic mediator has long been known to induce anti-inflammatory activity (Kowaluk et al., 1998; Linden, 2001). Along these lines, adenosine has been reported to reduce central and peripheral inflammation. Using $A_1R^{-/-}$ genetically engineered mice and a pretreatment with the specific A_1R agonist 2-chloro-2'-C-methyl-N6-cyclopentyladenosine (CCPA) in wild-type mice, it was shown that A_1R modulates LPS-induced transmigration of polymorphonuclear cells and reduced levels of TNF-α, IL-6, and chemokine (C-X-C motif) ligand 2 and 3 in the lung (Ngamsri et al., 2010). There are also data suggesting that A_1Rs are upregulated in acute forms of neuroinflammation and downregulated in chronic forms. Activation of cerebral A_1R acts as a brake for the microglial response after traumatic brain injury (Haselkorn et al., 2010). Both A_1Rs and $A_{2A}Rs$ appear to be involved in the inflammatory response, and pharmacologic interventions might mitigate this (Lukashev et al., 2005; Sitkovsky & Ohta, 2005). However, $A_{2A}Rs$ as well as pharmacologic intervention targeting $A_{2A}Rs$ might have bidirectional effects on neuroinflammation. Specifically, the local glutamate level after brain injury is one of the crucial factors that determines the direction of an $A_{2A}R$-mediated effect on neuroinflammation (Dai & Zhou, 2011).

ROS Reduction, Uncoupling Proteins, and Mitochondrial Membrane Potential

Both βHB and AcAc have been shown to induce neuroprotective effects. These effects have been linked to reduction of ROS through enhanced NADH oxidation and inhibition of mitochondrial permeability transition (Kim et al., 2007, 2010; Maalouf et al., 2007). Furthermore, the KD has been shown to enhance mitochondrial biogenesis (Bough et al., 2006). The ROS and inflammation are tightly linked through a strong reciprocal relationship; ROS generated by inflammatory cells act as inflammatory signaling molecules and participate in the inflammatory response. Furthermore, ROS play a key role in the control of NF-κB, activator protein-1 (AP-1), and other transcription factors involved in gene expression of both inflammatory and immune mediators. When sustained, oxidative stress can lead to a chronic inflammatory state and inflammation can aggravate ROS production (Harijith et al., 2014).

The KD can reduce both ROS production and inflammation. Recently, it has been shown that ROS can activate the NLRP3 inflammasome protein, a molecular platform activated on signs of cellular "danger" to trigger innate immune defenses through the maturation of pro-inflammatory cytokines, such as IL-1β and IL-18 (Zhou et al., 2011). Moreover, oxidative stress can act as a central regulator of high-mobility group box 1 (HMGB1) translocation, release, and activity in inflammation and cell death. Thus, modulation of HMGB1 can limit inflammation and reduce tissue damage during infection as well as sterile inflammation (Yu et al., 2015). Thus, ketone bodies appear to have the ability to target the inflammatory pathways through direct action on NLRP3 (Youm et al., 2015) and by causing a decrease in ROS production and levels (Kim et al., 2007, 2015; Maalouf et al., 2007).

CLINICAL EVIDENCE AND FUTURE INDICATIONS

There is currently no clinical open-label study or controlled trial that demonstrates that the effects of the KD are mediated through an anti-inflammatory mechanism. Notwithstanding this lack of data, it is intriguing to note once again that the KD is an effective treatment for a condition associated with both inflammation and medically refractory seizures—namely, FIRES (Nabbout et al., 2010; Peng et al., 2019; Singh et al., 2014). At present, whether the KD would indeed be useful for diverse conditions associated with neuroinflammation—for example, pain, multiple sclerosis, and Parkinson's disease, among others—remains unclear, but the current evidence pointing to broad anti-inflammatory effects of the KD is compelling, as this metabolism-based treatment could constitute a readily available therapy for neurologic disorders associated with inflammation. Detailed preclinical studies in relevant animal models of neurologic disease are no doubt of paramount importance to uncover the underlying biology of KD action. Ultimately, though, well-designed clinical trials must be implemented to validate readily available therapeutic approaches like the KD.

REFERENCES

Asrih, M., Altirriba, J., Rohner-Jeanrenaud, F., & Jornayvaz, F. R. (2015). Ketogenic diet impairs FGF21 signaling and promotes differential inflammatory responses in the liver and white adipose tissue. *PLOS ONE, 10*, Article e0126364.

Austin, G. L., Dalton, C. B., Hu, Y., Morris, C. B., Hankins, J., Weinland, S. R., Westman, E. C., Yancy, W. S., Jr., & Drossman, D. A. (2009). A very low-carbohydrate diet improves symptoms and quality of life in diarrhea-predominant irritable bowel syndrome. *Clinical Gastroenterology and Hepatology, 7*, 706–708.e701.

Baborka, C. J. (1930). Migraine: Results of treatment by ketogenic diet in fifty cases. *Mayo Clinic Proceedings, 5*, 190–191.

Benlloch, M., López-Rodríguez, M. M., Cuerda-Ballester, M., Drehmer, E., Carrera, S., Ceron, J. J., Tvarijonaviciute, A., Chirivella, J., Fernández-García, D., & de la Rubia Ortí, J. E. (2019). Satiating effect of a ketogenic diet and its impact on muscle improvement and oxidation state in multiple sclerosis patients. *Nutrients, 11*, 1156.

Blanquart, C., Barbier, O., Fruchart, J. C., Staels, B., & Glineur, C. (2003). Peroxisome proliferator-activated receptors: Regulation of transcriptional activities and roles in inflammation. *Journal of Steroid Biochemistry and Molecular Biology, 85*, 267–273.

Bock, M., Karber, M., & Kuhn, H. (2018). Ketogenic diets attenuate cyclooxygenase and lipoxygenase gene expression in multiple sclerosis. *EBioMedicine, 36*, 293–303.

Bough, K. J., Wetherington, J., Hassel, B., Pare, J. F., Gawryluk, J. W., Greene, J. G., Shaw, R., Smith, Y., Geiger, J. D., & Dingledine, R. J. (2006). Mitochondrial biogenesis in the anticonvulsant mechanism of the ketogenic diet. *Annals of Neurology, 60*, 223–235.

Bullón, P., Alcocer-Gómez, E., Carrión, A. M., Marín-Aguilar, F., Garrido-Maraver, J., Román-Malo, L.,

Ruiz-Cabello, J., Culic, O., Ryffel, B., Apetoh, L., Ghiringhelli, F., Battino, M., Sanchez-Alcazar, J. A., & Cordero, M. D. (2016). AMPK phosphorylation modulates pain by activation of NLRP3 inflammasome. *Antioxidants & Redox Signaling, 24*, 157–170.

Cheng, B., Yang, X., An, L., Gao, B., Liu, X., & Liu, S. (2009). Ketogenic diet protects dopaminergic neurons against 6-OHDA neurotoxicity via up-regulating glutathione in a rat model of Parkinson's disease. *Brain Research, 1286*, 25–31.

Choi, I. Y., Piccio, L., Childress, P., Bollman, B., Ghosh, A., Brandhorst, S., Suarez, J., Michalsen, A., Cross, A. H., Morgan, T. E., Wei, M., Paul, F., Bock, M., & Longo, V. D. (2016). A diet mimicking fasting promotes regeneration and reduces autoimmunity and multiple sclerosis symptoms. *Cell Reports, 15*, 2136–2146.

Choong, C. J., & Mochizuki, H. (2017). Gene therapy targeting mitochondrial pathway in Parkinson's disease. *Journal of Neural Transmission (Vienna), 124*, 193–207.

Cintra, D. E., Ropelle, E. R., Moraes, J. C., Pauli, J. R., Morari, J., Souza, C. T., Grimaldi, R., Stahl, M., Carvalheira, J. B., Saad, M. J., & Velloso, L. A. (2012). Unsaturated fatty acids revert diet-induced hypothalamic inflammation in obesity. *PLOS ONE, 7*, Article e30571.

Cooper, M. A., Menta, B. W., Perez-Sanchez, C., Jack, M. M., Kahn, Z. W., Ryals, J. M., Winter, M., & Wright, D. E. (2018). A ketogenic diet reduces metabolic syndrome-induced allodynia and promotes peripheral nerve growth in mice. *Experimental Neurology, 306*, 149–157.

Cooper, M. A., Ryals, J. M., Wu, P.-Y., Wright, K. D., Walter, K. R., & Wright, D. E. (2017). Modulation of diet-induced mechanical allodynia by metabolic parameters and inflammation. *Journal of the Peripheral Nervous System, 22*, 39–46.

Covington, D. K., Briscoe, C. A., Brown, A. J., & Jayawickreme, C. K. (2006). The G-protein-coupled receptor 40 family (GPR40-GPR43) and its role in nutrient sensing. *Biochemical Society Transactions, 34*, 770–773.

Cuzzocrea, S., Mazzon, E., Dugo, L., Patel, N. S., Serraino, I., Di Paolo, R., Genovese, T., Britti, D., De Maio, M., Caputi, A. P., & Thiemermann, C. (2003). Reduction in the evolution of murine type II collagen-induced arthritis by treatment with rosiglitazone, a ligand of the peroxisome proliferator-activated receptor γ. *Arthritis and Rheumatism, 48*, 3544–3556.

Cuzzocrea, S., Pisano, B., Dugo, L., Ianaro, A., Maffia, P., Patel, N. S., Di_Paola, R., Ialenti, A., Genovese, T., Chatterjee, P. K., Di Rosa, M., Caputi, A. P., & Thiemermann, C. (2004). Rosiglitazone, a ligand of the peroxisome proliferator-activated receptor-γ, reduces acute inflammation. *European Journal of Pharmacology, 483*, 79–93.

Dai, S. S., & Zhou, Y. G. (2011). Adenosine 2A receptor: A crucial neuromodulator with bidirectional effect in neuroinflammation and brain injury. *Reviews in Neuroscience, 22*, 231–239.

Di Lorenzo, C., Pinto, A., Ienca, R., Coppola, G., Sirianni, G., Di Lorenzo, G., Parisi, V., Serrao, M., Spagnoli, A., Vestri, A., Schoenen, J., Donini, L. M., & Pierelli, F. (2019). A randomized double-blind, cross-over trial of very low-calorie diet in overweight migraine patients: A possible role for ketones? *Nutrients, 11*, 1742.

Dupuis, N., & Auvin, S. (2015). Inflammation and epilepsy in the developing brain: Clinical and experimental evidence. *CNS Neuroscience & Therapeutics, 21*, 141–151.

Dupuis, N., Curatolo, N., Benoist, J.-F., & Auvin, S. (2015). Ketogenic diet exhibits anti-inflammatory properties. *Epilepsia, 56*, e95–e98.

Freitag, C. M., & Miller, R. J. (2014). Peroxisome proliferator-activated receptor agonists modulate neuropathic pain: A link to chemokines? *Frontiers in Cellular Neuroscience, 8*, 238.

Goldberg, R. J., & Katz, J. (2007). A meta-analysis of the analgesic effects of omega-3 polyunsaturated fatty acid supplementation for inflammatory joint pain. *Pain, 129*, 210–223.

Hafström, I., Ringertz, B., Gyllenhammar, H., Palmblad, J., & Harms-Ringdahl, M. (1988). Effects of fasting on disease activity, neutrophil function, fatty acid composition, and leukotriene biosynthesis in patients with rheumatoid arthritis. *Arthritis and Rheumatism, 31*, 585–592.

Harada, S., Haruna, Y., Aizawa, F., Matsuura, W., Nakamoto, K., Yamashita, T., Kasuya, F., & Tokuyama, S. (2014). Involvement of GPR40, a long-chain free fatty acid receptor, in the production of central post-stroke pain after global cerebral ischemia. *European Journal of Pharmacology, 744*, 115–123.

Hargraves, W. A., & Hentall, I. D. (2005). Analgesic effects of dietary caloric restriction in adult mice. *Pain, 114*, 455–461.

Harijith, A., Ebenezer, D. L., & Natarajan, V. (2014). Reactive oxygen species at the crossroads of inflammasome and inflammation. *Frontiers in Physiology, 5*, 352.

Haselkorn, M. L., Shellington, D. K., Jackson, E. K., Vagni, V. A., Janesko-Feldman, K., Dubey, R. K., Gillespie, D. G., Cheng, D., Bell, M. J., Jenkins, L. W., Homanics, G. E., Schnermann, J., & Kochanek, P. M. (2010). Adenosine A$_1$ receptor activation as a brake on the microglial response after experimental traumatic brain injury in mice. *Journal of Neurotrauma, 27*, 901–910.

Higami, Y., Barger, J. L., Page, G. P., Allison, D. B., Smith, S. R., Prolla, T. A., & Weindruch, R. (2006). Energy restriction lowers the expression of genes linked to inflammation, the cytoskeleton, the extracellular matrix, and angiogenesis in mouse adipose tissue. *Journal of Nutrition, 136*, 343–352.

Hirsch, E. C., & Hunot, S. (2009). Neuroinflammation in Parkinson's disease: A target for neuroprotection? *Lancet Neurology, 8*, 382–397.

Holland, W. L., Adams, A. C., Brozinick, J. T., Bui, H. H., Miyauchi, Y., Kusminski, C. M., Bauer, S. M., Wade, M., Singhal, E., Cheng, C. C., Volk, K., Kuo, M.-S., Gordillo, R., Kharitonenkov, A., & Scherer, P. E. (2013). An FGF21-adiponectin-ceramide axis controls energy expenditure and insulin action in mice. *Cell Metabolism, 17*, 790–797.

Hong, S., Gronert, K., Devchand, P. R., Moussignac, R. L., & Serhan, C. N. (2003). Novel docosatrienes and 17S-resolvins generated from docosahexaenoic acid in murine brain, human blood, and glial cells: Autacoids in anti-inflammation. *Journal of Biological Chemistry, 278*, 14677–14687.

Joniec-Maciejak, I., Wawer, A., Turzyńska, D., Sobolewska, A., Maciejak, P., Szyndler, J., Mirowska-Guzel, D., & Płaźnik, A. (2018). Octanoic acid prevents reduction of striatal dopamine in the MPTP mouse model of Parkinson's disease. *Pharmacological Reports, 70*, 988–992.

Jung, K. J., Lee, E. K., Kim, J. Y., Zou, Y., Sung, B., Heo, H. S., Kim, M. K., Lee, J., Kim, N. D., Yu, B. P., & Chung, H. Y. (2009). Effect of short term calorie restriction on pro-inflammatory NF-κB and AP-1 in aged rat kidney. *Inflammation Research, 58*, 143–150.

Jurcovicova, J., Stanciková, M., Svík, K., Ondrejicková, O., Krsova, D., Seres, J., & Rokyta, R. (2001). Stress of chronic food restriction attenuates the development of adjuvant arthritis in male Long Evans rats. *Clinical and Experimental Rheumatology, 19*, 371–376.

Karki, P., Kurihara, T., Nakamachi, T., Watanabe, J., Asada, T., Oyoshi, T., Shioda, S., Yoshimura, M., Arita, K., & Miyata, A. (2015). Attenuation of inflammatory and neuropathic pain behaviors in mice through activation of free fatty acid receptor GPR40. *Molecular Pain, 11*, 6.

Kersten, S., Desvergne, B., & Wahli, W. (2000). Roles of PPARs in health and disease. *Nature, 405*, 421–424.

Kim, D. Y., Davis, L. M., Sullivan, P. G., Maalouf, M., Simeone, T. A., van Brederode, J., & Rho, J. M. (2007). Ketone bodies are protective against oxidative stress in neocortical neurons. *Journal of Neurochemistry, 101*, 1316–1326.

Kim, D. Y., Hao, J., Liu, R., Turner, G., Shi, F.-D., Rho, J. M. (2012). Inflammation-mediated memory dysfunction and effects of a ketogenic diet in a murine model of multiple sclerosis. *PLOS ONE, 7*, Article e35476.

Kim, D. Y., Simeone, K. A., Simeone, T. A., Pandya, J. D., Wilke, J. C., Ahn, Y., Geddes, J. W., Sullivan,

P. G., & Rho, J. M. (2015). Ketone bodies mediate anti-seizure effects through mitochondrial permeability transition. *Annals of Neurology, 78*, 77–87.

Kim, D. Y., Vallejo, J., & Rho, J. M. (2010). Ketones prevent synaptic dysfunction induced by mitochondrial respiratory complex inhibitors. *Journal of Neurochemistry, 114*, 130–141.

Kowaluk, E. A., Bhagwat, S. S., & Jarvis, M. F. (1998). Adenosine kinase inhibitors. *Current Pharmaceutical Design, 4*, 403–416.

Koyuncu, H., Fidan, V., Toktas, H., Binay, O., & Celik, H. (2020). Effect of ketogenic diet versus regular diet on voice quality of patients with Parkinson's disease. *Acta Neurologica Belgica,* in press, doi. org/10.1007/s13760-020-01486-0.

Kramer, U., Chi, C. S., Lin, K. L., Specchio, N., Sahin, M., Olson, H., Nabbout, R., Kluger, G., Lin, J. J., & van Baalen, A. (2011). Febrile infection-related epilepsy syndrome (FIRES): Pathogenesis, treatment, and outcome; A multicenter study on 77 children. *Epilepsia, 52*, 1956–1965.

Kroker, G. F., Stroud, R. M., Marshall, R., Bullock, T., Carroll, F. M., Greenberg, M., Randolph, T. G., Rea, W. J., & Smiley, R. E. (1984). Fasting & rheumatoid arthritis: A multicenter study. *Clinical Ecology, 2*, 137–144.

Landaeta-Diaz, L., Fernandez, J. M., Da Silva-Grigoletto, M., Rosado-Alvarez, D., Gomez-Garduno, A., Gomez-Delgado, F., Lopez-Miranda, J., Perez-Jimenez, F., & Fuentes-Jimenez, F. (2013). Mediterranean diet, moderate-to-high intensity training, and health-related quality of life in adults with metabolic syndrome. *European Journal of Preventive Cardiology, 20*, 555–564.

Lee, I. S., Shin, G., & Choue, R. (2010). A 12-week regimen of caloric restriction improves levels of adipokines and pro-inflammatory cytokines in Korean women with BMIs greater than 23 kg/m^2. *Inflammation Research, 59*, 399–405.

Lee, Y. H., Bae, S. C., & Song, G. G. (2012). Omega-3 polyunsaturated fatty acids and the treatment of rheumatoid arthritis: A meta-analysis. *Archives of Medical Research, 43*, 356–362.

Lin, Q., Ruuska, S. E., Shaw, N. S., Dong, D., & Noy, N. (1999). Ligand selectivity of the peroxisome proliferator-activated receptor α. *Biochemistry, 38*, 185–190.

Lin, Z., Tian, H., Lam, K. S., Lin, S., Hoo, R. C., Konishi, M., Itoh, N., Wang, Y., Bornstein, S. R., Xu, A., & Li, X. (2013). Adiponectin mediates the metabolic effects of FGF21 on glucose homeostasis and insulin sensitivity in mice. *Cell Metabolism, 17*, 779–789.

Linden, J. (2001). Molecular approach to adenosine receptors: Receptor-mediated mechanisms of tissue protection. *Annual Review of Pharmacology and Toxicology, 41*, 775–787.

Liu, C., Zhang, N., Zhang, R., Jin, L., Petridis, A. K., Loers, G., Zheng, X., Wang, Z., & Siebert, H.-C. (2020). Cuprizone-induced demyelination in mouse hippocampus is alleviated by ketogenic diet. *Journal of Agriculture and Food Chemistry, 68*, 11215–11228.

LoVerme, J., Fu, J., Astarita, G., La Rana, G., Russo, R., Calignano, A., & Piomelli, D. (2005). The nuclear receptor peroxisome proliferator-activated receptor-alpha mediates the anti-inflammatory actions of palmitoylethanolamide. *Molecular Pharmacology, 67*, 15–19.

Lukashev, D. E., Ohta, A., & Sitkovsky, M. V. (2005). Physiological regulation of acute inflammation by A$_{2A}$ adenosine receptor. *Drug Development Research, 64*, 172–177.

Lutas, A., & Yellen, G. (2013). The ketogenic diet: Metabolic influences on brain excitability and epilepsy. *Trends in Neuroscience, 36*, 32–40.

Maalouf, M., Sullivan, P. G., Davis, L., Kim, D. Y., & Rho, J. M. (2007). Ketones inhibit mitochondrial production of reactive oxygen species production following glutamate excitotoxicity by increasing NADH oxidation. *Neuroscience, 145*, 256–264.

Maggioni, F., Margoni, M., & Zanchin, G. (2011). Ketogenic diet in migraine treatment: A brief but ancient history. *Cephalalgia, 31*, 1150–1151.

Masino, S. A., Li, T., Theofilas, P., Sandau, U., Ruskin, D. N., Fredholm, B. B., Geiger, J. D., Aronica, E., & Boison, D. (2011). A ketogenic diet suppresses seizures in mice through adenosine A$_1$ receptors. *Journal of Clinical Investigation, 121*, 2679–2683.

Masino, S. A., & Rho, J. M. (2012). Mechanisms of ketogenic diet action. In M. A. Rogawski, A. V. Delgado-Escueta, J. L. Noebels, M. Avoli, & R. W. Olsen (Eds.), *Jasper's basic mechanisms of the epilepsies* (pp. 1001–1022). National Center for Biotechnology Information.

Matta, J. A., Miyares, R. L., & Ahern, G. P. (2007). TRPV1 is a novel target for omega-3 polyunsaturated fatty acids. *Journal of Physiology, 578*, 397–411.

McDaniel, S. S., Rensing, N., Thio, L. L., Yamada, K. A., & Wong, M. (2011). The ketogenic diet inhibits the mammalian target of rapamycin (mTOR) pathway. *Epilepsia, 52*, e7–11.

Michalsen, A., Riegert, M., Lüdtke, R., Bäcker, M., Langhorst, J., Schwickert, M., & Dobos, G. J. (2005). Mediterranean diet or extended fasting's influence on changing the intestinal microflora, immunoglobulin A secretion and clinical outcome in patients with rheumatoid arthritis and fibromyalgia: An observational study. *BMC Complementary and Alternative Medicine, 5*, 22.

Morgenweck, J., Abdel-aleem, O. S., McNamara, K. C., Donahue, R. R., Badr, M. Z., & Taylor, B. K. (2010). Activation of peroxisome proliferator-activated receptor γ in brain inhibits inflammatory pain, dorsal horn expression of Fos, and local edema. *Neuropharmacology, 58,* 337–345.

Morgenweck, J., Griggs, R. B., Donahue, R. R., Zadina, J. E., & Taylor, B. K. (2013). PPARγ activation blocks development and reduces established neuropathic pain in rats. *Neuropharmacology, 70,* 236–246.

Nabbout, R., Mazzuca, M., Hubert, P., Peudennier, S., Allaire, C., Flurin, V., Aberastury, M., Silva, W., & Dulac, O. (2010). Efficacy of ketogenic diet in severe refractory status epilepticus initiating fever induced refractory epileptic encephalopathy in school age children (FIRES). *Epilepsia, 51,* 2033–2037.

Nabbout, R., Vezzani, A., Dulac, O., & Chiron, C. (2011). Acute encephalopathy with inflammation-mediated status epilepticus. *Lancet Neurology, 10,* 99–108.

Nakamoto, K., Nishinaka, T., Sato, N., Aizawa, F., Yamashita, T., Mankura, M., Koyama, Y., Kasuya, F., & Tokuyama, S. (2015). The activation of supraspinal GPR40/FFA1 receptor signalling regulates the descending pain control system. *British Journal of Pharmacology, 172,* 1250–1262.

Nakamoto, K., Nishinaka, T., Sato, N., Mankura, M., Koyama, Y., Kasuya, F., & Tokuyama, S. (2013). Hypothalamic GPR40 signaling activated by free long chain fatty acids suppresses CFA-induced inflammatory chronic pain. *PLOS ONE, 8,* Article e81563.

Ngamsri, K.-C., Wagner, R., Vollmer, I., Stark, S., & Reutershan, J. (2010). Adenosine receptor A$_1$ regulates polymorphonuclear cell trafficking and microvascular permeability in lipopolysaccharide-induced lung injury. *Journal of Immunology, 185,* 4374–4384.

Peng, P., Peng, J., Yin, F., Deng, X., Chen, C., He, F., Wang, X., Guang, S., & Mao, L. (2019). Ketogenic diet as a treatment for super-refractory status epilepticus in febrile infection-related epilepsy syndrome. *Frontiers in Neurology, 10,* 423.

Phillips, M. C. L., Murtagh, D. K. J., Gilbertson, L. J., Asztely, F. J. S., & Lynch, C. D. P. (2018). Low-fat versus ketogenic diet in Parkinson's disease: A pilot randomized controlled trial. *Movement Disorders, 33,* 1306–1314.

Porta, N., Vallee, L., Boutry, E., Fontaine, M., Dessein, A. F., Joriot, S., Cuisset, J. M., Cuvellier, J. C., & Auvin, S. (2009). Comparison of seizure reduction and serum fatty acid levels after receiving the ketogenic and modified Atkins diet. *Seizure, 18,* 359–364.

Rahman, M., Muhammad, S., Kahn, M. A., Chen, H., Ridder, D. A., Muller-Fielitz, H., Pokorna, B., Vollbrandt, T., Stolting, I., Nadrowitz, R., Okun, J. G., Offermanns, S., & Schwaninger, M. (2014). The β-hydroxybutyrate receptor HCA$_2$ activates a neuroprotective subset of macrophages. *Nature Communications, 5,* 3944.

Rees, D., Miles, E. A., Banerjee, T., Wells, S. J., Roynette, C. E., Wahle, K. W., & Calder, P. C. (2006). Dose-related effects of eicosapentaenoic acid on innate immune function in healthy humans: A comparison of young and older men. *American Journal of Clinical Nutrition, 83,* 331–342.

Roffey, D. M., Ashdown, L. C., Dornan, H. D., Creech, M. J., Dagenais, S., Dent, R. M., & Wai, E. K. (2011). Pilot evaluation of a multidisciplinary, medically supervised, nonsurgical weight loss program on the severity of low back pain in obese adults. *Spine Journal, 11,* 197–204.

Ruskin, D. N., Kawamura, M., Jr., & Masino, S. A. (2009). Reduced pain and inflammation in juvenile and adult rats fed a ketogenic diet. *PLOS ONE, 4,* Article e8349.

Ruskin, D. N., Sturdevant, I. C., Wyss, L. S., & Masino, S. A. (2021). Ketogenic diet effects on inflammatory allodynia and ongoing pain in rodents. *Scientific Reports, 11,* 725.

Ruskin, D. N., Suter, T. A. C. S., Ross, J. L., & Masino, S. A. (2013). Ketogenic diets and thermal pain: Dissociation of hypoalgesia, elevated ketones, and lowered glucose in rats. *Journal of Pain, 14,* 467–474.

Salas-Salvado, J., Bullo, M., Garcia-Lorda, P., Figueredo, R., Del Castillo, D., Bonada, A., & Balanza, R. (2006). Subcutaneous adipose tissue cytokine production is not responsible for the restoration of systemic inflammation markers during weight loss. *International Journal of Obesity, 30,* 1714–1720.

Sampath, H., & Ntambi, J. M. (2005). Polyunsaturated fatty acid regulation of genes of lipid metabolism. *Annual Review of Nutrition, 25,* 317–340.

Shaafi, S., Najmi, S., Aliasgharpour, H., Mahmoudi, J., Sadigh-Etemad, S., Farhoudi, M., & Baniasadi, N. (2016). The efficacy of the ketogenic diet on motor functions in Parkinson's disease: A rat model. *Iranian Journal of Neurology, 15,* 63–69.

Singh, R. K., Joshi, S. M., Potter, D. M., Leber, S. M., Carlson, M. D., & Shellhaas, R. A. (2014). Cognitive outcomes in febrile infection-related epilepsy syndrome treated with the ketogenic diet. *Pediatrics, 134,* e1431–e1435.

Sitkovsky, M. V., & Ohta, A. (2005). The 'danger' sensors that STOP the immune response: The A$_2$ adenosine receptors? *Trends in Immunology, 26,* 299–304.

Sköldstam, L., Larsson, L., & Lindström, F. D. (1979). Effect of fasting and lactovegetarian diet on rheumatoid arthritis. *Scandinavian Journal of Rheumatology, 8,* 249–255.

Smith, S. A. (2002). Peroxisome proliferator-activated receptors and the regulation of mammalian lipid metabolism. *Biochemical Society Transactions, 30,* 1086–1090.

Sung, B., Park, S., Yu, B. P., & Chung, H. Y. (2004). Modulation of PPAR in aging, inflammation, and calorie restriction. *The Journals of Gerontology. Series A, Biological Sciences and Medical Sciences, 59,* 997–1006.

Swindell, W. R. (2009). Genes and gene expression modules associated with caloric restriction and aging in the laboratory mouse. *BMC Genomics, 10,* 585.

Taha, A. Y., Burnham, W. M., & Auvin, S. (2010). Polyunsaturated fatty acids and epilepsy. *Epilepsia, 51,* 1348–1358.

Tieu, K., Perier, C., Caspersen, C., Teismann, P., Wu, D.-C., Yan, S.-D., Niani, A., Vila, M., Jackson-Lewis, V., Ramasamy, R., et al. (2003). D-β-Hydroxybutyrate rescues mitochondrial respiration and mitigates features of Parkinson disease. *Journal of Clinical Investigation, 112,* 892–901.

Traba, J., Kwarteng-Siaw, M., Okoli, T. C., Li, J., Huffstutler, R. D., Bray, A., Waclawiw, M. A., Han, K., Pelletier, M., Sauve, A. A., Siegel, R.M., & Sack, M.N. (2015). Fasting and refeeding differentially regulate NLRP3 inflammasome activation in human subjects. *Journal of Clinical Investigation, 125,* 4592–4600.

Uceyler, N., Rogausch, J. P., Toyka, K. V., & Sommer, C. (2007). Differential expression of cytokines in painful and painless neuropathies. *Neurology, 69,* 42–49.

Uceyler, N., Valenza, R., Stock, M., Schedel, R., Sprotte, G., & Sommer, C. (2006). Reduced levels of antiinflammatory cytokines in patients with chronic widespread pain. *Arthritis and Rheumatism, 54,* 2656–2664.

Udén, A. M., Trang, L., Venizelos, N., & Palmblad, J. (1983). Neutrophil functions and clinical performance after total fasting in patients with rheumatoid arthritis. *Annals of the Rheumatic Diseases, 42,* 45–51.

Wang, D., Couture, R., & Hong, Y. (2014). Activated microglia in the spinal cord underlies diabetic neuropathic pain. *European Journal of Pharmacology, 728,* 59–66.

White, D. K., Neogi, T., Rejeski, W. J., Walkup, M. P., Lewis, C. E., Nevitt, M. C., Foy, C. G., Felson, D. T., & Look, A. R. G. (2015). Can an intensive diet and exercise program prevent knee pain among overweight adults at high risk? *Arthritis Care Research, 67,* 965–971.

Yang, X., & Cheng, B. (2010). Neuroprotective and anti-inflammatory activities of ketogenic diet on MPTP-induced neurotoxicity. *Journal of Molecular Neuroscience, 42,* 145–153.

Ye, J., & Keller, J. N. (2010). Regulation of energy metabolism by inflammation: A feedback response in obesity and calorie restriction. *Aging, 2,* 361–368.

Youm, Y. H., Nguyen, K. Y., Grant, R. W., Goldberg, E. L., Bodogai, M., Kim, D., D'Agostino, D., Planavsky, N., Lupfer, C., Kanneganti, T. D., Kang, S., Horvath, T. L., Fahmy, T. M., Crawford, P. A., Biragyn, A., Alnemi, E., & Dixit, V. D. (2015). The ketone metabolite β-hydroxybutyrate blocks NLRP3 inflammasome-mediated inflammatory disease. *Nature Medicine, 21,* 263–269.

Yu, Y., Tang, D., & Kang, R. (2015). Oxidative stress-mediated HMGB1 biology. *Frontiers in Physiology, 6,* 93.

Zhou, R., Yazdi, A. S., Menu, P., & Tschopp, J. (2011). A role for mitochondria in NLRP3 inflammasome activation. *Nature, 469,* 221–225.

20

The Ketogenic Diet in the Treatment of Schizophrenia

ZOLTÁN SARNYAI, MD, PHD, ANN-KATRIN KRAEUTER, PHD,
AND CHRISTOPHER M. PALMER, MD

INTRODUCTION

Schizophrenia is a chronic, debilitating, lifelong mental disorder that usually has its onset around and after puberty. The disorder affects between 0.5% and 1% of the population worldwide (van Os & Kapur, 2009). Individuals with schizophrenia exhibit a variety of symptoms, which are classified into positive, negative, and cognitive symptom domains (Lieberman & First, 2018; Tamminga & Holcomb, 2005; van Os & Kapur, 2009). Positive or psychotic symptoms include auditory and sometimes visual hallucinations, disordered thoughts and speech, abnormal and disorganized behavior, and catatonia (Schultz & Andreasen, 1999). Negative symptoms are characterized by abnormal emotional responses, which may result in social withdrawal, anhedonia, and a lack of motivation (Andreasen, 1995). Cognitive symptoms include deficits in sustained attention and impaired working memory (van Os & Kapur, 2009). Most commonly, the disease starts in adolescence with positive, psychotic symptoms and progresses to negative and cognitive symptoms later in life (Dutta et al., 2007).

The most common pharmacologic treatment for schizophrenia includes the long-term use of antipsychotic agents that, in varying degrees, block D_2 type dopamine receptors in the brain (Howes & Kapur, 2009). The psychotic symptoms usually respond to antipsychotic treatment, but the negative and cognitive symptoms seem to be more resistant to such an approach (Lieberman & First, 2018). Furthermore, antipsychotic agents induce a wide range of side effects (Newcomer, 2005). The long-term use of the earlier, first-generation antipsychotics, such as chlorpromazine and haloperidol, result in Parkinson's disease-like symptoms, and the newer, second-generation drugs, such as olanzapine and clozapine, have

been shown to induce significant weight gain, type 2 diabetes, and metabolic syndrome, resulting in shortened life expectancy due to early cardiovascular death (Miyamoto et al., 2012; Newcomer, 2005; van Os & Kapur, 2009). Therefore, there is a dire need to develop more effective and safer therapeutic options for people with schizophrenia.

No significant advances have been made in developing conceptually novel pharmacologic approaches for schizophrenia. The original antipsychotic, chlorpromazine, was a serendipitous discovery, because it was not designed to treat schizophrenia. An effort to understand its mechanism of action uncovered its dopamine receptor-blocking properties, leading to the formulation of the dopamine hypothesis to explain the pathophysiology of schizophrenia (Howes & Kapur, 2009; Seeman, 2006, 2013; Sunahara et al., 1993; van Os & Kapur, 2009). According to this hypothesis, schizophrenia is caused by an overactive dopamine system, which is effectively blocked by antipsychotic agents acting as dopamine antagonists. Although relatively little direct evidence supported the theory, it resulted in the development of a series of compounds similarly acting as dopamine antagonists. Refinement of the original hypothesis led to the introduction of the newer antipsychotic agents with somewhat different receptor-binding profiles, which contributed to their somewhat mitigated side effects (Ballon et al., 2014; Girgis et al., 2008).

More recently, schizophrenia has been conceptualized as a neurodevelopmental disorder that originates during early fetal development due to combined genetic and environmental factors (Marenco & Weinberger, 2000). The abnormal brain developmental trajectory, which may particularly influence the maturation of the prefrontal cortex, results in the presentation of the psychotic symptoms in the patient's late teens/early twenties, around the time when the prefrontal cortex should fully integrate into functional circuits. However, others have argued that neurodegeneration is taking place during the course of the illness, leading to deterioration of the symptoms over time (Lieberman, 1999, 2006; Lieberman et al., 2006). Although these theories are intellectually more appealing and correspond with some recent neuroimaging and neuropathology findings, they have failed to identify pathways or targets that can be pharmacologically manipulated.

The lack of progress in identifying molecular pathways relevant to disease pathophysiology and new drug targets for medication development has prompted researchers to search for fundamentally different approaches. One such approach is the use of the ketogenic diet (KD), and possibly ketogenic agents, in the management of schizophrenia. This chapter describes a rationale for the use of the KD in schizophrenia and provides an overview of the recently emerging preclinical and clinical findings that support the introduction of the KD to treat schizophrenia. Furthermore, the potential mechanism of action of this nutritional intervention in schizophrenia and other psychotic disorders is outlined.

RATIONALE FOR KD THERAPY IN SCHIZOPHRENIA

There are three main lines of arguments that support the rationale for using the KD in schizophrenia. First are the bidirectional interactions between schizophrenia and the metabolic syndrome, such as obesity, type 2 diabetes, and cardiovascular disease, and the fact that the KD as a metabolic intervention has been proven to help some of these disorders. Second, the comorbidity between schizophrenia and epilepsy and the efficacy of some antiepileptic agents in the treatment of schizophrenia point toward shared disease mechanisms, which might be amenable for modification by the KD. Last, recent developments have identified glucose and energy metabolism abnormalities as a potential core pathophysiology of schizophrenia, which argues for the mechanistic relevance of the KD.

Bidirectional Interactions Between Schizophrenia and Metabolic Syndrome

Cardiovascular disease (CVD), which includes coronary artery, cerebrovascular, and peripheral vascular disease, is the leading cause of death in the United States and most developed countries, accounting for about 50% of all deaths (Virani et al., 2020). The major risk factors for CVD include obesity and its consequences, dyslipidemia, hypertension, insulin resistance leading to diabetes, and cigarette smoking. In patients with schizophrenia, however, CVD occurs more frequently and accounts for more premature deaths than suicide (Hennekens, 2007). Patients with schizophrenia have higher rates of obesity, dyslipidemia, hypertension, diabetes, and cigarette smoking than people in the general population (Hennekens, 2007; Hennekens et al., 2005). These risk factors are the major contributors to early cardiovascular death in people with schizophrenia (Hennekens et al., 2005). Metabolic syndrome—defined as a group of cardiovascular risk factors, including abdominal obesity, hypertriglyceridemia, low high-density lipoprotein-cholesterol (HDL-C) levels, high blood pressure, and elevated blood glucose levels (Alberti & Zimmet, 1998)—is associated with significantly worse cognitive performance in schizophrenia (Lindenmayer et al., 2012). Similarly, a correlation has been identified between metabolic syndrome and neurocognitive and social cognitive performance in people with schizophrenia (Chen et al., 2020). Dietary modification through caloric restriction has been shown to improve cognitive function in patients with schizophrenia having MS (Adamowicz et al., 2020). Recent clinical research shows that the KD is effective in managing cardiovascular risk factors (Kosinski & Jornayvaz, 2017; Li & Heber, 2020), including obesity (Abbasi, 2018; Muscogiuri et al., 2019), insulin resistance (Staverosky, 2016), and type 2 diabetes (Abbasi, 2018; Bolla et al., 2019; Ludwig et al., 2018; Westman et al., 2018). Collectively, these results strongly suggest that systemic metabolic abnormalities that contribute to the increased risk for cardiovascular disorders and schizophrenia may share common pathophysiologic mechanisms (Pillinger et al., 2018). Therefore, the KD may normalize not only the systemic metabolic alterations, such as obesity, insulin resistance, and type 2 diabetes, but also the core pathophysiology of schizophrenia.

Schizophrenia and Epilepsy Comorbidity

Epilepsy has long been considered a risk factor for psychosis (Roy et al., 2014) and there is a long-documented epidemiologic link between epilepsy and schizophrenia (Campbell et al., 2020; Chang et al., 2011). A recent systematic review found that up to 6% of individuals with epilepsy have a comorbid psychotic illness, and that epilepsy patients have an almost eightfold increased risk of psychosis (Clancy et al., 2014). Conversely, there is an increased incidence of epilepsy and seizures in schizophrenia (Hüfner et al., 2015). Shared genetic susceptibility between epilepsy and schizophrenia has been demonstrated (Cascella et al., 2009), although genetic overlap has not been clearly identified between epilepsy and schizophrenia (Campbell et al., 2020). However, shared underlying pathophysiology has been suggested (Kandratavicius et al., 2014). For example, inflammatory processes driven by pro-inflammatory cytokines have been proposed as a common mechanism underlying the links between epilepsy and schizophrenia (Paudel et al., 2018). Furthermore, abnormalities in the brain inhibitory GABAergic (Dienel & Lewis, 2019; Lewis et al., 2012; Wassef et al., 2003; Wenneberg et al., 2020) and excitatory glutamatergic (Coyle et al., 2012; Steiner et al., 2012, 2013; Tsai et al., 1995) systems have been identified in schizophrenia. Similarly, these neurotransmitter systems play a key role in the pathophysiology of epilepsy (Noebels et al., 2013). Not surprisingly, abnormalities of the excitatory/inhibitory balance (E/I) has been shown both in schizophrenia (Allen et al., 2019; Hjelmervik et al., 2020; Kang et al., 2019; Uhlhaas & Singer, 2013) and in epilepsy (Bonansco & Fuenzalida, 2016; Zhang & Sun, 2011). Beyond the shared underlying mechanisms, there is a strong body of clinical evidence showing that antiepileptic agents are effectively used as adjuncts in the treatment of schizophrenia (Hosák & Libiger, 2002; Okuma, 1994; Stahl, 2004). Importantly, as described in detail in other chapters of this book, the KD has been used effectively in the management of epilepsy for a century (Lutas & Yellen, 2013; Rho & Stafstrom, 2012; Rogawski et al., 2016). Therefore, based on the observed comorbidity, the shared pathophysiology, and pharmacologic treatment, as well as on the well-established efficacy of the KD in epilepsy, it is likely that metabolic intervention via the KD will produce therapeutic benefits in schizophrenia.

Schizophrenia as a Disease of Impaired Glucose and Energy Metabolism

An important recent advance that provides a strong mechanistic rationale for the therapeutic use of the KD is the emerging understanding of schizophrenia as a disease of abnormal systemic and brain glucose and energy metabolism. Elevated blood glucose levels and insulin resistance have been consistently shown in drug-naïve, first-episode patients (Harris et al., 2013; Herberth et al., 2011; Pillinger et al., 2017; Steiner et al., 2017, 2018), which indicates that an early metabolic syndrome-like abnormality seems to be a central part of the disorder. Polymorphisms in genes encoding glycolytic enzymes have been identified in schizophrenia (Stone et al., 2004). A series of transcriptomic and proteomic studies have uncovered changes that correspond with impaired glycolysis and an abnormally functioning tricarboxylic acid (TCA) cycle in the prefrontal cortex of people with schizophrenia (Bubber et al., 2011; Nascimento & Martins-de-Souza, 2015; Prabakaran et al., 2004; Sullivan et al., 2018a, 2019b; Zuccoli et al., 2017). In support of these postmortem findings, in vivo magnetic resonance spectroscopy analysis demonstrated abnormalities in bioenergetics and elevated brain lactate levels in the dorsolateral prefrontal cortex (Chouinard et al., 2017; Dogan et al., 2018; Du et al., 2014; Hagihara et al., 2018; Rowland et al., 2016; Sullivan et al., 2019a). Furthermore, deficits in mitochondrial oxidative phosphorylation (OXPHOS) have been consistently shown in the brains of people with schizophrenia (Ben-Shachar, 2017; Ben-Shachar & Karry, 2008; Ben-Shachar & Laifenfeld, 2004; Bergman & Ben-Shachar, 2016). In addition, recent studies using neurons differentiated from patient-derived inducible pluripotent stem cells (iPSCs) have provided further evidence for impaired mitochondrial OXPHOS and decreased adenosine triphosphate (ATP) production (Ni et al., 2019; Robicsek et al., 2013, 2018). Collectively, these results indicate the presence of bioenergetic deficits in schizophrenia (Sullivan et al., 2018b), which raises the possibility of using the KD to produce alternative fuels and/or to support different aspects of mitochondrial function for therapeutic benefit.

PRECLINICAL EVIDENCE FOR KD IN SCHIZOPHRENIA

The full spectrum of disease pathophysiology and the human-specific symptoms (delusions, hallucinations, and thought disorder) of schizophrenia cannot be modeled in animals. However, it is possible to utilize mechanistically driven and translationally validated animal models to study treatment efficacy (Sarnyai et al., 2011; Sarnyai & Guest, 2017; Sarnyai et al., 2015).

Effects of KD in Different Animal Models of Schizophrenia

Glutamate receptor (*N*-methyl-D-aspartate or NMDA-type) antagonist psychomimetic drugs, such as phencyclidine and ketamine, produce symptoms indistinguishable from schizophrenia in humans (Jentsch & Roth, 1999) and induce a behavioral profile in rodents that captures a wide spectrum of the schizophrenia-like phenotype (Cadinu et al., 2018). In addition, phencyclidine administration in rats also mimics the systemic insulin resistance and the brain glycolytic abnormalities seen in schizophrenia (Ernst et al., 2012). We, therefore, used the NMDA-type glutamate receptor antagonist dizocilpine (MK-801) to induce hyperactivity, stereotyped behavior, decreased sociability/social withdrawal, working memory deficit, and impaired pre-pulse inhibition of the acoustic startle reflex in mice (Kraeuter et al., 2015). Three weeks of the KD induced metabolic ketosis characterized by elevated levels of the main circulating ketone body, β-hydroxybutyrate (βHB), lower circulating blood glucose levels, and temporary weight loss in the KD-treated group compared to mice on standard diet (Kraeuter et al., 2015). The KD regimen resulted in a complete restoration of the normal behavioral phenotype in the MK-801-treated mice (Kraeuter et al., 2015). We further demonstrated that the efficacy of the KD is independent of the temporary caloric restriction and the resulting initial weight loss. We found that the beneficial effect of the KD on the MK-801-induced pre-pulse inhibition deficit, a translatable endophenotype of schizophrenia, persisted even when the weight loss was not present (Kraeuter et al., 2019c).

Converging evidence for the efficacy of the KD comes from the use of DBA/2 mice, which have been proposed to exhibit a variety of behavioral and metabolic features that resemble those found in schizophrenia (Olivier et al., 2001; Sarnyai et al., 2015). Recently examined were the effects of the KD on hippocampal P20/N40 gating in DBA/2 mice, a translational endophenotype that mirrors inhibitory deficits in P50 sensory gating in schizophrenia patients (Tregellas et al., 2015). Animals with the highest blood ketone levels showed the lowest P20/N40 gating ratios, suggesting that the KD may normalize sensory gating deficits (Tregellas et al., 2015). This preliminary result, together with the efficacy of the KD on MK-801-induced disruption of sensorimotor gating, measured as pre-pulse inhibition of startle (Kraeuter et al., 2019c), suggests that the KD may effectively target sensory gating deficits,

which are conceptualized as fundamental in the development of hallucinatory episodes in persons with schizophrenia.

Ready to Translate: The Questions of Sex-Specificity, Treatment Length, and Interactions with Antipsychotics

In a recent study, we addressed three issues—chronic KD administration, sex-specificity, and interactions with antipsychotic drugs—that are relevant to the potential translation of preclinical findings. We investigated the effect of a 6-month trial of the KD in female mice with and without chronic olanzapine treatment. We found that the KD is effective in normalizing the schizophrenia-like pre-pulse inhibition deficit in female mice with an efficacy similar to that of olanzapine (Kraeuter et al., 2019b). However, the combination of the KD and olanzapine did not result in stronger effects than the diet or the pharmacologic treatment alone (Kraeuter et al., 2019b). This suggests that the KD may be used together with antipsychotics without lessening their efficacy.

βHB Mimics the Effect of KD

As discussed in this chapter, the KD is likely to exert its effects through multiple mechanisms. One plausible mechanism is that during ketosis, the main endogenous circulating ketone body, βHB, produced during metabolic ketosis, plays a primary role in the mediation of the diet's effects. To investigate this potential mechanism in schizophrenia, we administered βHB to MK-801-treated mice for 3 weeks. We found that chronic βHB treatment mimicked the efficacy of the KD in normalizing the MK-801-induced pre-pulse inhibition deficit (Kraeuter et al., 2020b), which indicates that the production of βHB during the KD may be a major mechanism through which the diet exerts its therapeutic effects.

The preclinical results presented here persuasively argue for the potential efficacy of the KD in the treatment of schizophrenia and lend support for the use of the KD in the clinical setting (Kraeuter et al., 2019a, 2020a, 2020c; Sarnyai et al., 2019).

CLINICAL EVIDENCE: CASE STUDIES AND PILOT TRIALS IN SCHIZOPHRENIA AND SCHIZOAFFECTIVE DISORDER

As noted, animal models are useful in developing new treatments, but they cannot mimic the full spectrum of symptoms and pathophysiology known to occur in schizophrenia and schizoaffective disorder. Therefore, it is important to assess any evidence that the KD can be effective in people with the disorders. Although there are as yet no published randomized controlled trials of the KD in schizophrenia or schizoaffective disorder, results from small pilot trials and case studies have recently become available.

Before reviewing the existing evidence, it is essential to highlight some of the overarching issues with evaluating the efficacy of KD treatment for chronic psychotic disorders. First, it is important to assess whether the treatment works, and if so, how well. Does it alleviate all symptoms or just some of the symptoms? In addition to symptom improvement, does the treatment restore people's ability to function in life, a metric usually not included in standardized symptom rating scales? Also central is the issue of compliance, which poses a significant challenge for many people. Can people with schizophrenia or schizoaffective disorder comply with the KD? If so, for how long? In other words, is this a practical and sustainable treatment?

These are important issues, not only in people with chronic psychotic disorders, but in all people interested in implementing the KD. However, schizophrenia and schizoaffective disorder pose unique challenges to compliance. These disorders include symptoms of anhedonia, amotivation, and cognitive impairment, all of which can impede a person's ability to comply with a strict diet. Additionally, as already noted, people with schizophrenia and schizoaffective disorder have higher rates of obesity, cardiovascular disease, type 2 diabetes, and cigarette smoking, all issues related to lifestyle choices. These trends impose a significant challenge to adherence to healthy lifestyle choices.

The first human trial of the KD for schizophrenia dates back to 1965, when ten hospitalized women with schizophrenia (19 to 63 years old) who were already receiving medications and electroconvulsive therapy (ECT) were placed on a KD for 1 month (Pacheco et al., 1965). The study was poorly conducted, because it had no control group and three different rating scales were initially used, with results employing only one scale (the Beckomberga Rating Scale for the S-factor) being reported. The authors nonetheless reported that patients showed significant improvement in symptoms after 2 weeks on the diet and continued improvement at 1 week after stopping the diet. The authors did not objectively measure ketosis and did not have strict measures in place to

ensure compliance. No follow-up beyond 1 week after stopping the diet was reported.

In 2009, Kraft and Westman reported the case of a 70-year-old woman with schizophrenia, diagnosed at the age of 17 (Kraft & Westman, 2009). She had a classic symptom onset of schizophrenia, including paranoia, disorganized speech, auditory and visual hallucinations, and recurrent suicidal thoughts, with multiple suicide attempts. She began a KD for weight loss. Within 8 days, she noted improvement in her energy level and a marked reduction in hallucinations. She remained on the diet for a full year and lost about 22 pounds. She reported continued remission of her hallucinations for the remainder of the year.

In 2017, one of this chapter's authors (CP) published two case reports of the KD as a treatment for schizoaffective disorder (Palmer, 2017). The cases included a 33-year-old man diagnosed with schizoaffective disorder for 14 years and a 31-year-old woman diagnosed with schizoaffective disorder for 8 years. Both patients were also obese. They had each tried numerous psychotropic medications, and the woman also had a course of ECT, but symptoms remained treatment resistant. A standardized rating scale, the Positive and Negative Syndrome Scale (PANSS), was used to evaluate symptoms before and after the diet, and the longitudinal course of symptoms over 1 year was also evaluated. In both cases, dramatic reductions in PANSS total scores were noted after 6 weeks of the KD. However, both patients had episodes of dietary noncompliance while still compliant with medications, and psychotic and mood symptoms returned quickly. When the patients resumed the diet, the symptoms again abated, demonstrating an ABAB response pattern.

These cases illustrated that the KD can be an effective treatment for schizoaffective disorder and that it is possible for people with chronic psychotic disorders to follow the diet for up to 1 year. Furthermore, the effects of treatment were not sustained during noncompliance with the diet, comparable to the effects of psychotropic medications. Both patients also lost significant amounts of weight: the woman lost 30 pounds in 4 months and the man lost 104 pounds over 1 year. In particular, the male patient had a significant improvement in function, leading to successful completion of online college courses, development of new friendships, and being able to move from his father's home to an independent living situation.

A small pilot trial of the 3:1 ratio KD (3 parts fat to every 1 part of protein + carbohydrate) for

6 weeks in two Ecuadorian twins, both diagnosed with schizophrenia, was reported by Gilbert-Jaramillo et al. (2018). Their study used the PANSS as the primary outcome measure and used a blinded investigator. The fraternal twins were 22 years old—a male diagnosed with schizophrenia since the age of 18 and a female diagnosed with schizophrenia since the age of 14. Both had tried several medications yet their symptoms remained treatment resistant. Medications were continued during the trial. Both patients had difficulty with compliance, but they were able to achieve ketosis for at least short periods. Total PANSS scores decreased during times of compliance but were close to baseline scores during periods of noncompliance and after the study ended. Both patients lost weight, albeit only a few pounds.

Finally, in 2019, CP published two additional case studies demonstrating the long-term potential of the KD as an effective and sustainable treatment for schizophrenia that can induce full remission of symptoms, at least in some people (Palmer, 2019). The first case was a follow-up of the 70-year-old woman first reported by Kraft and Westman. At age 82, she remained alive and well on the KD. She had lost a total of 150 pounds over the 12 years, was completely off all psychotropic medications, no longer saw a psychiatrist or mental health provider, and remained free of psychotic symptoms. She was able to regain her independence and no longer required a guardian or the home health team that she had used before starting the diet. She reported that she no longer thought about suicide and that she was happy to be alive.

The second case was a 39-year-old woman who had suffered from chronic psychotic symptoms, anxiety, depression, and anorexia nervosa for 20 years. She tried numerous psychotropic medications, including clozapine and injectable antipsychotic medications, without benefit. At the recommendation of a healthcare professional, she started a KD for gastrointestinal complaints. Within 1 month, she noted improvement in symptoms, but she abruptly stopped the 14 medications she had been taking, including antipsychotic and other psychotropic medications, which precipitated a severe episode of psychosis. She was hospitalized and placed on Haldol decanoate, and her symptoms stabilized and within months went into full remission. She remained on the KD. Over the following year, she tapered off the Haldol decanoate and remained symptom-free. Four years later, she remained on the KD, remained off all antipsychotic medications, and remained free of psychotic symptoms. She lost 70 pounds over this time, which exacerbated her anorexia nervosa. However, with continued psychotherapy, she was able to regain 30 pounds while remaining on the KD and was able to maintain a healthy weight for the remainder of the follow-up period. She also regained functional status, achieving a master's degree and working full-time by the end of the follow-up period.

This small body of literature suggests that the KD can be an effective and sustainable treatment for chronic psychotic disorders, at least in some people. More research is needed to validate its efficacy and safety in larger samples of people with schizophrenia or schizoaffective disorder. However, these small studies and case reports support the pursuit of more substantial, controlled trials.

POTENTIAL MECHANISMS OF ACTION OF THE KD IN SCHIZOPHRENIA

Like many other nutritional interventions, the KD differs from classic pharmacologic interventions, which are designed to target a specific molecule, a receptor, an enzyme, or other proteins. In contrast, diet-based therapeutics are likely to act through multiple mechanisms. The mechanism of action of the KD has been intensively studied in the context of its antiseizure effects for a long time. As expected, a variety of potential mechanisms have been highlighted, including the modulation of excitatory and inhibitory neurotransmission, support of brain bioenergetics, reduction of oxidative stress, and even alteration of the gut microbiome (Boison, 2017; Bough, 2008; D'Andrea Meira et al., 2019; Koppel & Swerdlow, 2018; Lutas & Yellen, 2013; Olson et al., 2018; Rho & Stafstrom, 2012; Rogawski et al., 2016). Some of these mechanisms are discussed in other chapters of this volume. Here, we focus on potential mechanisms of action of the KD in the context of schizophrenia, including its role as an alternative fuel source, targeting mitochondrial impairments, acting through molecular targets of βHB, and altering the gut microbiome. Since no study to date has directly investigated how the KD exerts its beneficial effects in schizophrenia, we consider what is known about its mechanisms of action in the context of the proposed pathophysiology of schizophrenia.

Alternative Fuel Provision

Healthy synaptic communication requires appropriate formation of dendritic spines and the synthesis, release, and recycling of neurotransmitters. Constantly forming and remodeling dendritic spines and maintaining neurotransmission are fundamentally energy demanding (Harris et al., 2012). Glucose is the primary energy substrate for the brain (Dienel, 2019). From glucose, the high-energy molecule ATP is produced through glycolysis in the cytoplasm and the TCA cycle and OXPHOS in the mitochondria (Dienel, 2019). Reversing the ion movements that generate postsynaptic responses consumes the majority of the energy used from ATP (Magistretti & Pellerin, 1999). Glucose is not only the major substrate for ATP, but glucose metabolism also results in the production of glutamate and subsequently GABA (Dienel, 2019). Therefore, deficits in glucose and synaptic energy supply lead to impaired synaptic communication and can ultimately result in abnormal brain function and behavior (Kann, 2016). Impaired glycolysis has been demonstrated in the brain of people with schizophrenia (Du et al., 2014; Prabakaran et al., 2004; Sullivan et al., 2018a, 2018b). This impairment results in insufficient ATP production, which may contribute to abnormal synaptic communication and the psychopathology observed in schizophrenia, such as hallucinations and impaired cognitive functions.

During ketosis, the availability of glucose as the fuel for ATP production decreases dramatically as production of the ketone bodies acetoacetate and βHB increases. βHB and acetoacetate can be transported into the brain via the monocarboxylic acid transporters (Leino et al., 2001). Within the brain, βHB is enzymatically converted by β-hydroxybutyrate dehydrogenase into acetoacetate. Acetoacetate receives a coenzyme A from succinyl-CoA from the Krebs cycle to form acetoacetate-CoA. Acetoacetate-CoA will spontaneously degrade to acetyl-CoA, which can fuel the Krebs cycle without using glucose through its metabolite pyruvate. In this manner, the KD can provide alternative fuel sources (acetoacetate and βHB) to circumvent the impaired glycolysis in schizophrenia. The acetyl-CoA derived from the ketone bodies feeds the Krebs cycle to produce reducing equivalents for OXPHOS and ultimately supports the generation of ATP and restored synaptic communication, resulting in symptom improvement.

βHB as Mediator

The main circulating ketone body, βHB, serves several important biologic functions beyond the alternative provision of acetyl-CoA. βHB has a variety of molecular targets, including the nod-like receptor family pyrin domain-containing 3 (NLRP3) inflammasome, RNA-binding proteins, and G-protein-coupled receptors (Achanta & Rae, 2017). In addition, βHB has also been identified as an epigenetic modifier that can target DNA and histones. For example, βHB is an endogenous inhibitor of many protein deacetylases (HDACs) and is a β-hydroxybutyrylation modulator (Han et al., 2020). Several of the βHB targets may play a role in different aspects of schizophrenia pathophysiology.

βHB as an NLRP3-Inflammosome Inhibitor

Mitochondrial complex I dysfunction (Ben-Shachar, 2016), oxidative stress (Bitanihirwe & Woo, 2011), and immune activation (Meyer, 2013) are consistently reported in schizophrenia. Mitochondrial production of reactive oxygen species was linked to the activation of an inflammatory redox sensor, the NLRP3. Upon its activation, NLRP3 recruits apoptosis-associated speck-like protein (ASC) and caspase-1 to form the NLRP3 inflammasome, activating IL-1β (Kim et al., 2016). Furthermore, elevated levels of IL-1β have been shown in schizophrenia (Momtazmanesh et al., 2019). βHB effectively suppresses activation of the NLRP3 inflammasome (Youm et al., 2015), and it may curtail the activity of pro-inflammatory cytokines and related inflammatory processes in the brain, resulting in symptom improvement.

βHB as an HDAC Inhibitor

Postmortem brain studies have provided evidence for dysregulated expression of HDAC1 and HDAC2 as a central feature in schizophrenia (Benes et al., 2007; Sharma et al., 2008). It has been shown recently in a large postmortem sample that the HDAC2 transcript expression is significantly downregulated in the dorsolateral prefrontal cortex (DLPFC) of people with schizophrenia compared to controls (Schroeder et al., 2017). Positron emission tomography (PET) imaging using [11C]Martinostat labeling has provided the first in vivo data to show that the relative HDAC expression was lower in the DLPFC of patients with schizophrenia compared with controls, and HDAC expression positively correlated with cognitive performance scores across groups (Gilbert et al., 2019). These findings provide evidence of HDAC dysregulation in patients with schizophrenia and suggest that altered HDAC expression may impact cognitive function. This raises the possibility for the therapeutic use of HDAC modifiers in schizophrenia (Guidotti & Grayson, 2014; Qiu et al., 2017). Considering the potent HDAC-inhibitor properties of βHB, the KD may exert some of its beneficial effects in schizophrenia through epigenetic mechanisms, which involve histone acetylation by βHB.

The KD Targets Impaired Mitochondrial Function

Mitochondrial impairments have long been recognized in schizophrenia (Ben-Shachar & Laifenfeld, 2004; Bergman & Ben-Shachar, 2016; Ni & Chung, 2020; Suárez-Méndez et al., 2020; Valiente-Pallejà et al., 2020). Complex I (type I NADH dehydrogenase) within the electron transport chain in the mitochondria, which catalyzes the transfer of electrons from NADH to coenzyme Q10 and translocates protons across the inner mitochondrial membrane, is particularly affected, resulting in impaired OXPHOS and decreased ATP production (Ben-Shachar, 2017; Ben-Shachar & Karry, 2008; Ben-Shachar et al., 1999; Bergman & Ben-Shachar, 2016; Bergman et al., 2018; Holper et al., 2019). Therefore, this protein complex has been suggested as a potential drug target in schizophrenia (Ben-Shachar & Ene, 2018; Brenner-Lavie et al., 2009). A large body of research indicates that the mitochondria are likely targets for the effects of the KD in a number of neuropsychiatric disorders and other conditions, including cancer (Branco et al., 2016; Fogle et al., 2019; Hasan-Olive et al., 2019; Koppel & Swerdlow, 2018; Kovács et al., 2019; Seyfried et al., 2014; Vidali et al., 2015). Although there is no direct evidence currently available to indicate that the KD may act through this target in schizophrenia, results from the efficacy of the KD in a rare disorder provide some promising clues (Storoni et al., 2019). Leber hereditary optic neuropathy (LHON) is a maternally inherited, bilateral, sequential optic neuropathy that usually affects young males. LHON arises from a defect in complex I of the OXPHOS chain that generates increased reactive oxygen species and causes a decline in cellular ATP production (Emperador et al., 2018). A recent in vitro study provides evidence that ketogenic treatment produces changes in the mitochondria that are in line with a potential therapeutic improvement in patients (Emperador et al., 2019). Based on the wide-ranging effects of the KD on the mitochondria, it stands to reason that other features of multiple mitochondrial abnormalities in schizophrenia

(Ni & Chung, 2020), including increased reactive oxygen species (Prabakaran et al., 2004), inflammatory processes induced by mtDNA fragments (Suárez-Méndez et al., 2020), and deficient intracellular Ca^{2+} management (Monteiro et al., 2020), may also be amenable to KD-induced improvements.

Potential Role of the Gut Microbiome

As a dietary intervention, the KD is expected to alter the gut microbiome. Recent studies have revealed that the KD has a profound effect on the bacterial composition of the gut (Ang et al., 2020; Cabrera-Mulero et al., 2019; De Caro et al., 2019; Hampton, 2018; Nagpal et al., 2019; Olson et al., 2018), which may mediate its effects on epilepsy and other neuropsychiatric disorders.

The gut microbiome is thought to play a role in the neurodevelopmental pathophysiology of schizophrenia (Kelly et al., 2020; Petra et al., 2015). A recent study (Zhu et al., 2020) identified metagenome-wide associations of gut microbiome features and schizophrenia, including differences in short-chain fatty acid synthesis, tryptophan metabolism, and synthesis/degradation of neurotransmitters. Transplantation of a schizophrenia-enriched bacterium, *Streptococcus vestibularis*, produced deficits in social behaviors and altered neurotransmitter levels in peripheral tissues in recipient mice. Shotgun metagenomic sequencing and 16S rRNA sequencing have revealed that patients with schizophrenia had significantly reduced gut microbial richness compared with that of healthy controls. The composition of gut microbiota clearly distinguished the patients with schizophrenia from the healthy controls (Xu et al., 2020). Schwarz et al. (2018) demonstrated that numbers of *Lactobacillus*-group bacteria were elevated in patients with first-episode psychosis (FEP) and significantly correlated with severity along different symptom domains, which suggests a functional link between microbiome changes and symptomatology. Furthermore, a subgroup of FEP patients with the most substantial microbiota differences also showed weaker treatment response, specifically, a lack of significant improvement of symptoms (Schwarz et al., 2018). In unmedicated and medicated patients with schizophrenia, a decreased microbiome α-diversity index (local species pool) and marked gut microbial composition disturbances were identified (Zheng et al., 2019). Several unique bacterial taxa (e.g., Veillonellaceae and Lachnospiraceae) were associated with disease severity. A specific microbial panel (Aerococcaceae, Bifidobacteriaceae, Brucellaceae, Pasteurellaceae, and Rikenellaceae) enabled discrimination of patients from healthy controls. In addition, germ-free mice receiving microbiome fecal transplants from patients with schizophrenia had lower glutamate and higher glutamine and GABA in the hippocampus and displayed schizophrenia-relevant behaviors, consistent with findings in other mouse models of the disorder involving glutamatergic hypofunction. These results suggest that the microbiome itself can alter neurochemistry and neurologic function in ways that may be relevant to schizophrenia pathology (Zheng et al., 2019).

In the landmark study by Olson et al. (2018), the antiseizure effects of the KD in animal models was shown to result from diet-induced changes in the gut microbiome—specifically through alterations in the GABA:glutamate ratios in the brain. Thus, one could assume that the KD may have similar effects through correcting the disease-relevant dysbiosis in schizophrenia and normalizing aberrant neurochemical alterations in the brain. These results collectively suggest the potential for the KD to improve the pathophysiologic processes underlying the cognitive and behavioral symptoms of schizophrenia by altering the gut microbiome.

In summary, the KD may exert its therapeutic effects in schizophrenia through multiple mechanisms involving glucose metabolism, βHB-driven alterations in inflammatory and epigenetic processes, mitochondrial functions, and the gut microbiome. This does not rule out the possibility that other mechanisms shared by schizophrenia and metabolic ketosis may participate. More research is needed to specifically study the mechanism of action of KD intervention in schizophrenia.

CONCLUSION AND FUTURE DIRECTIONS

There are growing interest and excitement in exploring the use of the KD as a treatment for schizophrenia and schizoaffective disorder. As reviewed in this chapter, numerous theoretical underpinnings support further exploration of this treatment. Some are based on epidemiologic and clinical data, such as higher rates of metabolic disorders found in people with psychotic disorders. Others are based on basic science that links mechanisms of KD action to known abnormalities found in people with chronic psychotic

disorders. These include abnormalities in metabolism, immune system function, neurotransmitter imbalances, and the gut microbiome. In addition to these theoretical underpinnings, growing preclinical and clinical data support the feasibility, effectiveness, and sustainability of KD treatment.

Clearly, more research is needed. Controlled clinical trials are required to demonstrate efficacy, safety, and tolerability. One challenge is compliance with the diet. Most clinicians and researchers are not familiar with the KD and are also not skilled at motivating people to change behaviors. Attention to this critical aspect of clinical trials is of paramount importance. Otherwise, clinical trials will predictably conclude that they cannot get people to adhere to the dietary intervention. Working with clinicians and researchers with a proven track record of achieving compliance with the diet in the target population will be important in designing and implementing such trials.

Exogenous ketone supplements offer an alternative to the strict KD and should certainly be explored. However, it is not clear that exogenous ketones induce all known effects of the KD, so this line of research should progress alongside using the KD itself.

This field of scientific enquiry presents exciting opportunities for better understanding the pathophysiology of schizophrenia and schizoaffective disorder and for developing novel treatments based on new ways of understanding these illnesses. The treatments may very well include dietary interventions but will also likely include new medications and supplements that could be developed based on this research. Millions of people are desperate for more effective solutions.

REFERENCES

Abbasi, J. (2018). Interest in the ketogenic diet grows for weight loss and type 2 diabetes. *JAMA, 319,* 215–217.

Achanta, L. B., & Rae, C. D. (2017). β-Hydroxybutyrate in the brain: One molecule, multiple mechanisms. *Neurochemistry Research, 42,* 35–49.

Adamowicz, K., Mazur, A., Mak, M., Samochowiec, J., & Kucharska-Mazur, J. (2020). Metabolic syndrome and cognitive functions in schizophrenia—Implementation of dietary intervention. *Frontiers in Psychiatry, 11,* 359.

Alberti, K. G. M. M., & Zimmet, P. Z. (1998). Definition, diagnosis and classification of diabetes mellitus and its complications. Part 1: Diagnosis and classification of diabetes mellitus; Provisional report of a WHO consultation. *Diabetic Medicine, 15,* 539–553.

Allen, P., Sommer, I. E., Jardri, R., Eysenck, M. W., & Hugdahl, K. (2019). Extrinsic and default mode networks in psychiatric conditions: Relationship to excitatory-inhibitory transmitter balance and early trauma. *Neuroscience & Biobehavorial Reviews, 99*, 90–100.

Andreasen, N. C. (1995). Symptoms, signs, and diagnosis of schizophrenia. *Lancet, 346*, 477–481.

Ang, Q. Y., Alexander, M., Newman, J. C., Tian, Y., Cai, J., Upadhyay, V., Turnbaugh, J. A., Verdin, E., Hall, K. D., Leibel, R. L., Ravussin, E., Rosenbaum, M., Patterson, A. D., & Turnbaugh, P. J. (2020). Ketogenic diets alter the gut microbiome resulting in decreased intestinal Th17 cells. *Cell, 181*, 1263–1275.

Ballon, J. S., Pajvani, U., Freyberg, Z., Leibel, R. L., & Lieberman, J. A. (2014). Molecular pathophysiology of metabolic effects of antipsychotic medications. *Trends in Endocrinology & Metabolism, 25*, 593–600.

Ben-Shachar, D. (2017). Mitochondrial multifaceted dysfunction in schizophrenia: Complex I as a possible pathological target. *Schizophrenia Research, 187*, 3–10.

Ben-Shachar, D., & Ene, H. M. (2018). Mitochondrial targeted therapies: Where do we stand in mental disorders? *Biological Psychiatry, 83*, 770–779.

Ben-Shachar, D., & Karry, R. (2008). Neuroanatomical pattern of mitochondrial complex I pathology varies between schizophrenia, bipolar disorder and major depression. *PLOS ONE, 3*, Article e3676.

Ben-Shachar, D., & Laifenfeld, D. (2004). Mitochondria, synaptic plasticity, and schizophrenia. *International Review of Neurobiology, 59*, 273–296.

Ben-Shachar, D., Zuk, R., Gazawi, H., Reshef, A., Sheinkman, A., & Klein, E. (1999). Increased mitochondrial complex I activity in platelets of schizophrenic patients. *International Journal of Neuropsychopharmacology, 2*, 245–253.

Benes, F. M., Lim, B., Matzilevich, D., Walsh, J. P., Subburaju, S., & Minns, M. (2007). Regulation of the GABA cell phenotype in hippocampus of schizophrenics and bipolars. *Proceedings of the National Academy of Sciences of the United States of America, 104*, 10164–10169.

Bergman, O., & Ben-Shachar, D. (2016). Mitochondrial oxidative phosphorylation system (OXPHOS) deficits in schizophrenia: Possible interactions with cellular processes. *Canadian Journal of Psychiatry, 61*, 457–469.

Bergman, O., Karry, R., Milhem, J., & Ben-Shachar, D. (2018). NDUFV2 pseudogene (NDUFV2P1) contributes to mitochondrial complex I deficits in schizophrenia. *Molecular Psychiatry, 25*, 805–820.

Bitanihirwe, B. K., & Woo, T. U. (2011). Oxidative stress in schizophrenia: An integrated approach. *Neuroscience & Biobehavorial Reviews, 35*, 878–893.

Boison, D. (2017). New insights into the mechanisms of the ketogenic diet. *Current Opinion in Neurology, 30*, 187–192.

Bolla, A. M., Caretto, A., Laurenzi, A., Scavini, M., & Piemonti, L. (2019). Low-carb and ketogenic diets in type 1 and type 2 diabetes. *Nutrients, 11*, 962.

Bonansco, C., & Fuenzalida, M. (2016). Plasticity of hippocampal excitatory-inhibitory balance: Missing the synaptic control in the epileptic brain. *Neural Plasticity, 2016*, 8607038.

Bough, K. (2008). Energy metabolism as part of the anticonvulsant mechanism of the ketogenic diet. *Epilepsia, 49*(Suppl. 8), 91–93.

Branco, A. F., Ferreira, A., Simoes, R. F., Magalhaes-Novais, S., Zehowski, C., Cope, E., Silva, A. M., Pereira, D., Sardao, V. A., & Cunha-Oliveira, T. (2016). Ketogenic diets: From cancer to mitochondrial diseases and beyond. *European Journal of Clinical Investigation, 46*, 285–298.

Brenner-Lavie, H., Klein, E., & Ben-Shachar, D. (2009). Mitochondrial complex I as a novel target for intraneuronal DA: Modulation of respiration in intact cells. *Biochemical Pharmacology, 78*, 85–95.

Bubber, P., Hartounian, V., Gibson, G. E., & Blass, J. P. (2011). Abnormalities in the tricarboxylic acid (TCA) cycle in the brains of schizophrenia patients. *European Neuropsychopharmacology, 21*, 254–260.

Cabrera-Mulero, A., Tinahones, A., Bandera, B., Moreno-Indias, I., Macías-González, M., & Tinahones, F. J. (2019). Keto microbiota: A powerful contributor to host disease recovery. *Reviews in Endocrine and Metabolic Disorders, 20*, 415–425.

Cadinu, D., Grayson, B., Podda, G., Harte, M. K., Doostdar, N., & Neill, J. C. (2018). NMDA receptor antagonist rodent models for cognition in schizophrenia and identification of novel drug treatments: An update. *Neuropharmacology, 142*, 41–62.

Campbell, C., Cavalleri, G. L., & Delanty, N. (2020). Exploring the genetic overlap between psychiatric illness and epilepsy: A review. *Epilepsy & Behavior, 102*, 106669.

Cascella, N. G., Schretlen, D. J., & Sawa, A. (2009). Schizophrenia and epilepsy: Is there a shared susceptibility? *Neuroscience Research, 63*, 227–235.

Chang, Y. T., Chen, P. C., Tsai, I. J., Sung, F. C., Chin, Z. N., Kuo, H. T., Tsai, C. H., & Chou, I. C. (2011). Bidirectional relation between schizophrenia and epilepsy: A population-based retrospective cohort study. *Epilepsia, 52*, 2036–2042.

Chen, S., Xia, X., Deng, C., Wu, X., Han, Z., Tao, J., & Wu, X. (2020). The correlation between metabolic syndrome and neurocognitive and social cognitive performance of patients with schizophrenia. *Psychiatry Research, 288*, 112941.

Chouinard, V. A., Kim, S. Y., Valeri, L., Yuksel, C., Ryan, K. P., Chouinard, G., Cohen, B. M., Du, F., & Ongur, D. (2017). Brain bioenergetics and redox state measured by ^{31}P magnetic resonance spectroscopy in unaffected siblings of patients with psychotic disorders. *Schizophrenia Research, 187*, 11–16.

Clancy, M. J., Clarke, M. C., Connor, D. J., Cannon, M., & Cotter, D. R. (2014). The prevalence of psychosis in epilepsy: A systematic review and meta-analysis. *BMC Psychiatry, 14*, 75.

Coyle, J. T., Basu, A., Benneyworth, M., Balu, D., & Konopaske, G. (2012). Glutamatergic synaptic dysregulation in schizophrenia: Therapeutic implications. *Handbook of Experimantal Pharmacology, 2012*(213), 267–295.

D'Andrea Meira, I., Romao, T. T., Pires do Prado, H. J., Kruger, L. T., Pires, M. E. P., & da Conceicao, P. O. (2019). Ketogenic diet and epilepsy: What we know so far. *Frontiers in Neuroscience, 13*, 5.

De Caro, C., Iannone, L. F., Citraro, R., Striano, P., De Sarro, G., Constanti, A., Cryan, J. F., & Russo, E. (2019). Can we 'seize' the gut microbiota to treat epilepsy? *Neuroscience & Biobehavorial Reviews, 107*, 750–764.

Dienel, G. A. (2019). Brain glucose metabolism: Integration of energetics with function. *Physiological Reviews, 99*, 949–1045.

Dienel, S. J., & Lewis, D. A. (2019). Alterations in cortical interneurons and cognitive function in schizophrenia. *Neurobiology of Disease, 131*, 104208–104208.

Dogan, A. E., Yuksel, C., Du, F., Chouinard, V.-A., & Öngür, D. (2018). Brain lactate and pH in schizophrenia and bipolar disorder: A systematic review of findings from magnetic resonance studies. *Neuropsychopharmacology, 43*, 1681–1690.

Du, F., Cooper, A. J., Thida, T., Sehovic, S., Lukas, S. E., Cohen, B. M., Zhang, X., & Ongur, D. (2014). In vivo evidence for cerebral bioenergetic abnormalities in schizophrenia measured using ^{31}P magnetization transfer spectroscopy. *JAMA Psychiatry, 71*, 19–27.

Dutta, R., Greene, T., Addington, J., McKenzie, K., Phillips, M., & Murray, R. M. (2007). Biological, life course, and cross-cultural studies all point toward the value of dimensional and developmental ratings in the classification of psychosis. *Schizophrenia Bulletin, 33*, 868–876.

Emperador, S., López-Gallardo, E., Hernández-Ainsa, C., Habbane, M., Montoya, J., Bayona-Bafaluy, M. P., & Ruiz-Pesini, E. (2019). Ketogenic treatment reduces the percentage of a LHON heteroplasmic mutation and increases mtDNA amount of a LHON homoplasmic mutation. *Orphanet Journal of Rare Diseases, 14*, 150.

Emperador, S., Vidal, M., Hernández-Ainsa, C., Ruiz-Ruiz, C., Woods, D., Morales-Becerra, A., Arruga, J., Artuch, R., López-Gallardo, E., Bayona-Bafaluy, M. P., Montoya, J., & Ruiz-Pesini, E. (2018). The decrease in mitochondrial DNA mutation load parallels visual recovery in a Leber hereditary optic neuropathy patient. *Frontiers in Neuroscience, 12*, 61.

Ernst, A., Ma, D., Garcia-Perez, I., Tsang, T. M., Kluge, W., Schwarz, E., Guest, P. C., Holmes, E., Sarnyai, Z., & Bahn, S. (2012). Molecular validation of the acute phencyclidine rat model for schizophrenia: Identification of translational changes in energy metabolism and neurotransmission. *Journal of Proteome Research, 11*, 3704–3714.

Fogle, K. J., Smith, A. R., Satterfield, S. L., Gutierrez, A. C., Hertzler, J. I., McCardell, C. S., Shon, J. H., Barile, Z. J., Novak, M. O., & Palladino, M. J. (2019). Ketogenic and anaplerotic dietary modifications ameliorate seizure activity in *Drosophila* models of mitochondrial encephalomyopathy and glycolytic enzymopathy. *Molecular Genetics and Metabolism, 126*, 439–447.

Gilbert-Jaramillo, J., Vargas-Pico, D., Espinosa-Mendoza, T., Falk, S., Llanos-Fernandez, K., Guerrero-Haro, J., Orellana-Roman, C., Poveda-Loor, C., Valdevila-Figueira, J., & Palmer, C. (2018). The effects of the ketogenic diet on psychiatric symptomatology, weight and metabolic dysfunction in schizophrenia patients. *Journal of Clinical Nutrition and Metabolism, 5*, 1–5.

Gilbert, T. M., Zürcher, N. R., Wu, C. J., Bhanot, A., Hightower, B. G., Kim, M., Albrecht, D. S., Wey, H. Y., Schroeder, F. A., Rodriguez-Thompson, A., Morin, T. M., Hart, K. L., Pellegrini, A. M., Riley, M. M., Wang, C., Stufflebeam, S. M., Haggarty, S. J., Holt, D. J., Loggia, M. L., . . . Hooker, J. M. (2019). PET neuroimaging reveals histone deacetylase dysregulation in schizophrenia. *Journal of Clinical Investigation, 129*, 364–372.

Girgis, R. R., Javitch, J. A., & Lieberman, J. A. (2008). Antipsychotic drug mechanisms: Links between therapeutic effects, metabolic side effects and the insulin signaling pathway. *Molecular Psychiatry, 13*, 918–929.

Guidotti, A., & Grayson, D. R. (2014). DNA methylation and demethylation as targets for antipsychotic therapy. *Dialogues in Clinical Neuroscience, 16*, 419–429.

Hagihara, H., Catts, V. S., Katayama, Y., Shoji, H., Takagi, T., Huang, F. L., Nakao, A., Mori, Y., Huang, K. P., Ishii, S., Graef, I. A., Nakayama, K. I., Shannon Weickert, C., & Miyakawa, T. (2018). Decreased brain pH as a shared endophenotype of psychiatric disorders. *Neuropsychopharmacology, 43*, 459–468.

Hampton, T. (2018). Gut microbes may account for the anti-seizure effects of the ketogenic diet. *JAMA, 320*, 1307.

Han, Y. M., Ramprasath, T., & Zou, M. H. (2020). β-Hydroxybutyrate and its metabolic effects on age-associated pathology. *Experimental & Molecular Medicine*, *52*, 548–555.

Harris, J. J., Jolivet, R., & Attwell, D. (2012). Synaptic energy use and supply. *Neuron*, *75*, 762–777.

Harris, L. W., Guest, P. C., Wayland, M. T., Umrania, Y., Krishnamurthy, D., Rahmoune, H., & Bahn, S. (2013). Schizophrenia: Metabolic aspects of aetiology, diagnosis and future treatment strategies. *Psychoneuroendocrinology*, *38*, 752–766.

Hasan-Olive, M. M., Lauritzen, K. H., Ali, M., Rasmussen, L. J., Storm-Mathisen, J., & Bergersen, L. H. (2019). A ketogenic diet improves mitochondrial biogenesis and bioenergetics via the PGC1alpha-SIRT3-UCP2 axis. *Neurochemistry Research*, *44*, 22–37.

Hennekens, C. H. (2007). Increasing global burden of cardiovascular disease in general populations and patients with schizophrenia. *Journal of Clinical Psychiatry*, *68*(Suppl. 4), 4–7.

Hennekens, C. H., Hennekens, A. R., Hollar, D., & Casey, D. E. (2005). Schizophrenia and increased risks of cardiovascular disease. *American Heart Journal*, *150*, 1115–1121.

Herberth, M., Koethe, D., Cheng, T. M., Krzyszton, N. D., Schoeffmann, S., Guest, P. C., Rahmoune, H., Harris, L. W., Kranaster, L., Leweke, F. M., & Bahn, S. (2011). Impaired glycolytic response in peripheral blood mononuclear cells of first-onset antipsychotic-naive schizophrenia patients. *Molecular Psychiatry*, *16*, 848–859.

Hjelmervik, H., Craven, A. R., Sinceviciute, I., Johnsen, E., Kompus, K., Bless, J. J., Kroken, R. A., Løberg, E. M., Ersland, L., Grüner, R., et al. (2020). Intra-regional Glu-GABA vs inter-regional Glu-Glu imbalance: A ^{1}H-MRS study of the neurochemistry of auditory verbal hallucinations in schizophrenia. *Schizophrenia Bulletin*, *46*, 633–642.

Holper, L., Ben-Shachar, D., & Mann, J. J. (2019). Multivariate meta-analyses of mitochondrial complex I and IV in major depressive disorder, bipolar disorder, schizophrenia, Alzheimer disease, and Parkinson disease. *Neuropsychopharmacology*, *44*, 837–849.

Hosák, L., & Libiger, J. (2002). Antiepileptic drugs in schizophrenia: A review. *European Psychiatry*, *17*, 371–378.

Howes, O. D., & Kapur, S. (2009). The dopamine hypothesis of schizophrenia: Version III—The final common pathway. *Schizophrenia Bulletin*, *35*, 549–562.

Hüfner, K., Frajo-Apor, B., & Hofer, A. (2015). Neurology issues in schizophrenia. *Current Psychiatry Reports*, *17*, 32.

Jentsch, J. D., & Roth, R. H. (1999). The neuropsychopharmacology of phencyclidine: From NMDA receptor hypofunction to the dopamine hypothesis of schizophrenia. *Neuropsychopharmacology*, *20*, 201–225.

Kandratavicius, L., Hallak, J. E., & Leite, J. P. (2014). What are the similarities and differences between schizophrenia and schizophrenia-like psychosis of epilepsy? A neuropathological approach to the understanding of schizophrenia spectrum and epilepsy. *Epilepsy & Behavior*, *38*, 143–147.

Kang, E., Song, J., Lin, Y., Park, J., Lee, J. H., Hussani, Q., Gu, Y., Ge, S., Li, W., Hsu, K. S., Berninger, B., Christian, K. M., Song, H., & Ming, G. L. (2019). Interplay between a mental disorder risk gene and developmental polarity switch of GABA action leads to excitation–inhibition imbalance. *Cell Reports*, *28*, 1419–1428.

Kann, O. (2016). The interneuron energy hypothesis: Implications for brain disease. *Neurobiology of Disease*, *90*, 75–85.

Kelly, J. R., Minuto, C., Cryan, J. F., Clarke, G., & Dinan, T. G. (2021). The role of the gut microbiome in the development of schizophrenia. *Schizophrenia Research*, *234*, 4–23.

Kim, H. K., Andreazza, A. C., Elmi, N., Chen, W., & Young, L. T. (2016). Nod-like receptor pyrin containing 3 (NLRP3) in the post-mortem frontal cortex from patients with bipolar disorder: A potential mediator between mitochondria and immune-activation. *Journal of Psychiatric Research*, *72*, 43–50.

Koppel, S. J., & Swerdlow, R. H. (2018). Neuroketotherapeutics: A modern review of a century-old therapy. *Neurochemistry International*, *117*, 114–125.

Kosinski, C., & Jornayvaz, F. R. (2017). Effects of ketogenic diets on cardiovascular risk factors: Evidence from animal and human studies. *Nutrients*, *9*, 517.

Kovács, Z., D'Agostino, D. P., Diamond, D., Kindy, M. S., Rogers, C., & Ari, C. (2019). Therapeutic potential of exogenous ketone supplement induced ketosis in the treatment of psychiatric disorders: Review of current literature. *Frontiers in Psychiatry*, *10*, 363.

Kraeuter, A.-K., Guest, P. C., & Sarnyai, Z. (2019a). The therapeutic potential of ketogenic diet throughout life: Focus on metabolic, neurodevelopmental and neurodegenerative disorders. *Advances in Experimental Medicine and Biology*, *1178*, 77–101.

Kraeuter, A. K., Archambault, N., van den Buuse, M., & Sarnyai, Z. (2019b). Ketogenic diet and olanzapine treatment alone and in combination reduce a pharmacologically-induced prepulse inhibition deficit in female mice. *Schizophrenia Research*, *212*, 221–224.

Kraeuter, A. K., Guest, P. C., & Sarnyai, Z. (2020a). Protocol for the use of the ketogenic diet in preclinical and clinical practice. *Methods in Molecular Biology*, *2138*, 83–98.

Kraeuter, A. K., Loxton, H., Lima, B. C., Rudd, D., & Sarnyai, Z. (2015). Ketogenic diet reverses behavioral abnormalities in an acute NMDA receptor hypofunction model of schizophrenia. *Schizophrenia Research, 169,* 491–493.

Kraeuter, A. K., Mashavave, T., Suvarna, A., van den Buuse, M., & Sarnyai, Z. (2020b). Effects of beta-hydroxybutyrate administration on MK-801-induced schizophrenia-like behaviour in mice. *Psychopharmacology, 237,* 1397–1405.

Kraeuter, A. K., Phillips, R., & Sarnyai, Z. (2020c). Ketogenic therapy in neurodegenerative and psychiatric disorders: From mice to men. *Progress in Neuro-psychopharmacology and Biological Psychiatry, 101,* 109913.

Kraeuter, A. K., van den Buuse, M., & Sarnyai, Z. (2019c). Ketogenic diet prevents impaired prepulse inhibition of startle in an acute NMDA receptor hypofunction model of schizophrenia. *Schizophrenia Research, 206,* 244–250.

Kraft, B. D., & Westman, E. C. (2009). Schizophrenia, gluten, and low-carbohydrate, ketogenic diets: A case report and review of the literature. *Nutrition & Metabolism, 6,* 10.

Leino, R. L., Gerhart, D. Z., Duelli, R., Enerson, B. E., & Drewes, L. R. (2001). Diet-induced ketosis increases monocarboxylate transporter (MCT1) levels in rat brain. *Neurochemistry International, 38,* 519–527.

Lewis, D. A., Curley, A. A., Glausier, J. R., & Volk, D. W. (2012). Cortical parvalbumin interneurons and cognitive dysfunction in schizophrenia. *Trends in Neuroscience, 35,* 57–67.

Li, Z., & Heber, D. (2020). Ketogenic diets. *JAMA, 323,* 386–386.

Lieberman, J. A. (1999). Is schizophrenia a neurodegenerative disorder? A clinical and neurobiological perspective. *Biological Psychiatry, 46,* 729–739.

Lieberman, J. A. (2006). Neurobiology and the natural history of schizophrenia. *Journal of Clinical Psychiatry, 67,* e14.

Lieberman, J. A., & First, M. B. (2018). Psychotic disorders. *New England Journal of Medicine, 379,* 270–280.

Lieberman, J. A., Malaspina, D., & Jarskog, L. F. (2006). Preventing clinical deterioration in the course of schizophrenia: The potential for neuroprotection. *CNS Spectrums, 11*(4), suppl 1–13; quiz suppl 14–5.

Lindenmayer, J. P., Khan, A., Kaushik, S., Thanju, A., Praveen, R., Hoffman, L., Cherath, L., Valdez, G., & Wance, D. (2012). Relationship between metabolic syndrome and cognition in patients with schizophrenia. *Schizophrenia Research, 142,* 171–176.

Ludwig, D. S., Willett, W. C., Volek, J. S., & Neuhouser, M. L. (2018). Dietary fat: From foe to friend? *Science, 362,* 764–770.

Lutas, A., & Yellen, G. (2013). The ketogenic diet: Metabolic influences on brain excitability and epilepsy. *Trends in Neuroscience, 36,* 32–40.

Magistretti, P. J., & Pellerin, L. (1999). Cellular mechanisms of brain energy metabolism and their relevance to functional brain imaging. *Philosophical Transactions of the Royal Society B: Biological Sciences, 354,* 1155–1163.

Marenco, S., & Weinberger, D. R. (2000). The neurodevelopmental hypothesis of schizophrenia: Following a trail of evidence from cradle to grave. *Development and Psychopathology, 12,* 501–527.

Meyer, U. (2013). Developmental neuroinflammation and schizophrenia. *Progress in Neuro-Psychopharmacoly and Biological Psychiatry, 42,* 20–34.

Miyamoto, S., Miyake, N., Jarskog, L. F., Fleischhacker, W. W., & Lieberman, J. A. (2012). Pharmacological treatment of schizophrenia: A critical review of the pharmacology and clinical effects of current and future therapeutic agents. *Molecular Psychiatry, 17,* 1206–1227.

Momtazmanesh, S., Zare-Shahabadi, A., & Rezaei, N. (2019). Cytokine alterations in schizophrenia: An updated review. *Frontiers in Psychiatry, 10,* 892.

Monteiro, J., Assis-de-Lemos, G., de-Souza-Ferreira, E., Marques, A. M., Neves, G. A., Silveira, M. S., & Galina, A. (2020). Energization by multiple substrates and calcium challenge reveal dysfunctions in brain mitochondria in a model related to acute psychosis. *Journal of Bioenergetics and Biomembranes, 52,* 1–15.

Muscogiuri, G., Barrea, L., Laudisio, D., Pugliese, G., Salzano, C., Savastano, S., & Colao, A. (2019). The management of very low-calorie ketogenic diet in obesity outpatient clinic: A practical guide. *Journal of Translational Medicine, 17,* 356.

Nagpal, R., Neth, B. J., Wang, S., Craft, S., & Yadav, H. (2019). Modified Mediterranean-ketogenic diet modulates gut microbiome and short-chain fatty acids in association with Alzheimer's disease markers in subjects with mild cognitive impairment. *EBioMedicine, 47,* 529–542.

Nascimento, J. M., & Martins-de-Souza, D. (2015). The proteome of schizophrenia. npj Schizophrenia 1, 14003.

Newcomer, J. W. (2005). Second-generation (atypical) antipsychotics and metabolic effects: A comprehensive literature review. *CNS Drugs, 19*(Suppl. 1), 1–93.

Ni, P., & Chung, S. (2020). Mitochondrial dysfunction in schizophrenia. *Bioessays, 42*(6), e1900202.

Ni, P., Noh, H., Park, G. H., Shao, Z., Guan, Y., Park, J. M., Yu, S., Park, J. S., Coyle, J. T., Weinberger, D. R., Straub, R. E., Cohen, B. M., McPhie, D. L., Yin, C., Huang, W., Kim, H. Y., & Chung, S. (2019). iPSC-derived homogeneous populations of developing schizophrenia cortical interneurons have compromised mitochondrial function. *Molecular Psychiatry, 25*(11), 3103–3104.

Noebels, J., Avoli, M., Rogawski, M., Olsen, R., & Delgado-Escueta, A. (2013). *Jasper's basic mechanisms of the epilepsies.* Oxford University Press.

Okuma, T. (1994). Use of antiepileptic drugs in schizophrenia. *CNS Drugs, 1,* 269–284.

Olivier, B., Leahy, C., Mullen, T., Paylor, R., Groppi, V. E., Sarnyai, Z., & Brunner, D. (2001). The DBA/2J strain and prepulse inhibition of startle: A model system to test antipsychotics? *Psychopharmacology, 156,* 284–290.

Olson, C. A., Vuong, H. E., Yano, J. M., Liang, Q. Y., Nusbaum, D. J., & Hsiao, E. Y. (2018). The gut microbiota mediates the anti-seizure effects of the ketogenic diet. *Cell, 173,* 1728–1741.

Pacheco, A., Easterling, W. S., & Pryer, M. W. (1965). A pilot study of the ketogenic diet in schizophrenia. *American Journal of Psychiatry, 121,* 1110–1111.

Palmer, C. M. (2017). Ketogenic diet in the treatment of schizoaffective disorder: Two case studies. *Schizophrenia Research, 189,* 208–209.

Palmer, C. M., Gilbert-Jaramillo, J., & Westman, E. C. (2019). The ketogenic diet and remission of psychotic symptoms in schizophrenia: Two case studies. *Schizophrenia Research, 208,* 439–440.

Paudel, Y. N., Shaikh, M. F., Shah, S., Kumari, Y., & Othman, I. (2018). Role of inflammation in epilepsy and neurobehavioral comorbidities: Implication for therapy. *European Journal of Pharmacology, 837,* 145–155.

Petra, A. I., Panagiotidou, S., Hatziagelaki, E., Stewart, J. M., Conti, P., & Theoharides, T. C. (2015). Gut-microbiota-brain axis and its effect on neuropsychiatric disorders with suspected immune dysregulation. *Clinical Therapeutics, 37,* 984–995.

Pillinger, T., Beck, K., Gobjila, C., Donocik, J. G., Jauhar, S., & Howes, O. D. (2017). Impaired glucose homeostasis in first-episode schizophrenia: A systematic review and meta-analysis. *JAMA Psychiatry, 74,* 261–269.

Pillinger, T., D'Ambrosio, E., McCutcheon, R., & Howes, O. D. (2018). Is psychosis a multisystem disorder? A meta-review of central nervous system, immune, cardiometabolic, and endocrine alterations in first-episode psychosis and perspective on potential models. *Molecular Psychiatry, 24,* 776–794.

Prabakaran, S., Swatton, J. E., Ryan, M. M., Huffaker, S. J., Huang, J. T., Griffin, J. L., Wayland, M., Freeman, T., Dudbridge, F., Lilley, K. S., Karp, N. A., Hester, S., Tkachev, D., Mimmack, M. L., Yolken, R. H., Webster, M. J., Torrey, E. F., & Bahn, S. (2004). Mitochondrial dysfunction in schizophrenia: Evidence for compromised brain metabolism and oxidative stress. *Molecular Psychiatry, 9,* 684–697.

Qiu, X., Xiao, X., Li, N., & Li, Y. (2017). Histone deacetylase inhibitors (HDACIs) as novel therapeutic application in various clinical diseases. *Progress in Neuro-Psychopharmacology & Biological Psychiatry, 72,* 60–72.

Rho, J. M., & Stafstrom, C. E. (2012). The ketogenic diet: What has science taught us? *Epilepsy Research, 100,* 210–217.

Robicsek, O., Ene, H. M., Karry, R., Ytzhaki, O., Asor, E., McPhie, D., Cohen, B. M., Ben-Yehuda, R., Weiner, I., & Ben-Shachar, D. (2018). Isolated mitochondria transfer improves neuronal differentiation of schizophrenia-derived induced pluripotent stem cells and rescues deficits in a rat model of the disorder. *Schizophrenia Bulletin, 44,* 432–442.

Robicsek, O., Karry, R., Petit, I., Salman-Kesner, N., Muller, F. J., Klein, E., Aberdam, D., & Ben-Shachar, D. (2013). Abnormal neuronal differentiation and mitochondrial dysfunction in hair follicle-derived induced pluripotent stem cells of schizophrenia patients. *Molecular Psychiatry, 18,* 1067–1076.

Rogawski, M. A., Loscher, W., & Rho, J. M. (2016). Mechanisms of action of antiseizure drugs and the ketogenic diet. *Cold Spring Harbor Perspectives in Medicine, 6,* a022780.

Rowland, L. M., Pradhan, S., Korenic, S., Wijtenburg, S. A., Hong, L. E., Edden, R. A., & Barker, P. B. (2016). Elevated brain lactate in schizophrenia: A 7 T magnetic resonance spectroscopy study. *Translational Psychiatry, 6,* e967.

Roy, K., Balon, R., Penumetcha, V., & Levine, B. H. (2014). Psychosis and seizure disorder: Challenges in diagnosis and treatment. *Current Psychiatry Reports, 16,* 509.

Sarnyai, Z., Alsaif, M., Bahn, S., Ernst, A., Guest, P. C., Hradetzky, E., Kluge, W., Stelzhammer, V., & Wesseling, H. (2011). Behavioral and molecular biomarkers in translational animal models for neuropsychiatric disorders. *International Review of Neurobiology, 101,* 203–238.

Sarnyai, Z., & Guest, P. C. (2017). Connecting brain proteomics with behavioural neuroscience in translational animal models of neuropsychiatric disorders. *Advances in Experimental Medicine and Biology, 974,* 97–114.

Sarnyai, Z., Jashar, C., & Olivier, B. (2015). Modeling combined schizophrenia-related behavioral and metabolic phenotypes in rodents. *Behavioural Brain Research, 276,* 130–142.

Sarnyai, Z., Kraeuter, A. K., & Palmer, C. M. (2019). Ketogenic diet for schizophrenia: Clinical implication. *Current Opinion in Psychiatry, 32,* 394–401.

Schroeder, F. A., Gilbert, T. M., Feng, N., Taillon, B. D., Volkow, N. D., Innis, R. B., Hooker, J. M., & Lipska, B. K. (2017). Expression of HDAC2 but not HDAC1 transcript is reduced in dorsolateral prefrontal cortex of patients with schizophrenia. *ACS Chemical Neuroscience, 8,* 662–668.

Schultz, S. K., & Andreasen, N. C. (1999). Schizophrenia. *Lancet, 353,* 1425–1430.

Schwarz, E., Maukonen, J., Hyytiäinen, T., Kieseppä, T., Orešič, M., Sabunciyan, S., Mantere, O., Saarela, M., Yolken, R., & Suvisaari, J. (2018). Analysis of microbiota in first episode psychosis identifies preliminary associations with symptom severity and treatment response. *Schizophrenia Research, 192,* 398–403.

Seeman, P. (2006). Targeting the dopamine D_2 receptor in schizophrenia. *Expert Opinion on Therapeutic Targets, 10,* 515–531.

Seeman, P. (2013). Schizophrenia and dopamine receptors. *European Neuropsychopharmacology, 23,* 999–1009.

Seyfried, T. N., Flores, R. E., Poff, A. M., & D'Agostino, D. P. (2014). Cancer as a metabolic disease: Implications for novel therapeutics. *Carcinogenesis, 35,* 515–527.

Sharma, R. P., Grayson, D. R., & Gavin, D. P. (2008). Histone deactylase 1 expression is increased in the prefrontal cortex of schizophrenia subjects: Analysis of the National Brain Databank microarray collection. *Schizophrenia Research, 98,* 111–117.

Stahl, S. M. (2004). Anticonvulsants as mood stabilizers and adjuncts to antipsychotics: Valproate, lamotrigine, carbamazepine, and oxcarbazepine and actions at voltage-gated sodium channels. *Journal of Clinical Psychiatry, 65,* 738–739.

Staverosky, T. (2016). Ketogenic weight loss: The lowering of insulin levels is the sleeping giant in patient care. *Journal of Medical Practice Management, 32,* 63–66.

Steiner, J., Berger, M., Guest, P. C., Dobrowolny, H., Westphal, S., Schiltz, K., & Sarnyai, Z. (2017). Assessment of insulin resistance among drug-naive patients with first-episode schizophrenia in the context of hormonal stress axis activation. *JAMA Psychiatry, 74,* 968–970.

Steiner, J., Bogerts, B., Sarnyai, Z., Walter, M., Gos, T., Bernstein, H. G., & Myint, A. M. (2012). Bridging the gap between the immune and glutamate hypotheses of schizophrenia and major depression: Potential role of glial NMDA receptor modulators and impaired blood-brain barrier integrity. *World Journal of Biological Psychiatry, 13,* 482–492.

Steiner, J., Fernandes, B. S., Guest, P. C., Dobrowolny, H., Meyer-Lotz, G., Westphal, S., Borucki, K., Schiltz, K., Sarnyai, Z., & Bernstein, H.-G. (2018). Glucose homeostasis in major depression and schizophrenia: A comparison among drug-naive first-episode patients. *European Archives of Psychiatry and Clinical Neuroscience, 269,* 373–377.

Steiner, J., Walter, M., Glanz, W., Sarnyai, Z., Bernstein, H. G., Vielhaber, S., Kastner, A., Skalej, M., Jordan, W., Schiltz, K., Klingbeil, C., Wandinger, K. P., Bogerts, B., & Stoecker, W. (2013). Increased prevalence of diverse N-methyl-D-aspartate glutamate receptor antibodies in patients with an initial diagnosis of schizophrenia: Specific relevance of IgG NR1a antibodies for distinction from N-methyl-D-aspartate glutamate receptor encephalitis. *JAMA Psychiatry, 70,* 271–278.

Stone, W. S., Faraone, S. V., Su, J., Tarbox, S. I., Van Eerdewegh, P., & Tsuang, M. T. (2004). Evidence for linkage between regulatory enzymes in glycolysis and schizophrenia in a multiplex sample. *Neuropsychiatric Genetics, Part B of the American Journal of Medical Genetics, 127B,* 5–10.

Storoni, M., Robert, M. P., & Plant, G. T. (2019). The therapeutic potential of a calorie-restricted ketogenic diet for the management of Leber hereditary optic neuropathy. *Nutritional Neuroscience, 22,* 156–164.

Suárez-Méndez, S., García-de la Cruz, D. D., Tovilla-Zárate, C. A., Genis-Mendoza, A. D., Ramón-Torres, R. A., González-Castro, T. B., & Juárez-Rojop, I. E. (2020). Diverse roles of mtDNA in schizophrenia: Implications in its pathophysiology and as biomarker for cognitive impairment. *Progress in Biophysics & Molecular Biology, 155,* 36–41.

Sullivan, C. R., Koene, R. H., Hasselfeld, K., O'Donovan, S. M., Ramsey, A., & McCullumsmith, R. E. (2018a). Neuron-specific deficits of bioenergetic processes in the dorsolateral prefrontal cortex in schizophrenia. *Molecular Psychiatry, 24,* 1319–1328.

Sullivan, C. R., Mielnik, C. A., Funk, A., O'Donovan, S. M., Bentea, E., Pletnikov, M., Ramsey, A. J., Wen, Z., Rowland, L. M., & McCullumsmith, R. E. (2019a). Measurement of lactate levels in postmortem brain, iPSCs, and animal models of schizophrenia. *Scientific Reports, 9,* 5087.

Sullivan, C. R., Mielnik, C. A., O'Donovan, S. M., Funk, A. J., Bentea, E., DePasquale, E. A., Alganem, K., Wen, Z., Haroutunian, V., Katsel, P., Ramsey, A. J., Meller, J., & McCullumsmith, R. E. (2019b). Connectivity analyses of bioenergetic changes in schizophrenia: Identification of novel treatments. *Molecular Neurobiology, 56,* 4492–4517.

Sullivan, C. R., O'Donovan, S. M., McCullumsmith, R. E., & Ramsey, A. (2018b). Defects in bioenergetic coupling in schizophrenia. *Biological Psychiatry, 83,* 739–750.

Sunahara, R. K., Seeman, P., Van Tol, H. H., & Niznik, H. B. (1993). Dopamine receptors and antipsychotic drug response. *British Journal of Psychiatry,* Suppl., *22,* 31–38.

Tamminga, C. A., & Holcomb, H. H. (2005). Phenotype of schizophrenia: A review and formulation. *Molecular Psychiatry, 10,* 27–39.

Tregellas, J. R., Smucny, J., Legget, K. T., & Stevens, K. E. (2015). Effects of a ketogenic diet on auditory gating in DBA/2 mice: A proof-of-concept study. *Schizophrenia Research, 169,* 351–354.

Tsai, G., Passani, L. A., Slusher, B. S., Carter, R., Baer, L., Kleinman, J. E., & Coyle, J. T. (1995). Abnormal excitatory neurotransmitter metabolism in schizophrenic brains. *Archives of General Psychiatry, 52,* 829–836.

Uhlhaas, P. J., & Singer, W. (2013). High-frequency oscillations and the neurobiology of schizophrenia. *Dialogues in Clinical Neuroscience, 15,* 301–313.

Valiente-Pallejà, A., Torrell, H., Alonso, Y., Vilella, E., Muntané, G., & Martorell, L. (2020). Increased blood lactate levels during exercise and mitochondrial DNA alterations converge on mitochondrial dysfunction in schizophrenia. *Schizophrenia Research, 220,* 61–68.

van Os, J., & Kapur, S. (2009). Schizophrenia. *Lancet, 374,* 635–645.

Vidali, S., Aminzadeh, S., Lambert, B., Rutherford, T., Sperl, W., Kofler, B., & Feichtinger, R. G. (2015). Mitochondria: The ketogenic diet—A metabolism-based therapy. *International Journal of Biochemistry and Cell Biology, 63,* 55–59.

Virani, S. S., Alonso, A., Benjamin, E. J., Bittencourt, M. S., Callaway, C. W., Carson, A. P., Chamberlain, A. M., Chang, A. R., Cheng, S., Delling, F. N., Elkind, M. S. V., Evenson, K. R., Ferguson, J. F., Gupta, D. K., Khan, S. S., Kissela, B. M., Knutson, K. L., Lee, C. D., Lewis, T. T., . . . American Heart Association Council on Epidemiology and Prevention Statistics Committee and Stroke Statistics Subcommittee. (2020). Heart disease and stroke statistics update: A report from the American Heart Association. *Circulation, 141,* e139–e596.

Wassef, A., Baker, J., & Kochan, L. D. (2003). GABA and schizophrenia: A review of basic science and clinical studies. *Journal of Clinical Psychopharmacology, 23,* 601–640.

Wenneberg, C., Glenthøj, B. Y., Hjorthøj, C., Buchardt Zingenberg, F. J., Glenthøj, L. B., Rostrup, E.,

Broberg, B. V., & Nordentoft, M. (2020). Cerebral glutamate and GABA levels in high-risk of psychosis states: A focused review and meta-analysis of ¹H-MRS studies. *Schizophrenia Research, 215,* 38–48.

Westman, E. C., Tondt, J., Maguire, E., & Yancy, W. S., Jr. (2018). Implementing a low-carbohydrate, ketogenic diet to manage type 2 diabetes mellitus. *Expert Review of Endocrinology & Metabolism, 13,* 263–272.

Xu, R., Wu, B., Liang, J., He, F., Gu, W., Li, K., Luo, Y., Chen, J., Gao, Y., Wu, Z., Wang, Y., Zhou, W., & Wang, M. (2020). Altered gut microbiota and mucosal immunity in patients with schizophrenia. *Brain, Behavior, and Immunity, 85,* 120–127.

Youm, Y. H., Nguyen, K. Y., Grant, R. W., Goldberg, E. L., Bodogai, M., Kim, D., D'Agostino, D., Planavsky, N., Lupfer, C., Kanneganti, T.D., Kang, S., Horvath, T. L., Fahmy, T. M., Crawford, P. A., Biragyn, A., Alnemri, E., & Dixit, V. D. (2015). The ketone metabolite β-hydroxybutyrate blocks NLRP3 inflammasome-mediated inflammatory disease. *Nature Medicine, 21,* 263–269.

Zhang, Z., & Sun, Q. Q. (2011). The balance between excitation and inhibition and functional sensory processing in the somatosensory cortex. *International Review of Neurobiology, 97,* 305–333.

Zheng, P., Zeng, B., Liu, M., Chen, J., Pan, J., Han, Y., Liu, Y., Cheng, K., Zhou, C., Wang, H., Zhou, X., Gui, S., Perry, S. W., Wong, M. L., Licinio, J., Wei, H., & Xie, P. (2019). The gut microbiome from patients with schizophrenia modulates the glutamate-glutamine-GABA cycle and schizophrenia-relevant behaviors in mice. *Science Advances, 5,* eaau8317.

Zhu, F., Ju, Y., Wang, W., Wang, Q., Guo, R., Ma, Q., Sun, Q., Fan, Y., Xie, Y., Yang, Z., Jie, Z., Zhao, B., Xiao, L., Yang, L., Zhang, T., Feng, J., Guo, L., He, X., Chen, Y., . . . Ma, X. (2020). Metagenome-wide association of gut microbiome features for schizophrenia. *Nature Communication, 11,* 1612.

Zuccoli, G. S., Saia-Cereda, V. M., Nascimento, J. M., & Martins-de-Souza, D. (2017). The energy metabolism dysfunction in psychiatric disorders postmortem brains: Focus on proteomic evidence. *Frontiers in Neuroscience, 11,* 493.

21

The Ketogenic Diet and the Gut Microbiome

CHUNLONG MU, PHD, JANE SHEARER, PHD, MORRIS H.
SCANTLEBURY, MD, AND WENDIE N. MARKS, PHD

INTRODUCTION

The gut microbiome is the collection of microorganisms, including bacteria, viruses, fungi, and other microorganisms, that colonize the gastrointestinal tract, as well as their genetic components. Collectively, the gut microbiome is the largest and most taxonomically diverse collection of microorganisms in the body, comprising approximately 23 million nonredundant genes (Tierney et al., 2019). Firmicutes, Bacteroidetes, Proteobacteria, and Actinobacteria are the most abundant phyla of microbiota within the human gut, with the highest density occurring in the colon (Mohajeri et al., 2018). Although the taxonomic composition of the gut microbiota varies between individuals, the contributions of diverse gut microbiota to metabolic pathway outcomes, such as carbohydrate metabolism and amino acid degradation, are relatively consistent (Cho & Blaser, 2012). Functionally, gut microbiota and their metabolites contribute to caloric extraction from otherwise inaccessible nutrients, vitamin synthesis, immune regulation, gut epithelial renewal, and the maintenance of mucosal integrity, thus playing an essential role in the preservation of human health (Zmora et al., 2019).

The gut microbiome is affected by host genetics, age, and environment, but diet is proposed to be the dominant factor in shaping the gut microbiome (Carmody et al., 2015). The ketogenic diet (KD) is a metabolism-based intervention that is widely used to treat drug-resistant childhood epilepsy syndromes, obesity, and a subset of neurodevelopmental disorders (Kraeuter et al., 2020). The KD was initially designed to mimic a state of fasting wherein adequate protein and calories are provided for growth, yet carbohydrate intake is sufficiently reduced to confer a state of ketosis by the production of β-hydroxybutyrate, acetate, and acetoacetate. A typical KD consists of a fixed ratio of fats to the combination of protein and carbohydrates at 3:1 to 4:1, respectively (Dhamija et al., 2013). It is proposed that the therapeutic effects of the KD are multifactorial, including effects on metabolism, inflammation, and neural pathways (for details, see Rho, 2017); however, these mechanisms have yet to be fully elucidated. Although previous research has focused on the neurologic benefits of the KD, research into the effects of the KD on the gut are gaining momentum. Several lines of research indicate that the KD alters the taxonomic composition of the gut microbiome, with potential functional consequences for a variety of neurologic and physiologic disorders. This chapter focuses on the association between alterations in the gut microbiome and the therapeutic effects of a KD within the context of neurologic and physiologic disorders.

THE EFFECT OF DIETARY MACRONUTRIENTS ON THE GUT MICROBIOME

Similar to the nutritional requirements of humans, gut microbes need essential macronutrients to survive, including carbohydrates, proteins, and lipids. Dietary composition can selectively enrich different microbial groups with an increase in dietary fats or proteins, at the expense of carbohydrates, leading to shifts in the gut microbiota. The effects of diet on the human gut microbiome have been reviewed extensively elsewhere (Li et al., 2019). Directly relevant to this chapter are the effects of a characteristic high-fat, low-carbohydrate KD on the gut microbiome. In humans, long-term adherence to a diet enriched with proteins and animal fats can boost a *Bacteroides*-dominated microbiome, while a diet enriched with carbohydrates will lead to a *Prevotella*-dominated microbiome (Wu et al., 2011). In Wistar rats, a high-protein, low-carbohydrate diet leads to an increase of *Escherichia coli* and a decrease of *Akkermansia muciniphila*,

Bifidobacterium, *Prevotella*, and *Ruminococcus bromii*, most of which are involved in carbohydrate fermentation (Mu et al., 2017). Gut microbes are also capable of metabolizing fibers and nondigestible polysaccharides that cannot be metabolized by host enzymes. Polysaccharide utilization is dependent on microbial composition. An increase in *Bacteroides* species is commonly observed following a diet high in fiber or polysaccharides. Bacteroidetes, such as *Bacteroides intestinalis*, *B. xylanisolvens*, and *B. thetaiotaomicron*, encode several glycoside hydrolases and polysaccharide lyases to metabolize polysaccharides, a phenomenon rarely observed in species of Firmicutes or Proteobacteria (El Kaoutari et al., 2013). The difference in gut microbe nutrient preference is largely the result of dissimilarities in the genetic composition of the gut microbes and the intestinal microenvironment created by different diets (Tramontano et al., 2018). As the gut microenvironment takes part in complex interactions with metabolic and immunologic pathways, microbial adaptation to different dietary macronutrients partially reflects the outcome of these host–microbe interactions.

EFFECTS OF THE KD ON THE GUT MICROBIOME IN NEUROLOGIC AND PHYSIOLOGIC DISORDERS

The gut microbiome is capable of regulating neurologic and physiologic disorders through the microbiome–gut–brain axis, a bidirectional communication between the gut and the brain (Mu et al., 2016). The metabolic, immunologic, endocrinologic, and vagus nerve pathways are the major mechanisms responsible for these interactions. A graphic representation of the pathways involved is shown in Figure 21.1. In the discussion of the known associations between the therapeutic effects of the KD and the gut microbiome that follows, where possible, attention is paid to the metabolic, immunologic, or endocrinologic mechanisms that may be involved in mediating the effects of the KD on the gut microbiome in neurologic and physiologic disorders.

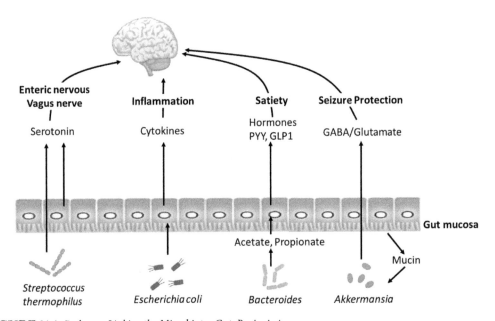

FIGURE 21.1 *Pathways Linking the Microbiota–Gut–Brain Axis*

The metabolic, immune, neural, and endocrine pathways are the major mechanisms mediating the microbiota–gut–brain axis. For example, *Streptococcus thermophilus* can produce serotonin that targets peripheral organs. Likewise, *Escherichia coli* secretes lipopolysaccharide, which induces cytokines and affects immune responses. The endocrine pathway is involved in gastrointestinal hormone secretion (e.g., PYY, GLP-1), regulated in part by the secretion of short-chain fatty acids, such as acetate and propionate. Both of these metabolites can signal the brain and stimulate satiety. Finally, *Akkermansia* can utilize mucin and affect the neural GABA/glutamate ratio, which confers seizure-protective activity. Abbreviations: PYY = peptide YY; GLP-1 = glucagonlike peptide-1; GABA = γ-aminobutyric acid.

Autism Spectrum Disorder

Autism spectrum disorder (ASD) is a neurodevelopmental condition characterized by alterations in social communication, as well as repetitive and stereotyped behaviors (Rho, 2017). The prevalence of ASD is 1 per 59 children in the United States, with boys four times more likely to be diagnosed than girls (Baio et al., 2018). Pharmacologic treatment strategies consist of antipsychotics, antidepressants, and anticonvulsants, as well as glutamatergic, GABAergic, cholinergic, and endocrinologic agents (Farmer et al., 2019; Goel et al., 2018). However, currently used medications are actually behavioral modifiers that are often ineffective at alleviating the core symptoms of ASD and can result in adverse effects, such as weight gain and sedation (Farmer et al., 2019; Goel et al., 2018). Medications are generally avoided unless symptoms are severe, such as extreme hyperactivity, anxiety, self-injurious behaviors, and epilepsy. Therefore, more effective treatment strategies are needed to ameliorate the symptoms of ASD. Nonpharmacologic interventions mainly focus on specific behaviors depending on individual conditions. Recent studies suggest that manipulation of the gut microbiome may serve as an alternative treatment strategy.

A growing number of studies suggests that children with ASD have an altered gut microbiome relative to typically developed controls. The causes of these alterations, whether due to restricted dietary patterns seen in some individuals with ASD, underlying pathology, or medication use, remain to be elucidated. Generally, the alterations include an increased abundance of *Clostridium*, *Desulfovibrio*, and *Lactobacillus* species and a decreased abundance of *Parabacteroides*, as reviewed in Bezawada et al. (2020). Further evidence for the involvement of the gut microbiome in ASD pathology has been derived from animal studies. Germ-free mice colonized by the microbiome from children with ASD manifested autism-related behaviors, while mice colonized by the microbiome from typically developed children did not (Sharon et al., 2019). Interestingly, Sharon and colleagues (2019) further identified a deficiency in taurine production in mice colonized by the ASD microbiome, with taurine supplementation improving repetitive and social behaviors in these mice, thus demonstrating a direct metabolic involvement of the gut microbiome in ASD via taurine.

The KD increasingly holds promise as an alternative or adjunctive treatment in ASD. The KD has been shown to improve behavioral outcomes in children with ASD (Lee et al., 2018), with similar improvements in behavior demonstrated in the BTBR mouse model of ASD (Ruskin et al., 2013). The therapeutic mechanisms of the KD in ASD are likely multifactorial (Cheng et al., 2017). However, there is evidence to support the view that the effects of the diet may work through reshaping the gut microbiota. In the BTBR mouse model of ASD, a KD administered for 10 to 14 days decreased the *Bacteroides:Prevotella* ratio, as well as the counts of *A. muciniphila*, *Bifidobacterium*, *Lactobacillus*, *Methanobrevibacter*, and *Roseburia* in both cecal and fecal compartments (Newell et al., 2016). Alternatively, the diet increased the counts of Enterobacteriaceae in feces (Newell et al., 2016). Metabolomics profiling in BTBR mice fed a KD further identified negative correlations between fecal *Clostridium leptum* and serum metabolites, such as betaine, acetoacetate, β-hydroxybutyrate, and glutathione, and positive correlations between *A. muciniphila* and lactate, taurine, and sarcosine (Klein et al., 2016). As the KD has been shown to normalize metabolic dysfunction in the mitochondria and to exert neuroprotective effects (Cheng et al., 2017), it will be important for future work to determine whether these identified relationships indicate a potential impact of gut microbes on host metabolism in ASD.

Clinical studies that examine the effects of the KD on the gut microbiome in children with ASD are in their infancy. Nevertheless, there is preliminary evidence in support of this association. In a clinical pilot study, children with ASD had higher concentrations of trimethylamine N-oxide (TMAO) than typically developed controls (Mu et al., 2020). TMAO is produced by hepatic oxidation of trimethylamine, which is produced by microbial metabolism and is transported from the gut to the liver (Subramaniam & Fletcher, 2018). Following 3 months of treatment with a modified, gluten-free KD with medium-chain triglyceride supplementation, autistic symptoms of social affect and nervousness were ameliorated (Lee et al., 2018). In another study using a similar diet, the relative concentration of TMAO was decreased (Mu et al., 2020) in ASD patients exposed to the KD versus controls. The alterations in TMAO observed in ASD children after treatment suggest a possible alteration in gut microbial function. However, the potential mechanisms mediating the effects of gut microbiota on neurologic function following the KD remain unknown.

Epilepsy

Epilepsy is a common neurologic disorder involving recurrent unprovoked seizures that affects 50 to 70 million people globally. Anticonvulsant medications are the first-line treatment, but they can fail in ~ 30% of patients, who then are diagnosed with the medically refractory form of the disorder (Lee & Kossoff, 2011). The KD is thought to reduce the severity of drug-resistant epilepsy by multiple mechanisms, including, but not limited to, neurotransmitter expression, ion channel activity, mitochondrial bioenergetics, and inflammation response (Rho, 2017). However, a growing body of evidence suggests a change in the composition of the gut microbiota is a contributing factor to the anticonvulsant effects of the diet.

Alterations in the gut microbiome have been observed in populations of epileptic patients. Relative to healthy controls, infants with refractory epilepsy have a higher abundance of Proteobacteria and a lower abundance of *Bacteroides* in their fecal content (Xie et al., 2017). Importantly, changes in the gut microbiota are also found after treatment with a KD. A 1-week KD reduced seizure frequency by 50% in 64% of the children who had been diagnosed with refractory epilepsy (Xie et al., 2017). In this clinical population, a decrease in the abundance of Proteobacteria and *Cronobacter* in feces to levels similar to those in healthy controls was observed (Xie et al., 2017). However, it is unknown whether the decrease in seizure frequency was due to alterations in the gut microbiota. In a separate population of children ages 1 to 10 years with refractory epilepsy, 50% of patients showed a 50% decrease in seizure severity after consuming the KD for 6 months (Zhang et al., 2018). Regardless of KD efficacy, increases in the abundance of *Bacteroides,* and a decrease in Ruminococcaceae, *Faecalibacterium*, Actinobacteria, *Coprobacter,* and *Leucobacter* were observed. When compared with nonresponders (< 50% seizure reduction) to the KD, responders had a lower abundance of *Clostridium* XIVa, *Alistipes, Helicobacter, Blautia, Eggerthella,* and *Steptococcus* (Zhang et al., 2018). In a population of children 2 to 15 years old with refractory epilepsy, 3 months of KD therapy reduced the abundance of *Bifidobacterium* and *Dialister* and the expression of genes that encode carbohydrate metabolism in the gut microbiome (Lindefeldt et al., 2019). However, the abundance of *Esherichia* was increased by the KD (Lindefeldt et al., 2019). In a pilot study consisting of six

patients 8 to 34 years old who had glucose transporter type 1 deficiency syndrome and concomitant seizure symptoms, a 3-month treatment with a KD significantly increased the abundance of *Desulfovibrio,* but it had no effects on Firmicutes, Bacteroidetes, *Bifidobacterium, Lactobacillus, Clostridium perfringens,* Enterobacteriaceae, *Clostridium* cluster XIV, or *Faecalibacterium prausnitzii* (Tagliabue et al., 2017). Taken together, these findings reveal an inconsistent alteration in microbial composition in different cohorts of clinical patients after KD treatment. It is possible that differences in age, host genetics, diet adherence, diet composition, and medication use all contributed to the observed variations in the gut microbiome. Profiling the gut microbiome following KD treatment is only the first step toward understanding how the gut microbiome interacts with the host. Future studies need to investigate how microbial metabolites change with shifts in microbial composition, and whether microbial metabolites affect epilepsy pathogenesis.

The mechanisms through which the gut microbiome regulate the severity of epilepsy require further investigation. Increasingly, though, studies point to the microbiota–gut–brain axis as an important factor in modulating neural activity. A recent study demonstrated that gut microbial changes induced by a KD mediate the diet's anticonvulsant effects by affecting hippocampal γ-aminobutyric acid:glutamate (GABA:glutamate) ratios (Olson et al., 2018). In this study, adult mice fed a KD had a significantly increased seizure threshold induced by a 6-Hz stimulation. Furthermore, the abundance of *A. muciniphila* and *Parabacteroides* in the feces was also increased. In addition, fecal transplantation from KD-fed to control diet-fed mice or treatment of control diet-fed mice with *A. muciniphila* and *Parabacteroides* species increased seizure thresholds. Both the KD and *A. muciniphila/Parabacteroides* supplementation led to a decrease in circulated γ-glutamyl amino acid and an increase in the GABA:glutamate ratio. Interestingly, treatment of control diet-fed mice with a γ-glutamyltranspeptidase inhibitor also increased the seizure threshold, thereby providing a neuroprotective effect. These findings suggest neurotransmitter modulation may be a key mediator linking the gut microbiota and the brain. This study showed that the gut microbiota mediated the anticonvulsant effects of the KD and may be useful in developing a novel therapeutic strategy for seizure treatment (Olson et al., 2018).

Alzheimer's Disease

Alzheimer's disease (AD) is the most common neurodegenerative disorder that results in chronic and progressive dementia (Power et al., 2019). Accumulations of amyloid protein and hyperphosphorylated tau protein are among the key mechanisms thought to be involved in the pathogenesis of the disorder (Power et al., 2019). Evidence suggests that the gut microbiome is also altered in patients with AD. In a cohort of 43 patients with AD and 43 age- and gender-matched cognitively normal controls, the fecal microbiome of patients was enriched with Actinobacteria, Ruminococcaceae, and *Subdoligranulum* but was lacking in Bacteroidetes, specifically *Bacteroides* (Zhuang et al., 2018). Given these alterations, the brain–gut–microbiota axis has been proposed as a contributing factor in the underlying etiology of AD (Kowalski & Mulak, 2019).

The KD has shown promise as an effective treatment for neurodegenerative diseases (Ota et al., 2019; Taylor et al., 2018), which may be mediated by the gut microbiome. A pilot study has revealed that a modified Mediterranean-KD is protective in elders with mild cognitive impairment, a common prodromal symptom of AD (Nagpal et al., 2019). In addition to the behavioral effects, an elevation in Enterobacteriaceae and *Akkermansia* as well as fecal butyrate concentrations, and a decrease in fecal *Bifidobacterium* species, were observed. In subjects with mild cognitive impairment after dietary intervention, the abundance of *Tenericutes* and an unclassified genus within Enterobacteriaceae was positively correlated with Aβ42 protein, while the alpha-diversity indexes (e.g., number of bacteria populations) and Shannon diversity (characterizing both the abundance and evenness of the bacterial species in the gut), were negatively correlated with phosphorylated tau expression (Nagpal et al., 2019). This pilot study provides a strong impetus for possible nutritional interventions in elderly populations with AD.

Although the mechanisms of the therapeutic effects of the KD in neurodegenerative disorders are unknown, there is evidence to suggest that the effects of the diet may be related to improved cerebral blood flow. In adult mice, a KD administered for 16 weeks enhanced neurovascular function by improving cerebral blood flow and P-glycoprotein expression, which improved clearance of amyloid protein (Ma et al., 2018). In addition, the diet increased the relative abundance of *A. muciniphila* and *Lactobacillus*, while it reduced *Desulfovibrio* (Ma et al., 2018). It is noteworthy that, as already discussed, Olson et al. (2018) identified a critical role of *A. muciniphila* in ameliorating epilepsy symptoms. Of future interest would be to investigate how *A. muciniphila* is related to the severity of AD.

OTHER CONDITIONS

Obesity and Related Comorbidities

The gut microbiome has been recognized as a contributing factor in the etiology of obesity. Direct evidence from fecal transplant experiments in germ-free mice show the phenotype can be transferred through the gut microbiome alone (Turnbaugh et al., 2008). Intestinal dysbiosis is often observed in obese individuals and is characterized by an increase in bacteria belonging to Firmicutes, *Clostridium*, *Eubacterium rectale*, *Clostridium coccoides*, *Lactobacillus reuteri*, and *A. muciniphila* (Gomes et al., 2018). Dysbiosis associated with obesity is linked to a reduction in the secretion of satiety hormones and a compromised gut barrier. A compromised gut barrier eases the ability of intestinal bacteria and pathogenic metabolites to pass through the gut, thereby exacerbating the systemic inflammation typically observed in obese individuals and ultimately triggering insulin resistance (Gomes et al., 2018). Additionally, the dysbiosis is also linked with a withdrawal of vagal afferents from the gut and the hindbrain (Sen et al., 2017). Manipulating the gut microbiota to treat obesity is a topic of intense investigation.

The KD is an effective, but often controversial, weight-management therapy (O'Neill & Raggi, 2020). A recent review by Castellana et al. (2019) on the very-low-calorie KD shows that it can be a promising option to achieve significant weight loss. The effectiveness of a KD in weight management may be tightly linked to the gut microbiome. The dynamics of fecal microbiota composition were tracked in an obese 40-year-old man following KD intervention (Durbán et al., 2013). Researchers found a change in microbial abundance within 24 hr of KD treatment. These changes were characterized by a decrease in the abundance of *Prevotella* and an increase in *Bacteroides* and *Sutterella*, as well as an overall increase in microbial diversity (Durbán et al., 2013). Following the supplementation of carbohydrates in the diet, the microbiome returned to its previous composition within 4 weeks (Durbán et al., 2013). Another recent study showed that a very-low-calorie KD (600–800 kcal per day) administered for 2 months in obese adults not only effectively reduced body weight, but also increased microbial diversity and the abundance of Firmicutes (Ruminococcaceae), with a reduction observed in Proteobacteria, such as Enterobacteriaceae (Gutierrez-Repiso et al., 2019). Whether the alterations in the gut microbiota observed in this study were the result of the reduced caloric consumption or the result of the KD is unknown.

In addition to obesity, there also appears to be benefits of the KD in mitigating some obesity-related comorbidities, including nonalcoholic fatty liver disease (Watanabe et al., 2020) and type 2 diabetes (Walsh et al., 2020). While there is no consensus regarding the direction and magnitude of changes in the microbiota with the KD in these comorbidities, there is some evidence that the KD plays a role in reducing the low-grade inflammation associated with these conditions (Bhanpuri et al., 2018).

Cancer

Many risk factors that affect cancer development (i.e., genetics, alcohol, diet, medication, and other environmental exposures) are also potent contributors to host–microbiome interactions. As such, it is not surprising that there is indirect evidence of the gut microbiome's contributing to cancer risk. For example, one such mechanism is the "estrobolome," bacterial genes and functional pathways that metabolize estrogens and modulate estrogen homeostasis (Kwa et al., 2016). β-Glucuronidase enzymes from gut microbes can reactivate estrogens from the inactive form, thus perpetuating estrogen-based carcinogenesis (Ervin et al., 2019; Shapira et al., 2013). Given this, the microbiome and its modulation through the KD in cancer is worthy of consideration.

Many cancers are highly dependent on glycolysis to generate ATP. Therefore, KDs selectively starve tumors in part by limiting glucose as a substrate (Tan-Shalaby, 2017). As such, the KD has been used as an adjuvant therapy for cancer, with positive outcomes observed in cancer subtypes where the prognosis is associated with metabolic status (Chung & Park, 2017). Although comprehensive human studies are lacking, there are some clues from animal work. In a mouse model of glioma, a KD administered for 21 days increased survival rate (McFarland et al., 2017). The mice also demonstrated an increase in the abundance of *Faecalibaculum rodentium* and the percentage

of T helper 17 cells (McFarland et al., 2017). There is further evidence to suggest that a probiotic consisting of *F. rodentium* may serve as an alternative glioma therapy. In a mouse model of intestinal tumors induced by exposure to azoxymethane and dextran sulfate sodium, the relative abundance of *F. rodentium* was greatly reduced during the early period of tumor induction (Zagato et al., 2020). Alternatively, the introduction of *F. rodentium* reduced tumor burden by inhibiting calcineurin, nuclear factor of activated T cells, and cytoplasmic 3 activation in tumor cells (Zagato et al., 2020). In contrast, in FVB/NJ mice that are susceptible to colorectal cancer, following tumor induction by 4 weeks of exposure to azoxymethane, a KD administered for 10 weeks significantly increased the colonic tumor load by threefold (Moore, 2016). A reduction in the relative abundance of *Clostridiales* and *Lactobacillales* and an increase in *Bacteroidales* and *Sphaerochaetales* in feces were also observed in these mice (Moore, 2016). Given these inconsistent findings, caution and further studies are needed to determine the factors that mediate whether a KD leads to positive or negative outcomes in cancer treatment.

The microbiome, and hence the KD, may also have the potential to alter the responsiveness of patients to treatment. Abdelwahab et al. (2012) demonstrated that the KD enhanced the antitumor impact of radiation in a mouse model of malignant glioma. Furthermore, studies in both children and adults suggest that gut microbiome composition predicts chemotherapy and radiation treatment responsiveness (Hakim et al., 2018; Jang et al., 2020; Singh et al., 2020). In summary, there is now general agreement that microbiome modulation via the KD has the potential to influence the susceptibility to, progression of, and treatment of certain forms of cancer.

Multiple Sclerosis

Multiple sclerosis (MS) is an autoimmune disease in which the immune system attacks the myelin sheaths that cover nerve fibers. Eventually, the cumulative damage results in communication deficits between the brain and the rest of the body. Relative to healthy individuals, the quantity and diversity of fecal microbiota are decreased in patients with MS (Berer et al., 2017), indicating that the gut microbiota may be involved in the pathogenesis of the disorder. Preclinical studies have demonstrated a direct link between the gut microbiota and myelin function. Comparison of germ-free and conventional mice show that the former have a higher expression of genes involved in myelination, greater myelin plasticity, and hypermyelinated axons in the prefrontal cortex (Hoban et al., 2016). Further evidence demonstrating a role of the gut microbiome in MS is derived from studies wherein transplantation of feces from patients with MS, characterized by an increase in *A. muciniphila*, to transgenic mice that express inflammatory demyelination, accelerated the incidence of autoimmunity in the mice (Berer et al., 2017).

The KD has been shown to be effective at reducing the symptoms of MS, with associative evidence that the gut microbiome plays a role in its efficacy (Swidsinski et al., 2017). In patients with MS, a 6-month KD intervention decreased *Bacteroides*, *F. prausnitzii*, and *Roseburia* during the early stages of the diet intervention (Swidsinski et al., 2017). At 12 weeks after treatment, the gut microbiota recovered to levels similar to those in healthy individuals, demonstrating a long-lasting effect of a KD in this disorder (Swidsinski et al., 2017). Unfortunately, alteration of clinical

symptoms of MS was not examined in this study. These findings imply that the KD may normalize gut microbial dysbiosis in patients with MS. However, it remains to be directly shown whether gut microbiota altered by the KD can be therapeutically beneficial in MS and the mechanisms involved.

CONCLUSIONS

The gut microbiome has long been recognized as an important regulator of metabolism and the immune system. Nevertheless, the important causal interactions between the gut microbiome and neural function are still under investigation. The available evidence on the effects of the KD on the gut microbiome indicates that there is little consensus in microbial alterations between cohorts when examining similar disease states. This is readily seen in Figure 21.2, which summarizes major changes with the KD in the various disease states discussed in this chapter. Lack of consensus is, in part, due to inherent interindividual variation of the gut microbiome (starting

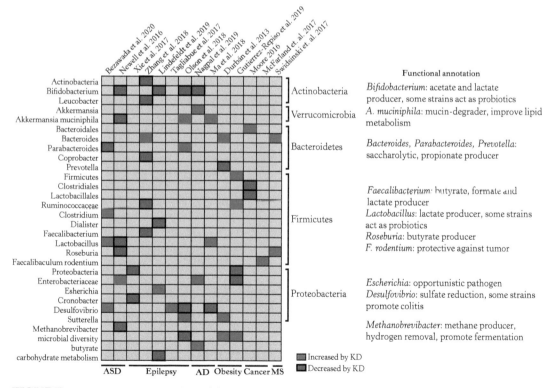

FIGURE 21.2 *Summary of the Effects of the Ketogenic Diet on the Gut Microbiota Composition across Numerous Independent Studies*

There is little agreement with respect to microbial alterations between cohorts examining similar disease states. Abbreviations: AD = Alzheimer's disease; ASD = autism spectrum disorder; MS = multiple sclerosis.

microbiome), individual age, variance in what defines the KD, length of dietary exposure, source of dietary components (e.g., plant- vs. animal-based foods), and timing of assessment (e.g., fed or fasted state), among other factors. It should also be recognized that there are interactions between the gut microbiome, the diet, and the pharmacotherapy common in many of the disease states discussed in this chapter.

Alterations in gut microbial composition are widely observed after the KD, but whether the gut microbiome mediates the therapeutic effects of a KD remains largely unknown. However, the literature summarized here provides strong support for the theory that key microbes and microbial metabolites are likely involved. With a growing body of literature demonstrating the benefits of the KD in disorders like ASD and epilepsy, further investigation into the role of the gut microbiome in mediating these effects is warranted.

REFERENCES

Abdelwahab, M. G., Fenton, K. E., Preul, M. C., Rho, J. M., Lynch, A., Stafford, P., & Scheck, A. C. (2012). The ketogenic diet is an effective adjuvant to radiation therapy for the treatment of malignant glioma. PLOS ONE, 7(5), Article e36197.

Baio, J., Wiggins, L., Christensen, D. L., Maenner, M. J., Daniels, J., Warren, Z., Kurzius-Spencer, M., Zahorodny, W., Rosenberg, C. R., White, T., Durkin, M.S., Imm, P., Nikolaou, L., Yeargin-Allsopp, M., Lee, L.C., Harrington, R., Lopez, M., Fitzgerald, R.T., Hewitt, A., . . . Dowling, N.F. (2018). Prevalence of autism spectrum disorder among children aged 8 years—Autism and Developmental Disabilities Monitoring Network, 11 sites, United States, 2014. MMWR Surveillance Summaries, 67(6), 1-23.

Berer, K., Gerdes, L. A., Cekanaviciute, E., Jia, X., Xiao, L., Xia, Z., Liu, C., Klotz, L., Stauffer, U., Baranzini, S. E., Kumpfel, T., Hohlfeld, R., Krishnamoorthy, G., & Wekerle, H. (2017). Gut microbiota from multiple sclerosis patients enables spontaneous autoimmune encephalomyelitis in mice. Proceedings of the National Academy of Sciences of the United States of America, 114(40), 10719–10724.

Bezawada, N., Phang, T. H., Hold, G. L., & Hansen, R. (2020). Autism spectrum disorder and the gut microbiota in children: A systematic review. Annals of Nutrition & Metabolism, 76(1), 16–29.

Bhanpuri, N. H., Hallberg, S. J., Williams, P. T., McKenzie, A. L., Ballard, K. D., Campbell, W. W., McCarter, J. P., Phinney, S. D., & Volek, J. S. (2018). Cardiovascular disease risk factor responses to a type 2 diabetes care model including nutritional ketosis induced by sustained carbohydrate restriction at 1 year: An open label, non-randomized, controlled study. Cardiovascular Diabetology, 17(1), Article 56.

Carmody, R. N., Gerber, G. K., Luevano, J. M., Jr., Gatti, D. M., Somes, L., Svenson, K. L., & Turnbaugh, P. J. (2015). Diet dominates host genotype in shaping the murine gut microbiota. Cell Host & Microbe, 17(1), 72–84.

Castellana, M., Conte, E., Cignarelli, A., Perrini, S., Giustina, A., Giovanella, L., Giorgino, F., & Trimboli, P. (2019). Efficacy and safety of very low calorie ketogenic diet (VLCKD) in patients with overweight and obesity: A systematic review and meta-analysis. Reviews in Endocrine and Metabolic Disorders, 21(1), 5–16.

Cheng, N., Rho, J. M., & Masino, S. A. (2017). Metabolic dysfunction underlying autism spectrum disorder and potential treatment approaches. Frontiers in Molecular Neuroscience, 10, Article 34.

Cho, I., & Blaser, M. J. (2012). The human microbiome: At the interface of health and disease. Nature Reviews Genetics, 13(4), 260–270.

Chung, H. Y., & Park, Y. K. (2017). Rationale, feasibility and acceptability of ketogenic diet for cancer treatment. Journal of Cancer Prevention, 22(3), 127–134.

Dhamija, R., Eckert, S., & Wirrell, E. (2013). Ketogenic diet. The Canadian Journal of Neurological Sciences, 40(2), 158–167.

Durbán, A., Abellán, J. J., Latorre, A., & Moya, A. (2013). Effect of dietary carbohydrate restriction on an obesity-related Prevotella-dominated human fecal microbiota. Metagenomics, 2, Article 235722.

El Kaoutari, A., Armougom, F., Gordon, J. I., Raoult, D., & Henrissat, B. (2013). The abundance and variety of carbohydrate-active enzymes in the human gut microbiota. Nature Reviews Microbiology, 11(7), 497–504.

Ervin, S. M., Li, H., Lim, L., Roberts, L. R., Liang, X., Mani, S., & Redinbo, M. R. (2019). Gut microbial β-glucuronidases reactivate estrogens as components of the estrobolome that reactivate estrogens. Journal of Biological Chemistry, 294(49), 18586–18599.

Farmer, C., Leon, J., & Hommer, R. (2019). Effective medications for treating individuals with autism spectrum disorder. In Carlson, J. S. & Barterian, J. A. (Eds.), School Psychopharmacology (pp. 83–98). Springer.

Goel, R., Hong, J. S., Findling, R. L., & Ji, N. Y. (2018). An update on pharmacotherapy of autism spectrum disorder in children and adolescents. International Review of Psychiatry, 30(1), 78–95.

Gomes, A. C., Hoffmann, C., & Mota, J. F. (2018). The human gut microbiota: Metabolism and perspective in obesity. Gut Microbes, 9(4), 308–325.

Gutierrez-Repiso, C., Hernandez-Garcia, C., Garcia-Almeida, J. M., Bellido, D., Martin-Nunez, G. M., Sanchez-Alcoholado, L., Alcaide-Torres, J., Sajoux, I., Tinahones, F. J., & Moreno-Indias, I. (2019). Effect of synbiotic supplementation in a very-low-calorie ketogenic diet on weight loss achievement and gut microbiota: A randomized controlled pilot study. *Molecular Nutrition & Food Research, 63*(19), Article e1900167.

Hakim, H., Dallas, R., Wolf, J., Tang, L., Schultz-Cherry, S., Darling, V., Johnson, C., Karlsson, E. A., Chang, T. C., Jeha, S., Pui, C. H., Sun, Y., Pounds, S., Hayden, R. T., Tuomanen, E., & Rosch, J. W. (2018). Gut microbiome composition predicts infection risk during chemotherapy in children with acute lymphoblastic leukemia. *Clinical Infectious Diseases, 67*(4), 541–548.

Hoban, A. E., Stilling, R. M., Ryan, F. J., Shanahan, F., Dinan, T. G., Claesson, M. J., Clarke, G., & Cryan, J. F. (2016). Regulation of prefrontal cortex myelination by the microbiota. *Translational Psychiatry, 6*(4), Article e774.

Jang, B. S., Chang, J. H., Chie, E. K., Kim, K., Park, J. W., Kim, M. J., Song, E. J., Nam, Y. D., Kang, S. W., Jeong, S. Y., & Kim, H. J. (2020). Gut microbiome composition is associated with a pathologic response after preoperative chemoradiation in rectal cancer patients. *International Journal of Radiation Oncology – Biology – Physics, 107*(4), 736–746.

Klein, M. S., Newell, C., Bomhof, M. R., Reimer, R. A., Hittel, D. S., Rho, J. M., Vogel, H. J., & Shearer, J. (2016). Metabolomic modeling to monitor host responsiveness to gut microbiota manipulation in the BTBR(T+tf/j) mouse. *Journal of Proteome Research, 15*(4), 1143–1150.

Kowalski, K., & Mulak, A. (2019). Brain-gut-microbiota axis in Alzheimer's disease. *Journal of Neurogastroenterology Motility, 25*(1), 48–60.

Kraeuter, A. K., Phillips, R., & Sarnyai, Z. (2020). Ketogenic therapy in neurodegenerative and psychiatric disorders: From mice to men. *Progress in Neuro-Psychopharmacology & Biological Psychiatry, 101*, Article 109913.

Kwa, M., Plottel, C. S., Blaser, M. J., & Adams, S. (2016). The intestinal microbiome and estrogen receptor–positive female breast cancer. *Journal of the National Cancer Institute, 108*(8), Article djw029.

Lee, P. R., & Kossoff, E. H. (2011). Dietary treatments for epilepsy: Management guidelines for the general practitioner. *Epilepsy & Behavior, 21*(2), 115–121.

Lee, R. W. Y., Corley, M. J., Pang, A., Arakaki, G., Abbott, L., Nishimoto, M., Miyamoto, R., Lee, E., Yamamoto, S., Maunakea, A. K., Lum-Jones, A., & Wong, M. (2018). A modified ketogenic gluten-free diet with MCT improves behavior in children

with autism spectrum disorder. *Physiology & Behavior, 188*, 205–211.

Li, D., Wang, P., Wang, P., Hu, X., & Chen, F. (2019). Targeting the gut microbiota by dietary nutrients: A new avenue for human health. *Critical Reviews in Food Science and Nutrition, 59*(2), 181–195.

Lindefeldt, M., Eng, A., Darban, H., Bjerkner, A., Zetterstrom, C. K., Allander, T., Andersson, B., Borenstein, E., Dahlin, M., & Prast-Nielsen, S. (2019). The ketogenic diet influences taxonomic and functional composition of the gut microbiota in children with severe epilepsy. *NPJ Biofilms and Microbiomes, 5*(1), Article 5.

Ma, D., Wang, A. C., Parikh, I., Green, S. J., Hoffman, J. D., Chlipala, G., Murphy, M. P., Sokola, B. S., Bauer, B., Hartz, A. M. S., & Lin, A. L. (2018). Ketogenic diet enhances neurovascular function with altered gut microbiome in young healthy mice. *Scientific Reports, 8*(1), Article 6670.

McFarland, B., Dees, K., Melo, N., Fehling, S., Gibson, S., Yan, Z., Kumar, R., Morrow, C., & Benveniste, E. (2017). EXTH-30. Therapeutic benefit of a ketogenic diet through altered gut microbiota in a mouse model of glioma. *Neuro-oncology, 19*(Suppl 6), vi78.

Mohajeri, M. H., La Fata, G., Steinert, R. E., & Weber, P. (2018). Relationship between the gut microbiome and brain function. *Nutrition Reviews, 76*(7), 481–496.

Moore, L. A. (2016). *Effect of diet and genetic background on the gut microbiome and colorectal cancer in mice.* Texas A&M University. Undergraduate Research Scholars Program. Available electronically from https://hdl.handle.net/1969.1/157664.

Mu, C., Corley, M. J., Lee, R. W. Y., Wong, M., Pang, A., Arakaki, G., Miyamoto, R., Rho, J. M., Mickiewicz, B., Dowlatabadi, R., Vogel, H. J., Korchemagin, Y., & Shearer, J. (2020). Metabolic framework for the improvement of autism spectrum disorders by a modified ketogenic diet: A pilot study. *Journal of Proteome Research, 19*(1), 382–390.

Mu, C., Yang, Y., Luo, Z., & Zhu, W. (2017). Temporal microbiota changes of high-protein diet intake in a rat model. *Anaerobe, 47*, 218–225.

Mu, C., Yang, Y., & Zhu, W. (2016). Gut microbiota: The brain peacekeeper. *Frontiers in Microbiology, 7*, Article 345.

Nagpal, R., Neth, B. J., Wang, S., Craft, S., & Yadav, H. (2019). Modified Mediterranean-ketogenic diet modulates gut microbiome and short-chain fatty acids in association with Alzheimer's disease markers in subjects with mild cognitive impairment. *EBioMedicine, 47*, 529–542.

Newell, C., Bomhof, M. R., Reimer, R. A., Hittel, D. S., Rho, J. M., & Shearer, J. (2016). Ketogenic diet modifies the gut microbiota in a murine model of autism spectrum disorder. *Molecular Autism*, 7(1), Article 37.

Olson, C. A., Vuong, H. E., Yano, J. M., Liang, Q. Y., Nusbaum, D. J., & Hsiao, E. Y. (2018). The gut microbiota mediates the anti-seizure effects of the ketogenic diet. *Cell*, 173(7), 1728–1741.

O'Neill, B., & Raggi, P. (2020). The ketogenic diet: Pros and cons. *Atherosclerosis*, 292, 119–126.

Ota, M., Matsuo, J., Ishida, I., Takano, H., Yokoi, Y., Hori, H., Yoshida, S., Ashida, K., Nakamura, K., Takahashi, T., & Kunugi, H. (2019). Effects of a medium-chain triglyceride-based ketogenic formula on cognitive function in patients with mild-to-moderate Alzheimer's disease. *Neuroscience Letters*, 690, 232–236.

Power, R., Prado-Cabrero, A., Mulcahy, R., Howard, A., & Nolan, J. M. (2019). The role of nutrition for the aging population: Implications for cognition and Alzheimer's disease. *Annual Review of Food Science Technology*, 10, 619–639.

Rho, J. M. (2017). How does the ketogenic diet induce anti-seizure effects? *Neuroscience Letters*, 637, 4–10.

Ruskin, D. N., Svedova, J., Cote, J. L., Sandau, U., Rho, J. M., Kawamura, M., Jr., Boison, D., & Masino, S. A. (2013). Ketogenic diet improves core symptoms of autism in BTBR mice. *PLOS ONE*, 8(6), Article e65021.

Sen, T., Cawthon, C. R., Ihde, B. T., Hajnal, A., DiLorenzo, P. M., Claire, B., & Czaja, K. (2017). Diet-driven microbiota dysbiosis is associated with vagal remodeling and obesity. *Physiology & Behavior*, 173, 305–317.

Shapira, I., Sultan, K., Lee, A., & Taioli, E. (2013). Evolving concepts: How diet and the intestinal microbiome act as modulators of breast malignancy. *ISRN Oncology*, 2013, Article 693920.

Sharon, G., Cruz, N. J., Kang, D. W., Gandal, M. J., Wang, B., Kim, Y. M., Zink, E. M., Casey, C. P., Taylor, B. C., Lane, C. J., Bramer, L. M., Isern, N. G., Hoyt, D. W., Noecker, C., Sweredoski, M. J., Moradian, A., Borenstein, E., Jansson, J. K., Knight, R., . . . Mazmanian, S. K. (2019). Human gut microbiota from autism spectrum disorder promote behavioral symptoms in mice. *Cell*, 177(6), 1600–1618.

Singh, A., Nayak, N., Rathi, P., Verma, D., Sharma, R., Chaudhary, A., Agarwal, A., Tripathi, Y. B., & Garg, N. (2020). Microbiome and host crosstalk: A new paradigm to cancer therapy. *Seminars in Cancer Biology*, 70, 71–84.

Subramaniam, S., & Fletcher, C. (2018). Trimethylamine N-oxide: Breathe new life. *British Journal of Pharmacology*, 175(8), 1344–1353.

Swidsinski, A., Dorffel, Y., Loening-Baucke, V., Gille, C., Goktas, O., Reisshauer, A., Neuhaus, J., Weylandt, K. H., Guschin, A., & Bock, M. (2017). Reduced mass and diversity of the colonic microbiome in patients with multiple sclerosis and their improvement with ketogenic diet. *Frontiers in Microbiology*, 8, Article 1141.

Tagliabue, A., Ferraris, C., Uggeri, F., Trentani, C., Bertoli, S., de Giorgis, V., Veggiotti, P., & Elli, M. (2017). Short-term impact of a classical ketogenic diet on gut microbiota in GLUT1 deficiency syndrome: A 3-month prospective observational study. *Clinical Nutrition ESPEN*, 17, 33–37.

Tan-Shalaby, J. (2017). Ketogenic diets and cancer: Emerging evidence. *Federal Practitioner*, 34(Suppl 1), 37S–42S.

Taylor, M. K., Sullivan, D. K., Mahnken, J. D., Burns, J. M., & Swerdlow, R. H. (2018). Feasibility and efficacy data from a ketogenic diet intervention in Alzheimer's disease. *Alzheimer's & Dementia*, 4, 28–36.

Tierney, B. T., Yang, Z., Luber, J. M., Beaudin, M., Wibowo, M. C., Baek, C., Mehlenbacher, E., Patel, C. J., & Kostic, A. D. (2019). The landscape of genetic content in the gut and oral human microbiome. *Cell Host & Microbe*, 26(2), 283–295.

Tramontano, M., Andrejev, S., Pruteanu, M., Klunemann, M., Kuhn, M., Galardini, M., Jouhten, P., Zelezniak, A., Zeller, G., Bork, P., Typas, A., & Patil, K. R. (2018). Nutritional preferences of human gut bacteria reveal their metabolic idiosyncrasies. *Nature Microbiology*, 3(4), 514–522.

Turnbaugh, P. J., Baeckhed, F., Fulton, L., & Gordon, J. I. (2008). Diet-induced obesity is linked to marked but reversible alterations in the mouse distal gut microbiome. *Cell Host & Microbe*, 3(4), 213–223.

Walsh, J. J., Myette-Cote, E., Neudorf, H., & Little, J. P. (2020). Potential therapeutic effects of exogenous ketone supplementation for type 2 diabetes: A review. *Current Pharmaceutical Design*, 26(9), 958–969.

Watanabe, M., Tozzi, R., Risi, R., Tuccinardi, D., Mariani, S., Basciani, S., Spera, G., Lubrano, C., & Gnessi, L. (2020). Beneficial effects of the ketogenic diet on nonalcoholic fatty liver disease: A comprehensive review of the literature. *Obesity Reviews*, 21(8), Article e13024.

Wu, G. D., Chen, J., Hoffmann, C., Bittinger, K., Chen, Y. Y., Keilbaugh, S. A., Bewtra, M., Knights, D., Walters, W. A., Knight, R., Sinha, R., Gilroy, E., Gupta, K., Baldassano, R., Nessel, L., Li, H., Bushman, F. D., & Lewis, J. D. (2011). Linking long-term dietary patterns with gut microbial enterotypes. *Science*, 334(6052), 105–108.

Xie, G., Zhou, Q., Qiu, C. Z., Dai, W. K., Wang, H. P., Li, Y. H., Liao, J. X., Lu, X. G., Lin, S. F., Ye, J. H., Ma, Z. Y., & Wang, W. J. (2017). Ketogenic diet poses a significant effect on imbalanced gut microbiota in infants with refractory epilepsy. *World Journal of Gastroenterology*, 23(33), 6164–6171.

Zagato, E., Pozzi, C., Bertocchi, A., Schioppa, T., Saccheri, F., Guglietta, S., Fosso, B., Melocchi, L., Nizzoli, G., Troisi, J., Marzano, M., Oresta, B., Spadoni, I., Atarashi, K., Carloni, S., Arioli, S., Fornasa, G., Asnicar, F., Segata, N., . . . Rescigno, M. (2020). Endogenous murine microbiota member *Faecalibaculum rodentium* and its human homologue protect from intestinal tumour growth. *Nature Microbiology, 5*(3), 511–524.

Zhang, Y., Zhou, S., Zhou, Y., Yu, L., Zhang, L., & Wang, Y. (2018). Altered gut microbiome composition in children with refractory epilepsy after ketogenic diet. *Epilepsy Research, 145,* 163–168.

Zhuang, Z.Q., Shen, L.L., Li, W.W., Fu, X., Zeng, F., Gui, L., Lü, Y., Cai, M., Zhu, C., Tan, Y.L., Zheng, P., Li, H. Y., Zhu, J., Zhou, H. D., Bu, X. L., & Wang Y. J. (2018). Gut microbiota is altered in patients with Alzheimer's disease. *Journal of Alzheimers Disease, 63*(4), 1337–1346.

Zmora, N., Suez, J., & Elinav, E. (2019). You are what you eat: Diet, health and the gut microbiota. *Nature Reviews Gastroenterology & Hepatology, 16*(1), 35–56.

SECTION III

Ketogenic Diet in the Laboratory

Overview: Ketogenic Diet in the Laboratory

Progress on Models and Mechanisms

DETLEV BOISON, PHD

Clinical and public interests in the ketogenic diet (KD) and metabolic treatments continue to spur research into mechanisms underlying their anticonvulsant, neuroprotective, and antiepileptogenic efficacy. Opportunities beyond seizure control are being explored and discovered in basic, translational, and clinical research paradigms. This section features known and new molecular targets and clinical applications.

The range of specific mechanisms includes transcription factors, enzymes, energy molecules, ion channels, and more. Clinical opportunities discussed in this section include neurodegenerative disease, seizure disorders, and psychiatric disorders, as well as pan-disease benefits, such as reduced inflammation and even increased longevity. Many of these benefits are likely due to a combination of acute and long-lasting effects of metabolic therapy.

As one example, the nutritionally regulated nuclear transcription factor peroxisome proliferator-activated receptor gamma (PPARγ) is a target molecule with neuroprotective and anti-seizure properties that regulates pathways mobilized by the KD. PPARγ is expressed in many neurons, and in Chapter 23 Simeone shows that pharmacologic or genetic inactivation of PPARγ blocks the anticonvulsant effect of KD feeding. PPARγ has been identified as a therapeutic target in neurodegenerative diseases.

Neuroprotection and seizure protection are also well-known properties of adenosine, a purine nucleoside that links cell energy metabolism and neuronal activity, and which is increased by a ketogenic diet. In Chapter 24, Kawamura highlights a number of paradigms used to explore the relationship between the KD and adenosine, including in vitro models and in vivo feeding protocols. Adenosine receptors are linked to K$^+$ channels, including K$_{ATP}$ channels, a mechanism

for decreasing neuronal excitability that has been implicated in multiple research paradigms examining mechanisms underlying KD and metabolic therapy.

Beyond ion channels, adenosine has been linked to epigenetic and antiepileptogenic properties of the KD. In Chapter 25, Murugan, Tescarollo, and Boison describe the relationship between epigenetic changes and the pathologies associated with epilepsy. They review the augmentation of the neuromodulator adenosine by KD and the ability of adenosine-based mechanisms to restore homeostasis. These actions of adenosine mobilized by the KD include antiepileptogenic effects through decreased DNA methylation.

Moving beyond seizures, ketosis in aged rats has been shown to have neuroprotective properties and to reduce neurodegeneration. Recovery from stroke and other pathophysiologic conditions in the aged is challenging, and in Chapter 26, Xu, Sethuraman, LaManna, and Puchowicz focus on investigating the mechanistic links to reduced inflammation and neuroprotection via ketosis in the aged. One target mechanism involves succinate-induced stabilization of hypoxic inducible factor-1α (HIF-1α). Ketone bodies play a role in the restoration of energy balance and act as signaling molecules though the upregulation of anti-inflammatory and pro-survival pathways targeted by HIF-1α.

Enhanced K$_{ATP}$ channel activity prevents neuronal action potentials and is a powerful mechanism for "metabolic seizure resistance." In Chapter 27, Martínez-François, Danial, and Yellen outline metabolic changes in brain cells mediated by the protein BAD (BCL-2-associated agonist of cell death). Abolishing BAD's role in metabolism reduces the capacity of cells to utilize glucose and increases the capacity to use ketone bodies. Blocking BAD also reduces seizure-like activity, and this seizure protection is mediated by K_{ATP} channels.

Sada and Inoue review the functions of the astrocyte/neuron lactate shuttle and their work in brain slices showing that lactate reverses ketone body-induced inhibition. A major breakthrough is that inhibition of lactate dehydrogenase, a metabolic enzyme in the lactate shuttle, can reduce seizures. Furthermore, new research has revealed that lactate dehydrogenase inhibition is one of the mechanisms targeted by an existing antiseizure drug, stiripentol. Stiripentol can be used to treat Dravet syndrome, a seizure disorder that can also often be treated effectively with a KD. This has been an interesting case of finding a metabolic mechanism unexpectedly in an approved antiseizure drug.

The neurovascular system is implicated in metabolic therapy several ways. In Chapter 29, Janigro describes how prolonged exposure of the endothelial cells of the blood–brain barrier to ketones induces expression of monocarboxylate transporters and enhances the brain uptake rate of ketones. In addition, cell migration and expression of gap junction proteins are upregulated by ketones. Altogether, these reports suggest that the beneficial effects of the KD may depend on increased brain uptake of ketones to match metabolic demand and repair of a disrupted blood–brain barrier. Therefore, it may be possible to develop alternative strategies to optimize the KD's therapeutic benefits in brain disorders where the blood–brain barrier is compromised.

Metabolic and redox alterations by the KD are outlined by Johnson and Patel, and these changes appear to work in concert to provide their therapeutic benefits. Many of the downstream alterations in metabolic signaling pathways and redox status are associated with the antiseizure effects of the KD. Some mechanisms include activation of the NF E2-related factor 2 (Nrf2) and Forkhead Box (FOXO) pathways. Additional research has identified tryptophan metabolism, nicotinamide adenine dinucleotide (NAD) regulation, and uncoupling protein upregulation.

Finally, in Chapter 31, Elamin, Ruskin, Masino, and Sacchetti propose NAD as a potential unifying mechanism and highlight some of the evidence linking an altered NAD^+:NADH ratio with reduced seizures and with a range of short- and long-term changes associated with the beneficial effects of a KD. Feeding rats a KD produced an early (within 2 days) and persistent elevation of hippocampal NAD^+, a marker of cellular health and a substrate for enzymes implicated in longevity and DNA damage repair. An increase in NAD^+:NADH is consistent with multiple lines of evidence and hypotheses and may be a common mechanism underlying the beneficial effects of KD therapy.

23

Ketogenic Diet and PPARγ

TIMOTHY A. SIMEONE, PHD

INTRODUCTION

Historical Overview of the Ketogenic Diet and PPARs

A switch from diet of low-fat and high-carbo-hydrate/protein consumption to a high-fat, low-carbohydrate, low-protein ketogenic diet (KD) necessitates an adjustment in the metabolic machinery to handle new primary fuel sources. As detailed elsewhere in this volume, the three prominent biochemical consequences of the KD are decreased glucose, increased free fatty acids, and increased ketone bodies (i.e., β-hydroxy-butyrate, acetoacetate, and acetone). The lower glucose and higher free fatty acids, of course, directly result from the formulation of the diet. The ketone bodies are a partial breakdown product from using fatty acids for fuel in a low-glucose environment, and they can be used as an efficient, deliverable fuel source. Ketone bodies skip glycol-ysis and enter the tricarboxylic acid cycle at the level of acetyl-CoA.

For fatty acids to be used for fuel and for ketogenesis to occur, a series of enzymes and proteins must be present and have increased expression. These include, but are not limited to, β-oxidation enzymes, such as long-chain acetyl-CoA synthetase 1 (ACS1), carnitine palmitoyl-transferase (CPT), which commits palmitate to mitochondrial entry, and the ketogenic enzyme mitochondrial 3-hydroxy-3-methylglutaryl-CoA synthase (HMGCS2). For animals that are on a KD, ketogenesis mainly occurs in the periphery in hepatocytes of the liver, but there is evidence that astrocytes are capable of local β-oxidation and ketogenesis (Auestad et al., 1991; Cullingford et al., 2002a, 2002b; Guzmán & Blázquez, 2004; Takahashi et al., 2014).

These findings have two immediate implica-tions. One is that dramatic dietary changes in fuel sources somehow coordinate the expression of large numbers of genes. The second implication is

that there are nutrient sensors that regulate the shift in gene expression. In hepatocytes, fatty acids are endogenous ligands for peroxisome proliferator-activated receptor α (PPARα), a nuclear receptor transcription factor that regulates genes involved in β-oxidation and ketogenesis. Logically, it has been hypothesized that the KD engages PPARα in the brain, providing increased ability to use fatty acids to produce ATP and ketone bodies, which may be critically important for KD-mediated neuroprotective and antiseizure effects. Indeed, PPARα agonists exert antiseizure effects in acute seizure models (Gavzan et al., 2018; Porta et al., 2009; Puligheddu et al., 2013). However, the KD also exhibits anti-inflammatory and antioxidant properties and promotes mitochondrial health, mechanisms with growing empirical support for their importance in controlling seizures in refrac-tory epilepsy. An alternative nutrient-sensing transcription factor that regulates genes in these pathways, as well as genes involved in β-oxidation and ketogenesis, is PPARγ. Remarkably, PPARγ, like the KD, is under intense investigation for therapeutic potential in Alzheimer's disease, Parkinson's disease, Huntington's disease, amyo-trophic lateral sclerosis, multiple sclerosis, stroke, and cancer (reviewed in Bhattamisra et al., 2020; Carta & Simuni, 2015; Collino et al., 2008; Corona & Duchen, 2015; Dineley et al., 2014; Heneke & Landreth, 2007; Johri et al., 2014; Lilamand et al., 2020; Mandrekar-Colucci & Landreth, 2011; Shen et al., 2015). This chapter reviews PPARγ function and its modulation and the evidence for PPARγ involvement in the KD mechanism of action.

What Are PPARs?

PPARs are ligand-inducible transcription factors that belong to the superfamily of nuclear recep-tors (NRs), which is comprised of 48 transcription factors, including receptors for endogenous ste-roid hormones, thyroid hormone, lipophilic vita-mins, and cholesterol metabolites (Burris et al.,

2013). Functional diversity among the 48 NRs is provided by distinct preferences for both ligands and DNA sequences recognized as response elements within the genome. In most cases, the NRs function as dimers, either homodimers or heterodimers, and bind response elements in the absence and presence of ligand. NR binding in the absence of ligand may have passive or active (i.e., constitutive basal transcription or silencing) consequences on target gene regulation (Burris et al., 2013). As a group, NRs are a significant and important therapeutic target for human disease, which is illustrated by the fact that 10% to 15% of Food and Drug Administration-approved drugs target NRs (Overington et al., 2006).

There are three different PPAR isoforms, PPARα (also known as NR1C1), PPARβ (also known as PPARδ and NR1C2), and PPARγ (also known as NR1C3), which are encoded by genes located on human chromosomes 22, 6, and 3, respectively (Collino et al., 2008). PPARs are involved in several aspects of development, such as differentiation of adipose tissue, brain, placenta, and skin, and the three isoforms display unique tissue- and time-dependent expression patterns during development in cell types having ectodermal, mesodermal, and endodermal embryonic origins (Desvergne & Wahli, 1999). Postnatally, the three isoforms exhibit tissue-specific expression. PPARα is highly expressed in tissues that catabolize fatty acids (e.g., hepatocytes, cardiomyocytes, enterocytes, and kidney proximal tubule cells). PPARβ is expressed ubiquitously in all cell types, with higher levels in proliferating and differentiating cells. PPARγ is strongly expressed in adipose tissue and the immune system. All PPARs have roles in lipid and glucose metabolism and homeostasis, inflammation, cell proliferation and differentiation, and vascular biology (Braissant et al., 1996; Tontonoz & Spiegelman, 2008); however, their role in actual peroxisome proliferation is species-dependent, and it remains unclear whether PPARs are involved in this function in humans (Schrader et al., 2015).

Members of the NR superfamily contain four domains (Figure 23.1a). The N-terminal transactivation domain (activation function-1, AF-1) is involved in ligand-independent transactivation and in interaction with transcriptional coactivators and influences the ligand-binding affinity of the ligand-binding domain (LBD). The AF-1 sequence has minimal homology among PPAR isoforms, which underlies the differential biological functions of the isoforms. The DNA-binding domain (DBD) contains two highly conserved zinc fingers. There is a hinge region between the DBD and the C-terminal LBD, which is required for receptor dimerization. The LBD contains the ligand-dependent transactivation domain AF-2 and is less homologous among the isoforms, resulting in isoform specificity and sensitivity to ligands (Harmon et al., 2011; Kersten & Wahli, 2000). In the nucleus, PPARs form obligate heterodimers with retinoid X receptors (RXR).

Of the three isoforms, PPARγ is the most extensively studied. Two PPARγ isoforms, PPARγ1 and PPARγ2, result from alternative splicing and differential promoter use (Tontonoz et al., 1994). The PPARγ isoforms are identical except that PPARγ2 contains an additional 28 amino acids at its N terminus. This additional region conveys 5- to 10-fold more effective ligand-independent transactivation and increased ligand-binding affinity of the LBD to PPARγ2 relative to PPARγ1 (Bugge et al., 2009; Castillo et al., 1999; Shao et al., 1998; Werman et al., 1997). Expression of PPARγ1 appears to be ubiquitous. In contrast, PPARγ2 is restricted to adipose tissue; however, high-fat diets can induce the expression of PPARγ2 (Vidal-Puig et al., 1996, 1997).

PPARγ activation is initiated by ligand binding. The PPARγ ligand-binding pocket is large (130 nm^3), which allows structural promiscuity for a wide variety of endogenous or natural agonists (i.e., unsaturated fatty acids, eicosanoids, oxidized lipids, nitroalkenes), synthetic agonists (e.g., thiazolidinediones [TZDs]), and synthetic antagonists (currently there are no known endogenous antagonists; Fong et al., 2010; Itoh et al., 2008; Kroker & Bruning, 2015; Sauer, 2015; see Table 23.1). PPARγ's large LBD makes it an effective sensor and transducer of environmental nutritional and inflammatory states.

Ligand binding induces a conformational change in the receptor, leading to dissociation of corepressors, such as NCOR1 (nuclear receptor corepressor 1) and SMRT (silencing mediator of retinoic acid and thyroid hormone receptor), which normally keep basal levels of PPAR-mediated transcription low. Without corepressor complexes, the PPARγ-RXR heterodimer is free to bind specific recognition sequences called PPAR-response elements (PPREs) in the promoter regions of target genes. Once corepressors disengage, coactivators are recruited, and they alter chromatin structure and recruit transcriptional machinery to promote the commencement of transcription (Figure 23.1b). Coactivators of PPARγ include CREB-binding protein (CBP),

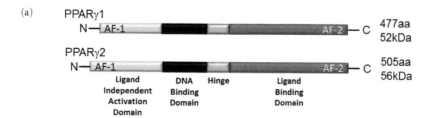

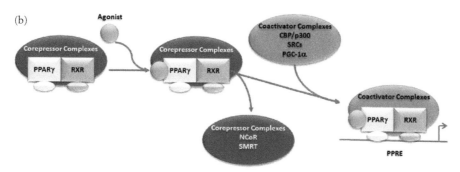

FIGURE 23.1 *PPARγ Splice Variants and Activity*

(a) PPARγ has two splice variants that have identical primary sequences except that the N terminal of PPARγ2 has an extension of 28 amino acids. PPARγ1 and PPARγ2 have an activation function-1 domain (AF-1) required for ligand-independent activation, a DNA-binding domain required for sequence-specific binding to genomic DNA at a peroxisome proliferator response element (PPRE), a hinge domain required for receptor dimerization, a ligand-binding domain required for ligand-dependent modulation, and an activation function-2 domain (AF-2) within the ligand-binding domain that is required for ligand-dependent activation, ligand-dependent dimerization, coactivator recruitment, and corepressor release. The extra 28 amino acids in the AF-1 of PPARγ2 confer 5- to 10-fold more ligand-independent activation and greater ligand-binding affinity than those of PPARγ1. (b) PPARγ forms a heterodimer with the retinoid X receptor (RXR), and in the absence of agonist, it is bound to corepressor complexes (e.g., NCOR1 and SMRT). Once an agonist is bound, the corepressors are released, PPARγ-RXR recruits coactivators (e.g., CBP/p300, SRCs, and PGC-1α), and the complex binds to PPREs in the promoter region of target genes, leading to initiation of transcription by RNA polymerase II and general transcription factors.

TABLE 23.1 PPARΓ AGONISTS

Type of Agonist	Agonist Class	Examples
Natural or Endogenous		
	Unsaturated fatty acids	DHA, EPA, linoleic acid, arachidonic acid, etc.
	Eicosanoids	15d-PGJ$_2$, 15d-PGD$_2$, PGA$_1$, etc.
	Oxidized lipids	9-HODE, 13-HODE, 4-HDHA, 5-5-HEPA, 4-oxoDHA, 6-oxoOTE, lysophosphatidic acid, etc.
	Nitroalkenes	LNO$_2$, OA-NO$_2$, etc.
Synthetic		
	Thiazolidinediones	Pioglitazone, rosiglitazone, etc.
	Non-thiazolidinediones	GW-347845, NSAIDs, indenones, etc.
	Dual alpha/gamma agonists	Muraglitazar, tesaglitazar, resveratrol
	Pan alpha/beta/gamma agonists	Benzafibrate, GW-677954, etc.
	Selective PPARγ modulators (SPPARMs or partial agonists)	Telmisartan, halofenate, MRL-24, SR1664, etc.

Note. DHA = Docosahexaenoic acid, EPA = Eicosapentaenoic acid, 15d-PGJ$_2$ = 15-Deoxy-Delta-12,14-prostaglandin J2, 15d-PGD$_2$ = 15-Deoxy-Delta-12,14-prostaglandin D2, PGA$_1$ = Prostaglandin A1, 9-HODE = 9-Hydroxyoctadecadienoic acid, 13-HODE = 13-Hydroxyoctadecadienoic acid, 4-HDHA = 4-hydroxy Docosahexaenoic, 5-HEPA = 5-hydroxy Eicosapentaenoic acid, 4-oxoDHA = 4-oxo Docosahexaenoic acid, 6-oxoOTE = 6-oxooctadecatrienoic acid, LNO$_2$ = Nitrolinoleate, OA-NO$_2$ = Nitro-oleic acid, NSAIDs = Nonsteroidal anti-inflammatory drugs.

Date from Fong et al. (2010), Itoh et al. (2008), Kroker and Bruning (2015), and Suer et al. (2015).

SRC1/2/3 (steroid receptor coactivator), and PPARγ coactivator 1α (PGC-1α; Auwerx, 1999; Katsouri et al., 2012; Kroker & Bruning, 2015). The PPARγ-RXR-corepressor or coactivator complexes are further regulated by several posttranslational modifications, such as phosphorylation, acetylation, SUMOylation, and ubiquitination, which can increase or decrease PPARγ transcriptional activity (Ahmadian et al., 2013).

PPARγ controls hundreds of genes, many of which are involved in lipid and glucose metabolism and homeostasis, insulin sensitization, fluid homeostasis, anti-inflammation, antioxidant effects, and mitochondrial health. Its most well-known role is as a master regulator of adipogenesis, where it coordinates gene expression necessary for adipocyte formation (Ahmadian et al., 2013; Auwerx, 1999; Fong et al., 2010; Krocker & Bruning, 2015). The insulin-sensitizing effects of TZDs, such as pioglitazone and rosiglitazone, are clinically useful in the treatment of metabolic disorders like type 2 diabetes mellitus. However, these full agonists can lead to weight gain, fluid retention, and bone loss due to PPARγ activation in a wide range of tissues (Ahmadian et al., 2013). Several strategies to reduce TZD side effects are under investigation, ranging from partial agonism to tissue-specific activation (Sujii & Evans, 2011).

Many of the PPARγ-regulated genes overlap with KD-responsive genes. However, determining the genes that PPARγ regulates at any one time is not straightforward. An additional level of complexity is that the gene sets regulated by PPARγ depend on tissue-dependent differential expression of types of corepressors and coactivators, the state of biochemical cascades that regulate posttranslational modifications, and the nature of the bound agonist (full or partial), which determines the degree of conformational change and the ability of PPARγ to interact with particular corepressors and coactivators (Ahmadian et al., 2013; Krocker & Bruning, 2015; Sauer, 2015). For example, the full agonist TZDs exert beneficial insulin-sensitizing effects as well as detrimental side effects, such as weight gain, whereas several partial agonists or so-called selective PPARγ modulators (SPPARMs) have been shown to retain antidiabetic effects while eliminating weight gain via attenuated and selective gene-regulatory activity in comparison to full agonists (Carmona et al, 2007; Tan et al., 2012). Additionally, phosphorylation of Ser273 in the LBD of PPARγ dysregulates a group of distinct genes, resulting in insulin insensitivity. TZDs prevent Ser273 phosphorylation, but their effectiveness in producing insulin sensitization in humans has been found to be inversely related to the degree of PPARγ phosphorylation (Choi et al., 2010). This implies that PPARγ activation may differentially regulate gene sets based on the state of the tissue (e.g., normal brain versus oxidatively stressed and inflamed epileptic brain). This is an intriguing prospect that warrants further investigation.

PPARγ IN THE BRAIN

Where Is PPARγ in the Brain?

PPARγ is regionally distinct, with high expression in neurons, astrocytes, and microglia in the cortex and moderate expression in neurons in the hippocampus (Cullingford et al., 1998; Lu et al., 2011; Moreno et al., 2004; Sarruf et al., 2009; Zhao et al., 2009). Moreno et al. (2004) have performed the most extensive study to date, cataloging the expression patterns throughout the brain of not only PPARγ, but also PPARα, PPARβ, and the three RXR isoforms. PPARγ has the most restrictive distribution in the CNS. For example, PPARγ is absent from neurons in the olfactory bulb, the perirhinal and entorhinal cortices, the temporal and occipital neocortices, the thalamic reticular nucleus, the ventral tegmental area, and cerebellar Purkinjie cells. It is highly expressed in neurons of the basal ganglia, thalamic rhomboid, centromedial, and parafascicular nuclei, nuclei of the reticular formation and cerebellar stellate, and basket and Golgi cells. PPARγ has moderate to weak expression in neurons of the hypothalamic nuclei, septohippocampal nucleus, and the hippocampal formation. Oligodendrocytes do not express PPARγ, but it is expressed in some astrocytes (Moreno et al., 2004). These descriptions are in broad agreement with findings in studies using neuron-specific PPARγ knockout mice (Lu et al., 2011; Sarruf et al., 2009). Sarruf et al. (2009) confirmed moderate expression in the hypothalamus but found expression in the ventral tegmental area, in contrast to the previous study. They also reported that neuronal loss of PPARγ resulted in 90% reduction of PPARγ mRNA in brain, indicating that most PPARγ in the brain is expressed in neurons (Sarruf et al., 2009). A subsequent study found that in normal mice, PPARγ mRNA was greatest in cortex, followed by cerebellum, hippocampus, diencephalon, and hypothalamus (Lu et al., 2011). Knockout of PPARγ from neurons reduced mRNA in all CNS regions except cerebellum. The reduction was greatest in the hippocampus and least in cortex (Lu et al., 2011). If the residual mRNA is from expression in glia, then we can infer that hippocampal glia express minimal levels of PPARγ.

Only one study has attempted to discern differential expression of the two PPARγ isoforms in the hippocampal CA1 region of mice (Gahring et al., 2005). The PPARγ antibody, which recognizes both isoforms, stained essentially all cells of the CA1 pyramidal layer and some associated cells, including presumed astrocytes. However, using an antibody that recognized an epitope within the extra 28 N-terminal amino acids of PPARγ2, it was found that only a small subset of neurons associated with the pyramidal cell layer were stained, suggesting that PPARγ1 is the primary isoform in the hippocampus. The PPARγ2-positive cells lacked astrocytic morphology, but they did co-label with nicotinic acetylcholine receptors' alpha4 and beta4 subunits; thus, the authors concluded that PPARγ2 was exclusively expressed in putative interneurons (Gahring et al., 2005). This intriguing finding warrants confirmation and expansion to other brain regions.

What Is the Function of PPARγ in the Brain?

The role of PPARγ in the brain during normal conditions remains largely unknown, but it most likely involves minimal activity in order to maintain lipid and glucose homeostasis. PPARγ may also have a role in neuronal development and neurogenesis. PPARγ is highly expressed in mouse embryonic brain and neural stem cells (NSCs) compared to the relatively low levels expressed in adult mouse brain (Wada et al., 2006) and may have differential roles in NSC differentiation during development and adulthood. Activation of PPARγ in embryonic NSCs promotes NSC proliferation and inhibits NSC differentiation. In contrast, the ever-interesting compound cannabidiol (CBD) increased adult rat hippocampal neurogenesis via interaction with a PPARγ pathway (Espisito et al., 2011). PPARγ has also been implicated in promoting neurite outgrowth and dendritic spine density (Brodbeck et al., 2008; Quintanilla et al., 2013).

PPARγ's primary action appears to be neuroprotective in environments that involve inflammation and oxidative stress, as in Alzheimer's disease, Parkinson's disease, Huntington's disease, amyotrophic lateral sclerosis, multiple sclerosis, and stroke. Multiple reviews detail PPARγ's effects in each of these neurodegenerative

disorders (Carta & Simuni, 2015; Collino et al., 2008; Corona & Duchen, 2015; Dineley et al., 2014; Heneke & Landreth, 2007; Johri et al., 2014; Mandrekar-Colucci & Landreth, 2011; Shen et al., 2015). Here, an overview of PPARγ's major effects that most likely contribute to neuroprotection is briefly presented.

PPARγ has low expression in the brain and primarily in neurons; however, in in vitro and in vivo models of various neurodegenerative disorders, PPARγ expression increases in neurons, astrocytes, and microglia (Diab et al., 2002; Fong et al., 2010; Kitamura et al., 1999; Victor et al., 2006; Wang et al., 2012). It is hypothesized that the inflammatory response and increase in oxidative stress results in the generation of fatty acid metabolites, such as eicosanoids, oxidized lipids, and nitroalkenes, which are all potent endogenous PPARγ agonists (Figure 23.2a; Fong et al., 2010). In a positive feedforward loop, PPARγ increases expression of itself and coactivators, such as PGC-1α (Figure 23.2b). Experimental evidence has proven that this endogenous neuroprotective mechanism is important in limiting damage, because when it is absent, mice experience significantly more brain damage and oxidative stress in response to an insult like middle cerebral artery occlusion (Victor et al., 2006; Zhao et al., 2009).

The neuroprotective properties of PPARγ activation in all of the above-mentioned neurodegenerative disorders have consistently been found to involve three general areas: prevention of mitochondrial apoptosis signaling pathways (Figure 23.2c), suppression of inflammatory mediators (reactive oxygen species [ROS]; Figure 23.2d), and limitation of ROS (Figure 23.2e). Mitochondrial membrane potential depends on several factors, an important one being the balanced presence of anti-apoptotic Bcl-2 and Bcl-xl and pro-apoptotic Bad and Bax. Upon injury, Bad and Bax translocate to mitochondria, bind Bcl-2 and Bcl-xl, and depolarize mitochondria. Significant depolarization of the mitochondrial membrane potential can lead to the release of pro-apoptotic factors, such as cytochrome *c*, caspase-9, and caspase-3 (Youle & Strasser, 2008). PPARγ activation increases neurotrophic alpha-1 transcription, which leads to activation of Akt signaling pathways, resulting in increased Bcl-2 expression and phosphorylation of Bad (p-Bad). PPARγ activation also upregulates 14-3-3 epsilon expression, which sequesters p-Bad and prevents Bad translocation into mitochondria (Fuenzalida et al., 2007; Thouennon et al., 2015; Wu et al., 2009a, 2009b).

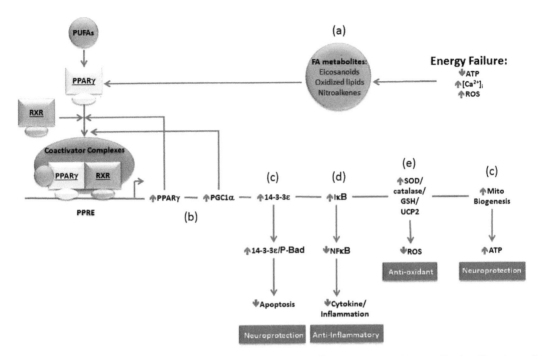

FIGURE 23.2 *Hypothetical Homeostatic Neuroprotection by Endogenous PPARγ Agonists During Situations of Energy Failure Experienced During Epilepsy, Stroke, and Other Neurodegenerative Disorders*
(a) During extended periods of high oxidative stress, metabolites of fatty acids (FA) are generated that have higher affinities for PPARγ than their parent lipids, resulting in an increased activation of PPARγ. (b) In a positive feedforward loop, PPARγ upregulates expression of itself and the coactivator PGC-1α. Neuroprotection is achieved through multiple pathways. (c) PPARγ decreases apoptosis by increasing the expression of 14-3-3 epsilon, which prevents the translocation of p-Bad into the mitochondria and the release of pro-apoptotic factors, and it increases mitochondrial biogenesis, which provides neurons with increased ATP and additional calcium buffering. (d) Inflammation is dampened by PPARγ-mediated inhibition of the pro-inflammatory transcription factor NF-κB and (e) oxidative stress is controlled by upregulation of the expression of antioxidants, such as superoxide dismutase (SOD), catalase, glutathione (GSH), and uncoupling protein 2 (UCP2).

PPARγ activation suppresses pro-inflammatory gene expression by inhibiting the transcription factor NF-κB. PPARγ accomplishes this by increasing the expression of IκBα and IκBβ, which prevent the nuclear translocation and DNA binding of NF-κB (Heneka et al., 2003). PPARγ may also inhibit NF-κB activity by direct physical interaction, steric inhibition, or cofactor competition (Sauer et al., 2015). The end effect is that PPARγ activation decreases inflammatory cytokine production (TNF-α, interleukin-6, IFN-γ), iNOS and COX2 expression, astrogliosis, and microglial activation (Breidert et al., 2002; Combs et al., 2000; Dehmer et al., 2004; Heneka et al., 2000; Lim et al., 2000; Sundararajan et al., 2005; Yan et al., 2003; Zhao et al., 2005).

Cellular injury and inflammation can increase the production of ROS, which further causes cellular damage by oxidizing proteins, lipids, and DNA.

This results in altered neuronal signaling, further neuroinflammation, and the initiation of apoptosis. PPARγ activation limits ROS by increasing gene expression for the antioxidants SOD, catalase, glutathione, and uncoupling protein 2 (UCP2; Chen et al., 2006; Diano et al., 2011; Doonan et al., 2009; Girnun et al., 2002; Zhao et al., 2006). As mentioned previously, PPARγ increases PGC-1α. PGC-1α also acts as a coactivator of the oxidative stress-induced transcription factor Nrf2, which is a master regulator of antioxidant gene sets as well as mitochondrial biogenesis (Clark & Simon, 2009; Milder et al., 2010; St. Pierre et al., 2006). Deficiency in PPARγ is linked to reduced expression of antioxidants (superoxide dismutase 1, catalase, glutathione S-transferase, uncoupling protein-1 [UCP1]), lipid metabolism enzymes (lipoprotein lipase), and the transcription factor liver X receptor-α (Victor et al., 2006; Zhao et al., 2009).

KD'S REGULATION OF PPARγ

PPARγ in Epilepsy

PPARγ was first cloned from *Xenopus laevis* and mouse liver in the early 1990s (Dreyer et al., 1992; Elbrecht et al., 1996; Zhu et al., 1993). Since then, thousands of studies have addressed PPARγ's structure/function, regulation, pharmacology, expression, and importance in disease, primarily in peripheral organs. At the turn of the 21st century, neuroscientists began investigating PPARγ's therapeutic potential for neurodegenerative diseases, in which a role for neuroinflammation and oxidative stress in disease processes has long been recognized (Combs et al., 2000; Kitamura et al., 1999) and has been investigated in hundreds of publications.

The epilepsy community's interest in PPARγ has had a late and slow start. The first research study appeared in 2006, and the total count of studies by the time of the preparation of the second edition of this book was a little over two dozen (Abdallah, 2010; Adabi Mohazab et al., 2012; Boes et al., 2015; Chuang et al., 2012; Han et al., 2011; Hong et al., 2008, 2011, 2013; Hughes et al., 2014; Hung et al., 2019; Hussein et al., 2019; Jeong et al., 2011; Jin et al., 2020; Knowles et al., 2018; Lucchi et al., 2017; Luna-Medina et al., 2007; Maurois et al., 2008; Okada et al., 2006; Peng et al., 2019; San et al., 2015; Simeone et al., 2017a, 2017b; Tan et al., 2020; Wong et al., 2015; Yu et al., 2008). The studies span acute seizure models, post-status epilepticus (SE) models, kindling and genetic models of chronic epilepsy, and, for the most part, they consistently support beneficial neuroprotective and antiseizure effects of PPARγ agonists in epilepsy.

Comparable to findings in chronic neurodegenerative disorders and acute stroke models, the expression of brain PPARγ increases subsequent to SE induced by lithium-pilocarpine, unilateral intrahippocampal kainic acid, intraperitoneal injection of kainic acid, and electrically induced self-sustaining SE (Boes et al., 2015; Chuang et al., 2012; Hong et al., 2008; Jeong et al., 2011; Yu et al., 2008). Similar increases also occur after 6-Hz corneal stimulation-induced acute seizures and after penelenyltetrazole (PTZ) treatment of zebrafish (Jin et al., 2020; Lucchi et al., 2017). Concomitantly, the products of the PPARγ-regulated genes *Pgc-1alpha* and *Ucp2* are increased after lithium-pilocarpine and intrahippocampal kainic acid (Chuang et al., 2012; Han et al., 2011). In a recent study, we examined the nuclear content of

both splice variants, PPARγ1 and PPARγ2, in the brains of wild-type mice and epileptic littermates that lack the Kv1.1 potassium channel (*Kcna1*-null). *Kcna1*-null mice develop severe spontaneous recurrent seizures (SRS) and are a model of temporal lobe epilepsy and sudden unexpected death in epilepsy (SUDEP; Fenoglio-Simeone et al., 2009a,b; Glasscock et al., 2010; Kim et al., 2015; Simeone et al., 2013, 2014a, 2014b, 2017b; Smart et al., 1998; Wenzel et al., 2007;). Similar to previous reports, we found that PPARγ1 predominated in wild-type brain. In contrast, in epileptic *Kcna1*-null brain, we found that PPARγ2 was the dominant form. The total nuclear PPARγ did not change, but the PPARγ2:PPARγ1 ratio increased threefold in *Kcna1*-null brains (Simeone et al., 2017). Further studies are needed to determine the mechanism of this flip in isoform nuclear content. Potential causes that preferentially enhance nuclear translocation of PPARγ2 over PPARγ1 may be generation of isoform-specific ligands, altered expression of isoform-specific cofactors, or posttranslational modifications. Alternatively, transcription, translation, or splicing of PPARγ2 could be increased in epilepsy. Recently, it was found that at the initial stage of adipogenesis, another nuclear receptor, glucocorticoid receptor (GR), is transiently recruited along with the transcription factor C/EBPβ to a complex consisting of PBP/MED1/TRAP220 and p300 to enhancer regions of the *Pparg2* isoform. In response to glucocortocoids, this results in a transient increase in H3K9 acetylation and enhances the induction of PPARγ2, which becomes the principal driver of adipogenesis (Steger et al., 2010). Intriguingly, both C/EBPβ and glucocorticoids increase in the brain with seizures (Engel et al., 2013; Lu et al., 2013; Maguire & Salpekar, 2013). PGC-1α activation of PPARγ also enhances interactions with p300/CBP (Puigserver et al., 1999). Whether PPARγ2 regulates distinct gene sets is unclear, but it has been shown to upregulate catalase expression to a greater degree than PPARγ1 and is important in providing protection against lipotoxicity (Medina-Gomez et al., 2007a, 2007b; Yakunin et al., 2014).

Assuming that the seizure/injury-induced changes in PPARγ expression are part of an endogenous neuroprotective mechanism that limits damage in a way similar to that proposed for other neurodegenerative disorders, then loss of PPARγ should exacerbate markers of injury and possibly seizures. Chuang et al. (2012) found that pretreatment with bilateral focal injections of the PPARγ antagonist

GW9662 (150 nl of a 12-mM solution or 1.5 to 2 mg/kg) reduces UCP2 and exacerbates intra-hippocampal kainic acid SE-induced increases in ROS, oxidized proteins, mitochondrial Bax, cytosolic cytochrome *c*, and DNA fragmentation, and decreases in mitochondrial respiratory complex I (MRCI) activity. Unfortunately, the authors failed to report the details of SE, so it is not known whether PPARγ antagonism worsened the SE (Chuang et al., 2012). We administered GW9662 (1 mg/kg/day in the drinking water for 2 weeks) to *Kcna1*-null mice and wild-type littermates; however, contrary to expectations, inhibiting PPARγ did not increase SRS in *Kcna1*-null mice nor did it lower the seizure threshold in wild-type mice (Simeone et al., 2017b). A possible explanation for the lack of effect on *Kcna1*-null seizures may be that the dose of GW9662 was too low. Supporting this hypothesis, we found that GW9662 had no effect on the nuclear PPARγ2:PPARγ1 ratio in non-epileptic wild-type brain. It did reduce the PPARγ2:PPARγ1 ratio in epileptic *Kcna1*-null brain, but only from threefold to twofold of the wild-type ratio (Simeone et al., 2017b). A greater reduction may be needed to observe an effect on SRS. We also found that seizure thresholds of *Pparg2*-null mice and neuron-specific-PPARγ knockout mice were no different than those in control littermates (Simeone et al., 2017b). From these experimental results we can draw the tentative conclusions that PPARγ itself is somehow involved in increasing nuclear PPARγ2 and that the seizure-induced increase affords some neuroprotection against injury but may not raise the seizure threshold per se.

PPARγ Agonism in Epilepsy

The PPARγ agonists pioglitazone and rosiglitazone have been clinically useful in the management of type 2 diabetes mellitus since 1999, but as of today there are no published reports, case reports or otherwise, describing epilepsy patients with comorbid type 2 diabetes who have been prescribed pioglitazone or rosiglitazone. Nevertheless, experimental evidence from animal studies supports that PPARγ agonists will have antiseizure, neuroprotective, and possibly disease-modifying effects in epilepsy. Even though this field of research is small and there are relatively few studies, there is wide diversity in treatment protocol (agonist, dose, and pretreatment and posttreatment) and endpoints (acute seizures, SRS, inflammatory markers, cell death,

cognitive comorbidities) and it is worth detailing the similarities and differences to gain a sense of the robustness of PPARγ effects.

PPARγ Agonist Pretreatment Raises Thresholds in Acute Seizure Models

Abdallah (2010) and Adabi Mohazab et al. (2012) utilized PTZ to induce seizures in mice according to three different paradigms. Abdallah (2010) pretreated mice with pioglitazone (10 mg/kg, orally) 30 min prior to an intraperitoneal (IP) injection of PTZ and measured latency to stage 4/5 clonic-tonic seizures. All vehicle controls reached stage 4/5, whereas only 20% of the pioglitazone group reached stage 4/5, and those that did took twice as long as the control group. Adabi Mohazab et al. (2012) injected PTZ intravenously and measured the threshold dose required to induce a whole-body clonic seizure. They found that a 1-hr pretreatment with pioglitazone was ineffective, whereas a 4-hr pretreatment provided a dose-dependent (10–80 mg/kg, orally) increase in the seizure threshold dose. Maurois et al. (2008) also found that the PPARγ agonist FMOC-L-leucine—(*N*-[9-fluorenylmethoxycarbonyl]-)-L-leucine (up to 100 mg/kg, IP)—was not effective in the 6-Hz seizure test with 1-hr pretreatment. We have found similar effects when exposing mice to flurothyl gas and measuring latency to clonus and generalized tonic-clonic seizures. A 1-hr pretreatment with pioglitazone had inconsistent effects, whereas a 4-hr pretreatment dose-dependently (1–80 mg/kg, IP) increased the latency to generalized tonic-clonic seizures but had no effect on clonic seizures (Simeone et al., 2017a).

PPARγ Agonists Raise Thresholds in Seizure-Susceptible and Kindling Models

EL mice develop susceptibility to stress-induced tonic-clonic seizures beginning 12 weeks postnatally. Providing pioglitazone (20 mg/kg/day) from 5 to 11 weeks postnatally delayed the age of onset and duration of stress-induced seizures (Okada et al., 2006). Maurois et al. (2008) used a dietary-induced magnesium deficiency-dependent audiogenic seizure model. Mice were pretreated with either FOMC-L-leucine or rosiglitazone (up to 100 mg/kg, IP) 1 hr before acoustic stimuli. FOMC-L-leucine dose-dependently reduced the number of mice responding to acoustic stimuli by 50%, whereas rosiglitazone was ineffective. The FOMC-L-leucine effects were blocked by co-administration of the PPARγ antagonist GW9662 (1 and 2 mg/kg IP; Maurois et al., 2008). Finally,

Abdallah (2010) kindled mice with daily IP injections of subconvulsive PTZ (40 mg/kg) until the mice exhibited stage 4/5 clonic-tonic seizures on 3 consecutive days. Pretreatment with pioglitazone (10 mg/kg, orally) 30 min prior to each PTZ injection resulted in only 30% of mice reaching stage 4/5 seizures by day 17 (Abdullah, 2010). However, because pioglitazone was administered before PTZ and most pioglitazone-treated mice did become kindled as defined by the author, it is difficult to determine whether pioglitazone exerted any antiepileptogenic effect in addition to its anticonvulsant effect.

PPARγ Agonists Reduce SRS and Improve Spatial Learning

Multiple studies have used SE models to later investigate neuropathology during the latent period and after development of SRS (discussed in the next section), however, limited studies have provided information concerning the effect of PPARγ agonists on either seizures during SE or the development of SRS. Luna-Medina et al. (2007) pretreated rats with a thiadiazolidine compound, NP031112 (50 mg/kg, orally), 1 hr before kainic acid injection (10 mg/kg, IP) and monitored the development of behavioral seizures and SE. NP031112 had no effect on SE. Similarly, Hong et al. (2013) found that rosiglitazone had no effect on the development of lithium-pilocarpine SE. Rats were pretreated with rosiglitazone (0.1 mg/kg; Intracerebroventricular, ICV) 24 hr and 1 hr prior to pilocarpine hydrochloride (30 mg/kg, IP) administration. Rats then received repeated injections of pilocarpine (10 mg/kg, IP) every 30 min until they developed convulsive seizures, which were scored behaviorally according to the Racine scale. Rosiglitazone had no effect on SE. The authors continued daily administration of rosiglitazone and examined development of SRS by performing video-EEG recordings beginning 2 weeks post-SE for 6 weeks. They found that 50% of rosiglitazone-treated rats developed SRS, compared to 83% of vehicle-treated rats. Moreover, rosiglitazone nearly doubled the latency to SRS development and decreased the frequency and duration of SRS (Hong et al., 2013). An earlier study by this group demonstrated that the same protocol improved the SE rats' spatial learning as assessed in the Morris water maze (Hong et al., 2011). In contrast, rosiglitazone (3 mg/kg, IP) administered to rats daily immediately following the end of self-sustained SE had no effect on the development and occurrence of SRS; however,

the rosiglitazone-treated rats did have improved spatial learning in the Morris water maze (Boes et al., 2015).

As the presumed effect of PPARγ agonism is genetic regulation, the lack of effect on an intense insult like SE may be related to the short length of pretreatment. Accordingly, San et al. (2015) repeatedly injected rats with declining doses of PTZ to induce SE and found that pretreatment with pioglitazone (10 mg/kg, orally) for 5 days delayed the onset of SE. Similarly, a 4-day pretreatment of rat pups with pioglitazone (5–20 mg/kg/day, IP) dose-dependently increased the latency to febrile-SE and reduced its duration (Hussein et al., 2019). Pioglitazone also alleviated memory deficits as measured by the novel object recognition task in the rats exposed to early-life febrile-SE. Hung et al. (2019) found that 14 days of daily pioglitazone treatment (10 mg/kg/day, orally) reduced the percentage of mice experiencing pilocarpine-induced SE, the severity of SE, and SE-related mortality. Finally, we have found that administration of pioglitazone (10 mg/kg, IP) for 5 days decreases SRS and seizure severity in epileptic *Kcna1*-null mice by 75% (Simeone et al., 2017b).

PPARγ Agonists Are Neuroprotective After SE and During SRS

Within hours to days, intrahippocampal kainic acid-induced SE results in increases in UCP2, ROS, oxidized proteins, mitochondrial Bax, cytosolic cytochrome *c*, DNA fragmentation, and decreases in MRCI activity in rat hippocampi (Chuang et al., 2012). Pretreatment with bilateral focal injections of rosiglitazone (150 nl of a 4-mM solution or 0.7–0.8 mg/kg) further increased UCP2 and prevented all other changes. In fact, MRCI activity was improved compared to that in the sham controls (Chuang et al., 2012). In a similar study, Luna-Medina et al. (2007) found that intrahippocampal injection of kainic acid results in significant cerebral edema, hippocampal cell loss, astrogliosis, and the induction of TNF-α in astrocytes, microglia, and neurons. Co-injection of NP031112 (5–8 ng/kg) prevented edema, cell loss, and TNF-α induction and reduced astrogliosis. Furthermore, pretreatment with NP031112 (50 mg/kg, orally) 1 hr before kainic acid injection (10 mg/kg, IP) also prevented hippocampal neuronal loss as quantified 72 hr after SE (Luna-Medina et al., 2007). San et al. (2015) demonstrated that pretreatment with pioglitazone (10 mg/kg/day, orally) for 5 days before PTZ-induced

SE reduced hippocampal neuronal loss, mTOR activation, and the proinflammatory cytokines IL-1β and IL-6 as quantified 72 hr after SE.

In the rat pilocarpine SE model, post-SE daily administration of rosiglitazone has antioxidant and anti-inflammatory effects. Rosiglitazone increases hippocampal neuronal survival, decreases ROS and lipid peroxidation, increases SOD and GSH, and decreases microglia and astrocytic activation, iNOS, TNF-α, IL-1β, IL-6, and BDNF (Hong et al., 2008, 2012, 2013; Peng et al., 2019; Yu et al., 2008). Similarly, in the febrile-SE model, pioglitazone reduced hippocampal iNOS, TNF-α, IL-1β, and neuronal neurodegeneration (Hussein et al., 2019). In EL mice and the PTZ-kindling model, pioglitazone also decreased TNF-α, IL-1β, IL-6, IL-10, and caspase-3 (Abdallah, 2010; Okada et al., 2006). However, rosiglitazone did not reduce hippocampal cell death in the self-sustained SE model (Boes et al., 2015).

Evidence for KD Activation of PPARγ

Although the possibility of a role for PPARγ in the mechanism of action of the KD has been speculated about in review articles for the past several years (Gano et al., 2014; Kobow et al., 2012; Masino & Rho, 2012), there have been only two studies published exploring this possibility, one using an acute SE model and one using a chronic epilepsy model and acute seizure threshold model (Jeong et al., 2011; Simeone et al., 2017b). Jeong et al. (2011) fed wild-type mice a KD (4:1 ratio of fats to carbohydrate + protein) for 4 weeks and found a threefold increase of PPARγ protein in cell lysate from hippocampal tissue compared to that from standard diet (SD)-fed mice. The mice were injected with kainic acid (30 mg/kg) to induce status and tissue was collected at 2 and 6 hr after the kainic acid injection. The KD delayed the onset of generalized tonic-clonic seizures, but the overall seizure burden that the mice experienced during the 2 and 6 hr post-kainic acid was not reported. In the SD-fed mice, there was a 4-fold and 2-fold increase of PPARγ at the 2- and 6-hr time points after injection, respectively. In contrast, the KD-induced elevated PPARγ levels fell to normal-diet control levels by 6 hr after kainic acid. Hippocampal TNF-α followed the same pattern as PPARγ, whereas the KD blunted the SE-induced increases in NF-κB, microglial CD11b, and COX2 expression. From the studies mentioned previously detailing the effect of injury or

degeneration and PPARγ agonists on the expression of PPARγ, one would expect that PPARγ would be further increased, not decreased, by SE in the KD-fed mice. The authors did not address this discrepancy (Jeong et al., 2011). Nevertheless, the authors presented evidence that the KD does have effects on PPARγ and downstream markers of inflammation known to be regulated by PPARγ.

In another study, we aimed to determine whether the KD changes PPARγ expression in the brains of epileptic and normal mice, and, if so, whether it is necessary for the antiseizure effects of the KD. As already described, we have found that in nuclear extracts from wild-type mouse brain, PPARγ1 is the dominant isoform, whereas PPARγ2 is dominant in epileptic *Kcna1*-null brain (Simeone et al., 2017b). Treating *Kcna1*-null mice for 2 weeks with a KD (6:1 ratio) reduced seizure incidence and severity by ~75%, as we have reported previously (Fenoglio-Simeone et al., 2009b; Kim et al. 2015; Simeone et al., 2017b). KD treatment increased PPARγ2 in both genotypes, resulting in PPARγ2:PPARγ1 ratios that were 2-fold and 6-fold higher for wild-type and *Kcna1*-null brain, respectively, compared to SD-fed wild-type mice.

To determine whether the effect of the KD on PPARγ was necessary for KD antiseizure efficacy, we performed pharmacologic and genetic experiments. Co-administering the PPARγ antagonist GW9662 (1 mg/kg/day) in the drinking water for the 2-week KD treatment prevented the increase in nuclear PPARγ2 and prevented KD-mediated seizure reduction in *Kcna1*-null mice. To further test the importance of PPARγ in the KD mechanism, we obtained *Pparg2*-null mice and conditional neuron-specific PPARγ knockout mice. Previous studies have demonstrated that KD treatment raises the threshold for flurothyl seizures (Dutton et al., 2011; Rho et al., 1999). Similarly, we found that KD treatment effectively raised the seizure thresholds of control mice. However, KD treatment was unable to raise the seizure threshold of *Pparg2*-null mice and conditional neuron-specific PPARγ knockout mice. Furthermore, the pharmacologic and genetic manipulations of PPARγ expression/function did not affect the stereotypic KD-related increase of blood β-hydroxybutyrate or decrease of glucose (Simeone et al., 2017b). Results from this study strongly support that central actions of PPARγ, specifically PPARγ2, play a critical role in the antiseizure mechanism of the KD.

What Does the KD Provide That Could Be Activating PPARγ?

The selective increase of nuclear PPARγ2 over PPARγ1 may be due to the additional 30 amino acids in the PPARγ2 AF-1 that convey a 5- to 10-fold more effective ligand-independent transactivation and increased ligand binding affinity to the LBD relative to PPARγ1 (Bugge et al., 2009; Castillo et al., 1999; Shao et al., 1998; Werman et al., 1997). PPARγ2 is the only PPARγ isoform regulated at the transcriptional level by nutrition (Medina-Gomez et al., 2007a). The PPARγ2-expanded AF-1 also confers differential interaction with transcriptional cofactors and posttranslational modifications that would most likely result in tissue-specific differences in the regulation of gene sets by the PPARγ splice variants. This is evident in the periphery, where PPARγ2, but not PPARγ1, is induced during high-fat diets and initiates adipogenesis, increases lipid-buffering, and reduces lipotoxicity (Medina-Gomez et al., 2007b). Therefore, the most likely mechanisms for the isoform-specificity of the KD probably involve either regulation of signaling cascades responsible for posttranslational modifications that contribute to selective nuclear translocation or transcription of PPARγ2 and/or providing a PPARγ ligand, possibly selective for PPARγ2.

The KD provides plenty of fat, of course, and unsaturated fatty acids, such as omega-3 and omega-6 long-chain polyunsaturated fatty acids, are notably increased in blood serum of patients (Fraser et al., 2003). Importantly, long-chain polyunsaturated fatty acids and their metabolites, eicosanoids, oxidized lipids, and nitroalkenes, are natural ligands for PPARγ (Fong et al., 2010; Yamamoto et al., 2005). Also, it was recently determined that the saturated fatty acid decanoic acid (a.k.a. capric acid), a primary constituent of the medium-chain triglyceride KD, is a ligand for PPARγ at physiologically relevant concentrations (Malapaka et al., 2012).

In vivo treatment suggests that decanoic acid is a selective PPARγ modulator (i.e., partial agonist) because it improves glucose sensitivity and lipid profiles without weight gain in diabetic mice (Malapaka et al., 2012). In vitro experiments in hippocampal slices found that decanoic acid decreases PTZ-induced epileptiform activity in a concentration-dependent manner (Chang et al., 2013). Furthermore, decanoic acid-induced increases in citrate synthase, catalase, and MRCI activity in SH-SY5Y neuronal cultures

were inhibited by a PPARγ antagonist (Hughes et al., 2014). In follow-up in vivo seizure experiments, decanoic acid increased seizure thresholds in the maximal electroshock seizure threshold (MEST), flurothyl, and 6-Hz seizure-threshold tests, but it failed to provide protection against IV PTZ seizures (Tan et al., 2017; Wlaź et al., 2015). Alternatively, Jeong et al. (2012) found that treatment of cultured HT22 cells (a hippocampal neuronal cell line) with the ketone body acetoacetate (5 mM) increased PPARγ over a 12-hr period; however, we have been unable to replicate this finding in primary hippocampal neuronal cultures, and in fact this concentration of acetoacetate results in significant neuronal death within 24 and 48 hr (Simeone et al., 2015). Therefore, at the moment it seems that the unsaturated and saturated fatty acids provided by a KD may be the ligands for PPARγ, and that PPARγ may be involved in the antiseizure mechanism of the various formulations of the KD regardless of the type of fat content.

FUNCTIONAL CONSEQUENCES OF PPARγ ACTIVATION RELEVANT TO EPILEPSY

PPARγ agonists and the KD regulate similar anti-inflammatory, antioxidant, and pro-mitochondrial pathways. These include, but are not limited to, upregulation of IκB; inhibition of NF-κB; reduction of cytokines, such as IL-1β, IL-6, and TNF-α; upregulation of genes encoding mitochondrial enzymes involved in oxidative phosphorylation (e.g., multiple subunits of complexes I, II, IV, and V); induction of mitochondrial biogenesis; and upregulation of UCP2, catalase, and glutathione, all of which have been suggested as possible disease-modifying targets for epilepsy (Abdallah, 2010; Adabi Mohazab et al., 2012; Bernardo et al., 2006; Bough et al., 2006; Chuang et al., 2012; Fong et al., 2010; Heneka & Landreth, 2007; Hong et al., 2008, 2012, 2013; Mandrekar-Colucci et al., 2013; Masino & Rho, 2012; Miglio et al., 2009; Sullivan et al., 2004; Yang & Cheng, 2010; Yu et al., 2008).

Mitochondria are of particular interest in temporal lobe epilepsy. In human epilepsies and animal chemoconvulsant seizure models, brain tissue from seizure foci exhibit mitochondrial ROS and oxidative damage, reduced ATP-producing complex I activity, and diminished antioxidant systems (Bruce & Baudry, 1995; DiMauro et al., 1999; Kim et al., 2015; Kudin et al., 2009;

Kunz et al., 2000; Malthankar-Phatak et al., 2006; Mueller et al., 2001; Ryan et al., 2012; Simeone et al., 2014a; Sudha et al., 2001; Sullivan et al., 2003; Vielhaber et al., 2008; Wallace, 1999; Simeone et al., unpublished observation). Oxidative stress and mitochondrial overload likely contribute to the neuronal cell loss in severe epilepsy associated with sclerosis. In this circumstance, it is clear that the proposed actions of PPARγ would be neuroprotective and would increase the number of surviving cells. But this illustrates only one outcome of unhealthy mitochondria and does not address the potential consequences that chronic mitochondrial dysfunction has for neuronal hyperexcitability and seizure severity.

Several elegant studies have demonstrated that mitochondria regulate synaptic transmission via three properties: production of ATP, production of ROS, and sequestration of cytosolic calcium (Harris et al., 2012; Lee et al., 2007, 2012). Thus, any perturbation of mitochondrial health will send ripples of dysregulation across synaptic, neuronal, and network activity. Stabilizing synaptic mitochondria could be another mechanism by which PPARγ and the KD reduce seizure activity.

To test this hypothesis, we turned once again to the Kcna1-null mouse model of epilepsy, because it has mitochondrial pathology similar to that reported for human epilepsies (Kim et al., 2015; Simeone et al., 2014a; Simeone et al., unpublished observations). Mitochondria isolated from cortical and hippocampal tissue from epileptic Kcna1-null mice have reduced ATP-producing MRCI-driven respiration, increased ROS, and decreased UCP2 (Simeone et al., 2014a). The decrease of UCP2, a mitochondrial protein with downstream antioxidant effects, may contribute to the rise in ROS. The MRCI inhibition appears to be due to posttranslational inhibition by elevated ROS, because acute addition of an antioxidant like ascorbic acid restores Kcna1-null MRCI-driven respiration to wild-type levels, whereas exogenous H_2O_2 mimics the MRCI dysfunction of Kcna1-null mitochondria (Simeone et al., 2014a). In addition, the mitochondrial membrane potential is depolarized, and mitochondrial calcium sequestration capacity is reduced (Kim et al., 2015; Simeone et al., 2014a; Simeone et al., unpublished observation).

Thus, the three properties of mitochondria that play a role in synaptic transmission (ATP, ROS, and calcium) are dysfunctional in Kcna1-null mitochondria and predict widespread effects on synaptic and network activity. This is exactly what we observed using a multi-electrode array to record extracellular potentials from in vitro hippocampal slices from Kcna1-null brains (Simeone et al., 2013). We found that Kcna1-null hippocampi generate spontaneous network activity originating in the CA3 region in the form of sharp waves (SPWs) and ripples (80–200 Hz bandwidth) with an increased incidence and duration compared to slices from wild-type hippocampi. Also present in Kcna1-null hippocampi were epilepsy-associated pathologic high-frequency oscillations in the fast ripple bandwidth (200–600 Hz), which can be viewed as biomarkers of hyperexcitable networks. Furthermore, Kcna1-null CA3 has enhanced coupling of excitatory inputs and population spike generation, and CA3 principal cells have reduced spike-timing reliability. Removing the influence of granule cell mossy fiber path inputs by microdissecting the Kcna1-null CA3 region mostly rescued the network oscillatory behavior and improved spike timing. We found that Kcna1-null mossy fibers are hyperexcitable and have reduced paired pulse ratios, suggesting increased neurotransmitter release at these terminals (Simeone et al., 2013). Collectively, these data indicate enhanced synaptic release in the Kcna1-null CA3 region reduces spike-timing precision of individual neurons, leading to disorganization of network oscillatory activity and promotion of the emergence of fast ripples.

This synaptic phenotype is mimicked by acute application of the MRCI inhibitor rotenone to wild-type hippocampal slices. Experimental inhibition of MRCI results in increased SPWs, ripples, and fast ripples (Simeone et al., 2014a; Heruye & Simeone, unpublished observations). Moreover, rotenone provoked seizurelike events in vitro, supporting a possible role in worsening in vivo seizures (Simeone et al., 2014a).

We have further demonstrated that in vivo treatment of Kcna1-null mice with either pioglitazone, or a KD, or a cocktail of ascorbic acid, alpha-tocopherol, and pyruvate designed to target mitochondrial health rescues MRCI respiration, restores mossy fiber neurotransmitter release probabilities, and dampens network hyperexcitability (i.e., reduces the incidence of SPWs, ripples, and fast ripples; Simeone et al., 2014a, 2014b, 2017b). We have recently found that the KD increases hippocampal mRNA and protein of the antioxidant catalase, and that inhibition of catalase or genetic loss of PPARγ2 results in loss of KD protection against PTZ seizures (Knowles et al., 2018). Therefore, we speculate that, in Kcna1-null mice, one important antiseizure mechanism resulting from KD modulation of PPARγ is restoration of MRCI function, possibly by increasing endogenous antioxidant pathways and decreasing ROS. Chuang et al. (2012) implicated just such a pathway in the neuroprotective effects of rosiglitazone in the intrahippocampal kainate model of SE. Specifically, rosiglitazone increased UCP2, decreased ROS, and restored MRCI function.

The notion that PPARγ activation also underlies neuronal ketogenesis is a recently proposed, intriguing PPARγ-mediated mechanism (Tan et al., 2020). Through a series of pharmacologic and genetic experiments using in vitro and in vivo models, the authors demonstrated that pioglitazone activation of PPARγ initiates PPARγ binding to the promoter region of the *AZGP1* gene, which encodes the zinc-α2-glycoprotein (ZAG) protein. This results in increased ZAG, which is transferred to mitochondria, where it binds to long-chain L-3-hydroxyacyl-CoA dehydrogenase and promotes β-oxidation and ketogenesis of acetoacetate. Acute overexpression of ZAG via viral transfection provided a modest, but significant, reduction in seizure severity in the PTZ kindling model (Tan et al., 2020). The implications for the KD are clearly significant. The KD not only improves mitochondrial function via PPARγ, but

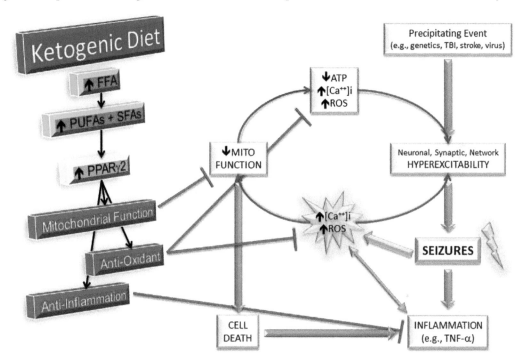

FIGURE 23.3 *Proposed Mechanisms of Action of PPARγ2 Activation Underlying the Antiseizure Efficacy of the Ketogenic Diet (KD)*

Right: A depiction of the interactions of oxidative stress, inflammation, and mitochondrial dysfunction that may participate in worsening seizure severity and genesis. Seizures are generated by a precipitating factor, such as a genetic predisposition, injury, stroke, or viral infection, that results in neuronal, synaptic, and network hyperexcitability. The ictal events lead to increases in production of reactive oxygen species (ROS) and intracellular calcium, which can overload cellular buffering capacities. Seizures can also initiate the release of pro-inflammatory cytokines that can further increase ROS and calcium. The ROS and excess calcium cause dysregulation of mitochondrial function, most notably at complex I, resulting in decreased ATP generation, increased ROS production, mitochondrial membrane depolarization, and a further increase in cytosolic calcium as mitochondria lose their capacity to sequester calcium. Extreme mitochondrial damage will lead to release of pro-apoptotic factors and cell death, which will increase inflammatory processes. Chronic mitochondrial dysfunction in neurons will dysregulate neuronal, synaptic, and network excitability and exacerbate the precipitating event-induced hyperexcitability. Left: The KD increases free fatty acids. Whether the increase is in polyunsaturated fatty acids, such as docahexaenoic acid and eicosapentaenoic acid, or medium-chain saturated fatty acids, such as decanoic acid, depends on the formulation of the diet. Nevertheless, the increase in fatty acids represents an increase in natural agonists for the nuclear transcription factor PPARγ. In particular, enrichment of nuclear PPARγ2 is important for the KD's antiseizure efficacy. Upregulation of gene sets involved in promoting mitochondrial function, antioxidation, and anti-inflammation may contribute to not only the KD's neuroprotective properties but also the KD's ability to dampen hyperexcitabilty.

also promotes the pathways to convert the KD into fuel to generate ATP, ultimately restoring functional reliability to neurons and networks and preventing cell death and seizures.

CONCLUDING REMARKS

The development of epilepsy necessarily originates with a precipitating factor (e.g., genetic predisposition, traumatic brain injury, virus, etc.) that lowers the seizure threshold or moves the baseline activity of the brain closer to the seizure threshold so that previously nonsignificant internal or external stimuli are capable of synchronizing large networks into high-frequency oscillatory activity. If the resulting seizure phenotype is severe, then a chronic inflammatory and oxidative state develops, with concomitant mitochondrial dysfunction. The result is not only death of vulnerable cell types, but also dysregulation of cellular, synaptic, and network excitability, which further lowers the seizure threshold and exacerbates the seizure phenotype (Figure 23.3, *left*).

Experimental evidence indicates that the KD prevents cell death and hyperexcitability by promoting mitochondrial health and anti-inflammatory and antioxidant pathways. Limited, but strong, evidence reviewed here suggests that the KD regulates PPARγ to achieve these effects (Figure 23.3, *right*). This discovery presents multiple opportunities for both researchers and clinicians. The immediate translational potential resides in the availability of the PPARγ agonists pioglitazone and rosiglitazone, which are FDA-approved for therapeutic use in type 2 diabetes mellitus. The TZDs are not perfect and can have significant side effects. The good news is that the diabetes academic and industry communities have undertaken active research efforts into developing PPARγ partial agonists (SPPARMs) with improved side-effect profiles. These may also prove useful in epilepsy. Furthermore, additional targets with therapeutic potential in epilepsy may be identified by focusing on the upstream pathways or ligands leading to PPARγ activation and the downstream effectors that result in increasing the seizure threshold and/or dampening hyperexcitability and improved neuroprotection. Recent examples validating the potential importance of PPARγ are the identification that PPARγ is involved in the antiseizure effects of the ghrelin receptor antagonist EP-80317 and the plant-derived α-asaronol (Jin et al., 2020; Lucchi et al., 2017).

The identification of PPARγ as a potential mediator of KD efficacy in epilepsy does not preclude the other mechanisms discussed in this volume. Some, such as ketone bodies, may work synergistically with PPARγ, and others may be downstream effectors of PPARγ, such as adenosine.

ACKNOWLEDGMENTS

This work was supported by an award from Citizens United for Research in Epilepsy Foundation, Nebraska State Scientific Research Funding LB692, and the NIH NINDS (NS085389). Dr. Kristina A. Simeone is thanked for many insightful discussions and comments on this manuscript.

REFERENCES

Abdallah, D. M. (2010). Anticonvulsant potential of the peroxisome proliferator-activated receptor γ agonist pioglitazone in pentylenetetrazole-induced acute seizures and kindling in mice. *Brain Research*, 1351, 246–253.

Adabi Mohazab, R., Javadi-Paydar, M., Delfan, B., & Dehpour, A.R. (2012). Possible involvement of PPAR-gamma receptor and nitric oxide pathway in the anticonvulsant effect of acute pioglitazone on pentylenetetrazole-induced seizures in mice. *Epilepsy Research*, 101, 28–35.

Ahmadian, M., Suh, J. M., Hah, N., Liddle, C., Atkins, A. R., Downes, M., & Evans, R. M. (2013). PPARγ signaling and metabolism: The good, the bad and the future. *Nature Medicine*, 19, 557–566.

Auestad, N., Korsak, R. A., Morrow, J. W., & Edmond, J. (1991) Fatty acid oxidation and ketogenesis by astrocytes in primary culture. *Journal of Neurochemistry*, 56, 1376–1386.

Auwerx, J. (1999). PPARγ, the ultimate thrifty gene. *Diabetologia*, 42, 1033–1049.

Bhattamisra, S. K., Shin, L. Y., Saad, H. I. B. M., Rao, V., Candasamy, M., Pandey, M., & Choudhury, H. (2020). Interlink between insulin resistance and neurodegeneration with an update on current therapeutic approaches. *CNS & Neurological Disorders—Drug Targets*, 19(3), 174–183. https://doi.org/10.2174/1871527319666200518102130.

Bernardo, A., & Minghetti, L. (2006). PPAR-gamma agonists as regulators of microglial activation and brain inflammation. *Current Pharmaceutical Design*, 12, 93–109.

Boes, K., Russmann, V., Ongerth, T., Licko, T., Salvamoser, J. D., Siegl, C., & Potschka, H. (2015). Expression regulation and targeting of the peroxisome proliferator-activated receptor γ following electrically-induced status epilepticus. *Neuroscience Letters*, 604, 151–156.

Bough, K. J., Wetherington, J., Hassel, B., Pare, J. F., Gawryluk, J. W., Greene, J. G., Shaw, R., Smith, Y., Geiger, J. D., & Dingledine, R. J. (2006). Mitochondrial biogenesis in the anticonvulsant mechanism of the ketogenic diet. *Annals of Neurology, 60,* 223–235.

Braissant, O., Foufelle, F., Scotto, C., Dauça, M., & Wahli, W. (1996). Differential expression of peroxisome proliferator-activated receptors (PPARs): Tissue distribution of PPAR-alpha, -beta, and -gamma in the adult rat. *Endocrinology, 137,* 354–66.

Breidert, T., Callebert, J., Heneka, M. T., Landreth, G., Launay, J. M., & Hirsch, E. C. (2002). Protective action of the peroxisome proliferator-activated receptor-gamma agonist pioglitazone in a mouse model of Parkinson's disease. *Journal of Neurochemistry, 82,* 615–624.

Brodbeck, J., Balestra, M. E., Saunders, A. M., Roses, A. D., Mahley, R. W., & Huang, Y. (2008). Rosiglitazone increases dendritic spine density and rescues spine loss caused by apolipoprotein E4 in primary cortical neurons. *Proceedings of the National Academy of Sciences of the United States of America, 105,* 1343–1346.

Bruce, A. J., & Baudry, M. (1995). Oxygen free radicals in rat limbic structures after kainate-induced seizures. *Free Radical Biology and Medicine, 18,* 993–1002.

Bugge, A., Grontved, L., Aagaard, M. M., Borup, R., & Mandrup, S. (2009). The PPARγ2 A/B-domain plays a gene-specific role in transactivation and cofactor recruitment. *Molecular Endocrinology, 23,* 794–808.

Burris, T. P., Solt, L. A., Wang, Y, Crumbley, C., Banerjee, S., Griffett, K., Lundasen, T., Hughes, T., & Kojetin, D. J. (2013). Nuclear receptors and their selective pharmacologic modulators. Pharmacol Rev. *65,* 710–778.

Carmona, M. C., Louche, K., Lefebvre, B., Pilon, A., Hennuyer, N., Audinot-Bouchez, V., Fievet, C., Torpier, G., Formstecher, P., Renard, P., Lefebvre, P., Dacquet, C., Staels, B., Casteilla, L., Pénicaud, L., & Consortium of the French Ministry of Research and Technology. (2007). S 26948: A new specific peroxisome proliferator activated receptor gamma modulator with potent antidiabetes and antiatherogenic effects. *Diabetes, 56,* 2797–2808.

Carta, A. R., & Simuni, T. (2015). Thiazolidinediones under preclinical and early clinical development for the treatment of Parkinson's disease. *Expert Opinion on Investigational Drugs, 24,* 219–227.

Castillo, G., Brun, R. P., Rosenfield, J. K., Hauser, S., Park, C. W., Troy, A. E., Wright, M. E., & Spiegelman, B. M. (1999). An adipogenic cofactor bound by the differentiation domain of PPARγ. *EMBO Journal, 18,* 3676–3687.

Chang, P., Terbach, N., Plant, N., Chen, P. E., Walker, M. C., & Williams, R. S. (2013). Seizure control by ketogenic diet-associated medium chain fatty acids. *Neuropharmacology, 69,* 105–114.

Chen, S. D., Wu, H. Y., Yang, D. I., Lee, S. Y., Shaw, F. Z., Lin, T. K., Liou, C. W., & Chuang, Y. C. (2006). Effects of rosiglitazone on global ischemia-induced hippocampal injury and expression of mitochondrial uncoupling protein 2. *Biochemical and Biophysical Research Communications, 351,* 198–203.

Choi, J. H., Banks, A. S., Estall, J. L., Kajimura, S., Boström, P., Laznik, D., Ruas, J. L., Chalmers, M. J., Kamenecka, T. M., Blüher, M., Griffin, P. R., & Spiegelman, B. M. (2010). Anti-diabetic drugs inhibit obesity-linked phosphorylation of PPARγ by Cdk5. *Nature, 466,* 451–456.

Chuang, Y. C., Lin, T. K., Huang, H. Y., Chang, W. N., Liou, C. W., Chen, S. D., Chang, A. Y. W., & Chan, S. H. H. (2012). Peroxisome proliferator-activated receptors gamma/mitochondrial uncoupling protein 2 signaling protects against seizure-induced neuronal cell death in the hippocampus following experimental status epilepticus. *Journal of Neuroinflammation, 9,* 184.

Clark, J., & Simon, D. K. (2009). Transcribe to survive: Transcriptional control of antioxidant defense programs for neuroprotection in Parkinson's disease. *Antioxidants & Redox Signaling, 11,* 509–528.

Collino, M., Patel, N. S., & Thiemermann, C. (2008). PPARs as new therapeutic targets for the treatment of cerebral ischemia/reperfusion injury. *Therapeutic Advances in Cardiovascular Disease, 2,* 179–197.

Combs, C. K., Johnson, D. E., Karlo, J. C., Cannady, S. B., & Landreth, G. E. (2000). Inflammatory mechanisms in Alzheimer's disease: Inhibition of beta amyloid-stimulated proinflammatory responses and neurotoxicity by PPARγ agonists. *Journal of Neuroscience, 20,* 558–567.

Corona, J. C., & Duchen, M. R. (2015). PPARγ and PGC-1α as therapeutic targets in Parkinson's. *Neurochemistry Research, 40,* 308–316.

Cullingford, T. E., Bhakoo, K., Peuchen, S., Dolphin, C. T., Patel, R., & Clark, J. B. (1998). Distribution of mRNAs encoding the peroxisome proliferator-activated receptor alpha, beta, and gamma and the retinoid X receptor alpha, beta, and gamma in rat central nervous system. *Journal of Neurochemistry, 70,* 1366–1375.

Cullingford, T. E., Dolphin, C. T., & Sato, H. (2002a). The peroxisome proliferator-activated receptor alpha-selective activator ciprofibrate upregulates expression of genes encoding fatty acid oxidation and ketogenesis enzymes in rat brain. *Neuropharmacology, 42,* 724–730.

Cullingford, T. E., Eagles, D. A., & Sato, H. (2002b). The ketogenic diet upregulates expression of the gene encoding the key ketogenic enzyme mitochondrial 3-hydroxy-3-methylglutaryl-CoA synthase in rat brain. *Epilepsy Research, 49,* 99–107.

Dehmer, T., Heneka, M. T., Sastre, M., Dichgans, J., & Schulz, J. B. (2004). Protection by pioglitazone in the MPTP model of Parkinson's disease correlates with I kappa B alpha induction and block of NF kappa B and iNOS activation. *Journal of Neurochemistry, 88,* 494–501.

Desvergne, B., & Wahli, W. (1999) Peroxisome proliferator-activated receptors: Nuclear control of metabolism. *Endocrine Reviews, 20,* 649–688.

Diab, A., Deng, C., Smith, J. D., Hussain, R. Z., Phanavanh, B., Lovett-Racke, A. E., Drew, P. D., & Racke, M. K. (2002). Peroxisome proliferator-activated receptor-gamma agonist 15-deoxy-Delta(12,14)-prostaglandin J(2) ameliorates experimental autoimmune encephalomyelitis. *Journal of Immunology, 168,* 2508–2515.

Diano, S., Liu, Z. W., Jeong, J. K., Dietrich, M. O., Ruan, H. B., Kim, E., Suyama, S., Kelly, K., Gyengesi, E., Arbiser, J. L., Belsham, D. D., Sarruf, D. A., Schwartz, M. W., Bennett, A. M., Shanabrough, M., Mobbs, C. V., Yang, X., Gao, X. B., & Horvath, T. L. (2011). Peroxisome proliferation-associated control of reactive oxygen species sets melanocortin tone and feeding in diet-induced obesity. *Nature Medicine, 17,* 1121–1127.

DiMauro, S., Kulikova, R., Tanji, K., Bonilla, E., & Hirano, M. (1999). Mitochondrial genes for generalized epilepsies. *Advances in Neurology, 79,* 411–419.

Dineley, K. T., Jahrling, J. B., & Denner, L. (2014). Insulin resistance in Alzheimer's disease. *Neurobiology of Disease, 72,* 92–103.

Doonan, F., Wallace, D. M., O'Driscoll, C., & Cotter, T. G. (2009). Rosiglitazone acts as a neuroprotectant in retinal cells via up-regulation of sestrin-1 and SOD-2. *Journal of Neurochemistry, 109,* 631–643.

Dreyer, C., Krey, G., Keller, H., Givel, F., Helftenbein, G., & Wahli, W. (1992). Control of the peroxisomal beta-oxidation pathway by a novel family of nuclear hormone receptors. *Cell, 68,* 879–887.

Dutton, S. B., Sawyer, N. T., Kalume, F., Jumbo-Lucioni, P., Borges, K., Catterall, W. A., & Escayg, A. (2011). Protective effect of the ketogenic diet in Scn1a mutant mice. *Epilepsia, 52,* 2050–2056.

Elbrecht, A., Chen, Y., Cullinan, C. A., Hayes, N., Leibowitz, M. D., Moller, D. E., & Berger, J. (1996). Molecular cloning, expression and characterization of human peroxisome proliferator activated receptors gamma 1 and gamma 2. *Biochemical and Biophysical Research Communications, 224,* 431–437.

Engel, T., Sanz-Rodriguez, A., Jimenez-Mateos, E. M., Concannon, C. G., Jimenez-Pacheco, A., Moran, C., Mesuret, G., Petit, E., Delanty, N.,

Farrell, M. A., O'Brien, D. F., Prehn, J. H., Lucas, J. J., & Henshall, D. C. (2013). CHOP regulates the p53-MDM2 axis and is required for neuronal survival after seizures. *Brain, 136,* 577–592.

Esposito, G., Scuderi, C., Valenza, M., Togna, G. I., Latina, V., De Filippis, D., Cipriano, M., Carratù, M. R., Iuvone, T., & Steardo, L. (2011). Cannabidiol reduces Aβ-induced neuroinflammation and promotes hippocampal neurogenesis through PPARγ involvement. *PLOS ONE, 6,* Article e28668.

Fenoglio-Simeone, K., Mazarati, A., Sefidvash-Hockley, S., Shin, D., Wilke, J., Milligan, H., Sankar, R., Rho, J. M., & Maganti, R. (2009a). Anticonvulsant effects of the selective melatonin receptor agonist ramelteon. *Epilepsy Behavior, 16,* 52–57.

Fenoglio-Simeone, K. A., Wilke, J. C., Milligan, H. L., Allen, C. N., Rho, J. M., & Maganti, R. K. (2009b). Ketogenic diet treatment abolishes seizure periodicity and improves diurnal rhythmicity in epileptic Kcna1-null mice. *Epilepsia, 50,* 2027–2034.

Fong, W. H., Tsai, H. D., Chen, Y. C., Wu, J. S., & Lin, T. N. (2010). Anti-apoptotic actions of PPAR-gamma against ischemic stroke. *Molecular Neurobiology, 41,* 180–186.

Fraser, D. D., Whiting, S., Andrew, R. D., Macdonald, E. A., Musa-Veloso, K., & Cunnane, S. C. (2003). Elevated polyunsaturated fatty acids in blood serum obtained from children on the ketogenic diet. *Neurology, 60,* 1026–1029.

Fuenzalida, K., Quintanilla, R., Ramos, P., Piderit, D., Fuentealba, R. A., Martinez, G., Inestrosa, N. C., & Bronfman, M. (2007). Peroxisome proliferator-activated receptor gamma up-regulates the Bcl-2 anti-apoptotic protein in neurons and induces mitochondrial stabilization and protection against oxidative stress and apoptosis. *Journal of Biological Chemistry, 282,* 37006–37015.

Gahring, L. C., Persiyanov, K., Days, E. L., & Rogers, S. W. (2005). Age-related loss of neuronal nicotinic receptor expression in the aging mouse hippocampus corresponds with cyclooxygenase-2 and PPAR gamma expression and is altered by long-term NS398 administration. *Journal of Neurobiology, 62,* 453–468.

Gano, L. B., Patel, M., & Rho, J. M. (2014). Ketogenic diets, mitochondria, and neurological diseases. *Journal of Lipid Research, 55,* 2211–2228.

Gavzan, H., Hashemi, F., Babaei, J., & Sayyah, M. (2018). A role for peroxisome proliferator-activated receptor α in anticonvulsant activity of docosahexaenoic acid against seizures induced by pentylenetetrazole. *Neuroscience Letters, 681,* 83–86.

Girnun, G. D., Domann, F. E., Moore, S. A., & Robbins, M. E. (2002). Identification of a functional peroxisome proliferator-activated receptor response element in the rat catalase promoter. *Molecular Endocrinology, 16,* 2793–2801.

Guzmán, M., & Blázquez, C. (2004). Ketone body synthesis in the brain: Possible neuroprotective effects. *Prostaglandins, Leukotrienes and Essential Fatty Acids, 70,* 287–292.

Han, Y., Xie, N., Cao, L., Zhao, X., Liu, X., Jiang, H., & Chi, Z. (2011). Adenosine monophosphate-activated protein kinase and peroxisome proliferator-activated receptor gamma coactivator 1α signaling provides neuroprotection in status epilepticus in rats. *Neuroscience Letters, 500,* 133–138.

Harmon, G. S., Lam, M. T., & Glass, C. K. (2011). PPARs and lipid ligands in inflammation and metabolism. *Chemical Reviews, 111*(10), 6321–6340. doi:10.1021/cr2001355. PMID: 21988241; PMCID: PMC3437919.

Harris, J. J., Jolivet, R., & Attwell, D. (2012). Synaptic energy use and supply. *Neuron, 75,* 762–777.

Heneka, M. T., Gavrilyuk, V., Landreth, G. E., O'Banion, M. K., Weinberg, G., & Feinstein, D. L. (2003). Noradrenergic depletion increases inflammatory responses in brain: Effects on IκB and HSP70 expression. *Journal of Neurochemistry, 85,* 387–398.

Heneka, M. T., Klockgether, T., & Feinstein, D. L. (2000). Peroxisome proliferator-activated receptor-gamma ligands reduce neuronal inducible nitric oxide synthase expression and cell death *in vivo*. *Journal of Neuroscience, 20,* 6862–6867.

Heneka, M. T., & Landreth, G. E. (2007). PPARs in the brain. *Biochimica et Biophysica Acta, 1771,* 1031–1045.

Hong, S., Huang, Y., Yu, X., Li, Y., Yang, J., Li, R., Deng, Y., & Zhao, G. (2008). Peroxisome proliferator-activated receptor gamma agonist, rosiglitazone, suppresses CD40 expression and attenuates inflammatory responses after lithium pilocarpine-induced status epilepticus in rats. *International Journal of Developmental Neuroscience, 26,* 505–515.

Hong, S., Xin, Y., HaiQin, W., GuiLian, Z., Ru, Z., ShuQin, Z., HuQing, W., Li, Y., & Yun, D. (2012). The PPARγ agonist rosiglitazone prevents cognitive impairment by inhibiting astrocyte activation and oxidative stress following pilocarpine-induced status epilepticus. *Neurological Sciences, 33,* 559–566.

Hong, S., Xin, Y., HaiQin, W., GuiLian, Z., Ru, Z., ShuQin, Z., HuQing, W., Li, Y., Ning, B., & YongNan, L. (2013). The PPARγ agonist rosiglitazone prevents neuronal loss and attenuates development of spontaneous recurrent seizures through BDNF/TrkB signaling following pilocarpine-induced status epilepticus. *Neurochemistry International, 63,* 405–412.

Hughes, S. D., Kanabus, M., Anderson, G., Hargreaves, I. P., Rutherford, T., O'Donnell, M., Cross, J. H., Rahman, S., Eaton, S., & Heales, S. J. (2014) The ketogenic diet component decanoic acid increases mitochondrial citrate synthase and complex I activity in neuronal cells. *Journal of Neurochemistry, 129,* 426–433.

Hung, T. Y., Chu, F. L., Wu, D. C., Wu, S. N., & Huang, C. W. (2019) The protective role of peroxisome proliferator-activated receptor-gamma in seizure and neuronal excitotoxicity. *Molecular Neurobiology, 56,* 5497–5506.

Hussein, H. A., Moghimi, A., & Roohbakhsh, A. (2019) Anticonvulsant and ameliorative effects of pioglitazone on cognitive deficits, inflammation and apoptosis in the hippocampus of rat pups exposed to febrile seizure. *Iranian Journal of Basic Medical Science, 22,* 267–276.

Itoh, T., Fairall, L., Amin, K., Inaba, Y., Szanto, A., Balint, B. L., Nagy, L., Yamamoto, K., & Schwabe, J. W. (2008). Structural basis for the activation of PPARγ by oxidized fatty acids. *Nature Structural & Molecular Biology, 15,* 924–931.

Jarrett, S. G., Milder, J. B., Liang, L. P., & Patel, M. (2008). The ketogenic diet increases mitochondrial glutathione levels. *Journal of Neurochemistry, 106,* 1044–1051.

Jeong, E. A., Jeon, B. T., Shin, H. J., Kim, N., Lee, D. H., Kim, H. J., Kang, S. S., Cho, G. J., Choi, W. S., & Roh, G. S. (2011). Ketogenic diet-induced peroxisome proliferator-activated receptor-γ activation decreases neuroinflammation in the mouse hippocampus after kainic acid-induced seizures. *Experimental Neurology, 232,* 195–202.

Jin, M., Zhang, B., Sun, Y., Zhang, S., Li, X., Sik, A., Bai, Y., Zheng, X., & Liu, K. (2020) Involvement of peroxisome proliferator-activated receptor γ in anticonvulsant activity of α-asaronol against pentylenetetrazole-induced seizures in zebrafish. *Neuropharmacology, 162,* 107760. https://doi.org/10.1016/j.neuropharm.2019.107760

Johri, A., Chandra, A., & Beal, M. F. (2013). PGC-1α, mitochondrial dysfunction, and Huntington's disease. *Free Radical Biology and Medicine, 62,* 37–46.

Katsouri, L., Blondrath, K., & Sastre, M. (2012). Peroxisome proliferator-activated receptor-γ cofactors in neurodegeneration. *IUBMB Life, 64,* 958–964.

Kersten, S., & Wahli, W. (2000). Peroxisome proliferator activated receptor agonists. *Experientia Supplementum, 89,* 141–151

Kim, D. Y., Simeone, K. A., Simeone, T. A., Pandya, J. D., Wilke, J. C., Ahn, Y., Geddes, J. W., Sullivan, P. G., & Rho, J. M. (2015). Ketone bodies mediate anti-seizure effects through mitochondrial permeability transition. *Annals of Neurology, 78,* 77–87.

Kitamura, Y., Shimohama, S., Koike, H., Kakimura, J., Matsuoka, Y., Nomura, Y., Gebicke-Haerter, P. J., & Taniguchi, T. (1999). Increased expression of cyclooxygenases and peroxisome proliferator-activated receptor-gamma in Alzheimer's disease brains. *Biochemical and Biophysical Research Communications*, *254*, 582–586.

Knowles, S., Budney, S., Deodhar, M., Matthews, S. A., Simeone, K. A., & Simeone, T. A. (2018). Ketogenic diet regulates the antioxidant catalase via the transcription factor PPARγ2. *Epilepsy Research*, *147*, 71–74.

Kobow, K., Auvin, S., Jensen, F., Löscher, W., Mody, I., Potschka, H., Prince, D., Sierra, A., Simonato, M., Pitkänen, A., Nehlig, A., & Rho, J. M. (2012). Finding a better drug for epilepsy: Antiepileptogenesis targets. *Epilepsia*, *53*, 1868–1876.

Kroker, A. J., & Bruning, J. B. (2015). Review of the structural and dynamic mechanisms of PPARγ partial agonism. *PPAR Research*, *2015*, Article ID 816856, 15 pages. https://doi.org/10.1155/2015/816856

Kudin, A. P., Zsurka, G., Elger, C. E., & Kunz, W. S. (2009). Mitochondrial involvement in temporal lobe epilepsy. *Experimental Neurology*, *218*, 326–332.

Kunz, W. S., Kudin, A. P., Vielhaber, S., Blümcke, I., Zuschratter, W., Schramm, J., Beck, H., & Elger, C. E. (2000). Mitochondrial complex I deficiency in the epileptic focus of patients with temporal lobe epilepsy. *Annals of Neurology*, *48*, 766–773.

Lee, D., Lee, K. H., Ho, W. K., & Lee, S. H. (2007). Target cell-specific involvement of presynaptic mitochondria in post-tetanic potentiation at hippocampal mossy fiber synapses. *Journal of Neuroscience*, *27*, 13603–13613.

Lee, S. H., Kim, K. R., Ryu, S. Y., Son, S., Hong, H. S., Mook-Jung, I., Lee, S. H., & Ho, W. K. (2012). Impaired short-term plasticity in mossy fiber synapses caused by mitochondrial dysfunction of dentate granule cells is the earliest synaptic deficit in a mouse model of Alzheimer's disease. *Journal of Neuroscience*, *32*, 5953–5963.

Lilamand, M., Porte, B., Cognat, E., Hugon, J., Mouton-Liger, F., & Paquet, C. (2020). Are ketogenic diets promising for Alzheimer's disease? A translational review. *Alzheimer's Research & Therapy*, *12*, 42.

Lim, G. P., Yang, F., Chu, T., Chen, P., Beech, W., Teter, B., Tran, T., Ubeda, O., Ashe, K. H., Frautschy, S. A., & Cole, G. M. (2000). Ibuprofen suppresses plaque pathology and inflammation in a mouse model for Alzheimer's disease. *Journal of Neuroscience*, *20*, 5709–5714.

Lu, M., Sarruf, D. A., Talukdar, S., Sharma, S., Li, P., Bandyopadhyay, G., Nalbandian, S., Fan, W., Gayen, J. R., Mahata, S. K., Webster, N. J., Schwartz, M. W., & Olefsky, J. M. (2011). Brain PPAR-γ promotes obesity and is required for the insulin-sensitizing effect of thiazolidinediones. *Nature Medicine*, *17*, 618–622.

Lu, J., Wu, D. M., Zheng, Y. L., Hu, B., Cheng, W., Zhang, Z. F., & Li, M. Q. (2013). Troxerutin counteracts domoic acid-induced memory deficits in mice by inhibiting CCAAT/enhancer binding protein beta-mediated inflammatory response and oxidative stress. *Journal of Immunology*, *190*, 3466–3479.

Lucchi, C., Costa, A. M., Giordano, C., Curia, G., Piat, M., Leo, G., Vinet, J., Brunel, L., Fehrentz, J. A., Martinez, J., Torsello, A., & Biagini, G. (2017). Involvement of PPARγ in the anticonvulsant activity of EP-80317, a ghrelin receptor antagonist. *Frontiers in Pharmacology*, *8*, 676. https://doi.org/10.3389/fphar.2017.00676

Luna-Medina, R., Cortes-Canteli, M., Sanchez-Galiano, S., Morales-Garcia, J. A., Martinez, A., Santos, A., & Perez-Castillo, A. (2007). NP031112, a thiadiazolidinone compound, prevents inflammation and neurodegeneration under excitotoxic conditions: Potential therapeutic role in brain disorders. *Journal of Neuroscience*, *27*, 5766–5776.

Maguire, J., & Salpekar, J. A. (2013). Stress, seizures, and hypothalamic-pituitary-adrenal axis targets for the treatment of epilepsy. *Epilepsy & Behavior*, *26*, 352–362.

Malapaka, R. R., Khoo, S., Zhang, J., Choi, J. H., Zhou, X. E., Xu, Y., Gong, Y., Li, J., Yong, E. L., Chalmers, M. J., Chang, L., Resau, J. H., Griffin, P. R., Chen, Y. E., & Xu, H. E. (2012). Identification and mechanism of 10-carbon fatty acid as modulating ligand of peroxisome proliferator-activated receptors. *Journal of Biological Chemistry*, *287*, 183–195.

Malthankar-Phatak, G. H., de Lanerolle, N., Eid, T., Spencer, D. D., Behar, K. L., Spencer, S. S., Kim, J. H., & Lai, J. C. (2006). Differential glutamate dehydrogenase (GDH) activity profile in patients with temporal lobe epilepsy. *Epilepsia*, *47*, 1292–1299.

Mandrekar-Colucci, S., & Landreth, G. E. (2011). Nuclear receptors as therapeutic targets for Alzheimer's disease. *Expert Opinion on Therapeutic Targets*, *15*, 1085–1097.

Mandrekar-Colucci, S., Sauerbeck, A., Popovich, P. G., & McTigue, D. M. (2013). PPAR agonists as therapeutics for CNS trauma and neurological diseases. *ASN Neuro*, *5*, e00129.

Masino, S. A., & Rho, J. M. (2012). Mechanisms of ketogenic diet action. In J. L. Noebels, M. Avoli, M. A. Rogawski, R. W. Olsen, & A. V. Delgado-Escueta (Eds.), *Jasper's basic mechanisms of the epilepsies* (4th ed.). National Center for Biotechnology Information.

Maurois, P., Rocchi, S., Pages, N., Bac, P., Stables, J. P., Gressens, P., & Vamecq, J. (2008). The PPARγ agonist FMOC-L-leucine protects both mature and immature brain. *Biomedicine & Pharmacotherapy, 62,* 259–63.

Medina-Gomez, G., Gray, S. L., Yetukuri, L., Shimomura, K., Virtue, S., Campbell, M., Curtis, R. K., Jimenez-Linan, M., Blount, M., Yeo, G. S., Lopez, M., Seppänen-Laakso, T., Ashcroft, F. M., Oresic, M., & Vidal-Puig, A. (2007a). PPAR gamma 2 prevents lipotoxicity by controlling adipose tissue expandability and peripheral lipid metabolism. *PLOS Genetics, 3,* Article e64.

Medina-Gomez, G., Gray, S., & Vidal-Puig, A. (2007b). Adipogenesis and lipotoxicity: Role of peroxisome proliferator-activated receptor gamma (PPARγ) and PPARγcoactivator-1 (PGC1). *Public Health Nutrition,10,* 1132–1137.

Miglio, G., Rosa, A. C., Rattazzi, L., Collino, M., Lombardi, G., & Fantozzi, R. (2009). PPARγ stimulation promotes mitochondrial biogenesis and prevents glucose deprivation-induced neuronal cell loss. *Neurochemistry International, 55,* 496–504.

Milder, J. B., Liang, L. P., & Patel, M. (2010). Acute oxidative stress and systemic Nrf2 activation by the ketogenic diet. *Neurobiology of Disease, 40,* 238–244.

Moreno, S., Farioli-Vecchioli, S., & Cerù, M. P. (2004). Immunolocalization of peroxisome proliferator-activated receptors and retinoid X receptors in the adult rat CNS. *Neuroscience, 123,* 131–145.

Mueller, S. G., Kollias, S. S., Trabesinger, A. H., Buck, A., Boesiger, P., & Wieser, H. G. (2001). Proton magnetic resonance spectroscopy characteristics of a focal cortical dysgenesis during status epilepticus and in the interictal state. *Seizure, 10,* 518–524.

Okada, K., Yamashita, U., & Tsuji, S. (2006). Ameliorative effect of pioglitazone on seizure responses in genetically epilepsy-susceptible EL mice. *Brain Research, 1102,* 175–178.

Overington, J. P., Al-Lazikani, B., & Hopkins, A. L. (2006) How many drug targets are there? *Nature Reviews Drug Discovery, 5,* 993–996.

Peng, J., Wang, K., Xiang, W., Li, Y., Hao, Y., & Guan, Y. (2019). Rosiglitazone polarizes microglia and protects against pilocarpine-induced status epilepticus. *CNS Neuroscience & Therapeutics, 25,* 1363–1372.

Porta, N., Vallee, L., Lecointe, C., Bouchaert, E., Staels, B., Bordet, R., & Auvin, S. (2009). Fenofibrate, a peroxisome proliferator-activated receptor-α agonist, exerts anticonvulsive properties. *Epilepsia, 50,* 943–948.

Puigserver, P., Adelmant, G., Wu, Z., Fan, M., Xu, J., O'Malley, B., & Spiegelman, B. (1999). Activation of PPARγ coactivator-1 through transcription factor docking. *Science, 286,* 1368–1371.

Puligheddu, M., Pillolla, G., Melis, M., Lecca, S., Marrosu, F., De Montis, M. G., Scheggi, S., Carta, G., Murru, E., Aroni, S., Muntoni, A. L., & Pistis, M. (2013). PPAR-alpha agonists as novel antiepileptic drugs: Preclinical findings. *PLOS ONE, 8,* Article e64541.

Quintanilla, R. A., Godoy, J. A., Alfaro, I., Cabezas, D., von Bernhardi, R., Bronfman, M., & Inestrosa, N. C. (2013). Thiazolidinediones promote axonal growth through the activation of the JNK pathway. *PLOS ONE, 8,* Article e65140.

Quintanilla, R. A., Utreras, E., & Cabezas-Opazo, F. A. (2014). Role of PPAR γ in the differentiation and function of neurons. *PPAR Research.* vol. 2014, Article ID 768594, 9 pages. https://doi.org/10.1155/2014/768594

Rho, J. M., Kim, D. W., Robbins, C. A., Anderson, G. D., & Schwartzkroin, P. A. (1999). Age-dependent differences in flurothyl seizure sensitivity in mice treated with a ketogenic diet. *Epilepsy Research, 37,* 233–240.

Ryan, K., Backos, D. S., Reigan, P., & Patel, M. (2012). Post-translational oxidative modification and inactivation of mitochondrial complex I in epileptogenesis. *Journal of Neuroscience, 32,* 11250–11258.

San, Y. Z., Liu, Y., Zhang, Y., Shi, P. P., & Zhu, Y. L. (2015) Peroxisome proliferator-activated receptor-γ agonist inhibits the mammalian target of rapamycin signaling pathway and has a protective effect in a rat model of status epilepticus. *Molecular Medicine Reports, 12,* 1877–1883.

Sarruf, D. A., Yu, F., Nguyen, H. T., Williams, D. L., Printz, R. L., Niswender, K. D., & Schwartz, M. W. (2009). Expression of peroxisome proliferator-activated receptor-gamma in key neuronal subsets regulating glucose metabolism and energy homeostasis. *Endocrinology, 150,* 707–712.

Sauer, S. (2015). Ligands for the nuclear peroxisome proliferator-activated receptor gamma. *Trends in Pharmacological Sciences, 36,* 688–704.

Schrader, M., Costello, J. L., Godinho, L. F., Azadi, A. S., & Islinger, M. (2015). Proliferation and fission of peroxisomes—An update. *Biochimica et Biophysica Acta, 1863*(5), 971–983. https://doi.org/10.1016/j.bbamcr.2015.09.024

Shao, D., Rangwala, S. M., Bailey, S. T., Krakow, S. L., Reginato, M. J., & Lazar, M. A. (1998). Interdomain communication regulating ligand binding by PPARγ. *Nature, 396,* 377–380.

Shen, Y., Lu, Y., Yu, F., Zhu, C., Wang, H., & Wang, J. (2015). Peroxisome proliferator-activated receptor-γ and its ligands in the treatment of tumors in the nervous system. *Current Stem Cell*

Research & Therapy, 11(3), 208–215. https://doi.org/10.2174/1574888X10666150728122034

Simeone, K. A., Matthews, S. A., Samson, K. K., & Simeone, T. A. (2014a). Targeting deficiencies in mitochondrial respiratory complex I and functional uncoupling exerts anti-seizure effects in a genetic model of temporal lobe epilepsy and in a model of acute temporal lobe seizures. *Experimental Neurology, 251*, 84–90.

Simeone, T. A., Matthews S. A., & Simeone K. A. (2015). [Unpublished raw data]. Creighton University.

Simeone, T. A., Matthews, S. A., Samson, K. K., & Simeone, K. A. (2017b). Regulation of brain PPARγ2 contributes to ketogenic diet anti-seizure efficacy. *Experimental Neurology, 287*(Part 1), 54–64.

Simeone, T. A., Matthews, S. A., & Simeone, K.A. (2017a). Synergistic protection against acute flurothyl-induced seizures by adjuvant treatment of the ketogenic diet with the type 2 diabetes drug pioglitazone. *Epilepsia, 58*, 1440–1450.

Simeone, T. A., Samson, K. K., Matthews, S. A., & Simeone, K. A. (2014b). *In vivo* ketogenic diet treatment attenuates pathologic sharp waves and high frequency oscillations in *in vitro* hippocampal slices from epileptic *Kv1.1α* knockout mice. *Epilepsia, 55*, e44–e49.

Simeone, T. A., Simeone, K. A., Samson, K. K., Kim, D. Y., & Rho, J. M. (2013). Loss of the Kv1.1 potassium channel promotes pathologic sharp waves and high frequency oscillations in *in vitro* hippocampal slices. *Neurobiology of Disease, 54*, 68–81.

Smart, S. L., Lopantsev, V., Zhang, C. L., Robbins, C. A., Wang, H., Chiu, S. Y., Schwartzkroin, P. A., Messing, A., & Tempel, B. L. (1998). Deletion of the K(V)1.1 potassium channel causes epilepsy in mice. *Neuron, 20*, 809–819.

Steger, D. J., Grant, G. R., Schupp, M., Tomaru, T., Lefterova, M. I., Schug, J., Manduchi, E., Stoeckert, C. J., Jr., & Lazar, M. A. (2010). Propagation of adipogenic signals through an epigenomic transition state. *Genes & Development, 24*, 1035–1044.

St-Pierre, J., Drori, S., Uldry, M., Silvaggi, J. M., Rhee, J., Jäger, S., Handschin, C., Zheng, K., Lin, J., Yang, W., Simon, D. K., Bachoo, R., & Spiegelman, B. M. (2006). Suppression of reactive oxygen species and neurodegeneration by the PGC-1 transcriptional coactivators. *Cell, 127*, 397–408.

Sudha, K., Rao, A. V., & Rao, A. (2001). Oxidative stress and antioxidants in epilepsy. *Clinica Chimica Acta, 303*, 19–24.

Sugii, S., & Evans, R. M. (2011). Epigenetic codes of PPARγ in metabolic disease. *FEBS Letters, 585*, 2121–2128.

Sullivan, P. G., Dube, C., Dorenbos, K., Steward, O., & Baram, T. Z. (2003). Mitochondrial uncoupling protein-2 protects the immature brain from excitotoxic neuronal death. *Annals of Neurology, 53*, 711–717.

Sullivan, P. G., Rippy, N. A., Dorenbos, K., Concepcion, R. C., Agarwal, A. K., & Rho, J. M. (2004). The ketogenic diet increases mitochondrial uncoupling protein levels and activity. *Annals of Neurology, 55*, 576–580.

Sundararajan, S., Gamboa, J. L., Victor, N. A., Wanderi, E. W., Lust, W. D., & Landreth, G. E. (2005). Peroxisome proliferator-activated receptor-gamma ligands reduce inflammation and infarction size in transient focal ischemia. *Neuroscience, 130*, 685–696.

Takahashi, S., Iizumi, T., Mashima, K., Abe, T., & Suzuki, N. (2014). Roles and regulation of ketogenesis in cultured astroglia and neurons under hypoxia and hypoglycemia. *ASN Neuro, 6*(5), 1759091414550997. https://doi.org/10.1177/1759091414550997

Tan, C., Liu, X., Peng, W., Wang, H., Zhou, W., Jiang, J., Wei, X., Mo, L., Chen, Y., & Chen, L. (2020). Seizure-induced impairment in neuronal ketogenesis: Role of zinc-α2-glycoprotein in mitochondria. *Journal of Cellular and Molecular Medicine, 24*(12), 6833–6845. https://doi.org/10.1111/jcmm.15337

Tan, K. N., Carrasco-Pozo, C., McDonald, T. S., Puchowicz, M., & Borges, K. (2017). Tridecanoin is anticonvulsant, antioxidant, and improves mitochondrial function. *Journal of Cerebral Blood Flow and Metabolism, 37*, 2035–2048.

Tan, Y., Muise, E. S., Dai, H., Raubertas, R., Wong, K. K., Thompson, G. M., Wood, H. B., Meinke, P. T., Lum, P. Y., Thompson, J. R., & Berger, J. P. (2012). Novel transcriptome profiling analyses demonstrate that selective peroxisome proliferator-activated receptor γ (PPARγ) modulators display attenuated and selective gene regulatory activity in comparison with PPARγ full agonists. *Molecular Pharmacology, 82*, 68–79.

Thouennon, E., Cheng, Y., Falahatian, V., Cawley, N. X., & Loh, Y. P. (2015). Rosiglitazone-activated PPARγ induces neurotrophic factor-α1 transcription contributing to neuroprotection. *Journal of Neurochemistry, 134*, 463–470.

Tontonoz, P., Hu, E., Graves, R. A., Budavari, A. I., & Spiegelman, B. M. (1994). mPPAR gamma 2: Tissue-specific regulator of an adipocyte enhancer. *Genes & Development, 8*, 1224–1234.

Tontonoz, P., & Spiegelman, B. M. (2008). Fat and beyond: The diverse biology of PPARγ. *Annual Review of Biochemistry, 77*, 289–312.

Victor, N. A., Wanderi, E. W., Gamboa, J., Zhao, X., Aronowski, J., Deininger, K., Lust, W. D., Landreth, G. E., & Sundararajan, S. (2006). Altered PPARγ expression and activation after transient focal ischemia in rats. *European Journal of Neuroscience, 24*, 1653–1663.

Vidal-Puig, A., Jimenez-Liñan, M., Lowell, B. B., Hamann, A., Hu, E., Spiegelman, B., Flier, J. S., & Moller, D. E. (1996). Regulation of PPAR gamma gene expression by nutrition and obesity in rodents. *Journal of Clinical Investigation, 97,* 2553–2561.

Vidal-Puig, A. J., Considine, R. V., Jimenez-Liñan, M., Werman, A., Pories, W. J., Caro, J. F., & Flier, J. S. (1997). Peroxisome proliferator-activated receptor gene expression in human tissues. Effects of obesity, weight loss, and regulation by insulin and glucocorticoids. *Journal of Clinical Investigation, 99,* 2416–2422.

Vielhaber, S., Niessen, H. G., Debska-Vielhaber, G., Kudin, A. P., Wellmer, J., Kaufmann, J., Schönfeld, M. A., Fendrich, R., Willker, W., Leibfritz, D., Schramm, J., Elger, C. E., Heinze, H. J., & Kunz, W. S. (2008). Subfield-specific loss of hippocampal N-acetyl aspartate in temporal lobe epilepsy. *Epilepsia, 49,* 40–50.

Wada, K., Nakajima, A., Katayama, K., Kudo, C., Shibuya, A., Kubota, N., Terauchi, Y., Tachibana, M., Miyoshi, H., Kamisaki, Y., Mayumi, T., Kadowaki, T., & Blumberg, R. S. (2006). Peroxisome proliferator-activated receptor gamma-mediated regulation of neural stem cell proliferation and differentiation. *Journal of Biological Chemistry, 281,* 12673–12681.

Wallace, D. C. (1999). Mitochondrial diseases in man and mouse. *Science, 283,* 1482–1488.

Wang, H., Jiang, R., He, Q., Zhang, Y., Zhang, Y., Li, Y., Zhuang, R., Luo, Y., Li, Y., Wan, J., Tang, Y., Yu, H., Jiang, Q., & Yang, J. (2012). Expression pattern of peroxisome proliferator-activated receptors in rat hippocampus following cerebral ischemia and reperfusion injury. *PPAR Research.* vol. 2012, Article ID 596394, 10 pages. https://doi.org/10.1155/2012/596394

Wenzel, H. J., Vacher, H., Clark, E., Trimmer, J. S., Lee, A. L., Sapolsky, R. M., Tempel, B. L., & Schwartzkroin, P. A. (2007). Structural consequences of *Kcna1* gene deletion and transfer in the mouse hippocampus. *Epilepsia, 48,* 2023–2046.

Werman, A., Hollenberg, A., Solanes, G., Bjorbaek, C., Vidal-Puig, A. J., & Flier, J. S. (1997). Ligand-independent activation domain in the N terminus of peroxisome proliferator-activated receptor gamma (PPARγ). Differential activity of PPARγ1 and -2 isoforms and influence of insulin. *Journal of Biological Chemistry, 272,* 20230–20235.

Wlaź, P., Socała, K., Nieoczym, D., Żarnowski, T., Żarnowska, I., Czuczwar, S. J., & Gasior, M. (2015). Acute anticonvulsant effects of capric acid in seizure tests in mice. *Progress in Neuro-Psychopharmacology & Biological Psychiatry, 57,* 110–116.

Wong, S. B., Cheng, S. J., Hung, W. C., Lee, W. T., & Min, M. Y. (2015). Rosiglitazone suppresses in vitro seizures in hippocampal slice by inhibiting presynaptic glutamate release in a model of temporal lobe epilepsy. *PLOS ONE, 10,* Article e0144806.

Wu, J. S., Cheung, W. M., Tsai, Y. S., Chen, Y. T., Fong, W. H., Tsai, H. D., Chen, Y. C., Liou, J. Y., Shyue, S. K., Chen, J. J., Chen, Y. E., Maeda, N., Wu, K. K., & Lin, T. N. (2009a). Ligand-activated peroxisome proliferator activated receptor-gamma protects against ischemic cerebral infarction and neuronal apoptosis by 14-3-3 epsilon upregulation. *Circulation, 119,* 1124–1134.

Wu, J. S., Lin, T. N., & Wu, K. K. (2009b). Rosiglitazone and PPAR-gamma overexpression protect mitochondrial membrane potential and prevent apoptosis by upregulating anti-apoptotic Bcl-2 family proteins. *Journal of Cellular Physiology, 220,* 58–71.

Yakunin, E., Kisos, H., Kulik, W., Grigoletto, J., Wanders, R. J., & Sharon, R. (2014). The regulation of catalase activity by PPAR γ is affected by α-synuclein. *Annals of Clinical and Translational Neurology, 1,* 145–159.

Yamamoto, K., Itoh, T., Abe, D., Shimizu, M., Kanda, T., Koyama, T., Nishikawa, M., Tamai, T., Ooizumi, H., & Yamada, S. (2005). Identification of putative metabolites of docosahexaenoic acid as potent PPARγ agonists and antidiabetic agents. *Bioorganic & Medicinal Chemistry Letters, 15,* 517–522.

Yan, Q., Zhang, J., Liu, H., Babu-Khan, S., Vassar, R., Biere, A. L., Citron, M., & Landreth, G. (2003). Antiinflammatory drug therapy alters β-amyloid processing and deposition in an animal model of Alzheimer's disease. *Journal of Neuroscience, 23,* 7504–7509.

Yang, X., & Cheng, B. (2010). Neuroprotective and anti-inflammatory activities of ketogenic diet on MPTP-induced neurotoxicity. *Journal of Molecular Neuroscience, 42,* 145–153.

Youle, R. J., & Strasser, A. (2008). The Bcl-2 protein family: Opposing activities that mediate cell death. *Nature Reviews Molecular Cell Biology, 9,* 47–59

Yu, X., Shao, X. G., Sun, H., Li, Y. N., Yang, J., Deng, Y. C., & Huang, Y. G. (2008). Activation of cerebral peroxisome proliferator-activated receptors gamma exerts neuroprotection by inhibiting oxidative stress following pilocarpine-induced status epilepticus. *Brain Research, 1200,* 146–158.

Zhao, X., Strong, R., Zhang, J., Sun, G., Tsien, J. Z., Cui, Z., Grotta, J. C., & Aronowski, J. (2009). Neuronal PPARγ deficiency increases susceptibility to brain damage after cerebral ischemia. *Journal of Neuroscience, 29,* 6186–6195.

Zhao, Y., Patzer, A., Gohlke, P., Herdegen, T., & Culman, J. (2005). The intracerebral application of the PPARγ-ligand pioglitazone confers neuroprotection against focal ischaemia in the rat brain. *European Journal of Neuroscience, 22,* 278–282.

Zhao, Y., Patzer, A., Herdegen, T., Gohlke, P., & Culman, J. (2006). Activation of cerebral peroxisome proliferator-activated receptors gamma promotes neuroprotection by attenuation of neuronal cyclooxygenase-2 overexpression after focal cerebral ischemia in rats. *FASEB Journal, 20,* 1162–1175.

Zhu, Y., Alvares, K., Huang, Q., Rao, M. S., & Reddy, J. K. (1993). Cloning of a new member of the peroxisome proliferator-activated receptor gene family from mouse liver. *Journal of Biological Chemistry, 268,* 26817–26820.

Zolezzi, J. M., Bastías-Candia, S., Santos, M. J., & Inestrosa, N. C. (2014). Alzheimer's disease: Relevant molecular and physiopathological events affecting amyloid-β brain balance and the putative role of PPARs. *Frontiers in Aging Neuroscience, 6,* 176. https://doi.org/10.3389/fnagi.2014.00176

Ketogenic Diet and Adenosine in Epilepsy

Models and Mechanisms

MASAHITO KAWAMURA JR., MD, PHD

ANIMAL MODELS FOR KETOGENIC DIET RESEARCH

The ketogenic diet (KD) was developed to mimic fasting, which alleviates epileptic seizures (Wilder, 1921). KD increases ketone bodies—β-hydroxy-butyrate (βHB), acetoacetate (AA), acetone—which are synthesized from free fatty acids in the liver (Masino & Rho, 2012) and then are used for energy in the brain instead of glucose (Masino et al., 2009). In recent decades, KD has increasingly been used as a therapy for medically refractory epilepsy (Hallbook et al., 2007). Despite 100 years of the KD's clinical use, the mechanisms underlying the success of KD therapy are not fully understood. However, recent detailed studies have shown the various mechanisms of action of the KD, including ATP-sensitive potassium (K_{ATP}) channels (Ma et al., 2007), BCL-2-associated agonist of cell death (Gimenez-Cassina et al., 2012), vesicular glutamate transporters (VGLUT; Juge et al., 2010), voltage-dependent calcium channels (VDCC; Kadowaki et al., 2017), lactate dehydrogenase (LDH; Sada et al., 2015), gut microbiome (Olson et al., 2018), glucolysis (Shao et al., 2018), mitochondrial biogenesis (Bough et al., 2006), and adenosine (Kawamura et al., 2014; Masino et al., 2011). These mechanisms were found mainly by using in vivo and in vitro animal models of KD. Therefore, animal models and experiments are essential for understanding the antiseizure mechanisms of the KD in detail. To elucidate antiseizure mechanisms, behavioral measures, such as seizure score, number of seizures, and latency to seizure events, are usually characterized in vivo in animal models. Behavioral tests are not able to be used in vitro. Because epilepsy is caused by abnormal neuronal discharges in neural networks, in vitro models of the KD usually use acute brain slices or brain-slice cultures.

Electrophysiologic measurements are the most direct and useful approach for researching seizures and seizure treatments both in vivo and in vitro. In vivo electrophysiologic recording of brain is usually done by extracellular recording of electrically evoked activity (Stewart & Reid, 1993), continuous recording of spontaneous field activity (Li et al., 2008), or multiple unit activity (Lin et al., 2006); these preparations can be acute or chronic. In vitro electrophysiologic recording is done using single-cell intracellular sharp electrodes (Abe & Ogata, 1981), patch-clamp electrodes (Oyama et al., 2020), extracellular field recording with single electrodes (Kawamura et al., 2019), or electrode arrays (Knowles et al., 1987) using acute slices of brain. From using these behavioral tests and electrophysiologic recordings, several KD mechanisms were found in animal models. This chapter focuses on animal models for KD research in vivo and in vitro, reviewing adenosine-based mechanisms underlying KD that were found in the animal models.

IN VIVO ANIMAL MODELS OF KD RESEARCH

Because applying a diet therapy necessarily involves whole animals, in vivo animal models are useful for investigating KD mechanisms. The KD can be used successfully in animal models, including rodents. Rodents can be fed a KD for several weeks (Lusardi et al., 2015). Calorie and water intake with the KD are similar to intake with a normal control diet in rodents (Likhodii et al., 2000). Body weights are limited in young rodents but not in adults (Ruskin et al., 2009). The KD increases blood ketone body levels and decreases blood sugar levels, findings suggesting that the KD causes ketosis in animal models (Bough et al., 2006). Ketosis with the KD is controlled by the ketogenic ratio of fat:(protein +

carbohydrate). A higher ketogenic ratio is known to increase the ketosis level (Ruskin et al., 2017). Ketogenic ratios from 3:1 to 6.3:1 are usually used for animal models (see Table 24.1). The next step is how to cause seizures in KD-fed animals. Three seizure models have been used in KD-fed animals: (1) electrical shock-induced seizure models, (2) drug-induced seizure models, and (3) genetically modified seizure models. The KD has been reported to have antiseizure effects in all three types of seizure models (Table 24.1).

Electrical Shock-Induced Seizure Models

Electroshock is a classical method for inducing seizures in rodents. The shock is applied to the eyes or ears and the seizures are compared by threshold of electroshock intensity or duration to cause seizure behavior. Three groups reported that ~ 2 weeks feeding of KD (ketogenic ratio of 3:1 or 6:1) to mice caused suppression of electroshock-induced seizures (Hartman et al., 2008; Martillotti et al., 2006; Nakazawa et al., 1983). Interestingly, Hartman et al. showed 12 days or 16 days of KD (6.3:1 ratio) feeding increased the current intensity needed for producing seizures in 50% of mice tested with the 6-Hz seizure model, but the antiseizure effects disappeared at 21 days, suggesting a time limit for the KD's effects on electroshock-induced seizures (Hartman et al., 2008). Amygdala kindling is also a well-known electrical shock-induced seizure model for rodents, which develop spontaneous recurrent seizures and are used for investigating epileptogenesis. KD (4:1 ratio) delayed kindling-induced seizure development in mice and rats, which suggests that the KD inhibits amygdala kindling-induced epileptogenesis (Hu et al., 2011; Jiang et al., 2012).

Drug-Induced Seizure Models

Several kinds of drugs that cause seizures as adverse effects are used for animal seizure models. Pentylenetetrazole (PTZ) is a well-known drug for inducing seizures in animals. A KD (6.3:1) was reported to increase the PTZ seizure threshold in rats (Bough & Eagles, 1999; Bough et al., 2006). Flurothyl-induced seizures are also known as an animal model of epilepsy. A KD (4.3:1 or 6.3:1 ratio) increased the latency to flurothyl-induced generalized clonic seizures (Bough et al., 2006; Rho et al., 1999). A small number of drugs, such as kainic acid, are known to cause spontaneous recurrent seizures. A KD (4.3:1 or 5:1 ratio) was

reported to reduce kainic acid-induced spontaneous recurrent seizures in both mice and rats (Kwon et al., 2008; Muller-Schwarze et al., 1999; Su et al., 2000). Like amygdala kindling, PTZ kindling is used for investigating epileptogenesis. A KD (6.3:1 ratio) suppressed PTZ kindling-induced seizure development (Lusardi et al., 2015). Interestingly, the suppression was maintained until 4 days after reversal of the KD. Pilocarpine is also used as a clinically relevant model of progressive epilepsy. A KD (6.3:1 ratio) reduced progression of seizures in pilocarpine-induced epileptic rats, and the suppression persisted until 8 weeks after KD reversal (Lusardi et al., 2015). These results suggest that the KD prevents epileptogenesis in PTZ-kindling and pilocarpine-induced animal models.

Genetically Modified Seizure Models

Genetically modified animals (mainly mice) are also used for KD research. The rationale for using genetically modified models is that all the animals exhibit spontaneous seizures. The EL/Suz mouse was discovered in an outbred DDY mouse colony and is used as a model of multifactorial idiopathic epilepsy. Seizure susceptibility in EL/Suz mice is known to be age-dependent, and the KD (4.75:1 ratio) increases the age of onset of seizures (Todorova et al., 2000). Interestingly, Mantis et al. reported that calorie restriction to achieve a 15% to 18% body weight reduction combined with a KD (4.1 ratio) enhanced antiseizure effects in EL/Suz mice (Mantis et al., 2014). Calorie restriction increased ketosis and hypoglycemia in KD-fed EL/Suz mice, and glucose application attenuated the enhancement of the antiseizure effect, suggesting that calorie restriction promotes the shift from glucose-based to ketone body-based metabolism (Mantis et al., 2014). The *Kcna1*-null mouse (C3HeB/FeJ background) lacks voltage-gated potassium (Kv 1.1) channels and is thought to be a model for several types of epilepsy, including human temporal lobe epilepsy. A KD (6.3:1 ratio) reduced the number of daily seizures in *Kcna1*-null mice (Kim do et al., 2015). Adenosine kinase transgenic (ADK-Tg) mice overexpressing the ADK target gene have electrographic hippocampal seizures consistent with decreased extracellular adenosine levels. A KD (6.3:1 ratio) reduced the frequency and duration of electrographic seizures in these mice (Masino et al., 2011).

Exogenous Ketone Body Application

Chronic ketosis is a hallmark of the KD. Therefore, one approach for reproducing a KD is direct

TABLE 24.1 IN VIVO ANIMAL MODELS OF KETOGENIC DIET

Electroshock-induced seizure models

Reference	Animal	Manipulation	Seizure	Effect
Nakazawa et al., 1983	DDY mouse	KD (3:1 ratio) for 2 weeks	Electroshock via cornea electrode	Increasing the electroconvulsive threshold
Martillotti et al., 2006	C57BL/6 mouse	KD (6:1 ratio) for 2 weeks	Electroshock via ear-clip electrode	Reducing the duration of hindlimb extension
Hartman et al., 2008	NIH Swiss mouse	KD (6.3:1 ratio) for 2–21 days	6-Hz seizure via cornea electrode	Increasing current intensity producing seizures in 50% of mice tested
Hu et al., 2011	C57BL/6 background mouse	KD (4.3:1 ratio) for 2 weeks	Amygdala kindling	Delaying kindling development
Jiang et al., 2012	SD rat	KD (4:1 ratio) for 28–48 days	Amygdala kindling	Delaying kindling development

Drug-induced seizure models

Reference	Animal	Manipulation	Seizure	Effect
Bough & Eagles, 1999	*SD rat*	KD (6.3:1 ratio) for 35–60 days	PTZ	Increasing seizure threshold
Bough et al., 2006	*SD rat*	KD (6.3:1 ratio) for 0–31 days	PTZ or flurothyl	Increasing seizure threshold
Rho et al., 1999	C3Heb/Fej mice	KD (4.3:1 ratio) for 3–15 days	Flurothyl	Increasing the latency to generalized clonic seizure
Muller-Schwarze et al., 1999	SD rat	KD (5:1 ratio) for 8 weeks	Kainic acid	Reducing spontaneous recurrent seizures
Su et al., 2000	SD rat	KD (5:1 ratio) for 12 weeks	Kainic acid	Reducing spontaneous recurrent seizures
Kwon et al., 2008	ICR mouse	KD (4.3:1 ratio) for 4 weeks	Kainic acid	Delaying the KA-induced seizure onset time
Lusardi et al., 2015	CD-1 mouse or Wistar rat	KD (6.3:1 ratio) for 13 (mice) or 15 (rats) weeks	PTZ kindling (mice) or pilocarpine (rats)	Delaying kindling development (rats) and reducing seizure count (mice)

Genetically modified animal models

Reference	Animal	Manipulation	Seizure	Effect
Todorova et al., 2000	EL/Suz mouse	KD (4.75:1 ratio) for 1–10 weeks	Genetic model	Delaying age at seizure onset
Mantis et al., 2014	EL/Suz mouse	KD (4:1 ratio) with calorie restriction for 9 weeks	Genetic model	Decreasing seizure susceptibility
Kim et al., 2015	*Kcna1*-null mouse	KD (6.3:1 ratio) for 3 weeks	Genetic model	Reducing mean daily seizure count
Masino et al., 2011	*Adk-Tg* mouse	KD (6.3:1 ratio) for 3–4 weeks	Genetic model	Reducing seizure frequency and duration

(continued)

TABLE 24.1 CONTINUED

Endogenous ketone body applications

D'Agostino et al., 2013	SD rat	Oral gavage of ketone ester at 30 min before test	Central nervous system O$_2$ toxicity seizures	Increasing latency to seizure
Kovács et al., 2017	Wistar Albino Glaxo/Rijswijk rat	Oral gavage of ketone ester for 7 days	Genetic model	Decreasing number of spike-wave discharges
Kadowaki et al., 2017	ICR mouse	2-phenylbutyrate (acetoacetate analog) intraperitoneal administration at 1 hr before test	Kainate applied into hippocampus	Reducing number and total duration of paroxysmal discharges
Kim et al., 2015	*Kcna1*-null mouse	βHB (5 mM) administration using subcutaneously implanted osmotic minipumps for 10–14 days	Genetic model	Reducing mean daily seizure count
Juge et al., 2010	Wistar rat	AA (10 mM) administration into hippocampus directly for 4 hr	4-AP applied into hippocampus	Reducing total seizure severity score

Note. AA = acetoacetate, βHB = β-hydroxybutyrate, ICR mouse = Institute for Cancer Research mouse, KD = ketogenic diet, PTZ = pentylenetetrazole, SD rat = Sprague–Dawley rat.

application of ketone bodies. Exogenous ketone body application works successfully in vivo in animal models. Kim et al. applied βHB directly into the brains of *Kcna1*-null mice via subcutaneously implanted osmotic minipumps, and they reported that administration of this ketone body reduced the number of seizures (Kim do et al., 2015). Juge et al. also reported that seizures in Wistar rats induced by intrahippocampal 4-aminopyridine were moderated by intrahippocampal 10 mM AA, both infused by microdialysis (Juge et al., 2010). Obviously, it is difficult to use direct brain administration in patients. Moreover, oral administration of free acid forms of βHB or AA is ineffective in causing ketosis (D'Agostino et al., 2013). Oral administration of ketone esters and intraperitoneal administration of analogs of ketone bodies were also investigated. Ketone esters are reported to induce a rapid and sustained ketosis (Brunengraber, 1997; Desrochers et al., 1995). Oral administration of ketone esters once, 40 min before oxygen toxicity seizures, increased latency to seizure events (D'Agostino et al., 2013). Ketone ester gavage daily for 7 days also reduced the number of electrographic seizure events in a genetically modified animal model, Wistar Albino Glaxo/Rijswijk rats (Kovacs et al., 2017). These reports suggest gavage application of ketone esters can be used successfully to suppress seizures in animal models. An analog of AA (2-phenylbutyrate) is another possibility for direct ketone body application. Kadowaki et al. reported 2-phenylbutyrate administered intraperitoneally crossed the blood–brain barrier and reduced the number of kainate-induced seizure events (Kadowaki et al., 2017).

IN VITRO MODELS IN KD RESEARCH

Several in vivo studies elucidated the anticonvulsant effects of the KD. On the other hand, more detailed investigations are required for understanding the antiseizure mechanisms of the KD at the molecular level. Therefore, in vitro models are useful for detailed experiments. Studies of in vitro animal models were done mainly by using hippocampal slice preparations. The advantages of using hippocampal slices for in vitro studies are several. First, the hippocampus is the key region underlying mesial temporal lobe epilepsy, so hippocampal slices can serve as a model of temporal lobe epilepsy. In a majority of patients, mesial temporal lobe epilepsies are associated with hippocampal sclerosis (Watson, 2003), which is atrophy combined with global gliosis

and loss of CA1 and/or CA3 pyramidal neurons in the hippocampus (Thom, 2009). The structure of the hippocampus is simple. It includes principal cells (granular cells of dentate gyrus and CA1-4 pyramidal neurons) and surrounding interneurons. The principal cells form an excitatory circuit that is modulated by inhibitory interneurons. Interestingly, CA3 pyramidal neurons are connected to each other by excitatory recurrent collaterals. Thus, the hippocampal circuit is regulated by a balance between excitation from recurrent collaterals and inhibition from interneurons. When the balance collapses, the hippocampal circuit becomes hyperexcitable and causes seizures easily. Therefore, the atrophy in the hippocampus is thought to be one of the main focuses of mesial temporal lobe epilepsy, and excision of hippocampal sclerosis with selective amygdalohippocampectomy successfully improves ~ 70% of surgical patients (Paglioli et al., 2006; Wiebe et al., 2001). Therefore, the hippocampus is thought be a good experimental target for investigating epileptogenesis and therapy for temporal lobe epilepsy (Kawamura et al., 2016). Second, hippocampal slices have demonstrated ease of use. Acute brain slices must be maintained by perfusion with oxygenated artificial cerebrospinal fluid (Sakmann et al., 1989), and continuous perfusion allows the extracellular fluid to be changed easily. Thus, it is easy to apply and wash out several agonists and/or antagonists of various proteins, such as channels, receptors, and transporters, and it is easy to examine the detail of functional mechanisms of neuronal activities at the molecular level. Third, we usually make 3 to 6 brain slices from one rodent and get 3 to 6 recordings from them, allowing us to reduce the number of animals used. Last, a huge number of electrophysiologic experiments have been done using hippocampal slice preparations in the last half-century. Several methods for causing seizure-like bursts in vitro have been used in the hippocampal slice preparation, including kindling (Sayin et al., 1999), kainic acid treatment (Congar et al., 2000; Smith & Dudek, 2001), inhibition of GABA receptors (Kohling et al., 2000; Stafstrom et al., 2009), inhibition of potassium ion channels (Stafstrom et al., 2009), and neuronal hyperexcitability due to changing extracellular ion concentrations (Congar et al., 2000; Dulla et al., 2005; Kojima et al., 1989; Stafstrom et al., 2009). All these approaches support the use of hippocampal slice preparations to elucidate epileptic mechanisms. The major difficulty in using acute hippocampal slices for KD research is the

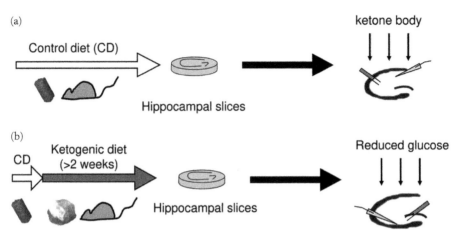

FIGURE 24.1 *Approaches for Reproducing the Conditions of Ketogenic Diet Feeding in Hippocampal Slices*
(a) The first approach is the direct application of ketone bodies to hippocampal slices from control diet-fed animals.
(b) The second approach is recording hippocampal slices made from ketogenic diet-fed animals. Extracellular glucose
is reduced during incubation and recording to maintain the in vivo effect of the ketogenic diet.

inability to precisely reproduce or maintain the condition of diet therapy in the in vitro preparation. In vivo recording clearly does not have this problem, because it uses the whole body of the laboratory animal and diet-altered metabolism is maintained (Table 24.1). Therefore, special strategies must be implemented for examining mechanisms of the KD using hippocampal slice preparations (Figure 24.1).

Direct Application of Ketone Bodies

The first approach for reproducing KD conditions in hippocampal slices is direct application of ketone bodies, similar to application of ketone esters or ketone body analogs in vivo. In this paradigm, hippocampal slices are taken from control diet-fed animals and dissolved ketone bodies are applied in an extracellular solution, such as artificial cerebrospinal fluid (Figure 24.1a). However, results of direct application of ketone bodies in hippocampal slices are contradictory.

Thio et al. reported that direct application of ketone bodies had no effect on synaptic activity in acute hippocampal slices from Sprague-Dawley (SD) rats. They recorded evoked field excitatory postsynaptic potentials (fEPSP) and population spikes (PS) in the CA1 region stimulated by Schaffer collateral fibers and applied mixed ketone bodies (1 mM AA and 2 mM βHB) to the slices (Thio et al., 2000). A 20-min application of ketone bodies did not change either fEPSP slope or PS amplitude. The investigators also recorded the potassium channel blocker 4-aminopyridine-induced epileptiform discharge

from the dentate granule cell layer and CA3 region and reported that application of ketone bodies for 105 min did not change the frequency or duration of the ictal events. Kimura et al. also reported that application of mixed ketone bodies (1 mM each AA and βHB) for 20 min did not change fEPSP slope, and an 80-min application did not change the high-frequency tetanic stimulation-induced long-term potentiation (LTP) recorded from the CA1 region in acute hippocampal slices from Wistar rats (Kimura et al., 2012). Similar results were reported that mixed ketone bodies (1 mM AA and 2 mM βHB) had no effect on CA1 region synaptic transmission or theta burst-induced LTP in SD rat acute hippocampal slices (Youssef, 2015). A unique approach was used by Samoilova et al. (2010). They made organotypic hippocampal slices, which were cultured with low-glucose and 10-mM βHB medium for at least 3 days. This chronic in vitro ketosis, however, did not alleviate intrinsic or induced epileptiform discharges (but it was neuroprotective). All these studies concluded that ketone bodies do not directly affect synaptic transmission in the rat hippocampus.

Other studies, however, have found positive results. Juge et al. (2010) made acute hippocampal slices from C57Bl/6 mice and incubated the slices with 10-mM AA for over 2 hr, after which they recorded EPSPs from CA1 pyramidal neurons using the whole-cell patch-clamp technique. The frequency and amplitude of miniature EPSPs (mEPSP) from AA-incubated slices were significantly reduced compared to those in control slices. Ketone bodies inhibited valinomycin-evoked glutamate uptake by purified VGLUT, suggesting that ketone bodies inhibit synaptic transmission, with reduction of glutamate release via direct ketone body-induced suppression of glutamate uptake into vesicles. Juge and colleagues also reported that in vivo direct application of AA into hippocampus reduced seizure behaviors (Table 24.1). These results clearly show that direct application of ketone bodies modulates synaptic transmission in hippocampal slices and reduces seizure activity in vivo (Juge et al., 2010). In addition, Kadowaki et al. reported 15-min application of 10-mM AA or AA analog (2-phenylbutyrate) inhibited the VDCCs of CA1 pyramidal neurons in acute hippocampal slices in ICR mice (Kadowaki et al., 2017). Moreover, 10-mM 2-phenylbutyrate decreased the amplitude of Schaffer collateral-evoked EPSPs of CA1 pyramidal neurons (Kadowaki et al., 2017). The same group reported that direct administration of 2.5-mM βHB caused hyperpolarization in neurons in slices from the subthalamic nucleus of the basal ganglia by inhibition of LDH in ICR mice (Sada et al., 2015). Tanner et al. recorded single-channel activity from dentate granule neurons after incubating acute hippocampal slices from C57Bl/6 mice with 2-mM βHB for over 40 min (Tanner et al., 2011). Preincubation with this ketone body increased steady-state and stimulus-elevated open probability of K_{ATP} channels, which contribute to the slow afterhyperpolarization after action potential bursts to modulate spontaneous firing, suggesting that direct ketone body-mediated opening of K_{ATP} channels in dentate granule neurons may act as a seizure gate in the hippocampus. Similar results were reported from neurons of the substantia nigra in coronal midbrain slices of rats and mice from the same laboratory (Ma et al., 2007). Kim et al. recorded from organotypic hippocampal slices that were cultured with 5-mM βHB and 1-mM AA medium for 2 weeks (Kim et al., 2015). Extracellular multielectrode array recordings showed spontaneous seizure-like events in organotypic hippocampal slice cultures from *Kcna1*-null mice. The application of ketone bodies for 2 weeks attenuated the seizure-like events generated by the mutant tissue. The authors also reported that in vivo administration of ketone bodies reduced the number of seizures (Table 24.1).

In sum, several studies have used direct application of ketone bodies in hippocampal acute slices or organotypic cultures, and both positive and negative results have been found (Table 24.2). Negative and positive studies used rats and mice, respectively, so a simple explanation is that the discrepancy arises from species differences. However, this is unlikely because KD or direct in vivo application of ketone bodies is known to reduce behavioral seizures in both rats and mice (Table 24.1). The methods for applying ketone bodies varied in these reports, including concentration of ketone bodies, time of application, and application pathway (perfusion or preincubation), and these factors might contribute to interstudy variation. Using similar protocols for direct application of ketone bodies would be useful for finding common mechanisms.

Acute Hippocampal Slices from KD-Fed Animals

A second approach is possibly the most direct and useful way for investigating mechanisms of KD because it uses acute hippocampal slices from KD-fed animals (Figure 24.1b, Table 24.2). The question about this approach is whether the intra- and extracellular milieu produced by KD feeding can be maintained after making and incubating brain slices. However, four reports show that it can work successfully. Stafstrom et al. (1999) reported that a KD (4.8:1 ratio) induced antiseizure effects in acute hippocampal slices from kainic acid-treated rats. The authors recorded fEPSP and PS from area CA1 from SD rats fed a KD for 6 to 8 weeks. Synaptic transmission was not significantly different between slices from control rats and KD-fed rats. The frequency of kainic acid-induced spontaneous seizures was significantly lower in slices from KD-fed rats than from control diet-fed rats. Similar results were reported by Simeone et al. (2014) using extracellular multielectrode array recordings in acute hippocampal slices from KD-fed *Kcna1*-null mice. The pathologic seizure-like events generated in *Kcna1*-null slices were diminished by KD treatment (6.3:1 ratio) for 11 to 15 days. However, mossy fiber-CA3 dendritic field potential slopes and fiber volley amplitudes of mossy fiber are not significantly different between slices from control diet-fed and KD-fed *Kcna1*-null mice (Simeone et al., 2014). Bough et al. (2006) recorded medial perforant pathway-evoked fEPSPs from the dentate molecular layer in acute hippocampal slices from SD rats fed a KD (6.3:1 ratio) for over 20 days. Reducing extracellular glucose concentration from 10 mM to 2 mM depressed the slope of fEPSPs reversibly in slices from control diet-fed

TABLE 24.2 IN VITRO ANIMAL MODELS OF KETONE BODIES

Direct application of ketone bodies

Reference	Animal	Manipulation	Recording	Effect
Thio et al., 2000	SD rat	1 mM AA and 2 mM βHB for 20 min	fEPSP and PS recordings	No change
Kimura et al., 2012	Wistar rat	1 mM AA and 1 mM βHB for 20 min	fEPSP recording	No change
Youssef, 2015	SD rat	1 mM AA and 2 mM βHB	fEPSP recording	No change
Samoilova et al., 2010	Wistar rat	10 mM βHB for 3 days (slice culture)	PS recording	No change
Juge et al., 2010	C57BL/6 mouse	10 mM AA for 2 hr	Whole-cell patch clamp recording	Reducing frequency and amplitude of mEPSC in CA1 pyramidal neurons
Tanner et al., 2011	C57BL/6 mouse	2 mM βHB for 40 min	Single channel recording	Increasing open probability of K$_{ATP}$ channels in granule cells
Kim et al., 2015	Kcna1-null mouse	5 mM βHB and 1 mM AA for 2 weeks (slice culture)	Multielectrode recordings	Reducing spontaneous seizure-like events
Kadowaki et al., 2017	ICR mouse	10 mM AA or 10 mM 2-phenylbutyrate for 15 min	Whole-cell patch clamp recording	Inhibiting VDCC and EPSP in CA1 pyramidal neurons

Acute hippocampal slices from KD-fed animals

Reference	Animal	Manipulation	Recording	Effect
Stafstrom et al., 1999	SD rat	KD (4.8:1 ratio) for 6–8 weeks	fEPSP and PS recordings	Reducing spontaneous seizure-like events
Simeone et al., 2015	Kcna1-null mouse	KD (6.3:1 ratio) for 11–15 days	Multielectrode recordings	Reducing spontaneous seizure-like events
Bough et al., 2006	SD rat	KD (6.3:1 ratio) for 20 days	fEPSP recording	Inhibiting reduced glucose-induced depression
Kawamura et al., 2014	SD rat and C57BL/6 mouse	KD (6.3:1 ratio) for 13–18 days	PS recording	Reducing evoked seizure-like bursting

Note. AA = acetoacetate, βHB = β-hydroxybutyrate, fEPSP = field excitatory postsynaptic potentials, ICR mouse = Institute for Cancer Research mouse, K$_{ATP}$ channels = ATP-sensitive potassium channels, KD = ketogenic diet, mEPSC = miniature excitatory postsynaptic currents, PS = population spikes, SD rat = Sprague–Dawley rat, VDCC, voltage-dependent calcium channels.

rats and this depression was inhibited in slices from KD-fed rats. The effects were lost after slices were incubated in 10-mM glucose for over 3.5 hr. The investigators concluded that synaptic transmission in hippocampal slices from KD-fed rats was more resistant to reduced glucose than that in slices from control diet-fed rats (Bough et al., 2006). Kawamura et al. (2014) also reported that a KD had antiseizure effects in acute hippocampal slices from rats and mice. They recorded PS and GABA receptor blocker bicuculline-induced seizure-like bursts in the CA3 region in acute hippocampal slices from SD rats or C57BL/6 mice fed a KD (6.3:1 ratio) for 13 to 18 days. Excitability and bicuculline-induced bursts were significantly inhibited by reduced extracellular glucose concentration in slices from KD-fed rats and mice but were not changed by reduced extracellular glucose in slices from control diet-fed rodents. These four studies successfully used acute hippocampal slices from KD-fed rodents to elucidate the changes in neuronal activities underlying the treatment. Interestingly, the reduced extracellular glucose concentration is thought be one of the most important points for reproducing the effects of a KD in this approach. It is well known that the KD causes a stable, mild hypoglycemia in humans (Huttenlocher, 1976) and rodents (Bough et al., 2006). Moreover, plasma glucose level correlates with the antiepileptic effect of the KD (Mantis et al., 2004), and endogenous administration of glucose reverses KD-induced antiseizure effects (Mantis et al., 2014; Masino et al., 2011), indicating that extracellular glucose is mechanistically relevant. Synaptic transmission in hippocampal slices from KD-fed rodents was not different from that in slices from control diet-fed rodents when extracellular glucose concentration in artificial cerebrospinal fluid was standard in all three reports; however, evidence is mounting that the standard glucose concentration for acute brain slices is higher than physiologic brain glucose levels (Kealy et al., 2013; Lowry & Fillenz, 2001; Shram et al., 1997). Reduced glucose revealed the difference between KD-fed and control diet-fed animals in two of the studies (Bough et al., 2006; Kawamura et al., 2014), which parallels the finding that the antiseizure effect of the KD is correlated with plasma glucose levels (Mantis et al., 2004). Therefore, it would be useful to make extracellular glucose concentrations lower than standard to reproduce or maintain effects of the KD in acute hippocampal slices.

ADENOSINE-BASED MECHANISMS UNDERLIE THE KD'S EFFECTS

Through use of in vivo and in vitro animal models, adenosine-based mechanisms were found to be key for the antiseizure effects of the KD. Adenosine is a core molecule of ATP and works as an energy source in the central nervous system. Adenosine is released from the intracellular to the extracellular space directly by adenosine transporters, such as equilibrative nucleoside transporters and concentrative nucleoside transporters (King et al., 2006; Latini & Pedata, 2001). The extracellular adenosine concentration is also increased by breakdown of extracellular ATP through activation of ectonucleotidases, such as the ectonucleoside triphosphate diphosphohydrolase family, the ectonucleotide pyrophosphatase/phosphodiesterase family, alkaline phosphatases, and ecto-5′-nucleotidase (Zimmermann, 2000). Extracellular ATP is known to be released by several ATP-releasing sites, including gap junction hemichannels, pannexin channels, chloride channels, and vesicular release (Kawamura & Ruskin, 2012). Extracellular adenosine can activate four types of adenosine receptors (ARs): A_1R, $A_{2A}R$, $A_{2B}R$, and A_3R (Fredholm et al., 2000). All subtypes of ARs are functionally expressed to modulate neuroactivity in the central nervous system (Dunwiddie & Masino, 2001). Activation of A_1Rs is well known to suppress neuronal activity by inhibiting synaptic transmission through closing presynaptic VDCC (Gundlfinger et al., 2007; Wu & Saggau, 1994) and by hyperpolarizing membrane potential through opening potassium channels (Greene & Haas, 1991; Kawamura et al., 2010). The activation of $A_{2A}Rs$ has been reported to enhance neuronal activity by increasing the influx of calcium through presynaptic VDCCs (Goncalves et al., 1997) and depolarizing membrane potential (Chamberlain et al., 2013). It has also been reported that activation of $A_{2B}Rs$ (Fusco et al., 2018) or A_3Rs (Dunwiddie et al., 1997) modulates synaptic transmission. These neuronal modulations by ARs regulate seizure activity. Activation of A_1Rs has been reported to reduce seizures in both in vivo (Malhotra & Gupta, 1997; Zhang et al., 1994) and in vitro (Thompson et al., 1992). Importantly, A_1R knockout mice have spontaneous electrographic seizures (Li et al., 2007) and selective antagonists of A_1R cause seizure-like bursts in acute hippocampal slices (Hill et al., 2020; Thummler & Dunwiddie, 2000), suggesting that endogenous adenosine prevents the hyperexcitability underlying seizures through activation of A_1R. Moreover, selective agonists of A_1R have antiseizure effects in animal seizure models (Barraco et al., 1984; Dunwiddie & Worth, 1982; Klaft et al., 2020; Zeraati et al., 2006); however, these adenosine agonists have not proved useful in clinical treatment because of peripheral adverse effects (Dunwiddie & Masino, 2001). On the other hand, antagonists and genetic deficiency of $A_{2A}R$ reduce seizure activity (El Yacoubi et al., 2008; Zeraati et al., 2006), which suggests that $A_{2A}R$ works as "proconvulsant." These findings indicate that endogenous adenosine regulates seizure activity through activation of ARs. Therefore, adenosine can directly link cellular metabolism to seizure controls. The KD modulates brain metabolism through supply of ketone bodies as an energy source for the brain, and the final product of brain energy metabolism is ATP. Several studies have reported that the KD increases brain ATP levels in humans (Pan et al., 1999) and rodents (DeVivo et al., 1978; Nakazawa et al., 1983; Nylen et al., 2009). The altered brain bioenergetics may modulate neuronal activity through purinergic signaling, such as activation of ARs (Masino & Geiger, 2008).

An investigation of adenosine-based mechanisms was done by mimicking the altered metabolism during KD treatment using single-cell patch-clamp recording. Fasting and KD are thought to have their anticonvulsant effect by changing brain metabolism. Extracellular glucose levels are known to be reduced by KD-altered metabolism and intracellular ATP conditions are also thought to be increased by a KD. The combination of reducing extracellular glucose and increasing intracellular ATP might reproduce mechanistically important KD conditions in acute hippocampal slices. As already mentioned, it is easy to change the extracellular solution for an in vitro brain slice (including moderately lowering glucose), but it is trickier to change the intracellular milieu. The whole-cell patch-clamp technique is a method for recording from a single cell (Oyama et al., 2020), and this technique allows physical exchange between the intracellular fluid and the artificial intracellular solution in the recording pipette. This allows the researcher to modify the intracellular fluid composition of the recorded neuron experimentally, including elevating intracellular ATP. Kawamura et al. (2010) found that increased intracellular ATP and reduced extracellular glucose caused hyperpolarization in hippocampal neurons. They recorded from CA3 pyramidal neurons

with the whole-cell patch-clamp technique in acute hippocampal slices from control diet-fed rats and mice. Reduced extracellular glucose and increased intracellular ATP caused outward current (or hyperpolarization when recording membrane potential) in CA3 pyramidal neurons. This outward current was dose-dependent for both extracellular glucose and intracellular ATP, and importantly it was found in both rats and mice. Pharmacologic and genetic experiments demonstrated that when intracellular ATP was sufficient or increased, reduced extracellular glucose opened pannexin-1 channels and released intracellular ATP to the extracellular space. Released ATP was rapidly hydrolyzed to adenosine, which activated the A_1R, with subsequent opening of K_{ATP} channels. Opening of these potassium channels caused hyperpolarization and reduced excitability. These results indicate that mimicking the KD condition with increased ATP and reduced glucose reduces excitability in hippocampal CA3 pyramidal neurons, with autocrine modulation via A_1R, and this might be one of the key mechanisms of the anticonvulsant effects of the KD (Figure 24.2). The same mechanisms were found using acute hippocampal slices from KD-fed rats and mice (Kawamura et al., 2014). KD (6.3:1 ratio)-induced suppression of bicuculline-induced bursts (Table 24.2) was inhibited by A_1R antagonist and did not occur in slices from A_1R knockout mice. Antagonism of K_{ATP} channels or pannexin-1 channels inhibited the KD-induced suppression of bicuculline-induced bursts. These results suggest that the KD has antiseizure effects through a pannexin-1 channel–A_1R–K_{ATP} channel autocrine pathway (Figure 24.2). Adenosine-based mechanisms were also found by using in vivo animal models. Masino et al. (2011) used ADK-Tg mice and reported that A_1R-induced antiseizure effects underlie the KD. ADK is the astroglially expressed enzyme for adenosine clearance (Yamada et al., 1980) and works to decrease the extracellular adenosine level. Epilepsy is known to cause progressive astrogliosis (Dossi et al., 2018) and upregulation of the ADK level (Aronica et al., 2011; de Groot et al., 2012; Gouder et al., 2004). ADK upregulation leads to a reduced adenosine level and increased seizure activity. In fact, overexpression of ADK (ADK-Tg mice lacking endogenous astrocytic ADK, but with the target gene for ADK inserted ubiquitously) causes spontaneous electrographic seizures (Fedele et al., 2005). Masino et al. (2011) reported that a KD (6.3:1 ratio) reduced the frequency and duration of electrographic seizures in

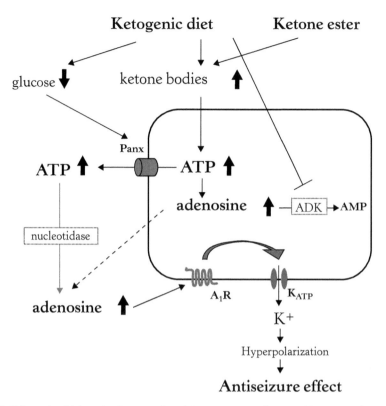

FIGURE 24.2 *Schematic of Adenosine Receptor-Based Antiseizure Regulation in Hippocampal Pyramidal Neurons and Relationship to Ketogenic Diet*

The ketogenic diet (KD) increases ketone body levels and reduces glucose levels. Ketone ester also increases the levels of ketone bodies in the central nervous system. Ketone bodies might increase intracellular ATP production, and increased ATP is released to the extracellular space due to opening of pannexin-1 channels (panx) caused by lowered extracellular glucose. Extracellular adenosine is increased after breakdown of ATP by nucleotidases. Extracellular adenosine is also increased by inhibition of adenosine kinase (ADK) by the KD. Increased extracellular adenosine activates adenosine A_1 receptors (A_1R) and opens K_{ATP} channels (K_{ATP}), which hyperpolarizes hippocampal pyramidal neurons. This hyperpolarization reduces neuronal hyperexcitability and causes the KD's antiseizure effects.

ADK-Tg mice (Table 24.1). The effect of the KD was inhibited by intraperitoneal injection of A_1R antagonist. Importantly, the KD had no effect on induced electrographic seizures in A_1R knockout mice. Masino et al. (2011) also reported that the KD reduced ADK expression, suggesting that the KD increases the intracellular adenosine level by inhibiting ADK activity, and increased adenosine levels might link to activation of A_1Rs (Figure 24.2). Kovacs et al. (2017) also reported that the ketone ester-induced antiseizure effect was caused by activation of A_1Rs. Intraperitoneal application of A_1R antagonist suppressed the ketone ester gavage-induced reduction of the number of electrographic seizure events in Wistar Albino Glaxo/Rijswijk rats.

Recently, AR-independent mechanisms have been investigated. Williams-Karnesky et al. (2013)

reported that a deficit of adenosine combined with overexpression of ADK led to DNA hypermethylation in an AR-independent manner, suggesting that cytosolic adenosine blocks DNA methylation. Importantly, increases in DNA methylation contributed to the progression of the epileptic phenotype. The authors also reported that adenosine augmentation therapy reduced DNA hypermethylation and prevented kainic acid-induced epileptogenesis in rats (Williams-Karnesky et al., 2013). The KD has the same effects. Pilocarpine-induced epileptic rats had a decreased adenosine level and increased DNA methylation in the hippocampus (Lusardi et al., 2015). A KD (6.3:1 ratio) increased adenosine and suppressed DNA hypermethylation. The KD also reduced seizure progression in pilocarpine-induced epileptic rats, suggesting that KD prevents epileptogenesis by epigenetic modulation through AR-independent function (Lusardi et al., 2015).

Altogether, these reports indicate that AR-dependent and AR-independent pathways play a significant role in the antiseizure and/or antiepileptogenesis effects of the KD.

CONCLUSIONS

Research on the antiseizure mechanisms of the KD uses both in vivo and in vitro models. In vivo animal models are useful for direct measurements of KD-induced effects. The usefulness of in vitro models is that they make it easy to elucidate the details of neuronal modulation by the KD at the molecular level. However, the pitfall of in vitro recording is that the environment of acute brain slice preparations is different from the environment in vivo. A slice is made by cutting brain tissue, and that causes traumatic injury, so reactive gliosis occurs in the acute hippocampal slice (Takano et al., 2014). Also, artificial cerebrospinal fluid does not exactly reproduce actual cerebrospinal fluid, which might be changed by KD treatment. Thus, results from in vitro brain slice preparations should be confirmed by in vivo electrophysiologic recordings or behavioral tests as much as possible. For that reason, both in vivo and in vitro electrophysiologic recordings are useful, and both are essential for KD research. A combination of both in vivo and in vitro recordings should provide further data about the complex mechanisms underlying KD treatment and new ketone body and/or ketone analog treatment in detail. This chapter also describes adenosine-based mechanisms underlying the KD, such as ATP release from pannexin channels, activation of A_1R, K_{ATP} channel opening, inhibition of ADK activity, and suppression of DNA hypermethylation. Adenosine plays an important role in the anticonvulsant effects of the KD through both AR-dependent and AR-independent pathways.

ACKNOWLEDGMENTS

Dr. David N. Ruskin is thanked for comments on this manuscript. The support of JSPS KAKENHI Grant Number JP20K07745 to MK is gratefully acknowledged.

REFERENCES

Abe, H., & Ogata, N. (1981). Effects of penicillin on electrical activities of neurons in guinea-pig hippocampal slices. *The Japanese Journal of Pharmacology*, 31, 661–675.

Aronica, E., Zurolo, E., Iyer, A., de Groot, M., Anink, J., Carbonell, C., van Vliet, E. A., Baayen, J. C.,

Boison, D., & Gorter, J. A. (2011). Upregulation of adenosine kinase in astrocytes in experimental and human temporal lobe epilepsy. *Epilepsia*, 52, 1645–1655.

Barraco, R. A., Swanson, T. H., Phillis, J. W., & Berman, R. F. (1984). Anticonvulsant effects of adenosine analogues on amygdaloid-kindled seizures in rats. *Neuroscience Letters*, 46, 317–322.

Bough, K. J., & Eagles, D. A. (1999). A ketogenic diet increases the resistance to pentylenetetrazole-induced seizures in the rat. *Epilepsia*, 40, 138–143.

Bough, K. J., Wetherington, J., Hassel, B., Pare, J. F., Gawryluk, J. W., Greene, J. G., Shaw, R., Smith, Y., Geiger, J. D., & Dingledine, R. J. (2006). Mitochondrial biogenesis in the anticonvulsant mechanism of the ketogenic diet. *Annals of Neurology*, 60, 223–235.

Brunengraber, H. (1997). Potential of ketone body esters for parenteral and oral nutrition. *Nutrition*, 13, 233–235.

Chamberlain, S. E., Sadowski, J. H., Teles-Grilo Ruivo, L. M., Atherton, L. A., & Mellor, J. R. (2013). Long-term depression of synaptic kainate receptors reduces excitability by relieving inhibition of the slow afterhyperpolarization. *Journal of Neuroscience*, 33, 9536–9545.

Congar, P., Gaiarsa, J. L., Popovici, T., Ben-Ari, Y., & Crepel, V. (2000). Permanent reduction of seizure threshold in post-ischemic CA3 pyramidal neurons. *Journal of Neurophysiology*, 83, 2040–2046.

D'Agostino, D. P., Pilla, R., Held, H. E., Landon, C. S., Puchowicz, M., Brunengraber, H., Ari, C., Arnold, P., & Dean, J. B. (2013). Therapeutic ketosis with ketone ester delays central nervous system oxygen toxicity seizures in rats. *American Journal of Physiology Regulatory, Integrative and Comparative Physiology*, 304, R829–R836.

de Groot, M., Iyer, A., Zurolo, E., Anink, J., Heimans, J. J., Boison, D., Reijneveld, J. C., & Aronica, E. (2012). Overexpression of ADK in human astrocytic tumors and peritumoral tissue is related to tumor-associated epilepsy. *Epilepsia*, 53, 58–66.

Desrochers, S., Dubreuil, P., Brunet, J., Jette, M., David, F., Landau, B. R., & Brunengraber, H. (1995). Metabolism of (R,S)-1,3-butanediol acetoacetate esters, potential parenteral and enteral nutrients in conscious pigs. *American Journal of Physiology*, 268, E660–E667.

DeVivo, D. C., Leckie, M. P., Ferrendelli, J. S., & McDougal, D. B., Jr. (1978). Chronic ketosis and cerebral metabolism. *Annals of Neurology*, 3, 331–337.

Dossi, E., Vasile, F., & Rouach, N. (2018). Human astrocytes in the diseased brain. *Brain Research Bulletin*, 136, 139–156.

Dulla, C. G., Dobelis, P., Pearson, T., Frenguelli, B. G., Staley, K. J., & Masino, S. A. (2005). Adenosine and ATP link PCO_2 to cortical excitability via pH. *Neuron*, 48, 1011–1023.

Dunwiddie, T. V., Diao, L., Kim, H. O., Jiang, J. L., & Jacobson, K. A. (1997). Activation of hippocampal adenosine A_3 receptors produces a desensitization of A_1 receptor-mediated responses in rat hippocampus. *Journal of Neuroscience, 17,* 607–614.

Dunwiddie, T. V., & Masino, S. A. (2001). The role and regulation of adenosine in the central nervous system. *Annual Review of Neuroscience, 24,* 31–55.

Dunwiddie, T. V., & Worth, T. (1982). Sedative and anticonvulsant effects of adenosine analogs in mouse and rat. *Journal of Pharmacology and Experimental Therapeutics, 220,* 70–76.

El Yacoubi, M., Ledent, C., Parmentier, M., Costentin, J., & Vaugeois, J. M. (2008). Evidence for the involvement of the adenosine A_{2A} receptor in the lowered susceptibility to pentylenetetrazol-induced seizures produced in mice by long-term treatment with caffeine. *Neuropharmacology, 55,* 35–40.

Fedele, D. E., Gouder, N., Guttinger, M., Gabernet, L., Scheurer, L., Rulicke, T., Crestani, F., & Boison, D. (2005). Astrogliosis in epilepsy leads to overexpression of adenosine kinase, resulting in seizure aggravation. *Brain, 128,* 2383–2395.

Fredholm, B. B., Arslan, G., Halldner, L., Kull, B., Schulte, G., & Wasserman, W. (2000). Structure and function of adenosine receptors and their genes. *Naunyn-Schmiedeberg's Archives of Pharmacology, 362,* 364–374.

Fusco, I., Ugolini, F., Lana, D., Coppi, E., Dettori, I., Gaviano, L., Nosi, D., Cherchi, F., Pedata, F., Giovannini, M. G., & Pugliese A. M. (2018). The selective antagonism of adenosine A_{2B} receptors reduces the synaptic failure and neuronal death induced by oxygen and glucose deprivation in rat CA1 hippocampus in vitro. *Frontiers in Pharmacology, 9,* 399.

Gimenez-Cassina, A., Martinez-Francois, J. R., Fisher, J. K., Szlyk, B., Polak, K., Wiwczar, J., Tanner, G. R., Lutas, A., Yellen, G., & Danial, N. N. (2012). BAD-dependent regulation of fuel metabolism and K_{ATP} channel activity confers resistance to epileptic seizures. *Neuron, 74,* 719–730.

Goncalves, M. L., Cunha, R. A., & Ribeiro, J. A. (1997). Adenosine A_{2A} receptors facilitate $^{45}Ca^{2+}$ uptake through class A calcium channels in rat hippocampal CA3 but not CA1 synaptosomes. *Neuroscience Letters, 238,* 73–77.

Gouder, N., Scheurer, L., Fritschy, J. M., & Boison, D. (2004). Overexpression of adenosine kinase in epileptic hippocampus contributes to epileptogenesis. *Journal of Neuroscience, 24,* 692–701.

Greene, R. W., & Haas, H. L. (1991). The electrophysiology of adenosine in the mammalian central nervous system. *Progress in Neurobiology, 36,* 329–341.

Gundlfinger, A., Bischofberger, J., Johenning, F. W., Torvinen, M., Schmitz, D., & Breustedt, J. (2007).

Adenosine modulates transmission at the hippocampal mossy fibre synapse via direct inhibition of presynaptic calcium channels. *Journal of Physiology, 582,* 263–277.

Hallbook, T., Kohler, S., Rosen, I., & Lundgren, J. (2007). Effects of ketogenic diet on epileptiform activity in children with therapy resistant epilepsy. *Epilepsy Research, 77,* 134–140.

Hartman, A. L., Lyle, M., Rogawski, M. A., & Gasior, M. (2008). Efficacy of the ketogenic diet in the 6-Hz seizure test. *Epilepsia, 49,* 334–339.

Hill, E., Hickman, C., Diez, R., & Wall, M. (2020). Role of A_1 receptor-activated GIRK channels in the suppression of hippocampal seizure activity. *Neuropharmacology, 164,* 107904.

Hu, X. L., Cheng, X., Fei, J., & Xiong, Z. Q. (2011). Neuron-restrictive silencer factor is not required for the antiepileptic effect of the ketogenic diet. *Epilepsia, 52,* 1609–1616.

Huttenlocher, P. R. (1976). Ketonemia and seizures: Metabolic and anticonvulsant effects of two ketogenic diets in childhood epilepsy. *Pediatric Research, 10,* 536–540.

Jiang, Y., Yang, Y., Wang, S., Ding, Y., Guo, Y., Zhang, M. M., Wen, S. Q., & Ding, M. P. (2012). Ketogenic diet protects against epileptogenesis as well as neuronal loss in amygdaloid-kindling seizures. *Neuroscience Letters, 508,* 22–26.

Juge, N., Gray, J. A., Omote, H., Miyaji, T., Inoue, T., Hara, C., Uneyama, H., Edwards, R. H., Nicoll, R. A., & Moriyama, Y. (2010). Metabolic control of vesicular glutamate transport and release. *Neuron, 68,* 99–112.

Kadowaki, A., Sada, N., Juge, N., Wakasa, A., Moriyama, Y., & Inoue, T. (2017). Neuronal inhibition and seizure suppression by acetoacetate and its analog, 2-phenylbutyrate. *Epilepsia, 58,* 845–857.

Kawamura, M., Jr., & Ruskin, D. (2012). Adenosine and autocrine metabolic regulation of neuronal activity. In S. Masino & D. Boison (Eds.), *Adenosine* (pp. 71–85). Springer.

Kawamura, M., Jr., Ruskin, D. N., Geiger, J. D., Boison, D., & Masino, S. A. (2014). Ketogenic diet sensitizes glucose control of hippocampal excitability. *Journal of Lipid Research, 55,* 2254–2260.

Kawamura, M., Jr., Ruskin, D. N., & Masino, S. A. (2010). Metabolic autocrine regulation of neurons involves cooperation among pannexin hemichannels, adenosine receptors, and K_{ATP} channels. *Journal of Neuroscience, 30,* 3886–3895.

Kawamura, M., Jr., Ruskin, D. N., & Masino, S. A. (2019). Adenosine A_1 receptor-mediated protection of mouse hippocampal synaptic transmission against oxygen and/or glucose deprivation: A comparative study. *Journal of Neurophysiology, 122,* 721–728.

Kawamura, M. J., Ruskin, D. N., & Masino, S. A. (2016). Metabolic therapy for temporal lobe epilepsy in a dish: Investigating mechanisms of ketogenic diet using electrophysiological recordings in hippocampal slices. *Frontiers in Molecular Neuroscience, 9,* 112.

Kealy, J., Bennett, R., & Lowry, J. P. (2013). Simultaneous recording of hippocampal oxygen and glucose in real time using constant potential amperometry in the freely-moving rat. *Journal of Neuroscience Methods, 215,* 110–120.

Do Young Kim, D. V. M., Simeone, K. A., Simeone, T. A., Pandya, J. D., Wilke, J. C., Ahn, Y., Geddes, J. W., Sullivan, P. G., & Rho, J. M. (2015). Ketone bodies mediate antiseizure effects through mitochondrial permeability transition. *Annals of Neurology, 78,* 77–87.

Kimura, R., Ma, L. Y., Wu, C., Turner, D., Shen, J. X., Ellsworth, K., Wakui, M., Maalouf, M., & Wu, J. (2012). Acute exposure to the mitochondrial complex I toxin rotenone impairs synaptic long-term potentiation in rat hippocampal slices. *CNS Neuroscience & Therapeutics, 18,* 641–646.

King, A. E., Ackley, M. A., Cass, C. E., Young, J. D., & Baldwin, S. A. (2006). Nucleoside transporters: From scavengers to novel therapeutic targets. *Trends in Pharmacological Sciences, 27,* 416–425.

Klaft, Z. J., Duerrwald, L. M., Gerevich, Z., & Dulla, C. G. (2020). The adenosine A_1 receptor agonist WAG 994 suppresses acute kainic acid-induced status epilepticus in vivo. *Neuropharmacology, 176,* 108213.

Knowles, W. D., Traub, R. D., & Strowbridge, B. W. (1987). The initiation and spread of epileptiform bursts in the in vitro hippocampal slice. *Neuroscience, 21,* 441–455.

Kohling, R., Vreugdenhil, M., Bracci, E., & Jefferys, J. G. (2000). Ictal epileptiform activity is facilitated by hippocampal $GABA_A$ receptor-mediated oscillations. *Journal of Neuroscience, 20,* 6820–6829.

Kojima, H., Kowada, M., & Katsuta, Y. (1989). Cellular substrates for epileptiform activity induced by repeated tetanic stimulation in hippocampal slices. *Neurologia medico-chirurgica, 29,* 1–5.

Kovacs, Z., D'Agostino, D. P., Dobolyi, A., & Ari, C. (2017). Adenosine A_1 receptor antagonism abolished the anti-seizure effects of exogenous ketone supplementation in Wistar Albino Glaxo Rijswijk rats. *Frontiers in Molecular Neuroscience, 10,* 235.

Kwon, Y. S., Jeong, S. W., Kim, D. W., Choi, E. S., & Son, B. K. (2008). Effects of the ketogenic diet on neurogenesis after kainic acid-induced seizures in mice. *Epilepsy Research, 78,* 186–194.

Latini, S., & Pedata, F. (2001). Adenosine in the central nervous system: Release mechanisms and extracellular concentrations. *Journal of Neurochemistry, 79,* 463–484.

Li, T., Quan Lan, J., Fredholm, B. B., Simon, R. P., & Boison, D. (2007). Adenosine dysfunction in astrogliosis: Cause for seizure generation? *Neuron Glia Biology, 3,* 353–366.

Li, T., Ren, G., Lusardi, T., Wilz, A., Lan, J. Q., Iwasato, T., Itohara, S., Simon, R. P., & Boison, D. (2008). Adenosine kinase is a target for the prediction and prevention of epileptogenesis in mice. *Journal of Clinical Investigation, 118,* 571–582.

Likhodii, S. S., Musa, K., Mendonca, A., Dell, C., Burnham, W. M., & Cunnane, S. C. (2000). Dietary fat, ketosis, and seizure resistance in rats on the ketogenic diet. *Epilepsia, 41,* 1400–1410.

Lin, L., Chen, G., Xie, K., Zaia, K. A., Zhang, S., & Tsien, J. Z. (2006). Large-scale neural ensemble recording in the brains of freely behaving mice. *Journal of Neuroscience Methods, 155,* 28–38.

Lowry, J. P., & Fillenz, M. (2001). Real-time monitoring of brain energy metabolism in vivo using microelectrochemical sensors: The effects of anesthesia. *Bioelectrochemistry, 54,* 39–47.

Lusardi, T. A., Akula, K. K., Coffman, S. Q., Ruskin, D. N., Masino, S. A., & Boison, D. (2015). Ketogenic diet prevents epileptogenesis and disease progression in adult mice and rats. *Neuropharmacology, 99,* 500–509.

Ma, W., Berg, J., & Yellen, G. (2007). Ketogenic diet metabolites reduce firing in central neurons by opening K_{ATP} channels. *Journal of Neuroscience, 27,* 3618–3625.

Malhotra, J., & Gupta, Y. K. (1997). Effect of adenosine receptor modulation on pentylenetetrazole-induced seizures in rats. *British Journal of Pharmacology, 120,* 282–288.

Mantis, J. G., Centeno, N. A., Todorova, M. T., McGowan, R., & Seyfried, T. N. (2004). Management of multifactorial idiopathic epilepsy in EL mice with caloric restriction and the ketogenic diet: Role of glucose and ketone bodies. *Nutrition & Metabolism, 1,* 11.

Mantis, J. G., Meidenbauer, J. J., Zimick, N. C., Centeno, N. A., & Seyfried, T. N. (2014). Glucose reduces the anticonvulsant effects of the ketogenic diet in EL mice. *Epilepsy Research, 108,* 1137–1144.

Martillotti, J., Weinshenker, D., Liles, L. C., & Eagles, D. A. (2006). A ketogenic diet and knockout of the norepinephrine transporter both reduce seizure severity in mice. *Epilepsy Research, 68,* 207–211.

Masino, S. A., & Geiger, J. D. (2008). Are purines mediators of the anticonvulsant/neuroprotective effects of ketogenic diets? *Trends in Neuroscience, 31,* 273–278.

Masino, S. A., Kawamura, M., Wasser, C. A., Pomeroy, L. T., & Ruskin, D. N. (2009). Adenosine, ketogenic diet and epilepsy: The emerging therapeutic relationship between metabolism and brain activity. *Current Neuropharmacology, 7,* 257–268.

Masino, S. A., Li, T., Theofilas, P., Sandau, U. S., Ruskin, D. N., Fredholm, B. B., Geiger, J. D., Aronica, E., & Boison, D. (2011). A ketogenic diet suppresses seizures in mice through adenosine A₁ receptors. *Journal of Clinical Investigation, 121,* 2679–2683.

Masino, S. A., & Rho, J. M. (2012). Mechanisms of ketogenic diet action. In J. L. Noebels, M. Avoli, M. A. Rogawski, R. W. Olsen, & A. V. Delgado-Escueta (Eds.), *Jasper's basic mechanisms of the epilepsies* (pp. 1001–1022). National Center for Biotechnology Information.

Muller-Schwarze, A. B., Tandon, P., Liu, Z., Yang, Y., Holmes, G. L., & Stafstrom, C. E. (1999). Ketogenic diet reduces spontaneous seizures and mossy fiber sprouting in the kainic acid model. *Neuroreport, 10,* 1517–1522.

Nakazawa, M., Kodama, S., & Matsuo, T. (1983). Effects of ketogenic diet on electroconvulsive threshold and brain contents of adenosine nucleotides. *Brain and Development, 5,* 375–380.

Nylen, K., Velazquez, J. L., Sayed, V., Gibson, K. M., Burnham, W. M., & Snead, O. C., III. (2009). The effects of a ketogenic diet on ATP concentrations and the number of hippocampal mitochondria in Aldh5a1⁻/⁻ mice. *Biochimica et Biophysica Acta, 1790,* 208–212.

Olson, C. A., Vuong, H. E., Yano, J. M., Liang, Q. Y., Nusbaum, D. J., & Hsiao, E. Y. (2018). The gut microbiota mediates the anti-seizure effects of the ketogenic diet. *Cell, 173,* 1728–1741.

Oyama, Y., Ono, K., & Kawamura, M., Jr. (2020). Mild hypothermia protects synaptic transmission from experimental ischemia through reduction in the function of nucleoside transporters in the mouse hippocampus. *Neuropharmacology, 163,* 107853.

Paglioli, E., Palmini, A., Portuguez, M., Azambuja, N., da Costa, J. C., da Silva Filho, H. F., Martinez, J. V., & Hoeffel, J. R. (2006). Seizure and memory outcome following temporal lobe surgery: Selective compared with nonselective approaches for hippocampal sclerosis. *Journal of Neurosurgery, 104,* 70–78.

Pan, J. W., Bebin, E. M., Chu, W. J., & Hetherington, H. P. (1999). Ketosis and epilepsy: ³¹P spectroscopic imaging at 4.1 T. *Epilepsia, 40,* 703–707.

Rho, J. M., Kim, D. W., Robbins, C. A., Anderson, G. D., & Schwartzkroin, P. A. (1999). Age-dependent differences in flurothyl seizure sensitivity in mice treated with a ketogenic diet. *Epilepsy Research, 37,* 233–240.

Ruskin, D. N., Kawamura, M., & Masino, S. A. (2009). Reduced pain and inflammation in juvenile and adult rats fed a ketogenic diet. *PLOS ONE, 4,* Article e8349.

Ruskin, D. N., Murphy, M. I., Slade, S. L., & Masino, S. A. (2017). Ketogenic diet improves behaviors in a maternal immune activation model of autism spectrum disorder. *PLOS ONE, 12,* Article e0171643.

Sada, N., Lee, S., Katsu, T., Otsuki, T., & Inoue, T. (2015). Epilepsy treatment: Targeting LDH enzymes with a stiripentol analog to treat epilepsy. *Science, 347,* 1362–1367.

Sakmann, B., Edwards, F., Konnerth, A., & Takahashi, T. (1989). Patch clamp techniques used for studying synaptic transmission in slices of mammalian brain. *Quarterly Journal of Experimental Physiology, 74,* 1107–1118.

Samoilova, M., Weisspapir, M., Abdelmalik, P., Velumian, A. A., & Carlen, P. L. (2010). Chronic in vitro ketosis is neuroprotective but not anti-convulsant. *Journal of Neurochemistry, 113,* 826–835.

Sayin, Ü, Rutecki, P., & Sutula, T. (1999). NMDA-dependent currents in granule cells of the dentate gyrus contribute to induction but not permanence of kindling. *Journal of Neurophysiology, 81,* 564–574.

Shao, L. R., Rho, J. M., & Stafstrom, C. E. (2018). Glycolytic inhibition: A novel approach toward controlling neuronal excitability and seizures. *Epilepsia Open, 3,* 191–197.

Shram, N. F., Netchiporouk, L. I., Martelet, C., Jaffrezic-Renault, N., & Cespuglio, R. (1997). Brain glucose: Voltammetric determination in normal and hyperglycaemic rats using a glucose microsensor. *Neuroreport, 8,* 1109–1112.

Simeone, T. A., Samson, K. K., Matthews, S. A., & Simeone, K. A. (2014). In vivo ketogenic diet treatment attenuates pathologic sharp waves and high frequency oscillations in in vitro hippocampal slices from epileptic Kv 1.1alpha knockout mice. *Epilepsia, 55,* e44–e49.

Smith, B. N., & Dudek, F. E. (2001). Short- and long-term changes in CA1 network excitability after kainate treatment in rats. *Journal of Neurophysiology, 85,* 1–9.

Stafstrom, C. E., Ockuly, J. C., Murphree, L., Valley, M. T., Roopra, A., & Sutula, T. P. (2009). Anticonvulsant and antiepileptic actions of 2-deoxy-D-glucose in epilepsy models. *Annals of Neurology, 65,* 435–447.

Stafstrom, C. E., Wang, C., & Jensen, F. E. (1999). Electrophysiological observations in hippocampal slices from rats treated with the ketogenic diet. *Developmental Neuroscience, 21,* 393–399.

Stewart, C., & Reid, I. (1993). Electroconvulsive stimulation and synaptic plasticity in the rat. *Brain Research, 620,* 139–141.

Su, S. W., Cilio, M. R., Sogawa, Y., Silveira, D. C., Holmes, G. L., & Stafstrom, C. E. (2000). Timing of ketogenic diet initiation in an experimental epilepsy model. *Developmental Brain Research, 125,* 131–138.

Takano, T., He, W., Han, X., Wang, F., Xu, Q., Wang, X., Oberheim Bush, N. A., Cruz, N., Dienel, G. A., & Nedergaard, M. (2014). Rapid manifestation of reactive astrogliosis in acute hippocampal brain slices. *Glia, 62,* 78–95.

Tanner, G. R., Lutas, A., Martinez-Francois, J. R., & Yellen, G. (2011). Single K_{ATP} channel opening in response to action potential firing in mouse dentate granule neurons. *Journal of Neuroscience, 31,* 8689–8696.

Thio, L. L., Wong, M., & Yamada, K. A. (2000). Ketone bodies do not directly alter excitatory or inhibitory hippocampal synaptic transmission. *Neurology, 54,* 325–331.

Thom, M. (2009). Hippocampal sclerosis: Progress since Sommer. *Brain Pathology, 19,* 565–572.

Thompson, S. M., Haas, H. L., & Gahwiler, B. H. (1992). Comparison of the actions of adenosine at pre- and postsynaptic receptors in the rat hippocampus in vitro. *Journal of Physiology, 451,* 347–363.

Thummler, S., & Dunwiddie, T. V. (2000). Adenosine receptor antagonists induce persistent bursting in the rat hippocampal CA3 region via an NMDA receptor-dependent mechanism. *Journal of Neurophysiology, 83,* 1787–1795.

Todorova, M. T., Tandon, P., Madore, R. A., Stafstrom, C. E., & Seyfried, T. N. (2000). The ketogenic diet inhibits epileptogenesis in EL mice: A genetic model for idiopathic epilepsy. *Epilepsia, 41,* 933–940.

Watson, C. (2003). Hippocampal sclerosis and the syndrome of medial temporal lobe epilepsy. *Expert Review of Neurotherapeutics, 3,* 821–828.

Wiebe, S., Blume, W. T., Girvin, J. P., & Eliasziw, M. (2001). A randomized, controlled trial of surgery for temporal-lobe epilepsy. *New England Journal of Medicine, 345,* 311–318.

Wilder, R. M. (1921). The effects of ketonemia on the course of epilepsy. *Mayo Clinic Proceedings, 2,* 307–308.

Williams-Karnesky, R. L., Sandau, U. S., Lusardi, T. A., Lytle, N. K., Farrell, J. M., Pritchard, E. M., Kaplan, D. L., & Boison, D. (2013). Epigenetic changes induced by adenosine augmentation therapy prevent epileptogenesis. *Journal of Clinical Investigation, 123,* 3552–3563.

Wu, L. G., & Saggau, P. (1994). Adenosine inhibits evoked synaptic transmission primarily by reducing presynaptic calcium influx in area CA1 of hippocampus. *Neuron, 12,* 1139–1148.

Yamada, Y., Goto, H., & Ogasawara, N. (1980). Purification and properties of adenosine kinase from rat brain. *Biochimica et Biophysica Acta, 616,* 199–207.

Youssef, F. F. (2015). Ketone bodies attenuate excitotoxic cell injury in the rat hippocampal slice under conditions of reduced glucose availability. *Neurological Research, 37,* 211–216.

Zeraati, M., Mirnajafi-Zadeh, J., Fathollahi, Y., Namvar, S., & Rezvani, M. E. (2006). Adenosine A_1 and A_{2A} receptors of hippocampal CA1 region have opposite effects on piriform cortex kindled seizures in rats. *Seizure, 15,* 41–48.

Zhang, G., Franklin, P. H., & Murray, T. F. (1994). Activation of adenosine A_1 receptors underlies anticonvulsant effect of CGS21680. *European Journal of Pharmacology, 255,* 239–243.

Zimmermann, H. (2000). Extracellular metabolism of ATP and other nucleotides. *Naunyn-Schmiedeberg's Archives of Pharmacology, 362,* 299–309.

25

Ketogenic Diet and Epigenetic Mechanisms of Epileptogenesis

MADHUVIKA MURUGAN, PHD, FABIO C. TESCAROLLO, PHD,
AND DETLEV BOISON, PHD

INTRODUCTION

Fasting has been known as a means for controlling epilepsy for thousands of years. Formal studies of fasting in the early years of the 20th century led to the critical observation that elevated ketone bodies were excreted during fasting, and diets tailored to elevate ketones were established (Peterman, 1924, 1925; Wheless, 2008). The ketogenic diet (KD) and its antiseizure effects were first reported in the early 1920s (Wilder, 1921; Wilder & Winter, 1922) However, the difficulty of compliance with the KD, in combination with the availability of modern antiseizure drugs, diminished enthusiasm for the KD throughout much of the 20th century, but studies in patients with seizures refractory to conventional drugs have demonstrated the KD's clear efficacy for seizure suppression. While the earliest studies suggested efficacy of the KD only in children, several studies show similar therapeutic effects in adults (Barborka, 1930; Coppola et al., 2002; Sirven et al., 1999).

Beneficial effects of the KD can manifest clinically as quickly as several days after diet initiation or may take as long as 8 months. Diet reversal yields even more perplexing outcomes. In some individuals, seizures return within hours of glucose reintroduction, suggesting a transient antiseizure mechanism, while others were able to return to a "normal" diet and remain seizure-free, suggesting an antiepileptogenic mechanism that outlasts treatment duration. A detailed review of the proposed antiepileptogenic and neuroprotective mechanisms of the KD has been published previously (Masino & Rho, 2012), illustrating that the metabolic influences of the diet are broad. Indeed, the broad range of metabolic influences suggests that the therapeutic benefits of the KD are not limited to epilepsy but might extend to other neurologic disorders (Kossoff & Hartman, 2012; Stafstrom & Rho, 2012).

The dramatic reduction or elimination of seizures in up to 40% of individuals with epilepsy on a KD is a strong argument for continued use of the diet. This is particularly compelling when considering that individuals in controlled trials of the diet are refractory to conventional antiseizure drugs and have been suffering from epilepsy for many years at the time the diet is initiated. A more comprehensive understanding of the underlying mechanisms could yield evidence for predictive biomarkers that can identify patients who are most likely to respond well to the KD and that could perhaps augment responsiveness in nonresponders.

EPILEPTOGENESIS

According to recent data, approximately 60% of all epilepsy cases occur as a consequence of acute insults to the brain, such as traumatic brain injury, cerebrovascular insult, or infections (Clossen & Reddy, 2017; Klein et al., 2018). Following an insult, the brain enters a period during which progressive neurobiologic alterations convert a nonepileptic brain into a brain capable of generating spontaneous and recurrent seizures, which are defined as epilepsy (Pitkanen et al., 2015; Sloviter & Bumanglag, 2013). The series of events that lead to the development of epilepsy is known as epileptogenesis. During this period, pathophysiologic alterations are observed in brains of both patients and animal models of temporal lobe epilepsy (TLE), including metabolic impairments, increased inflammatory processes, microglial and astroglial activation, alterations in ligand- and voltage-gated ion channels, altered expression of ionotropic and metabotropic receptors, astrogliosis, neurogenesis, aberrant synaptic plasticity, remodeling of neuronal circuits, axonal sprouting, neuronal loss, and epigenetic reprogramming (Clossen & Reddy, 2017; Klein et al., 2018).

EPIGENETIC MECHANISMS IN EPILEPTOGENESIS

Heritable factors confer a small but appreciable increased risk of epilepsy development (Kullmann, 2002). Genetic loci have been identified in subpopulations of specific epilepsy syndromes, but they account for only a fraction of the incidence and are not well correlated with seizure severity and comorbidities (Myers & Mefford, 2015). In general, large-scale genome-wide studies have not identified broadly applicable genomic variations that would indicate a common genetic risk in epilepsy (Cavalleri et al., 2007; Kasperaviciute et al., 2010; Mefford et al., 2010). However, a recent study suggests that genetic variants of the adenosine kinase (*Adk*) gene are associated with an increased risk for the development of posttraumatic epilepsy (Diamond et al., 2015).

While the role of genetics in epilepsy and epileptogenesis needs further investigation, changes in gene expression and regulation might play an additional role. Studies of gene expression changes following seizures, in the clinically latent phase of epileptogenesis before spontaneous seizures develop, and in the epileptic brain agree that many genes are (dys)regulated in the epileptogenic brain (Lukasiuk & Pitkanen, 2004). However, the specific genes regulated are not consistent across studies, regardless of species or model specificity (Aronica & Gorter, 2007). Pathway analyses across multiple epilepsy studies have revealed that despite variations in the specific genes regulated, certain functional pathways are commonly identified across studies (Aronica & Gorter, 2007). Thus, expression changes that target intra- and extracellular signaling, transcription, protein biosynthesis, and immune responses are all well represented in all time windows evaluated (Aronica & Gorter, 2007). This network view of epilepsy risk and development presents a model that can account for the confounding factors in genomic studies of epilepsy, including phenotypic inconsistencies associated with heritable risk factors, and the variable susceptibility and disease progression in acquired epilepsies.

Epigenetic changes are biochemical alterations of the DNA or the chromatin structure that do not affect the coding sequence of the DNA but contribute to the regulation of gene transcription and entire networks, affecting the neuronal excitability, including interictal discharges, high-frequency oscillations, and increased response to stimuli, which are determinants of seizures and of epilepsy progression (Klein et al., 2018; Sloviter et al., 1991). Epigenetic changes include DNA methylation, histone modifications, and expression of noncoding RNA (Figure 25.1; Boison & Rho, 2019;

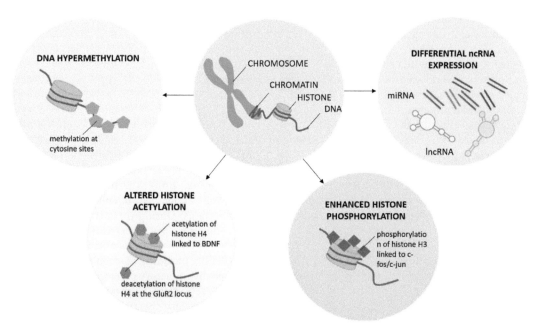

FIGURE 25.1 *Epigenetic Mechanisms in Epilepsy and Epileptogenesis*

The epigenetic modifications implicated in epilepsy and epileptogenesis include: DNA hypermethylation, altered histone acetylation, enhanced histone phosphorylation, and differential expression of noncoding RNA, such as lncRNA and microRNA (miRNA).

Jaenisch & Bird, 2003; Kiefer, 2007). Importantly, epigenetic changes may simultaneously affect several genes thought to represent a risk factor for epilepsy. In contrast to genetic mutations, epigenetic changes are potentially reversible and may constitute a novel target for therapeutic intervention. This chapter highlights the epigenetic mechanisms implicated in epileptogenesis and expands on existing mechanisms by which the KD influences the epigenetic mechanisms.

DNA Methylation

DNA methylation, the most commonly investigated epigenetic mechanism, is known to play a critical role in epilepsy (Boison & Rho, 2019; Hauser et al., 2018; Henshall, 2018; Henshall & Kobow, 2015; Miller-Delaney et al., 2015). It depends on the transmethylation pathway catalyzed by DNA methyltransferase (DNMT). DNA methylation involves the transfer of a methyl group from S-adenosylmethionine (SAM) to a cytosine base of DNA, resulting in 5-methylcytosine (5-mC). The methylation pathway finally results in the obligatory products, adenosine and homocysteine, the prompt removal of which is essential for continuous DNA methylation to occur (Figure 25.2; Boison et al., 2002; Gouder et al., 2004; Williams-Karnesky et al., 2013). Concurrently, adenosine deficiency shifts the equilibrium of the S-adenosylhomocysteine (SAH) hydrolase reaction away from

the formation of SAH (Mandaviya et al., 2014), which is also known to block DNMT activity by product inhibition (James et al., 2002), thereby reinforcing the increase in DNA methylation in the epileptic brain. Seizures resulting from the proconvulsant methionine sulfoximine, which increases the methylation flux by increasing the SAM:SAH ratio, can be blocked by adenosine and homocysteine (Gill & Schatz, 1985; Schatz et al., 1983; Sellinger et al., 1984).

The first evidence for abundant DNA methylation changes in epileptic tissue was observed in microdissected human dentate gyrus taken from TLE specimens (Kobow et al., 2009). Other clinical studies reported upregulated DNMT activity and associated global hypermethylation in patients with TLE (Miller-Delaney et al., 2015). Similar patterns of DNA hypermethylation were also observed in rodent experimental models of status epilepticus (Boison & Rho, 2019; Kobow & Blumcke, 2012; Kobow et al., 2009, 2013; Miller-Delaney et al., 2015; Williams-Karnesky et al., 2013). Since methylation of DNA is linked to the repression of gene expression, a recent study confirmed that differential gene expression changes were associated with DNA methylation during early epileptogenesis and occurred in a cell-specific manner (Berger et al., 2019). In earlier work, bisulfite sequencing of DNA from epileptic hippocampus revealed increased reelin promoter methylation in specimens with granule cell dispersion

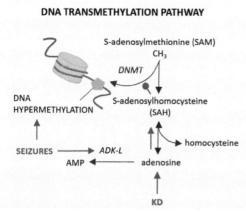
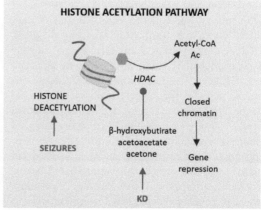

FIGURE 25.2 *Regulation of Epigenetic and Antiepileptogenesis Mechanisms by the Ketogenic Diet*

The diagram represents the two major epigenetic alterations by which the KD confers antiepileptogenesis in clinical and animal models of temporal lobe epilepsy (TLE). (1) Global DNA hypermethylation induced by seizures is restored by the KD via adenosine augmentation, a shift in SAH and SAM homeostasis, and reducing DNA methylation by inhibiting DNA methyltransferases (DNMT). (2) Seizure-induced histone deacetylation is catalyzed by histone deacetylases (HDACs), resulting in closed chromatin structure and transcriptional gene repression. The KD-induced increase in ketone bodies (β-hydroxybutyrate, acetoacetate, and acetone) inhibits HDACs and prevents histone deacetylation.

(Haas et al., 2002; Zhao et al., 2006). These studies together have led to the methylation hypothesis of epileptogenesis, which suggests that seizures by themselves can induce epigenetic chromatin modifications, thereby aggravating the epileptogenic condition (Kobow & Blumcke, 2012).

In the context of epileptogenesis, adenosine has been identified as a key regulator of DNA methylation (Williams-Karnesky et al., 2013). Enhanced adenosine kinase (ADK) and the respective decrease in adenosine levels shifts the reaction equilibrium toward increasing the flux of methyl groups through the transmethylation pathway, resulting in a global DNA hypermethylation, which is implicated in the progression and maintenance of epilepsy (Boison & Rho, 2019; Williams-Karnesky et al., 2013). Thus, adenosine deficiency and related DNA hypermethylation result in a vicious cycle associated with the onset of epileptogenesis, spontaneous seizures, progression of epilepsy, and chronic pharmacoresistant epilepsy (Boison, 2016). In line with this, a transient dose of adenosine delivered by an adenosine-releasing silk-based polymer to the hippocampus prevented epilepsy progression long term in the systemic kainic acid model of TLE (Williams-Karnesky et al., 2013).

Histone Modifications

Histones are important proteins that maintain the chromatin structure in eukaryotic cells and regulate gene expression by allowing DNA transcription. Histone modifications, including histone acetylation and phosphorylation, are associated with epilepsy and epileptogenesis (Boison & Rho, 2019; Hartman & Rho, 2014; Hauser et al., 2018). Histone deacetylation is an essential part of gene regulation and is mediated by histone deacetylase (HDAC; Simeone et al., 2017). Epileptic seizures triggered the deacetylation of histone H4 at the GluR2 locus (Huang et al., 2002; Tsankova et al., 2004), which is associated with increased neuronal excitability and the initiation of epileptogenesis (Tsankova et al., 2004). Increased H4 acetylation was linked with upregulated brain-derived neurotrophic factor (BDNF) expression, another possible mechanism for epileptogenesis (Huang et al., 2002).

In addition to histone deacetylation, histone phosphorylation has also been associated with epilepsy. In both pilocarpine and kainic acid-induced seizures, increased H3 phosphorylation was reported across multiple studies (Crosio et al., 2003; Sng et al., 2006). H3 phosphorylation is believed to facilitate the underlying mechanism that promotes the expression of c-fos/c-jun genes that are implicated in cellular growth, differentiation, and neuronal survival (Sng et al., 2006).

Noncoding RNA

Noncoding RNAs are a class of RNA transcripts without protein-coding capacity. Based on their size, they are classified as long-noncoding RNA (lncRNA; > 200 nucleotides) or microRNA (miRNA; < 200 nucleotides) and are capable of acting as epigenetic modulators. For example, lncRNAs are known to participate in the regulation of pathologic processes of epilepsy and are dysregulated during epileptogenesis. Moreover, aberrant expression of lncRNAs linked to epilepsy has been observed both in patients and in animal models (Lee et al., 2015; Xiao et al., 2018). With regard to epileptogenesis, an altered methylation profile of lncRNAs was associated with the development and progression of TLE (Xiao et al., 2018). Aberrant methylated lncRNAs specifically affected ion-gated channel activity, synaptic transmission, and γ-aminobutyric acid (GABA) receptor activity, mechanisms commonly associated with epileptogenesis (Xiao et al., 2018). In line with this, lncRNAs have been implicated in the regeneration of GABAergic neurons (Qureshi & Mehler, 2013).

In addition to lncRNA, miRNAs have also been linked to epilepsy development and progression. Certain miRNAs, such as miR-9, miR-124a, and miR-132, which target NRSF/RE1-silencing transcription factor (REST), which has a direct role in epigenetics (Wu & Xie, 2006), were also found to be altered in epilepsy (Jimenez-Mateos et al., 2011; Peng et al., 2013; Pichardo-Casas et al., 2012). However, the functional role of noncoding RNAs in epileptogenesis is elusive and warrants further investigation.

KETOGENIC DIET, EPIGENETICS, AND ANTIEPILEPTOGENESIS

TLE, the most common form of focal epilepsy, with about 80% of seizures originating in the hippocampus—a critical structure for consolidation, storage, and retrieval of memories—is refractory to conventional antiseizure drugs in up to 40% of patients, leaving removal of the hippocampus as the antiseizure treatment of last resort for many. The growing field of epigenetic research has led to the discovery that significant epigenetic changes occur in the epileptic hippocampus.

This finding, combined with the potential of the KD to influence epigenetic mechanisms, presents a unique therapeutic opportunity. The KD, although regaining its importance, is used only as a last resort for the treatment of highly refractory patients. This makes it very difficult to investigate the KD's antiepileptogenic mechanisms in a clinical setting. Therefore, much of the mechanistic understanding of the antiepileptogenic potential of the KD, particularly its effects on epigenetic mechanisms, comes from animal studies. It is important to understand how the KD can prevent or reverse the epigenetic mechanisms that lead to the development of epilepsy.

Although the mechanisms are not yet well understood, strict adherence to a KD reduces seizures, and in a consistent 10% to 20% of cases, it prevents seizure progression. It is known that the antiseizure effects of the KD are based on multiple mechanisms (Elamin & Masino, 2020; Masino & Rho, 2012), including an adenosine receptor-dependent mechanism (Masino et al., 2011), whereas the antiepileptogeneic effect of the diet is likely due to the effect it has on the adenosine-dependent transmethylation pathway (Lusardi et al., 2015; Williams-Karnesky et al., 2013). As described previously, adenosine plays a key role in regulating DNA methylation (Figure 25.2; Boison et al., 2002; Mato et al., 2008). As predicted by the underlying biochemistry, exogenous application of either adenosine or pharmacologic inhibition of ADK with 5-iodotubercidin (ITU) inhibited the reaction and reduced DNA methylation, whereas addition of the methyl-group donor SAM increased DNA methylation in the naive rodent brain (Williams-Karnesky et al., 2013). These findings show that global DNA methylation levels are under the direct control of adenosine, and that disruption of adenosine homeostasis (due to ADK upregulation at the epileptogenic focus) affected DNA methylation levels and altered gene expression in the epileptic brain. Moreover, the restoration of DNA methylation was directly linked to reduced epilepsy progression, including the progressive increase of spontaneous convulsive seizures and additional mossy fiber sprouting, lasting well after the conclusion of the adenosine delivery (Williams-Karnesky et al., 2013). In a kindling model of epileptogenesis, the KD also delayed the acquisition of kindling in mice, an effect that persisted even after a return to a standard lab diet, while the conventional antiepileptogenic drug valproic acid attenuated only the seizures without blocking the kindling process. These data demonstrate persistent effects of the

KD that are not merely due to seizure suppression (Lusardi et al., 2015). When a KD was fed to rats after status epilepticus, the diet not only reduced spontaneous seizure development but also reduced DNA methylation levels both during diet administration and after a return to standard diet (Kobow et al., 2013; Lusardi et al., 2015). Though a direct link between the KD and DNA methylation levels must still be demonstrated, when evaluated together, these results show that the lasting effects of the KD may be conferred via adenosine regulation of the DNA methylome, suggesting a key mechanism implicated in epilepsy and epileptogenesis (Basu et al., 2019; Hartman & Rho, 2014; Reddy et al., 2018; Tanaka et al., 2000).

The KD also confers antiepileptogenic properties via the inhibition of histone deacetylation (Figure 25.2). Experimental findings support the idea that the KD, as well as its ketone body byproducts resulting from fatty acid oxidation, such as β-hydroxybutyrate (BHB), acetoacetate (AcAc), and acetone, may have antiepileptogenic potential by inhibiting HDACs (Hartman & Rho, 2014). Recent experimental findings show that the inhibition of HDAC by chronic administration of butyrate, a ketone body product of anaerobic fermentation in bacteria, retarded the development of limbic epileptogenesis and prevented epileptogenic mossy fiber axonal sprouting in mice submitted to the hippocampal kindling model of TLE (Reddy et al., 2018). In another study using TSC2$^{+/-}$ mice, a genetically modified mouse model of tuberous sclerosis complex, which leads to developmental delays, cognitive defects, autism, and epilepsy by altered mTORC1 signaling and aberrant hippocampal synaptic plasticity, the inhibition of HDAC by trichostatin A resulted in normalization in synaptic plasticity and restored mTORC1 signaling (Basu et al., 2019). Overall, the evidence shows a great involvement of alterations in histone acetylation in epileptogenesis. There is much to be explored about the mechanisms of action of the KD as well as single ketone bodies in seizure and epileptogenesis suppression and the involvement of adenosine in these mechanisms, especially histone (de)acetylation.

A recent study showed global changes in miRNA expression in pediatric epilepsy patients after KD therapy (Olaso-González et al., 2018). However, many of the miRNAs were involved in antioxidant pathways and were not linked to epigenetic mechanisms. Another study showed that a high-energy diet caused differential regulation of the lncRNA transcriptome in a model of non-alcoholic steatohepatitis in minipigs (Xia et al.,

2016). Although there is no direct evidence linking the KD and epigenetic mechanisms controlled by noncoding RNA, research in other areas has suggested that it warrants further investigation.

CONCLUSION

With up to 35% of persons with epilepsy considered to have seizures refractory to treatment and with no therapies available that prevent epilepsy or its progression, the novel epigenetic functions of KD therapy discussed here may be of therapeutic value not only in relieving the seizure burden in patients with epilepsy but also in modifying the development of epilepsy, thereby preventing the sequelae of drug resistance and epilepsy-associated comorbidities. The KD represents a powerful adjunct to existing pharmacologic and surgical approaches to seizure relief. Renewed interest in the KD has led to refinements in the diet's formulation and administration (Kossoff et al., 2009; Wibisono et al., 2015) and better understanding of the potential positive and negative interactions with conventional antiepileptic drugs (Morrison et al., 2009; van der Louw et al., 2015), improving compliance and seizure suppression rates. However, the diet requires close monitoring by physicians and dietitians, and seemingly minor deviations from the ketogenic regimen can negate its beneficial effects. While a "ketogenic diet in a pill" may be unlikely, ongoing studies to understand the biochemical mechanisms of the KD are an essential step in the continued refinement of antiseizure and antiepileptogenic therapies. The neuroprotective mechanisms of the KD are varied, and diet efficacy may rely on their combined influences. Among the metabolites regulated by the KD, however, adenosine has both a direct relevance to seizure suppression by A1R activation and an indirect influence on epilepsy and epileptogenesis via regulation of DNA methylation. A clearer understanding of how KD therapy affects adenosine metabolism and its epigenetic sequelae may aid the understanding of adenosine dysregulation in epilepsy and may guide the development of therapies designed to directly restore adenosine homeostasis, with the goal of developing a novel class of antiepileptogenic drugs.

REFERENCES

Aronica, E., & Gorter, J. A. (2007). Gene expression profile in temporal lobe epilepsy. *Neuroscientist*, 13, 100–108.

Barborka, C. J. (1930). Epilepsy in adults—Results of treatment by ketogenic diet in one hundred cases. *Archives of Neurology and Psychiatry*, 23, 904–914.

Basu, T., O'Riordan, K. J., Schoenike, B. A., Khan, N. N., Wallace, E. P., Rodriguez, G., Maganti, R. K., & Roopra, A. (2019). Histone deacetylase inhibitors restore normal hippocampal synaptic plasticity and seizure threshold in a mouse model of tuberous sclerosis complex. *Scientific Reports*, 9, 5266.

Berger, T. C., Vigeland, M. D., Hjorthaug, H. S., Etholm, L., Nome, C. G., Tauboll, E., Heuser, K., & Selmer, K. K. (2019). Neuronal and glial DNA methylation and gene expression changes in early epileptogenesis. *PLOS ONE*, 14, Article e0226575.

Boison, D. (2016). Adenosinergic signaling in epilepsy. *Neuropharmacology*, 104, 131–139.

Boison, D., & Rho, J. M. (2020). Epigenetics and epilepsy prevention: The therapeutic potential of adenosine and metabolic therapies. *Neuropharmacology*, 107741.

Boison, D., Scheurer, L., Zumsteg, V., Rulicke, T., Litynski, P., Fowler, B., Brandner, S., & Mohler, H. (2002). Neonatal hepatic steatosis by disruption of the adenosine kinase gene. *Proceedings of the National Academy of Sciences of the United States of America*, 99, 6985–6990.

Cavalleri, G. L., Weale, M. E., Shianna, K. V., Singh, R., Lynch, J. M., Grinton, B., Szoeke, C., Murphy, K., Kinirons, P., O'Rourke, D., Ge, D., Depondt, C., Claeys, K. G., Pandolfo, M., Gumbs, C., Walley, N., McNamara, J., Mulley, J. C., Linney, K. N., . . . Goldstein, D. B. (2007). Multicentre search for genetic susceptibility loci in sporadic epilepsy syndrome and seizure types: A case-control study. *Lancet Neurology*, 6, 970–980.

Clossen, B. L., & Reddy, D. S. (2017). Novel therapeutic approaches for disease-modification of epileptogenesis for curing epilepsy. *Biochimica and Biophysica Acta Molecular Basis of Disease*, 1863, 1519–1538.

Coppola, G., Veggiotti, P., Cusmai, R., Bertoli, S., Cardinali, S., Dionisi-Vici, C., Elia, M., Lispi, M. L., Sarnelli, C., Tagliabue, A., Toraldo, C., & Pascotto, A. (2002). The ketogenic diet in children, adolescents and young adults with refractory epilepsy: An Italian multicentric experience. *Epilepsy Research*, 48, 221–227.

Crosio, C., Heitz, E., Allis, C. D., Borrelli, E., & Sassone-Corsi, P. (2003). Chromatin remodeling and neuronal response: Multiple signaling pathways induce specific histone H3 modifications and early gene expression in hippocampal neurons. *Journal of Cell Science*, 116, 4905–4914.

Diamond, M. L., Ritter, A. C., Jackson, E. K., Conley, Y. P., Kochanek, P. M., Boison, D., & Wagner, A. K. (2015). Genetic variation in the adenosine regulatory cycle is associated with posttraumatic epilepsy development. *Epilepsia*, 56, 1198–1206.

Elamin, M., & Masino, S. (2020). KD mechanisms. *Epilepsy Research, This issue.*

Gill, M. W., & Schatz, R. A. (1985). The effect of diazepam on brain levels of S-adenosyl-L-methionine and S-adenosyl-L-homocysteine: Possible correlation with protection from methionine sulfoximine seizures. *Research Communications in Chemical Pathology and Pharmacology, 50,* 349–363.

Haas, C. A., Dudeck, O., Kirsch, M., Huszka, C., Kann, G., Pollak, S., Zentner, J., & Frotscher, M. (2002). Role for reelin in the development of granule cell dispersion in temporal lobe epilepsy. *Journal of Neuroscience, 22,* 5797–5802.

Hartman, A. L., & Rho, J. M. (2014). The new ketone alphabet soup: BHB, HCA, and HDAC. *Epilepsy Currents, 14,* 355–357.

Hauser, R. M., Henshall, D. C., & Lubin, F. D. (2018). The epigenetics of epilepsy and its progression. *Neuroscientist, 24,* 186–200.

Henshall, D. C. (2018). Epigenetic changes in status epilepticus. *Epilepsia,* Suppl 2, 82–86.

Henshall, D. C., & Kobow, K. (2015). Epigenetics and epilepsy. *Cold Spring Harbor Perspectives in Medicine, 5*(12), a022731.

Huang, Y., Doherty, J. J., & Dingledine, R. (2002). Altered histone acetylation at glutamate receptor 2 and brain-derived neurotrophic factor genes is an early event triggered by status epilepticus. *Journal of Neuroscience, 22,* 8422–8428.

Jaenisch, R., & Bird, A. (2003). Epigenetic regulation of gene expression: how the genome integrates intrinsic and environmental signals. *Nature Genetics, 33*(Suppl.), 245–254.

James, S. J., Melnyk, S., Pogribna, M., Pogribny, I. P., & Caudill, M. A. (2002). Elevation in S-adenosylhomocysteine and DNA hypomethylation: Potential epigenetic mechanism for homocysteine-related pathology. *Journal of Nutrition, 132,* 2361S–2366S.

Jimenez-Mateos, E. M., Bray, I., Sanz-Rodriguez, A., Engel, T., McKiernan, R. C., Mouri, G., Tanaka, K., Sano, T., Saugstad, J. A., Simon, R. P., Stallings, R. L., & Henshall, D. C. (2011). miRNA expression profile after status epilepticus and hippocampal neuroprotection by targeting miR-132. *American Journal of Pathology, 179,* 2519–2532.

Kasperaviciute, D., Catarino, C. B., Heinzen, E. L., Depondt, C., Cavalleri, G. L., Caboclo, L. O., Tate, S. K., Jamnadas-Khoda, J., Chinthapalli, K., Clayton, L. M., Shianna, K. V., Radtke, R. A., Mikati, M. A., Gallentine, W. B., Husain, A. M., Alhusaini, S., Leppert, D., Middleton, L. T., Gibson, R. A., . . . Sisodiya, S. M. (2010). Common genetic variation and susceptibility to partial epilepsies: A genome-wide association study. *Brain, 133,* 2136–2147.

Kiefer, J. C. (2007). Epigenetics in development. *Developmental Dynamics, 236,* 1144–1156.

Klein, P., Dingledine, R., Aronica, E., Bernard, C., Blumcke, I., Boison, D., Brodie, M. J., Brooks-Kayal, A. R., Engel, J., Jr., Forcelli, P. A., Hirsch, L. J., Kaminski, R. M., Klitgaard, H., Kobow, K., Lowenstein, D. H., Pearl, P. L., Pitkanen, A., Puhakka, N., Rogawski, M. A., . . . Loscher, W. (2018). Commonalities in epileptogenic processes from different acute brain insults: Do they translate? *Epilepsia, 59,* 37–66.

Kobow, K., & Blumcke, I. (2012). The emerging role of DNA methylation in epileptogenesis. *Epilepsia, 53*(Suppl. 9), 11–20.

Kobow, K., Jeske, I., Hildebrandt, M., Hauke, J., Hahnen, E., Buslei, R., Buchfelder, M., Weigel, D., Stefan, H., Kasper, B., Pauli, E., & Blumcke, I. (2009). Increased reelin promoter methylation is associated with granule cell dispersion in human temporal lobe epilepsy. *Journal of Neuropathology and Experimental Neurology, 68,* 356–364.

Kobow, K., Kaspi, A., Harikrishnan, K. N., Kiese, K., Ziemann, M., Khurana, I., Fritzsche, I., Hauke, J., Hahnen, E., Coras, R., Muhlebner, A., El-Osta, A., & Blumcke, I. (2013). Deep sequencing reveals increased DNA methylation in chronic rat epilepsy. *Acta Neuropathologica, 126*(5), 741–756.

Kossoff, E. H., & Hartman, A. L. (2012). Ketogenic diets: New advances for metabolism-based therapies. *Current Opinion in Neurology, 25,* 173–178.

Kossoff, E. H., Zupec-Kania, B. A., Amark, P. E., Ballaban-Gil, K. R., Christina Bergqvist, A. G., Blackford, R., Buchhalter, J. R., Caraballo, R. H., Helen Cross, J., Dahlin, M. G., Donner, E. J., Klepper, J., Jehle, R. S., Kim, H. D., Christiana Liu, Y. M., Nation, J., Nordli, D. R., Jr., Pfeifer, H. H., Rho, J. M., . . . Vining, E. P. (2009). Optimal clinical management of children receiving the ketogenic diet: recommendations of the International Ketogenic Diet Study Group. *Epilepsia, 50,* 304–317.

Kullmann, D. M. (2002). Genetics of epilepsy. *Journal of Neurolology, Neurosurgery, and Psychiatry, 73*(Suppl. 2), 32–35.

Lee, D. Y., Moon, J., Lee, S. T., Jung, K. H., Park, D. K., Yoo, J. S., Sunwoo, J. S., Byun, J. I., Lim, J. A., Kim, T. J., Jung, K. Y., Kim, M., Jeon, D., Chu, K., & Lee, S. K. (2015). Dysregulation of long noncoding RNAs in mouse models of localization-related epilepsy. *Biochemical and Biophysical Research Communications, 462,* 433–440.

Lukasiuk, K., & Pitkanen, A. (2004). Large-scale analysis of gene expression in epilepsy research: Is synthesis already possible? *Neurochemical Research, 29,* 1169–1178.

Lusardi, T. A., Akula, K. K., Coffman, S. Q., Ruskin, D. N., Masino, S. A., & Boison, D. (2015). Ketogenic diet prevents epileptogenesis and disease progression in adult mice and rats. *Neuropharmacology, 99,* 500–509.

Mandaviya, P. R., Stolk, L., & Heil, S. G. (2014). Homocysteine and DNA methylation: A review of animal and human literature. *Molecula Genetics and Metabolism*, 113, 243–252.

Masino, S. A., Li, T., Theofilas, P., Sandau, U. S., Ruskin, D. N., Fredholm, B. B., Geiger, J. D., Aronica, E., & Boison, D. (2011). A ketogenic diet suppresses seizures in mice through adenosine A1 receptors. *Journal of Clinical Investigation*, 21(7), 2679–2683.

Masino, S. A., & Rho, J. M. (2012). Mechanisms of ketogenic diet action. In J. L. Noebels, M. Avoli, M. A. Rogawski, R. W. Olsen, & A. V. Delgado-Escueta (Eds.), *Jasper's Basic mechanisms of the epilepsies*. https://www.ncbi.nlm.nih.gov/books/NBK98219/

Mato, J. M., Martinez-Chantar, M. L., & Lu, S. C. (2008). Methionine metabolism and liver disease. *Annual Review of Nutrition*, 28, 273–293.

Mefford, H. C., Muhle, H., Ostertag, P., von Spiczak, S., Buysse, K., Baker, C., Franke, A., Malafosse, A., Genton, P., Thomas, P., Gurnett, C. A., Schreiber, S., Bassuk, A. G., Guipponi, M., Stephani, U., Helbig, I., & Eichler, E. E. (2010). Genome-wide copy number variation in epilepsy: Novel susceptibility loci in idiopathic generalized and focal epilepsies. *PLOS Genetics*, 6, Article e1000962.

Miller-Delaney, S. F., Bryan, K., Das, S., McKiernan, R. C., Bray, I. M., Reynolds, J. P., Gwinn, R., Stallings, R. L., & Henshall, D. C. (2015). Differential DNA methylation profiles of coding and non-coding genes define hippocampal sclerosis in human temporal lobe epilepsy. *Brain*, 138, 616–631.

Morrison, P. F., Pyzik, P. L., Hamdy, R., Hartman, A. L., & Kossoff, E. H. (2009). The influence of concurrent anticonvulsants on the efficacy of the ketogenic diet. *Epilepsia*, 50, 1999–2001.

Myers, C. T., & Mefford, H. C. (2015). Advancing epilepsy genetics in the genomic era. *Genome Medicine*, 7, 91.

Olaso-González, G., Serna, E., Herrero, J. R., Martínez, C., Gómez-Cabrera, M. C., Pedrón, C., & Vina, J. (2018). MiRNome of epileptic children suggests the involvement of antioxidant pathways in the neuroprotective role of ketogenic diet. *Free Radical Biology and Medicine*, 120, S80–S81.

Peng, J., Omran, A., Ashhab, M. U., Kong, H., Gan, N., He, F., & Yin, F. (2013). Expression patterns of miR-124, miR-134, miR-132, and miR-21 in an immature rat model and children with mesial temporal lobe epilepsy. *Journal of Molecular Neuroscience*, 50, 291–297.

Peterman, M. G. (1924). The ketogenic diet in the treatment of epilepsy: A preliminary report. *American Journal of Diseases of Children*, 28, 28–33.

Peterman, M. G. (1925). The ketogenic diet in epilepsy. *JAMA*, 84, 1979–1983.

Pichardo-Casas, I., Goff, L. A., Swerdel, M. R., Athie, A., Davila, J., Ramos-Brossier, M., Lapid-Volosin, M., Friedman, W. J., Hart, R. P., & Vaca, L. (2012). Expression profiling of synaptic microRNAs from the adult rat brain identifies regional differences and seizure-induced dynamic modulation. *Brain Research*, 1436, 20–33.

Pitkanen, A., Lukasiuk, K., Dudek, F. E., & Staley, K. J. (2015). Epileptogenesis. *Cold Spring Harbor Perspectives in Medicine*, 18;5(10), a022822.

Qureshi, I. A., & Mehler, M. F. (2013). Long non-coding RNAs: Novel targets for nervous system disease diagnosis and therapy. *Neurotherapeutics*, 10, 632–646.

Reddy, S. D., Clossen, B. L., & Reddy, D. S. (2018). Epigenetic histone deacetylation inhibition prevents the development and persistence of temporal lobe epilepsy. *Journal of Pharmacology and Experimental Therapeutics*, 364, 97–109.

Schatz, R. A., Wilens, T. E., Tatter, S. B., Gregor, P., & Sellinger, O. Z. (1983). Possible role of increased brain methylation in methionine sulfoximine epileptogenesis: Effects of administration of adenosine and homocysteine thiolactone. *Journal of NeuroscienceResearch*, 10, 437–447.

Sellinger, O. Z., Schatz, R. A., Porta, R., & Wilens, T. E. (1984). Brain methylation and epileptogenesis: The case of methionine sulfoximine. *Annals of Neurology*, 16(Suppl.), 115–120.

Simeone, T. A., Simeone, K. A., & Rho, J. M. (2017). Ketone bodies as anti-seizure agents. *Neurochemical Research*, 42, 2011–2018.

Sirven, J., Whedon, B., Caplan, D., Liporace, J., Glosser, D., O'Dwyer, J., & Sperling, M. R. (1999). The ketogenic diet for intractable epilepsy in adults: Preliminary results. *Epilepsia*, 40, 1721–1726.

Sloviter, R. S., & Bumanglag, A. V. (2013). Defining "epileptogenesis" and identifying "antiepileptogenic targets" in animal models of acquired temporal lobe epilepsy is not as simple as it might seem. *Neuropharmacology*, 69, 3–15.

Sloviter, R. S., Sollas, A. L., Barbaro, N. M., & Laxer, K. D. (1991). Calcium-binding protein (calbindin-D28K) and parvalbumin immunocytochemistry in the normal and epileptic human hippocampus. *Journal of Comparative Neurology*, 308, 381–396.

Sng, J. C., Taniura, H., & Yoneda, Y. (2006). Histone modifications in kainate-induced status epilepticus. *European Journal of Neuroscience*, 23, 1269–1282.

Stafstrom, C. E., & Rho, J. M. (2012). The ketogenic diet as a treatment paradigm for diverse neurological disorders. *Frontiers in Pharmacology*, 3, 59.

Tanaka, H., Grooms, S. Y., Bennett, M. V., & Zukin, R. S. (2000). The AMPAR subunit GluR2: Still front and center-stage. *Brain Research*, 886, 190–207.

Tsankova, N. M., Kumar, A., & Nestler, E. J. (2004). Histone modifications at gene promoter regions in rat hippocampus after acute and chronic electroconvulsive seizures. *Journal of Neuroscience, 24,* 5603–5610.

van der Louw, E. J., Desadien, R., Vehmeijer, F. O., van der Sijs, H., Catsman-Berrevoets, C. E., & Neuteboom, R. F. (2015). Concomitant lamotrigine use is associated with decreased efficacy of the ketogenic diet in childhood refractory epilepsy. *Seizure, 32,* 75–77.

Wheless, J. W. (2008). History of the ketogenic diet. *Epilepsia, 49*(Suppl. 8), 3–5.

Wibisono, C., Rowe, N., Beavis, E., Kepreotes, H., Mackie, F. E., Lawson, J. A., & Cardamone, M. (2015). Ten-year single-center experience of the ketogenic diet: Factors influencing efficacy, tolerability, and compliance. *Journal of Pediatrics, 166,* 1030–1036.

Wilder, R. M. (1921). The effects of ketonemia on the course of epilepsy. *Mayo Clin Bull, 2,* 307–308.

Wilder, R. M., & Winter, M. D. (1922). The threshold of ketogenesis. *Journal of Biological Chemistry, 52,* 393–401.

Williams-Karnesky, R. L., Sandau, U. S., Lusardi, T. A., Lytle, N. K., Farrell, J. M., Pritchard, E. M., Kaplan, D. L., & Boison, D. (2013). Epigenetic changes induced by adenosine augmentation therapy prevent epileptogenesis. *Journal of Clinical Investigation, 123*(8), 3552–3563.

Wu, J., & Xie, X. (2006). Comparative sequence analysis reveals an intricate network among REST, CREB and miRNA in mediating neuronal gene expression. *Genome Biology, 7,* R85.

Xia, J., Xin, L., Zhu, W., Li, L., Li, C., Wang, Y., Mu, Y., Yang, S., & Li, K. (2016). Characterization of long non-coding RNA transcriptome in high-energy diet induced nonalcoholic steatohepatitis minipigs. *Scientific Reports, 6,* 30709.

Xiao, W., Cao, Y., Long, H., Luo, Z., Li, S., Deng, N., Wang, J., Lu, X., Wang, T., Ning, S., Wang, L., & Xiao, B. (2018). Genome-wide DNA methylation patterns analysis of noncoding RNAs in temporal lobe epilepsy patients. *Molecular Neurobiology, 55,* 793–803.

Zhao, S., Chai, X., Bock, H. H., Brunne, B., Forster, E., & Frotscher, M. (2006). Rescue of the reeler phenotype in the dentate gyrus by wild-type coculture is mediated by lipoprotein receptors for Reelin and Disabled 1. *Journal of Comparative Neurology, 495,* 1–9.

26

Ketogenic Diet, Aging, and Neurodegeneration

KUI XU, MD, PHD, AARTI SETHURAMAN, PHD, JOSEPH C. LAMANNA, PHD, AND MICHELLE A. PUCHOWICZ, PHD

OVERVIEW

It has been established for over 50 years that brain can utilize ketone bodies under carbohydrate (glucose)-sparing conditions (Cahill & Owen, 1967; Owen et al., 1967; Randle et al., 1963). Use of the ketogenic diet (KG) to treat intractable epilepsy in children was established nearly a century ago and continues to be an option for clinicians (DeVivo et al., 1978; Freeman et al., 1998; Lennox, 1928; Millichap et al., 1964; Tallian et al., 1998; Schwartzkroin, 1999; Wilder, 1921), but the KG's mechanisms of action remain diverse and unclear (Bridge, 1931; Jarrett et al., 2008; Lund et al., 2009; Maalouf et al., 2007, 2009a; Masino & Rho, 2012; Milder & Patel, 2012; Millichap et al., 1964; Nakazawa et al., 1983; Prins & Hovda, 2009; Stafstrom & Rho, 2012; Yudkoff et al., 2007). To date, the mechanistic link of ketosis and neuroprotection continues to be investigated. The mechanisms appear to be related to the change in the regulation of the cell's stress responses (Milder et al., 2010), as well as changes in oxidative (glucose) metabolism (Bough & Rho, 2007; Masino & Rho, 2012; Prins & Hovda, 2009; Puchowicz et al., 2008; Zhang et al., 2018). Neuroprotection by ketosis has been described to be associated with improved mitochondrial function, decreased reactive oxygen species (ROS) and apoptotic and inflammatory mediators, and increased protective pathways (Guo et al., 2018; Julio-Amilpas et al., 2015; Veech, 2004; Yang et al., 2017).

This chapter focuses on two potential mechanisms that elucidate the neuroprotective effects of ketosis in the brain. It also concentrates on the applications of ketosis in the treatment of the aged brain and presents current data from rodent studies where the KG was used to induce a chronic state of ketosis and neuroprotection was assessed. The neuroprotection associated with diet-induced ketosis appears to be mainly through stabilization of glucose metabolism and the regulation of downstream metabolic pathways, such as the citric acid cycle and cytosolic-mitochondrial redox shuttle systems. It is also apparent that ketone bodies can act as signaling molecules that target hypoxia-inducible factor 1α (HIF-1α)-related cellular defenses and regulatory systems independent of oxygen deprivation. It is known that HIF-1α activation can result in stabilization of the "redox state" of the cell (Semenza, 2011), and that there are two regulatory sides of HIF-1α, angiogenic and metabolic (Semenza, 2007b). We have previously shown neuroprotection by ketosis in the rat and mouse model of middle cerebral artery occlusion (MCAO) Xu et al., 2017). The hypothesis that the mechanistic link between ketosis and neuroprotection is through HIF-1α and its downstream effects on metabolic enzymes has been presented (Puchowicz et al., 2008).

KETONE BODIES ARE ALTERNATE ENERGY SUBSTRATES TO GLUCOSE

Ketone bodies (or the state of ketosis) have been shown to be neuroprotective after oxidative stress and metabolic challenges, such as those associated with stroke, ischemia, injury, Alzheimer's disease, Parkinson's disease, glucose transporter deficiency, and seizures (Cunnane et al., 2011; Kashiwaya et al., 2000; Maalouf et al., 2009a; Prins & Hovda, 2009). Ketone bodies are alternatives to glucose as energy substrates, and thus they have the potential to restore energy balance via stabilization of ATP supply. They are thought to be more efficient energy substrates than glucose for utilization by brain (Cahill & Veech, 2003; Kashiwaya et al., 2000; Sato et al., 1995; Veech, 2004; Veech et al., 2001). One application for the use of ketone bodies as an alternative substrate is for those with aging-related defects in glucose metabolism. Hypometabolism is a clinical presentation in some patients with Alzheimer's disease and is thought to be associated with defects in glucose metabolism (Cunnane et al., 2011). Studies measuring the ^{13}C-amino acid:^{13}C-lactate ratio in brain showed the fraction of amino acid carbon derived from glucose decreased with ketosis, reflecting the utilization of ketones as carbon precursors for synthesis of aspartate, glutamine, glutamate, and gamma-aminobutyric acid (GABA; Yudkoff et al., 2007). The neuroprotective role of ketone bodies may be through improvement in metabolic efficiency, by sparing glucose and the degradation of muscle-derived amino acids for substrates.

Ketone body utilization has properties that are considered metabolically favorable over glucose metabolism, including:

- The direct generation of NADH, FADH$_2$, and succinate, which makes these substrates readily available (compartmentalized) to the mitochondria for energy production.
- The direct generation of acetyl-CoA, which enters the citric acid cycle via the citrate synthase reaction, thus relieving oxidative stress induced by pyruvate dehydrogenase inhibition, as well as making available ATP and lactate generated from glycolysis for other functions, such as the shuttling of substrates between neurons and glia.
- The potential reduction of mitochondrial ROS production associated with reperfusion injury.
- Stabilization of HIF-1α independent of hypoxia.

USE OF THE KG TO INDUCE KETOSIS: A MODEL OF STABILIZED CHRONIC KETOSIS

The efficacy of ketosis in metabolic modulations and cellular protection remains debated. The action of ketosis (or ketone bodies) on metabolic adaptations requires stable ketosis, which relates to the duration and level of ketosis. The KG-induced ketosis is a way to establish chronic stable ketosis. The diet-induced approach avoids the constraints (sodium or fluid overload, pH imbalance, or starvation with chronic fasting) of using alternate modes of inducing ketosis, such as by infusions of ketone bodies or ketone body precursors (sodium salts or acids), or long-term fasting (Desrochers et al., 1995; Puchowicz et al., 2000). Ketosis induction by diet (in rodents and humans) requires at least 3 weeks of maintaining the KG (Leino et al., 2001; Pan et al., 2000; Puchowicz et al., 2007). This regime can be viewed as a preconditioning state where blood

concentrations of ketone bodies remain stable over time. We have previously reported that 3 weeks of diet-induced stable ketosis is necessary to induce metabolic adaptations in the brains of rats and mice (Puchowicz et al., 2007, 2008; Xu et al., 2017). Metabolic adaptations associated with chronic ketosis include the upregulation of monocarboxylate transporters (MCT1) at the blood–brain barrier, as well as upregulation of cytoprotective pathways involving HIF-1α, protein kinase B (pAKT), and AMP-activated protein kinase (AMPK). We have established in our rat model of ketosis that metabolic adaptations also include a correlation between cerebral metabolic rate for glucose (CMRglu) and blood ketone levels (Zhang et al., 2013), as well as decreased glucose shunting toward neurotransmitters, GABA, glutamate, and glutamine (Zhang et al., 2015). Positron emission tomography (PET) showed a 10% decrease in CMRglu for each 1 mM increase of total plasma ketone bodies in cortical and cerebellar brain regions. Together with our meta-analysis, these data revealed that the degree and duration of ketosis played major roles in determining the corresponding change in CMRglu with ketosis and that preconditioning with the KG resulted in significant glucose sparing and a concomitant increase in ketone body utilization in cortical brain (Zhang et al., 2013, 2015).

OXIDATIVE STRESS-INDUCED ALTERED GLUCOSE METABOLISM

Supply of energy substrate to the mitochondria is critical, especially during conditions of high energy demand where glucose metabolism may be deficient, such as with oxidative injury. The ability of the central nervous system to recover from an ischemic and/or hypoxic event is its capacity to recover from metabolic stress. It is well known that the status of cellular bioenergetics of the neurovascular unit is a major determinant of the pathophysiologic outcome. Stoichiometric analysis predicts that glycolysis cannot sustain NADH demand (energy demand) for more than a few hours, depending on glycogen stores. Thus, increased risk for sudden cell death remains problematic.

Under pathologic conditions, the brain's energy demand and supply are mismatched, resulting in energy inefficiency. For example, survival and recovery of neurologic function after cardiac arrest and resuscitation is limited by the ability of the brain to recover from an ischemic event due to metabolic stress. After cardiac arrest and resuscitation, increased glycolytic rates are associated with lactic acidosis and downstream metabolic blocks in energetics. After 24 hr of reperfusion, there is an "apparent" defect in glucose metabolism that may continue as a secondary response to oxidative stress-induced injury (Selman et al., 1990). At this stage of oxidative damage, there is a decrease in CMRglu (Bentourkia et al., 2000; DiVivo et al., 1973; Willis et al., 2002). Mitochondria are among the organelles most susceptible to oxidative stress. Brain mitochondrial function is known to decrease 2 days after ischemia/reperfusion injury (Xu et al., 2008a), which more often results in delayed neuronal death 4 days after recovery (Xu et al., 2006). The degree of neurologic deficit is highly dependent on the length of time to restored blood flow and on the severity of oxidative damage. The generation of ROS and cytotoxic products of lipid peroxidation, such as 4-hydroxy-2-nonenal (HNE) and glutathione (GSH/GSSH), also plays a major role in the cell's ability to recover. In a previous study, we showed that KG-induced ketosis resulted in overall survival rates 4 days after cardiac arrest and resuscitation that were significantly higher in the KG-fed group than in the standard diet group (86% versus 55%, $p < 0.05$, Figure 26.1). The protective effect of the

KG on postresuscitation survival is comparable to the effect of postresuscitation treatment with adenosine (ADO) in 3-month-old rats (Xu et al., 2006) and the postresuscitation treatment with N-tert-butyl-α-phenylnitrone (PBN, a spin trapping agent reacts with unstable free radicals) in 24-month-old rats (Xu et al., 2010). These data support the idea that diet-induced ketosis is neuroprotective when glucose utilization is limited (Xu et al., 2012).

Research continues to show that altered energy metabolism is associated with aging and/ or oxidative damage to key enzymes that regulate glucose metabolism (Cunnane et al., 2011; Gibson et al., 1998). The imbalance between non-oxidative and oxidative-derived ATP is recognized but not clearly understood (Hemmila & Drewes, 1993; Hempel et al., 1977; Hoxworth et al., 1999; Xu et al., 2006, 2008a). One explanation may be the lack of glucose carbon entry (flux) into the citric acid cycle (i.e., via the pyruvate dehydrogenase complex) that results in a dysregulation or "leakiness" of the citric acid cycle (cataplerosis). These consequences can lead to irreversible neurologic deficit. Anaplerosis, a process that balances cataplerosis, ordinarily maintains/supplies intermediates to the citric acid cycle, which become vital during increased leakiness associated with ischemia/

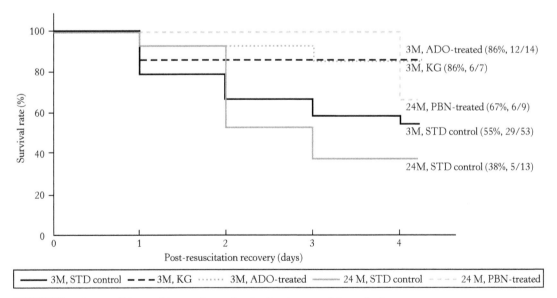

FIGURE 26.1 *Overall Survival Rates 4 Days after Cardiac Arrest and Resuscitation*

The 3-month-old (3M) rats fed with 3 weeks of ketogenic (KG) diet had a significantly higher survival rates than the control rats fed a standard diet (86% vs. 55%, $p < 0.05$, Wilcoxon survival analysis; Xu et al., 2012). The KG diet provided protection similar to that provided by the post-resuscitation treatment with adenosine (ADO) in 3-month-old rats (Xu et al., 2006) and the post-resuscitation treatment with N-tert-butyl-α-phenylnitrone (PBN, a spin-trapping agent that reacts with free radicals) in the 24-month-old (24M) rats (Xu et al., 2010). Cardiac arrest occurred at about 12 min and 7 min in the 3M and 24M rats, respectively. Data adapted from Xu et al. (2006, 2010, 2012).

reperfusion injury (Brunengraber & Roe, 2006; Kasumov et al., 2007) and other neuropathologies. The balance between cataplerosis and anaplerosis is essential to maintaining energy balance and, therefore, mitochondrial function. Using stable isotopomer analysis, we investigated the role of ketosis in the partitioning of glucose and ketones as substrates at the level of acetyl-CoA and the citric acid cycle in vivo in cortical brain (Zhang et al., 2015). The study revealed that glucose entry into the citric acid cycle was decreased with ketosis, whereas acetoacetate (AcAc) entry was increased. The increased contribution of AcAc to central metabolism suggests that the carbon backbone from ketones plays a role in balancing the citric acid cycle. The possibility of increased pyruvate carboxylation via malic enzyme should also be considered as a mechanism of ketosis in energy stabilization (Hassel, 2000).

DIET-INDUCED KETOSIS AS A NEUROPROTECTIVE STRATEGY IN THE AGED: CLINICAL RELEVANCE

The aging population is at risk for increased morbidity and mortality following ischemic or hypoxic events, such as those related to stroke or other neurodegenerative conditions. Stroke is a common pathology and the leading cause of disability in the United States, because there are few (if any) clinical treatment strategies that can reverse cellular damage. All brain cells are susceptible to infarction after ischemia/reperfusion (Pundik et al., 2012). Another example of a condition that results in moderate to severe ischemia/ reperfusion injury to brain is cardiac arrest and resuscitation. In the United States, about one million cardiac arrests occur per year; about half of individuals (elderly or adult) having first-time cardiac arrest will not survive the first few days. Of those who do survive, about 90% will have short- or long-term neurologic deficits. These deficits are often related to oxidative stress-induced postresuscitation mortality and delayed selective neuronal cell loss (Hoxworth et al., 1999; Xu et al., 2006, 2008a). In the elderly, failure to recover is especially pronounced, because the aged brain is susceptible to oxidative stress damage as result of declines in repair systems and decreased antioxidant capacity. Brain pathophysiology associated with oxidative stress and injury, such as with ischemia/reperfusion injury, often results in energy imbalances related to dysregulation of glucose (oxidative) metabolism. It could be that ketones are effective against pathology associated

with altered glucose metabolism (Cahill & Veech, 2003; Prins & Hovda, 2009; Sato et al., 1995; Veech, 2004; Veech et al., 2001, 2012). Ketones may also play a role as signaling molecules that directly or indirectly act through the regulation of cell salvation pathways, such as HIF-1α.

Previously, we reported that the HIF-1α response to hypoxia is suppressed in the aged rat brain, and we proposed that this was an explanation for why the aged are more susceptible to an oxidative insult (Ndubuizu et al., 2010; Xu et al., 2010). Consistent with our previous study in rats, HIF-1α accumulation and vascular endothelial growth factor (VEGF) expression were attenuated in cortical brain of hypoxia-exposed aged mice (Benderro & LaManna, 2011). In another study, we showed that ketosis is induced in aged rats (18 months old) fed a KG for 3 weeks, and that diet-induced ketosis was neuroprotective against focal cerebral ischemia (MCAO; Figure 26.2). We consistently found lower levels of ketosis (~ 40% plasma ketones, mM) in aged rats after 3 weeks of the KG than in young adult rats, with no differences in plasma glucose or lactate between aged versus young KG groups (Zhang et al., 2018). To determine the partitioning of glucose and ketones in aged brain, cortical CMRglu was measured by [¹⁸F]FDG PET. The results showed that he aged rats fed the KG, the CMRglu was similar to the young and aged rats fed standard chow (STD). These findings are similar to what was previously reported by Roy et al. in their study of aged rats (Roy et al., 2012). However, in our studies in the young adult rat, cortical CMRglu in the KG-fed was significantly lower than in the STD-fed rat (Zhang et al., 2013, 2018). These differences may be attributed to lower cortical βHB levels (nmol/ g tissue) in the KG-fed aged rats compared to KG-fed young rats.

NEUROPROTECTION THROUGH STABILIZATION OF HIF-1A

The notion that ketone bodies can act as metabolic signaling molecules in addition to being alternate oxidative substrates to glucose has received considerable attention (Bough & Rho, 2007; Gano et al., 2014; Maalouf et al., 2009b; Milder et al., 2010b; Shimazu et al., 2013; Tannahill et al., 2013). The role of HIF-1α as a key regulator of oxygen homeostasis during hypoxia is well described (Agani et al., 2002; Chavez et al., 2000, 2006; Semenza, 2007a, 2011; Semenza et al., 2000; Sharp et al., 2001). However, the metabolic role of HIF-1α in neuroprotection remains unclear.

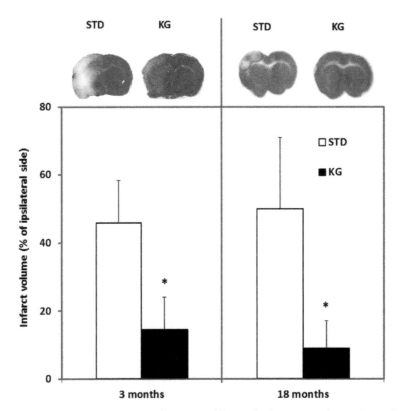

FIGURE 26.2 *Total Brain Infarct Volume Following Middle Cerebral Artery Occlusion (MCAO) in 3- and 18-Month-Old Rats Fed Ketogenic or Standard Diets*

Rats were randomly assigned to two diet groups, fed ad libitum, ketogenic (high fat, no carbohydrate; KG) or standard lab-chow (STD) diet for 3 weeks prior to ischemic stroke. Rats underwent 90 min of MCAO (distal MCAO in the 18-month-old rats and proximal MCAO in the 3-month-old rats). The total infarct volumes were evaluated by triphenyltetrazolium chloride (TTC) staining 24 hr after reperfusion. Results: After rats were fed for 3 weeks of KG diet, plasma ketone bodies (mM) were increased 5-fold in the 18-month-old rats (3.1 ± 0.8 vs. 0.6 ± 0.1, KG vs. STD; $n = 4$ each). After 24 hr of reperfusion after MCAO, the infarct volumes in the aged rats were 5-fold lower in the KG group than in the STD diet group and 3-fold lower in the 3-month-old KG group than in the STD group ($N = 9$, $N = 11$, respectively; adapted from Puchowicz et al., 2008). Data are presented as $M \pm SEM$, % infarct volume of the ipsilateral hemisphere.

HIF-1α is a nuclear factor associated with neuroprotection via regulation of energy metabolism and is a key regulator of oxygen homeostasis during hypoxia, but it may also play a role in neuroprotection after ischemia through gene regulation (Guo et al., 2008; Shi, 2009). HIF-1α activation can also promote cell survival (Bergeron et al., 2000). Understanding the mechanistic role of ketone bodies as metabolic regulators of HIF-1α can help researchers target treatment strategies critically needed for neurodegenerative disorders. Since the aged population has an increased risk for ischemic events, such as those associated with transient global or focal stroke, the development of treatment strategies that incorporate ketosis may be useful.

The mechanism of HIF-1α stabilization through ketosis has been proposed (Puchowicz et al., 2008a) to be most likely through changes in cytoplasmic/mitochondrial redox state (Guo et al., 2008). This is consistent with reports of stabilization of HIF-1α through impairment of proteasome function, as a result of very low ratios of α-ketoglutarate/fumarate (Serra-Perez et al., 2010). A mechanism that explains diet-induced HIF-1α stabilization (via the KG) is feedback inhibition of the prolyl-hydroxylase (PHD) reaction by succinate, an intermediate of mitochondrial metabolism, as a result of ketone body utilization (see Figure 26.3). Elevated cellular levels of succinate and fumarate compete with α-ketoglutarate PHD binding, resulting in inhibition of PHD

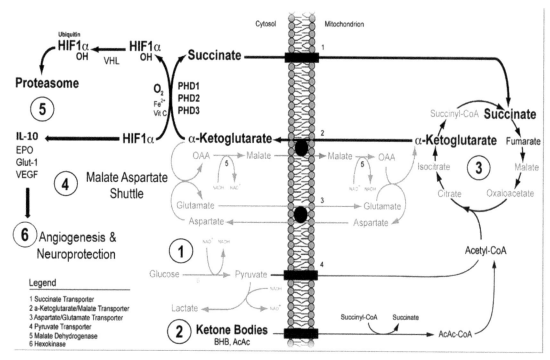

FIGURE 26.3 *Scheme of Proposed Mechanism of Neuroprotection by Diet-Induced Ketosis*

Our scheme emphasizes that cytosolic generated succinate—via prolyl-hydroxylase (PHD) activity—must be balanced by mitochondrial redox of the citric acid cycle. Thus, if there is an accumulation of succinate, as a result of an imbalance of redox, HIF-1α would then be stabilized through inhibition of PHD (Puchowicz et al., 2008a). Pathway of ketosis to induce HIF-1α accumulation, cell redox via malate-aspartate shuttle (scheme below), emphasizes cytosolic generated succinate (via PHD) must be balanced by mitochondrial redox of the citric acid cycle. Steps 1–6 (circled): A link to the stabilization of HIF-1α is through feedback product inhibition of PHD via elevated tissue succinate (Semenza, 2007a) or reduced α-ketoglutarate (steps 3 and 4; McFate et al., 2008). Thus, an accumulation of succinate (or reduction in α-ketoglutarate) would result in an altered redox state via the malate aspartate shuttle (step 4) and stabilization of HIF-1α (via inhibition of PHD; step 5), as well as HIF-1α-mediated angiogenesis and neuroprotection through HIF-1α target genes (step 6). Other intermediates of energy metabolism acting on HIF-1α regulation have been described (Chen et al., 2015; Mills & O'Neill, 2014; Tannahill et al., 2013). The potential mechanism by which ketosis stabilizes HIF-1α is through a shift in "redox state" of the cell via changes in carbon flux into/out of the malate-aspartate shuttle (Semenza, 2011); a target would include changes in succinate:α-ketoglutarate ratio.

and thus stabilization of HIF-1α (Hou et al., 2014; Mills & O'Neill, 2014), independent of hypoxia. The mechanisms of ketosis that are relevant to neuroprotection and stabilization of HIF-1α (via succinate), need to be further studied.

We propose that PHD inhibition occurs as a result of ketone body utilization by the cell via the activation of acetoacetate to acetoacetyl-CoA (via 3-ketoacyl-CoA transferase), which involves the generation of succinate in the mitochondria. Once activated, HIF-1α modulates energy metabolism through downstream regulation of metabolism and related target genes. HIF-1α target genes include those related to angiogenesis, erythropoiesis, glucose metabolism, and cell survival (Agani et al., 2002; Baranova et al., 2007; Chavez

et al., 2006; Chen et al., 2015; Helton et al., 2005; Puchowicz et al., 2008b; Semenza, 2001; Sharp et al., 2001), as well as genes related to inflammation. It has been suggested that HIF-1α may also play a role in promoting apoptosis (Helton et al., 2005; Serra-Perez et al., 2010); however, little is known about this mechanism.

We have reported that the HIF-1α response to hypoxia is blunted in the aged brain due to increased PHD levels (Ndubuizu et al., 2010). The lack of HIF-1α induction after an oxidative insult, such as with reperfusion injury and/or the aging process, increases vulnerability to oxidative damage that can result in poor recovery or cell death (Xu et al., 2007, 2008b). These findings are consistent with other reports on mice with neuron-specific knockdown of HIF-1α that were subjected to transient focal cerebral ischemia; the results showed increased tissue damage and reduced cell survival (Baranova et al., 2007).

The neuroprotective roles of for HIF-1α and related target genes, such as erythropoietin, have been described (Barteczek et al., 2017; Chong et al., 2003b; Ghezzi et al., 2010). As a neuroprotective agent, erythropoietin has many functions: antagonizing glutamate's cytotoxic action, enhancing antioxidant enzyme expression, reducing the free radical production rate, and affecting neurotransmitter release (Bartesaghi et al., 2005; Leist et al., 2004). It exerts its neuroprotective effect indirectly through restoration of blood flow or directly by activating transmitter molecules in neurons that play a role in erythrogenesis. Although the mechanism is unclear, it is apparent that erythropoietin has antiapoptotic action after central and peripheral nerve injury (Chong et al., 2003b). Although apoptosis is not reversible, early intervention with therapeutic procedures, such as erythropoietin administration or preconditioning with the KG, may reduce the number of neurons that undergo apoptosis and may improve outcome.

An additional target gene of HIF-1α is the gene for VEGF. VEGF is an endothelial cell-specific growth factor (Storkebaum et al., 2004), but recent evidence indicates that VEGF also has direct effects on glial cell types (Silverman et al., 1999). A neuroprotective mechanism of VEGF in ischemic brain insults is thought to be through increased perfusion of the penumbra via vasodilatation and angiogenesis (Zhang et al., 2002). We have previously reported that preconditioning with the KG diet results in an angiogenic response similar to what was found with mild hypoxic exposure (Puchowicz et al., 2007). However, we found no changes in cerebral regional blood flow with KG-induced ketosis in adult rats. Thus, the KG may be a therapeutic strategy that targets neuroprotective mechanisms through HIF-regulated VEGF, independent of modifications in perfusion (Chong et al., 2003a).

DISCUSSION

The mechanism of HIF-1α regulation under various metabolic conditions, such as with stroke, inflammation and altered glucose metabolism, needs to be further explored. There are two mechanisms that explain neuroprotection through diet-induced ketosis. First, ketone bodies are alternate energy substrates to glucose, thus

reducing oxidative stress by relieving metabolic blocks downstream of glycolysis at the level of the citric acid cycle, thereby enabling mitochondrial electron transfer and generation of ATP (Julio-Amilpas et al., 2015; Prins, 2008; Sato et al., 1995; Semenza, 2011; Veech, 2004). Second, ketosis induces the stabilization of HIF-1α and upregulation of its downstream target genes.

There is feedback regulation of HIF-1α activation through shifts in metabolic redox, such as with the KG or fasting, that is independent of hypoxia-induced stabilization of HIF-1α (Mills & O'Neill, 2014). Thus, HIF-1α acts as a metabolic sensor through a continuous feedback loop directly coupled to oxidative metabolism via the citric acid cycle and malate aspartate shuttle systems (Figure 26.3). The link between ketosis and the stabilization of HIF-1α is through a feedback product inhibition of PHD via elevated tissue succinate (Semenza, 2007a). Succinate is an intermediate of the catabolism of ketone bodies and thus we purport stabilization of HIF-1α is through a metabolic couple between mitochondrial and cytosolic redox states. Thus, changes in redox state may result in stabilization of HIF-1α (Guo et al., 2008; Mills & O'Neill, 2014; Serra-Perez et al., 2010). This concept is consistent with a study where mitochondrial redox in hippocampal tissue was improved via the activation of Nrf2 by the KG (Milder et al., 2010b). On the other hand, oxidizing environments (high levels of ROS) may suppress stabilization of HIF-1α (Guo et al., 2008). A study where HIF-1α played a role in N-acetylcysteine-mediated neuroprotection in rats subjected to MCAO (Zhang et al., 2014) supported the notion that reduced oxidizing environments may result in HIF stabilization.

Neuroprotection by HIF-1α may be cell-specific (Vangeison et al., 2008). It has been reported that neuron-specific inactivation of HIF-1α results in increased brain injury, as studied in a mouse model of transient focal cerebral ischemia (Baranova et al., 2007). These findings suggest that HIF-1α and its target genes are regulated distinctly, especially under pathologic conditions. Although HIF-1α is expressed in both neurons and glia, the neuroprotective efficacy of the KG (via HIF-1α) may be cell-specific and conditional (Barteczek et al., 2017; Bergeron et al., 2000; Chavez & LaManna, 2002). The suppression of the HIF-1α response to hypoxia in the aged may explain the greater risk for morbidity and mortality after an oxidative insult (Ndubuizu et al., 2010; Xu et al., 2010).

In a study where ischemic preconditioning with the KG in mice was implemented, the neuroprotection by the diet was mediated through adenosine A1 receptor activation of Akt and Erk1/2 prosurvival proteins (Yang et al., 2017). The potential role of KG therapy on HIF-2α should also be explored. It has been shown that HIF-2α mediates the transcriptional activation of erythropoietin in astrocytes, thereby promoting downstream paracrine-dependent neuronal survival (Chavez et al., 2006). Studies have also shown that neuronal HIF-1α and HIF-2α may act together in cellular preservation after ischemic stroke (Barteczek et al., 2017); however, the benefits during the very acute phase versus prolonged recovery phase remain to be determined.

Reports have shown that HIF-1α accumulation elicits a neuroprotective response through modification of inflammatory pathways via modulation of cytokine regulation (Speer et al., 2013; Yang et al., 2018). We have shown activation of HIF-1α in cortical brain in rats results in upregulation of the anti-inflammatory cytokine interleukin-10 (IL-10) and downregulation of the pro-inflammatory cytokines IL-6 and

tumor necrosis factor α (TNF-α; data unpublished). Figure 26.4 offers a proposed scheme of how HIF-1α mediates downstream inflammatory pathways through JAK-STAT3 or the NLRP3 inflammasome, resulting in neuroprotection. The mechanisms for how modulated cytokines lead to neuroprotection are still under investigation. Other mechanisms include IL-10-mediated inactivation of the NLRP3 inflammation (Gurung et al., 2015), which is a pathway associated with neuroprotection (Guo et al., 2018; Ismael et al., 2018). IL-10 is also known to involve transcriptional downregulation of pro-inflammatory cytokines via the JAK1-STAT3 pathway (Riley et al., 1999).

Overall, HIF-1α plays an important role in ketosis-mediated neuroprotection. Unravelling the underlying mechanisms can offer new therapeutic interventions to minimize neural damage by oxidative injury, such as with stroke, as well as to reduce the need for preconditioning therapies. Understanding the central role of ketosis on regulation of HIF-1α as a signaling molecule in brain under pathophysiologic conditions will help to delineate the role of HIF-1α in inflammation and neuroprotection.

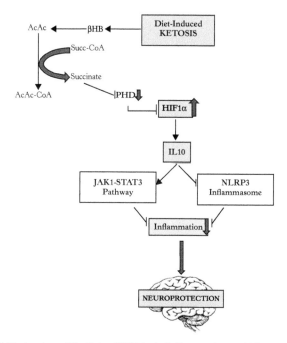

FIGURE 26.4 *Proposed Mechanism of the Role of HIF-1α in Inflammation and Neuroprotection*

HIF-1α modulates downstream inflammatory pathways through JAK-STAT3 or the NLRP3 inflammasome, resulting in neuroprotection. Another mechanism includes IL-10-mediated inactivation of NLRP3 inflammation. IL-10 is also known to involve transcriptional downregulation of pro-inflammatory cytokines via the JAK1-STAT3 pathway.

CONCLUSION AND FUTURE DIRECTION

Research has consistently shown that ketosis is neuroprotective against ischemic insults in rats (Puchowicz et al., 2008b) and mice. Studies in ketotic rats showed significantly decreased infarct volumes (with the MCAO model) and improved survival and recovery after cardiac arrest and resuscitation (Xu et al., 2012). The mechanisms of action of ketosis include glucose sparing and ketone body utilization in brain, as well as a shift in metabolic redox, which plays a role in energy balance and the downstream innate signaling of HIF-1α. The mechanism of neuroprotection by KG-induced HIF-1α stabilization is the regulation and activation of genes associated with inflammation, salvation pathways, and stabilization of energy metabolism. Furthermore, the KG has been associated with less oxidative damage through reduction of glucose carbon shunting toward oxidative pathways (Zhang et al., 2013, 2018) and disposal of HNE through increased oxidation of HNE's toxic intermediates—this novel mechanism has been described in livers of KG-fed rats (Jin et al., 2014; Li et al., 2012). Neuroprotection by ketosis may also occur through pathways independent of HIF-1α regulation, such as AKT-modulation of Nrf2 and NF-kB, but these mechanisms remain to be elucidated.

REFERENCES

Agani, F. H., Puchowicz, M., Chavez, J. C., Pichiule, P., & LaManna, J. (2002). Role of nitric oxide in the regulation of HIF-1α expression during hypoxia. *American Journal of Physiology-Cell Physiology, 283*, C178–C186.

Baranova, O., Miranda, L. F., Pichiule, P., Dragatsis, I., Johnson, R. S., & Chavez, J. C. (2007a). Neuron-specific inactivation of the hypoxia inducible factor 1alpha increases brain injury in a mouse model of transient focal cerebral ischemia. *Journal of Neuroscience, 27*, 6320–6332.

Barteczek, P., Li, L., Ernst, A. S., Bohler, L. I., Marti, H. H., & Kunze, R. (2017). Neuronal HIF-1α and HIF-2α deficiency improves neuronal survival and sensorimotor function in the early acute phase after ischemic stroke. *Journal of Cerebral Blood Flow and Metabolism, 37*, 291–306.

Bartesaghi, S., Marinovich, M., Corsini, E., Galli, C. L., & Viviani, B. (2005). Erythropoietin: A novel neuroprotective cytokine. *Neurotoxicology, 26*, 923–928.

Benderro, G. F., & LaManna, J. C. (2011). Hypoxia-induced angiogenesis is delayed in aging mouse brain. *Brain Research, 1389*, 50–60.

Bentourkia, M., Bol, A., Ivanoiu, A., Labar, D., Sibomana, M., Coppens, A., Michel, C., Cosnard, G., & De Volder, A. G. (2000). Comparison of regional cerebral blood flow and glucose metabolism in the normal brain: Effect of aging. *Journal of Neurological Sciences, 181*, 19–28.

Bergeron, M., Gidday, J. M., Yu, A. Y., Semenza, G. L., Ferriero, D. M., & Sharp, F. R. (2000). Role of hypoxia-inducible factor-1 in hypoxia-induced ischemic tolerance in neonatal rat brain. *Annals of Neurology, 48*, 285–296.

Bough, K. J., & Rho, J. M. (2007). Anticonvulsant mechanisms of the ketogenic diet. *Epilepsia, 48*, 43–58.

Bridge, E. M. (1931). The mechanism of the ketogenic diet in epilepsy. *Bulletin of Johns Hopkins Hospital, 48*, 373–389.

Brunengraber, H., & Roe, C. R. (2006). Anaplerotic molecules: Current and future. *Journal of Inherited Metabolic Disorders, 29*, 327–331.

Cahill, G. F., Jr., & Owen, O. E. (1967). Starvation and survival. *Transactions of the American Clinical and Climatological Association, 79*, 13–18.

Cahill, G. F., Jr., & Veech, R. L. (2003). Ketoacids? Good medicine? *Transactions of the American Clinical and Climatological Association, 114*, 149–161.

Chavez, J. C., Agani, F., Pichiule, P., & LaManna, J. C. (2000). Expression of hypoxia-inducible factor-1alpha in the brain of rats during chronic hypoxia. *Journal of Applied Physiology, 89*, 1937–1942.

Chavez, J. C., Baranova, O., Lin, J., & Pichiule, P. (2006). The transcriptional activator hypoxia inducible factor 2 (HIF-2/EPAS-1) regulates the oxygen-dependent expression of erythropoietin in cortical astrocytes. *Journal of Neuroscience, 26*, 9471–9481.

Chavez, J. C., & LaManna, J. C. (2002). Activation of hypoxia-inducible factor-1 in the rat cerebral cortex after transient global ischemia: Potential role of insulin-like growth factor-1. *Journal of Neuroscience, 22*, 8922–8931.

Chen, T. T., Maevsky, E. I., & Uchitel, M. L. (2015). Maintenance of homeostasis in the aging hypothalamus: The central and peripheral roles of succinate. *Frontiers in Endocrinology, 6*, 7.

Chong, Z. Z., Kang, J. Q., & Maiese, K. (2003a). Apaf-1, Bcl-xL, cytochrome c, and caspase-9 form the critical elements for cerebral vascular protection by erythropoietin. *Journal of Cerebral Blood Flow and Metabolism, 23*, 320–330.

Chong, Z. Z., Kang, J. Q., & Maiese, K. (2003b). Erythropoietin fosters both intrinsic and extrinsic neuronal protection through modulation of microglia, Akt1, Bad, and caspase-mediated pathways. *British Journal of Pharmacology, 138*, 1107–1118.

Cunnane, S., Nugent, S., Roy, M., Courchesne-Loyer, A., Croteau, E., Tremblay, S., Castellano, A., Pifferi, F., Bocti, C., Paquet, N., Begdouri, H., Bentourkia, M., Turcotte, E., Allard, M., Barberger-Gateau, P., Fulop, T., & Rapoport, S. I. (2011). Brain fuel metabolism, aging, and Alzheimer's disease. *Nutrition, 27,* 3–20.

Desrochers, S., Dubreuil, P., Brunet, J., Jetté, M., David, F., Landau, B. R., & Brunengraber, H. (1995). Metabolism of (*R,S*)-1,3-butanediol acetoacetate esters, potential parenteral and enteral nutrients in conscious pigs. *American Journal of Physiology, 268*(Pt. 1), E660–E667.

DeVivo, D. C., Leckie, M. P., Ferrendelli, J. S., & McDougal, D. B., Jr. (1978). Chronic ketosis and cerebral metabolism. *Annals of Neurology, 3,* 331–337.

DeVivo, D. C., Pagliara, A. S., & Prensky, A. L. (1973). Ketotic hypoglycemia and the ketogenic diet therapy. *Neurology, 23,* 640–649.

Freeman, J. M., Vining, E. P. G., Pillas, D. J., Pyzik, P. L., Casey, J. C., & Kelly, M. T. (1998). The efficacy of the ketogenic diet—1998: A prospective evaluation of intervention in 150 children. *Pediatrics, 102,* 1358–1363.

Gano, L. B., Patel, M., & Rho, J. M. (2014). Ketogenic diets, mitochondria, and neurological diseases. *Journal of Lipid Research, 55,* 2211–2228.

Ghezzi, P., Bernaudin, M., Bianchi, R., Blomgren, K., Brines, M., Campana, W., Cavaletti, G., Cerami, A., Chopp, M., Coleman, T., Digicaylioglu, M., Ehrenreich, H., Erbayraktar, S., Erbayraktar, Z., Gassmann, M., Genc, S., Gokmen, N., Grasso, G., Juul, S., . . . Zhu, C. (2010). Erythropoietin: Not just about erythropoiesis. *Lancet, 375,* 2142.

Gibson, G. E., Sheu, K. F., & Blass, J. P. (1998). Abnormalities of mitochondrial enzymes in Alzheimer disease. *Journal of Neural Transmission, 105,* 855–870.

Guo, M., Wang, X., Zhao, Y., Yang, Q., Ding, H., Dong, Q., Chen, X., & Cui, M. (2018). Ketogenic diet improves brain ischemic tolerance and inhibits NLRP3 inflammasome activation by preventing Drp1-mediated mitochondrial fission and endoplasmic reticulum stress. *Frontiers in Molecular Neuroscience, 11,* 86.

Guo, S., Bragina, O., Xu, Y., Cao, Z., Chen, H., Zhou, B., Morgan, M., Lin, Y., Jiang, B. H., Liu, K. J., & Shi, H. (2008). Glucose up-regulates HIF-1α expression in primary cortical neurons in response to hypoxia through maintaining cellular redox status. *Journal of Neurochemistry, 105,* 1849–1860.

Gurung, P., Li, B., Subbarao Malireddi, R. K., Lamkanfi, M., Geiger, T. L., & Kanneganti, T. D. (2015). Chronic TLR stimulation controls NLRP3 inflammasome activation through IL-10 mediated regulation of NLRP3 expression and caspase-8 activation. *Scientific Reports, 5,* 14488.

Hassel, B. (2000). Carboxylation and anaplerosis in neurons and glia. *Molecular Neurobiology, 22,* 21–40.

Helton, R., Cui, J., Scheel, J. R., Ellison, J. A., Ames, C., Gibson, C., Blouw, B., Ouyang, L., Dragatsis, I., Zeitlin, S., Johnson, R. S., Lipton, S. A., & Barlow, C. (2005). Brain-specific knock-out of hypoxia-inducible factor-1α reduces rather than increases hypoxic-ischemic damage. *Journal of Neuroscience, 25,* 4099–4107.

Hemmila, J. M., & Drewes, L. R. (1993). Glucose transporter (GLUT1) expression by canine brain microvessel endothelial cells in culture: An immunocytochemical study. *Advances in Experimental Medicine and Biology, 331,* 13–18.

Hempel, F. G., Jobsis, F. F., LaManna, J. L., Rosenthal, M. R., & Saltzman, H. A. (1977). Oxidation of cerebral cytochrome aa3 by oxygen plus carbon dioxide at hyperbaric pressures. *Journal of Applied Physiology, 43,* 873–879.

Hou, P., Kuo, C. Y., Cheng, C. T., Liou, J. P., Ann, D. K., & Chen, Q. (2014). Intermediary metabolite precursor dimethyl-2-ketoglutarate stabilizes hypoxia-inducible factor-1alpha by inhibiting prolyl-4-hydroxylase PHD2. *PLOS ONE, 9,* Article e113865.

Hoxworth, J. M., Xu, K., Zhou, Y., Lust, W. D., & LaManna, J. C. (1999). Cerebral metabolic profile, selective neuron loss, and survival of acute and chronic hyperglycemic rats following cardiac arrest and resuscitation. *Brain Research, 821,* 467–479.

Ismael, S., Zhao, L., Nasoohi, S., & Ishrat, T. (2018). Inhibition of the NLRP3-inflammasome as a potential approach for neuroprotection after stroke. *Science Reports, 8,* 5971.

Jarrett, S. G., Milder, J. B., Liang, L. P., & Patel, M. (2008). The ketogenic diet increases mitochondrial glutathione levels. *Journal of Neurochemistry, 106,* 1044–1051.

Jin, Z., Berthiaume, J. M., Li, Q., Henry, F., Huang, Z., Sadhukhan, S., Gao, P., Tochtrop, G. P., Puchowicz, M. A., & Zhang, G. F. (2014). Catabolism of (2E)-4-hydroxy-2-nonenal via omega- and omega-1-oxidation stimulated by ketogenic diet. *Journal of Biological Chemistry, 289,* 32327–32338.

Julio-Amilpas, A., Montiel, T., Soto-Tinoco, E., Geronimo-Olvera, C., & Massieu, L. (2015). Protection of hypoglycemia-induced neuronal death by beta-hydroxybutyrate involves the preservation of energy levels and decreased production of reactive oxygen species. *Journal of Cerebral Blood Flow and Metabolism, 35,* 851–860.

Kashiwaya, Y., Takeshima, T., Mori, N., Nakashima, K., Clarke, K., & Veech, R. L. (2000). D-β-Hydroxybutyrate protects neurons in models of

Alzheimer's and Parkinson's disease. *Proceedings of the National Academy of Sciences, U. S. A, 97*(10), 5440–5444.

Kasumov, T., Cendrowski, A. V., David, F., Jobbins, K. A., Anderson, V. E., & Brunengraber, H. (2007). Mass isotopomer study of anaplerosis from propionate in the perfused rat heart. *Archives of Biochemistry and Biophysics, 463,* 110–117.

Leino, R. L., Gerhart, D. Z., Duelli, R., Enerson, B. E., & Drewes, L. R. (2001). Diet-induced ketosis increases monocarboxylate transporter (MCT1) levels in rat brain. *Neurochemistry International, 38*(6), 519–527.

Leist, M., Ghezzi, P., Grasso, G., Bianchi, R., Villa, P., Fratelli, M., Savino, C., Bianchi, M., Nielsen, J., Gerwien, J., Kallunki, P., Larsen, A. K., Helboe, L., Christensen, S., Pedersen, L. O., Nielsen, M., Torup, L., Sager, T., Sfacteria, A., . . . Brines, M. (2004). Derivatives of erythropoietin that are tissue protective but not erythropoietic. *Science, 305,* 239–242.

Lennox, W. B. (1928). Ketogenic diet in the treatment of epilepsy. *New England Journal of Medicine, 199,* 74–75.

Li, Q., Tomcik, K., Zhang, S., Puchowicz, M. A., & Zhang, G. F. (2012). Dietary regulation of catabolic disposal of 4-hydroxynonenal analogs in rat liver. *Free Radical Biology and Medicine, 52,* 1043–1053.

Lund, T. M., Risa, O., Sonnewald, U., Schousboe, A., & Waagepetersen, H. S. (2009). Availability of neurotransmitter glutamate is diminished when beta-hydroxybutyrate replaces glucose in cultured neurons. *Journal of Neurochemistry, 110,* 80–91.

Maalouf, M., Rho, J. M., & Mattson, M. P. (2009a). The neuroprotective properties of calorie restriction, the ketogenic diet, and ketone bodies. *Brain Research Reviews, 59,* 293–315.

Maalouf, M., Sullivan, P. G., Davis, L., Kim, D. Y., & Rho, J. M. (2007). Ketones inhibit mitochondrial production of reactive oxygen species production following glutamate excitotoxicity by increasing NADH oxidation. *Neuroscience, 145,* 256–264.

Masino, S. A., & Rho, J. M. (2012). Mechanisms of ketogenic diet action. In J. L. Noebels, M. Avoli, M. A. Rogawski, R. W. Olsen, & A. V. Delgado-Escueta (Eds.), *Jasper's basic mechanisms of epilepsies* (pp. 1001–1022). National Center for Biotechnology Information.

McFate, T., Mohyeldin, A., Lu, H., Thakar, J., Henriques, J., Halim, N. D., Wu, H., Schell, M. J., Tsang, T. M., Teahan, O., Zhou, S., Califano, J. A., Jeoung, N. H., Harris, R. A., & Verma, A. (2008). Pyruvate dehydrogenase complex activity controls metabolic and malignant phenotype in cancer cells. *Journal of Biological Chemistry, 283,* 22700–22708.

Milder, J., & Patel, M. (2012). Modulation of oxidative stress and mitochondrial function by the ketogenic diet. *Epilepsy Research, 100,* 295–303.

Milder, J. B., Liang, L. P., & Patel, M. (2010). Acute oxidative stress and systemic Nrf2 activation by the ketogenic diet. *Neurobiology Disease, 40,* 238–244.

Millichap, J. G., Jones, J. D., & Rudis, B. P. (1964). Mechanism of anti-convulsant actin of ketogenic diet. *American Journal of Diseases of Children, 107,* 593–604.

Mills, E., & O'Neill, L. A. (2014). Succinate: A metabolic signal in inflammation. *Trends in Cell Biology, 24,* 313–320.

Nakazawa, M., Kodama, S., & Matsuo, T. (1983). Effects of ketogenic diet on electroconvulsive threshold and brain contents of adenosine nucleotides. *Brain and Development, 5,* 375–380.

Ndubuizu, O. I., Tsipis, C. P., Li, A., & LaManna, J. C. (2010). Hypoxia-inducible factor-1 (HIF-1)-independent microvascular angiogenesis in the aged rat brain. *Brain Research, 1366,* 101–109.

Owen, O. E., Morgan, A. P., Kemp, H. G., Sullivan, J. M., Herrera, M. G., & Cahill, G. F., Jr. (1967). Brain metabolism during fasting. *Journal of Clinical Investigation, 46,* 1589–1595.

Pan, J. W., Rothman, T. L., Behar, K. L., Stein, D. T., & Hetherington, H. P. (2000). Human brain beta-hydroxybutyrate and lactate increase in fasting-induced ketosis. *Journal of Cerebral Blood Flow and Metabolism, 20,* 1502–1507.

Prins, M. L. (2008). Cerebral metabolic adaptation and ketone metabolism after brain injury. *Journal of Cerebral Blood Flow and Metabolism, 28,* 1–16.

Prins, M. L., & Hovda, D. A. (2009). The effects of age and ketogenic diet on local cerebral metabolic rates of glucose after controlled cortical impact injury in rats. *Journal of Neurotrauma, 26,* 1083–1093.

Puchowicz, M. A., Smith, C. L., Bomont, C., Koshy, J., David, F., & Brunengraber, H. (2000). Dog model of therapeutic ketosis induced by oral administration of R,S-1,3-butanediol diacetoacetate. *Journal of Nutritional Biochemistry, 11,* 281–287.

Puchowicz, M. A., Xu, K., Sun, X., Ivy, A., Emancipator, D., & LaManna, J. C. (2007). Diet-induced ketosis increases capillary density without altered blood flow in rat brain. *American Journal of Physiology-Endocrinology and Metabolism, 292,* E1607–E1615.

Puchowicz, M. A., Zechel, J. L., Valerio, J., Emancipator, D. S., Xu, K., Pundik, S., LaManna, J. C., & Lust, W. D. (2008). Neuroprotection in diet-induced ketotic rat brain after focal ischemia. *Journal of Cerebral Blood Flow and Metabolism, 28,* 1907–1916.

Pundik, S., Xu, K., & Sundararajan, S. (2012). Reperfusion brain injury: Focus on cellular bioenergetics. *Neurology, 79,* S44–S51.

Randle, P. J., Garland, P. B., Hales, C. N., & Newsholme, E. A. (1963). The glucose-fatty acid cycle: Its role in insulin sensitivity and the metabolic disturbances of diabetes mellitus. *Lancet*, 785–789.

Riley, J. K., Takeda, K., Akira, S., & Schreiber, R. D. (1999). Interleukin-10 receptor signaling through the JAK-STAT pathway: Requirement for two distinct receptor-derived signals for anti-inflammatory action. *Journal of Biological Chemistry, 274*, 16513–16521.

Roy, M., Nugent, S., Tremblay-Mercier, J., Tremblay, S., Courchesne-Loyer, A., Beaudoin, J. F., Tremblay, L., Descoteaux, M., Lecomte, R., & Cunnane, S. C. (2012). The ketogenic diet increases brain glucose and ketone uptake in aged rats: A dual tracer PET and volumetric MRI study. *Brain Research, 1488*, 14–23.

Sato, K., Kashiwaya, Y., Keon, C. A., Tsuchiya, N., King, M. T., Radda, G. K., Chance, B., Clarke, K., & Veech, R. L. (1995). Insulin, ketone bodies, and mitochondrial energy transduction. *FASEB Journal, 9*, 651–658.

Schwartzkroin, P. A. (1999). Mechanisms underlying the anti-epileptic efficacy of the ketogenic diet. *Epilepsy Research, 37*, 171–180.

Selman, W. R., Ricci, A. J., Crumrine, R. C., LaManna, J. C., Ratcheson, R. A., & Lust, W. D. (1990). The evolution of focal ischemic damage: A metabolic analysis. *Metabolic Brain Disease, 5*, 33–44.

Semenza, G. L. (2001). Hypoxia-inducible factor 1: Oxygen homeostasis and disease pathophysiology. *Trends in Molecular Medicine, 7*, 345–350.

Semenza, G. L. (2007a). Hypoxia-inducible factor 1 (HIF-1) pathway. *Science's STKE, volume 2007, issue 407*, pp. cm8.

Semenza, G. L. (2007b). Life with oxygen. *Science, 318*, 62–64.

Semenza, G. L. (2011). Regulation of metabolism by hypoxia-inducible factor 1. *Cold Spring Harbor Symposia on Quantitative Biology, 76*, 347–353.

Semenza, G. L., Agani, F., Feldser, D., Iyer, N., Kotch, L., Laughner, E., & Yu, A. (2000). Hypoxia, HIF-1, and the pathophysiology of common human diseases. *Advances in Experimental Medicine and Biology, 475*, 123–130.

Serra-Perez, A., Planas, A. M., Nunez-O'Mara, A., Berra, E., Garcia-Villoria, J., Ribes, A., & Santalucia, T. (2010). Extended ischemia prevents HIF1α degradation at reoxygenation by impairing prolyl-hydroxylation: Role of Krebs cycle metabolites. *Journal of Biological Chemistry, 285*, 18217–18224.

Sharp, F. R., Bergeron, M., & Bernaudin, M. (2001). Hypoxia-inducible factor in brain. *Advances in Experimental Medicine and Biology, 502*, 273–291.

Shi, H. (2009). Hypoxia inducible factor 1 as a therapeutic target in ischemic stroke. *Current Medicinal Chemistry, 16*, 4593–4600.

Shimazu, T., Hirschey, M. D., Newman, J., He, W., Shirakawa, K., Le, M. N., Grueter, C. A., Lim, H., Saunders, L. R., Stevens, R. D., Newgard, C. B., Farese, R. V., Jr., de Cabo, R., Ulrich, S., Akassoglou, K., & Verdin, E. (2013). Suppression of oxidative stress by beta-hydroxybutyrate, an endogenous histone deacetylase inhibitor. *Science, 339*, 211–214.

Silverman, W. F., Krum, J. M., Mani, N., & Rosenstein, J. M. (1999). Vascular, glial and neuronal effects of vascular endothelial growth factor in mesencephalic explant cultures. *Neuroscience, 90*, 1529–1541.

Speer, R. E., Karuppagounder, S. S., Basso, M., Sleiman, S. F., Kumar, A., Brand, D., Smirnova, N., Gazaryan, I., Khim, S. J., & Ratan, R. R. (2013). Hypoxia-inducible factor prolyl hydroxylases as targets for neuroprotection by "antioxidant" metal chelators: From ferroptosis to stroke. *Free Radical Biology and Medicine, 62*, 26–36.

Stafstrom, C. E., & Rho, J. M. (2012). The ketogenic diet as a treatment paradigm for diverse neurological disorders. *Frontiers in Pharmacology, 3*, 59.

Storkebaum, E., Lambrechts, D., & Carmeliet, P. (2004). VEGF: Once regarded as a specific angiogenic factor, now implicated in neuroprotection. *Bioessays, 26*, 943–954.

Tallian, K. B., Nahata, M. C., & Tsao, C.-Y. (1998). Role of the ketogenic diet in children with intractable seizures. *Annals of Pharmacotherapy, 32*, 349–385.

Tannahill, G. M., Curtis, A. M., Adamik, J., Palsson-McDermott, E. M., McGettrick, A. F., Goel, G., Frezza, C., Bernard, N. J., Kelly, B., Foley, N. H., Zheng, L., Gardet, A., Tong, Z., Jany, S. S., Corr, S. C., Haneklaus, M., Caffrey, B. E., Pierce, K., Walmsley, S., . . . O'Neill, L. A. (2013). Succinate is an inflammatory signal that induces IL-1β through HIF-1α. *Nature, 496*, 238–242.

Vangeison, G., Carr, D., Federoff, H. J., & Rempe, D. A. (2008). The good, the bad, and the cell type-specific roles of hypoxia inducible factor-1alpha in neurons and astrocytes. *Journal of Neuroscience, 28*, 1988–1993.

Veech, R. L. (2004). The therapeutic implications of ketone bodies: The effects of ketone bodies in pathological conditions; ketosis, ketogenic diet, redox states, insulin resistance, and mitochondrial metabolism. *Prostaglandins, Leukotrienes and Essential Fatty Acids, 70*, 309–319.

Veech, R. L., Chance, B., Kashiwaya, Y., Lardy, H. A., & Cahill, G. F., Jr. (2001). Ketone bodies, potential therapeutic uses. *IUBMB Life, 51*, 241–247.

Veech, R. L., Valeri, C. R., & Vanitallie, T. B. (2012). The mitochondrial permeability transition pore provides a key to the diagnosis and treatment of traumatic brain injury. *IUBMB Life, 64*, 203–207.

Wilder, R. M. (1921). The effect of ketonemia on the course of epilepsy. *Mayo Clinic Bulletin, 2,* 307–308.

Willis, M. W., Ketter, T. A., Kimbrell, T. A., George, M. S., Herscovitch, P., Danielson, A. L., Benson, B. E., & Post, R. M. (2002). Age, sex and laterality effects on cerebral glucose metabolism in healthy adults. *Psychiatry Research, 114,* 23–37.

Xu, K., LaManna, J. C., & Puchowicz, M. A. (2012). Neuroprotective properties of ketone bodies. *Advances in Experimental Medicine and Biology, 737,* 97–102.

Xu, K., Puchowicz, M. A., Lust, W. D., & LaManna, J. C. (2006). Adenosine treatment delays postischemic hippocampal CA1 loss after cardiac arrest and resuscitation in rats. *Brain Research, 1071,* 208–217.

Xu, K., Puchowicz, M. A., Sun, X., & LaManna, J. C. (2008). Mitochondrial dysfunction in aging rat brain following transient global ischemia. *Advances in Experimental Medicine and Biology, 614,* 379–386.

Xu, K., Puchowicz, M. A., Sun, X., & LaManna, J. C. (2010). Decreased brainstem function following cardiac arrest and resuscitation in aged rat. *Brain Research, 1328,* 181–189.

Xu, K., Sun, X., Puchowicz, M. A., & LaManna, J. C. (2007). Increased sensitivity to transient global ischemia in aging rat brain. *Advances in Experimental Medicine and Biology, 599,* 199–206.

Xu, K., Ye, L., Sharma, K., Jin, Y., Harrison, M. M., Caldwell, T., Berthiaume, J. M., Luo, Y., LaManna, J. C., & Puchowicz, M. A. (2017). Diet-induced ketosis protects against focal cerebral ischemia in mouse. *Advances in Experimental Medicine and Biology, 977,* 205–213.

Yang, J., Liu, C., Du, X., Liu, M., Ji, X., Du, H., & Zhao, H. (2018). Hypoxia inducible factor 1α plays a key role in remote ischemic preconditioning against stroke by modulating inflammatory responses in rats. *Journal of the American Heart Association, 24,* 7(5).

Yang, Q., Guo, M., Wang, X., Zhao, Y., Zhao, Q., Ding, H., Dong, Q., & Cui, M. (2017). Ischemic preconditioning with a ketogenic diet improves brain ischemic tolerance through increased extracellular adenosine levels and hypoxia-inducible factors. *Brain Research, 1667,* 11–18.

Yudkoff, M., Daikhin, Y., Melo, T. M., Nissim, I., Sonnewald, U., & Nissim, I. (2007). The ketogenic diet and brain metabolism of amino acids: Relationship to the anticonvulsant effect. *Annual Review of Nutrition, 27,* 415–430.

Zhang, Y., Kuang, Y., Xu, K., Harris, D., Lee, Z., LaManna, J., & Puchowicz, M. A. (2013). Ketosis proportionately spares glucose utilization in brain. *Journal of Cerebral Blood Flow and Metabolism, 33,* 1307–1311.

Zhang, Y., Xu, K., Kerwin, T., LaManna, J. C., & Puchowicz, M. (2018). Impact of aging on metabolic changes in the ketotic rat brain: Glucose, oxidative and 4-HNE metabolism. *Advances in Experimental Medicine and Biology, 1072,* 21–25.

Zhang, Y., Zhang, S., Marin-Valencia, I., & Puchowicz, M. A. (2015). Decreased carbon shunting from glucose toward oxidative metabolism in diet-induced ketotic rat brain. *Journal of Neurochemistry, 132,* 301–312.

Zhang, Z., Yan, J., Taheri, S., Liu, K. J., & Shi, H. (2014). Hypoxia-inducible factor 1 contributes to N-acetylcysteine's protection in stroke. *Free Radical Biology and Medicine, 68,* 8–21.

Zhang, Z. G., Zhang, L., Tsang, W., Soltanian-Zadeh, H., Morris, D., Zhang, R., Goussev, A., Powers, C., Yeich, T., & Chopp, M. (2002). Correlation of VEGF and angiopoietin expression with disruption of blood-brain barrier and angiogenesis after focal cerebral ischemia. *Journal of Cerebral Blood Flow and Metabolism, 22,* 379–392.

Metabolic Seizure Resistance via BAD and K_{ATP} Channels

JUAN RAMÓN MARTÍNEZ-FRANÇOIS, PHD, NIKA DANIAL, PHD, AND GARY YELLEN, PHD

The mechanisms of action of the ketogenic diet (KD) are poorly understood, but it has been used for almost a century and is arguably the most effective single treatment for epilepsy (Hartman et al., 2007; Neal et al., 2009; Thiele, 2003). This diet, when adhered to strictly, may reduce seizures in children by up to 50%, with 10% to 15% of children becoming seizure-free. Unfortunately, maintaining the KD's strict regimen is challenging. Thus, it would be very valuable to understand the KD's mechanisms of action and to harness them to create better epilepsy therapies.

On a KD, the liver produces the ketone bodies β-hydroxybutyrate (βHB) and acetoacetate from fatty acids, elevating ketone bodies to millimolar concentrations in the blood. Under these conditions, ketone bodies provide an alternative fuel source to tissues, including the brain, which otherwise would primarily utilize glucose (DeVivo et al., 1978; Mergenthaler et al., 2013; Owen et al., 1967; Zielke et al., 2009). The remarkable antiepileptic effect of increased ketone body metabolism points to a link between fuel utilization and neuronal excitability. However, the molecular mechanisms of this link are poorly understood (Danial et al., 2013; Hartman et al., 2007; Lutas & Yellen, 2013). Some proposed mechanisms include increased adenosine signaling through A_1 purinergic receptors (Masino et al., 2011), changes in gene expression after glycolysis reduction (Garriga-Canut et al., 2006), suppression of glutamate release (Juge et al., 2010), and changes in excitability mediated by lactate dehydrogenase activity (Sada et al., 2015).

A mouse model with altered metabolism reminiscent of the KD produces similar antiseizure effects, and this nondietary manipulation provides a better opportunity to dissect the mechanisms involved in metabolic seizure resistance (Giménez-Cassina et al., 2012). The model involves metabolic changes in brain cells mediated by the protein BAD (BCL-2-associated agonist of cell death). Abolishing BAD's role in metabolism reduces the capacity of cells to utilize glucose and increases their capacity to use ketone bodies. Seizure protection appears to come from switching away from glucose as the preferred energy source toward utilization of other fuels, rather than elevation of circulating ketone bodies. In addition, BAD alteration leads to increased activity of metabolically sensitive ATP-sensitive potassium (K_{ATP}) channels in the brain. Modulation of K_{ATP} channel activity may also play an important role in the antiseizure actions of the KD.

BAD MODULATES GLUCOSE AND KETONE BODY METABOLISM

BAD is best-known as a proapoptotic protein that is a member of the BCL-2 family of proteins (Czabotar et al., 2014; Danial & Korsmeyer, 2004; Moldoveanu et al., 2014). Besides its role in apoptosis, BAD modulates glucose metabolism in multiple cell types, including hepatocytes, pancreatic β-cells, and fibroblasts (Giménez-Cassina & Danial, 2015). The switch between BAD's apoptotic and metabolic roles is mediated through phosphorylation of its serine 155 (equivalent to serine 118 in human BAD), located within an α-helical segment known as the BH-3 domain (Danial et al., 2008; Datta et al., 2000). In hepatocytes and pancreatic β-cells, serine 155 phosphorylation promotes mitochondrial metabolism of glucose. In the presence of apoptotic signals, dephosphorylated BAD promotes apoptosis.

The reduction in glucose metabolism provoked by BAD modification is reminiscent of metabolic changes associated with the KD, that is, reduced glycolysis and increased ketone body metabolism. Thus, modifying BAD may be a productive avenue for studying the mechanisms that underlie the antiseizure effects of changes in metabolism. Given the systemic, nonspecific effects of dietary manipulation, the study of BAD alteration enables the study of metabolic seizure-resistance mechanisms in a more specific manner and without the use of dietary interventions.

METABOLIC CHANGES IN BAD-ALTERED PRIMARY NEURONS AND ASTROCYTES

Two key mouse models have been used to study the effects of BAD on neurons and astrocytes: a *Bad* knockout and a *Bad* knockin. The knockin mouse expresses a mutant of BAD that contains a nonphosphorylatable residue, alanine, at position 155 (BAD^{S155A}). In knockin animals, BAD's metabolic role is altered while leaving its apoptotic role intact, because BAD^{S155A} cannot be phosphorylated (Danial et al., 2008; Giménez-Cassina et al., 2014). Importantly, the mutant mice display neither gross neuroanatomic nor neurobehavioral abnormalities. Therefore, it is unlikely that genetic modification in these mouse models substantially impairs normal brain function.

To elucidate whether BAD has similar effects on metabolism in the brain as it does in other tissues, Giménez-Cassina et al. measured the mitochondrial oxygen consumption rates in primary cultures of neurons and astrocytes using mitochondrial respirometry (Giménez-Cassina et al., 2012). *Bad*-ablated cells exhibited reduced glucose metabolism and elevated capacity to metabolize ketone bodies compared to wild-type (WT) cells. Similar changes in brain metabolism are produced by the presence of ketone bodies. In hippocampal brain slices, βHB competes with glucose, lactate, and pyruvate for the generation of acetyl-CoA, inhibiting total glycolytic flux upstream of pyruvate kinase (Valente-Silva et al., 2015). Additionally, in humans, glucose flux in the brain is inversely correlated with the degree of ketosis, allowing ketone bodies to partially replace glucose in cerebral metabolism (Haymond et al., 1983; Owen et al., 1967). These observations cement the idea that disruption of BAD function may mimic the changes in brain metabolism produced by the KD and is a useful model to study the cellular mechanisms linking metabolism to excitability.

To corroborate that the effects of *Bad* disruption in the metabolism of cultured neurons and astrocytes were due to the metabolic, and not the apoptotic, role of BAD, mitochondrial respirometry was also performed in *Bad*^{S155A} cells (Giménez-Cassina et al., 2012). Indeed, *Bad*^{S155A} neurons and astrocytes also preferentially utilize βHB over glucose, like the BAD knockout. Conversely, BAD phosphorylation on serine 155 inhibits ketone body utilization resistance. This confirms that BAD, through its metabolic role, changes the ability of brain cells to metabolize different fuels.

ALTERATION OF BAD FUNCTION PRODUCES SEIZURE RESISTANCE

Disruption of BAD's metabolic role, by either knockout of the protein or knockin of a phosphorylation-resistant mutant variant, leads to altered metabolism without dietary manipulations. This metabolic switch from brain glucose to ketone body utilization also influences excitability and produces seizure resistance in vivo (Giménez-Cassina et al., 2012). The seizure resistance has been studied in two acute chemoconvulsant models of seizure, involving intraperitoneal injection of kainate (Ben-Ari et al., 1980) or subcutaneous injection of pentylenetretrazole (PTZ; Ferraro et al., 1999).

When injected with kainate, WT mice display a series of seizures of increasing severity that peak 1 to 2 hr after kainate injection and then slowly decay (Giménez-Cassina et al., 2012; Figure 27.1a). Most WT mice experience status epilepticus, with very severe tonic-clonic seizures, and many die. In contrast, seizure severity in *Bad*$^{-/-}$ mice is much milder than in WT mice, and mutant mice rarely go into status epilepticus or die (Figure 27.1). Electrographic seizures are also substantially milder (Figure 27.2). The in vivo seizure protection is due to BAD's metabolic, not apoptotic, role, because *Bad*^{S155A} mice were similarly resistant to kainate-induced seizures. Thus, disruption of the metabolic function of BAD alleviates both forebrain seizure activity and generalized behavioral seizures during status epilepticus.

BAD deletion is similarly protective against PTZ-induced seizures (Figure 27.1c); PTZ produces seizures by a different mechanism than kainate, by inhibiting GABA action rather than by stimulating glutamate receptors (Bough & Eagles, 1999; Ferraro et al., 1999). Thus, the effectiveness of BAD to protect from seizures remains, even

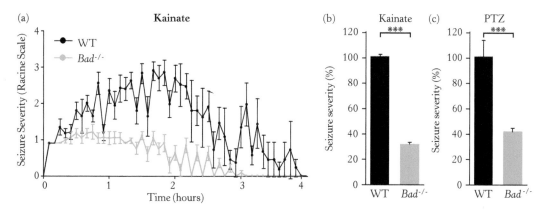

FIGURE 27.1 *Bad$^{-/-}$ Mice Are Resistant to Kainite- or Pentylenetetrazole-induced Acute Seizures*

(a) Raw seizure scores (Ferraro et al., 1997) in *Bad$^{-/-}$* 8- to 10-week-old male mice compared to wild-type (WT) mice over a 4-hr period after a single intraperitoneal injection of kainate (30 mg/kg). (b) Kainate-induced seizure severity calculated as Σ(all scores of a given mouse)/(time of experiment) for WT ($N = 42$) or *Bad$^{-/-}$* ($N = 13$) mice. The mean of the seizure severity values from WT mice was assigned a value of 100%. This value was then used to normalize the severity of the other tested genotypes and/or conditions within the same scale. (c) Integrated seizure severity (calculated as in B) in *Bad$^{-/-}$* and WT mice ($N = 16$) subjected to a single subcutaneous injection of pentylenetetrazole (PTZ) at 80 mg/kg monitored over a 70-min period. Data in A–C are presented as $M \pm$ SEM. *** $p < 0.001$; two-tailed Student's t-test. (Adapted from Giménez-Cassina, A., Martínez-François, J. R., Fisher, J. K., Szlyk, B., Polak, K., Wiwczar, J., Tanner, G. R., Lutas, A., Yellen, G., & Danial, N. N. (2012). BAD-dependent regulation of fuel metabolism and K_{ATP} channel activity confers resistance to epileptic seizures. *Neuron, 74*, 719–730. Figure 3.)

when the molecular and cellular mechanisms triggering acute seizures are different.

Additionally, *Bad* deletion can also be protective in a genetic model of chronic epilepsy. Mice with targeted deletion of *Kcna1*, a voltage-gated potassium channel gene, display spontaneous seizures and neuronal hyperexcitability (Lopantsev et al., 2003; Smart et al., 1998). In humans, loss-of-function mutations in this gene can cause epilepsy (Zuberi et al., 1999). Double-knockout, *Kcna1$^{-/-}$ · Bad$^{-/-}$*, mice spend less time in seizure compared to *Kcna1$^{-/-}$* mice. Additionally, double-knockout mice live approximately 2 weeks longer than control *Kcna1$^{-/-}$* mice (Foley et al., 2018). Interestingly, modifying metabolism by other means, such as a KD or subcutaneous administration of βHB, can also decrease seizures and increase longevity in *Kcna1*-null mice (Fenoglio-Simeone et al., 2009; Kim et al., 2015; Simeone et al., 2016, 2017).

BAD EFFECTS ON SEIZURE ARE UNLIKE THE EFFECTS OF OTHER BCL-2 FAMILY PROTEINS

Due to their apoptotic roles, certain BCL-2 family proteins, such as BIM and PUMA, have been implicated in protection against neuronal loss and seizure damage after prolonged periods of status epilepticus (Engel et al., 2010, 2011; Murphy et al., 2010). In a chronic seizure model (intra-amygdala microinjection of kainate), neuronal death in the hippocampus 24 hr after seizure initiation is decreased in *Bim$^{-/-}$* or *Puma$^{-/-}$* mice, demonstrating a role for these pro-apoptotic proteins in cell death after chronic seizures. In contrast, loss of BIM or PUMA is not seizure protective immediately after kainate injection (Engel et al., 2010; Murphy et al., 2010). Similarly, knockout of BIM or another BH3-only protein, BID, does not produce resistance to acute seizures elicited by intraperitoneal kainate injection (Giménez-Cassina et al., 2012). Unlike BAD, neither of these proteins affects glucose metabolism (Giménez-Cassina & Danial, 2015). Therefore, it appears that certain BCL-2 family members may play a role in epileptogenesis by promoting hippocampal neuron death, but this is distinct from the role of BAD in altering acute seizure susceptibility, which involves a switch in fuel preference, rather than apoptosis.

BAD has also been implicated in regulating synaptic transmission. The BAD-BAX-caspase-3 cascade can induce long-term depression in CA1 hippocampal neurons (Jiao & Li, 2011). Additionally, ABT-737, an inhibitor of BCL-2, BCL-X$_L$, and BCL-w survival proteins, slows the recovery of neurotransmission after intense synaptic activity and decreases hypoxia-triggered

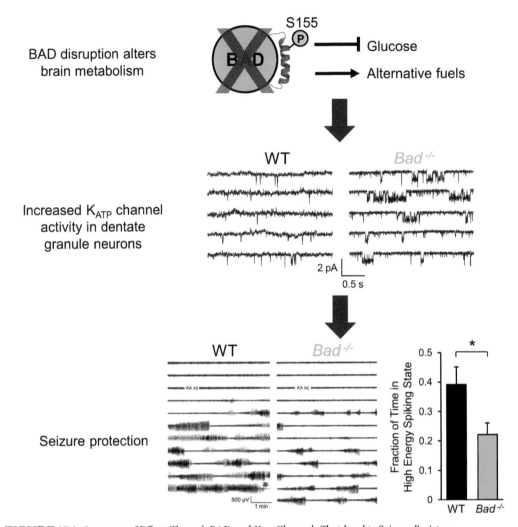

FIGURE 27.2 *Summary of Effects Through BAD and K_{ATP} Channels That Lead to Seizure Resistance*

Ablation of *Bad* leads to decreased glucose metabolism and increased consumption of alternative fuels (top panel). This metabolic switch increases K_{ATP} channel activity, as seen in cell-attached recordings of K_{ATP} channels in dentate granule neurons in hippocampal brain slices (middle panel). Compared to wild-type (WT) mice, *Bad*[-/-] mice are resistant to acute kainate-induced seizures, exhibiting reduced cortical seizure activity recorded by electroencephalogram (EEG) traces of approximately 1 hr for WT or *Bad*[-/-] mice (bottom left and middle panels), and reduced fraction of time spent in high-energy spiking state (bottom right panel). WT, $N = 17$; *Bad*[-/-], $N = 20$; $M \pm SEM$, * $p < 0.05$ by two-tailed Student's *t*-test. (Adapted from Giménez-Cassina, A., Martínez-François, J. R., Fisher, J. K., Szlyk, B., Polak, K., Wiwczar, J., Tanner, G. R., Lutas, A., Yellen, G., & Danial, N. N. (2012). BAD-dependent regulation of fuel metabolism and K_{ATP} channel activity confers resistance to epileptic seizures. *Neuron, 74*, 719–730. Figures 4 and 5.)

damage to synaptic function (Hickman et al., 2008). This effect of ABT-737 could result from BAD function, since this compound is likely acting on downstream signaling partners of BAD. However, ABT-737 also blocks binding of other BH3-only proteins to BCL-2 and BCL-X$_L$, which involves the same binding pocket used by BAD. Thus, disruption of these protein interactions by ABT-737 is not indicative of specific actions of BAD in synaptic transmission. In any case, the synaptic changes are unlikely to be part of the anticonvulsant action of BAD deletion. For these synaptic effects, *Bad*[-/-] and *Bad*[S155A] mice would have opposite phenotypes, because the alterations are dependent on the interaction of nonphosphorylated BAD with the downstream BCL-2 proteins; but, in fact, both genotypes produce seizure protection. These observations highlight the varied and complex roles of BAD in neuronal physiology and uniquely distinguish the switch in fuel preference as a potent mechanism to produce seizure protection.

THE METABOLIC SEIZURE RESISTANCE OF *BAD*[-/-] MICE LIKELY OCCURS IN THE BRAIN

As opposed to dietary manipulations that affect the whole organism, seizure protection arising from BAD modification seems to specifically originate from metabolic changes in the brain. Adenovirus-produced shRNA knockdown of BAD in the liver, the major source of ketone body production, does not protect against kainate-induced seizures, although it does produce the same metabolic effects observed in the liver of *Bad*[-/-] animals (Giménez-Cassina et al., 2012, 2014).

Interestingly, circulating levels of ketone bodies are similar in *Bad*[-/-] and WT mice, but βHB levels are increased in whole-brain tissue derived from *Bad*[-/-]. This suggests that, in the knockout animals, ketogenesis is being increased specifically in the brain; it also argues that changes in brain metabolism upon BAD alteration are unlikely to be generated by systemic modifications in metabolism. The precise changes in metabolism responsible for BAD's antiseizure effect remain to be established. Given that the KD's antiseizure effect can be reversed in patients promptly after carbohydrate consumption (Huttenlocher, 1976; Pfeifer et al., 2008), it seems likely that the transition in fuel type utilization is the crucial factor. Metabolomic studies comparing WT to *Bad*-altered genotypes could shed light on the metabolic pathways implicated in BAD's effect.

K_{ATP} CHANNELS LINK METABOLISM WITH EXCITABILITY

One likely candidate for linking altered brain metabolism with altered excitability, in the KD and in BAD-altered animals, is the ATP-sensitive potassium (K_{ATP}) channel. K_{ATP} channels are inhibited by intracellular ATP, are activated by intracellular ADP, and are widely expressed throughout the body, including the brain (Liss & Roeper, 2001; Nichols, 2006; Proks & Ashcroft, 2009). Their role linking metabolism with cell excitability has been best studied in insulin release by pancreatic β-cells (Ashcroft, 2005; Ashcroft et al., 1984). In these cells, the intracellular ATP:ADP ratio determines K_{ATP} channel activity. In basal conditions, K_{ATP} channels are spontaneously active, allowing K[+] efflux, maintaining the cell's resting membrane potential near the potassium equilibrium potential (i.e., hyperpolarized). Upon an increase in extracellular glucose concentration, and consequently an increase in the intracellular ATP concentration, K_{ATP} channels are inhibited.

This decrease in K_{ATP} channel activity depolarizes the cell and leads to insulin release. This exemplifies how K_{ATP} channels can link metabolism to cell excitability, but the effect is likely not unique to glucosensing neurons or other glucosensing cells like pancreatic β-cells.

Two brain regions that are particularly enriched in K_{ATP} channels are the hippocampus and the substantia nigra pars reticulata (SNr) (Dunn-Meynell et al., 1998; Karschin et al., 1997; Ma et al., 2007; Tanner et al., 2011; Yamada et al., 2001; Zawar et al., 1999). K_{ATP} channels present in these two areas are octamers comprised of two types of subunits: four Kir6.2 pore-forming subunits and four SUR1 regulatory subunits. Both of these brain regions are involved in the generation and propagation of seizure activity (Depaulis et al., 1994; Heinemann et al., 1992; Hsu, 2007; Iadarola & Gale, 1982; Krook-Magnuson et al., 2015; Lothman et al., 1992; McNamara et al., 1984), and excitability of neurons in these areas can be modulated by K_{ATP} channels (Forte et al., 2016; Lutas et al., 2014; Martínez-François et al., 2018; Stanford & Lacey, 1996; Tanner et al., 2011; Yamada et al., 2001; Zawar et al., 1999).

Neuronal K_{ATP} channel activity appears generally to be low, implying that the intracellular ATP concentration in neurons is often sufficiently high to inhibit these channels (Giménez-Cassina et al., 2012; Haller et al., 2001; Pelletier et al., 2000; Schwanstecher & Panten, 1993; Tanner et al., 2011; Yamada et al., 2001). Substantial metabolic insults to the brain are known to be capable of activating the channels; for instance, in brain ischemia, intracellular ATP and ATP:ADP markedly decrease after ~ 2 min (Katsura et al., 1992). In the CA1 area of the hippocampus, a brain region particularly susceptible to ischemic insult (Davolio & Greenamyre, 1995; Schmidt-Kastner & Freund, 1991; Smith et al., 1984), hypoxia triggers neuronal hyperpolarization by activating potassium conductances, including K_{ATP} channel currents (Yamada & Inagaki, 2005; Yamada et al., 2001). Consistent with this, K_{ATP} channel inhibitors, such as the sulfonylurea drugs glibenclamide or tolbutamide, can suppress the hypoxia-induced hyperpolarization. Furthermore, mice lacking either *Kcnj11* (gene encoding Kir6.2; hereafter referred to as *Kir6.2*) or *SUR1* exhibit a markedly reduced threshold for generalized seizures upon a hypoxic insult, that is, they are hypersensitive to hypoxia-induced seizures (Hernández-Sánchez et al., 2001; Yamada et al., 2001). Similar to *Bad*-altered mice, mice overexpressing SUR1 display a decrease in kainate-induced seizure susceptibility. These observations indicate that K_{ATP} channels play a crucial role in mediating antiseizure effects provoked by metabolic insufficiency or hypoxia.

Besides ischemic/hypoxic insult, other metabolic changes in brain regions implicated in seizure activity can also modulate K_{ATP} channel activity. Poisoning of GABAergic neurons in the SNr or hippocampal CA1 neurons with cyanide activates K_{ATP} channels (Matsumoto et al., 2002; Schwanstecher & Panten, 1993). In addition, in dentate granule neurons (DGNs) of the hippocampus, a much more subtle energetic challenge can lead to K_{ATP} channel opening: neuronal firing elicited by antidromic stimulation (Tanner et al., 2011). Firing of action potentials produces metabolic changes by activating the pumps, for example the Na^+/K^+-ATPase, that maintain intracellular ionic concentrations (Ivannikov et al., 2010; Mercer & Dunham, 1981). Activation of these pumps triggers ATP consumption, leading to an opening of K_{ATP} channels (Haller et al., 2001; Tanner et al., 2011). It has also been shown that K_{ATP} channel open probability in DGNs increases by extracellular application of βHB (Tanner et al., 2011). These observations are consistent with the idea that K_{ATP} channels could mediate the anticonvulsant effect of the KD. First, K_{ATP} channels

might open in conditions of hyperexcitability, such as during a seizure. Second, elevated levels of circulating ketone bodies could also increase K_{ATP} channel activity. These effects are synergistic, and the resulting increase in K_{ATP} channel current would reduce excitability and produce seizure resistance.

BAD DISRUPTION INCREASES K_{ATP} CHANNEL ACTIVITY

Can K_{ATP} channels mediate the seizure resistance elicited by BAD disruption? In single-channel, cell-attached experiments in DGNs in hippocampal brain slices, the basal K_{ATP} channel open probability is dramatically increased in $Bad^{-/-}$ mouse DGNs, from ~ 0.5% in WT to ~ 20% in $Bad^{-/-}$ (Figure 27.2). Confirming this increase in basal K_{ATP} channel activity in DGNs with disrupted BAD function, whole-cell K_{ATP} current is also inhibited by dialyzing the intracellular medium of either $Bad^{-/-}$ or Bad^{S155A} DGNs with high ATP (4 mM)—a phenomenon denominated "washdown" (Figure 27.3). On the other hand, washdown does not occur in WT DGNs (because K_{ATP} channels are mostly closed in this case) or in DGNs

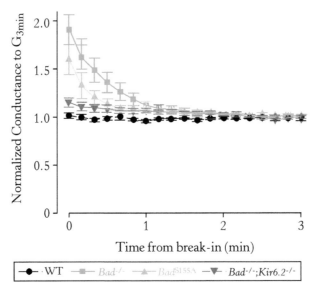

FIGURE 27.3 *BAD Modification Leads to Opening of K_{ATP} Channels*

Whole-cell conductance recorded from dentate granule neurons (DGNs) in acute hippocampal slices showing "washdown" of an initially high K_{ATP} channel conductance with high ATP (4 mM) in the recording pipette. Washdown is observed in $Bad^{-/-}$ ($N = 8$) and Bad^{S155A} ($N = 7$) DGNs but not in wild-type (WT; $N = 7$) or $Bad^{-/-};Kir6.2^{-/-}$ double-mutant ($N = 6$) DGNs. The time course of slope conductance during whole-cell recording was normalized to the value 3 min after break-in. (Adapted from Giménez-Cassina, A., Martínez-François, J. R., Fisher, J. K., Szlyk, B., Polak, K., Wiwczar, J., Tanner, G. R., Lutas, A., Yellen, G., & Danial, N. N. (2012). BAD-dependent regulation of fuel metabolism and K_{ATP} channel activity confers resistance to epileptic seizures. *Neuron, 74*, 719–730. Figure 5) lacking both BAD and Kir6.2. Additionally, the number of functional K$_{ATP}$ channels in DGNs is not affected by altering BAD's metabolic role. The maximal K$_{ATP}$ conductance, observed in whole-cell recordings dialyzing the neuron's intracellular medium with a low concentration of ATP (0.3 mM), is unchanged between WT and *Bad$^{-/-}$* or *Bad^{S155A}* DGNs (Giménez-Cassina et al., 2012).

Genetic deletion of *Bad* leads to increased activity of K$_{ATP}$ channels only in *Bad*-null cells, that is, the effect of BAD knockout on K$_{ATP}$ channels is cell autonomous and does not depend on other types of cells, such as astrocytes. Martínez-François et al. reconstituted BAD expression in *Bad$^{-/-}$* DGNs (Martínez-François et al., 2018). The expression of BAD in DGNs was achieved

by intracranial injection of an Adeno-associated virus (AAV) coding for BAD and a red fluorescent protein, mCherry, to visualize the transduced cells. In whole-cell experiments, transduced neurons expressing BAD lacked K$_{ATP}$ channel washdown, thus, the effect of *Bad* deletion on K$_{ATP}$ channels was indeed reversed. However, *Bad$^{-/-}$* neurons that had not been transduced still displayed washdown, confirming the effect is cell-autonomous (Figure 27.4).

Increased K$_{ATP}$ channel activity in *Bad*-altered DGNs suggests that K$_{ATP}$ channels might lead to decreased neuronal excitability. Indeed, fewer action potentials are elicited in response to current injection in *Bad$^{-/-}$* DGNs compared to WT neurons. Further, pharmacologic inhibition of

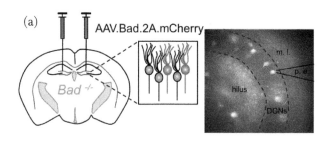

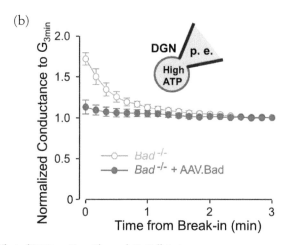

FIGURE 27.4 *The Effect of BAD on K$_{ATP}$ Channels Is Cell Autonomous*

(a) Left: Schematic representation of intracranial injection of AAV coding for BAD and mCherry in the hippocampus of *Bad$^{-/-}$* mice. Cells with reconstituted BAD expression display red fluorescence. Right: Epifluorescence picture of an acute hippocampal *Bad$^{-/-}$* slice with BAD-reconstituted cells. A DGN with red fluorescence is being recorded with a patch electrode (p.e.) in whole-cell mode. Regions observed in the picture: hilus, dentate granule cell layer (DGNs), and molecular layer (m.l.). (b) "Washdown" of an initially high K$_{ATP}$ channel conductance, with high ATP (4 mM) in the patch electrode, in *Bad$^{-/-}$* (*N* = 10) but not BAD-reconstituted *Bad$^{-/-}$* cells (*N* = 9). The time course of slope conductance measured during whole-cell recording was normalized to the value 3 min after break-in. Data are *M* ± *SEM*. (Adapted from Martínez-François, J. R., Fernández-Agüera, M. C., Nathwani, N., Lahmann, C., Burnham, V. L., Danial, N. N., & Yellen, G. (2018). BAD and K$_{ATP}$ channels regulate neuron excitability and epileptiform activity. *eLife, 7*, Article e32721. Figure 1.)

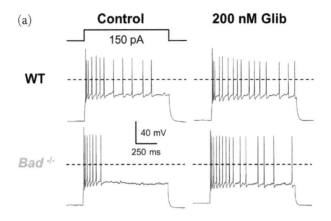

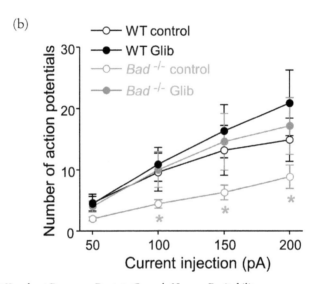

FIGURE 27.5 *BAD Knockout Decreases Dentate Granule Neuron Excitability*

(a) *Bad⁻/⁻* DGNs fire fewer action potentials than wild-type (WT) neurons fire. Pharmacologic inhibition of K_{ATP} channels with glibenclamide (200 nM) reverses the BAD-knockout effect on DGN excitability. Representative perforated-patch voltage recordings in response to a 1-s, 150-pA current pulse for WT (top traces) and *Bad⁻/⁻* (bottom traces) DGNs, in the presence or absence of 200 nM glibenclamide, as indicated. Dotted lines indicate 0 mV. (b) Glibenclamide application increases number of action potentials fired of *Bad⁻/⁻* ($N = 7$) DGNs but not that of WT ($N = 7$). Number of action potentials ($M \pm SEM$) is plotted against the magnitude of the current injection pulse. * $p < 0.05$; 1-way ANOVA. (Adapted from Martínez-François, J. R., Fernández-Agüera, M. C., Nathwani, N., Lahmann, C., Burnham, V. L., Danial, N. N., & Yellen, G. (2018). BAD and K_{ATP} channels regulate neuron excitability and epileptiform activity. *eLife, 7*, Article e32721. Figure 2.)

K_{ATP} channels acutely reverses the *Bad* knockout effect on the excitability of DGNs (Figure 27.5). Similarly, opening of K_{ATP} channels can rapidly decrease hippocampal neuron excitability in various other preparations (Forte et al., 2016; Huang et al., 2006, 2007). Thus, K_{ATP} channels can acutely modulate neuron excitability, and this could be a central mechanism in the KD's anticonvulsive effects.

K_{ATP} CHANNELS MEDIATE SEIZURE PROTECTION ELICITED BY BAD DISRUPTION

Lack of BAD leads to a remarkable increase in K_{ATP} channel activity and produces seizure protection. These two effects appear to be causally related: eliminating *Kir6.2* in a *Bad⁻/⁻* background nearly abolishes the seizure resistance produced by *Bad* ablation (Figure 27.6). This is not due to

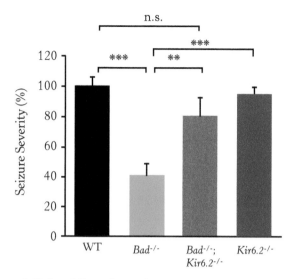

FIGURE 27.6 K_{ATP} *Channels Mediate Effects of BAD Alteration on Seizures in Vivo*

Integrated seizure severity in *Bad*$^{-/-}$ or *Kir6.2*$^{-/-}$ single mutants, or *Bad*$^{-/-}$; *Kir6.2*$^{-/-}$ double-mutant mice compared with WT mice after a single intraperitoneal injection of kainate monitored and analyzed as in Figure 27.1. Data are presented as mean ± *SEM.* ** $p < 0.01$; *** $p < 0.001$; n.s., nonsignificant; two-tailed Student's *t*-test. (Adapted from Giménez-Cassina, A., Martínez-François, J. R., Fisher, J. K., Szlyk, B., Polak, K., Wiwczar, J., Tanner, G. R., Lutas, A., Yellen, G., & Danial, N. N. (2012). BAD-dependent regulation of fuel metabolism and K_{ATP} channel activity confers resistance to epileptic seizures. *Neuron, 74,* 719–730. Figure 6.)

an increase in seizure severity produced by lack of *Kir6.2*; single deletion of *Kir6.2* does not increase the seizure sensitivity of these genetically-altered mice compared to WT animals (Giménez-Cassina et al., 2012). These results constitute genetic evidence that K_{ATP} channels are necessary in mediating BAD's effect on seizure protection.

As previously mentioned, K_{ATP} channels are well-known mediators between changes in metabolism and neuronal excitability. Indeed, either glucose deprivation or ketone body metabolism can increase K_{ATP} channel activity. The mechanism by which a metabolic fuel switch could increase K_{ATP} channel activity is unknown. Given that ATP and ADP directly control the open probability of K_{ATP} channels, BAD's metabolic effects may produce changes in ATP:ADP concentrations local to K_{ATP} channels.

Why would ATP:ADP levels change in the presence of abundant alternative fuels? One possibility is that K_{ATP} channel activity is controlled by local glycolysis. Glycolysis is bypassed and inhibited by mitochondrial metabolism of ketone bodies (DeVivo et al., 1978; Haymond et al., 1983; Valente-Silva et al., 2015). This metabolic change would increase ATP produced by mitochondria and decrease ATP produced by glycolysis. In fact, K_{ATP} channels and glycolytic enzymes can be found associated in large complexes in the

plasma membrane (Dhar-Chowdhury et al., 2007; Dubinsky et al., 1998; Hong et al., 2011), and these glycolytic enzyme complexes may produce ATP compartmentation in the cell (Chu et al., 2012; Hoffman et al., 2009; Proverbio & Hoffman, 1977). Furthermore, glycolysis inhibition can trigger the opening of K_{ATP} channels (Forte et al., 2016; Matsumoto et al., 2002; Schwanstecher & Panten, 1993; Tantama et al., 2013). Another possibility is that glucose metabolism is special in its ability to respond rapidly to acute energy challenges, as might occur in the elevated brain activity leading to seizures. Thus, BAD alteration, by switching metabolism away from glucose consumption, may produce a decrease in the ATP concentration at the plasma membrane, which could then trigger K_{ATP} channel opening and reduced neuronal excitability.

Although modulation of K_{ATP} channel activity by ATP/ADP is a straightforward explanation, K_{ATP} channel regulation is complex, and other processes, such as PIP_2 binding or phosphorylation, can also alter K_{ATP} channel activity (Nichols, 2006; Proks & Ashcroft, 2009). In addition, βHB levels are increased in *Bad*$^{-/-}$ compared to WT brains, and, as mentioned above, this can induce K_{ATP} channel opening. While it is unlikely that the effects of ketone bodies on K_{ATP} channel activity explain the totality of the observed K_{ATP} channel

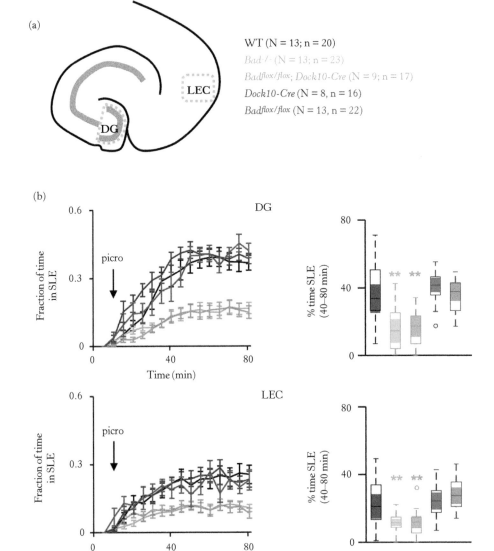

(a)

WT (N = 13; n = 20)
Bad⁻/⁻ (N = 13; n = 23)
Bad^flox/flox; Dock10-Cre (N = 9; n = 17)
Dock10-Cre (N = 8, n = 16)
Bad^flox/flox (N = 13, n = 22)

FIGURE 27.7 *Genetic Deletion of* Bad *Exclusively in the Dentate Gyrus Is Sufficient to Reduce Seizurelike Activity*

(a) Schematic representation of an acute brain slice containing the entorhinal cortex and hippocampus. Regions of interest depicted are the dentate gyrus and hilus (DG) and the lateral entorhinal cortex (LEC). (b) Deleting *Bad* in the whole animal (*Bad⁻/⁻*; green) or only in DGNs (*Bad^flox/flox*; *Dock10-Cre*, orange) decreases time spent in seizurelike events (SLEs) in the hippocampus or entorhinal cortex (for which the DG and LEC are representative examples, respectively). Left column: Fraction of time spent in SLEs (*M ± SEM*) for genotypes indicated versus time. Right column: Percent time spent in SLEs calculated from the 40- to 80-min range when seizurelike activity reaches a plateau for each region of interest. Shaded area represents 95% confidence interval. ** $p < 0.01$; 1-way ANOVA. (Adapted from Martínez-François, J. R., Fernández-Agüera, M. C., Nathwani, N., Lahmann, C., Burnham, V. L., Danial, N. N., & Yellen, G. (2018). BAD and K_{ATP} channels regulate neuron excitability and epileptiform activity. *eLife, 7*, Article e32721. Figure 6.)

activation, these metabolites may constitute part of multiple actions needed to exert the full effect observed upon BAD alteration.

TARGETED DELETION OF *BAD* IN DGNS IS SUFFICIENT TO ALLEVIATE SEIZURELIKE ACTIVITY IN VITRO

Whole-body BAD knockout reduces seizures and neuronal excitability through K$_{ATP}$ channels, and this effect likely occurs in the brain. To further study the effects in the brain of *Bad* deletion, epileptiform activity was studied in acute brain slices containing the hippocampus and the entorhinal cortex. Seizurelike events (SLEs) were triggered by application of picrotoxin, a GABA$_A$ receptor antagonist. The SLEs were monitored by intracellular calcium imaging using the fluorescent biosensor GCaMP6f. *Bad$^{-/-}$* slices spent less time in SLEs than WT slices did (Figure 27.7). Furthermore, BAD's alleviation of epileptiform activity can be reversed by genetic deletion or acute pharmacologic inhibition of K$_{ATP}$ channels (Martínez-François et al., 2018). These results recapitulate the antiseizure effect of *Bad* deletion in vivo and its requirement for K$_{ATP}$ channels.

The in vitro model was then used to assess whether *Bad* deletion exclusively in DGNs is sufficient to alleviate picrotoxin-induced epileptiform activity. The dentate gyrus is thought to prevent the propagation of epileptiform activity that may initiate in the entorhinal cortex from spreading to the hippocampus and producing many types of seizures, as in temporal lobe epilepsy (Dengler & Coulter, 2016; Heinemann et al., 1992; Hsu, 2007; Krook-Magnuson et al., 2013, 2015; Lothman et al., 1992). In principle, strengthening the "seizure gate" property of the dentate gyrus by decreasing DGN excitability could prevent seizures.

To test if ablating *Bad* solely in DGNs is sufficient to alleviate picrotoxin-induced SLEs, conditional knockout BAD mice (*Bad$^{flox/flox}$*) were crossed with transgenic mice (*Dock10-Cre*) that express Cre recombinase exclusively in DGNs (Kohara et al., 2014). These mice (*Bad$^{flox/flox}$; Dock10-Cre*) lack *Bad* in the dentate gyrus but not in any other area of the entorhinal-hippocampal slices (Martínez-François et al., 2018). Remarkably, epileptiform activity in slices that lack BAD only in the dentate gyrus is significantly reduced compared to either of the parental lines. In fact, *Bad$^{flox/flox}$;Dock10-Cre* slices spend an amount of time in SLEs comparable to that spent by *Bad$^{-/-}$* slices (Figure 27.7). This demonstrates that ablating *Bad* in a DGN-specific manner is sufficient to decrease seizurelike activity equivalent to whole-brain BAD knockout.

To assess whether alleviation of seizurelike activity via BAD and K$_{ATP}$ channels in the entorhinal-hippocampal circuit elicits seizure protection in vivo, further experiments in acute or chronic seizure models using genetically modified animals, such as the *Bad$^{flox/flox}$;Dock10-Cre* mice, are necessary. These experiments would support the idea that K$_{ATP}$ channel opening in specific brain regions, such as the dentate gyrus, elicits seizure protection. In this scenario, elevated neuronal activity, which would ordinarily lead to seizures in a susceptible individual, would produce an increase in K$_{ATP}$ channel current. This would then reduce subsequent neuronal activity by hyperpolarizing neurons.

It will also be important to reveal other relevant brain regions associated with the antiseizure effect. For instance, besides being present in DGNs in the hippocampus, K$_{ATP}$ channels are also present in GABAergic neurons of the SNr. It has been shown that reducing neuronal firing in either of these two brain areas inhibits seizure activity (Akman et al., 2015; Coulter & Carlson, 2007; Krook-Magnuson et al., 2013; Paz et al., 2007; Vercueil et al., 1998). Studies on K$_{ATP}$ channel activity or in vivo seizure models in conditional Kir6.2 knockout lines could be used to define the brain regions and brain cell types implicated in seizure resistance.

CONCLUSION

In summary, elimination of BAD's metabolic role switches brain cells away from glucose utilization toward consumption of alternative fuels. These metabolic changes are reminiscent of those elicited by a KD. Remarkably, BAD disruption produces robust seizure protection in the absence of dietary treatments. At the cellular level, it appears that K$_{ATP}$ channels mediate BAD's anticonvulsant effect. Disruption of BAD function increases K$_{ATP}$ channel activity in neurons in the dentate gyrus, a brain region that is likely a gate for seizure activity. Selective elimination of BAD in this brain region is sufficient to alleviate seizure-like activity in vitro. The mechanisms by which BAD modulates brain metabolism and how these metabolic changes affect excitability have just started to be revealed. The mechanisms leading to seizure reduction will ideally serve as the basis for development of more effective therapies for epilepsy.

ACKNOWLEDGMENTS
We thank members of the Yellen lab for critical review and discussion of the manuscript. This work was supported by grants from the National Institutes of Health (R01 NS083844 to G.Y. and N.N.D. and R01 NS055031 to G.Y.).

REFERENCES
Akman, O., Gulcebi, M. I., Carcak, N., Ketenci Ozatman, S., Eryigit, T., Moshé, S. L., Galanopoulou, A. S., & Onat, F. Y. (2015). The role of the substantia nigra pars reticulata in kindling resistance in rats with genetic absence epilepsy. *Epilepsia, 56,* 1793–1802.

Ashcroft, F. M. (2005). ATP-sensitive potassium channelopathies: Focus on insulin secretion. *Journal of Clinical Investigation, 115,* 2047–2058.

Ashcroft, F. M., Harrison, D. E., & Ashcroft, S. J. (1984). Glucose induces closure of single potassium channels in isolated rat pancreatic beta-cells. *Nature, 312,* 446–448.

Ben-Ari, Y., Tremblay, E., Ottersen, O. P., & Meldrum, B. S. (1980). The role of epileptic activity in hippocampal and "remote" cerebral lesions induced by kainic acid. *Brain Research, 191,* 79–97.

Bough, K. J., & Eagles, D. A. (1999). A ketogenic diet increases the resistance to pentylenetetrazole-induced seizures in the rat. *Epilepsia, 40,* 138–143.

Chu, H., Puchulu-Campanella, E., Galan, J. A., Tao, W. A., Low, P. S., & Hoffman, J. F. (2012). Identification of cytoskeletal elements enclosing the ATP pools that fuel human red blood cell membrane cation pumps. *Proceedings of the National Academy of Sciences of the United States of America,109,* 12794–12799.

Coulter, D. A., & Carlson, G. C. (2007). Functional regulation of the dentate gyrus by GABA-mediated inhibition. *Progress in Brain Research, 163,* 235–243.

Czabotar, P. E., Lessene, G., Strasser, A., & Adams, J. M. (2014). Control of apoptosis by the BCL-2 protein family: Implications for physiology and therapy. *Nature Reviews Molecular Cell Biology,15,* 49–63.

Danial, N. N., Hartman, A. L., Stafstrom, C. E., & Thio, L. L. (2013). How does the ketogenic diet work? Four potential mechanisms. *Journal of Child Neurology, 28,* 1027–1033.

Danial, N. N., & Korsmeyer, S. J. (2004). Cell death: Critical control points. *Cell, 116,* 205–219.

Danial, N. N., Walensky, L. D., Zhang, C. Y., Choi, C. S., Fisher, J. K., Molina, A. J., Datta, S. R., Pitter, K. L., Bird, G. H., Wikstrom, J. D., Deeney, J. T., Robertson, K., Morash, J., Kulkarni, A., Neschen, S., Kim, S., Greenberg, M. E., Corkey, B. E., Shirihai, O. S., Shulman, G. I., . . . Korsmeyer, S. J. (2008). Dual role of proapoptotic BAD in insulin secretion and beta cell survival. *Nature Medicine, 14,* 144–153.

Datta, S. R., Katsov, A., Hu, L., Petros, A., Fesik, S. W., Yaffe, M. B., & Greenberg, M. E. (2000). 14-3-3 proteins and survival kinases cooperate to inactivate BAD by BH3 domain phosphorylation. *Molecular Cell, 6,* 41–51.

Davolio, C., & Greenamyre, J. T. (1995). Selective vulnerability of the CA1 region of hippocampus to the indirect excitotoxic effects of malonic acid. *Neuroscience Letters, 192,* 29–32.

Dengler, C. G., & Coulter, D. A. (2016). Normal and epilepsy-associated pathologic function of the dentate gyrus. *Progress in Brain Research, 226,* 155–178.

Depaulis, A., Vergnes, M., & Marescaux, C. (1994). Endogenous control of epilepsy: The nigral inhibitory system. *Progress in Neurobiology, 42,* 33–52.

DeVivo, D. C., Leckie, M. P., Ferrendelli, J. S., & McDougal, D. B. (1978). Chronic ketosis and cerebral metabolism. *Annals of Neurology, 3,* 331–337.

Dhar-Chowdhury, P., Malester, B., Rajacic, P., & Coetzee, W. A. (2007). The regulation of ion channels and transporters by glycolytically derived ATP. *Cellular and Molecular Life Sciences, 64,* 3069–3083.

Dubinsky, W. P., Mayorga-Wark, O., & Schultz, S. G. (1998). Colocalization of glycolytic enzyme activity and K_{ATP} channels in basolateral membrane of *Necturus* enterocytes. *American Journal of Physiology, 275,* C1653–C1659.

Dunn-Meynell, A. A., Rawson, N. E., & Levin, B. E. (1998). Distribution and phenotype of neurons containing the ATP-sensitive K^+ channel in rat brain. *Brain Research, 814,* 41–54.

Engel, T., Hatazaki, S., Tanaka, K., Prehn, J. H. M., & Henshall, D. C. (2010). Deletion of Puma protects hippocampal neurons in a model of severe status epilepticus. *Neuroscience, 168,* 443–450.

Engel, T., Plesnila, N., Prehn, J. H. M., & Henshall, D. C. (2011). In vivo contributions of BH3-only proteins to neuronal death following seizures, ischemia, and traumatic brain injury. *Journal of Cerebral Blood Flow & Metabolism, 31,* 1196–1210.

Fenoglio-Simeone, K. A., Wilke, J. C., Milligan, H. L., Allen, C. N., Rho, J. M., & Maganti, R. K. (2009). Ketogenic diet treatment abolishes seizure periodicity and improves diurnal rhythmicity in epileptic Kcna1-null mice. *Epilepsia, 50,* 2027–2034.

Ferraro, T. N., Golden, G. T., Smith, G. G., St. Jean, P., Schork, N. J., Mulholland, N., Ballas, C., Schill, J., Buono, R. J., & Berrettini, W. H. (1999). Mapping loci for pentylenetetrazol-induced seizure susceptibility in mice. *Journal of Neuroscience, 19,* 6733–6739.

Foley, J., Burnham, V., Tedoldi, M., Danial, N. N., & Yellen, G. (2018). BAD knockout provides metabolic seizure resistance in a genetic model of epilepsy with sudden unexplained death in epilepsy. *Epilepsia*, 59, e1–e4.

Forte, N., Medrihan, L., Cappetti, B., Baldelli, P., & Benfenati, F. (2016). 2-Deoxy-D-glucose enhances tonic inhibition through the neurosteroid-mediated activation of extrasynaptic GABA$_A$ receptors. *Epilepsia*, 57, 1987–2000.

Garriga-Canut, M., Schoenike, B., Qazi, R., Bergendahl, K., Daley, T. J., Pfender, R. M., Morrison, J. F., Ockuly, J., Stafstrom, C., Sutula, T., & Roopra, A. (2006). 2-Deoxy-D-glucose reduces epilepsy progression by NRSF-CtBP-dependent metabolic regulation of chromatin structure. *Nature Neuroscience*, 9, 1382–1387.

Giménez-Cassina, A., & Danial, N. N. (2015). Regulation of mitochondrial nutrient and energy metabolism by BCL-2 family proteins. *Trends in Endocrinology & Metabolism, 26*, 165–175.

Giménez-Cassina, A., Martínez-François, J. R., Fisher, J. K., Szlyk, B., Polak, K., Wiwczar, J., Tanner, G. R., Lutas, A., Yellen, G., & Danial, N. N. (2012). BAD-dependent regulation of fuel metabolism and K$_{ATP}$ channel activity confers resistance to epileptic seizures. *Neuron, 74*, 719–730.

Giménez-Cassina, A., Garcia-Haro, L., Choi, C. S., Osundiji, M. A., Lane, E. A., Huang, H., Yildirim, M. A., Szlyk, B., Fisher, J. K., Polak, K., Patton, E., Wiwczar, J., Godes, M., Lee, D. H., Robertson, K., Kim, S., Kulkarni, A., Distefano, A., Samuel, V., Cline, G., . . . Danial, N. N (2014). Regulation of hepatic energy metabolism and gluconeogenesis by BAD. *Cell Metabolism, 19*, 272–284.

Haller, M., Mironov, S. L., Karschin, A., & Richter, D. W. (2001). Dynamic activation of K$_{ATP}$ channels in rhythmically active neurons. *Journal of Physiology, 537*, 69–81.

Hartman, A. L., Gasior, M., Vining, E. P. G., & Rogawski, M. A. (2007). The neuropharmacology of the ketogenic diet. *Pediatric Neurology, 36*, 281–292.

Haymond, M. W., Howard, C., Ben-Galim, E., & DeVivo, D. C. (1983). Effects of ketosis on glucose flux in children and adults. *American Journal of Physiology, 245*, E373–E378.

Heinemann, U., Beck, H., Dreier, J. P., Ficker, E., Stabel, J., & Zhang, C. L. (1992). The dentate gyrus as a regulated gate for the propagation of epileptiform activity. *Epilepsy Research, 7*(Suppl.), 273–280.

Hernández-Sánchez, C., Basile, A. S., Fedorova, I., Arima, H., Stannard, B., Fernandez, A. M., Ito, Y., & LeRoith, D. (2001). Mice transgenically overexpressing sulfonylurea receptor 1 in forebrain resist seizure induction and excitotoxic neuron death. *Proceedings of the National Academy of Sciences of the United States of America, 98*, 3549–3554.

Hickman, J. A., Hardwick, J. M., Kaczmarek, L. K., & Jonas, E. A. (2008). Bcl-xL inhibitor ABT-737 reveals a dual role for Bcl-xL in synaptic transmission. *Journal of Neurophysiology, 99*, 1515–1522.

Hoffman, J. F., Dodson, A., & Proverbio, F. (2009). On the functional use of the membrane compartmentalized pool of ATP by the Na$^+$ and Ca^{++} pumps in human red blood cell ghosts. *Journal of General Physiology, 134*, 351–361.

Hong, M., Kefaloyianni, E., Bao, L., Malester, B., Delaroche, D., Neubert, T. A., & Coetzee, W. A. (2011). Cardiac ATP-sensitive K$^+$ channel associates with the glycolytic enzyme complex. *FASEB Journal, 25*, 2456–2467.

Hsu, D. (2007). The dentate gyrus as a filter or gate: A look back and a look ahead. *Progress in Brain Research, 163*, 601–613.

Huang, C.-W., Huang, C.-C., & Wu, S.-N. (2006). The opening effect of pregabalin on ATP-sensitive potassium channels in differentiated hippocampal neuron-derived H19-7 cells. *Epilepsia, 47*, 720–726.

Huang, C.-W., Huang, C.-C., Cheng, J.-T., Tsai, J.-J., & Wu, S.-N. (2007). Glucose and hippocampal neuronal excitability: Role of ATP-sensitive potassium channels. *Journal of Neuroscience Research, 85*, 1468–1477.

Huttenlocher, P. R. (1976). Ketonemia and seizures: Metabolic and anticonvulsant effects of two ketogenic diets in childhood epilepsy. *Pediatric Research, 10*, 536–540.

Iadarola, M. J., & Gale, K. (1982). Substantia nigra: Site of anticonvulsant activity mediated by gamma-aminobutyric acid. Science 218, 1237–1240.

Ivannikov, M. V., Sugimori, M., & Llinás, R. R. (2010). Calcium clearance and its energy requirements in cerebellar neurons. *Cell Calcium, 47*, 507–513.

Jiao, S., & Li, Z. (2011). Nonapoptotic function of BAD and BAX in long-term depression of synaptic transmission. *Neuron, 70*, 758–772.

Juge, N., Gray, J. A., Omote, H., Miyaji, T., Inoue, T., Hara, C., Uneyama, H., Edwards, R. H., Nicoll, R. A., & Moriyama, Y. (2010). Metabolic control of vesicular glutamate transport and release. *Neuron, 68*, 99–112.

Karschin, C., Ecke, C., Ashcroft, F. M., & Karschin, A. (1997). Overlapping distribution of K$_{ATP}$ channel-forming Kir6.2 subunit and the sulfonylurea receptor SUR1 in rodent brain. *FEBS Letters, 401*, 59–64.

Katsura, K., Minamisawa, H., Ekholm, A., Folbergrová, J., & Siesjö, B. K. (1992). Changes of labile metabolites during anoxia in moderately hypo- and hyperthermic rats: Correlation to membrane fluxes of K$^+$. *Brain Research, 590*, 6–12.

Kim, D. Y., Simeone, K. A., Simeone, T. A., Pandya, J. D., Wilke, J. C., Ahn, Y., Geddes, J. W., Sullivan, P. G., & Rho, J. M. (2015). Ketone bodies mediate antiseizure effects through mitochondrial permeability transition. *Annals of Neurology, 78,* 77–87.

Kohara, K., Pignatelli, M., Rivest, A. J., Jung, H. Y., Kitamura, T., Suh, J., Frank, D., Kajikawa, K., Mise, N., Obata, Y., Wickersham, I. R., & Tonegawa, S. (2014). Cell type-specific genetic and optogenetic tools reveal hippocampal CA2 circuits. *Nature Neuroscience, 17,* 269–279.

Krook-Magnuson, E., Armstrong, C., Bui, A., Lew, S., Oijala, M., & Soltesz, I. (2015). In vivo evaluation of the dentate gate theory in epilepsy. *Journal of Physiology, 593,* 2379–2388.

Krook-Magnuson, E., Armstrong, C., Oijala, M., & Soltesz, I. (2013). On-demand optogenetic control of spontaneous seizures in temporal lobe epilepsy. *Nature Communications, 4,* 1376.

Liss, B., & Roeper, J. (2001). Molecular physiology of neuronal K_{ATP} channels (review). *Molecular Membrane Biology, 18,* 117–127.

Lopantsev, V., Tempel, B. L., & Schwartzkroin, P. A. (2003). Hyperexcitability of CA3 pyramidal cells in mice lacking the potassium channel subunit Kv1.1. *Epilepsia, 44,* 1506–1512.

Lothman, E. W., Stringer, J. L., & Bertram, E. H. (1992). The dentate gyrus as a control point for seizures in the hippocampus and beyond. *Epilepsy Research, 7,* 301–313.

Lutas, A., Birnbaumer, L., & Yellen, G. (2014). Metabolism regulates the spontaneous firing of substantia nigra pars reticulata neurons via K_{ATP} and nonselective cation channels. *Journal of Neuroscience, 34,* 16336–16347.

Lutas, A., & Yellen, G. (2013). The ketogenic diet: Metabolic influences on brain excitability and epilepsy. *Trends in Neuroscience, 36,* 32–40.

Ma, W., Berg, J., & Yellen, G. (2007). Ketogenic diet metabolites reduce firing in central neurons by opening K_{ATP} channels. *Journal of Neuroscience, 27,* 3618–3625.

Martínez-François, J. R., Fernández-Agüera, M. C., Nathwani, N., Lahmann, C., Burnham, V. L., Danial, N. N., & Yellen, G. (2018). BAD and K_{ATP} channels regulate neuron excitability and epileptiform activity. *eLife, 7,* Article e32721.

Masino, S. A., Li, T., Theofilas, P., Sandau, U. S., Ruskin, D. N., Fredholm, B. B., Geiger, J. D., Aronica, E., & Boison, D. (2011). A ketogenic diet suppresses seizures in mice through adenosine A_1 receptors. *Journal of Clinical Investigation, 121,* 2679–2683.

Matsumoto, N., Komiyama, S., & Akaike, N. (2002). Pre- and postsynaptic ATP-sensitive potassium channels during metabolic inhibition of rat hippocampal CA1 neurons. *Journal of Physiology, 541,* 511–520.

McNamara, J. O., Galloway, M. T., Rigsbee, L. C., & Shin, C. (1984). Evidence implicating substantia nigra in regulation of kindled seizure threshold. *Journal of Neuroscience, 4,* 2410–2417.

Mercer, R. W., & Dunham, P. B. (1981). Membrane-bound ATP fuels the Na/K pump: Studies on membrane-bound glycolytic enzymes on inside-out vesicles from human red cell membranes. *Journal of General Physiology, 78,* 547–568.

Mergenthaler, P., Lindauer, U., Dienel, G. A., & Meisel, A. (2013). Sugar for the brain: The role of glucose in physiological and pathological brain function. *Trends in Neurosciences, 36,* 587–597.

Moldoveanu, T., Follis, A. V., Kriwacki, R. W., & Green, D. R. (2014). Many players in BCL-2 family affairs. *Trends in Biochemical Sciences, 39,* 101–111.

Murphy, B. M., Engel, T., Paucard, A., Hatazaki, S., Mouri, G., Tanaka, K., Tuffy, L. P., Jimenez-Mateos, E. M., Woods, I., Dunleavy, M., Bonner, H. P., Meller, R., Simon, R. P., Strasser, A., Prehn, J. H., & Henshall, D. C. (2010). Contrasting patterns of Bim induction and neuroprotection in Bim-deficient mice between hippocampus and neocortex after status epilepticus. *Cell Death & Differentiation, 17,* 459–468.

Neal, E. G., Chaffe, H., Schwartz, R. H., Lawson, M. S., Edwards, N., Fitzsimmons, G., Whitney, A., & Cross, J. H. (2009). A randomized trial of classical and medium-chain triglyceride ketogenic diets in the treatment of childhood epilepsy. *Epilepsia, 50,* 1109–1117.

Nichols, C. G. (2006). K_{ATP} channels as molecular sensors of cellular metabolism. *Nature, 440,* 470–476.

Owen, O. E., Morgan, A. P., Kemp, H. G., Sullivan, J. M., Herrera, M. G., & Cahill, G. F. (1967). Brain metabolism during fasting. *Journal of Clinical Investigation, 46,* 1589–1595.

Paz, J. T., Chavez, M., Saillet, S., Deniau, J.-M., & Charpier, S. (2007). Activity of ventral medial thalamic neurons during absence seizures and modulation of cortical paroxysms by the nigrothalamic pathway. *Journal of Neuroscience, 27,* 929–941.

Pelletier, M. R., Pahapill, P. A., Pennefather, P. S., & Carlen, P. L. (2000). Analysis of single K_{ATP} channels in mammalian dentate gyrus granule cells. *Journal of Neurophysiology, 84,* 2291–2301.

Pfeifer, H. H., Lyczkowski, D. A., & Thiele, E. A. (2008). Low glycemic index treatment: Implementation and new insights into efficacy. *Epilepsia, 49*(Suppl. 8), 42–45.

Proks, P., & Ashcroft, F. M. (2009). Modeling K_{ATP} channel gating and its regulation. *Progress in Biophysics and Molecular Biology, 99,* 7–19.

Proverbio, F., & Hoffman, J. F. (1977). Membrane compartmentalized ATP and its preferential use by the Na,K-ATPase of human red cell ghosts. *Journal of General Physiology, 69,* 605–632.

Sada, N., Lee, S., Katsu, T., Otsuki, T., & Inoue, T. (2015). Epilepsy treatment: Targeting LDH enzymes with a stiripentol analog to treat epilepsy. *Science, 347,* 1362–1367.

Schmidt-Kastner, R., & Freund, T. F. (1991). Selective vulnerability of the hippocampus in brain ischemia. *Neuroscience, 40,* 599–636.

Schwanstecher, C., & Panten, U. (1993). Tolbutamide- and diazoxide-sensitive K$^+$ channel in neurons of substantia nigra pars reticulata. *Naunyn-Schmiedeberg's Archives of Pharmacology, 348*, 113–117.

Simeone, K. A., Matthews, S. A., Rho, J. M., & Simeone, T. A. (2016). Ketogenic diet treatment increases longevity in Kcna1-null mice, a model of sudden unexpected death in epilepsy. *Epilepsia, 57*, e178–e182.

Simeone, T. A., Matthews, S. A., Samson, K. K., & Simeone, K. A. (2017). Regulation of brain PPARγ2 contributes to ketogenic diet anti-seizure efficacy. *Experimental Neurology, 287*, 54–64.

Smart, S. L., Lopantsev, V., Zhang, C. L., Robbins, C. A., Wang, H., Chiu, S. Y., Schwartzkroin, P. A., Messing, A., & Tempel, B. L. (1998). Deletion of the K$_V$1.1 potassium channel causes epilepsy in mice. *Neuron, 20*, 809–819.

Smith, M. L., Auer, R. N., & Siesjö, B. K. (1984). The density and distribution of ischemic brain injury in the rat following 2–10 min of forebrain ischemia. *Acta Neuropathologica, 64*, 319–332.

Stanford, I. M., & Lacey, M. G. (1996). Electrophysiological investigation of adenosine trisphosphate-sensitive potassium channels in the rat substantia nigra pars reticulata. *Neuroscience, 74*, 499–509.

Tanner, G. R., Lutas, A., Martínez-François, J. R., & Yellen, G. (2011). Single K$_{ATP}$ channel opening in response to action potential firing in mouse dentate granule neurons. *Journal of Neuroscience, 31*, 8689–8696.

Tantama, M., Martínez-François, J. R., Mongeon, R., & Yellen, G. (2013). Imaging energy status in live cells with a fluorescent biosensor of the intracellular ATP-to-ADP ratio. *Nature Communications, 4*, 2550.

Thiele, E. A. (2003). Assessing the efficacy of antiepileptic treatments: The ketogenic diet. *Epilepsia, 44*(Suppl. 7), 26–29.

Valente-Silva, P., Lemos, C., Köfalvi, A., Cunha, R. A., & Jones, J. G. (2015). Ketone bodies effectively compete with glucose for neuronal acetyl-CoA generation in rat hippocampal slices. *NMR in Biomedicine, 28*, 1111–1116.

Vercueil, L., Benazzouz, A., Deransart, C., Bressand, K., Marescaux, C., Depaulis, A., & Benabid, A. L. (1998). High-frequency stimulation of the subthalamic nucleus suppresses absence seizures in the rat: Comparison with neurotoxic lesions. *Epilepsy Research, 31*, 39–46.

Yamada, K., & Inagaki, N. (2005). Neuroprotection by K$_{ATP}$ channels. *Journal of Molecular and Cellular Cardiology, 38*, 945–949.

Yamada, K., Ji, J. J., Yuan, H., Miki, T., Sato, S., Horimoto, N., Shimizu, T., Seino, S., & Inagaki, N. (2001). Protective role of ATP-sensitive potassium channels in hypoxia-induced generalized seizure. *Science, 292*, 1543–1546.

Zawar, C., Plant, T. D., Schirra, C., Konnerth, A., & Neumcke, B. (1999). Cell-type specific expression of ATP-sensitive potassium channels in the rat hippocampus. *Journal of Physiology, 514*(Part 2), 327–341.

Zielke, H. R., Zielke, C. L., & Baab, P. J. (2009). Direct measurement of oxidative metabolism in the living brain by microdialysis: A review. *Journal of Neurochemistry, 109*(Suppl. 1), 24–29.

Zuberi, S. M., Eunson, L. H., Spauschus, A., De Silva, R., Tolmie, J., Wood, N. W., McWilliam, R. C., Stephenson, J. B., Kullmann, D. M., & Hanna, M. G. (1999). A novel mutation in the human voltage-gated potassium channel gene (Kv1.1) associates with episodic ataxia type 1 and sometimes with partial epilepsy. *Brain: A Journal of Neurology, 122*(Part 5), 817–825.

Lactate Dehydrogenase

A Novel Metabolic Target

NAGISA SADA, PHD AND TSUYOSHI INOUE, PHD

THE KETOGENIC DIET FOR DRUG-RESISTANT EPILEPSY

Epilepsy is a neurologic disorder that is characterized by the hyperexcitation of electrical activities in the brain. Approximately 1% of the world's population has epilepsy, and one third of patients with epilepsy have seizures that are resistant to currently available antiepileptic drugs (Kwan & Brodie, 2000). Therefore, it is important to develop new antiepileptic drugs that can treat drug-resistant epilepsy. Toward this goal, we first need to identify "endogenous proteins" that have the ability to suppress epileptic seizures so that they can be target molecules for the development of antiepileptic drugs. We then need to identify "chemical compounds" that act on the target molecules and suppress seizures, so that the compounds can be candidate antiepileptic drugs. Thus, the exploration for new target molecules in basic neuroscience will ultimately lead to drug development for drug-resistant epilepsy.

Epileptic seizures are caused by the hyperexcitation of electrical activities in the brain; therefore, antiepileptic drugs must suppress neuronal hyperexcitation. Because electrical activities in the brain are generated by ion channels and synaptic receptors, currently used antiepileptic drugs have been designed to act on the molecules generating electrical currents (Meldrum & Rogawski, 2007). For example, multiple antiepileptic drugs inhibit voltage-gated Na^+ channels, gabapentin and pregabalin inhibit L-type Ca^{2+} channels, and benzodiazepines and barbiturates activate $GABA_A$ receptors (see Figure 1 in Bialer & White, 2010). However, these antiepileptic drugs are not effective in one third of patients with epilepsy (Kwan & Brodie, 2000). New target molecules are required for the treatment of drug-resistant seizures.

It is noteworthy that treatment using the ketogenic diet (KD) is effective for some patients with drug-resistant epilepsy (Freeman et al., 1998; Neal et al., 2008). Thus, target molecules of the KD are obviously different from the targets of currently used antiepileptic drugs. Accordingly, neuroscientists have recently focused on the molecular mechanisms underlying the antiepileptic effects of the KD (Boison, 2017; Lutas & Yellen, 2013; Rho, 2017; Sada & Inoue, 2018; Simeone et al., 2018).

MECHANISMS RESPONSIBLE FOR THE ANTIEPILEPTIC EFFECTS OF THE KD

KD treatment was first developed in the 1920s (Wilder, 1921), and its modified version using the medium-chain triglyceride (MCT) KD was developed in the 1970s (Huttenlocher et al., 1971). The KD consists of high-fat and low-carbohydrate nutrients, which consequently increase ketone bodies, β-hydroxybutyrate (βHB) and acetoacetate, and mildly decrease glucose in patients with epilepsy (Huttenlocher et al., 1976). These two metabolic changes, as well as the KD's antiepileptic effects, are also observed in rodents (Bough et al., 2006). Therefore, electrical regulation by the two metabolic changes has been actively studied via electrophysiology in rodents (Lutas & Yellen, 2013; Sada & Inoue, 2018).

In terms of increases in ketone bodies, rodent studies have revealed that the KD increases the plasma level of βHB to 1 to 8 mM and has antiseizure effects in pentylenetetrazole models (Bough & Eagles, 1999; Bough et al., 1999, 2006). It is also known that an intraperitoneal injection of ketone bodies directly suppresses seizures in vivo in audiogenic seizure-susceptible mice (Rho et al., 2002). At the molecular and cellular levels, ketone bodies decrease the firing rate of neurons in the substantia nigra via adenosine 5'-triphosphate (ATP)-sensitive K^+ channels (K_{ATP} channels; Ma et al., 2007). Single-channel recordings have revealed that ketone bodies open K_{ATP} channels in the dentate granule cells of the hippocampus

(Tanner et al., 2011). Acetoacetate inhibits vesicular glutamate transporters (VGLUTs; Juge et al., 2010). Since VGLUTs fill synaptic vesicles with glutamate, the VGLUTs' inhibition by acetoacetate reduces miniature excitatory postsynaptic currents (EPSCs) and suppresses 4-aminopyridine-induced acute seizures in vivo (Juge et al., 2010). Acetoacetate also inhibits voltage-dependent Ca^{2+} channels and reduces EPSCs in pyramidal cells of the hippocampus (Kadowaki et al., 2017). Using patch-clamp recordings from hippocampal slices, researchers reported that acetoacetate reduces EPSCs in epileptiform slices more potently than in normal slices. In addition to ketone bodies, decanoic acid is supplied by the MCT KD in patients with epilepsy (Haidukewych et al., 1982; Sills et al., 1986). Recent electrophysiologic studies have shown that decanoic acid reduces EPSCs via AMPA-type glutamate receptors and suppresses epileptiform activity in entorhinal cortex-hippocampal slices (Chang et al., 2013, 2016).

With reference to decreases in glucose, seizures are known to be suppressed by 2-deoxy-D-glucose, a glycolytic inhibitor (Garriga-Canut et al., 2006). BAD (BCL-2-associated agonist of cell death) knockout mice exhibit energy metabolism similar to that on the KD, that is, decreases in glucose metabolism and increases in ketone body metabolism (Giménez-Cassina et al., 2012). Knockout of BAD opens metabolically sensitive K_{ATP} channels, reduces epileptiform activity in brain slices, and protects against kainic acid and pentylenetetrazol-induced seizures in vivo (Giménez-Cassina et al., 2012; Martínez-François et al., 2018). In addition, the KD suppresses seizures in mice by activation of adenosine A_1 receptors (Masino et al.,

2011). Recordings from hippocampal slices have revealed that reductions in glucose hyperpolarize pyramidal neurons, which is mediated by adenosine A_1 receptors and K_{ATP} channels (Kawamura et al., 2010). Consistent with this, the direct activation of adenosine A_1 receptors suppresses chronic seizures in a chronic model of temporal lobe epilepsy (Gouder et al., 2003).

These extensive studies have uncovered the molecules that exert the antiepileptic effects of the KD. However, these are not molecules in energy metabolic systems like glycolysis and the TCA cycle. Since the KD changes energy metabolites, we hypothesized that the brain has "metabolic pathways" responsible for the antiepileptic effects of the KD. In more detail, we assumed there are "metabolic enzymes" that regulate electrical activities in neurons and suppress seizures in vivo, and which work in the same manner as the KD. In order to explore such metabolic pathways and enzymes, we focused on the astrocyte–neuron lactate shuttle in the brain, because this shuttle was known to be a metabolic pathway involved in the regulation of brain electrical activity (Parsons & Hirasawa, 2010; Rouach et al., 2008).

ASTROCYTE–NEURON LACTATE SHUTTLE

Glucose is the main energy source in the brain, and it produces ATP in neurons and glial cells. The concentration of glucose in vivo is approximately 2.5 mM in the brain (Silver & Erecińska, 1994) and is maintained at a lower concentration than that in the blood. Glucose is directly transported into neurons and is then converted to pyruvate by glycolysis, which produces ATP

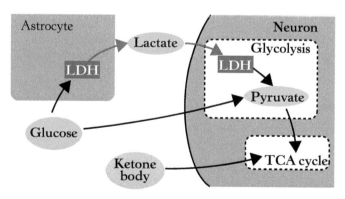

FIGURE 28.1. *The Astrocyte–Neuron Lactate Shuttle*
Glucose is directly transported into neurons and then is converted to pyruvate by glycolysis. As an alternative pathway, glucose is transported into astrocytes and is converted to lactate by LDH, and the lactate is released into extracellular spaces: lactate is then transported into neurons and is converted to pyruvate by glycolysis. This pathway is called the astrocyte–neuron lactate shuttle (red arrows). Decreases in glucose and increases in ketone bodies are elicited by the ketogenic diet. Ketone bodies are transported into neurons, which bypass glycolysis and directly enter the TCA cycle in neurons.

in the TCA cycle (Figure 28.1). Astrocytes are a type of glial cell, and their role as energy supplier has received increasing attention (Bélanger et al., 2011). As shown in Figure 28.1, glucose is initially transported into astrocytes and converted to lactate by lactate dehydrogenase (LDH). The lactate is then released to extracellular spaces, transported into neurons, and converted to pyruvate by LDH in glycolysis, which produces ATP in the TCA cycle (Figure 28.1). This metabolic pathway is called the astrocyte–neuron lactate shuttle (Bélanger et al., 2011).

Several lines of evidence support that the astrocyte–neuron lactate shuttle is used in the supply of energy to neurons. First, astrocytes show lower rates of oxidative metabolism than neurons, and consequently release a large amount of lactate to the extracellular spaces (Bouzier-Sore et al., 2006; Itoh et al., 2003). Second, lactate appears to an energy source preferred over glucose in the brain (Larrabee, 1995; Smith et al., 2003). Third, although glucose uptake rates into neurons and astrocytes are similar in the resting state of the brain (Chuquet et al., 2010; Nehlig et al., 2004), increased neural activities elicit higher glucose uptake in astrocytes (Chuquet et al., 2010) and enhance lactate release to extracellular spaces (Hu & Wilson, 1997). Thus, the energy supply to neurons is achieved not only by the direct glucose pathway to neurons, but also by the astrocyte–neuron lactate shuttle (see Figure 28.1).

There is also growing evidence to show that the astrocyte–neuron lactate shuttle regulates electrical activity in neurons. First, inhibition of glycolysis reduces synaptic transmission in the hippocampus, and this is rescued by the presence of lactate (Schurr et al., 1988), which demonstrates that the metabolism of lactate to pyruvate in neurons contributes to the maintenance of synaptic transmission. Second, the inhibition of monocarboxylate transporters, which transport lactate into neurons, also reduces synaptic transmission in the hippocampus (Izumi et al., 1997). Third, orexin-containing neurons in the hypothalamus are hyperpolarized by the inhibition of monocarboxylate transporters (Parsons & Hirasawa, 2010). Importantly, they are also hyperpolarized by fluoroacetate, a glial toxin, and the hyperpolarization is reversed by the application of lactate (Parsons & Hirasawa, 2010). These findings suggest that lactate released from astrocytes regulates membrane potentials in neurons.

Rouach and colleagues provided more direct evidence to show that electrical activities in neurons are regulated by the metabolic pathway from astrocytes (Rouach et al., 2008).

Astrocytes in the hippocampus are connected to one another by gap junctions; therefore, small molecules injected into single astrocytes using patch pipettes diffuse into many neighboring astrocytes (D'Ambrosio et al., 1998). Based on this property, a group of nearby astrocytes can be controlled by selective filling of active small molecules into single astrocytes using patch pipettes (Henneberger et al., 2010; Rouach et al., 2008). By filling glucose into single astrocytes in glucose-deprived hippocampal slices, the researchers demonstrated that the deprivation of extracellular glucose reduces synaptic transmission, and this reduction is rescued by the selective filling of glucose into astrocytes (Rouach et al., 2008). The data show that hippocampal synaptic transmission is regulated by metabolic communication from astrocytes.

LDH: A METABOLIC TARGET FOR EPILEPSY

These studies prompted us to investigate electrical regulation by the astrocyte–neuron lactate shuttle, and we found that this lactate shuttle is involved in the antiepileptic effects of the KD (Sada et al., 2015). The KD is known to increase ketone bodies and to decrease glucose in rodents (Bough et al., 2006). Therefore, we made patch-clamp recordings from neurons in the subthalamic nucleus of mouse brain slices, and we switched the glucose in the extracellular perfusate (artificial cerebrospinal fluid; ACSF) to ketone bodies. The metabolic switch hyperpolarized neurons, and this hyperpolarization was recovered by the addition of lactate in ACSF (Sada et al., 2015). Based on the metabolic pathways shown in Figure 28.1, it is likely that the hyperpolarization is elicited by the decrease in extracellular lactate, which is elicited by the metabolic switch from glucose to ketone bodies. Thus, it is suggested that the astrocyte–neuron lactate shuttle regulates membrane potential in neurons.

To confirm this idea, we focused on LDH. LDH is a metabolic enzyme located in the astrocyte–neuron lactate shuttle (Figure 28.1), and therefore the lactate shuttle can be suppressed by inhibiting LDH. We used oxamate, an LDH inhibitor that has been used to inhibit LDH in the brain (Lam et al., 2005), and examined the effects of the LDH inhibitor on membrane potential in neurons (Sada et al., 2015; see Figure 28.2). Inhibition of LDH hyperpolarized neurons in the subthalamic nucleus and hyperpolarized pyramidal cells in the hippocampus (Figure 28.2a). Furthermore, the hyperpolarization elicited by the LDH inhibition was not recovered by the addition of lactate, but it was recovered by the addition of pyruvate (Figure 28.2b). Lactate is an upstream metabolite of LDH in neurons, whereas pyruvate is a downstream metabolite in neurons (see Figure 28.1). Thus, neuronal LDH in the lactate shuttle regulates membrane potential in neurons (Figure 28.2c).

We also obtained direct evidence to show that membrane potentials in neurons are regulated by lactate released from astrocytes (Sada et al., 2015; see Figure 28.3). Patch-clamp recordings were obtained from neighboring pairs of pyramidal cells and astrocytes in hippocampal slices, and oxamate was selectively applied to

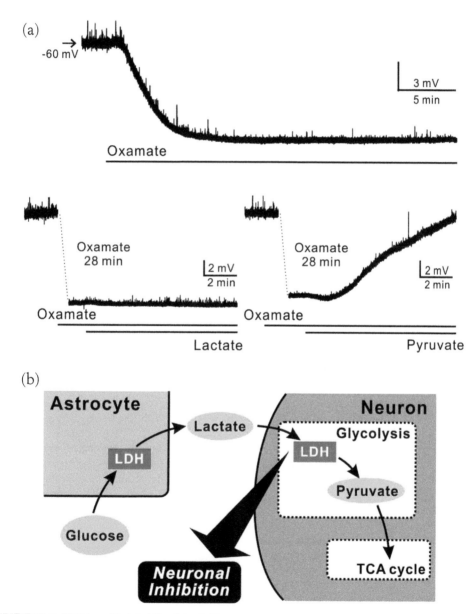

FIGURE 28.2 *LDH is an Electrical Regulator in Neurons*

(a) Pyramidal cells in the hippocampus are hyperpolarized by oxamate, an LDH inhibitor. (b) The hyperpolarization elicited by the LDH inhibitor is reversed by pyruvate, but not by lactate. Lactate and pyruvate are located upstream and downstream of neuronal LDH on the astrocyte–neuron lactate shuttle, respectively. Thus, the lactate-to-pyruvate conversion via LDH in neurons is critical for this electrical regulation. (c) The summary scheme showing the neuronal inhibition by inhibiting LDH in neurons. Reproduced from Sada et al. (2015).

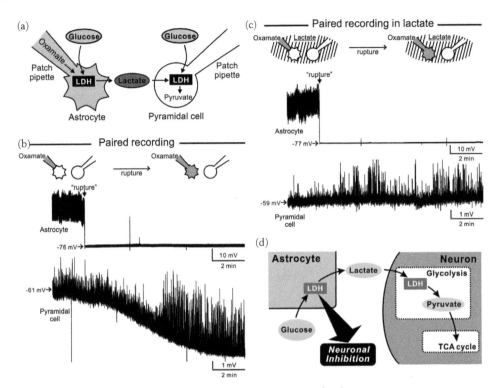

FIGURE 28.3. *Electrical Regulation by the Astrocyte–Neuron Lactate Shuttle*

(a) The experimental design of simultaneous recordings from pyramidal cells and astrocytes in the hippocampus. LDH in astrocytes is selectively inhibited by the intracellular application of oxamate via patch pipettes. (b) Pyramidal cells are hyperpolarized by LDH inhibition in astrocytes. Neurons are recorded in the whole-cell mode using normal intracellular solution, whereas astrocytes are recorded in the cell-attached mode using intracellular solution including oxamate. Oxamate is selectively applied by rupturing the patch membranes in astrocytes. (c) Pyramidal cells are not hyperpolarized by the LDH inhibition in astrocytes when lactate is present extracellularly. Thus, lactate is a mediator for this astrocyte-induced electrical regulation in neurons. (d) The summary scheme showing the neuronal inhibition by inhibiting LDH in astrocytes. Reproduced from Sada et al. (2015).

recorded astrocytes through the patch pipette (Figure 28.3a). The selective inhibition of LDH in astrocytes elicited hyperpolarization in neighboring pyramidal cells (Figure 28.3b), indicating that LDH in astrocytes regulates membrane potentials in neurons. To further confirm that the hyperpolarization was due to reductions in the release of lactate from astrocytes (see Figure 28.3a), we performed the same experiments under the extracellular perfusion of lactate. The hyperpolarization induced by oxamate in astrocytes (see Figure 28.3b) was not observed when lactate was present in the extracellular perfusate (Figure 28.3c). Thus, astrocytic LDH in the lactate shuttle also regulates membrane potential in neurons (Figure 28.3d).

These in vitro studies show that lactate release from astrocytes to neurons via LDH regulates membrane potential in neurons. We further clarified the regulation of brain lactate in vivo by

epileptic seizures, LDH inhibition, and the KD (Sada et al., 2015, 2020; see Figure 28.4). LDH enzymes consist of two subunits, LDHA and LDHB, and our biochemical analyses revealed that LDHA expression in the hippocampus was upregulated in a chronic model of temporal lobe epilepsy (Sada et al., 2020). Because LDHA is present in astrocytes but not in neurons (Bittar et al., 1996), the upregulation of LDHA led to higher lactate levels in the hippocampus of this seizure model (Sada et al., 2020; Figure 28.4a). Lactate levels in the hippocampus were lowered by inhibition of LDHA (Sada et al., 2020; Figure 28.4b), and also were lowered by ingestion of the KD (Sada et al., 2015; Figure 28.4c). Thus, the astrocyte–neuron lactate shuttle can be manipulated by inhibiting LDH in the brain.

Finally, we found that seizures in vivo were suppressed by the inhibition of LDH (Sada et al., 2015, 2020). Microinjection of kainic acid into

(a) ***Chronic Seizures***

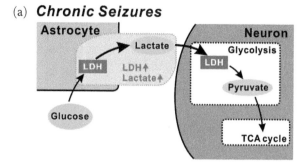

(b) ***LDHA Inhibition***

(c) ***Ketogenic Diet***

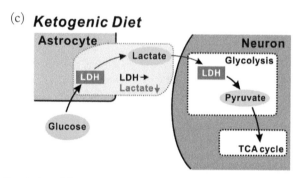

FIGURE 28.4 *In Vivo Regulation of the Astrocyte–Neuron Lactate Shuttle*

(a) The scheme showing the lactate shuttle in a chronic model of temporal lobe epilepsy. The Lactate dehydrogenase A (LDHA) expression in the hippocampus is upregulated, and then the lactate levels are elevated in the chronic seizure model (Sada et al., 2020). (b) The scheme showing the lactate shuttle during inhibition of LDHA. Since LDHA is present in astrocytes (Bitter et al., 1996), lactate levels in the hippocampus are lowered by the LDHA inhibition (Sada et al., 2020). (c) The scheme showing the lactate shuttle during treatment with the ketogenic diet. Lactate levels in the hippocampus are lowered by ingestion of the ketogenic diet (Sada et al., 2015).

the mouse hippocampus is known to produce a chronic model of temporal lobe epilepsy, which exhibits spontaneous paroxysmal discharges with abnormal morphology in the hippocampus (Gouder et al., 2003; Heinrich et al., 2006; Riban et al., 2002). The LDH inhibitor oxamate and LDHA inhibitor NHI-1 (Granchi et al., 2011) suppressed the paroxysmal discharges in the hippocampus of this chronic seizure model (Sada et al., 2015, 2020). Overall, our findings show that chronic seizures increase LDH and activate the astrocyte–neuron lactate shuttle, and conversely, inhibition of LDH weakens the

lactate shuttle and suppresses chronic seizures in vivo.

FUTURE DIRECTIONS IN DRUG DEVELOPMENT

Our recent studies (Sada et al., 2015, 2020) indicate that LDH is a metabolic target in epilepsy, and they indicate that inhibition of LDH mimics the antiepileptic effects of the KD. LDH is a metabolic enzyme in glycolysis, and it is clearly different from molecules that have been already identified in previous studies of the KD: ATP-sensitive K$^+$ channels (Ma et al., 2007; Tanner et al., 2011), voltage-dependent Ca^{2+} channels (Kadowaki et al., 2017), adenosine A_1 receptors (Masino et al., 2011), AMPA-type glutamate receptors (Chang et al., 2013, 2016), vesicular glutamate transporters (Juge et al., 2010), and BAD (Giménez-Cassina et al., 2012). Thus, LDH is a novel metabolic target in epilepsy, and it will be useful in the development of antiepileptic drugs.

The next step in drug development is to identify chemical compounds that act on LDH. Although many antiepileptic drugs are clinically used, no antiepileptic drug has been designed to act on LDH. Therefore, we explored clinically used antiepileptic drugs and found that stiripentol, a drug used for Dravet syndrome (Chiron et al., 2000), is an LDH inhibitor (Sada et al., 2015). By modifying its chemical structure, we further identified isosafrole as a smaller compound than stiripentol that could inhibit LDH and suppress seizures in vivo (Sada et al., 2015). This smaller compound will be useful as a scaffold for compound screening. Thus, new antiepileptic drugs to mimic the KD can be developed by targeting LDH with stiripentol derivatives.

In order to develop new antiepileptic drugs, it will be important to create more powerful and selective LDH inhibitors. The design and synthesis of selective inhibitors for each LDH subunit (LDHA or LDHB) will be useful for drug development. For example, LDHA-selective inhibitors will enable us to develop antiepileptic drugs targeting astrocytes. To date, LDH inhibitors have been synthesized to create antimalarial compounds (Cameron et al., 2004; Deck et al., 1998). More importantly, LDHA is known to be involved in antitumor actions based on the Warburg effect (Fantin et al., 2006; Xie et al., 2014), and many LDHA inhibitors have been synthesized as antitumor agents (Billiard et al., 2013; Chen et al., 2016; Farabegoli et al., 2012; Granchi et al., 2011; Kim et al., 2019; Le et al., 2010). Drug development for epilepsy that targets LDH, which is based on the antiepileptic mechanism of the KD, may also lead to new antitumor drugs based on the Warburg effect.

REFERENCES

Bélanger, M., Allaman, I., & Magistretti, P. J. (2011). Brain energy metabolism: Focus on astrocyte-neuron metabolic cooperation. *Cell Metabolism, 14*, 724–728.

Bialer, M., & White, H. S. (2010). Key factors in the discovery and development of new antiepileptic drugs. *Nature Reviews Drug Discovery, 9*, 68–82.

Billiard, J., Dennison, J. B., Briand, J., Annan, R. S., Chai, D., Colón, M., Dodson, C. S., Gilbert, S. A., Greshock, J., Jing, J., Lu, H., McSurdy-Freed, J. E., Orband-Miller, L. A., Mills, G. B., Quinn, C. J., Schneck, J. L., Scott, G. F., Shaw, A. N., Waitt, G. M., . . . Duffy, K. J. (2013). Quinoline 3-sulfonamides inhibit lactate dehydrogenase A and reverse aerobic glycolysis in cancer cells. *Cancer & Metabolism, 1*, 19.

Bittar, P. G., Charnay Y., Pellerin, L., Bouras, C., & Magistretti, P. J. (1996). Selective distribution of lactate dehydrogenase isoenzymes in neurons and astrocytes of human brain. *Journal of Cerebral Blood Flow & Metabolism, 16*, 1079–1089.

Boison, D. (2017). New insights into the mechanisms of the ketogenic diet. *Current Opinion in Neurology, 30*, 187–192.

Bough, K. J., & Eagles, D. A. (1999). Ketogenic diet increases the resistance to pentylenetetrazole-induced seizures in the rat. *Epilepsia, 40*, 138–143.

Bough, K. J., Valiyil, R., Han, F. T., & Eagles, D. A. (1999). Seizure resistance is dependent upon age and calorie restriction in rats fed a ketogenic diet. *Epilepsy Research, 35*, 21–28.

Bough, K. J., Wetherington, J., Hassel, B., Pare, J. F., Gawryluk, J. W., Greene, J. G., Shaw, R., Smith, Y., Geiger, J. D., & Dingledine, R. J. (2006). Mitochondrial biogenesis in the anticonvulsant mechanism of the ketogenic diet. *Annals of Neurology, 60*, 223–235.

Bouzier-Sore, A. K., Voisin, P., Bouchaud, V., Bezancon, E., Franconi, J. M., & Pellerin, L. (2006). Competition between glucose and lactate as oxidative energy substrates in both neurons and astrocytes: A comparative NMR study. *European Journal of Neuroscience, 24*, 1687–1694.

Cameron, A., Read, J., Tranter, R., Winter, V. J., Sessions, R. B., Brady, R. L., Vivas, L., Easton, A., Kendrick, H., Croft, S. L., Barros, D., Lavandera, J. L., Martin, J. J., Risco, F., García-Ochoa, S., Gamo, F. J., Sanz, L., Leon, L., Ruiz, J. R., . . . Gómez de las Heras, F. (2004). Identification and activity of a series of azole-based compounds with lactate dehydrogenase-directed anti-malarial activity. *Journal of Biological Chemistry, 279*, 31429–31439.

Chang, P., Augustin, K., Boddum, K., Williams, S., Sun, M., Terschak, J. A., Hardege, J. D., Chen, P. E., Walker, M. C., & Williams, R. S. (2016). Seizure control by decanoic acid through direct AMPA receptor inhibition. *Brain, 139*, 431–443.

Chang, P., Terbach, N., Plant, N., Chen, P. E., Walker, M. C., & Williams, R. S. (2013). Seizure control by ketogenic diet-associated medium chain fatty acids. *Neuropharmacology, 69*, 105–114.

Chen, C. Y., Feng, Y., Chen, J. Y., & Deng, H. (2016). Identification of a potent inhibitor targeting human lactate dehydrogenase A and its metabolic modulation for cancer cell line. *Bioorganic & Medicinal Chemistry Letters, 26,* 72–75.

Chiron, C., Marchand, M. C., Tran, A., Rey, E., d'Athis, P., Vincent, J., Dulac, O., & Pons, G. (2000). Stiripentol in severe myoclonic epilepsy in infancy: A randomised placebo-controlled syndrome-dedicated trial; STICLO study group. *Lancet, 356,* 1638–1642.

Chuquet, J., Quilichini, P., Nimchinsky, E.A., & Buzsáki G. (2010). Predominant enhancement of glucose uptake in astrocytes versus neurons during activation of the somatosensory cortex. *Journal of Neuroscience, 30,* 15298–15303.

D'Ambrosio, R., Wenzel, J., Schwartzkroin, P.A., McKhann, G. M., II, & Janigro, D. (1998). Functional specialization and topographic segregation of hippocampal astrocytes. *Journal of Neuroscience, 18,* 4425–4438.

Deck, L. M., Royer, R. E., Chamblee, B. B., Hernandez, V. M., Malone, R. R., Torres, J. E., Hunsaker, L. A. Piper, R. C., Makler, M. T., & Vander Jagt, D. L. (1998). Selective inhibitors of human lactate dehydrogenases and lactate dehydrogenase from the malarial parasite Plasmodium falciparum. *Journal of Medicinal Chemistry, 41,* 3879–3887.

Fantin, R. F., St-Pierre, J., & Leder, P. (2006). Attenuation of LDH-A expression uncovers a link between glycolysis, mitochondrial physiology, and tumor maintenance. *Cancer Cell, 9,* 425–434.

Farabegoli, F., Vettraino, M., Manerba, M., Fiume, L., Roberti, M., & Di Stefano, G. (2012). Galloflavin, a new lactate dehydrogenase inhibitor, induces the death of human breast cancer cells with different glycolytic attitude by affecting distinct signaling pathways. *European Journal of Pharmaceutical Sciences, 47,* 729–738.

Freeman, J. M., Vining, E. P., Pillas, D. J., Pyzik, P. L., Casey, J. C., & Kelly, L. M. (1998). The efficacy of the ketogenic diet—1998: A prospective evaluation of intervention in 150 children. *Pediatrics, 102,* 1358–1363.

Garriga-Canut, M., Schoenike, B., Qazi, R., Bergendahl, K., Daley, T. J., Pfender, R. M., Morrison, J. F., Ockuly, J., Stafstrom, C., Sutula, T., & Roopra, A. (2006). 2-Deoxy-D-glucose reduces epilepsy progression by NRSF-CtBP-dependent metabolic regulation of chromatin structure. *Nature Neuroscience, 9,* 1382–1387.

Giménez-Cassina, A., Martínez-François J. R., Fisher, J. K., Szlyk, B., Polak, K., Wiwczar, J., Tanner, G. R., Lutas, A., Yellen, G., & Danial, N. N. (2012). BAD-dependent regulation of fuel metabolism and K_{ATP} channel activity confers resistance to epileptic seizures. *Neuron, 74,* 719–730.

Gouder, N., Fritschy, J. M., & Boison, D. (2003). Seizure suppression by adenosine A_1 receptor activation in a mouse model of pharmacoresistant epilepsy. *Epilepsia, 44,* 877–885.

Granchi, C., Roy, S., Giacomelli, C., Macchia, M., Tuccinardi, T., Martinelli, A., Lanza, M., Betti, L., Giannaccini, G., Lucacchini, A., Funel, N., León L. G., Giovannetti, E., Peters, G. J., Palchaudhuri, R., Calvaresi, E. C., Hergenrother, P. J., & Minutolo, F. (2011). Discovery of N-hydroxyindole-based inhibitors of human lactate dehydrogenase isoform A (LDH-A) as starvation agents against cancer cells. *Journal of Medicinal Chemistry, 54,* 1599–1612.

Haidukewych, D., Forsythe, W. I., & Sills, M. (1982). Monitoring octanoic and decanoic acids in plasma from children with intractable epilepsy treated with medium-chain triglyceride diet. *Clinical Chemistry, 28,* 642–645.

Heinrich, C., Nitta, N., Flubacher, A., Müller, M., Fahrner, A., Kirsch, M., Freiman, T., Suzuki, F., Depaulis, A., Frotscher, M., & Haas, C. A. (2006). Reelin deficiency and displacement of mature neurons, but not neurogenesis, underlie the formation of granule cell dispersion in the epileptic hippocampus. *Journal of Neuroscience, 26,* 4701–4713.

Henneberger, C., Papouin, T., Oliet, S. H., & Rusakov, D. A. (2010). Long-term potentiation depends on release of D-serine from astrocytes. *Nature, 463,* 232–236.

Hu, Y., & Wilson, G. S. (1997). A temporary local energy pool coupled to neuronal activity: Fluctuations of extracellular lactate levels in rat brain monitored with rapid-response enzyme-based sensor. *Journal of Neurochemistry, 69,* 1484–1490.

Huttenlocher, P. R. (1976). Ketonemia and seizures: Metabolic and anticonvulsant effects of two ketogenic diets in childhood epilepsy. *Pediatric Research, 10,* 536–540.

Huttenlocher, P. R., Wilbourn, A. J., & Signore, J. M. (1971). Medium-chain triglycerides as a therapy for intractable childhood epilepsy. *Neurology, 21,* 1097–1103.

Itoh, Y., Esaki, T., Shimoji, K., Cook, M., Law, M. J., Kaufman, E., & Sokoloff, L. (2003). Dichloroacetate effects on glucose and lactate oxidation by neurons and astroglia in vitro and on glucose utilization by brain in vivo. *Proceedings of the National Academy of Sciences of the United States of America, 100,* 4879–4884.

Izumi, Y., Benz, A. M., Katsuki, H., & Zorumski, C. F. (1997). Endogenous monocarboxylates sustain hippocampal synaptic function and morphological integrity during energy deprivation. *Journal of Neuroscience, 17,* 9448–9457.

Juge, N., Gray, J. A., Omote, H., Miyaji, T., Inoue, T., Hara, C., Uneyama, H., Edwards, R. H., Nicoll, R. A., & Moriyama, Y. (2010). Metabolic control of vesicular glutamate transport and release. *Neuron, 68,* 99–112.

Kadowaki, A., Sada, N., Juge, N., Wakasa, A., Moriyama, Y., & Inoue, T. (2017). Neuronal inhibition and seizure suppression by acetoacetate and its analog, 2-phenylbutyrate. *Epilepsia, 58,* 845–857.

Kawamura, M., Jr., Ruskin, D. N., & Masino, S. A. (2010). Metabolic autocrine regulation of neurons involves cooperation among pannexin hemichannels, adenosine receptors, and K_{ATP} channels. *Journal of Neuroscience, 30,* 3886–3895.

Kim, E. Y., Chung, T. W., Han, C. W., Park, S. Y., Park, K. H., Jang, S. B., & Ha, K. T. (2019). A novel lactate dehydrogenase inhibitor, 1-(phenylseleno)-4-(trifluoromethyl) benzene, suppresses tumor growth through apoptotic cell death. *Scientific Reports, 9,* 3969.

Kwan, P., & Brodie, M. J. (2000). Early identification of refractory epilepsy. *New England Journal of Medicine, 342,* 314–319.

Lam, T.K., Gutierrez-Juarez, R., Pocai, A., & Rossetti, L. (2005). Regulation of blood glucose by hypothalamic pyruvate metabolism. *Science, 309,* 943–947.

Larrabee, M. G. (1995). Lactate metabolism and its effects on glucose metabolism in an excised neural tissue. *Journal of Neurochemistry, 64,* 1734–1741.

Le, A., Cooper, C. R., Gouw, A. M., Dinavahi, R., Maitra, A., Deck, L. M., Royer, R. E., Vander Jagt, D. L., Semenza, G. L., & Dang, C. V. (2010). Inhibition of lactate dehydrogenase A induces oxidative stress and inhibits tumor progression. *Proceedings of the National Academy of Sciences of the United States of America, 107,* 2037–3042.

Lutas, A., & Yellen, G. (2013). The ketogenic diet: Metabolic influences on brain excitability and epilepsy. *Trends in Neurosciences, 36,* 32–40.

Ma, W., Berg, J., & Yellen, G. (2007). Ketogenic diet metabolites reduce firing in central neurons by opening K_{ATP} channels. *Journal of Neuroscience, 27,* 3618–3625.

Martínez-François, J. R., Fernández-Agüera, M. C., Nathwani, N., Lahmann, C., Burnham, V. L., Danial, N. N., & Yellen, G. (2018). BAD and K_{ATP} channels regulate neuron excitability and epileptiform activity. *Elife, 7,* Article e32721.

Masino, S. A., Li, T., Theofilas, P., Sandau, U. S., Ruskin, D. N., Fredholm, B. B., Geiger, J. D., Aronica, E., & Boison, D. (2011). A ketogenic diet suppresses seizures in mice through adenosine A_1 receptors. *Journal of Clinical Investigation, 121,* 2679–2683.

Meldrum, B. S., & Rogawski, M. A. (2007). Molecular targets for antiepileptic drug development. *Neurotherapeutics, 4,* 18–61.

Neal, E. G., Chaffe, H., Schwartz, R. H., Lawson, M. S., Edwards, N., Fitzsimmons, G., Whitney, A., & Cross, J. H. (2008). The ketogenic diet for the treatment of childhood epilepsy: A randomised controlled trial. *Lancet Neurology, 7,* 500–506.

Nehlig, A., Wittendorp-Rechenmann, E., & Lam, C. D. (2004). Selective uptake of [^{14}C]2-deoxyglucose by neurons and astrocytes: High-resolution microautoradiographic imaging by cellular ^{14}C-trajectography combined with immunohistochemistry. *Journal of Cerebral Blood Flow & Metabolism, 24,* 1004–1014.

Parsons, M. P., & Hirasawa, M. (2010). ATP-sensitive potassium channel-mediated lactate effect on orexin neurons: Implications for brain energetics during arousal. *Journal of Neuroscience, 30,* 8061–8070.

Rho, J. M. (2017). How does the ketogenic diet induce anti-seizure effects? *Neuroscience Letters, 637,* 4–10.

Rho, J. M., Anderson, G. D., Donevan, S. D., & White, H. S. (2002). Acetoacetate, acetone, and dibenzylamine (a contaminant in L-(+)-β-hydroxybutyrate) exhibit direct anticonvulsant actions in vivo. *Epilepsia, 43,* 358–361.

Riban, V., Bouilleret, V., Pham-Lê, B. T., Fritschy, J. M., Marescaux, C., & Depaulis, A. (2002). Evolution of hippocampal epileptic activity during the development of hippocampal sclerosis in a mouse model of temporal lobe epilepsy. *Neuroscience, 112,* 101–111.

Rouach, N., Koulakoff, A., Abudara, V., Willecke, K., & Giaume, C. (2008). Astroglial metabolic networks sustain hippocampal synaptic transmission. *Science, 322,* 1551–1555.

Sada, N., & Inoue, T. (2018). Electrical control in neurons by the ketogenic diet. *Frontiers in Cellular Neuroscience, 12,* 208.

Sada, N., Lee, S., Katsu, T., Otsuki, T., & Inoue, T. (2015). Targeting LDH enzymes with a stiripentol analog to treat epilepsy. *Science, 347,* 1362–1367.

Sada, N., Suto, S., Suzuki, M., Usui, S., & Inoue, T. (2020). Upregulation of lactate dehydrogenase A in a chronic model of temporal lobe epilepsy. *Epilepsia, 61,* e37–e42.

Schurr, A., West, C. A., & Rigor, B. M. (1988). Lactate-supported synaptic function in the rat hippocampal slice preparation. *Science, 240,* 1326–1328.

Sills, M. A., Forsythe, W. I., & Haidukewych, D. (1986). Role of octanoic and decanoic acids in the control of seizures. *Archives of Disease in Childhood, 61,* 1173–1177.

Silver, I. A., & Erecińska, M. (1994). Extracellular glucose concentration in mammalian brain: Continuous monitoring of changes during increased neuronal activity and upon limitation in oxygen supply in normo-, hypo-, and hyperglycemic animals. *Journal of Neuroscience, 14,* 5068–5076.

Simeone, T. A., Simeone, K. A., Stafstrom, C. E., & Rho, J. M. (2018). Do ketone bodies mediate the anti-seizure effects of the ketogenic diet? *Neuropharmacology, 133,* 233–241.

Smith, D., Pernet, A., Hallett, W. A., Bingham, E., Marsden, P. K., & Amiel, S.A. (2003). Lactate: A preferred fuel for human brain metabolism in vivo. *Journal of Cerebral Blood Flow & Metabolism, 23,* 658–664.

Tanner, G. R., Lutas, A., Martínez-François, J. R., & Yellen, G. (2011). Single K_{ATP} channel opening in response to action potential firing in mouse dentate granule neurons. *Journal of Neuroscience, 31,* 8689–8696.

Wilder, R. M. (1921). The effects of ketonemia on the course of epilepsy. *Mayo Clinic Proceedings, 2,* 307–308.

Xie, H., Hanai, J., Ren, J. G., Kats, L., Burgess, K., Bhargava, P., Signoretti, S., Billiard, J., Duffy, K. J., Grant, A., Wang, X., Lorkiewicz, P. K., Schatzman, S., Bousamra, M., II, Lane, A. N., Higashi, R. M., Fan, T. W., Pandolfi, P. P., Sukhatme, V. P., & Seth, P. (2014). Targeting lactate dehydrogenase-A inhibits tumorigenesis and tumor progression in mouse models of lung cancer and impacts tumor-initiating cells. *Cell Metabolism, 19,* 795–809.

Effects of the Ketogenic Diet on the Blood–Brain Barrier

DAMIR JANIGRO, PHD

THE BLOOD–BRAIN BARRIER

The blood–brain barrier (BBB) is a selectively permeable cellular boundary that protects the mammalian brain from systemic factors (Daneman & Prat, 2015; Kaplan et al., 2020; Lochhead et al., 2020). Although the microvessel endothelial cells (ECs) have a primary role in the formation of the BBB, several other cells are equally important to maintain BBB integrity. ECs, astrocytes, pericytes, neurons, and other glial cells form a "neurovascular unit" (Figure 29.1; Abbott et al., 2006; Grant & Janigro, 2010; Kaplan et al., 2020; Kisler et al., 2020; Neuwelt et al., 2011). In addition to the layer of capillary ECs, other layers exist between blood and brain. These include a basement membrane (BM), consisting of type IV collagen, fibronectin, and laminin that cover capillaries completely, pericytes embedded in the BM, and astrocytes whose processes surround the BM (Figure 29.1). Each of these layers has potential to restrict the movement of solutes (Hawkins et al., 2006). Thus, the microenvironment of the BBB acts in concert with tight junctions to maintain the selective permeability of the neurovascular unit barrier.

Simply stated, BBB integrity is essential to the maintenance of brain homeostasis. Disruption of the BBB occurs in various conditions, such as neoplasia, trauma, epilepsy, Alzheimer's disease, infections (e.g., meningitis), and sterile inflammation (e.g., multiple sclerosis; Huber et al., 2001; Nation et al., 2019; Sweeney et al., 2018, 2019; Zlokovic, 2008). Thus, in these conditions it is highly desirable to reverse the disruption of the BBB. However, a highly restricted BBB is a huge challenge for the delivery of drugs into the diseased brain (Gloor et al., 2001). This dual nature of the BBB has been reviewed by Saunders et al. (2014).

CELLULAR ASSOCIATIONS AT THE BBB

The BBB maintains the proper ionic composition of the brain interstitial fluid, which is essential for optimal neuronal function. The BBB serves as a "transport barrier" by facilitating the uptake of necessary nutrients while at the same time preventing the uptake or actively exporting other molecules. Additionally, the BBB functions as a "metabolic barrier," possessing intracellular (e.g., cytochrome P450) and extracellular (e.g., peptidases and nucleotidases) enzymes (Abbott et al., 2010; Ghosh et al., 2011a, 2011b, 2013). The functions of the individual cells in brain microvessels are discussed in detail below.

ECs

ECs line the interior of blood vessels. The membranes of the capillary ECs are divided into two distinct sides: luminal (blood side) and abluminal (brain side; Daneman & Prat, 2015). ECs form blood vessels and mural cells sit on the abluminal side of the EC. The brain ECs are less "leaky" than those of the peripheral vessels. However, it has been shown that brain ECs become leaky when they are allowed to vascularize peripheral tissue, while peripheral ECs form tight junctions resembling the BBB when allowed to vascularize the brain parenchyma (Rubin et al., 1991). Central nervous system (CNS) microvascular ECs are 39% thinner than muscle ECs (Coomber & Stewart, 1985).

The type and amount of membrane lipids and proteins vary between luminal and abluminal sides of the blood vessel (Tewes & Galla, 2001). Thus, nutrients must transverse two sheaths of membrane; their combined characteristics determine which particles cross the barrier, and how fast. EC transporters are divided into two major categories: efflux transporters and nutrient transporters. Efflux transporters are polarized to the luminal surface and transport a broad variety of

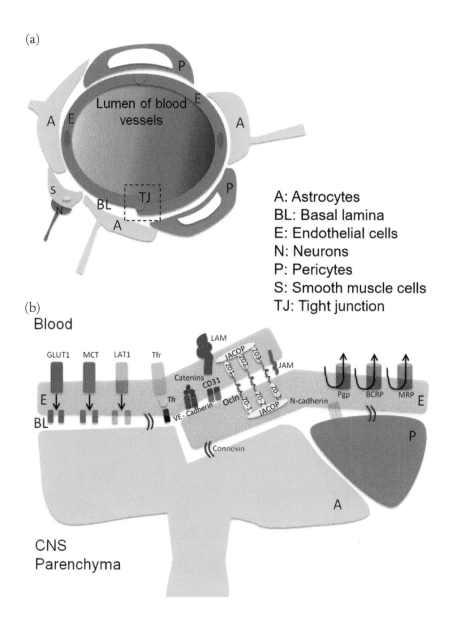

FIGURE 29.1 *Schematic of a Brain Capillary*

(a) Cell-to-cell interaction at the BBB. The endothelial cells (E) are joined together by tight junctions (TJ) and surrounded by a basal lamina (BL). Pericytes (P) reside within the BL and are distributed discontinuously along the length of cerebral capillaries. Astrocytic foot processes or end-feet from astrocytes (A) surround cerebral capillaries. Axonal projections from neurons (N) containing vasoactive neurotransmitters and peptide extend onto arteriolar smooth muscle cells (S). BBB permeability may be regulated by the molecules released from cells associated with endothelium (e.g., microglia, astrocytes). (b) Schematic representation of structural and transport components at the BBB. GLUT1, glucose transporter type 1; MCT, monocarboxylate transporter; LAT1, L-type amino acid transporter 1; Tfr, transferrin receptor; JAM, junctional adhesion molecules; LAM, leukocyte adhesion molecules; ZO-1/2/3, zonula occludin-1/2/3; JACOP, junction-associated coiled-coil protein; Ocln, occludin; CD31, cluster of differentiation 31; Pgp, P-glycoprotein; BCRP, breast cancer resistant protein; MRP, multidrug resistance-associated protein.

lipophilic molecules (Cordon-Cardo et al., 1989; Thiebaut et al., 1987). Nutrient transporters are specific for the transport of nutrients into, and the removal of waste products ou of, the CNS (Mittapalli et al., 2010). The ECs of the BBB contain high numbers of mitochondria, which are important for generating a large amount of adenosine triphosphate (ATP) to maintain ion gradients critical for the function of transporters. In addition, CNS ECs express low levels of leukocyte adhesion molecules, which ultimately limits the number of immune cells that can enter the CNS (Daneman et al., 2010). Furthermore, these ECs are thought to have distinctive metabolism; this generates a barrier by altering the physical properties of molecules, which then can modulate their solubility, reactivity, and transport properties. These metabolic properties are regulated by luminal flow and the resulting shear stress (Cucullo et al., 2011; Desai et al., 2002). The combination of a physical barrier (e.g., tight junctions and low transcytosis), a molecular barrier (e.g., low leukocyte adhesion molecules, efflux transporters, and specific metabolism), and presence of specific nutrient transporters (e.g., GLUT1; McAllister et al., 2001) allows CNS ECs to firmly regulate CNS homeostasis (Daneman & Prat, 2015; Ghosh et al., 2010). The specific nutrient transporters are probably topographically organized for the development or function of specific brain regions or particular subclasses of neurons. A major unanswered question regarding the BBB and ECs is whether they possess unique properties in different brain regions.

The following features distinguish BBB ECs from those in peripheral vasculature (Arcangeli et al., 1999; Dalvi et al., 2014; Gloor et al., 2001; Hawkins & Davis, 2005; Rubin et al., 1991):

i. Presence of a large number of tight junctions to limit the paracellular movement of macromolecules (Figures 29.1 and 29.2).

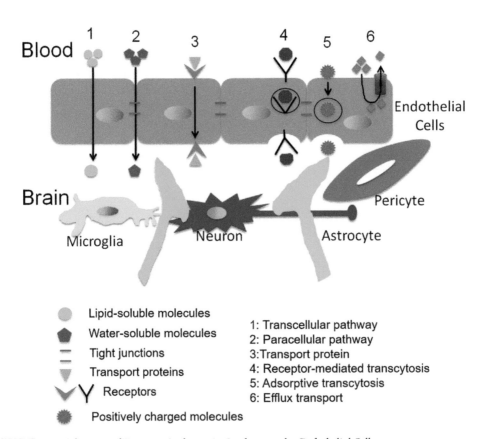

FIGURE 29.2 *Schematic of Transport Pathways in Cerebrovascular Endothelial Cells*

The transport of diverse molecules from the circulation across the BBB may include (1) the transcellular lipophilic pathway, (2) the paracellular aqueous pathway across tight junctions, (3) transport proteins, (4) receptor-mediated transcytosis, (5) adsorptive transcytosis, and (6) efflux transporters.

ii. Controlled fluid-phase endocytosis rate to limit transcellular passage of macromolecules.
iii. Presence of highly specific transporters and carrier molecules.
iv. Absence of fenestrations.
v. Few cytoplasmic vesicles.
vi. Increased mitochondrial content.

Astrocytes

Astrocytes are important glial cells that help in conditioning and developing the brain microvessel ECs. Interactions of ECs and astrocytes are known to regulate the phenotype of the BBB under (patho)physiologic conditions (Prat et al., 2001). Astrocytes are known to alter the properties of endothelial cells in multiple ways (Grant et al., 1998; Haseloff et al., 2005; Janzer & Raff, 1987; Lee et al., 2007; Stanness et al., 1996, 1997), such as:

i. Tightening the BBB, as evidenced by the decreased paracellular permeability of sucrose.
ii. Elevating trans-endothelial electrical resistance.
iii. Increasing the activity of barrier-related marker enzymes, such as alkaline phosphatase and γ-glutamyltranspeptidase.
iv. Enhancing the number, length, and complexity of tight junctions.
v. Increasing the expression of glucose transporters.
vi. Secreting angiogenic factors like vascular endothelial growth factor (VEGF), which is essential for the formation and remodeling of embryonic blood vessels and decreasing vascular stability in adult blood vessels.

Angiotensin-converting enzyme I produced by astrocytes converts angiotensin I into angiotensin II, which in turn acts on type 1 angiotensin receptors expressed by brain ECs. Angiotensin II promotes the recruitment of junctional proteins into the lipid raft, restricting BBB permeability (Wosik et al., 2007). Furthermore, retinoic acid (RA) secreted by radial glial cells acts on RA receptor β expressed in the developing vasculature, which increases trans-endothelial electrical resistance by enhancing the expression of vascular endothelial cadherin, P-glycoprotein, and zonula occludin-1 (Figure 29.1; Mizee et al., 2013). Other factors, such as transforming growth factor β, glial cell-derived neurotrophic factor, and

src-suppressed C-kinase substrate, are postulated to play a role in maintaining tightness of the BBB (Haseloff et al., 2005).

Pericytes

Pericytes, the mural cells of blood microvessels, are specialized cells of mesenchymal lineage that surround the surface of the vascular tube. They are on the abluminal side of the microvascular endothelial tube and are embedded on the vascular BM (Abbott et al., 2010; Kisler et al., 2020; Sweeney et al., 2018, 2019). The CNS microvasculature has a higher pericyte:endothelial ratio (1:3 to 1:1) than muscle (1:100; Shepro & Morel, 1993). Major functions of pericytes in the BBB include (Armulik et al., 2011; Hall et al., 2014; Kisler et al., 2020; Lai & Kuo, 2005; Sweeney et al., 2018, 2019):

i. Formation and maintenance of tight junctions.
ii. Autoregulation of cerebrovascular blood flow.
iii. Secretion of angiopoietin 1 and brain angiogenesis.
iv. Initiation of extrinsic blood coagulation pathway after cerebrovascular injury.
v. Regulation of inflammation by the secretion of cytokines (e.g., IL-1β and IL-6), leukocyte transmigration, antigen presentation, and T-cell activation.
vi. Contraction of capillary diameter by contractile proteins in pericytes.

A lack of a pericyte-specific markers, however, often leads to misidentification of pericytes as other cells occupying the perivascular space.

All blood vessels, including those of the brain, are ensheathed by the extracellular BMs. The inner vascular BM and outer parenchymal BM are two BMs that surround the vascular tube (Daneman & Prat, 2015; Sorokin, 2010). The BM is an extracellular matrix secreted specially by ECs and pericytes in vascular BM, and by astrocytic processes in parenchymal BM. Type IV collagens, nidogen, heparan sulfate proteoglycans, and laminin are some molecules present in BMs. These membranes anchor many signaling processes and provide an additional barrier that molecules and cells must cross prior to accessing neural tissue. The degradation of BMs by matrix metalloproteinases is observed in different neurologic diseases, allowing the infiltration of leukocytes (Daneman & Prat, 2015; Sorokin, 2010).

MOLECULES AT THE BBB

Tight Junctions

The tight junction (TJ) consists of membrane and cytoplasmic proteins (Figure 29.1). Identification of molecules expressed by CNS ECs led to an understanding of the structural and transport components of the BBB (Ohtsuki et al., 2014). Claudins, occludin, and junctional adhesion molecules (JAM) are the integral membrane proteins. Cingulin, zonula occludin proteins (ZO-1, 2, and 3), AF6, 7H6 antigen, and symplekin are the cytoplasmic accessory proteins that form plaque and function as adaptor proteins. The TJ complexes are dynamic entities that can "bend without breaking," thereby sustaining structural integrity (Huber et al., 2001).

Claudins are the largest family of transmembrane phosphoproteins; so far, 24 members of the family (claudins 1–24) have been characterized (Ballabh et al., 2004). Among these, claudins 1, 3, 5, and 12 have a role in TJ formation at the BBB. Claudin 1 is an integral component of TJs, and its absence is associated with several pathologic conditions, such as stroke, inflammatory diseases, and tumors (Liebner et al., 2000).

Occludin is another transmembrane phosphoprotein, and its subcellular localization parallels that of claudin. In adult brain microvessel ECs, occludin expression is higher than in the peripheral ECs that interact with claudins. Jointly, they form channels to regulate the paracellular flow of ions and other hydrophilic molecules (Hirase et al., 1997; Huber et al., 2001; Morita et al., 1999).

JAMs are members of the immunoglobulin superfamily that form homotypic interactions at the endothelial and epithelial cells' TJ, which are known to regulate leukocyte extravasation and paracellular permeability (Aurrand-Lions et al., 2001).

Several cytoplasmic proteins are also essential components of the TJs. Actin is the cytoskeletal protein that plays a major role in maintenance of the TJ. Actin-degrading molecules (e.g., cytochalasin-D and phalloidin) can disrupt the actin cytoskeleton, compromising the TJ (Huber et al., 2001). Zonula occludin proteins (ZO-1, 2, and 3) are also important. These proteins make direct contact with claudins, occludins, and JAMs on one side and the actin cytoskeleton on the other (Ballabh et al., 2004). Cingulin is another protein that links the TJ accessory proteins with the cytoskeleton (Huber et al., 2001). Several intracellular processes involving calcium signaling, phosphorylation, G-proteins, proteases, and inflammatory cytokine secretion can modulate TJ proteins (Huber et al., 2001; Kniesel & Wolburg, 2000).

Leukocyte Adhesion Molecules

The CNS of healthy individuals has an extremely low immune surveillance, lacking neutrophils and lymphocytes in the parenchyma (Galea et al., 2007). Entry of leukocytes into the brain parenchyma requires multiple steps, including rolling adhesion, firm adhesion, and extravasation. This requires several leukocyte adhesion molecules (LAMs) that include selectins (E-, P-selectin) for rolling adhesion and immunoglobulin family members for firm adhesion (Huang et al., 2006). In a normal brain, the expression of these adhesion molecules is much lower in CNS ECs than peripheral ECs. However, LAMs are elevated in neuroinflammatory conditions like stroke and multiple sclerosis (Daneman et al., 2010; Huang et al., 2006).

Transporters

The paracellular junctions that have low permeability control the transport of molecules and ions between the blood and brain. ECs of the CNS are highly polarized and have distinct luminal and abluminal compartments. As mentioned, there are two major transporter types that are expressed in CNS ECs: efflux transporters and nutrient transporters (Figures 29.1 to 29.4).

Efflux transporters (e.g., multidrug resistance protein 1, MDR1; breast cancer resistance protein, BCRP; multidrug resistance proteins, MRPs) hydrolyze ATP to transport substrates against their concentration gradient (Ha et al., 2007). Many efflux transporters are localized on the luminal surface in order to transport substrates into the blood compartment. These transporters facilitate the movement of a diverse range of substrates and provide a barrier to many small lipophilic molecules, which would otherwise passively diffuse through the membrane of ECs. MDR1, also called P-gp, is a well-studied transporter that is associated with drug-resistant epilepsy (Dombrowski et al., 2001; Marchi et al., 2004) and tumors (Abbott et al., 2001). Endogenous substrates of efflux transporters are still not well studied.

Nutrient transporters facilitate the movement of nutrients according to their concentration gradients. A wide variety of such transporters are expressed in CNS ECs to deliver specific nutrients into the brain parenchyma. Most of these

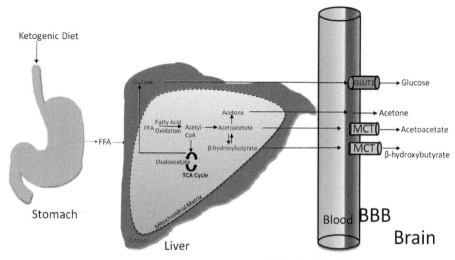

FIGURE 29.3 *Ketogenic Diet Metabolism and Brain Uptake*

The ketogenic diet is deficient in carbohydrates but provides large amount of long-chain free fatty acids (FFA). The acetyl-CoA produced by fatty acid oxidation goes into the Krebs/tricarboxylic acid (TCA) cycle or is converted to the ketone body (KB) acetoacetate (AcAc), which spontaneously degrades to acetone (Ac). AcAc is further converted to β-hydroxybutyrate (βHB) in a reversible reaction. The KBs represent alternative energy substrates for the brain. GLUT1, glucose transporter type 1; MCT, monocarboxylate transporter.

nutrient transporters are in the solute carrier class of facilitated transporters (SLC2A1 transports glucose, SLC16A1 transports lactate and pyruvate, SLC7A1 transports cationic amino acids, and SLC7A5 transports neural amino acids and L-DOPA; Zlokovic, 2008). SLC2A1, also called glucose transporter type 1 (GLUT1), is a well-studied nutrient transporter that provides glucose to the CNS (Figure 29.4). It is more frequently expressed by brain ECs than by non-brain ECs (Cornford et al., 1994). In humans, GLUT1 deficiency leads to an epileptic syndrome that can be treated with a high-ketone diet (De Vivo et al., 1991, 2002). Most of the transporters provide nutrients to the brain; however, some receptors assist in transporting waste from brain to blood (e.g., receptor for advanced glycation end products to transport amyloid β; Daneman & Prat, 2015).

Other Components

The rate of transcytosis is lower in brain ECs; however, it is upregulated upon BBB dysfunction during brain injury and disease. In ECs, transcytosis is mediated via caveolin-based vesicle trafficking (Figure 29.2; Gu et al., 2012). Additionally, the plasmalemmal vesicle-associated protein number is lower in the ECs of a healthy BBB than the ECs of a BBB after traumatic brain injury (TBI; Shue et al., 2008). The significance of these changes in the context of disease etiology is unknown.

FUNCTIONS OF THE BBB

Regulation of Ion Concentration

The BBB provides a suitable environment for neural functions because it regulates ionic composition in the brain. The combination of ion-specific channels and transporters at the BBB regulates the composition and quantity of ions in the CNS. The concentration of potassium in mammalian brain cerebrospinal fluid (CSF) and interstitial fluid (ISF) is maintained at around 2.5 to 2.9 mM, although it is approximately 4.5 mM in plasma. Even though the plasma K+ concentration changes following exercise or meal, it remains within the 2.5- to 2.9-mM range in the brain (see Janigro, 1999, 2012). In addition, Ca^+, Mg^{2+}, and pH are actively regulated in the BBB (Abbott et al., 2010; Jeong et al., 2006; Nischwitz et al., 2008; Somjen, 2004).

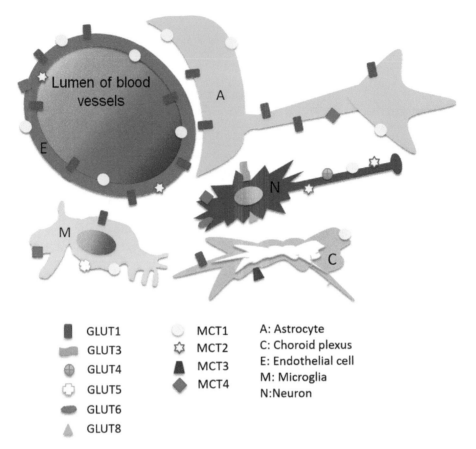

FIGURE 29.4 *Glucose and Monocarboxylate Transporters in the Brain*

Multiple types of glucose transporters (GLUTs) and monocarboxylate transporters (MCTs) are responsible for transporting glucose and monocarboxylic acids (ketone bodies, lactate, and pyruvate), respectively.

Entry of Macromolecules

The BBB acts as a shield to prevent the entry of most macromolecules into the brain. The total protein content in plasma is much higher than in the CSF, and the individual protein composition is distinctly different (Abbott et al., 2010). Proteins that are markedly high in plasma (e.g., albumin, prothrombin, and plasminogen) are detrimental to nervous tissue, since they can trigger cell apoptosis (Gingrich & Traynelis, 2000). Factor Xa and tissue plasminogen activator are widely expressed in the CNS and can convert prothrombin and plasminogen to thrombin and plasmin, respectively. If present, thrombin and plasmin can initiate cascades that result in seizures, glial activation, glial cell division, and cell death (Abbott et al., 2010). Hence, the ingress of these macromolecules upon BBB disruption can have serious pathologic consequences.

Regulation of Neurotransmitters

After meals, blood levels of a neuroexcitatory amino acid, glutamate, are elevated. If glutamate is freely transported into the brain ISF, it can be detrimental. For example, in a patient with an ischemic stroke, uncontrolled glutamate release into the brain can cause permanent neuroexcitatory damage of neural tissue. The peripheral and central nervous systems share many of the same neurotransmitters; the BBB, however, keeps them separate and minimizes the crosstalk (Abbott et al., 2006, 2010; Bernacki et al., 2008).

Elimination of Neurotoxins

The BBB is a protective barricade that shields the brain from neurotoxic substances circulating in the blood (e.g., endogenous metabolites or proteins, and xenobiotics ingested in food or acquired from the environment). ECs in the CNS express several energy-dependent efflux transporters (Figures 29.2 and 29.3) that actively extrude neurotoxins out of the brain (Abbott et al., 2010). These transporters also prevent neuronal cell death when neurons are exposed to toxins (Marchi et al., 2004).

Transport of Nutrients to the Brain

Most of the essential water-soluble nutrients and metabolites required for neuronal survival and differentiation are transported into the brain by specific transport systems (Figures 29.2 to 29.4) at the BBB. The endothelium begins to differentiate into a barrier layer from the embryonic angiogenesis stage and is maintained in adults by its association with other cell types, especially the endfeet of astroglial cells. Astrocytic glial cells promote the upregulation of TJ proteins and the differential expression of luminal and abluminal membrane-specific transporters (Abbott et al., 2006; Wolburg et al., 2009). Other cell types, namely pericytes, microglia, and nerve terminals, play supporting roles in barrier induction, maintenance, and function (Abbott et al., 2006; Nakagawa et al., 2009; Shimizu et al., 2008).

Together with oxygen, glucose is the obligatory nutrient for the human brain. The BBB regulates the transport of glucose in the CNS and prevents equalization of plasma levels (~ 5 mM) to the CSF and ISF levels (< 2.5 mM; McAllister et al., 2001). The glucose is used for ATP production, which is primarily used for ion transport and the maintenance of the ion gradient (Magistretti & Pellerin, 1995). However, a small fraction of glucose ATP is also used for biosynthetic processes. The diffusion of glucose across the BBB is facilitated by GLUT1. In the brain, GLUT1 interacts with other GLUT1 isoforms that mediate glucose transport into neurons and astrocytes (Figure 29.4; Klepper, 2008).

Brain glucose levels in a healthy and normally active person are kept adequate by a complex regulatory mechanism to ensure an appropriate supply to neurons, in spite of massive drops in plasma levels. Glucose is controlled by intracellular enzymes (e.g., hexokinase) and GLUT1 proteins that are expressed asymmetrically in the ECs (lower concentration in abluminal membrane than in luminal membrane; McAllister et al., 2001). Thus, glucose levels in the brain parenchyma and CSF ultimately depend on the "barrier" nature of the brain endothelium.

Under normal conditions, asymmetrically distributed GLUT1 in the BBB transports blood glucose into the brain, in which barrier integrity is maintained by TJs, preventing potassium leakage in the brain (Figure 29.5). However, under pathologic conditions, GLUT1 expression is altered (Cornford et al., 1998a, 1998c). Cerebral blood flow also fails to meet the brain metabolic demand when the BBB is damaged (Bruehl et al., 1998), and in such cases, potassium leaks across the open TJs in the brain (Cornford et al., 1998a, 1998b, 1998c). The elevated extracellular [K+] further increases the metabolic demand leading to exaggerated neuronal firing and further loss of homeostasis.

However, increased plasma ketone levels produced in starvation, exercise, or the ketogenic diet provide an alternative energy source to fulfill the energy demand in BBB-damaged conditions (Figures 29.3 and 29.5). In addition, KBs directly enhance GLUT1 activity (Janigro, 1999).

KETOGENIC DIET

The ketogenic diet (KD) is a strict high-fat, low-carbohydrate, and low-protein diet. On the KD, the body receives a minimal dietary source of glucose, which is required for all metabolic needs (Freeman et al., 2006). Fatty acids become an obligatory source of cellular energy production; however, they do not readily cross the BBB due to the presence of TJs (Mitchell et al., 2009). Whether their transport into the brain is by diffusion or via specific protein-mediated transport is still debated and controversial (Abumrad et al., 1998; Hamilton, 1998). The KD is characterized by elevated serum levels of circulating KBs: acetoacetate (AcAc), β-hydroxybutyrate (βHB), and acetone (Ac), which are mainly produced by the liver. The plasma concentration of KBs increases to 3 to 4 times basal levels (AcAc: 100 μmol/L, βHB: 200 μmol/L; Musa-Veloso et al., 2002). KBs are utilized by extrahepatic tissues as an energy source, but Ac is not an energy source and is exhaled or excreted as a waste. In the absence of glucose, KBs are the preferred source of brain energy. They are transported into the brain by simple diffusion (Ac) or facilitated diffusion (AcAc and βHB) mediated by monocarboxylate transporters (MCTs; Figures 29.3 to 29.5; Cremer, 1982; Klepper, 2008). The MCTs are expressed in the plasma membrane of choroid plexus and BBB cells (endothelial and epithelial), glia, and neurons, which ultimately oxidize ketones in the mitochondrial matrix, releasing acetyl-CoA that enters into the tricarboxylic acid (TCA) or Krebs cycle (Morris, 2005; Figures 29.3 and 29.4).

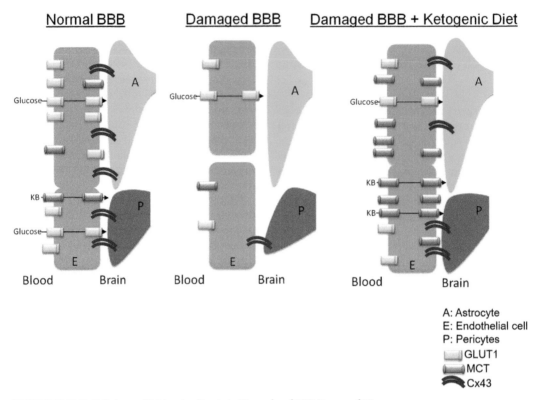

FIGURE 29.5 *Cellular and Molecular Events in Normal and BBB Damaged Tissue*

The ketogenic diet potentially has a role in re-establishing physiologic metabolic supply and repairing damaged BBB by inducing the expression levels of monocarboxylate transporter (MCT) and connexin 43 (Cx43) and enhancing glucose transporter type 1 (GLUT1) activity.

Once KBs cross the BBB, brain cells take up KBs via diffusion or a carrier-mediated process to support cellular energy requirements. Although neurons and glial cells express MCTs, since KBs must transverse the BBB first, the role of MCTs appears to be more significant at the BBB.

Regulation of Cerebral Ketone Uptake

In the absence of glucose, monocarboxylic acids (e.g., ketones, lactate, and pyruvate) generate a substantial amount of energy for the brain (Pierre & Pellerin, 2005). Prolonged fasting elevates normal circulating KB concentrations from ~ 5.8 mM/L to 9 mM/L (White & Venkatesh, 2011). The plasma concentration of KBs is a major factor regulating the rate of cerebral uptake. Since KBs are hydrophilic compounds in the blood, specific transporters are required to facilitate KB diffusion across the BBB and to maintain proper levels of these metabolic products in the brain (Pierre & Pellerin, 2005). Monocarboxylic acid transporters (e.g., MCT1 and MCT2) involved in transporting monocarboxylic acids (e.g., lactic acid

and pyruvate) are thought to facilitate the transport of KBs. MCT1 was the first monocarboxylic acid transporter identified in brain ECs (Leino et al., 1999; Pierre et al., 2000). Additionally, small amounts of MCT1 are found in astrocytic endfeet surrounding the capillaries. Interestingly, MCT2 is found only in BBB ECs and neurons, but not in astrocytes (Pierre et al., 2000). On the other hand, MCT4 is present exclusively in the astrocytes and glial cells (Pierre et al., 2000). Glucose and MCTs expressed in the major brain cells are summarized in Figure 29.4. The distribution of MCTs is associated with distinct functional characteristics. Brain MCT1 and MCT4 facilitate the release of monocarboxylates into the extracellular space and allow cells to maintain a high glycolytic rate (Pierre & Pellerin, 2005). The monocarboxylates produced and released by astrocytes in the extracellular space are an energy substrate for active neurons; monocarboxylates are taken up by MCT2 expressed in the dendrites and axons of neurons (Pierre & Pellerin, 2005; Takimoto & Hamada, 2014).

At a given arterial concentration, AcAc uptake is double that of βHB; however, it is not yet understood how the expression of MCT is regulated (White & Venkatesh, 2011). Prolonged fasting increases BBB uptake of KBs by increasing the expression of MCT1 as high as eightfold in mice (Leino et al., 2001). Similarly, another report in human subjects showed a 13-fold increase in cerebral βHB uptake following several days of fasting (Hasselbalch et al., 1994). Interestingly, a rapid increase in plasma ketone levels, following an intravenous infusion of βHB, does not induce cerebral uptake as significantly as prolonged fasting; this suggests that MCT upregulation is partially dependent upon the length of exposure to increased plasma KBs (Pan et al., 2000, 2001). Thus, a prolonged high-fat diet increases blood ketone concentrations, leading to an elevated expression of MCT and cerebral uptake of KBs (Figure 29.5).

Anti-inflammatory Effects of KBs

Neuroinflammation is defined as inflammation of the CNS that occurs upon invasion of pathogens, with trauma, and/or in neurodegeneration. Cells like macrophages, astrocytes, and oligodendrocytes and molecules like cytokines, complement, and pattern-recognition components are the known contributors to neuroinflammation (de Vries et al., 2012; Glass et al., 2010; Marchi et al., 2014). Pro-inflammatory molecules are either generated locally within the CNS or transported from the peripheral system upon BBB disruption (Limatola & Ransohoff, 2014; Ransohoff & Brown, 2012). Moreover, inflammatory mediators have been shown to influence TJs and to activate astrocytes and microglia (David et al., 2009; Ivens et al., 2007; Tomkins et al., 2008), ultimately compromising BBB integrity. An optimal amount of neuroinflammation is considered neuroprotective, and it generally occurs for a short period of time. Chronic neuroinflammation is often detrimental, inducing further cell and tissue damage. However, the opposing mechanisms of the ostensibly paradoxical exacerbation or amelioration of parenchymal brain injury are largely unknown (Cederberg & Siesj, 2010; Finnie, 2013).

The therapeutic efficacy of large-spectrum anti-neuroinflammatory drugs is limited by their side effects after even transient immunosuppression. Studies suggest that, in contrast to these drugs, the KD could be useful, particularly in patients with recent worsening of epilepsy and inflammation (Janigro, 1999; Marchi et al., 2012; Nabbout et al., 2011). The KD has been used as an effective treatment in patients with inflammation-induced epileptic encephalopathies (e.g., fever-induced refractory epileptic encephalopathy in school-age children; Nabbout et al., 2011). Additionally, polysaturated fatty acids, mostly eicosapentaenoic acid and docosahexaenoic acid, are thought to have anti-inflammatory actions, mediated typically by their hydroxylated metabolites (Grimble, 1998; Porta et al., 2009). Furthermore, KD attenuated thermal nociception and decreased peripheral edema, indicating an anti-inflammatory effect (Ruskin et al., 2009).

A systemic review published by Gibson et al., which analyzed 16 independent reports containing a total of 733 rodent studies, demonstrated a significant protective (both pathologic and functional) effect of KD or exogenous administration of KBs ($p < 0.001$) on outcomes of cerebral ischemia. Moreover, regardless of dietary intervention or administration-induced ketogenic state, ketones were found to have beneficial/anti-inflammatory effects on functional/behavioral tests, lesion volume, and brain water content (Gibson et al., 2012).

In TBI models, concussion (or mild TBI) models, and spinal cord injury, KD intervention (pretreatment or administration to postinjury animals) was associated with improved structural and functional outcomes (Prins, 2008; Prins & Matsumoto, 2014). Within minutes after injury, the ionic equilibrium across the neuronal membrane is disrupted, which requires cellular energy to re-establish homeostasis. Thus, the cerebral glucose uptake is increased in both rodents and humans within 30 min after fluid percussion and within 8 days after TBI, respectively (Bergsneider et al., 1997). However, this transient "hyperglycolysis" is followed by a prolonged period of reduction in glucose metabolism. Hence, utilizing brain ketone metabolism after TBI as a therapeutic approach is appealing because it can bypass the early glucose metabolic derangements and offers multiple consequences that are beneficial to the brain (Prins & Matsumoto, 2014). Ketone metabolism is particularly advantageous to TBI patients because it decreases the production of free radicals in mitochondria and cytosol (Sullivan et al., 2004; Ziegler et al., 2003). In addition, animals on the KD produced less Bcl-2-associated protein, ultimately decreasing cellular apoptosis and brain swelling. Furthermore, KD-induced decrease in mitochondrial release of cytochrome c into the cytosol inhibits the stimulation of the apoptotic signaling cascade (Hu et al., 2009a, 2009b).

It has also been shown that the KD can modulate lipopolysaccharide-induced fever by decreasing peripheral inflammation and CNS IL-1β expression (Dupuis et al., 2015). These properties potentially contribute to the beneficial effect of the KD in neuroinflammatory conditions (e.g., epilepsy, Alzheimer's disease, Parkinson's disease, multiple sclerosis) and/or brain trauma.

The NOD-like receptor P3 (NLRP3) inflammasome is a multiprotein complex of the innate immune system that is primarily responsible for IL-1β-derived autoinflammatory disorders, such as gout, obesity, atherosclerosis, and neurodegenerative diseases (Levy et al., 2015). βHB, but not the structurally similar AcAc or butyrate, was shown to limit cytokine production by inhibiting the activation of the NLRP3 inflammasome in human monocytes in vitro (Yasui et al., 2011). Since NLRP3 is a common factor in sterile neuroinflammation, the identification of βHB as an NLRP3 inhibitor provides a rationale for further investigating the effectiveness of KD treatment for neuroinflammatory diseases.

Neuroprotective Effects of KBs

Ketones, an alternative energy source for normal or injured brain, may also have neuroprotective effects (Prins, 2008). Ketones are considered neuroprotective because:

i. βHB is a more efficient energy source than glucose. It can also stimulate mitochondrial biogenesis by upregulating mitochondrial enzymes and genes that stimulate energy metabolism (Veech et al., 2001).

ii. KBs protect cells against glutamate-mediated apoptosis and necrosis by attenuating the formation of reactive oxygen species (Ziegler et al., 2003). They also attenuate apoptosis by reducing the activation of caspase-3 (Gasior et al., 2006).

iii. KBs enhance the conversion of glutamate to γ-aminobutyric acid (GABA) and boost GABA-mediated inhibition by interneurons (Gasior et al., 2006).

iv. Cerebral blood flow elevation by ketone metabolism is often considered neuroprotective (Hasselbalch et al., 1996).

Although studies have demonstrated beneficial neuroprotective effects of the KD, further research is necessary to clarify issues like dosing, timing, and the route and duration of KD administration.

Effects of KBs on the BBB

Data on the effects of the KD and/or KBs on the BBB are based largely on animal studies. There is evidence of rapid changes in cerebral blood flow and cellular transporters (decreased GLUT1 expression) that favor KBs' uptake and metabolism in several neurologic conditions, such as TBI, hemorrhagic shock, ischemia, and hypoxia (Gasior et al., 2006; Gibson et al., 2012; Prins & Matsumoto, 2014; White & Venkatesh, 2011). It has also been hypothesized that children with attention-deficit/hyperactivity disorder (ADHD) display a hyperactive behavior in order to raise skeletal muscle lactate production, MCT1 expression, and flux over the BBB to supply the brain with lactate. This may compensate for the reduced transport of lactate by astrocytes (Medin et al., 2019).

Mechanisms indirectly associated with BBB function have also been revealed. Since KBs are neuroprotective in neurologic disorders like epilepsy, a study examined the acute effects of ketone infusion on human brain (Svart et al., 2018). During 3-hydroxybutyrate infusions, concentrations increased and cerebral glucose utilization decreased, oxygen consumption remained unchanged, and cerebral blood flow increased dramatically. Thus, it appears that acute 3-hydroxybutyrate infusion reduces cerebral glucose uptake and increases cerebral blood flow in all measured brain regions, without detectable effects on cerebral oxygen uptake, although oxygen extraction decreased. Increased oxygen supply concomitant with unchanged oxygen utilization may therefore contribute to the neuroprotective effects of KBs. In addition, the KD has been suggested as a therapy in Alzheimer's disease (Neth et al., 2020). The authors compared the effects of a modified Mediterranean-ketogenic diet (MMKD) and an American Heart Association Diet (AHAD) on CSF levels of Alzheimer's biomarkers, neuroimaging measures, peripheral metabolism, and cognition in older adults at risk for Alzheimer's. MMKD was associated with increased CSF Ab42 and decreased tau. After the MMKD, there was increased cerebral perfusion and increased cerebral KB uptake (^{11}C-acetoacetate PET, in subsample). Memory performance improved after both diets, but the improvement may have been due to practice effects. The results suggest that a ketogenic intervention targeted toward adults at risk for Alzheimer's may prove beneficial in the prevention of cognitive decline. Since the BBB is an etiologic factor in Alzheimer's disease (Nation et al., 2019), it is possible that improved BBB function may be responsible for the observed effects. In agreement with a BBB mechanism's underlying ketogenic effects in dementias is recent in vitro evidence that KBs promote amyloid-β clearance from the brain to blood (Versele et al., 2020).

Along the same lines, it has been hypothesized that KBs can be used as an alternative energy source by neurons with impaired glucose utilization. The ketogen caprylidene has been shown to improve cognition in patients with mild to moderate Alzheimer's disease who lacked an AD-predisposing allele (ε4) of the gene for apolipoprotein E. In a pilot study, Torosyan et al. examined the effects of caprylidene on regional cerebral blood flow (rCBF) in patients with mild to moderate Alzheimer's disease. Daily ingestion of caprylidene over 45 days was associated with increased blood flow in specific brain regions in patients lacking an apolipoprotein ε4 allele, a finding further supporting the hypothesis that ketones induce improvement of neurovascular function in Alzheimer's disease.

Prins et al. demonstrated an increase in expression of MCT (MCT1 and MCT2) levels and ketone transport after TBI in rats (Prins & Giza, 2006). Additionally, the ketone-metabolizing enzyme β-hydroxybutyrate dehydrogenase is elevated after cerebral injury, and it converts βHB to AcAc, which is scarce in adult brain (Tieu et al., 2003). This evidence suggests the brain's improved ability to utilize exogenous KBs. Thus, taking advantage of improved transport and cellular metabolism of ketones, the injured brain may shift its source of energy from glucose to KBs. This is particularly beneficial because hyperglycemia is deleterious to the injured brain (Salim et al., 2009).

Astrocyte endfeet lacking the gap junction protein connexin 43 (Cx43) are inefficient in transmembrane receptor anchoring. This weakens the BBB, which is further weakened by increased hydrostatic vascular pressure and shear stress (Ezan et al., 2012). Interestingly, higher concentrations of KBs, either alone or in combination, significantly upregulated the expression of Cx43 at both the mRNA and protein levels (Ho et al., 2013; Figure 29.5). Further, the upregulation of Cx43 protein in ECs and glial cells by KBs accelerated cell migration (Bates et al., 2007).

In a separate report, βHB (0.5 mM/L) has been shown to promote human EC proliferation (Cheng et al., 2006). This suggests that the KD plays a role in repairing damaged BBB and restoring normal brain function. In contrast, Freeman et al. demonstrated AcAc-induced inhibition of EC proliferation by elevation of oxidative stress (Freeman et al., 1998, 2006). Hence, the response of cell types to different KBs may vary depending on cell-specific characteristics.

In severely uncontrolled diabetes, KBs are produced in massive quantities, a condition that is described as ketoacidosis; this causes high concentrations of protons and overwhelms the buffering system of the body by activating a pH-sensitive sodium-proton pump (Bohn & Daneman, 2002). In contrast, during high-fat/low-carbohydrate intake, KBs are produced in a regulated manner, causing a harmless physiologic state called dietary ketosis. There are minimal data on the adverse effects of the KD on the BBB. Depending on concentrations, acute administration of KBs alters the pH, sodium level, lipids, and glucose in the blood. The acute intravenous infusion of βHB also significantly increases the pH and sodium concentrations in the brain (Hiraide et al., 1991). Thus, hypoglycemia and dehydration are two predicted side effects of continuous ketone consumption. The long-term consequences of reduction in glucose cerebral metabolism are thought to increase cerebral blood flow, increase expression levels of MCT, and enhance KB uptake and metabolism on the BBB; however, details are not yet known. In contrast, a report showed that the prolonged intake of the KD can significantly raise mean blood cholesterol levels, leading to lipid deposition in blood vessels (Freeman et al., 1998).

CONCLUDING REMARKS

It has long been recognized that the increased concentration of KBs associated with the KD is an efficient fuel supply for the brain. Dramatic effects of such high-fat dietary treatment were shown in patients with multiple neurologic disorders and GLUT1 deficiency syndrome. Studies suggest that the KD has the potential to re-establish physiologic metabolic supply by activating glucose transporters, enhancing the expression of ketone transporters, and repairing damaged BBB by inducing the expression of gap junction proteins. However, additional studies are essential to validate these initial observations and to explore further.

358 SECTION III: KETOGENIC DIET IN THE LABORATORY

REFERENCES

Abbott, N. J., Khan, E. U., Rollinson, C., Reichel, A., Janigro, D., Dombrowski, S., & Dobbie, M. B. D. J. (2001). Drug resistance in epilepsy: The role of the blood–brain barrier. In V. Ling (Ed.), *Mechanisms of drug resistance in epilepsy: Lessons from oncology* (pp. 38–47). John Wiley.

Abbott, N. J., Patabendige, A. A., Dolman, D. E., Yusof, S. R., & Begley, D. J. (2010). Structure and function of the blood–brain barrier. *Neurobiology of Disease, 37*, 13–25.

Abbott, N. J., Ronnback, L., & Hansson, E. (2006). Astrocyte-endothelial interactions at the blood–brain barrier. *Nature Reviews in Neuroscience, 7*, 41–53.

Abumrad, N., Harmon, C., & Ibrahimi, A. (1998). Membrane transport of long-chain fatty acids: Evidence for a facilitated process. *Journal of Lipid Research, 39*, 2309–2318.

Arcangeli, A., Rosati, B., Crociani, O., Cherubini, A., Fontana, L., Passani, B., Wanke, E., & Olivotto, M. (1999). Modulation of HERG current and *herg* gene expression during retinoic acid treatment of human neuroblastoma cells: Potentiating effects of BDNF. *Journal of Neurobiology, 40*, 214–225.

Armulik, A., Genov, G., & Betsholtz, C. (2011). Pericytes: Developmental, physiological, and pathological perspectives, problems, and promises. *Developmental Cell, 21*, 193–215.

Aurrand-Lions, M., Johnson-Leger, C., Wong, C., Du Pasquier, L., & Imhof, B. A. (2001). Heterogeneity of endothelial junctions is reflected by differential expression and specific subcellular localization of the three JAM family members. *Blood, 98*, 3699–3707.

Ballabh, P., Braun, A., & Nedergaard, M. (2004). The blood–brain barrier: An overview; Structure, regulation, and clinical implications. *Neurobiology of Disease, 16*, 1–13.

Bates, D. C., Sin, W. C., Aftab, Q., & Naus, C. C. (2007). Connexin43 enhances glioma invasion by a mechanism involving the carboxy terminus. *Glia, 55*, 1554–1564.

Bergsneider, M., Hovda, D. A., Shalmon, E., Kelly, D. F., Vespa, P. M., Martin, N. A., Phelps, M. E., McArthur, D. L., Caron, M. J., & Kraus, J. F. (1997). Cerebral hyperglycolysis following severe traumatic brain injury in humans: A positron emission tomography study. *Journal of Neurosurgery, 86*, 241–251.

Bernacki, J., Dobrowolska, A., Nierwiska, K., & Malecki, A. (2008). Physiology and pharmacological role of the blood–brain barrier. *Pharmacological Reports, 60*, 600–622.

Bohn, D., & Daneman, D. (2002). Diabetic ketoacidosis and cerebral edema. *Current Opinion in Pediatrics, 14*, 287–291.

Bruehl, C., Hagemann, G., & Witte, O. W. (1998). Uncoupling of blood flow and metabolism in epilepsy. *Epilepsia, 39*, 1235–1242.

Cederberg, D., & Siesj, P. (2010). What has inflammation to do with traumatic brain injury? *Child's Nervous System, 26*, 221–226.

Cheng, S., Chen, G. Q., Leski, M., Zou, B., Wang, Y., & Wu, Q. (2006). The effect of D, L-hydroxybutyric acid on cell death and proliferation in L929 cells. *Biomaterials, 27*, 3758–3765.

Coomber, B. L., & Stewart, P. A. (1985). Morphometric analysis of CNS microvascular endothelium. *Microvascular Research, 30*, 99–115.

Cordon-Cardo, C., O'Brien, J. P., Casals, D., Rittman-Grauer, L., Biedler, J. L., Melamed, M. R., & Bertino, J. R. (1989). Multidrug-resistance gene (P-glycoprotein) is expressed by endothelial cells at blood–brain barrier sites. *Proceedings of the National Academy of Sciences USA, 86*, 695–698.

Cornford, E. M., Hyman, S., Cornford, M. E., & Damian, R. T. (1998a). Glut1 glucose transporter in the primate choroid plexus endothelium. *Journal of Neuropathology and Experimental Neurology, 57*, 404–414.

Cornford, E. M., Hyman, S., Cornford, M. E., Damian, R. T., & Raleigh, M. J. (1998b). A single glucose transporter configuration in normal primate brain endothelium: Comparison with resected human brain. *Journal of Neuropathology and Experimental Neurology, 57*, 699–713.

Cornford, E. M., Hyman, S., Cornford, M. E., Landaw, E. M., & Delgado-Escueta, A. V. (1998c). Interictal seizure resections show two configurations of endothelial Glut1 glucose transporter in the human blood–brain barrier. *Journal of Cerebral Blood Flow & Metabolism, 18*, 26–42.

Cornford, E. M., Hyman, S., & Swartz, B. E. (1994). The human brain GLUT1 glucose transporter: Ultrastructural localization to the blood–brain barrier endothelia. *Journal of Cerebral Blood Flow & Metabolism, 14*, 106–112.

Cremer, J. E. (1982). Substrate utilization and brain development. *Journal of Cerebral Blood Flow & Metabolism, 2*, 394–407.

Cucullo, L., Hossain, M., Puvenna, V., Marchi, N., & Janigro, D. (2011). The role of shear stress in blood–brain barrier endothelial physiology. *BMC Neuroscience, 12*, 40.

Dalvi, S., On, N., Nguyen, H., Pogorzelec, M., Miller, D.W., & Hatch, G. M. (2014). The blood brain barrier—regulation of fatty acid and drug transport. In T. Heinbockel (Ed.), *Neurochemistry*. InTech.

Daneman, R., & Prat, A. (2015). The blood–brain barrier. *Cold Spring Harbor Perspectives in Biology, 7*, a020412.

Daneman, R., Zhou, L., Agalliu, D., Cahoy, J. D., Kaushal, A., & Barres, B. A. (2010). The mouse blood–brain barrier transcriptome: A new resource for understanding the development and function of brain endothelial cells. *PLOS ONE, 5,* Article e13741.

David, Y., Cacheaux, L. P., Ivens, S., Lapilover, E., Heinemann, U., Kaufer, D., & Friedman, A. (2009). Astrocytic dysfunction in epileptogenesis: Consequence of altered potassium and glutamate homeostasis? *Journal of Neuroscience, 29,* 10588–10599.

De Vivo, D. C., Leary, L., & Wang, D. O. N. G. (2002). Glucose transporter 1 deficiency syndrome and other glycolytic defects. *Journal of Child Neurology, 17,* 3S15–3S23.

De Vivo, D. C., Trifiletti, R. R., Jacobson, R. I., Ronen, G. M., Behmand, R. A., & Harik, S. I. (1991). Defective glucose transport across the blood–brain barrier as a cause of persistent hypoglycorrhachia, seizures, and developmental delay. *New England Journal of Medicine, 325,* 703–709.

de Vries, H. E., Kooij, G., Frenkel, D., Georgopoulos, S., Monsonego, A., & Janigro, D. (2012). Inflammatory events at blood-brain barrier in neuroinflammatory and neurodegenerative disorders: Implications for clinical disease. *Epilepsia, 53,* 45–52.

Desai, S. Y., Marroni, M., Cucullo, L., Krizanac-Bengez, L., Mayberg, M. R., Hossain, M. T., Grant, G. G., & Janigro, D. (2002). Mechanisms of endothelial survival under shear stress. *Endothelium, 9,* 89–102.

Dombrowski, S. M., Desai, S. Y., Marroni, M., Cucullo, L., Goodrich, K., Bingaman, W., Mayberg, M. R., Bengez, L., & Janigro, D. (2001). Overexpression of multiple drug resistance genes in endothelial cells from patients with refractory epilepsy. *Epilepsia, 42,* 1501–1506.

Dupuis, N., Curatolo, N., Benoist, J. F., & Auvin, S. (2015). Ketogenic diet exhibits anti-inflammatory properties. *Epilepsia,* e95–e98. doi:10.1111/epi.13038

Ezan, P., Andr, P., Cisternino, S., Saubama, B., Boulay, A. C., Doutremer, S., Thomas, M. A., Quenech'du, N., Giaume, C., & Cohen-Salmon, M. (2012). Deletion of astroglial connexins weakens the blood–brain barrier. *Journal of Cerebral Blood Flow & Metabolism, 32,* 1457–1467.

Finnie, J. W. (2013). Neuroinflammation: Beneficial and detrimental effects after traumatic brain injury. *Inflammopharmacology, 21,* 309–320.

Freeman, J., Veggiotti, P., Lanzi, G., Tagliabue, A., & Perucca, E. (2006). The ketogenic diet: From molecular mechanisms to clinical effects. *Epilepsy Research, 68,* 145–180.

Freeman, J. M., Vining, E. P., Pillas, D. J., Pyzik, P. L., & Casey, J. C. (1998). The efficacy of the ketogenic diet—1998: A prospective evaluation of intervention in 150 children. *Pediatrics, 102,* 1358–1363.

Galea, I., Bechmann, I., & Perry, V. H. (2007). What is immune privilege (not)? *Trends in Immunology, 28,* 12–18.

Gasior, M., Rogawski, M. A., & Hartman, A. L. (2006). Neuroprotective and disease-modifying effects of the ketogenic diet. *Behavioural Pharmacology, 17,* 431.

Ghosh, C., Gonzalez-Martinez, J., Hossain, M., Cucullo, L., Fazio, V., Janigro, D., & Marchi, N. (2010). Pattern of P450 expression at the human blood–brain barrier: Roles of epileptic condition and laminar flow. *Epilepsia, 51,* 1408–1417.

Ghosh, C., Hossain, M., Puvenna, V., Martinez-Gonzalez, J., Alexopolous, A., Janigro, D., & Marchi, N. (2013). Expression and functional relevance of UGT1A4 in a cohort of human drug-resistant epileptic brains. *Epilepsia, 54,* 1562–1570.

Ghosh, C., Marchi, N., Desai, N. K., Puvenna, V., Hossain, M., Gonzalez-Martinez, J., Alexopoulos, A. V., & Janigro, D. (2011a). Cellular localization and functional significance of CYP3A4 in the human epileptic brain. *Epilepsia, 52,* 562–571.

Ghosh, C., Puvenna, V., Gonzalez-Martinez, J., Janigro, D., & Marchi, N. (2011b). Blood–brain barrier P450 enzymes and multidrug transporters in drug resistance: A synergistic role in neurological diseases. *Current Drug Metabolism, 12,* 742–749.

Gibson, C. L., Murphy, A. N., & Murphy, S. P. (2012). Stroke outcome in the ketogenic state-systematic review of the animal data. *Journal of Neurochemistry, 123,* 52–57.

Gingrich, M. B., & Traynelis, S. F. (2000). Serine proteases and brain damage—Is there a link? *Trends in Neuroscience, 23,* 399–407.

Glass, C. K., Saijo, K., Winner, B., Marchetto, M. C., & Gage, F. H. (2010). Mechanisms underlying inflammation in neurodegeneration. *Cell, 140,* 918–934.

Gloor, S. M., Wachtel, M., Bolliger, M. F., Ishihara, H., Landmann, R., & Frei, K. (2001). Molecular and cellular permeability control at the blood–brain barrier. *Brain Research Reviews, 36,* 258–264.

Grant, G. A., Abbott, N. J., & Janigro, D. (1998). Understanding the physiology of the blood–brain barrier: In vitro models. *News in Physiological Sciences, 13,* 287–293.

Grant, G. A., & Janigro, D. (2010). The blood–brain barrier. In H. R. Winn (Ed.), *Youmans neurological surgery.* Saunders.

Grimble, R. F. (1998). Nutritional modulation of cytokine biology. *Nutrition, 14,* 634–640.

Gu, Y., Zheng, G., Xu, M., Li, Y., Chen, X., Zhu, W., Tong, Y., Chung, S. K., Liu, K. J., & Shen, J. (2012). Caveolin-1 regulates nitric oxide-mediated matrix metalloproteinases activity and blood–brain barrier permeability in focal cerebral ischemia and reperfusion injury. *Journal of Neurochemistry, 120,* 147–156.

Ha, S. N., Hochman, J., & Sheridan, R. P. (2007). Mini review on molecular modeling of P-glycoprotein (Pgp). *Current Topics in Medicinal Chemistry, 7,* 1525–1529.

Hall, C. N., Reynell, C., Gesslein, B., Hamilton, N. B., Mishra, A., Sutherland, B. A., Farrell, F. M., Buchan, A. M., Lauritzen, M., & Attwell, D. (2014). Capillary pericytes regulate cerebral blood flow in health and disease. *Nature, 508,* 55–60.

Hamilton, J. A. (1998). Fatty acid transport: Difficult or easy? *Journal of Lipid Research, 39,* 467–481.

Haseloff, R. F., Blasig, I. E., Bauer, H. C., & Bauer, H. (2005). In search of the astrocytic factor(s) modulating blood–brain barrier functions in brain capillary endothelial cells in vitro. *Cellular and Molecular Neurobiology, 25,* 25–39.

Hasselbalch, S. G., Knudsen, G. M., Jakobsen, J., Hageman, L. P., Holm, S., & Paulson, O. B. (1994). Brain metabolism during short-term starvation in humans. *Journal of Cerebral Blood Flow & Metabolism, 14,* 125–131.

Hasselbalch, S. G., Madsen, P. L., Hageman, L. P., Olsen, K. S., Justesen, N., Holm, S., & Paulson, O. B. (1996). Changes in cerebral blood flow and carbohydrate metabolism during acute hyperketonemia. *American Journal of Physiology-Endocrinology and Metabolism, 270,* E746–E751.

Hawkins, B. T., & Davis, T. P. (2005). The blood–brain barrier/neurovascular unit in health and disease. *Pharmacological Reviews, 57,* 173–185.

Hawkins, R. A., O'Kane, R. L., Simpson, I. A., & Via, J. R. (2006). Structure of the blood–brain barrier and its role in the transport of amino acids. *Journal of Nutrition, 136,* 218S–226S.

Hiraide, A., Katayama, M., Sugimoto, H., Yoshioka, T., & Sugimoto, T. (1991). Effect of 3-hydroxybutyrate on posttraumatic metabolism in man. *Surgery, 109,* 176–181.

Hirase, T., Staddon, J. M., Saitou, M., & Rubin, L. L. (1997). Occludin as a possible determinant of tight junction permeability in endothelial cells. *Journal of Cell Science, 110,* 1603–1613.

Ho, C. F., Chan, K. W., Yeh, H. I., Kuo, J., Liu, H. J., & Wang, C. Y. (2013). Ketone bodies upregulate endothelial connexin 43 (Cx43) gap junctions. *The Veterinary Journal, 198,* 696–701.

Hu, Z. G., Wang, H. D., Jin, W., & Yin, H. X. (2009a). Ketogenic diet reduces cytochrome *c* release and cellular apoptosis following traumatic brain injury in juvenile rats. *Annals of Clinical & Laboratory Science, 39,* 76–83.

Hu, Z. G., Wang, H. D., Qiao, L., Yan, W., Tan, Q. F., & Yin, H. X. (2009b). The protective effect of the ketogenic diet on traumatic brain injury-induced cell death in juvenile rats. *Brain Injury, 23,* 459–465.

Huang, J., Upadhyay, U. M., & Tamargo, R. J. (2006). Inflammation in stroke and focal cerebral ischemia. *Surgical Neurology, 66,* 232–245.

Huber, J. D., Egleton, R. D., & Davis, T. P. (2001). Molecular physiology and pathophysiology of tight junctions in the blood–brain barrier. *Trends in Neuroscience, 24,* 719–725.

Ivens, S., Kaufer, D., Flores, L. P., Bechmann, I., Zumsteg, D., Tomkins, O., Seiffert, E., Heinemann, U., & Friedman, A. (2007). TGF-beta receptor-mediated albumin uptake into astrocytes is involved in neocortical epileptogenesis. *Brain, 130,* 535–547.

Janigro, D. (1999). Blood-brain barrier, ion homeostasis and epilepsy: Possible implications towards the understanding of ketogenic diet mechanisms. *Epilepsy Research, 37,* 223–232.

Janigro, D. (2012). Are you in or out? Leukocyte, ion, and neurotransmitter permeability across the epileptic blood-brain barrier. *Epilepsia, 53*(Suppl. 1), 26–34.

Janzer, R. C., & Raff, M. C. (1987). Astrocytes induce blood–brain barrier properties in endothelial cells. *Nature, 325,* 253–257.

Jeong, S. M., Hahm, K. D., Shin, J. W., Leem, J. G., Lee, C., & Han, S. M. (2006). Changes in magnesium concentration in the serum and cerebrospinal fluid of neuropathic rats. *Acta Anaesthesiologica Scandinavica, 50,* 211–216.

Kaplan, L., Chow, B. W., & Gu, C. (2020). Neuronal regulation of the blood-brain barrier and neurovascular coupling. *Nature Reviews in Neuroscience, 21,* 416–432.

Kisler, K., Nikolakopoulou, A. M., Sweeney, M. D., Lazic, D., Zhao, Z., & Zlokovic, B. V. (2020). Acute ablation of cortical pericytes leads to rapid neurovascular uncoupling. *Frontiers Cell Neuroscience, 14,* 27.

Klepper, J. (2008). Glucose transporter deficiency syndrome (GLUT1DS) and the ketogenic diet. *Epilepsia, 49,* 46–49.

Kniesel, U., & Wolburg, H. (2000). Tight junctions of the blood–brain barrier. *Cellular and Molecular Neurobiology, 20,* 57–76.

Lai, C. H., & Kuo, K. H. (2005). The critical component to establish in vitro BBB model: Pericyte. *Brain Research Reviews, 50,* 258–265.

Lee, S., Chen, T. T., Barber, C. L., Jordan, M. C., Murdock, J., Desai, S., Ferrara, N., Nagy, A., Roos, K. P., & Iruela-Arispe, M. L. (2007). Autocrine VEGF signaling is required for vascular homeostasis. *Cell, 130,* 691–703.

Leino, R. L., Gerhart, D. Z., & Drewes, L. R. (1999). Monocarboxylate transporter (MCT1) abundance in brains of suckling and adult rats: A quantitative electron microscopic immunogold study. *Developmental Brain Research, 113,* 47–54.

Leino, R. L., Gerhart, D. Z., Duelli, R., Enerson, B. E., & Drewes, L. R. (2001). Diet-induced ketosis increases monocarboxylate transporter (MCT1) levels in rat brain. *Neurochemistry International, 38*, 519–527.

Levy, M., Thaiss, C. A., & Elinav, E. (2015). Taming the inflammasome. *Nature Medicine, 21*, 213–215.

Liebner, S., Fischmann, A., Rascher, G., Duffner, F., Grote, E. H., Kalbacher, H., & Wolburg, H. (2000). Claudin-1 and claudin-5 expression and tight junction morphology are altered in blood vessels of human glioblastoma multiforme. *Acta Neuropathologica Berlin, 100*, 323–331.

Limatola, C., & Ransohoff, R. M. (2014). Modulating neurotoxicity through CX3CL1/CX3CR1 signaling. *Frontiers Cell Neuroscience, 8*, 229.

Lochhead, J. J., Yang, J., Ronaldson, P. T., & Davis, T. P. (2020). Structure, function, and regulation of the blood–brain barrier tight junction in central nervous system disorders. *Frontiers Physiology, 11*, 914.

Magistretti, P. J., & Pellerin, L. (1995). Cellular basis of brain energy metabolism and their relevance to brain imaging—Evidence for a prominent role for astrocytes. *Cerebral Cortex, 5*, 301–306.

Marchi, N., Granata, T., Alexopoulos, A., & Janigro, D. (2012). The blood–brain barrier hypothesis in drug resistant epilepsy. *Brain, 135*, e211.

Marchi, N., Granata, T., & Janigro, D. (2014). Inflammatory pathways of seizure disorders. *Trends in Neuroscience, 37*, 55–65.

Marchi, N., Hallene, K. L., Kight, K. M., Cucullo, L., Moddel, G., Bingaman, W., Dini, G., Vezzani, A., & Janigro, D. (2004). Significance of MDR1 and multiple drug resistance in refractory human epileptic brain. *BMC Medicine, 2*, 37.

McAllister, M. S., Krizanac-Bengez, L., Macchia, F., Naftalin, R. J., Pedley, K. C., Mayberg, M. R., Marroni, M., Leaman, S., Stanness, K. A., & Janigro, D. (2001). Mechanisms of glucose transport at the blood–brain barrier: An in vitro study. *Brain Research, 904*, 20–30.

Medin, T., Medin, H., Hefte, M. B., Storm-Mathisen, J., & Bergersen, L. H. (2019). Upregulation of the lactate transporter monocarboxylate transporter 1 at the blood–brain barrier in a rat model of attention-deficit/hyperactivity disorder suggests hyperactivity could be a form of self-treatment. *Behavioral Brain Research, 360*, 279–285.

Mitchell, R. W., Edmundson, C. L., Miller, D. W., & Hatch, G. M. (2009). On the mechanism of oleate transport across human brain microvessel endothelial cells. *Journal of Neurochemistry, 110*, 1049–1057.

Mittapalli, R. K., Manda, V. K., Adkins, C. E., Geldenhuys, W. J., & Lockman, P. R. (2010). Exploiting nutrient transporters at the blood-brain barrier to improve brain distribution of small molecules. *Therapeutic Delivery, 1*, 775–784.

Mizee, M. R., Wooldrik, D., Lakeman, K. A., van het Hof, B., Drexhage, J. A., Geerts, D., Bugiani, M., Aronica, E., Mebius, R. E., & Prat, A. (2013). Retinoic acid induces blood–brain barrier development. *Journal of Neuroscience, 33*, 1660–1671.

Morita, K., Furuse, M., Fujimoto, K., & Tsukita, S. (1999). Claudine multigene family encoding four-transmembrane domain protein components of tight junction strands. *Proceeding of the National Academy of Sciences USA, 96*, 511–516.

Morris, A. A. M. (2005). Cerebral ketone body metabolism. *Journal of Inherited Metabolic Disease, 28*, 109–121.

Musa-Veloso, K., Likhodii, S. S., & Cunnane, S. C. (2002). Breath acetone is a reliable indicator of ketosis in adults consuming ketogenic meals. *American Journal of Clinical Nutrition, 76*, 65–70.

Nabbout, R., Vezzani, A., Dulac, O., & Chiron, C. (2011). Acute encephalopathy with inflammation-mediated status epilepticus. *Lancet Neurology, 10*, 99–108.

Nakagawa, S., Deli, M. A., Kawaguchi, H., Shimizudani, T., Shimono, T., Kittel, A., Tanaka, K., & Niwa, M. (2009). A new blood–brain barrier model using primary rat brain endothelial cells, pericytes and astrocytes. *Neurochemistry International, 54*, 253–263.

Nation, D. A., Sweeney, M. D., Montagne, A., Sagare, A. P., D'Orazio, L. M., Pachicano, M., Sepehrband, F., Nelson, A. R., Buennagel, D. P., Harrington, M. G., Benzinger, T. L. S., Fagan, A. M., Ringman, J. M., Schneider, L. S., Morris, J. C., Chui, H. C., Law, M., Toga, A. W., & Zlokovic, B. V. (2019). Blood–brain barrier breakdown is an early biomarker of human cognitive dysfunction. *Nature Medicine, 25*, 270–276.

Neth, B. J., Mintz, A., Whitlow, C., Jung, Y., Solingapuram, S. K., Register, T. C., Kellar, D., Lockhart, S. N., Hoscheidt, S., Maldjian, J., Heslegrave, A. J., Blennow, K., Cunnane, S. C., Castellano, C. A., Zetterberg, H., & Craft, S. (2020). Modified ketogenic diet is associated with improved cerebrospinal fluid biomarker profile, cerebral perfusion, and cerebral ketone body uptake in older adults at risk for Alzheimer's disease: A pilot study. *Neurobiology of Aging, 86*, 54–63.

Neuwelt, E. A., Bauer, B., Fahlke, C., Fricker, G., Iadecola, C., Janigro, D., Leybaert, L., Molnar, Z., O'Donnell, M. E., Povlishock, J. T., Saunders, N. R., Sharp, F., Stanimirovic, D., Watts, R. J., & Drewes, L. R. (2011). Engaging neuroscience to advance translational research in brain barrier biology. *Nature Reviews Neuroscience, 12*, 169–182.

Nischwitz, V., Berthele, A., & Michalke, B. (2008). Speciation analysis of selected metals and determination of their total contents in paired serum and cerebrospinal fluid samples: An approach to investigate the permeability of the human blood-cerebrospinal fluid-barrier. *Analytica Chimica Acta*, 627, 258–269.

Ohtsuki, S., Hirayama, M., Ito, S., Uchida, Y., Tachikawa, M., & Terasaki, T. (2014). Quantitative targeted proteomics for understanding the blood–brain barrier: Towards pharmacoproteomics. *Expert Review of Proteomics*, 11, 303–313.

Pan, J. W., Rothman, D. L., Behar, K. L., Stein, D. T., & Hetherington, H. P. (2000). Human brain β-hydroxybutyrate and lactate increase in fasting-induced ketosis. *Journal of Cerebral Blood Flow & Metabolism*, 20, 1502–1507.

Pan, J. W., Telang, F. W., Lee, J. H., de Graaf, R. A., Rothman, D. L., Stein, D. T., & Hetherington, H. P. (2001). Measurement of β-hydroxybutyrate in acute hyperketonemia in human brain. *Journal of Neurochemistry*, 79, 539–544.

Pierre, K., & Pellerin, L. (2005). Monocarboxylate transporters in the central nervous system: Distribution, regulation and function. *Journal of Neurochemistry*, 94, 1–14.

Pierre, K., Pellerin, L., Debernardi, R., Riederer, B. M., & Magistretti, P. J. (2000). Cell-specific localization of monocarboxylate transporters, MCT1 and MCT2, in the adult mouse brain revealed by double immunohistochemical labeling and confocal microscopy. *Neuroscience*, 100, 617–627.

Porta, N., Valle, L., Boutry, E., Fontaine, M., Dessein, A. F., Joriot, S., Cuisset, J. M., Cuvellier, J. C., & Auvin, S. (2009). Comparison of seizure reduction and serum fatty acid levels after receiving the ketogenic and modified Atkins diet. *Seizure*, 18, 359–364.

Prat, A., Biernacki, K., Wosik, K., & Antel, J. P. (2001). Glial cell influence on the human blood–brain barrier. *Glia*, 36, 145–155.

Prins, M. L. (2008). Cerebral metabolic adaptation and ketone metabolism after brain injury. *Journal of Cerebral Blood Flow & Metabolism*, 28, 1–16.

Prins, M. L., & Giza, C. C. (2006). Induction of monocarboxylate transporter 2 expression and ketone transport following traumatic brain injury in juvenile and adult rats. *Developmental Neuroscience*, 28, 447–456.

Prins, M. L., & Matsumoto, J. H. (2014). The collective therapeutic potential of cerebral ketone metabolism in traumatic brain injury. *Journal of Lipid Research*, 55, 2450–2457.

Ransohoff, R. M., & Brown, M. A. (2012). Innate immunity in the central nervous system. *Journal of Clinical Investigation*, 122, 1164–1171.

Rubin, L. L., Hall, D. E., Porter, S., Barbu, K., Cannon, C., Horner, H. C., Janatpour, M., Liaw, C. W.,

Manning, K., Morales, J., and et al. (1991). A cell culture model of the blood–brain barrier. *Journal of Cell Biology*, 115, 1725–1735.

Ruskin, D. N., Kawamura, M., & Masino, S. A. (2009). Reduced pain and inflammation in juvenile and adult rats fed a ketogenic diet. *PLOS ONE*, 4, Article e8349.

Salim, A., Hadjizacharia, P., Dubose, J., Brown, C., Inaba, K., Chan, L. S., & Margulies, D. (2009). Persistent hyperglycemia in severe traumatic brain injury: An independent predictor of outcome. *The American Surgeon*, 75, 25–29.

Saunders, N. R., Dreifuss, J. J., Dziegielewska, K. M., Johansson, P. A., Habgood, M. D., Moellgard, K., & Bauer, H. C. (2014). The rights and wrongs of blood–brain barrier permeability studies: A walk through 100 years of history. *Frontiers in Neuroscience*, 8. https://doi.org/10.3389/fnins.2014.00404

Shepro, D., & Morel, N. M. (1993). Pericyte physiology. *FASEB Journal*, 7, 1031–1038.

Shimizu, F., Sano, Y., Maeda, T., Abe, M., Nakayama, H., Takahashi, R., Ueda, M., Ohtsuki, S., Terasaki, T., & Obinata, M. (2008). Peripheral nerve pericytes originating from the blood–nerve barrier expresses tight junctional molecules and transporters as barrier-forming cells. *Journal of Cell Physiology*, 217, 388–399.

Shue, E. H., Carson-Walter, E. B., Liu, Y., Winans, B. N., Ali, Z. S., Chen, J., & Walter, K. A. (2008). Plasmalemmal vesicle associated protein-1 (PV-1) is a marker of blood–brain barrier disruption in rodent models. *BMC Neuroscience*, 9, 29.

Somjen, G. G. (2004). *Ions in the brain: Normal function, seizures, and stroke.* Oxford University Press.

Sorokin, L. (2010). The impact of the extracellular matrix on inflammation. *Nature Reviews Immunology*, 10, 712–723.

Stanness, K. A., Guatteo, E., & Janigro, D. (1996). A dynamic model of the blood–brain barrier "in vitro." *Neurotoxicology*, 17, 481–496.

Stanness, K. A., Westrum, L. E., Fornaciari, E., Mascagni, P., Nelson, J. A., Stenglein, S. G., Myers, T., & Janigro, D. (1997). Morphological and functional characterization of an in vitro blood–brain barrier model. *Brain Research*, 771, 329–342.

Sullivan, P. G., Rippy, N. A., Dorenbos, K., Concepcion, R. C., Agarwal, A. K., & Rho, J. M. (2004). The ketogenic diet increases mitochondrial uncoupling protein levels and activity. *Annals of Neurology*, 55, 576–580.

Svart, M., Gormsen, L. C., Hansen, J., Zeidler, D., Gejl, M., Vang, K., Aanerud, J., & Moeller, N. (2018). Regional cerebral effects of ketone body infusion with 3-hydroxybutyrate in humans: Reduced glucose uptake, unchanged oxygen consumption and increased blood flow by positron emission tomography; A randomized, controlled trial. *PLOS ONE*, 13, Article e0190556.

Sweeney, M. D., Kisler, K., Montagne, A., Toga, A. W., & Zlokovic, B. V. (2018). The role of brain vasculature in neurodegenerative disorders. *Nature Neuroscience, 21*, 1318–1331.

Sweeney, M. D., Zhao, Z., Montagne, A., Nelson, A. R., & Zlokovic, B. V. (2019). Blood–brain barrier: From physiology to disease and back. *Physiological Reviews, 99*, 21–78.

Takimoto, M., & Hamada, T. (2014). Acute exercise increases brain region-specific expression of MCT1, MCT2, MCT4, GLUT1, and COX IV proteins. *Journal of Applied Physiology, 116*, 1238–1250.

Tewes, B. J., & Galla, H. J. (2001). Lipid polarity in brain capillary endothelial cells. *Endothelium, 8*, 207–220.

Thiebaut, F., Tsuruo, T., Hamada, H., Gottesman, M. M., Pastan, I., & Willingham, M. C. (1987). Cellular localization of the multidrug resistance gene product in normal human tissues. *Proceedings of the National Academy of Sciences USA, 84*, 7735–7738.

Tieu, K., Perier, C., Caspersen, C., Teismann, P., Wu, D. C., Yan, S. D., Naini, A., Vila, M., Jackson-Lewis, V., & Ramasamy, R. (2003). D-β-Hydroxybutyrate rescues mitochondrial respiration and mitigates features of Parkinson disease. *Journal of Clinical Investigation, 112*, 892.

Tomkins, O., Shelef, I., Kaizerman, I., Eliushin, A., Afawi, Z., Misk, A., Gidon, M., Cohen, A., Zumsteg, D., & Friedman, A. (2008). Blood–brain barrier disruption in post-traumatic epilepsy. *Journal of Neurology Neurosurgery Psychiatry, 79*, 774–777.

Veech, R. L., Chance, B., Kashiwaya, Y., Lardy, H. A., & Cahill, G. F. (2001). Ketone bodies, potential therapeutic uses. *IUBMB Life, 51*, 241–247.

Versele, R., Corsi, M., Fuso, A., Sevin, E., Businaro, R., Gosselet, F., Fenart, L., & Candela, P. (2020). Ketone bodies promote amyloid-β1-40 clearance in a human in vitro blood–brain barrier model. *International Journal of Molecular Sciences, 21*.

White, H., & Venkatesh, B. (2011). Clinical review: Ketones and brain injury. *Critical Care, 15*, 219.

Wolburg, H., Noell, S., Mack, A., Wolburg-Buchholz, K., & Fallier-Becker, P. (2009). Brain endothelial cells and the glio-vascular complex. *Cell Tissue Research, 335*, 75–96.

Wosik, K., Cayrol, R., Dodelet-Devillers, A., Berthelet, F., Bernard, M., Moumdjian, R., Bouthillier, A., Reudelhuber, T. L., & Prat, A. (2007). Angiotensin II controls occludin function and is required for blood–brain barrier maintenance: Relevance to multiple sclerosis. *Journal of Neuroscience, 27*, 9032–9042.

Yasui, T., Hirose, J., Tsutsumi, S., Nakamura, K., Aburatani, H., & Tanaka, S. (2011). Epigenetic regulation of osteoclast differentiation: Possible involvement of Jmjd3 in the histone demethylation of Nfatc1. *Journal of Bone and Mineral Research, 26*, 2665–2671.

Ziegler, D. R., Ribeiro, L. C., Hagenn, M., Arajo, E., Torres, I. L., Gottfried, C., Netto, C. A., & Gonalves, C. A. (2003). Ketogenic diet increases glutathione peroxidase activity in rat hippocampus. *Neurochemical Research, 28*, 1793–1797.

Zlokovic, B. V. (2008). The blood–brain barrier in health and chronic neurodegenerative disorders. *Neuron, 57*, 178–201.

Metabolic and Redox Alterations by Ketogenic Diets

DEREK JOHNSON, BS AND MANISHA PATEL, PHD

METABOLIC CHANGES EXERTED BY KETOGENESIS

Under normal metabolic conditions, the human body utilizes glucose-derived acetyl-CoA (Aca) to create adenosine triphosphate (ATP) via the tricarboxylic acid (TCA) cycle and electron transport chain. When there is a shift from glucose utilization (glycolysis) caused by carbohydrate-restrictive diets, such as the ketogenic diet (KD), metabolic changes occur, and Aca is instead derived from the alternative parallel processes of gluconeogenesis and fatty acid oxidation.

During gluconeogenesis, mitochondrial pyruvate is utilized in the TCA cycle to produce oxaloacetate, which is transferred out of the mitochondria as malate. This malate is converted back to oxaloacetate in the cytoplasm and is then converted to phosphonyl pyruvate, followed by several more steps to ultimately create glucose and its downstream output, Aca. The second method, fatty acid oxidation, is a process by which both short- and long-chain fatty acids are broken down in the mitochondria to produce Aca. A critical regulator of this process is the lipid metabolite malonyl-CoA, which uniquely functions as both a precursor in long-chain fatty acid synthesis and as an inhibitor of the enzyme carnitine palmitoyltransferase, whose function is to transport long-chain fatty acids across the mitochondrial inner membrane. When glucose is present, malonyl-CoA is synthesized from citrate of the TCA cycle and is used to produce fatty acids, while in a glucose-deprived state, the glucagon:insulin ratio increases and not only reduces the production of malonyl-CoA in the cytoplasm but also stimulates its degradation (Foster, 2012). This in turn allows long-chain fatty acids to enter the mitochondria at a much faster rate (Foster, 2012).

Despite the increase in Aca by these two processes, the sequestering of oxaloacetate during gluconeogenesis restricts the ability of the TCA cycle to convert the Aca into citrate, requiring the diversion of Aca into ketone body synthesis for use. This process, known as ketogenesis, begins when two Aca molecules fuse to form acetoacetyl-CoA. Next, a third Aca molecule is added to create 3-hydroxy-3-methylglutaryl-CoA (HMG-CoA), followed by the removal of an Aca to produce the ketone body acetoacetate. While acetoacetate can be released into the bloodstream, it is typically reduced to β-hydroxybutyrate (βHB) via β-hydroxybutyrate dehydrogenase, and, to a lesser extent, it can be converted into acetone via acetoacetate decarboxylase. Importantly, although the liver is the major producer of ketone bodies, it is the only tissue that cannot utilize them; the liver lacks the enzyme succinyl CoA:3-ketoacid CoA transferase, a mitochondrial enzyme that is necessary for the conversion of acetoacetate to acetoacetyl-CoA during ketolysis (Fukao et al., 1997; Orii et al., 2008), and thus the liver disperses ketone bodies to extrahepatic tissues, such as the brain, which itself cannot undertake fatty acid oxidation (for schematic summary see Figure 30.1). In these tissues, βHB and acetoacetate are converted back into their Aca constituents and are either utilized in the TCA cycle or directly act upon the G-protein-coupled receptors to elicit other downstream effects. In the case of the latter, an interesting point is that the application of βHB has been shown to increase the expression of its G-protein-coupled receptor HCR2, but not the structurally similar HCR1 (Hasan-Olive et al., 2019).

KD-MEDIATED METABOLIC CHANGES

Metabolic alterations following ketogenesis have also been noted but not intensively studied. Unsurprisingly, given the KD's positive effects on energy production and the mechanism of ketogenesis induction, TCA cycle metabolites, such as α-ketoglutarate, isocitrate, and oxaloacetate, increase significantly in mice fed a short-term (8-week) KD compared to standard chow-fed

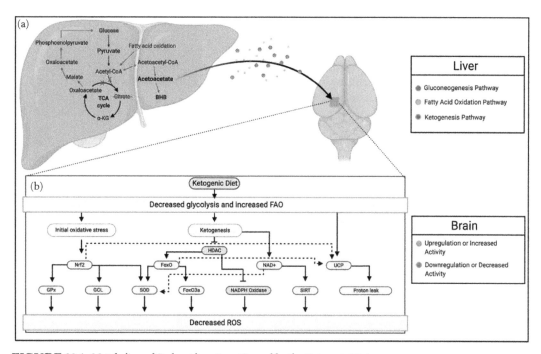

FIGURE 30.1 *Metabolic and Redox Alterations Caused by the Ketogenic Diet*

(a) Decreases in blood glucose stimulate gluconeogenesis and fatty acid oxidation pathways, and oxaloacetate utilized in gluconeogenesis in the liver contributes to shunting of acetyl-CoA into ketone synthesis. (b) Ketones are then transferred to the brain and facilitate decreases in ROS via a host of implicated mechanisms.

mice (Douris et al., 2015), and hippocampal gene expression analysis also shows upregulation of metabolic enzymes that contribute to increased ATP production (Noh et al., 2004). Additionally, mice given a KD display several distinct metabolic changes, particularly in pathways related to amino acid metabolism (Douris et al., 2015; Licha et al., 2019). Despite the fact that the mice were fed a diet consisting of only 8% protein, serum analysis showed amino acid metabolite levels to be either maintained (Douris et al., 2015) or upregulated (Licha et al., 2019) in these mice compared to standard diet-fed mice. This change is attributed to a decrease in the transcription of degrading enzymes (Douris et al., 2015) and possibly an increase in amino acid synthesis (Licha et al., 2019). Of particular note in relation to amino acid alterations, targeted and untargeted metabolomic analyses of rodent hippocampus, blood plasma, and serum indicated reductions in tryptophan levels and alterations in pathways regulating tryptophan degradation, specifically the kynurenine pathway that metabolizes tryptophan to nicotinamide adenine dinucleotide (NAD; Douris et al., 2015; Heischmann et al., 2018). Subsequent blood analysis of tryptophan, kynurenine, and kynurenine derivatives in children with refractory epilepsy on a KD also revealed significantly decreased levels of kynurenine, with a positive correlation between kynurenine levels and seizure frequency (Zarnowska et al., 2019). That is, as kynurenine levels decreased, so did seizure activity. The culmination of this line of research strongly suggests that tryptophan metabolism plays a role in the beneficial effects of the KD. More generally, alterations of amino acid metabolism and synthesis are also proposed to play a role in seizure modulation by providing an increase in glutamine. In this way, glutamate is more readily created and is able to be converted into GABA, thereby increasing inhibition and reducing excitability (Yudkoff et al., 2007). Although data exist to support this hypothesis, conflicting studies have also shown no change in glutamate despite increases in GABA, so further study is required (Calderon et al., 2017).

ALTERATION OF REACTIVE OXYGEN SPECIES PRODUCTION AND ANTIOXIDANT PATHWAYS BY KD

Reactive oxygen species (ROS) include free radicals, such as the superoxide radical and hydroxyl radical, as well as nonradicals, such as hydrogen peroxide (H_2O_2) and peroxynitrite. Low steady-state levels of ROS subserve a signaling role, whereas chronic elevated levels cause oxidative damage to cellular macromolecules and tissue injury. Cellular sources of ROS include mitochondria, NAD(P)H oxidase (NOX) enzymes, cytochrome P450, myeloperoxidase, xanthine oxidase, and nitric oxide synthase. Low steady-state levels of ROS are maintained by the existence of abundant and overlapping endogenous antioxidants. Superoxide dismutases (SODs) are primary antioxidants that catalyze the dismutation of superoxide to H_2O_2 and oxygen in the cytosol (SOD1), mitochondrial matrix (SOD2), mitochondrial inner membrane (SOD1), and extracellular space (SOD3). Catalases are heme peroxidases that catalyze the dismutation of H_2O_2 to water and oxygen and reside in peroxisomes (in most tissues) and mitochondria (notably in heart and liver). H_2O_2 is also detoxified by glutathione peroxidases (GPx) and thioredoxin/peroxiredoxins.

Although animals fed a chronic KD show decreased mitochondrial ROS levels in neural tissue, initially (1–3 days after diet commencement) an increase in mitochondrial ROS production in the hippocampus is observed; this ultimately results in an adaptive antioxidant mechanism (Milder et al., 2010). The early increase of KD-induced H_2O_2, glutathione disulfide, and 4-hydroxy-2-nonenal (4-HNE), an electrophile byproduct of lipid peroxidation, activated the NF E2-related factor 2 (Nrf2) pathway, which remained significantly elevated for at least 3 weeks (Milder et al., 2010). Thus, KD initiates low steady-state ROS production, which may serve as a redox signal to drive the activity of Nrf2 and provide long-term benefits in the form of increased antioxidants. Nrf2 pathway-mediated effects were later validated as an antiseizure mechanism using Nrf2 overexpression (Mazzuferi et al., 2013).

Several studies have shown an increase in antioxidant activity/transcription after a KD, with measurements varying depending on the location of interest. Early work by Ziegler and colleagues (2003) in rats demonstrated no differences in total brain antioxidant capacity after an 8-week KD regimen; however, specific assessment of the hippocampus and cerebellum revealed a significant increase and decrease in antioxidant capacity in these areas, respectively (Ziegler et al., 2003). Similar differences are seen in the periphery, with decreased ROS in the sciatic nerve (Cooper et al., 2018), liver, kidney, and heart after implementation of a KD. This work,

and many other studies since, have contributed to one of the most discussed aspects of the KD: the ability of ketones, specifically βHB and acetoacetate, to inhibit class I and II histone deacetylases in a dose-dependent fashion, and this finding has held true regardless of whether ketogenesis is induced by caloric restriction, fasting, or direct infusion (Shimazu et al., 2013). Histone acetylation plays an essential role in allowing chromatin to achieve an accessible state that is more conducive to gene transcription than its deacetylated state, allowing the upregulation of several oxidation-protective enzymes, including members of the Nrf2 and FoxO3a (Forkhead box O3a) pathways.

Nrf2 is a transcription factor and member of the Cap'n' collar family of proteins. It plays a pivotal role in detecting oxidative and electrophilic stressors and initiates the upregulation of several antioxidant enzymes, including SODs and catalase, in response to those stressors (Merry and Ristow, 2016; Zhu et al., 2005). Under normal cellular conditions, Nrf2 is bound in the cytosol by its upstream regulator kelch-like ECH-associated protein 1 (KEAP1), which facilitates its degradation through the ubiquitin proteasome pathway. However, when cysteine residues of the redox-sensitive KEAP1 interact with oxidants or electrophiles, Nrf2 is released (Shekh-Ahmad et al., 2018; Suzuki et al., 2019), allowing it to translocate to the nucleus to initiate transcription at antioxidant response elements (AREs; Shekh-Ahmad et al., 2018; Wilson et al., 2005). In the rodent hippocampus, increased activation and translocation of Nrf2 to the nucleus via the KD is responsible for the increased expression of numerous proteins, including GPx (Banning et al., 2005; Ziegler et al., 2003) and glutamate cysteine ligase (GCL; Milder et al., 2010), the rate-limiting enzyme in glutathione (GSH) synthesis. While the free radical scavenging ability of GPx is well documented (Ziegler et al., 2003), the increase in GCL is particularly critical, given that GSH is depleted after seizure activity (Liang & Patel, 2006) and increased GCL facilitates an increase in endogenous levels of GSH (Jarrett et al., 2008; Milder et al., 2010). The connection between Nrf2 and antioxidant regulation is also seen in the rodent kidney through application of the redox cycling agent paraquat. Paraquat redox cycles after receiving an electron from cellular sources in the presence of oxygen to generate superoxide and H_2O_2, which disrupt the electron transport chain, further generating substantial superoxide in addition to reducing nuclear Nrf2 and GSH levels, as well as activity of SOD and CAT (Wei et al., 2014). In congruence with previous studies, injection of βHB 5 to 7 days before infusion of paraquat in rats caused a decrease in lipid peroxidation, and interestingly maintained levels of nuclear Nrf2 and GSH in addition to maintaining activity of CAT and SOD (Wei et al., 2014). In summary, the effects of ketone bodies on the Nrf2 pathway are apparent in the central and peripheral nervous systems and have both high protective and therapeutic functions.

A second pathway that is altered by the KD is the Forkhead box (FoxO) pathway. A substantial quantity of literature outlines FoxO modulation of mitochondrial antioxidant enzyme transcription, and the FoxO pathway is thought to play a role in KD-facilitated ROS reduction. As mentioned previously, βHB has been shown to be an inhibitor of class I and II histone deacetylases, but notably not class III deacetylases, which include NAD$^+$-dependent sirtuins, which likely facilitate FoxO expression and antioxidant activity (Brunet et al., 2004; Kong et al., 2017). More specifically, βHB injected onto human embryonic kidney cells in vitro produced inhibition of class I and II histone deacetylase activity at histones H3$_{K9}$ and H3$_{K14}$ (Shimazu et al., 2013). Further analysis by the Shimazu group showed that the sites of increased acetylation corresponded to the promotor regions of the oxidative stress resistance genes of the FoxO3a pathway, with particular upregulation of the proteins FoxO3a and one of its target proteins, SOD (Shimazu et al., 2013). This finding was replicated in cardiomyocytes (Nagao et al., 2016) and PC12 neuronal culture cells (Kong et al., 2017); in the latter, βHB application not only produced an increase in FoxO3a but also provided a decrease in NOX2 and NOX4 in the rodent spinal cord (Kong et al., 2017). Conversely, FoxO-deficient hematopoietic stem cells display increased ROS as a result of altered expression of ROS-regulating genes, such as *SOD2* and *Gpx1* (Tothova et al., 2007); despite the increase in SOD activity following upregulation of FoxO3a, however, FoxO3a has since been shown to also produce antioxidant effects independent of SOD activity (Ferber et al., 2012).

REGULATION OF THE NAD$^+$:NADH RATIO BY KD

NAD is a cofactor present in all living cells that plays a role in several key cellular processes, including cellular respiration and DNA repair. Increases in the NAD$^+$:NADH ratio are expected, given the significant decrease in NAD$^+$ utilization during ketone metabolism compared to glucose metabolism, and it is proposed that the antiseizure effects of the KD may be explained in part by NAD$^+$:NADH-based alterations in redox status (Maalouf et al., 2007) and its modulation of potassium and calcium channel conductance (Elamin et al., 2017). Indeed, during increased oxidative stress, levels of NAD$^+$ are decreased (Hasan-Olive et al., 2019), and increasing the NAD$^+$:NADH ratio via exogenous application of NAD$^+$ diminishes ROS in cultured retinal pigment epithelium cells (Zhu et al., 2016). Ketone bodies specifically have also been shown to increase this ratio in the rodent hippocampus just 2 days after diet onset (Elamin et al., 2017), and KD-induced ketosis produces elevated nuclear SIRT1 expression in rats as a result of increased NAD$^+$ expression (Elamin et al., 2018). Furthermore, exogenous application of βHB in vitro facilitates increases in ATP production and ETC efficiency in addition to an increased NAD$^+$:NADH ratio (Hasan-Olive et al., 2019; Marosi et al., 2016). The mechanisms behind these positive outcomes may involve the increased activity of NAD-dependent deacetylases SIRT1 and SIRT3, which, as mentioned, are activators of the FoxO pathway.

INCREASED EXPRESSION OF UNCOUPLING PROTEINS BY KD

The transition of adenosine diphosphate (ADP) to ATP via ATP synthase is dependent upon the establishment of a proton gradient across the inner mitochondrial membrane. The production of superoxide is paired to the proton gradient, with increased negative potentials producing more ROS by restricting proton leak into the matrix (Sullivan et al., 2003); in turn, ROS-generated electrophiles, such as 4-HNE, may activate uncoupling proteins (UCPs) to dissipate the proton gradient in a negative feedback loop, thereby decreasing future ROS production (Echtay et al., 2003; Sullivan et al., 2003). The mechanisms that mediate this process are unclear; however, data on uncoupling protein 2 (UCP2) specifically suggest that interactions with GSH decrease proton conductance of the channel during basal conditions, while ROS-induced disruptions of this interaction activate UCP2 (Mailloux et al., 2011). In any case, despite varied distributions of uncoupling protein subtypes throughout the body, the KD has been shown to play a role in enhancing the expression of UCPs in various tissues, with noted elevations in UCP2 expression in the liver after only 8 weeks on the diet and persisting over several months

(Douris et al., 2015). Further, in the rodent hippocampus, the KD has been shown to increase the levels of UCP2, UCP4, and UCP5, concomitant with a 15% decrease in ROS (Sullivan et al., 2004), and in cardiac tissue not only has UCP3 been shown to be upregulated following H_2O_2 and 4-HNE exposure, but also the upregulation was dependent on activity of the Nrf2 pathway, as evident when siRNA knockdown of Nrf2 inhibited an increase in UCP3 expression (Anedda et al., 2013; Lopez-Bernardo et al., 2015). Interestingly, there are data that suggest that the FoxO transcription factors play a regulatory role in UCP expression; however, this avenue of research has not been explored fully (Liu et al., 2016).

CONCLUSIONS

Although the effectiveness of the KD in epilepsy has been known for over 100 years, the metabolic actions underlying its protective effects in epilepsy and other conditions are still being discovered. Several significant advances have led to key metabolic and redox-specific areas of focus that appear to work in concert to provide the therapeutic benefits of the KD (see figure 30.1). As the field of metabolism is revisited by epilepsy researchers, and animal models are guided by precision medicine, the connections between redox processes and metabolism will be further illuminated.

ACKNOWLEDGMENTS

The authors acknowledge the National Institutes of Neurological Disorders and Stroke for funding (NINDS grants R01NS039587 and R01NS086423) and BioRender for illustration support.

REFERENCES

Anedda, A., Lopez-Bernardo, E., Acosta-Iborra, B., Saadeh Suleiman, M., Landazuri, M. O., & Cadenas, S. (2013). The transcription factor Nrf2 promotes survival by enhancing the expression of uncoupling protein 3 under conditions of oxidative stress. *Free Radical Biology and Medicine, 61*, 395–407.

Banning, A., Deubel, S., Kluth, D., Zhou, Z., & Brigelius-Flohe, R. (2005). The *GI-GPx* gene is a target for Nrf2. *Molecular Cell Biology, 25*, 4914–4923.

Brunet, A., Sweeney, L. B., Sturgill, J. F., Chua, K. F., Greer, P. L., Lin, Y., Tran, H., Ross, S. E., Mostoslavsky, R., Cohen, H. Y., Hu, L. S., Cheng, H., Jedrychowski, M. P., Gygi, S. P., Sinclair, D. A., Alt, F. W., & Greenberg M. E. (2004). Stress-dependent regulation of FOXO transcription factors by the SIRT1 deacetylase. *Science, 303*, 2011–2015.

Calderon, N., Betancourt, L., Hernandez, L., & Rada, P. (2017). A ketogenic diet modifies glutamate, gamma-aminobutyric acid and agmatine levels in the hippocampus of rats: A microdialysis study. *Neuroscience Letters, 642*, 158–162.

Cooper, M. A., McCoin, C., Pei, D., Thyfault, J. P., Koestler, D., & Wright, D. E. (2018). Reduced mitochondrial reactive oxygen species production in peripheral nerves of mice fed a ketogenic diet. *Experimental Physiology, 103*, 1206–1212.

Douris, N., Melman, T., Pecherer, J. M., Pissios, P., Flier, J. S., Cantley, L. C., Locasale, J. W., & Maratos-Flier, E. (2015). Adaptive changes in amino acid metabolism permit normal longevity in mice consuming a low-carbohydrate ketogenic diet. *Biochimica et Biophysica Acta, 1852*, 2056–2065.

Echtay, K. S., Esteves, T. C., Pakay, J. L., Jekabsons, M. B., Lambert, A. J., Portero-Otin, M., Pamplona, R., Vidal-Puig, A. J., Wang, S., Roebuck, S. J., & Brand, M. D. (2003). A signalling role for 4-hydroxy-2-nonenal in regulation of mitochondrial uncoupling. *EMBO Journal, 22*, 4103–4110.

Elamin, M., Ruskin, D. N., Masino, S. A., & Sacchetti, P. (2017). Ketone-based metabolic therapy: Is increased NAD(+) a primary mechanism? *Frontiers in Molecular Neuroscience, 10*, 377.

Elamin, M., Ruskin, D. N., Masino, S. A., & Sacchetti, P. (2018). Ketogenic diet modulates NAD^+-dependent enzymes and reduces DNA damage in hippocampus. *Frontiers in Cellular Neuroscience, 12*, 263.

Ferber, E. C., Peck, B., Delpuech, O., Bell, G. P., East, P., & Schulze, A. (2012). FOXO3a regulates reactive oxygen metabolism by inhibiting mitochondrial gene expression. *Cell Death and Differentiation, 19*, 968–979.

Foster, D. W. (2012). Malonyl-CoA: The regulator of fatty acid synthesis and oxidation. *Journal of Clinical Investigation, 122*, 1958–1959.

Fukao, T., Song, X. Q., Mitchell, G. A., Yamaguchi, S., Sukegawa, K., Orii, T., & Kondo, N. (1997). Enzymes of ketone body utilization in human tissues: Protein and messenger RNA levels of succinyl-coenzyme A (CoA):3-ketoacid CoA transferase and mitochondrial and cytosolic acetoacetyl-CoA thiolases. *Pediatric Research, 42*, 498–502.

Hasan-Olive, M. M., Lauritzen, K. H., Ali, M., Rasmussen, L. J., Storm-Mathisen, J., & Bergersen, L. H. (2019). A ketogenic diet improves mitochondrial biogenesis and bioenergetics via the PGC1α-SIRT3-UCP2 axis. *Neurochemical Research, 44*, 22–37.

Heischmann, S., Gano, L. B., Quinn, K., Liang, L. P., Klepacki, J., Christians, U., Reisdorph, N., & Patel, M. (2018). Regulation of kynurenine metabolism by a ketogenic diet. *Journal of Lipid Research, 59*, 958–966.

Jarrett, S. G., Milder, J. B., Liang, L. P., & Patel, M. (2008). The ketogenic diet increases mitochondrial glutathione levels. *Journal of Neurochemistry, 106*, 1044–1051.

Kong, G., Huang, Z., Ji, W., Wang, X., Liu, J., Wu, X., Huang, Z., Li, R., & Zhu, Q. (2017). The ketone metabolite β-hydroxybutyrate attenuates oxidative stress in spinal cord injury by suppression of class I histone deacetylases. *Journal of Neurotrauma, 34*, 2645–2655.

Liang, L. P., & Patel, M. (2006). Seizure-induced changes in mitochondrial redox status. *Free Radical Biology and Medicine, 40*, 316–322.

Licha, D., Vidali, S., Aminzadeh-Gohari, S., Alka, O., Breitkreuz, L., Kohlbacher, O., Reischl, R. J., Feichtinger, R. G., Kofler, B., & Huber, C. G. (2019). Untargeted metabolomics reveals molecular effects of ketogenic diet on healthy and tumor xenograft mouse models. *International Journal of Molecular Science, 20*(16), 3873.

Liu, L., Tao, Z., Zheng, L. D., Brooke, J. P., Smith, C. M., Liu, D., Long, Y. C., & Cheng, Z. (2016). FoxO1 interacts with transcription factor EB and differentially regulates mitochondrial uncoupling proteins via autophagy in adipocytes. *Cell Death Discovery, 2*, 16066.

Lopez-Bernardo, E., Anedda, A., Sanchez-Perez, P., Acosta-Iborra, B., & Cadenas, S. (2015). 4-Hydroxynonenal induces Nrf2-mediated UCP3 upregulation in mouse cardiomyocytes. *Free Radical Biology and Medicine, 88*, 427–438.

Maalouf, M., Sullivan, P. G., Davis, L., Kim, D. Y., & Rho, J. M. (2007). Ketones inhibit mitochondrial production of reactive oxygen species production following glutamate excitotoxicity by increasing NADH oxidation. *Neuroscience, 145*, 256–264.

Mailloux, R. J., Seifert, E. L., Bouillaud, F., Aguer, C., Collins, S., & Harper, M. E. (2011). Glutathionylation acts as a control switch for uncoupling proteins UCP2 and UCP3. *Journal of Biological Chemistry, 286*, 21865–21875.

Marosi, K., Kim, S. W., Moehl, K., Scheibye-Knudsen, M., Cheng, A., Cutler, R., Camandola, S., & Mattson, M. P. (2016). 3-Hydroxybutyrate regulates energy metabolism and induces BDNF expression in cerebral cortical neurons. *Journal of Neurochemistry, 139*, 769–781.

Mazzuferi, M., Kumar, G., van Eyll, J., Danis, B., Foerch, P., & Kaminski, R. M. (2013). Nrf2 defense pathway: Experimental evidence for its protective role in epilepsy. *Annals of Neurology, 74*, 560–568.

Merry, T. L., & Ristow, M. (2016). Nuclear factor erythroid-derived 2-like 2 (NFE2L2, Nrf2) mediates exercise-induced mitochondrial biogenesis and the anti-oxidant response in mice. *Journal of Physiology, 594*, 5195–5207.

Milder, J. B., Liang, L. P., & Patel, M. (2010). Acute oxidative stress and systemic Nrf2 activation by the ketogenic diet. *Neurobiology of Disease, 40*, 238–244.

Nagao, M., Toh, R., Irino, Y., Mori, T., Nakajima, H., Hara, T., Honjo, T., Satomi-Kobayashi, S., Shinke, T., Tanaka, H., Ishida, T., & Hirata, K. (2016). β-Hydroxybutyrate elevation as a compensatory response against oxidative stress in cardiomyocytes. *Biochemical and Biophysical Research Communications, 475*, 322–328.

Noh, H. S., Lee, H. P., Kim, D. W., Kang, S. S., Cho, G. J., Rho, J. M., & Choi, W. S. (2004). A cDNA microarray analysis of gene expression profiles in rat hippocampus following a ketogenic diet. *Molecular Brain Research, 129*, 80–87.

Orii, K. E., Fukao, T., Song, X. Q., Mitchell, G. A., & Kondo, N. (2008). Liver-specific silencing of the human gene encoding succinyl-CoA:3-ketoacid CoA transferase. *The Tohoku Journal of Experimental Medicine, 215*, 227–236.

Shekh-Ahmad, T., Eckel, R., Dayalan Naidu, S., Higgins, M., Yamamoto, M., Dinkova-Kostova, A. T., Kovac, S., Abramov, A. Y., & Walker, M. C. (2018). KEAP1 inhibition is neuroprotective and suppresses the development of epilepsy. *Brain, 141*, 1390–1403.

Shimazu, T., Hirschey, M. D., Newman, J., He, W., Shirakawa, K., Le Moan, N., Grueter, C. A., Lim, H., Saunders, L. R., Stevens, R. D., Newgard, C. B., Farese, R. V., Cabo, R., Ulrich, S., Akassoglou, K., & Verdin, E. (2013). Suppression of oxidative stress by beta-hydroxybutyrate, an endogenous histone deacetylase inhibitor. *Science, 339*, 211–214.

Sullivan, P. G., Dube, C., Dorenbos, K., Steward, O., & Baram, T. Z. (2003). Mitochondrial uncoupling protein-2 protects the immature brain from excitotoxic neuronal death. *Annals of Neurology, 53*, 711–717.

Sullivan, P. G., Rippy, N. A., Dorenbos, K., Concepcion, R. C., Agarwal, A. K., & Rho, J. M. (2004). The ketogenic diet increases mitochondrial uncoupling protein levels and activity. *Annals of Neurology, 55*, 576–580.

Suzuki, T., Muramatsu, A., Saito, R., Iso, T., Shibata, T., Kuwata, K., Kawaguchi, S.I., Iwawaki, T., Adachi, S., Suda, H., Morita, M., Uchida, K., Baird, L., & Yamamoto, M. (2019). Molecular mechanism of cellular oxidative stress sensing by Keap1. *Cell Reports, 28*, 746–758.

Tothova, Z., Kollipara, R., Huntly, B. J., Lee, B. H., Castrillon, D. H., Cullen, D. E., McDowell, E. P., Lazo-Kallanian, S., Williams, I. R., Sears, C., Armstrong, S. A., Passegue, E., DePinho, R. A., & Gilliland, D. G. (2007). FoxOs are critical mediators of hematopoietic stem cell resistance to physiologic oxidative stress. *Cell, 128*, 325–339.

Wei, T., Tian, W., Liu, F., & Xie, G. (2014). Protective effects of exogenous beta-hydroxybutyrate on paraquat toxicity in rat kidney. *Biochemical and Biophysical Research Communications, 447,* 666–671.

Wilson, L. A., Gemin, A., Espiritu, R., & Singh, G. (2005). ets-1 is transcriptionally up-regulated by H_2O_2 via an antioxidant response element. *FASEB Journal, 19,* 2085–2087.

Yudkoff, M., Daikhin, Y., Melo, T. M., Nissim, I., Sonnewald, U., & Nissim, I. (2007). The ketogenic diet and brain metabolism of amino acids: Relationship to the anticonvulsant effect. *Annual Review of Nutrition, 27,* 415–430.

Zarnowska, I., Wrobel-Dudzinska, D., Tulidowicz-Bielak, M., Kocki, T., Mitosek-Szewczyk, K., Gasior, M., & Turski, W. A. (2019). Changes in tryptophan and kynurenine pathway metabolites in the blood of children treated with ketogenic diet for refractory epilepsy. *Seizure, 69,* 265–272.

Zhu, H., Itoh, K., Yamamoto, M., Zweier, J. L., & Li, Y. (2005). Role of Nrf2 signaling in regulation of antioxidants and phase 2 enzymes in cardiac fibroblasts: Protection against reactive oxygen and nitrogen species-induced cell injury. *FEBS Letters, 579,* 3029–3036.

Zhu, Y., Zhao, K. K., Tong, Y., Zhou, Y. L., Wang, Y. X., Zhao, P. Q., & Wang, Z. Y. (2016). Exogenous NAD^+ decreases oxidative stress and protects H_2O_2-treated RPE cells against necrotic death through the up-regulation of autophagy. *Scientific Reports, 6,* 26322.

Ziegler, D. R., Ribeiro, L. C., Hagenn, M., Siqueira, I. R., Araujo, E., Torres, I. L., Gottfried, C., Netto, C. A., & Goncalves, C. A. (2003). Ketogenic diet increases glutathione peroxidase activity in rat hippocampus. *Neurochemical Research, 28,* 1793–1797.

Nicotinamide Adenine Dinucleotide as a Central Mediator of Ketogenic Therapy

MARWA ELAMIN, MD, DAVID N. RUSKIN, PHD,
SUSAN A. MASINO, PHD, AND PAOLA SACCHETTI, PHD

INTRODUCTION

Appreciation of the ketogenic diet (KD) as an effective therapy depends in part on understanding the biologic mechanisms that can explain its beneficial effects and on the documentation of what improvements are a direct consequence of KD consumption. So far, it has been well established that the KD is effective and long lasting in the treatment of different forms of pediatric (Neal et al., 2008, 2009) and adult epileptic seizures (Cervenka et al., 2017; Sharma et al., 2013; Sirven et al., 1999). Evidence of success continues to accumulate as more centers globally prescribe the diet and support families in its implementation as well as strive to collect long-term data (Bertoli et al., 2014; Gerges et al., 2019; Groleau et al., 2014; Heussinger et al., 2018; Tian et al., 2019). Correlations have been found between ketone levels in the blood and the CSF and the degree of seizure control in KD-treated children with epilepsy (Gilbert et al., 2000; Ruskin et al., 2018).

In the laboratory, a variety of in vivo and in vitro models have been pursued, sometimes with mixed results. Overall, it has been determined that the success of the KD in reducing neuronal excitability may depend on species, seizure model, and glucose concentration in vitro (Kawamura et al., 2014, 2016). In general, chronic seizure models in rats and mice that offer more clinically relevant models show clear benefits of the KD. Overall, the KD does not have a marked effect on baseline activity but has a large effect in reducing high-intensity (i.e., ATP-consuming) electrical activity (Blaise et al., 2015; Koranda et al., 2011; Ma et al., 2007; Viggiano et al., 2016). The KD is also potentially effective against epileptogenesis, as shown in laboratory models (Lusardi et al., 2015), through hypermethylation of DNA (Boison, 2017). A clear mode of action has not been demonstrated in the laboratory, although various degrees of benefits have been obtained in chronic seizure models in rats and mice.

Applications of this therapy to a wide range of other conditions, ranging from neurodevelopmental disorders (Camberos-Luna & Massieu, 2020) to cancer (Khodadadi et al., 2017; Klement et al., 2016; Lussier et al., 2016; Schmidt et al., 2011; Seyfried & Mukherjee, 2005; Zuccoli et al., 2010), have shown promising results. In addition, the KD has been promoted for weight reduction (Gomez-Arbelaez et al., 2016; Jenkins et al., 2009; Paoli, 2014; Partsalaki et al., 2012) and for treatment or reversal of type 2 diabetes and metabolic syndrome (Hussain et al., 2012; McKenzie et al., 2017; Tay et al., 2015; Volek et al., 2008, 2009; Westman et al., 2008; Yancy et al., 2005).

Furthermore, healthy, disease-free cells and animals can also benefit from KD therapy. The use of ketone bodies as an energy source appears to be associated with a healthier metabolic phenotype that renders cells more resistant to external insults. Ketogenic treatment decreased myocardial damage after ischemic injury, reduced lung injury after hemorrhagic shock, enhanced kidney resistance to oxidative stress, and protected neurons against glutamate-induced toxicity (Koustova et al., 2003; Noh et al., 2006; Shimazu et al., 2013; Zou et al., 2002). At the cognitive level, beneficial effects on learning and memory were reported (Brownlow et al., 2017; Newman et al., 2017). A KD in mice started at 8 weeks of age did not affect longevity (Douris et al., 2015); however, a KD started at midlife extended longevity and healthspan (Newman et al., 2017; Roberts et al., 2017).

Nevertheless, there is a necessity to understand the underlying mechanisms of the diet to better target diseases and populations, and to further develop appropriate dietary regimens and coadjutant therapies to enhance its beneficial effects. Multiple mechanisms have been proposed to explain the antiseizure and neuroprotective effects of the diet, such as enhanced mitochondrial biogenesis (Bough et al., 2006), decreased formation of reactive oxygen radicals (Sullivan et al., 2004), increased adenosine (Masino et al., 2011b; Masino & Rho, 2012), and decreased DNA methylation (Kobow et al., 2013; Lusardi et al., 2015). The sum of all these effects could contribute to the beneficial effects of the KD. However, the positive effects observed across diseases could also be explained by the KD-induced alteration of fundamental cellular processes ubiquitously present that result in changes in a variety of cells and organs. One such generalized process is energy production and the availability of nicotinamide adenine dinucleotide (NAD), an essential cofactor for this process. NAD is an important metabolic coenzyme that acts with, and is essential for, the functioning of enzymes. NAD is especially important for many redox reactions, notably glycolysis and cellular respiration (Johnson & Imai, 2018; Rustin et al., 1996). It is also a signaling molecule, a marker for cellular health, and is considered an anti-aging molecule. Our research and research by others point to the oxidized form of NAD (NAD$^+$) as a central molecule for mechanisms that could explain the disparate beneficial effects obtained after a KD regimen in diverse contexts.

ENERGY PRODUCTION AND NAD REDOX STATE

Metabolism Overview

Effective energy production and consumption are central to cells' health and proper functioning. Although alternative metabolic pathways exist, the bulk of cellular energy production is accomplished via the breakdown of glucose through glycolysis and cellular respiration, a multistep process that results in production of adenosine triphosphate (ATP), the major source of energy for metabolic reactions. Carbohydrates are quickly processed and digested by the gastrointestinal tract and provide a readily available source of glucose that can be absorbed by cells and fuel metabolic processes. Through the process of glycolysis, a single 6-carbon glucose molecule is converted to two 3-carbon pyruvate molecules (Lodish et al., 2000), which are each then converted to acetyl-CoA via oxidative phosphorylation. Subsequently,

each acetyl-CoA molecule enters the citric acid cycle to generate ATP. Further production of ATP molecules results from the process of chemiosmosis, fueled by energy carriers accumulated during the previous steps.

In the absence of carbohydrates, when circulating levels of glucose drop, hormonal signaling triggers the breakdown of glycogen, a temporary form of glucose storage, or, in its absence, the breakdown of lipids. The breakdown of lipids yields far larger amounts of energy (9 kcal/g) than carbohydrates (4 kcal/g), and lipid reserves should allow maintenance of body functions for several days under proper hydration. Lipolysis generates fatty acids (FAs), which are broken down in the liver via β-oxidation to acetyl-CoA and are further metabolized to the ketone bodies acetoacetate (AcAc) and (βHB). Once released into the bloodstream, ketone bodies enter the cells and undergo ketolysis to produce intermediates like acetyl-CoA (Fukao et al., 2004), which subsequently enter the citric acid cycle to produce ATP (Izuta et al., 2018; Krebs, 1970), through the same steps as glucose. A diet low in sugar and starches (low in carbohydrates) accompanied by increased fat consumption, such as the KD, will shift the dependence of energy production from glucose to ketone bodies (Masino, 2017) and promote the metabolic changes just highlighted.

Glucose versus Ketone Body-Based Metabolism and NAD Reduction

When glucose is oxidized, the following changes in nicotinamide adenine dinucleotide hydride (NADH; the reduced form of NAD) and ATP occur: during glycolysis, eight ATP are produced (from two NADH + two ATP); during oxidative phosphorylation, six ATP are produced (from two NADH); and during the citric acid cycle, with two molecules of acetyl-CoA, 24 ATP are made from 12 NADH + four FADH$_2$ + four GTP. In total, 38 ATP molecules are produced.

Note that in the electron transport chain, NADH and FADH will produce approximately three and two ATP, respectively, while GTP will produce one ATP (Ahmad et al., 2020; Lodish et al., 2000).

When βHB is converted to AcAc, it reduces one NAD$^+$ molecule to NADH (Figure 31.1, right), while AcAc molecules are converted to two acetyl-CoA molecules without the need to reduce NAD$^+$ molecules. Therefore, the yield of ATP for a molecule of βHB is 27 (24 from acetyl-CoA and three from NADH produced during the conversion

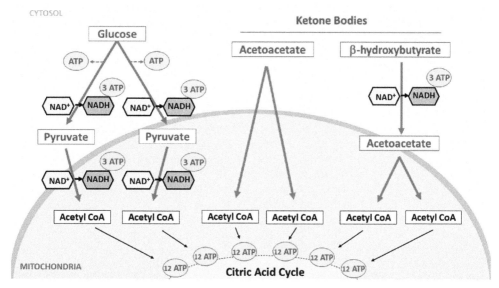

FIGURE 31.1 *Alternate Metabolic Pathways Whereby Glucose (left) Versus Ketone Bodies (right) Are Converted to ATP*

Note decreased NAD $^+$ consumption via ketone bodies versus glucose. See text for details. Used with permission from Elamin et al. (2020), *Epilepsy Research*. doi.org/10.1016/j.eplepsyres.2020.106469

step to AcAc), and the net yield of ATP for AcAc is 24 (from acetyl-CoA; Figure 31.1, right).

At first glance, glucose is more efficient in ATP production. To produce 1,000 ATP molecules, only 28 glucose molecules are needed, as compared to 37 βHB molecules and 42 AcAc molecules. But there are significant differences in NAD$^+$ reduction: glucose reduces 112 molecules of NAD$^+$, whereas βHB reduces 37, and AcAc reduces none. Accordingly, to produce comparable amounts of ATP, glucose-based metabolism reduces at least three times more NAD$^+$ molecules than ketone-based metabolism reduces. Considering that a single cortical neuron can consume 4.7 billion ATPs per second at rest (Zhu et al., 2012), it is reasonable to assume that the above-mentioned differences in NAD$^+$ utilization will have a significant effect on NAD redox state and the NAD$^+$/NADH ratio.

It is worth noting that studies have already shown that ketones are a more efficient fuel than glucose. A study looking at the hydraulic work and oxygen consumption of hearts metabolizing glucose versus ketone bodies uncovered that ketones increased fuel efficiency by 25% (Sato et al., 1995). Neurons grown in the presence of the ketone body βHB showed increased oxygen consumption and ATP production (Marosi et al., 2016). Multiple other studies also showed that

metabolizing ketone bodies in lieu of glucose led to significant increases in ATP production (Kim et al., 2010; Murray et al., 2016; Nylen et al., 2009), further confirming the higher efficiency of ketones as energy substrates.

Cellular Benefits of Increasing the NAD$^+$/NADH Ratio

Differential NAD$^+$ utilization is significant because NAD plays a central role as an oxidizing agent in a multitude of redox reactions. During redox reactions, NAD$^+$ accepts two electrons and a hydrogen and is converted to its reduced form, NADH. Electrons in NADH store energy that is utilized to run important reactions in the formation of ATP and, once the electrons are donated, NADH returns to its oxidized form, NAD$^+$.

The NAD$^+$/NADH redox couple regulates the cellular redox state and plays an essential role in glycolysis and oxidative phosphorylation, energy metabolism, mitochondrial function, and gene expression (Canto et al., 2015). Thus, alterations of the redox homeostasis can have tremendous impact on a multitude of biologic processes (Xiao et al., 2018). In particular, homeostasis of the NAD$^+$/NADH ratio is important to balance pro-oxidant and antioxidant factors in the cell. Oxidative eustress, a low level of oxidative stress, is beneficial to physiologic functions, and perturbation of the NAD^+/NADH balance induces an overproduction of reactive oxidative species (ROS). High levels of oxidative stress are detrimental and are linked to neuronal death and neurodegenerative diseases (Naoi et al., 2005). Overactive ROS damage macromolecules and affect cellular functions, with repercussion at the local and systemic levels (Dröge, 2002). Most ROS are produced in the mitochondria, with NADH as electron donor; thus, overreduction of NAD results in increased oxidative stress (Sies & Jones, 2020). In fact, it has been demonstrated that excess levels of cellular NADH can lead to ROS stress. For example, stress conditions like hypoxia increase cellular NADH levels and ROS production (Clanton, 2007; Oldham et al., 2015). Altering the NAD^+/NADH ratio can control the rate of ROS production (Kussmaul & Hirst, 2006) and impact downstream enzymatic levels and activities that regulate apoptosis and inflammation (Chen et al., 2008; Yeung et al., 2004; Zhu et al., 2011). Enhanced NAD^+/NADH should thus decrease inflammation, an effect observed in KD treatment (Dupuis et al., 2015; Forsythe et al., 2008; Nandivada et al., 2016; Ruskin et al., 2009, 2021; Yang & Cheng, 2010).

In general, catabolic reactions deplete NAD^+ pools, while anabolic reactions deplete NADH pools. Increasing the NAD^+/NADH ratio has multiple important implications: improved bioavailability of NAD^+ molecules has been linked to anti-aging (Scheibye-Knudsen et al., 2014), longevity (Van Der Veer et al., 2007; Zhang et al., 2016), and other potentially beneficial effects. For example, elevation in cellular NAD^+ levels in skeletal muscle and brown adipose tissue prevented high-fat diet-induced weight gain and obesity (Canto 2015). Conversely, aged mice showed a decrease in NAD^+ levels that correlated with mitochondrial dysfunction (Gomes AP, 2013). An increased NAD^+/NADH ratio was found to enhance mitochondrial function and protect against oxidative stress, and diverse research has shown that NAD molecules play an important role in cellular respiration, mitochondrial biogenesis, and redox reactions (Yang & Sauve, 2016). NAD^+ also serves as substrate for enzymes affecting cellular functions ranging from gene expression to posttranslational protein modifications, such as deacetylation and ADP-ribosylation (Belenky et al., 2007).

Overall, increasing the NAD^+/NADH ratio through ketone-enhancing treatments should protect against oxidative stress and enhance mitochondrial and cellular health.

KETOGENIC THERAPY MODULATES NAD^+ LEVELS

Fasting and ketosis induce an increase in the NAD^+/NADH ratio. We found clear evidence that metabolic therapy with a KD increases NAD^+/NADH, a mechanism that could compensate for metabolic dysregulation and serve as a common starting point for the diverse beneficial effects obtained with ketogenic treatments (Bough et al., 2008; Masino & Geiger, 2008). As already noted, a comparison of the metabolic pathways of glucose and ketone bodies (Figure 31.1) suggests that the use of ketone bodies as the main energy fuel requires fewer NAD^+ molecules than glucose (by a factor of four), which should lead to an increased cellular availability of this vital coenzyme. Experimental evidence suggests that ketone bodies are able to modulate NAD redox state in both health and disease. In vitro, dissociated neurons from C57BL/6 mice incubated with βHB for 24 hr showed increased NAD^+/NADH ratio and ATP production (Marosi et al., 2016), and treating rat hippocampal pyramidal neurons with ketone bodies resulted in an increase in NAD^+/NADH ratio and in oxygen consumption rate (Hasan-Olive et al., 2019). In vivo, the KD increases the hippocampal NAD^+/NADH ratio in healthy wild-type rats, and this increase appears to be rapid (within 2 days) and persistent (lasting at least 3 weeks; Elamin et al., 2017, 2018). Moreover, in healthy humans, nutritional ketosis achieved via ingestion of medium-chain triglyceride oils increases the NAD^+/NADH ratio (measured via ^{31}P magnetic resonance spectroscopy; Xin et al., 2018).

The relationship between the KD and NAD^+ is maintained under pathologic conditions. After 3 months of subcutaneous injections of ketone bodies, fresh cortical and hippocampal tissues extracted from mice with an Alzheimer-linked gene variant showed a significant increase in NAD^+/NADH ratio and ATP production (Yin et al., 2019). Application of the ketone bodies βHB and AcAc protected rat neocortical neurons from glutamate toxicity by increasing the NAD^+/NADH ratio (Maalouf et al., 2007). βHB or a ketone ester precursor showed protective effects by counterbalancing the decrease in NAD^+/NADH ratio in cases of neurotoxicity (Zhang et al., 2013). Furthermore, ketone ester treatment oxidized the cytoplasmic NAD^+/NADH couple in hippocampus and cortex in aged, affected Alzheimer's disease model mice, as well as reversed an apparent overoxidation of the mitochondrial couple in the hippocampus (Pawlosky et al., 2017), further confirming the ability of ketone bodies to modulate the NAD^+/NADH ratio. These studies suggest clear positive metabolic effects of ketolytic metabolism on NAD redox state.

Rapid increases in the NAD^+/NADH ratio could partially explain the ability of a KD to stop seizures in many patients within a few days of KD treatment (Freeman & Vining, 1999). For example, NAD^+ and NADH molecules can directly modulate the opening of ion channels important for neuronal excitability, such as ATP-sensitive and voltage-gated potassium channels (Dukes et al., 1994; Tipparaju et al., 2005). Accordingly, a rapid decrease in NAD^+ availability and consequent effect on neuronal excitability should be expected upon discontinuation of treatment. Interestingly, 15% of patients with refractory epilepsy experienced a rapid recurrence of seizures after KD discontinuation (Martinez et al., 2007); others remained seizure-free. The differential response among patients to treatment cessation indicates the existence of multiple downstream mechanisms and epigenetic changes (Lusardi et al., 2015; Masino & Rho, 2012) implicated in seizure control. Upregulation of key ketogenic enzymes, mainly mitochondrial 3-hydroxy-3-methylglutaryl-CoA synthase, after longer periods of ketogenic treatment (Cullingford et al., 2002) might also play a role in the maintenance of the beneficial effects even after discontinuation of the diet. More work is needed on downstream and lasting effects of metabolic therapy.

In summary, the metabolic pathways of glucose versus ketone bodies exert differential effects on NAD^+ reduction, and research has shown that a ketogenic treatment can modulate neuronal NAD redox state.

PROPOSED MECHANISMS OF KETOGENIC THERAPY AND THE CENTRAL ROLE OF NAD^+

The Importance of NAD for Mitochondrial Health

Replenishing or enhancing NAD^+ reserves seems to invigorate and restore cellular functions. Studies of aging have highlighted how the age-dependent decrease in NAD^+ impacts oxidative stress and metabolic and mitochondrial functions, and how replenishing NAD reserves improves aging processes. Depletion of NAD^+ levels resulting from accumulation of oxidative stress strongly correlates with age in both male and female human subjects (Massudi et al., 2012). In aged rats, the NAD^+/NADH ratio decreases, resulting in increased oxidative stress and diminished antioxidant capacities, but supplements return the ratio to young age levels and improve functions (Zhang et al. 2016).

The effects of NAD replenishment could be related to its beneficial role on mitochondrial function. NAD is an essential factor for mitochondrial ATP generation (Stein & Imai, 2012), and studies indicate NAD^+ is a rate-limiting factor for several mitochondrial processes (Alano et al., 2004; Bai et al., 2011). Indeed, increased NAD^+ levels were found to enhance mitochondrial function and to protect against oxidative stress damage (Kussmaul & Hirst, 2006; Pittelli et al., 2011). Cell lines and primary cultures exhibited an increase in mitochondrial ATP production and oxygen consumption after exogenous application of NAD (Kussmaul & Hirst, 2006; Lin & Guarente, 2003; Pittelli et al., 2011). Furthermore, circadian oscillations in mitochondrial NAD^+ synthesis were shown to be associated with enhanced mitochondrial respiration and ATP production (Peek et al., 2013).

Regarding the role of NAD^+ in ketogenic therapy, in vitro application of ketone bodies was shown to enhance mitochondrial respiration and to protect against excitotoxicity via increasing the NAD^+/NADH ratio in isolated cortical mitochondria (Maalouf et al., 2007). Neurons showed similar results, and the application of βHB increased the NAD^+/NADH ratio while enhancing mitochondrial oxygen consumption and ATP production (Marosi et al., 2016). As noted, ketone-based metabolism is associated with enhanced mitochondrial functions (Bough et al., 2006; Sook Noh et al., 2004) and upregulation of key mitochondrial enzymes (Cullingford et al., 2002), which can play a significant role in the control or prevention of epileptic seizures (Rahman, 2012; Waldbaum & Patel, 2010).

Considering the ability of NAD^+ to significantly enhance mitochondrial function in a manner similar to ketone-based metabolism (Kussmaul & Hirst, 2006; Maalouf et al., 2007; Marosi et al., 2016; Peek et al., 2013), it is reasonable to surmise that some of the beneficial effects of ketogenic therapy are mediated by NAD^+.

NAD+ as a Substrate for Key Cellular Enzymes

Low NAD+ levels could be due to a decrease in NAD+ production as well as increased consumption of NAD+ during cellular functions. In addition to being essential for redox reactions, NAD+ is central to pivotal enzymatic reactions where it is required as a substrate.

There are three main enzyme classes that consume NAD+: sirtuins, poly(ADP-ribose) polymerases (PARPs), and CD38. These NAD+-dependent enzymes affect multiple cellular functions, ranging from gene expression and posttranslational modification of proteins to deacetylation and ADP-ribosylation reactions in the cells (Belenky et al., 2007). The age-dependent depletion of NAD+ strongly correlated with overactivation of PARP and decreased sirtuin activity in male subjects (Massudi et al., 2012). Because sirtuins and PARPs are highly involved in epigenetic regulation, DNA repair, and RNA processing (Xie et al., 2020), they play an important role in diverse cell types and multiple organs.

It is worth noting that NAD+ is also a cofactor for CD38, or cyclic ADP ribose hydrolase, a glycoprotein found mostly on the surface of many immune cells (Cantó et al., 2013).

KD, NAD+, and Activation of Sirtuins

Sirtuins are a group of deacetylases (SIRT1–7) that use NAD+ as a main substrate (Michishita, 2005). Increasing the deacetylating activity of sirtuins can be achieved either by increasing gene expression levels, which subsequently increases the quantity of the enzymes, or by increasing cellular levels of NAD+ (Dali-Youcef et al., 2007; Landry et al., 2000; Revollo et al., 2004).

The most prominent and abundant member of this group is the nuclear SIRT1, whose main function is the deacetylation of several important targets that regulate apoptosis, inflammation, several growth factors, and transcription factors (Yang et al., 2006). SIRT2 is a cytosolic enzyme involved in the regulation of gluconeogenesis (Jiang et al., 2011) and central nervous system myelination (Beirowski et al., 2011), while SIRT4 is found to regulate fatty acid oxidation and mitochondrial gene expression (Nasrin et al., 2010). SIRT6 and SIRT7 are nuclear enzymes that are involved in decreasing age-associated DNA damage (McCord et al., 2009; Mostoslavsky et al., 2006; Vazquez et al., 2016). Hepatic SIRT6 is necessary for the ketogenic response to fasting and KD (Chen et al., 2019).

SIRT3 is the most abundant mitochondrial sirtuin (Michishita, 2005), and it plays a pivotal role in the regulation of mitochondrial respiration and fatty acid oxidation. In fact, mice lacking SIRT3 were phenotypically normal at baseline, but they exhibited severe metabolic irregularities during fasting, highlighting the role of SIRT3 in maintaining energy homeostasis (Hirschey et al., 2010). βHB application to cultured hippocampal neurons elevated SIRT3 expression that had been lowered by oxidative stress, part of a pathway enhancing mitochondrial bioenergetics (Hasan-Olive et al., 2019). βHB treatment in vivo also elevates SIRT3 levels lowered by human apolipoprotein E4 expression in the hippocampus and cortex of mice (Yin et al., 2019). Extracted hippocampi for Sprague-Dawley male rats treated with a KD exhibited a significant immediate (2 days) and persistent (3 weeks) increase in the NAD+/NADH ratio, associated with an increase in the collective activity of nuclear sirtuins (SIRT1, SIRT6, SIRT7), and a significant augmentation of *Sirt1* mRNA expression at 2 days (Elamin et al., 2018).

Increasing de novo NAD+ synthesis in *Caenorhabditis elegans* by inhibiting α-amino-β-carboxymuconate-ε-semialdehyde decarboxylase (an enzyme that limits NAD+ synthesis) increased SIRT1 activity, enhanced mitochondrial biogenesis, and increased oxygen consumption rate (Katsyuba et al., 2018), further affirming the link between NAD+, sirtuins, and mitochondrial health. Also, it has been hypothesized that one aspect of the neuroprotective effects of the KD is enhanced neuronal macroautophagy partially mediated by increased SIRT1 activity (McCarty et al., 2015).

Taken together, sirtuins impact a wide range of functions. Increasing NAD+ levels will have a direct effect on sirtuins' activity and may mediate the beneficial effects associated with all seven sirtuin subtypes (Dali-Youcef et al., 2007; Landry et al., 2000; Revollo et al., 2004). SIRT1 was shown to mediate the seizure-suppressing effects of the microRNA 199a-5p (Wang et al., 2016), highlighting the role of SIRT1 as a potential target for treating epilepsy. Administration of resveratrol, a well-known SIRT1 activator (Alcaín & Villalba, 2009), resulted in neuroprotection in a multitude of seizure models and showed synergistic effects with common antiepileptic drugs (Pallàs et al., 2014). In a temporal lobe epilepsy model, a decrease in NAD+ and a decrease in SIRT3 protein expression were uncovered in the acute and latent phases of epileptogenesis and are thought to contribute to disease pathogenesis (Gano et al., 2018). Hippocampal pyramidal neurons in KD-fed mice exhibited upregulation of SIRT3, and treatment of the dissociated cells with ketone bodies increased the $NAD^+/NADH$ ratio and oxygen consumption rates and improved mitochondrial biogenesis (Hasan-Olive et al., 2019).

It is important to note that sirtuin activity is not restricted to seizure inhibition but might also modulate neuronal death: in a model of acute acquired epilepsy, PARP1-mediated neuronal death exposed the compromised enzymatic activity of SIRT1. NAD repletion was able to enhance SIRT1 activity and resulted in decreased neuronal death (Wang et al., 2013). Taken together, these data affirm the positive role of sirtuins in the management of epilepsy and support the idea that NAD^+-driven activation of sirtuins is an important mechanism that may mediate the antiseizure effects of ketogenic therapy.

PARPs, DNA Damage, and Reactive Oxygen Species

The second NAD-dependent enzyme group is PARP, with PARP1 being the most abundantly expressed enzyme of the PARP family (Sodhi et al., 2010). This enzyme adds polymers of ADP-ribose into proteins, a process known as ADP-ribosylation that was first recognized for its important role in cell survival and DNA damage repair (de Murcia and de Murcia, 1994; Grube and Burkle, 1992). A steady-state level of DNA damage exists as a result of DNA oxidation by reactive oxygen species (ROS), a byproduct of normal cellular metabolism, and was reported to occur about 10,000 times per cell per day in humans and 50,000 times per cell per day in rats (Bernstein et al., 2013). PARP1 was previously described as a molecular sensor for this type of oxidative, naturally occurring, DNA damage (de Murcia & de Murcia, 1994), and it is considered as an important marker for damage, because levels of oxidative DNA damage were found to have an effect on both its activity (Dantzer et al., 2006) and protein levels (Shen et al., 2016). PARP1 was also found to play a role in gene transcription and programmed cell death (Kim et al., 2005).

PARP ribosylation reactions are major consumers of NAD^+ in the brain. Despite the fact that PARPs play a vital role in the DNA repair process, overactivation of PARPs (and the subsequent depletion of NAD^+) have been previously linked to several pathologic conditions, including MPTP-induced Parkinsonism, Alzheimer's disease, ischemic brain injury, and metalloproteinase-mediated neuronal death (Endres et al., 1997; Kauppinen & Swanson, 2005; Love et al., 1999; Mandir et al., 1999).

Inhibiting PARPs was previously shown to increase the cellular availability of NAD^+ (Hurtado-Bagès et al., 2020; Mendelsohn & Larrick, 2017). Animals treated with a KD for either 2 days or 3 weeks showed a significant decrease in hippocampal DNA damage and PARP1 protein levels (Elamin et al., 2018). This inhibition of PARP1 expression would be expected to augment the increase in NAD^+ that results from utilizing ketone bodies as an energy source (Figure 31.1) and further increase NAD^+ bioavailability. Indeed, KD-induced PARP inhibition was associated with increased NAD^+ (Elamin et al., 2018).

Ketogenic therapy decreased the formation of reactive oxygen radicals and reversed gene expression patterns of several genes that control ROS and oxidative stress in animal and cellular models (Maalouf et al., 2007; Stafford et al., 2010; Sullivan et al., 2004). Modification of cellular oxidative stress and ROS generation is important, since increased PARP1 activation and mitochondrial oxidative stress levels were shown to play a crucial role in epilepsy-associated neuronal death and to contribute to epileptogenesis (Waldbaum & Patel, 2010; Wang et al., 2013). Moreover, inhibition of PARP protected epileptic neurons in the hippocampus from cell death and preserved NAD^+ levels and mitochondrial respiration after status epilepticus (Lai et al., 2017; Yang et al., 2013).

The Interplay Among KD, NAD⁺, Sirtuins, and PARPs

In a positive feedback manner, KD-induced increases in NAD^+ should also mobilize other NAD^+-dependent mechanisms, such as sirtuins, to modify ROS generation and limit oxidative stress damage, which in turn should decrease PARP activity and protein levels, making more NAD^+ available. Sirtuins like SIRT2 can decrease oxidative stress by deacetylating FOXO3a, a well-known pro-apoptotic protein (Wang et al., 2007), and SIRT3 was found to mediate the decrease in ROS associated with caloric restriction (Qiu et al., 2010).

Hence, the collective paradigm of increasing NAD^+, inhibiting PARP1, and activating sirtuins might be a coherent strategy to protect neurons from epilepsy-induced cell death and a central part of the KD mechanism of action, mediating its observed effects in reducing oxidative stress and improving mitochondrial functions.

KD, NAD⁺, and Adenosine

The KD has been shown to increase activation of seizure-reducing adenosine A_1 receptors and to increase adenosine levels (Lusardi et al., 2015; Masino et al., 2011; Masino & Rho, 2012).

While there is no direct experimental evidence that we are aware of linking NAD^+, adenosine, and the KD, NAD^+ can be degraded into adenosine (Okuda et al., 2010; Zhang et al., 2018), possibly contributing to the increased adenosine levels, activation of adenosine A_1 receptors, and the seizure-suppressing effects (Kawamura et al., 2010; Masino et al., 2009, 2012).

Research has shown that S-adenosylhomocysteine hydrolase, an enzyme involved in adenosine biosynthesis, contains an NAD-binding domain that modulates its activity (Kloor et al., 2003). Last but not least, the NAD^+ precursor nicotinamide, in combination with adenosine, was shown to have strong protective effects against audiogenic seizures (Maitre et al., 1974), another potential link between NAD and adenosine that supports their role in working together to suppress seizures.

KD, NAD⁺, and Modulation of Ion Channels

A plethora of evidence suggests that the KD acts directly or indirectly on ion channels. In particular, multiple lines of evidence suggest that the KD can increase activation of ATP-sensitive K^+ channels (K_{ATP} channels) to decrease neuronal excitability (Giménez-Cassina et al., 2012; Kawamura et al., 2010, 2016; Tanner et al., 2011). In parallel, NAD is a known modulator of ionic transport, and several channels contain an NAD-binding domain (Kilfoil et al., 2013). Interestingly, NAD molecules can modulate K_{ATP} channels (Dukes et al., 1994) and directly interact with, and bind to, K_{ATP} channel subtypes (Dabrowski et al., 2003). Because of their ability to couple energy homeostasis to neuronal firing, K_{ATP} channels have been described as metabolic sensors (Olson & Terzic, 2010; Sun & Feng, 2013), and genetic defects of these channels can cause epilepsy, among other neurologic phenotypes (Olson & Terzic, 2010). Hence, it is not unreasonable to assume that NAD modulation of K_{ATP} is one of the mechanisms

through which ketogenic therapy exerts its antiepileptic effects.

Regarding other potassium channel subtypes, in vitro application of NAD^+ increased open time and open probability of the voltage-gated potassium channels Kvα1.5 and Kvβ1.3, which play a role in setting the resting membrane potential and regulating neuronal firing (Tipparaju et al., 2005; Yellen, 2002). The effects on Kvα1.5 and Kvβ1.3 currents appear to be specific to NAD^+ because application of NADH or NADPH did not achieve similar results (Tipparaju et al., 2005). Furthermore, physiologic concentrations of NAD^+, but not NADH, successfully modulated sodium-gated potassium channels (K_{Na}), Slack channels, and SLO potassium channels through direct binding (Kilfoil et al., 2013).

Finally, NAD^+ modulation of ion channels is not exclusive to potassium. Other channels that were shown to be directly modulated by NAD^+ include the calcium-permeable TRPM2 cation channel, the ryanodine receptor calcium release channel, and the voltage-gated $Na_v1.5$ sodium channels (Hara et al., 2002; Kilfoil et al., 2013; Liu et al., 2009; Zima et al., 2004). All of this supports the idea that the observed modulation of ion channel function with ketones or KD could be mediated via intracellular NAD^+.

SUMMARY AND PERSPECTIVE

Whereas glucose or ketone bodies can each produce molecules of ATP, ketone-based metabolism is associated with diverse cellular benefits and requires the conversion of far fewer (~ one third as many) molecules of NAD^+. Published research links ketone-based metabolism, altered levels of NAD^+, and multiple postulated antiseizure mechanisms mobilized by ketogenic therapies (Figure 31.2). A fundamental biochemical difference in NAD^+ may be a common starting point for multiple downstream mechanisms, and, therefore, it may explain the diverse beneficial effects of the KD in treating epilepsy and its emerging role in treating numerous additional disorders.

ACKNOWLEDGMENTS

Funding from the Schlumberger Foundation Faculty for the Future Award (ME), University of Hartford and Women's Advancement Initiative (PS), NIH grant AT008742 (DNR), and NIH grant NS065957 (SAM) is gratefully acknowledged.

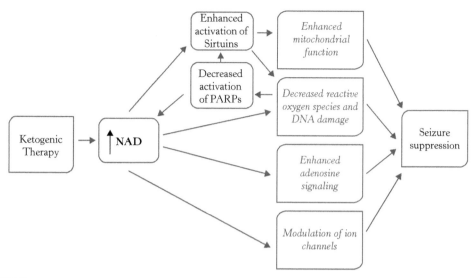

FIGURE 31.2 *Summary of the Proposed NAD-based Links Between Ketogenic Therapies and Suppression of Seizures*
See text for details. Used with permission from Elamin et al. (2020), *Epilepsy Research*. doi.org/10.1016/j.eplepsyres.2020.106469

REFERENCES

Aarhus, R., Graeff, R. M., Dickey, D. M., Walseth, T. F., & Lee, H. C. (1995). ADP-ribosyl cyclase and CD38 catalyze the synthesis of a calcium-mobilizing metabolite from NADP. *Journal of Biological Chemistry, 270*, 30327–30333. https://doi.org/10.1074/jbc.270.51.30327

Ahmad, M., Wolberg, A., & Kahwaji, C. I. (2020). Electron Transport Chain. In *Biochemistry* (Rev. ed.). StatPearls Publishing. https://www.ncbi.nlm.nih.gov/books/NBK526105/

Alano, C. C., Ying, W., & Swanson, R. A. (2004). Poly(ADP-ribose) polymerase-1-mediated cell death in astrocytes requires NAD+ depletion and mitochondrial permeability transition. *Journal of Biological Chemistry, 279*, 18895–18902. https://doi.org/10.1074/jbc.M313329200

Alcaín, F. J., & Villalba, J. M. (2009). Sirtuin activators. *Expert Opinion on Therapeutic Patents, 19*, 403–414. https://doi.org/10.1517/13543770902762893

Bai, P., Cantó, C., Oudart, H., Brunyánszki, A., Cen, Y., Thomas, C., Yamamoto, H., Huber, A., Kiss, B., Houtkooper, R. H., Schoonjans, K., Schreiber, V., Sauve, A. A., Menissier-De Murcia, J., & Auwerx, J. (2011). PARP-1 inhibition increases mitochondrial metabolism through SIRT1 activation. *Cell Metabolism, 13*, 461–468. https://doi.org/10.1016/j.cmet.2011.03.004

Beirowski, B., Gustin, J., Armour, S. M., Yamamoto, H., Viader, A., North, B. J., Michan, S., Baloh, R. H., Golden, J. P., Schmidt, R. E., Sinclair, D. A., Auwerx, J., & Milbrandt, J. (2011). Sir-two-homolog 2 (Sirt2) modulates peripheral myelination through polarity protein Par-3/atypical protein kinase C (aPKC) signaling. *Proceedings of the National Academy of Sciences, 108*, E952–E961. https://doi.org/10.1073/pnas.1104969108

Belenky, P., Bogan, K. L., & Brenner, C. (2007). NAD+ metabolism in health and disease. *Trends Biochemical Sciences, 32*, 12–19. https://doi.org/10.1016/j.tibs.2006.11.006

Bernstein, C. Prasad, A. R., Nfonsam, V., & Bernstei, H. (2013). DNA damage, DNA repair and cancer. In *New research directions in DNA repair* (pp. 413–466). Chen C. InTechOpen. https://doi.org/10.5772/53919

Bertoli, S., Trentani, C., Ferraris, C., De Giorgis, V., Veggiotti, P., & Tagliabue, A. (2014). Long-term effects of a ketogenic diet on body composition and bone mineralization in GLUT-1 deficiency syndrome: A case series. *Nutrition, 30*, 726–728. https://doi.org/10.1016/j.nut.2014.01.005

Blaise, J. H., Ruskin, D. N., Koranda, J. L., & Masino, S.A. (2015). Effects of a ketogenic diet on hippocampal plasticity in freely moving juvenile rats. *Physiological Reports, 3*, 12411. https://doi.org/10.14814/phy2.12411

Bough, K. J., Wetherington, J., Hassel, B., Pare, J. F., Gawryluk, J. W., Greene, J. G., Shaw, R., Smith, Y., Geiger, J. D., & Dingledine, R. J. (2006). Mitochondrial biogenesis in the anticonvulsant mechanism of the ketogenic diet. *Annals of Neurology, 60*, 223–235. https://doi.org/10.1002/ana.20899

Breen, L. T., Smyth, L. M., Yamboliev, I. A., & Mutafova-Yambolieva, V. N. (2006). β-NAD is a novel nucleotide released on stimulation of nerve terminals in human urinary bladder detrusor muscle. *American Journal of Physiology: Renal Physiology, 290,* F486–F495. https://doi.org/10.1152/ajprenal.00314.2005

Camberos-Luna, L., & Massieu, L. (2020). Therapeutic strategies for ketosis induction and their potential efficacy for the treatment of acute brain injury and neurodegenerative diseases. *Neurochemistry International, 133,* 104614. https://doi.org/10.1016/j.neuint.2019.104614

Cantó, C., Sauve, A. A., & Bai, P. (2013). Crosstalk between poly(ADP-ribose) polymerase and sirtuin enzymes. *Molecular Aspects of Medicine, 34,* 1168–1201. https://doi.org/10.1016/j.mam.2013.01.004

Cantó, C., Menzies, K. J., & Auwerx, J. (2015). NAD$^+$ metabolism and the control of energy homeostasis: A balancing act between mitochondria and the nucleus. *Cell Metabolism, 22,* 31–53. https://doi.org/10.1016/j.cmet.2015.05.023

Cervenka, M. C., Hocker, S., Koenig, M., Bar, B., Henry-Barron, B., Kossoff, E. H., Hartman, A. L., Probasco, J. C., Benavides, D. R., Venkatesan, A., Hagen, E. C., Dittrich, D., Stern, T., Radzik, B., Depew, M., Caserta, F. M., Nyquist, P., Kaplan, P. W., & Geocadin, R. G. (2017). Phase I/II multicenter ketogenic diet study for adult superrefractory status epilepticus. *Neurology, 88,* 938–943. https://doi.org/10.1212/WNL.0000000000003690

Chen, L., Liu, Q., Tang, Q., Kuang, J., Li, H., Pu, S., Wu, T., Yang, X., Li, R., Zhang, J., Zhang, Z., Huang, Y., Li, Y., Zou, M., Jiang, W., Li, T., Gong, M., Zhang, L., Wang, H., . . . He, J. (2019). Hepatocyte-specific Sirt6 deficiency impairs ketogenesis. *Journal of Biological Chemistry, 294,* 1579–1589. https://doi.org/10.1074/jbc.RA118.005309

Clanton, T. L. (2007). Hypoxia-induced reactive oxygen species formation in skeletal muscle. *Journal of Applied Physiology, 102,* 2379–2388. https://doi.org/10.1152/japplphysiol.01298.2006

Cullingford, T. E., Eagles, D. A., & Sato, H. (2002). The ketogenic diet upregulates expression of the gene encoding the key ketogenic enzyme mitochondrial 3-hydroxy-3-methylglutaryl-CoA synthase in rat brain. *Epilepsy Research, 49,* 99–107. https://doi.org/10.1016/S0920-1211(02)00011-6

Dabrowski, M., Trapp, S., & Ashcroft, F. M. (2003). Pyridine nucleotide regulation of the K_{ATP} channel Kir6.2/SUR1 expressed in *Xenopus* oocytes. *Journal of Physiology, 550,* 357–363. https://doi.org/10.1113/jphysiol.2003.041715

Dali-Youcef, N., Lagouge, M., Froelich, S., Koehl, C., Schoonjans, K., & Auwerx, J. (2007). Sirtuins: The "magnificent seven," function, metabolism and longevity. *Annals of Medicine, 39,* 335–345. https://doi.org/10.1080/07853890701408194

Dantzer, F., Amé, J., Schreiber, V., Nakamura, J., Ménissier-de Murcia, J., & de Murcia, G.

(2006). Poly(ADP-ribose) polymerase-1 activation during DNA damage and repair. *Methods in Enzymology, 409,* 493–510. https://doi.org/10.1016/S0076-6879(05)09029-4

de Murcia, G., & de Murcia, J. M. (1994). Poly(ADP-ribose) polymerase: A molecular nick-sensor. *Trends Biochemical Sciences, 19,* 172–176. https://doi.org/10.1016/0968-0004(94)90280-1

Dröge, W. (2002). Free radicals in the physiological control of cell function. *Physiological Reviews, 82,* 47–95. https://doi.org/10.1152/physrev.00018.2001

Dukes, L. D., McIntyre, M. S., Mertz, R. J., Philipson, L. H., Roe, M. W., Spencer, B., & Worley, J. F. (1994). Dependence on NADH produced during glycolysis for β-cell glucose signaling. *Journal of Biological Chemistry, 269,* 10979–10982.

Durnin, L., Dai, Y., Aiba, I., Shuttleworth, C. W., Yamboliev, I. A., & Mutafova-Yambolieva, V. N. (2012). Release, neuronal effects and removal of extracellular β-nicotinamide adenine dinucleotide (β-NAD$^+$) in the rat brain. *European Journal of Neuroscience, 35,* 423–435. https://doi.org/10.1111/j.1460-9568.2011.07957.x

Elamin, M., Ruskin, D. N., Masino, S. A., & Sacchetti, P. (2017). Ketone-based metabolic therapy: Is increased NAD$^+$ a primary mechanism? *Frontiers in Molecular Neuroscience, 10,* 377. https://doi.org/10.3389/fnmol.2017.00377

Elamin, M., Ruskin, D. N., Masino, S. A., & Sacchetti, P. (2018). Ketogenic diet modulates NAD$^+$-dependent enzymes and reduces DNA damage in hippocampus. *Frontiers in Cellular Neuroscience, 12,* 263. https://doi.org/10.3389/fncel.2018.00263

Endres, M., Wang, Z. Q., Namura, S., Waeber, C., & Moskowitz, M. A. (1997). Ischemic brain injury is mediated by the activation of poly(ADP-ribose) polymerase. *Journal of Cerebral Blood Flow & Metabolism, 17,* 1143–1151. https://doi.org/10.1097/00004647-199711000-00002

Freeman, J. M., & Vining, E. P. G. (1999). Seizures decrease rapidly after fasting: Preliminary studies of the ketogenic diet. *Archives of Pediatric and Adolescent Medicine, 153,* 946–949.

Fukao, T., Lopaschuk, G. D., & Mitchell, G. A. (2004). Pathways and control of ketone body metabolism: On the fringe of lipid biochemistry. *Prostaglandins, Leukotrienes & Essential Fatty Acids, 70,* 243–251. https://doi.org/10.1016/j.plefa.2003.11.001

Gano, L. B., Liang, L. P., Ryan, K., Michel, C. R., Gomez, J., Vassilopoulos, A., Reisdorph, N., Fritz, K. S., & Patel, M. (2018). Altered mitochondrial acetylation profiles in a kainic acid model of temporal lobe epilepsy. *Free Radical Biology And Medicine, 123,* 116–124. https://doi.org/10.1016/j.freeradbiomed.2018.05.063

Gerges, M., Selim, L., Girgis, M., El Ghannam, A., Abdelghaffar, H., & El-Ayadi, A. (2019).

Implementation of ketogenic diet in children with drug-resistant epilepsy in a medium resources setting: Egyptian experience. *Epilepsy and Behavior Case Reports, 11*, 35–38. https://doi.org/10.1016/j.ebcr.2018.11.001

Gilbert, D. L., Pyzik, P. L., & Freeman, J. M. (2000). The ketogenic diet: Seizure control correlates better with serum β-hydroxybutyrate than with urine ketones. *Journal of Child Neurology, 15*, 787–790. https://doi.org/10.1177/088307380001501203

Giménez-Cassina, A., Martínez-François, J. R., Fisher, J. K., Szlyk, B., Polak, K., Wiwczar, J., Tanner, G. R., Lutas, A., Yellen, G., & Danial, N. N. (2012). BAD-dependent regulation of fuel metabolism and K_{ATP} channel activity confers resistance to epileptic seizures. *Neuron, 74*, 719–730. https://doi.org/10.1016/j.neuron.2012.03.032

Groleau, V., Schall, J. I., Stallings, V. A., & Bergqvist, C. A. (2014). Long-term impact of the ketogenic diet on growth and resting energy expenditure in children with intractable epilepsy. *Developmental Medicine and Child Neurology, 56*, 898–904. https://doi.org/10.1111/dmcn.12462

Grube, K., & Burkle, A. (1992). Poly(ADP-ribose) polymerase activity in mononuclear leukocytes of 13 mammalian species correlates with species-specific life span. *Proceedings of the National Academy of Sciences, 89*, 11759–11763. https://doi.org/10.1073/pnas.89.24.11759

Haag, F., Adriouch, S., Braß, A., Jung, C., Möller, S., Scheuplein, F., Bannas, P., Seman, M., & Koch-Nolte, F. (2007). Extracellular NAD and ATP: Partners in immune cell modulation. *Purinergic Signalling, 3*, 71–81. https://doi.org/10.1007/s11302-006-9038-7

Hara, Y., Wakamori, M., Ishii, M., Maeno, E., Nishida, M., Yoshida, T., Yamada, H., Shimizu, S., Mori, E., Kudoh, J., Shimizu, N., Kurose, H., Okada, Y., Imoto, K., & Mori, Y. (2002). LTRPC2 Ca^{2+}-permeable channel activated by changes in redox status confers susceptibility to cell death. *Molecular Cell, 9*, 163–173. https://doi.org/10.1016/S1097-2765(01)00438-5

Hasan-Olive, M. M., Lauritzen, K. H., Ali, M., Rasmussen, L. J., Storm-Mathisen, J., & Bergersen, L. H. (2019). A ketogenic diet improves mitochondrial biogenesis and bioenergetics via the PGC1α-SIRT3-UCP2 axis. *Neurochemistry Research, 44*, 22–37. https://doi.org/10.1007/s11064-018-2588-6

Heussinger, N., Della Marina, A., Beyerlein, A., Leiendecker, B., Hermann-Alves, S., Dalla Pozza, R., & Klepper, J. (2018). 10 patients, 10 years—Long term follow-up of cardiovascular risk factors in Glut1 deficiency treated with ketogenic diet therapies: A prospective, multicenter case series. *Clinical Nutrition, 37*, 2246–2251. https://doi.org/10.1016/j.clnu.2017.11.001

Hewitt, J. Y. J. A. (1924). The metabolism of carbohydrates. Part III. The absorption of glucose, fructose and galactose from the small intestine. *Biochemical Journal, 18*, 161–170.

Hirschey, M. D., Shimazu, T., Goetzman, E., Jing, E., Schwer, B., Lombard, D. B., Grueter, C. A., Harris, C., Biddinger, S., Ilkayeva, O. R., Stevens, R. D., Li, Y., Saha, A. K., Ruderman, N. B., Bain, J. R., Newgard, C. B., Farese, R. V., Jr., Alt, F. W., Kahn, C. R., & Verdin, E. (2010). SIRT3 regulates mitochondrial fatty-acid oxidation by reversible enzyme deacetylation. *Nature, 464*, 121–125. https://doi.org/10.1038/nature08778

Hurtado-Bagès, S., Knobloch, G., Ladurner, A. G., & Buschbeck, M. (2020). The taming of PARP1 and its impact on NAD$^+$ metabolism. *Molecular Metabolism, 38*, 100950. https://doi.org/10.1016/j.molmet.2020.01.014

Izuta, Y., Imada, T., Hisamura, R., Oonishi, E., Nakamura, S., Inagaki, E., Ito, M., Soga, T., & Tsubota, K. (2018). Ketone body 3-hydroxybutyrate mimics calorie restriction via the Nrf2 activator, fumarate, in the retina. *Aging Cell, 17*, e12699. https://doi.org/10.1111/acel.12699

Johnson, S., & Imai, S. (2018). NAD$^+$ biosynthesis, aging, and disease. *F1000Research, 7*, 132. https://doi.org/10.12688/f1000research.12120.1

Kauppinen, T. M., & Swanson, R. A. (2005). Poly(ADP-ribose) polymerase-1 promotes microglial activation, proliferation, and matrix metalloproteinase-9-mediated neuron death. *Journal of Immunology, 174*, 2288–2296. https://doi.org/10.4049/jimmunol.174.4.2288

Kawamura, M., Ruskin, D. N., Geiger, J. D., Boison, D., & Masino, S. A. (2014). Ketogenic diet sensitizes glucose control of hippocampal excitability. *Journal of Lipid Research, 55*, 2254–2260. https://doi.org/10.1194/jlr.M046755

Kawamura, M., Ruskin, D. N., & Masino, S. A. (2010). Metabolic autocrine regulation of neurons involves cooperation among pannexin hemichannels, adenosine receptors, and KATP channels. *Journal of Neuroscience, 30*, 3886–3895. https://doi.org/10.1523/JNEUROSCI.0055-10.2010

Kawamura, M., Ruskin, D. N., & Masino, S. A. (2016). Metabolic therapy for temporal lobe epilepsy in a dish: Investigating mechanisms of ketogenic diet using electrophysiological recordings in hippocampal slices. *Frontiers in Molecular Neuroscience, 9*, 112. https://doi.org/10.3389/fnmol.2016.00112

Kilfoil, P. J., Tipparaju, S. M., Barski, O. A., & Bhatnagar, A. (2013). Regulation of ion channels by pyridine nucleotides. *Circulation Research, 112*, 721–741. https://doi.org/10.1161/CIRCRESAHA.111.247940

Kim, D. Y., Vallejo, J., & Rho, J. M. (2010). Ketones prevent synaptic dysfunction induced by mitochondrial respiratory complex inhibitors. *Journal of Neurochemistry, 114*, 130–141. https://doi.org/10.1111/j.1471-4159.2010.06728.x

Kim, J. E., Kim, Y. J., Kim, J. Y., & Kang, T. C. (2014). PARP1 activation/expression modulates regional-specific neuronal and glial responses to seizure in a hemodynamic-independent manner. *Cell Death & Disease*, 5, e1362–e1362. https://doi.org/10.1038/cddis.2014.331

Kim, M. Y., Zhang, T., & Kraus, W. L. (2005). Poly(ADP-ribosyl)ation by PARP-1: "PAR-laying" NAD+ into a nuclear signal. *Genes and Development*, 19, 1951–1967. https://doi.org/10.1101/gad.1331805

Kloor, D., Lüdtke, A., Stoeva, S., & Osswald, H. (2003). Adenosine binding sites at *S*-adenosyl-homocysteine hydrolase are controlled by the NAD⁺/NADH ratio of the enzyme. *Biochemical Pharmacology*, 66, 2117–2123. https://doi.org/10.1016/S0006-2952(03)00581-1

Koranda, J. L., Ruskin, D. N., Masino, S. A., & Harry Blaise, J. (2011). A ketogenic diet reduces long-term potentiation in the dentate gyrus of freely behaving rats. *Journal of Neurophysiology*, 106, 662–666. https://doi.org/10.1152/jn.00001.2011

Kossoff, E. H., Zupec-Kania, B. A., & Rho, J. M. (2009). Ketogenic diets: An update for child neurologists. *Journal of Child Neurology*, 24, 979–988. https://doi.org/10.1177/0883073809337162

Krebs, H. A. (1970). Rate control of the tricarboxylic acid cycle. *Advances in Enzyme Regulation*, 8, 335–353. https://doi.org/10.1016/0065-2571(70)90028-2

Kussmaul, L., & Hirst, J. (2006). The mechanism of superoxide production by NADH:ubiquinone oxidoreductase (complex I) from bovine heart mitochondria. *Proceedings in the National Academy of Sciences USA*, 103, 7607–7612. https://doi.org/10.1073/pnas.0510977103

Kuzmin, V. S., Pustovit, K. B., & Abramochkin, D. V. (2016). Effects of exogenous nicotinamide adenine dinucleotide (NAD⁺) in the rat heart are mediated by P_2 purine receptors. *Journal of Biomedical Sciences*, 23, 50. https://doi.org/10.1186/s12929-016-0267-y

Laffel, L. (1999). Ketone bodies: A review of physiology, pathophysiology and application of monitoring to diabetes. *Diabetes Metabolism Research and Reviews*, 15, 412–426. https://doi.org/10.1002/(sici)1520-7560(199911/12)15:6<412::aid-dmrr72>3.0.co;2-8.

Lai, Y. C., Scott Baker, J., Donti, T., Graham, B. H., Craigen, W. J., & Anderson, A. E. (2017). Mitochondrial dysfunction mediated by poly(ADP-ribose) polymerase-1 activation contributes to hippocampal neuronal damage following status epilepticus. *International Journal of Molecular Sciences*, 18, 1502. https://doi.org/10.3390/ijms18071502

Landry, J., Sutton, A., Tafrov, S. T., Heller, R. C., Stebbins, J., Pillus, L., & Sternglanz, R. (2000). The silencing protein SIR2 and its homologs are NAD-dependent protein deacetylases. *Proceedings in the National Academy of Sciences USA*, 97, 5807–11. https://doi.org/10.1073/pnas.110148297

Lefevre, F., & Aronson, N. (2000). Ketogenic diet for the treatment of refractory epilepsy in children: A systematic review of efficacy. *Pediatrics*, 105, e46. https://doi.org/10.1542/peds.105.4.e46

Lin, S. J., & Guarente, L. (2003). Nicotinamide adenine dinucleotide, a metabolic regulator of transcription, longevity and disease. *Current Opinions in Cellular Biology*, 15, 241–246. https://doi.org/10.1016/S0955-0674(03)00006-1

Liu, J., Yang, B., Zhou, P., Kong, Y., Hu, W., Zhu, G., Ying, W., Li, W., Wang, Y., & Li, S. (2017). Nicotinamide adenine dinucleotide suppresses epileptogenesis at an early stage. *Scientific Reports*, 7, 7321. https://doi.org/10.1038/s41598-017-07343-0

Liu, M., Sanyal, S., Gao, G., Gurung, I. S., Zhu, X., Gaconnet, G., Kerchner, L. J., Shang, L. L., Huang, C. L. H., Grace, A., London, B., & Dudley, S. C. (2009). Cardiac Na⁺ current regulation by pyridine nucleotides. *Circulation Research*, 105, 737–745. https://doi.org/10.1161/CIRCRESAHA.109.197277

Lodish, H., Berk, A., Matsudaira, P., Zipursky, L., Baltimore, D., & Darnell, J. (2000). *Molecular cell biology*. W. H. Freeman.

Love, S., Barber, R., & Wilcock, G. K. (1999). Increased poly(ADP-ribosyl)ation of nuclear proteins in Alzheimer's disease. *Brain*, 122, 247–253. https://doi.org/10.1093/brain/122.2.247

Lusardi, T. A., Akula, K. K., Coffman, S. Q., Ruskin, D. N., Masino, S. A., & Boison, D. (2015). Ketogenic diet prevents epileptogenesis and disease progression in adult mice and rats. *Neuropharmacology*, 99, 500–509. https://doi.org/10.1016/j.neuropharm.2015.08.007

Ma, W., Berg, J., & Yellen, G. (2007). Ketogenic diet metabolites reduce firing in central neurons by opening KATP channels. *Journal of Neuroscience*, 27, 3618–3625. https://doi.org/10.1523/JNEUROSCI.0132-07.2007

Maalouf, M., Sullivan, P. G., Davis, L., Kim, D. Y., & Rho, J. M. (2007). Ketones inhibit mitochondrial production of reactive oxygen species production following glutamate excitotoxicity by increasing NADH oxidation. *Neuroscience*, 145, 256–264. https://doi.org/10.1016/j.neuroscience.2006.11.065

Maher, F., Vannucci, S. J., & Simpson, I. A. (1994). Glucose transporter proteins in brain. *FASEB Journal*, 8, 1003–1011. https://doi.org/10.1096/fasebj.8.13.7926364

Maitre, M., Ciesielski, L., Lehmann, A., Kempf, E., & Mandel, P. (1974). Protective effect of adenosine and nicotinamide against audiogenic seizure. *Biochemical Pharmacology*, 23, 2807–2816. https://doi.org/10.1016/0006-2952(74)90054-9

Mandir, A. S., Przedborski, S., Jackson-Lewis, V., Wang, Z. Q., Simbulan-Rosenthal, C. M., Smulson, M. E., Hoffman, B. E., Guastella, D. B., Dawson, V. L., & Dawson, T. M. (1999). Poly(ADP-ribose) polymerase activation mediates 1-methyl-4-phenyl-1,2,3,6-tetrahydropyridine (MPTP)-induced parkinsonism. *Proceedings in the National Academy of Sciences USA, 96,* 5774–5779. https://doi.org/10.1165/rcmb.2004-0361OC

Marosi, K., Kim, S. W., Moehl, K., Scheibye-Knudsen, M., Cheng, A., Cutler, R., Camandola, S., & Mattson, M. P. (2016). 3-Hydroxybutyrate regulates energy metabolism and induces BDNF expression in cerebral cortical neurons. *Journal of Neurochemistry, 139,* 769–781. https://doi.org/10.1111/jnc.13868

Martinez, C. C., Pyzik, P. L., & Kossoff, E. H. (2007). Discontinuing the ketogenic diet in seizure-free children: Recurrence and risk factors. *Epilepsia, 48,* 187–190. https://doi.org/10.1111/j.1528-1167.2006.00911.x

Masino, S. A., Kawamura, M., Ruskin, D. N., Geiger, J. D., & Boison, D. (2012). Purines and neuronal excitability: Links to the ketogenic diet. *Epilepsy Research, 100,* 229–238. https://doi.org/10.1016/j.eplepsyres.2011.07.014

Masino, S., Kawamura, M., Jr., Wasser, C., Pomeroy, L., & Ruskin, D. (2009). Adenosine, ketogenic diet and epilepsy: The emerging therapeutic relationship between metabolism and brain activity. *Current Neuropharmacology, 7,* 257–268. https://doi.org/10.2174/157015909789152164

Masino, S. A., Li, T., Theofilas, P., Sandau, U. S., Ruskin, D. N., Fredholm, B. B., Geiger, J. D., Aronica, E., & Boison, D. (2011). A ketogenic diet suppresses seizures in mice through adenosine A_1 receptors. *Journal of Clinical Investigation, 121,* 2679–2683. https://doi.org/10.1172/JCI57813

Masino, S. A., & Rho, J. M. (2012). Mechanism of ketogenic diet action. In Noebels, J. L., Avoli, M., Rogawski, M. A., et al. (eds.), *Jasper's basic mechanisms of the epilepsies* (pp. 1003–1018). National Center for Biotechnology Information.

Masino, S. A., & Rho, J. M. (2019). Metabolism and epilepsy: Ketogenic diets as a homeostatic link. *Brain Research, 1703,* 26–30. https://doi.org/10.1016/j.brainres.2018.05.049

Massudi, H., Grant, R., Braidy, N., Guest, J., Farnsworth, B., & Guilleman, G. J. (2012). Age-associated changes in oxidative stress and NAD⁺ metabolism in human tissue. *PLOS ONE, 7,* Article e42357. https://doi.org/10.1371/journal.pone.0042357

McCarty, M. F., DiNicolantonio, J. J., & O'Keefe, J. H. (2015). Ketosis may promote brain macroautophagy by activating SIRT1 and hypoxia-inducible factor-1. *Medical Hypotheses, 85,* 631–639. https://doi.org/10.1016/j.mehy.2015.08.002

McCord, R. A., Michishita, E., Hong, T., Berber, E., Boxer, L. D., Kusumoto, R., Guan, S., Shi, X., Gozani, O., Burlingame, A. L., Bohr, V. A., & Chua, K. F. (2009). SIRT6 stabilizes DNA-dependent protein kinase at chromatin for DNA double-strand break repair. *Aging, 1,* 109–121. https://doi.org/10.18632/aging.100011

Mendelsohn, A. R., & Larrick, J. W. (2017). The NAD⁺/PARP1/SIRT1 axis in aging. *Rejuvenation Research, 20,* 244–247. https://doi.org/10.1089/rej.2017.1980

Michishita, E. (2005). Evolutionarily conserved and nonconserved cellular localizations and functions of human SIRT proteins. *Molecular Biology of the Cell, 16,* 4623–4635. https://doi.org/10.1091/mbc.E05-01-0033

Mostoslavsky, R., Chua, K. F., Lombard, D. B., Pang, W. W., Fischer, M. R., Gellon, L., Liu, P., Mostoslavsky, G., Franco, S., Murphy, M. M., Mills, K. D., Patel, P., Hsu, J. T., Hong, A. L., Ford, E., Cheng, H. L., Kennedy, C., Nunez, N., Bronson, R., . . . Alt, F. W. (2006). Genomic instability and aging-like phenotype in the absence of mammalian SIRT6. *Cell, 124,* 315–329. https://doi.org/10.1016/j.cell.2005.11.044

Murray, A. J., Knight, N. S., Cole, M. A., Cochlin, L. E., Carter, E., Tchabanenko, K., Pichulik, T., Gulston, M. K., Atherton, H. J., Schroeder, M. A., Deacon, R. M. J., Kashiwaya, Y., King, M. T., Pawlosky, R., Rawlins, J. N. P., Tyler, D. J., Griffin, J. L., Robertson, J., Veech, R. L., & Clarke, K. (2016). Novel ketone diet enhances physical and cognitive performance. *FASEB Journal, 30,* 4021–4032. https://doi.org/10.1096/fj.201600773R

Mutafova-Yambolieva, V. N., Sung, J. H., Hao, X., Chen, H., Zhu, M. X., Wood, J. D., Ward, S. M., & Sanders, K. M. (2007). β-Nicotinamide adenine dinucleotide is an inhibitory neurotransmitter in visceral smooth muscle. *Proceedings of the National Academy of Sciences USA, 104,* 16359–16364. https://doi.org/10.1073/pnas.0705510104

Nasrin, N., Wu, X., Fortier, E., Feng, Y., Bar, O. C., Chen, S., Ren, X., Wu, Z., Streeper, R. S., & Bordone, L. (2010). SIRT4 regulates fatty acid oxidation and mitochondrial gene expression in liver and muscle cells. *Journal of Biological Chemistry, 285,* 31995–32002. https://doi.org/10.1074/jbc.M110.124164

Neal, E. G., Chaffe, H., Schwartz, R. H., Lawson, M. S., Edwards, N., Fitzsimmons, G., Whitney, A., & Cross, J. H. (2008). The ketogenic diet for the treatment of childhood epilepsy: A randomised controlled trial. *Lancet Neurology, 7,* 500–506. https://doi.org/10.1016/S1474-4422(08)70092-9

Nylen, K., Velazquez, J. L. P., Sayed, V., Gibson, K. M., Burnham, W. M., & Snead, O. C. (2009). The effects of a ketogenic diet on ATP concentrations and the number of hippocampal mitochondria in Aldh5a1⁻/⁻ mice. *Biochimica et Biophysica Acta*

- *General Subjects, 1790,* 208–212. https://doi.org/10.1016/j.bbagen.2008.12.005

Okuda, H., Higashi, Y., Nishida, K., Fujimoto, S., & Nagasawa, K. (2010). Contribution of P2X7 receptors to adenosine uptake by cultured mouse astrocytes. *Glia, 58,* 1757–1765. https://doi.org/10.1002/glia.21046

Oldham, W. M., Clish, C. B., Yang, Y., & Loscalzo, J. (2015). Hypoxia-mediated increases in l-2-hydroxyglutarate coordinate the metabolic response to reductive stress. *Cell Metabolism, 22,* 291–303. https://doi.org/10.1016/j.cmet.2015.06.021

Olson, T. M., & Terzic, A. (2010). Human K_{ATP} channelopathies: Diseases of metabolic homeostasis. *Pflugers Archiv European Journal of Physiology, 460,* 295–306. https://doi.org/10.1007/s00424-009-0771-y

Pallàs, M., Ortuño-Sahagún, D., Andrés-Benito, P., Ponce-Regalado, M. D., & Rojas-Mayorquín, A. E. (2014). Resveratrol in epilepsy: Preventive or treatment opportunities? *Frontiers in Bioscience-Landmark, 19,* 1057–1064. https://doi.org/10.2741/4267

Paoli, A. (2014). Ketogenic diet for obesity: Friend or foe? *International Journal of Environmental Research and Public Health, 11,* 2092–2107. https://doi.org/10.3390/ijerph110202092

Peek, C. B., Affinati, A. H., Ramsey, K. M., Kuo, H. Y., Yu, W., Sena, L. A., Ilkayeva, O., Marcheva, B., Kobayashi, Y., Omura, C., Levine, D. C., Bacsik, D. J., Gius, D., Newgard, C. B., Goetzman, E., Chandel, N. S., Denu, J. M., Mrksich, M., & Bass, J. (2013). Circadian clock NAD^+ cycle drives mitochondrial oxidative metabolism in mice. *Science, 342,* 1243417. https://doi.org/10.1126/science.1243417

Pittelli, M., Felici, R., Pitozzi, V., Giovannelli, L., Bigagli, E., Cialdai, F., Romano, G., Moroni, F., & Chiarugi, A. (2011). Pharmacological effects of exogenous NAD on mitochondrial bioenergetics, DNA repair, and apoptosis. *Molecular Pharmacology, 80,* 1136–1146. https://doi.org/10.1124/mol.111.073916

Pulford, D. S. (1927). Ketogenic diets for epileptics. *Western Journal of Medicine,27,* 50–56.

Qiu, X., Brown, K., Hirschey, M. D., Verdin, E., & Chen, D. (2010). Calorie restriction reduces oxidative stress by SIRT3-mediated SOD2 activation. *Cell Metabolism, 12,* 662–667. https://doi.org/10.1016/j.cmet.2010.11.015

Rahman, S. (2012). Mitochondrial disease and epilepsy. *Developmental Medicine in Child Neurology, 54,* 397–406. https://doi.org/10.1111/j.1469-8749.2011.04214.x

Revollo, J. R., Grimm, A. A., & Imai, S. I. (2004). The NAD biosynthesis pathway mediated by nicotinamide phosphoribosyltransferase regulates Sir2 activity in mammalian cells. *Journal of Biological Chemistry, 279,* 50754–50763. https://doi.org/10.1074/jbc.M408388200

Ruskin, D. N., Kawamura, M., Jr., & Masino, S. A. (2009). Reduced pain and inflammation in juvenile and adult rats fed a ketogenic diet. *PLOS ONE, 4,* Article e8349. https://doi:10.1371/journal.pone.0008349

Ruskin, D. N., Sturdevant, I. C., Wyss, L. S., & Masino, S. A. (2021). Ketogenic diet effects on inflammatory allodynia and ongoing pain in rodents. *Scientific Reports, 11,* 725. https://doi.org/10.1038/s41598-020-80727-x

Rustin, P., Parfait, B., Chretien, D., Bourgeron, T., Djouadi, F., Bastin, J., Rötig, A., & Munnich, A. (1996). Fluxes of nicotinamide adenine dinucleotides through mitochondrial membranes in human cultured cells. *Journal of Biological Chemistry, 271,* 14785–14790. https://doi.org/10.1074/jbc.271.25.14785

Sato, K., Kashiwaya, Y., Keon, C. A., Tsuchiya, N., King, M. T., Radda, G. K., Chance, B., Clarke, K., & Veech, R. L. (1995). Insulin, ketone-bodies, and mitochondrial energy transduction. *FASEB Journal, 9,* 651–658.

Sharma, S., Sankhyan, N., Gulati, S., & Agarwala, A. (2013). Use of the modified Atkins diet for treatment of refractory childhood epilepsy: A randomized controlled trial. *Epilepsia, 54,* 481–486. https://doi.org/10.1111/epi.12069

Shen, Y., McMackin, M. Z., Shan, Y., Raetz, A., David, S., & Cortopassi, G. (2016). Frataxin deficiency promotes excess microglial DNA damage and inflammation that is rescued by PJ34. *PLOS ONE, 11,* Article e0151026. https://doi.org/10.1371/journal.pone.0151026

Sies, H., & Jones, D. P. (2020). Reactive oxygen species (ROS) as pleiotropic physiological signalling agents. *Nature Reviews in Molecular and Cellular Biology, 21,* 363–383. https://doi.org/10.1038/s41580-020-0230-3

Sirven, J., Whedon, B., Caplan, D., Liporace, J., Glosser, D., O'Dwyer, J., & Sperling, M. R. (1999). The ketogenic diet for intractable epilepsy in adults: Preliminary results. *Epilepsia, 40,* 1721–1726. https://doi.org/10.1111/j.1528-1157.1999.tb01589.x

Smyth, L. M., Bobalova, J., Mendoza, M. G., Lew, C., & Mutafova-Yambolieva, V. N. (2004). Release of β-nicotinamide adenine dinucleotide upon stimulation of postganglionic nerve terminals in blood vessels and urinary bladder. *Journal of Biological Chemistry, 279,* 48893–48903. https://doi.org/10.1074/jbc.M407266200

Sodhi, R. K., Singh, N., & Jaggi, A. S. (2010). Poly(ADP-ribose) polymerase-1 (PARP-1) and its therapeutic implications. *Vascular Pharmacology, 53,* 77–87. https://doi.org/10.1016/j.vph.2010.06.003

Sook Noh, H., Po Lee, H., Wook Kim, D., Soo Kang, S., Jae Cho, G., Rho, J. M., & Sung Choi, W. (2004). A cDNA microarray analysis of gene expression profiles in rat hippocampus following a ketogenic diet. *Molecular and Brain*

Research, *129*, 80–87. https://doi.org/10.1016/j.molbrainres.2004.06.020

Stafford, P., Abdelwahab, M. G., Kim, D. Y., Preul, M. C., Rho, J. M., & Scheck, A. C. (2010). The ketogenic diet reverses gene expression patterns and reduces reactive oxygen species levels when used as an adjuvant therapy for glioma. *Nutrition and Metabolism*, *7*, 74. https://doi.org/10.1186/1743-7075-7-74

Stein, L. R., & Imai, S. (2012). The dynamic regulation of NAD metabolism in mitochondria. *Trends in Endocrinology & Metabolism*, *23*, 420. https://doi.org/10.1016/J.TEM.2012.06.005

Sullivan, P. G., Rippy, N. A., Dorenbos, K., Concepcion, R. C., Agarwal, A. K., & Rho, J. M. (2004). The ketogenic diet increases mitochondrial uncoupling protein levels and activity. *Annals of Neurology*, *55*, 576–580. https://doi.org/10.1002/ana.20062

Sun, H. S., & Feng, Z. P. (2013). Neuroprotective role of ATP-sensitive potassium channels in cerebral ischemia. *Acta Pharmacologica. Sinica*, *34*, 24–32. https://doi.org/10.1038/aps.2012.138

Tanner, G. R., Lutas, A., Martínez-François, J. R., & Yellen, G. (2011). Single K_{ATP} channel opening in response to action potential firing in mouse dentate granule neurons. *Journal of Neuroscience*, *31*, 8689–8696. https://doi.org/10.1523/JNEUROSCI.5951-10.2011

Tian, X., Chen, J., Zhang, J., Yang, X., Ji, T., Zhang, Yao, Wu, Y., Fang, F., Wu, X., & Zhang, Y. (2019). The efficacy of ketogenic diet in 60 Chinese patients with Dravet syndrome. *Frontiers in Neurology*, *10*, 625. https://doi.org/10.3389/fneur.2019.00625

Tipparaju, S. M., Saxena, N., Liu, S.-Q., Kumar, R., & Bhatnagar, A. (2005). Differential regulation of voltage-gated K^+ channels by oxidized and reduced pyridine nucleotide coenzymes. *American Journal of Physiology- Cell Physiology*, *288*, C366–C376. https://doi.org/10.1152/ajpcell.00354.2004

Vazquez, B. N., Thackray, J. K., Simonet, N. G., Kane-Goldsmith, N., Martinez-Redondo, P., Nguyen, T., Bunting, S., Vaquero, A., Tischfield, J. A., & Serrano, L. (2016). SIRT7 promotes genome integrity and modulates non-homologous end joining DNA repair. *EMBO Journal*, *35*, 1488–1503. https://doi.org/10.15252/embj.201593499

Verderio, C., Bruzzone, S., Zocchi, E., Fedele, E., Schenk, U., De Flora, A., & Matteoli, M. (2001). Evidence of a role for cyclic ADP-ribose in calcium signalling and neurotransmitter release in cultured astrocytes. *Journal of Neurochemistry*, *78*, 646–657. https://doi.org/10.1046/j.1471-4159.2001.00455.x

Viggiano, A., Stoddard, M., Pisano, S., Operto, F. F., Iovane, V., Monda, M., & Coppola, G. (2016). Ketogenic diet prevents neuronal firing increase within the substantia nigra during pentylenetetrazole-induced seizure in rats. *Brain Research Bulletin*, *125*, 168–172. https://doi.org/10.1016/j.brainresbull.2016.07.001

Waldbaum, S., & Patel, M. (2010). Mitochondria, oxidative stress, and temporal lobe epilepsy. *Epilepsy Research*, *88*, 23–45. https://doi.org/10.1016/j.eplepsyres.2009.09.020

Wang, D., Li, Z., Zhang, Y., Wang, G., Wei, M., Hu, Y., Ma, S., Jiang, Y., Che, N., Wang, X., Yao, J., & Yin, J. (2016). Targeting of microRNA-199a-5p protects against pilocarpine-induced status epilepticus and seizure damage via SIRT1-p53 cascade. *Epilepsia*, *57*, 706–716. https://doi.org/10.1111/epi.13348

Wang, F., Nguyen, M., Qin, F. X. F., & Tong, Q. (2007). SIRT2 deacetylates FOXO3a in response to oxidative stress and caloric restriction. *Aging Cell*, *6*, 505–514. https://doi.org/10.1111/j.1474-9726.2007.00304.x

Wang, S., Yang, X., Lin, Y., Qiu, X., Li, H., Zhao, X., Cao, L., Liu, X., Pang, Y., Wang, X., & Chi, Z. (2013). Cellular NAD depletion and decline of SIRT1 activity play critical roles in PARP-1-mediated acute epileptic neuronal death in vitro. *Brain Research*, *1535*, 14–23. https://doi.org/10.1016/j.brainres.2013.08.038

Wigglesworth, V. B. (1924). Studies on ketosis: I. The relation between alkalosis and ketosis. *Biochemistry Journal*, *18*, 1203–1216.

Xiao, W., Wang, R.-S., Handy, D. E., & Loscalzo, J. (2018). NAD(H) and NADP(H) redox couples and cellular energy metabolism. *Antioxidant and Redox Signaling*, *28*, 251–272. https://doi.org/10.1089/ars.2017.7216.

Xie, N., Zhang, L., Gao, W., Huang, C., Huber, P. E., Zhou, X., Li, C., Shen, G., & Zou, B. (2020). NAD^+ metabolism: Pathophysiologic mechanisms and therapeutic potential. *Signal Transduction and Targeted Therapy*, *5*, 227. https://doi.org/10.1038/s41392-020-00311-7

Xin, L., Ipek, Ö., Beaumont, M., Shevlyakova, M., Christinat, N., Masoodi, M., Greenberg, N., Gruetter, R., & Cuenoud, B. (2018). Nutritional ketosis increases NAD^+/NADH ratio in healthy human brain: An in vivo study by ^{31}P-MRS. *Frontiers in Nutrition*, *5*, 62. https://doi.org/10.3389/fnut.2018.00062

Yang, T., Fu, M., Pestell, R., & Sauve, A. A. (2006). SIRT1 and endocrine signaling. *Trends in Endocrinology and Metabolism*, *17*, 186–191. https://doi.org/10.1016/j.tem.2006.04.002

Yang, X., Wang, S., Lin, Y., Han, Y., Qiu, X., Zhao, X., Cao, L., Wang, X., & Chi, Z. (2013). Poly(ADP-ribose) polymerase inhibition protects epileptic hippocampal neurons from apoptosis via suppressing Akt-mediated apoptosis-inducing factor translocation in vitro. *Neuroscience*, *231*, 353–362. https://doi.org/10.1016/j.neuroscience.2012.11.009

Yellen, G. (2002). The voltage-gated potassium channels and their relatives. *Nature, 419*, 35–42. https://doi.org/10.1038/nature00978

Yin, J., Nielsen, M., Li, S., & Shi, J. (2019). Ketones improve apolipoprotein E4-related memory deficiency via sirtuin 3. *Aging, 11*, 4579–4586. https://doi.org/10.18632/aging.102070

Zhang, H., Ryu, D., Wu, Y., Gariani, K., Wang, X., Luan, P., D'Amico, D., Ropelle, E. R., Lutolf, M. P., Aebersold, R., Schoonjans, K., Menzies, K. J., & Auwerx, J. (2016). NAD$^+$ repletion improves mitochondrial and stem cell function and enhances life span in mice. *Science, 352*, 1436–1443. https://dio.org/10.1126/science.aaf2693

Zhang, J., Wang, C., Shi, H., Wu, D., & Ying, W. (2018). Extracellular degradation into adenosine and the activities of adenosine kinase and AMPK mediate extracellular NAD$^+$-produced increases in the adenylate pool of BV2 microglia under basal conditions. *Frontiers in Cellular Neuroscience, 12*, 343. https://doi.org/10.3389/fncel.2018.00343

Zhu, X. H., Qiao, H., Du, F., Xiong, Q., Liu, X., Zhang, X., Ugurbil, K., & Chen, W. (2012). Quantitative imaging of energy expenditure in human brain. *Neuroimage, 60*, 2107–2117. https://doi.org/10.1016/j.neuroimage.2012.02.013

Zima, A. V., Copello, J. A., & Blatter, L. A. (2004). Effects of cytosolic NADH/NAD$^+$ levels on sarcoplasmic reticulum Ca^{2+} release in permeabilized rat ventricular myocytes. *Journal of Physiology, 555*, 727–741. https://doi.org/10.1113/jphysiol.2003.055848

SECTION IV

Ketone-Based Metabolism

*General Health and
Metabolic Alternatives*

32

Overview

Ketone-Based Metabolism—General Health and Metabolic Alternatives

DOMINIC P. D'AGOSTINO, PHD

Since 2010, there has been a sharp increase in basic science research on ketone-based therapies that has elucidated their roles in metabolic control and signaling. The rapid rise of high-impact peer-reviewed publications and public interest in this topic has advanced the science of ketone-based metabolism into many human clinical trials, but more federal funding is needed.

The ketone bodies β-hydroxybutyrate (BHB) and acetoacetate (AcAc) are produced from fatty acids in the liver and serve as alternative energy sources for the brain, heart, skeletal muscle, and peripheral tissues during prolonged fasting, calorie restriction, strenuous exercise, or adherence to a high-fat, low-carbohydrate ketogenic diet (KD; Cahill & Veech, 2003). Ketones have historically been labeled as abnormal metabolic byproducts of a pathologic state (VanItallie & Nufert, 2003), particularly due to their association with diabetic ketoacidosis (DKA) in uncontrolled type 1 diabetes, but emerging interest has focused on nutritional ketosis as a powerful metabolic therapy for general health and for a growing number of medical conditions in addition to drug-resistant epilepsy, where its use is well established (Stafstrom & Rho, 2012). Nutritional ketosis produces a nonpathologic hyperketonemia resulting from decreased glucose availability, lower insulin, and increased fat oxidation; however, long-term maintenance of the KD can be difficult for some and requires strict adherence. The restrictive nature of the KD has limited the clinical applicability of therapeutic ketosis due to practical considerations. Emerging data suggest that many of the benefits of the KD are mechanistically attributable to the ketone bodies or specific medium-chain triglycerides (MCTs), and this has motivated investigators to develop strategies to further augment the efficacy of the KD or to use metabolic-based supplements to circumvent the

need for dietary restriction, to improve compliance and the maintenance of the therapeutic state (Newman & Verdin, 2014; Veech, 2004). This section, "Ketone-Based Metabolism: General Health and Metabolic Alternatives," includes chapters that discuss the expanding medical and performance applications of nutritional ketosis and the emerging science of ketones and other related metabolites as alternative fuels and potent signaling molecules.

The physiologic shift into hyperketonemia through fasting or the KD is known to produce acute and chronic changes in metabolic physiology and molecular signaling pathways that provide therapeutic effects in varied disease states. Metabolic-based mechanisms of ketone therapies include an elevation of blood ketones and associated anaplerosis, with reduced blood glucose, increased insulin sensitivity, improved mitochondrial efficiency, suppressed oxidative stress, reduced inflammation, activation of signaling pathways, and epigenetic modulation. The reported benefits of hyperketonemia and similar metabolic alternatives have generated significant interest in the science and application of implementing strategies for inducing and sustaining blood levels of specific metabolites (Kesl et al., 2016). Most exogenous ketone supplements and engineered anaplerotic agents are currently under investigation for their potential benefits to both healthy and diseased individuals alike. It is likely that most of the conditions that are responsive to KD therapies would receive some benefit from exogenous ketone supplementation by elevating blood ketones and lowering blood glucose (Cahill & Veech, 2003). Currently, the most studied type of exogenous ketone would be ketone esters, which induce a dose-dependent hyperketonemia (1–7 mM) in rats, mice, dogs, pigs, and humans (Birkhahn & Border, 1978; Clarke et al.,

2012; Desrochers et al., 1995; Pascual et al., 2014). A case study of Alzheimer's disease highlighted the application in humans (Newport et al., 2015). There are a growing number of promising metabolic alternatives to ketone esters, and many of these agents and formulas are being evaluated for their therapeutic efficacy, practical application, and potential synergy with the KD (Borges & Sonnewald, 2012; Kesl et al., 2016). Importantly, ketone supplementation and metabolic alternatives provide a tool for achieving ketosis in patients who are unable, unwilling, or uninterested in consuming the KD or a low-carbohydrate diet.

Included in this section are chapters that discuss conditions for which ketones and metabolic alternatives have the most potential, including seizure disorders, glucose transporter type 1 deficiency syndrome (GLUT1DS), Alzheimer's disease (AD), brain tumors and metastatic cancer, insulin resistance and type 2 diabetes mellitus (T2DM), weight loss, and performance. GLUT1DS is a rare genetic disorder caused by a mutation in the *SLC2A1* gene, which encodes glucose transporter type 1. Patients with GLUT1DS have impaired glucose transport into the brain and other tissues, and thus alternative energy substrates in the form of ketones or other metabolic alternatives offer a means for the metabolic management of the disorder (Pascual et al., 2014). A known hallmark of AD is impaired brain glucose metabolism, which is associated with neurodegeneration and rapid progression (Cunnane et al., 2016). Preclinical data demonstrate that ketones protect against AD development and slow its progression (Kashiwaya et al., 2013). Cancer is another disorder potentially treated with nutritional ketosis due its metabolic phenotype, which is highly glycolytic, has abnormal mitochondrial structure and function (Seyfried et. al. 2014), and displays the Warburg effect, which is sometimes responsive to ketogenic therapies (Poff et al., 2017). This section discusses the research showing that ketone-based metabolism has pleotropic effects associated with enhanced insulin sensitivity (Kashiwaya et al., 1997), anticatabolic effects (Koutnik et al., 2019), antiseizure effects (Poff et al., 2019), and beneficial effects on brain signaling associated with behavior (Kovács, 2019). Indeed, the emerging literature shows that exogenous ketone supplementation can have a profound effect on metabolic control, inflammation, oxidative stress, and even cardiovascular function, especially in those with type 2 diabetes (Walsh et al., 2020).

Included in this section is a chapter by Poff et al. (Chapter 33) that describes the development and testing of exogenous ketone supplements, the diseases they are being investigated for use in, and the potential mechanisms of action of their therapeutic efficacy. The chapter by Kovács et al. (Chapter 34) takes a deep dive into how exogenous ketone supplements exert their beneficial effects on treatment-resistant neurodegenerative and behavioral disorders through modulation of mitochondrial function, ketone receptors, histone deacetylases, and inflammasome-linked signaling. The chapter by Hartman (Chapter 35) covers how specific amino acids (like D-leucine) influence molecular signaling to exert antiseizure effects. The chapter by Walker and Williams (Chapter 36) gives an overview of the acute in vitro and in vivo studies of the MCT decanoic acid, which imparts specific signaling effects by directly inhibiting AMPA receptors. Thus, the data demonstrate a novel metabolism-independent mechanism of MCTs, which were previously thought to be only a nutritional support for enhancing ketogenesis. Also included in this section is a chapter (Chapter 37) by Borges on triheptanoin, the triglyceride of heptanoate (C7 fatty acid), a safe and promising metabolic alternative that appears useful for a variety of conditions that respond to anaplerotic treatment. The chapter by Stafstrom et al. (Chapter 38) discusses inhibition of glycolysis as one way that the KD suppresses seizures and how 2-deoxy-D-glucose (2DG) is an antiglycolytic tool that has antiseizure effects in numerous seizure models. The chapter by Westman et al. (Chapter 39) reviews the rationale and recent clinical research supporting the use of ketogenic therapies for appetite reduction, weight loss, and improvements in glycemic and insulin control in individuals with obesity and T2DM. The chapter by Stubbs et al. (Chapter 40) discusses how exogenous ketones provide a promising tool for manipulating numerous processes implicated in exercise performance, recovery, and training adaptation. The last chapter in this section, by Beth Zupec-Kania and Jim Abrahams, reviews the genesis and ongoing efforts of the Charlie Foundation and Matthew's Friends in promoting the global awareness of ketogenic therapies for epilepsy, various cancers, and other neurologic and neurodegenerative disorders.

The chapters in this section aim to help the reader gain an appreciation for the science and emerging applications of nutritional ketosis, ketone supplementation, and other metabolic alternatives. As more basic science and clinical research trials (listed on clinicaltrials.gov) help to advance the science and human application of ketone metabolic therapies, it is inevitable that these metabolic tools will be utilized for the treatment and prevention of a broad range of disease states.

REFERENCES

Birkhahn, R. H., & Border, J. R. (1978). Intravenous feeding of the rat with short chain fatty acid esters: II. Monoacetoacetin. *American Journal of Clinical Nutrition, 31,* 436–441.

Borges, K., & Sonnewald, U. (2012). Triheptanoin: A medium chain triglyceride with odd chain fatty acids; A new anaplerotic anticonvulsant treatment? *Epilepsy Research, 100,* 239–244.

Cahill, G. F., Jr., & Veech, R. L. (2003). Ketoacids? Good medicine? *Transactions of the American Clinical and Climatological Association, 114,* 149–161; discussion 162–143.

Clarke, K., Tchabanenko, K., Pawlosky, R., Carter, E., Todd King, M., Musa-Veloso, K., Ho, M., Roberts, A., Robertson, J., Vanitallie, T. B., & Veech, R. L. (2012). Kinetics, safety and tolerability of (R)-3-hydroxybutyl (R)-3-hydroxybutyrate in healthy adult subjects. *Regulatory Toxicology and Pharmacology, 63,* 401–408.

Cunnane, S. C., Courchesne-Loyer, A., St-Pierre, V., Vandenberghe, C., Pierotti, T., Fortier, M., Croteau, E., & Castellano, C. A. (2016). Can ketones compensate for deteriorating brain glucose uptake during aging? Implications for the risk and treatment of Alzheimer's disease. *Annals of the New York Academy of Sciences, 1367*(1), 12–20.

Desrochers, S., Dubreuil, P., Brunet, J., Jette, M., David, F., Landau, B. R., & Brunengraber, H. (1995). Metabolism of (R,S)-1,3-butanediol acetoacetate esters, potential parenteral and enteral nutrients in conscious pigs. *American Journal of Physiology, 268,* E660–E667.

Kashiwaya, Y., King, M. T., & Veech, R. L. (1997). Substrate signaling by insulin: A ketone bodies ratio mimics insulin action in heart. *American Journal of Cardiology, 80,* 50A–64A.

Kashiwaya, Y., Bergman, C., Lee, J. H., Wan, R., King, M. T., Mughal, M. R., Okun, E., Clarke, K., Mattson, M. P., & Veech, R. L. (2013). A ketone ester diet exhibits anxiolytic and cognition-sparing properties, and lessens amyloid and tau pathologies in a mouse model of Alzheimer's disease. *Neurobiology of Aging, 34,* 1530–1539.

Kesl, S. L., Poff, A. M., Ward, N. P., Fiorelli, T. N., Ari, C., Van Putten, A. J., Sherwood, J. W., Arnold, P., & D'Agostino, D. P. (2016). Effects of exogenous ketone supplementation on blood ketone, glucose, triglyceride, and lipoprotein levels in Sprague-Dawley rats. *Nutrition & Metabolism, 13,* 9.

Koutnik, A. P., D'Agostino, D. P., & Egan, B. (2019). The anti-catabolic effects of ketone bodies. *Trends in Endocrinology and Metabolism, 30*(4), 227–229. https://doi.org/10.1016/j.tem.2019.01.006

Kovács, Z., D'Agostino, D. P., Diamond, D., Kindy, M. S., Rogers, C. Q., & Ari, C. (2019). Therapeutic potential of exogenous ketone supplement induced ketosis in the treatment of psychiatric disorders: Review of current literature. *Frontiers in Psychiatry, 10,* 363. https://doi.org/10.3389/fpsyt.2019.0036

Newman, J. C., & Verdin, E. (2014). Ketone bodies as signaling metabolites. *Trends in Endocrinology and Metabolism, 25,* 42–52.

Newport, M. T., VanItallie, T. B., Kashiwaya, Y., King, M. T., & Veech, R. L. (2015). A new way to produce hyperketonemia: Use of ketone ester in a case of Alzheimer's disease. *Alzheimer's and Dementia, 11,* 99–103.

Pascual, J. M., Liu, P., Mao, D., Kelly, D. I., Hernandez, A., Sheng, M., Good, L. B., Ma, Q., Marin-Valencia, I., Zhang, X., Park, J. Y., Hynan, L. S., Stavinoha, P., Roe, C. R., & Lu, H. (2014). Triheptanoin for glucose transporter type I deficiency (G1D): Modulation of human ictogenesis, cerebral metabolic rate, and cognitive indices by a food supplement. *JAMA Neurology, 71,* 1255–1265.

Poff, A. M., Koutnik, A. P., Egan, K. M., Sahebjum, S., D'Agostino, D. P., & Kumar, N. B. (2017). Targeting the Warburg effect: Implications for management of glioma. *Seminars in Cancer Biology, 56,* 135–148. https://doi.org/10.1016/j.semcancer.2017.12.011

Poff, A. M., Rho, J. M., & D'Agostino, D. P. (2019). Ketone administration for seizure disorders: History and rationale for ketone esters and metabolic alternatives. *Frontiers in Neuroscience, 13,* 1041. https://doi.org/10.3389/fnins.2019.0104

Seyfried, T. N., Flores, R. E., Poff, A. M., & D'Agostino, D. P. (2014). Cancer as a metabolic disease: Implications for novel therapeutics. *Carcinogenesis, 35*(3), 515–527.

Stafstrom, C. E., & Rho, J. M. (2012). The ketogenic diet as a treatment paradigm for diverse neurological disorders. *Frontiers in Pharmacology, 3,* 59.

VanItallie, T. B., & Nufert, T. H. (2003). Ketones: Metabolism's ugly duckling. *Nutrition Reviews, 61,* 327–341.

Veech, R. L. (2004). The therapeutic implications of ketone bodies: The effects of ketone bodies in pathological conditions; Ketosis, ketogenic diet, redox states, insulin resistance, and mitochondrial metabolism. *Prostaglandins, Leukotrienes, and Essential Fatty Acids, 70,* 309–319.

Walsh, J. J., Myette-Côté, É., Neudorf, H., & Little, J. P. (2020). Potential therapeutic effects of exogenous ketone supplementation for type 2 diabetes: A review. *Current Pharmaceutical Design, 26*(9), 958–969.

Ketone Supplementation for Health and Disease

ANGELA M. POFF, PHD, SHANNON L. KESL, PHD,
ANDREW P. KOUTNIK, PHD, SARA E. MOSS, BS,
CHRISTOPHER Q. ROGERS, PHD, AND
DOMINIC P. D'AGOSTINO, PHD

INDUCING THERAPEUTIC KETOSIS WITH KETONE SUPPLEMENTATION

Ketones are typically produced in the liver only under certain physiologic conditions associated with the suppression of the hormone insulin: starvation, fasting, calorie restriction, prolonged exercise, or during the consumption of the high-fat, low-carbohydrate ketogenic diet (KD). The restrictive nature of these states has limited the clinical applicability of therapeutic ketosis due to practical considerations. In an effort to circumvent this dilemma, researchers have developed exogenous ketogenic supplements—ketogenic precursors that are metabolized to produce a dose-dependent elevation of β-hydroxybutyrate (βHB) and acetoacetate (AcAc) in the blood (Clarke et al., 2012b; D'Agostino et al., 2013; Kesl, 2016; Puchowicz et al., 2000). The ketone supplements allow for a rapid and controlled induction of physiologic ketosis without the need for severe dietary restrictions. Since many of the benefits of ketosis are mechanistically attributable to ketone bodies, it is possible that exogenous ketone supplementation could mimic the therapeutic efficacy of the KD or provide similar benefits for health optimization or performance—although key differences do exist (Poff et al., 2020). In addition, the adjuvant use of exogenous ketone supplements for patients consuming a KD could enhance the upregulation of ketone receptors and ketolytic utilization, potentially speeding up keto-adaptation and inducing an easier transition to, and sustainment of, ketosis, and perhaps even helping return a sense of normalcy to patients and their caregivers. Furthermore, in some scenarios, a ketone-supplemented KD may be more effective than the KD or ketone supplementation alone.

DEVELOPMENT AND TESTING OF KETONE SUPPLEMENTS

Numerous sources of ketones and ketogenic precursors are being developed and tested, including medium-chain triglycerides (MCTs), diols, salts, and esters, which have all been shown to elevate blood ketone levels independently of caloric or carbohydrate restriction (Kesl et al., 2016). The investigation of natural and synthetic ketogenic precursors to establish nutritional ketosis without the need for dietary restriction has revealed that each formulation has distinct properties in terms of extent and duration of ketosis as well as metabolic signaling properties, including anticonvulsant effects (D'Agostino et al., 2013; Kesl et al., 2016). Most of the developed ketone supplements are currently under investigation for safety and efficacy in disease states.

MCTs

MCTs contain a glycerol backbone esterified to medium-chain fatty acids (MCFAs), which are fatty acids with hydrocarbon side chains 6 to 12 carbons long. MCFAs include caproic acid (C6:0, hexanoic acid), caprylic acid (C8:0, octanoic acid), capric acid (C10:0, decanoic acid), and lauric acid (C12:0, dodecanoic acid). MCTs are naturally found in coconut oil (~ 60%), palm kernel oil (~ 30%), cheese (7.3%), whole milk (6.9%), butter (6.8%), and full-fat yogurt (6.6%; Karen & Welma, 2015; Nagao & Yanagita, 2010). Compared to long-chain fatty acids (LCFAs), MCFAs have a lower melting point and a smaller molecule size and are less calorically dense (8.3 kcal/g, versus 9.2). These distinct physiochemical properties allow MCTs to be absorbed directly into the bloodstream through the hepatic portal vein without the need for bile or pancreatic enzymes for degradation. Additionally, MCTs do not require carnitine to enter the mitochondria, but quickly cross the double mitochondrial matrix, where they are metabolized to acetyl-CoA, and subsequently to ketone bodies (Papamandjaris et al., 1998). Thus, they are easily and rapidly digested, are transferred to the liver, and are used for energy rather than stored as fat. In comparison, LCFAs require re-esterification in the small intestine, transport by chylomicrons via the lymphatic and vascular systems, and oxidation in the liver for energy or storage. MCTs are metabolized as rapidly as glucose but have roughly twice the energy density (Stagey et al., 1997). In the early 1980s, Vigen K. Babayan of the Nutrition Laboratory at Harvard University developed a method for producing MCTs in large quantities (Bach & Babayan, 1982). These commercialized MCTs are acquired through lipid fractionation from natural fats, such as coconut oil and milk, and are predominantly comprised of C:8 and C:10 MCTs (Babayan, 1987; Hashim & Tantibhedyangkul, 1987).

Since the 1970s, MCTs have been used in a modification of the classic KD as an alternative fat source (Huttenlocher et al., 1971). The ketogenic properties of MCTs allow patients to eat less total fat in their diet and to include more carbohydrate and protein without sacrificing their nutritional ketosis. Although MCTs have the potential to be an efficient and beneficial ketogenic fat, they are currently limited in clinical usage due to gastrointestinal (GI) side effects stimulated by the large dose needed to induce ketonemia (typically greater than 40 g/day; Stagey et al., 1997). The original modified KD with MCT allowed 60% of dietary energy to be derived from MCTs; however, this caused GI distress in some children (Huttenlocher, 1976; Mak et al., 1999; Sills et al., 1986; Trauner, 1985). For this reason, an additional modified KD with MCT was developed that derived only 30% of its energy from MCTs; however, it induced much lower levels of ketosis (Elizabeth et al., 2009; Ruby et al., 1989). In a recent study, juvenile Sprague-Dawley rats were given a daily intragastric bolus of MCT oil (10 g/kg) that rapidly elevated blood βHB levels (4 mM βHB, < 30 min), which remained significantly elevated for up to 12 hr (Kesl et al., 2016). In addition to its metabolic effects, emerging data suggest that octanoic acid (C8) has specific anticonvulsant and neuroprotective properties independent of ketones (Chang et al., 2015). Research and development have been conducted to formulate a powder combining MCT oil with soluble fiber compounds that may delay gastric emptying and enhance absorption, thereby improving tolerability and ketogenic potential.

1,3-Butanediol

1,3-Butanediol (BD; also known as 1,3-butylene glycol) is an FDA-approved organic diol naturally present in some species of pepper (*C. annuum*) that is used as a food flavoring solvent, an intermediate in the manufacture of certain polyester plasticizers, and a humectant for cosmetics and that has been considered as a synthetic food for long-duration space missions (Budavari, 1989; Dymsza, 1975; Falbe et al., 1985). When ingested orally, BD is metabolized by the liver via alcohol dehydrogenase (ADH) to β-hydroxybutyraldehyde, which is rapidly oxidized to βHB by aldehyde dehydrogenase (Tate et al., 1971). BD contributes approximately 6 kcal/g of energy and can produce dose-dependent millimolar concentrations of ketones in the blood in a ratio of 6:1 of βHB to AcAc (D'Agostino et al., 2013; Desrochers et al., 1992; Drackley et al., 1990; Tobin et al., 1972). Extensive toxicology studies have concluded that BD is safe, with very few adverse health effects in humans or animals (Dymsza, 1975; Hess et al., 1981; Opitz, 1958; Scala & Paynter, 1967).

In a 28-day study, a daily 5 g/kg dose of BD administered via intragastric gavage in Sprague-Dawley rats caused a significant elevation of blood ketones (1 mM βHB, < 30 min) without an effect on blood glucose, triglyceride, or lipoprotein levels (Kesl et al., 2016). Recently, BD has been investigated as a backbone of ketone mono- and diesters, which are discussed later in this chapter in the section titled Ketone Esters.

Ketone Salts

Originally, researchers attempted to administer βHB and AcAc in their free acid forms; however, this was shown to be too expensive and ineffective at producing sustained ketosis. Subsequently, buffering the free acid of βHB with sodium was suggested, but this causes potentially harmful sodium overload and mineral imbalance at therapeutic levels of ketosis, and it has been shown that βHB alone is largely ineffective at preventing seizures in animal models (Bough & Rho, 2007). A study showed that oral administration of Na⁺/βHB in doses from 80 to 900 mg/kg/day elevated blood ketone levels to 0.19 to 0.36 mM, which was therapeutic in children with acyl-CoA dehydrogenase deficiency (Hove et al., 2003). However, for a 70-kg man to achieve these levels of ketosis would require ingesting between 5.6 and 6.3

g/day. Considering the potential effects of such a large sodium load, chronic administration of pure Na$^+$/βHB salts to achieve ketosis has been viewed unfavorably (Veech, 2004).

More recently, ketone salts (KS) with a balanced electrolyte formulation to prevent sodium overload have been developed and tested, and they can include potassium, calcium, magnesium, lithium, arginine, lysine, zinc, histidine, ornithine, creatine, agmatine, or citrulline. Maintaining a balanced electrolyte ratio should help offset any potential adverse effects of sodium on blood pressure. It is speculated that this formulation will be especially beneficial for elderly patients, who are most susceptible to sodium-induced hypertension (Veech, 2014). Furthermore, when first attempting to follow a KD, many people experience headaches and lethargy during the initial stages of "keto-adaptation," a term that describes the adaptive changes in metabolic physiology associated with transitioning toward fat and ketone metabolism. The symptoms are largely a result of reduced glucose availability to the brain and a transient depletion of minerals, especially sodium, potassium, and magnesium, in the plasma (Zhang et al., 2013b). These symptoms can be attenuated or reversed with sufficient supplementation of sodium, potassium, calcium, and magnesium, and thus a ketone supplement that delivers ketones with these electrolytes would be favorable.

Several mineral KS combinations are currently being tested for safety and efficacy. In a recent study, neither a 5 g/kg nor a 10 g/kg intragastric gavage of a Na$^+$/K$^+$ βHB salts significantly elevated blood ketone levels or reduced blood glucose levels in juvenile Sprague-Dawley rats (Kesl, 2016). However, there appears to be interspecies variability in absorption: in a recent case study, a 100-kg male patient was administered a 4% Na$^+$/K$^+$ βHB salt solution (containing 11 g of sodium and 7.1 g of βHB) and his plasma levels of βHB were significantly elevated at 30 to 60 min after administration. After receiving the same dose for 3 days, the patient had sustained elevated blood ketone levels from 15 to 120 min after administration. Similar results were seen in a 70-kg male who fasted 3 days before administration of the KS supplement (D'Agostino et al., 2014). In a 15-week study, Sprague-Dawley rats were administered Na$^+$/Ca^{2+} KS 20% by weight (~ 25 g/kg/day) in their food fed ad libitum. The Na$^+$/Ca^{2+} βHB-supplemented rats exhibited sustained elevated blood ketone levels (1 mM βHB) at 1, 4, 8, 10, and 13

weeks of chronic feeding that did not affect blood glucose levels compared to controls (Poff, 2016).

Combination KS and MCTs

Considering the variety of ketogenic precursors available, researchers are investigating unique combinations of the individual supplements in hopes of optimizing their benefits. A combination of βHB salts and MCT oil has been administered in mixtures with ratios of 1:1 to 1:2. Formulating in this way allows for rapid and sustained elevation of ketosis by delivering exogenous ketones while simultaneously stimulating endogenous ketogenesis with MCTs. In addition, the combination formulation allows for a lower dose of the components than with administration of the individual compounds, thus reducing the potential for side effects (gastric hyperosmolality) and resulting in a distinct blood ketone profile that is sustained over a longer time (D'Agostino et al., 2014).

In a 28-day study, the combination of a 50% Na$^+$/K$^+$ βHB salt mixed in a 1:1 solution with MCT oil (KS + MCT) significantly elevated and sustained blood ketone levels and reduced blood glucose levels in a dose-dependent manner (Kesl et al., 2016). Additionally, the study demonstrated a significant correlation between elevated blood ketone levels and reduced blood glucose levels after intragastric gavage administration, with no effect on blood triglyceride or lipoprotein levels. A noteworthy observation from the study revealed that, in rats, MCT caused a rise in ketones (> 3 mM) that exceeds what is possible in humans due to gastrointestinal intolerance. This is likely because rats have higher rates of absorption of MCT and higher rates of hepatic fat metabolism, which stimulate greater ketone production. Considering these results, it is important to take into account interspecies variability in the metabolic response to ketone supplements, which will need to be further characterized to fully understand how we can extrapolate findings and translate into human dosing equivalents. In the rats, the KS + MCT supplement elevated blood ketones similarly to MCT alone; however, the gastric side effects were not observed, suggesting a potential method for avoiding these adverse effects (Kesl, 2016). In a case study, a 100-kg male was administered a combination of a 4% Na$^+$/K$^+$ βHB salt solution (containing 11 g of sodium and 7.1 g of βHB) + 20 ml MCT oil. This combination induced a higher elevation of blood ketone levels than either βHB salts or MCT oil alone, starting 15 min after consumption and lasting for 4 hr. Similar results were observed in a 70-kg male who fasted 3 days prior to administration; however, elevated blood ketone levels were observed sooner after supplementation and were sustained for a considerably longer time (8 hr) after administration (D'Agostino, 2015). This effect was accompanied by a reduction in blood glucose and a lower starting blood glucose concentration on each subsequent day of supplementation (D'Agostino et al., 2014). In a 15-week study, Sprague-Dawley rats were administered a 1:1 mixture of Na^+/Ca^{2+} KS + MCT oil (20% by weight, ~ 25 g/kg/day) in their food fed ad libitum. The combination-supplemented rats had significantly sustained and elevated blood ketone levels at weeks 3, 4, 8, 10, and 13, without significantly effects on blood glucose levels during the study (Kesl, 2014).

Ketone Esters

Researchers have developed and investigated several synthetic ketone mono- and diesters to induce nutritional ketosis independent of dietary calorie or carbohydrate restriction. When ketone esters (KE) are administered, gastric esterases liberate ketones (βHB and AcAc) as free acid from a backbone molecule, which varies depending upon the specific formulation, but is favorably a ketogenic precursor, such as BD. As previously discussed, BD is subsequently metabolized by the liver to produce βHB (D'Agostino et al., 2013). Thus, the KEs currently available are unique among the ketone supplements in that they can directly elevate ketones in a dose-dependent manner and can supply ketogenic precursors that can further sustain ketogenesis. Additionally, synthetically derived KEs are currently the most potent form of exogenous ketones available, but their potency also necessitates a thorough investigation of their long-term safety and toxicity.

In the late 1970s, Birkhahn et al. were the first to synthesize a monoester of glycerol and AcAc (monoacetoacetin) for parenteral nutrition. Their studies demonstrated that monoacetoacetin induced hyperketonemia comparable to that in fasted rats at a dose of 50 g/kg/day (Birkhahn & Border, 1978; Birkhahn et al., 1977, 1979). In attempts to increase the caloric density of monoacetoacetin, they synthesized both a monoester and triester of glycerol and βHB. These esters are hydrolyzed to release free βHB in a way that elevates and sustains blood ketones. Later, Desrochers and colleagues synthesized mono- and diesters of AcAc with BD that elevated both AcAc and βHB (Desrochers et al., 1995b). These and other KEs developed by, or in collaboration with, Henri Brunengraber and Richard Veech have demonstrated an ability to induce a dose-dependent hyperketonemia (1–7 mM) in rats, mice, dogs, pigs, and humans (Brunengraber, 1997; Ciraolo et al., 1995; Desrochers et al., 1995a; Puchowicz et al., 2000; Srivastava et al., 2012; Sylvain et al., 1995). Clarke and colleagues demonstrated the safety of a KE in rats and humans, and this has also been documented in a recent case study of Alzheimer's disease (Clarke et al., 2012a, 2012b; Newport et al., 2015). The ketone ester R,S-1,3-butanediol acetoacetate diester (BD-AcAc$_2$), given as an intragastric gavage, elevated both AcAc and βHB blood levels to > 3 mM in rats (D'Agostino et al., 2013). The induction of therapeutic ketosis was rapid (within 30 min) and was sustained at high levels for over 4 hr. In a 28-day study, a daily intragastric gavage (5 g/kg body weight) of BD-AcAc$_2$ induced significantly elevated blood ketone levels and significantly reduced blood glucose levels without significantly altering blood triglyceride or lipoprotein levels (Kesl et al., 2016). In a 15-week chronic feeding study, BD-AcAc$_2$ was administered to Sprague-Dawley rats in a low dose (5% food weight, 10 g/kg/day; LKE) and a high dose (20% food weight, 25 g/kg/day; HKE) ad libitum. Both doses significantly elevated blood ketone levels without reducing blood glucose levels. Serum clinical chemistry of both LKE and HKE did not reveal any alterations in markers of kidney and liver function (Stubbs et al., 2018b) in the test rats compared to rats fed standard chow (Poff, 2016). Use of the pure ketone diester formulation has been studied in athletes and has been shown to increase ketone levels (Leckey, 2017); however, due to significant obstacles surrounding its preliminary nature—such as its unrefined taste formulation, potential for gastric side effects, and unknown pharmacokinetic profile—further development and analysis are required before the agent can be successfully tested in human subjects (Stubbs et al., 2018b).

POTENTIAL THERAPEUTIC MECHANISMS OF KETONE SUPPLEMENTATION

Induction of hyperketonemia produces acute and chronic changes in metabolic physiology and molecular signaling pathways that provide therapeutic effects in varied disease states. Metabolism-based mechanisms of ketone therapies include an elevation of blood ketones and associated anaplerosis, with simultaneous suppression of blood glucose, enhancement of insulin sensitivity, improvement of mitochondrial efficiency, suppression of specific inflammatory mediators, inhibition of oxidative stress, and preservation of mitochondrial health and function, among other effects.

Suppression of Blood Glucose

Hyperglycemia and hyperinsulinemia are pathologically linked to numerous disorders, including cancer, cardiovascular disease, obesity, type 2 diabetes, impaired wound healing, and neurodegenerative diseases, among others (Laakso & Kuusisto, 2014; Ryu et al., 2014). These states are associated with chronic systemic inflammation, oxidative stress, impairment of the immune system, and vascular and metabolic dysfunction (Bornfeldt & Tabas, 2011; de Carvalho Vidigal et al., 2012; Turina et al., 2005). Exogenous ketone supplements may provide therapeutic benefits in diseases characterized by hyperglycemia, because many reports have demonstrated that ketone administration, delivered either by infusion or by oral exogenous ketone supplements, consistently lowers blood glucose by approximately 10% to 20% (Ari et al., 2019c). One early report suggested that this effect may be due in part to an enhancement of insulin sensitivity. Male rats were fed a standard diet with 30% of calories replaced with the R-3-hydroxybutyrate-R-1,3-butanediol monoester (ketone monoester, KME) for 14 days. The KME-supplemented diet induced nutritional ketosis (3.5 mM βHB), and both plasma glucose and insulin were decreased by approximately 50% (Srivastava et al., 2012). Glucose was decreased from 5 mM to 2.8 mM, and insulin was decreased from 0.54 ng/ml to 0.26 ng/ml. In a similar study by the same group, mice receiving a KME diet exhibited a 73% increase in the Quantitative Insulin-Sensitivity Check Index (QUICKI), a surrogate marker of insulin sensitivity, compared to control, calorie-matched mice (Srivastava et al., 2012). Fasting plasma glucose levels were not altered in these mice, but fasting plasma insulin levels were reduced by approximately 85% in the KME-fed mice compared to controls, demonstrating that exogenous ketones enhanced insulin sensitivity in this model.

More recent work has led investigators to suggest the suppression of glucose after exogenous ketone administration is due at least in part to reduced hepatic glucose output. In 2018, Myette-Côté and colleagues published results from a double-blind randomized crossover trial in 10 male and 10 female healthy adults who had performed an oral glucose tolerance test (OGTT) 30 min after water or KME consumption (Myette-Cote et al., 2018). KME pretreatment reduced the 2-hr plasma glucose area under the curve (AUC) by 16% and the 2-hr serum free fatty acid AUC by 44%. This occurred without further elevation of insulin, suggesting that KME may suppress glucose elevation by reducing hepatic glucose output. Similar results have been demonstrated in animal models of infused exogenous ketone bodies, further supporting this potential underlying mechanism.

In a study examining the potential use of ketogenic supplements as a cancer therapy, mice consuming a standard high-carbohydrate diet mixed with the ketone ester $BD\text{-}AcAc_2$ at 20% by weight had approximately 30% lower blood glucose than control animals (Poff et al., 2014). BD did not significantly elevate blood ketones in this study, nor did it decrease blood glucose. This result is likely due in part to the comparatively small dose of BD being consumed at any time due to the route of administration, because BD in higher doses is known to elevate ketones. Insulin levels were not investigated in this study. In a study designed to assess the dose-dependent effects of exogenous ketone supplements on blood glucose, ketones, and lipids, healthy male rats were administered one of five ketogenic agents daily via intragastric gavage (Kesl et al., 2016). The ketogenic agents investigated included BD, $BD\text{-}AcAc_2$, a sodium/potassium β-hydroxybutyrate KS, MCT oil, and KS + MCT 1:1 mixture (BMS + MCT). $BD\text{-}AcAc_2$, KS, MCT oil, and KS + MCT-treated rats demonstrated a decrease in blood glucose after ketone supplement administration given as an acute bolus. As in the previously mentioned mouse study, BD did not lower blood glucose in these animals, although it is known to be a hypoglycemic agent. The duration of the reduction in blood glucose varied between supplements and lasted anywhere from 30 min to 12 hr, suggesting that ketone supplementation could potentially provide a novel method of glycemic control.

Enhanced Metabolic Efficiency

The superior metabolic efficiency of ketone bodies has been demonstrated since the 1940s, when Henry Lardy compared the energetic efficiency of 16 major carbohydrate, lipid, and intermediary metabolites (Lardy, 1945). He demonstrated that βHB and AcAc were unique among the panel of metabolites tested in their ability to increase bull-sperm mobility while simultaneously decreasing oxygen consumption. Nearly 50 years later, Richard Veech and colleagues confirmed Lardy's observation and elucidated the molecular mechanisms underlying the phenomenon in the working perfused rat heart (Kashiwaya et al., 1994). They demonstrated that supplementation of 5 mM ketones (4 mM βHB, 1 mM AcAc) to glucose-containing perfusate (10 mM glucose) increased cardiac hydraulic work by approximately 25% while simultaneously reducing oxygen consumption (Kashiwaya et al., 1994). Their study revealed that this effect was mediated by a reduction of the mitochondrial NAD couple and an oxidation

of the coenzyme Q couple, which increases the energy of the redox span between these sites, as shown in Figure 33.1. This results in an increase in energy released by electrons in the electron transport chain (ETC), causing more protons to be pumped into the inner mitochondrial space, thus enhancing the electrochemical gradient established there and increasing the energy of ATP hydrolysis. Indeed, thermodynamic tables for heat of combustion, calculated with bomb calorimeter experiments, show that βHB produces more energy than glucose per 2-carbon moiety (Cahill & Veech, 2003). These results are supported by human studies that demonstrated a reduction in blood flow and oxygen consumption

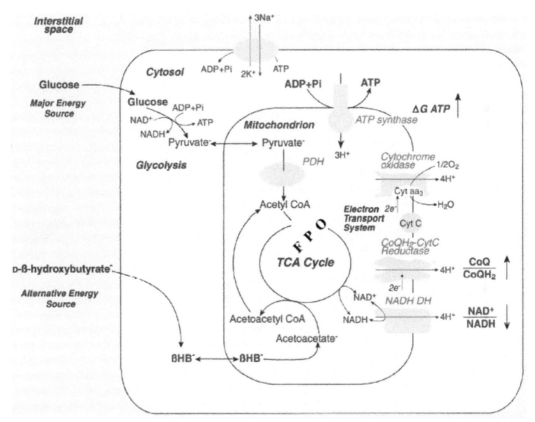

FIGURE 33.1 *Ketone Bodies Added in the Presence of Glucose Fundamentally Enhance Mitochondrial Metabolism*
When added to glucose, a physiologic level of ketone bodies reduces the mitochondrial NAD couple, oxidizes the co-enzyme Q couple, and increases the ΔG0 of ATP hydrolysis. These changes are shown on the right side of the figure. The arrows illustrate the effects of ketone bodies compared to glucose alone. Ketone bodies provide an alternative metabolic fuel that can preserve ATP production during the impairment of glycolysis, as occurs in diabetes or insulin resistance, or during inhibition of pyruvate dehydrogenase complex (PDH), as occurs in the presence of amyloid. Oxidation of the co-enzyme Q couple decreases superoxide anion production. Increases in the ΔG0 of ATP hydrolysis widen the extra/intracellular ionic gradients leading to hyperpolarization of cells, which may play a role in treating certain forms of epilepsy. The actions of ketone bodies mimic the acute effects of insulin in insulin-sensitive tissue and tissues with high metabolic demands, including heart and brain. Figure used with permission from Veech et al., (2001) Ketone bodies—potential therapeutic uses. *IUBMB Life* 51(4):241-7

in the brains of fasted obese subjects in ketosis (McHenry, 1966). Thus, ketones appear to be a superior mitochondrial fuel for ATP production per unit oxygen compared to glucose and can be considered among the most metabolically efficient energy metabolites at the biochemical level.

Anti-Inflammatory Effects

The physiologic state of ketosis has known anti-inflammatory properties, as several studies have demonstrated that the KD reduces circulating inflammatory markers in animals and in humans (Forsythe et al., 2008; Sharman & Volek, 2004; Torres-Gonzalez et al., 2008). Evidence suggests that this effect is, at least in part, directly mediated by the ketone bodies, indicating that exogenous ketone supplementation could be used to suppress inflammation. Dixit and colleagues reported that βHB inhibits the NLRP3 inflammasome, an important component of the innate immune system that controls activation of caspase-1 and production of the pro-inflammatory cytokines IL-1β and IL-18 by macrophages (Youm et al., 2015). This effect was mediated specifically by βHB, as neither AcAc nor the structurally related fatty acids butyrate and acetate elicited this response. βHB-induced inhibition of the NLRP3 inflammasome occurs without its being oxidized in the TCA cycle and is thus independent of its function as an energy metabolite. Furthermore, the anti-inflammatory changes associated with βHB were not dependent on alterations in AMPK, reactive oxygen species (ROS), glycolytic inhibition, UCP, or SIRT2 signaling, further validating its function as a signaling metabolite. To investigate the in vivo translatability of this finding, researchers administered the BD-AcAc$_2$ to a familial cold anti-inflammatory syndrome (FCAS) mouse model with an induced missense mutation in NLRP3. The KE protected the mice from neutrophilia and hyperglycemia and did not affect infiltration of peritoneal macrophages or overall frequency of splenic T cells, macrophages, or neutrophils, leading the authors to conclude that elevating blood ketones could be a therapeutic option for patients with NLRP3-mediated chronic inflammatory diseases. This same group went on to show that this signaling property of ketones could attenuate gout flares, and that βHB could deactivate neutrophil-induced IL-1B production regardless of animal age (Goldberg et al., 2017). Indeed, other research has shown that inhibition of the NLRP3 inflammasome mitigates the severity of numerous inflammatory diseases, including

atherosclerosis, type 2 diabetes, Alzheimer's disease, and inflammatory dermatologic conditions, among others (Duewell et al., 2010; Fomin et al., 2017; Heneka et al., 2013; Martinon et al., 2006; Vandanmagsar et al., 2011; Youm et al., 2013, 2015).

βHB has also been shown to bind HCAR2/GPR109a and to reduce NF-κB nuclear translocation (Taggart et al., 2005). NF-κB is a known regulator of pro-inflammatory proteins, and inhibition of its nuclear localization has anti-inflammatory implications. βHB has been shown to cause an anti-inflammatory response via the HCAR2/GPR109a receptor (Rahman et al., 2014). Interestingly, exogenous administration of BD-AcAc$_2$ also inhibited LPS-induced seizure modeling, demonstrating that exogenous ketone administration attenuated the adverse consequences of inflammation in the brain of Wistar Albino Glaxo/Rijswijk (WAG/Rij) rats, a rodent model of absence epilepsy (Kovacs et al., 2019b). However, seemingly conflicting responses have been demonstrated when exogenous ketones were administered to patients who were acutely infused with LPS (Thomsen et al., 2018) or had monocytes stimulated ex vivo with LPS (Neudorf et al., 2019). However, the βHB-augmented inflammatory response in patients with systemic infection was accompanied by a potent anticatabolic response in the skeletal muscle, demonstrating that these pro-inflammatory responses may be context dependent and might accompany positive effects in critical tissue (Koutnik et al., 2019; Thomsen et al., 2018). Encouragingly, the KD reduces expression of COX-1 and COX-2 enzymes in patients with multiple sclerosis (Bock et al., 2018), an effect that has been ascribed to ketone-induced HCAR-2 signaling because of the known inhibitory effect of HCAR-2 on COX activation (Fu et al., 2014; Gambhir, 2012).

Inhibition of Oxidative Stress

The KD has been reported to reduce oxidative stress in vivo in several preclinical and clinical reports (Jarrett et al., 2008). Studies suggest that this effect is mediated by the ketone bodies themselves, and therefore the effect would likely be recapitulated with exogenous ketone supplementation (Waldman, 2020). Some important molecular mechanisms underlying the effects of ketone metabolism on oxidative stress were delineated by studies investigating the bioenergetic efficiency and mitochondrial respiration in the working perfused rat heart following administration of a glucose-containing perfusate supplemented with exogenous 5-mM βHB (Kashiwaya et al., 1994). As described previously, ketone metabolism increases the oxidation of ubiquinol in the electron transport chain, reducing semiquinone radical, an intermediate in the reduction of ubiquinone that is sensitive to oxidation by molecular oxygen, to produce superoxide anion. Superoxide anion is an important precursor for the generation of many ROS; thus, ketone metabolism suppresses mitochondrial ROS production (Kashiwaya et al., 1994). Simultaneously, ketone metabolism suppresses oxidative stress by enhancing endogenous antioxidant capacity. Ketone metabolism induces reduction of the mitochondrial NAD and cytoplasmic NADP couples. NADH and NADPH are necessary for the regeneration of reduced glutathione (GSH), which is required for the neutralization of ROS by glutathione peroxidase, an important endogenous antioxidant enzyme. These molecular effects are observed in vivo, as the KD has been shown to increase the ratio of reduced to oxidized mitochondrial glutathione (GSH:GSSG) in rat brains (Jarrett et al., 2008). These effects appear to be ubiquitous in various tissues; however, the brain has been the most well characterized in this regard. For example, in vitro treatment with βHB and AcAc decreases neuronal ROS production after glutamate exposure (Maalouf et al., 2007) and inhibits apoptosis in cortical slices exposed to hydrogen peroxide (H_2O_2; Kim et al., 2007).

Eric Verdin and colleagues demonstrated that βHB functions as an endogenous histone deacetylase inhibitor (HDACI) in vitro and in vivo at physiologic concentrations easily achievable with exogenous ketone supplementation (Shimazu et al., 2013). Fasting, calorie restriction, and exogenous βHB administration all increased global histone acetylation in mice and induced the transcriptional activation of the oxidative stress resistance factors FOXO3a and MT2. This effect was found to be mediated directly by inhibition of class I and II HDACs. Furthermore, the authors demonstrated that exogenous ketone supplementation could prevent oxidative stress. Mice were administered βHB via a subcutaneous pump for 24 hr before receiving an injection of paraquat, which induces the production and accumulation of ROS. Protein carbonylation was suppressed by 54%, and lipid peroxidation was completely suppressed, in the kidneys of βHB pretreated mice. Immunoblotting of kidney tissue from these animals revealed a significant increase in the mitochondrial superoxide dismutase and catalase endogenous antioxidant systems. This study strongly supports the feasibility and applicability of exogenous ketone supplements for the prevention of oxidative stress.

Other studies have demonstrated that ketosis-induced HDAC inhibition may have widespread implications for diseases characterized by oxidative stress. For example, a KD reduced lipid peroxidation and spinal cord injury in rats, in association with an increase in histone acetylation and an increase in antioxidant stress genes *FOXO3a* and *MT2* and their related protein targets, superoxide dismutase and catalase in the spinal cord (Kong et al., 2017; Wang et al., 2017). While these studies utilized a KD to elicit HDAC inhibitory activity, our understanding of the signaling role of βHB in mediating these therapeutic effects strongly supports investigation of exogenous ketone supplements as a tool for this and similar pathologies.

Preservation of Mitochondrial Health and Function

Ketone metabolism is generally recognized to support or enhance mitochondrial health (Veech, 2004). As previously described, ketones suppress mitochondrial ROS production and enhance endogenous antioxidant systems. The resultant reduction in oxidative stress protects the mitochondrial DNA and mitochondrial membranes from damage that would impair respiratory and mitochondrial function. Interestingly, exogenous ketone supplementation with KE has been shown to induce mitochondrial biogenesis (Srivastava et al., 2012). For 1 month, mice in this study were fed a diet in which approximately 30% of calories were derived from KME. The mitochondrial content and expression of electron transport chain proteins were significantly increased in the intrascapular brown adipose tissue of KME-fed mice as compared to control mice, although calorie intake was matched between the two groups. These effects may elicit therapeutic benefit in specific conditions characterized by mitochondrial deficits, such as in the aging heart. It has been proposed that ketone metabolism in aging myocytes may stimulate mitophagy, a protective mechanism against mitochondrial damage (Thai et al., 2019). Thai and colleagues studied this possibility in a rabbit model, demonstrating that ketone bodies were able to stimulate mitophagy and myocyte repair in young and aged myocytes, but not in aged myocytes from rabbits with heart failure induced by aortic insufficiency and stenosis (Thai et al., 2019).

CONDITIONS WHERE KETONE SUPPLEMENTATION IS LIKELY BENEFICIAL

Because of the previously described therapeutic mechanisms of ketone metabolism, exogenous ketone supplementation is being investigated as a potential treatment for several disorders. The focus here is on some conditions for which ketone supplements have been most well demonstrated to be useful, including epilepsy and seizure disorders, glucose transporter type 1 deficiency syndrome, Alzheimer's disease, cancer, insulin resistance, type 2 diabetes mellitus, and weight loss. It is worth noting that exogenous ketone supplements are being studied in a far greater number of conditions, although they are not explored here, including COVID-19, with new research and potential applications emerging almost monthly (Ari et al., 2018, 2019a; Bradshaw et al., 2020; Gross et al., 2019; Jensen et al., 2020; Kovacs et al., 2019a, 2020; Lennerz et al., 2021; Monzo et al., 2021; Selvaraj & Margulies, 2021; Stubbs et al., 2020, 2021; Tan et al., 2020; Walsh et al., 2020a).

Epilepsy/Seizure Disorders

The KD is a proven, effective therapy for epilepsy in children and adults (Klein et al., 2014; Li et al., 2013; McDonald & Cervenka, 2019). In many cases, it is more effective than antiepileptic drugs (AED) and is therefore routinely used as a frontline treatment for children with intractable (drug-resistant) epilepsy (Levy et al., 2012). Although the mechanisms of KD therapy are largely unknown, achieving and sustaining therapeutic ketonemia (>1 mM blood ketones) or ketonuria (> 40 mg/dl) is generally associated with antiseizure efficacy. Despite its success, the dietary requirements of the KD can be unpalatable for some patients and difficult for caregivers, and they can contribute to noncompliance or cessation of treatment (Klein et al., 2014; Levy et al., 2012). Exogenous ketogenic supplementation mimics the metabolic and physiologic effects of the KD, including enhancing mitochondrial biogenesis, anaplerosis, suppression of glycolysis, and increasing ATP and adenosine production, all thought to mediate the therapeutic effects of the KD in epilepsy (Kesl, 2014, 2016; Kovac et al., 2013; Masino & Geiger, 2009; Srivastava et al., 2012; Stafstrom et al., 2008, 2009).

One of the earliest studies of the antiseizure efficacy of exogenous ketogenic supplementation was performed in a unique seizure model that uses hyperbaric hyperoxia (HBO) to reliably induce epileptic-like (tonic-clonic) seizures in wild-type rats, a condition known as central nervous system oxygen toxicity (CNS-OT). A single oral dose of the KE BD-AcAc$_2$ induced rapid (within 30 min) and sustained (> 4 hr) ketosis (> 3 mM βHB and > 3mM AcAc) and prolonged the latency to seizure by 574% (D'Agostino et al., 2013). An elevation in AcAc and acetone appears to be required for the anticonvulsant effects of ketosis. BD elevated blood βHB (> 5 mM) but did not elevate AcAc or acetone, nor did it affect latency to seizure. More recently, we demonstrated that adding MCT to KE could provide a similar therapeutic effect in this model while requiring a lower dose of KE, a method that could improve the safety and tolerability profiles (Ari et al., 2019b). This encouraging response prompted preliminary investigation into preventing or delaying seizures with ketogenic supplements in a variety of transgenic rodent and chemical-induced seizure models. Pentylenetetrazole (PTZ) is a GABA antagonist and epileptogenic agent that is used to induce seizures in rodents for preclinical analysis of anticonvulsant therapies. In 2015, Coppola and colleagues tested the dosage threshold for seizure induction by PTZ in control (water-treated) and KE-treated rats (Viggiano et al., 2015). Encouragingly, a single oral dose (4 g/kg body weight) of BD-AcAc$_2$ elevated blood βHB (2.7 mM) and increased the threshold of PTZ seizure from 122 ± 6 mg/kg to 140 ± 11 mg/kg. Since then, an anticonvulsant effect of KE treatment has also been demonstrated in the WAG/Rij rat model of absence epilepsy, the Ube3a m$^-$/p$^+$ mouse model of Angelman syndrome, and the kainic acid-induced mouse seizure model (Ciarlone et al., 2016; Kovacs et al., 2017, 2019b). This preclinical work is beginning to be translated into humans, as evidenced by an ongoing clinical trial examining the use of exogenous ketone supplements for Angelman syndrome (Herber et al., 2020). There is emerging evidence that ketone bodies alone exert antiseizure effects through a multiplicity of mechanisms, including, but not limited to, activation of inhibitory adenosine and ATP-sensitive potassium channels, enhancement of mitochondrial function, reduction in oxidative stress, attenuation of excitatory neurotransmission, and enhancement of central γ-aminobutyric acid (GABA) synthesis (GAD enzyme). Other novel actions more recently reported include inhibition of NLRP3 inflammasome assembly and activation of peripheral immune cells, as well as epigenetic effects via decreasing the activity of histone deacetylases (HDACs). The current preclinical evidence supports the role of ketone supplementation (as an ester or balanced electrolyte formulation) for epilepsy and a broad range of seizure disorders, especially those linked to neurometabolic dysregulation (Poff et al., 2019).

Interestingly, preclinical studies have suggested that specific MCFAs, such as C10:0 capric acid, may elicit antiseizure effects through mechanisms independent of ketone metabolism and signaling (Augustin et al., 2018; Chang et al., 2015). For example, capric acid increased the seizure threshold in the 6-Hz psychomotor and maximal electroshock test seizure models; however, it did not affect PTZ-induced seizures (Wlaz et al., 2015). Interestingly, caprylic acid (C8:0 MCFA) increased the seizure threshold in the 6-Hz psychomotor and intravenous PTZ-induced seizure models, but not in the MEST model (Wlaz et al., 2012).

Glucose Transporter Type 1 Deficiency Syndrome

Glucose transporter type 1 deficiency syndrome (GLUT1DS) is a rare genetic disorder caused by a mutation in the *SLC2A1* gene, which encodes the glucose transporter type 1 (GLUT1). This mutation results in a glucose deficiency in the brain, which causes seizures as well as cognitive and physical developmental delay. In a seminal study in 1967, Cahill and colleagues discovered that ketones replace glucose as the predominant energy substrate for the brain during prolonged fasting and starvation (Cahill, 2006a). Therefore, GLUT1DS is treated with the KD, which circumvents the metabolic blockade by inducing ketosis and is effective at suppressing seizures and enhancing cognitive and motor development in most patients. Maintaining therapeutic levels of ketosis is critical to support the development of children with GLUT1DS. Thus, it is clear how an exogenous ketone supplement could be useful in this patient population. Triheptanoin is a triglyceride containing three heptanoates, a 7-carbon fatty acid whose metabolism produces the 5-carbon ketone bodies β-ketopentanoate and β-hydroxypentanoate. Because it possesses odd-carbon fatty acids, heptanoate is metabolized through β-oxidation to produce propionyl-CoA, which can be subsequently carboxylated to succinyl-CoA, replenishing the TCA cycle via anaplerosis (Borges & Sonnewald, 2012). Triheptanoin has shown therapeutic efficacy in

children and adults with GLUT1DS, reducing seizure activity and improving neuropsychologic performance and cerebral metabolic rate (Pascual et al., 2014). There are ongoing studies investigating the therapeutic effects of KS and KE in a GLUT1DS mouse model, and they may provide an alternative or adjunctive treatment to the KD.

Kabuki Syndrome

Kabuki syndrome is a rare genetic disorder that leads to many developmental abnormalities. Its pathology is associated with a heterozygous mutation in either the *KMT2D* gene (Type 1) or *KDM6A* gene (Type 2), which leads to a loss of function (Bjornsson et al., 2014). Products of both genes play a role in gene regulation via histone modification. *KMT2D* codes for the protein kmt2d, which is a lysine methyltransferase responsible for methylating H3K4 (Rea et al., 2000). *KDM6A* codes for the protein kdm6a, which is a demethylase responsible for demethylating H3K27 (Lan et al., 2007). While these two functions seem contradictory, they both contribute to the opening of chromatin (Benjamin et al., 2017). When either of the two proteins is deficient, craniofacial, skeletal, mental, and dermatologic development is severely affected (Niikawa et al., 1988). Other developmental processes are affected, but to varying degrees across patients (Niikawa et al., 1988). So far, studies have been done only in relation to Type 1 Kabuki syndrome, as it is the most common form of the disorder. It has been shown that using βHB as an HDACI (via the KD as well as exogenous administration) increased acetylation of histone H3 in the model, indicating an increase in transcription and resulting in an increase in neurogenesis (Benjamin et al., 2017). Both H3K4 and H3K27 also have β-hydroxybutyrylation sites; however, further studies are required to understand the role they play in the disorder (Xie et al., 2016).

Alzheimer's Disease

In the early stages of Alzheimer's disease (AD), the brain exhibits a deficiency in glucose metabolism that contributes to the neurodegeneration and progression of the disorder (Chu & Jiao, 2015; de la Monte, 2012). Patients with preclinical and clinical AD have decreased cerebral glucose metabolism as visualized by fluorodeoxyglucose positron emission tomography (FDG-PET; Mosconi, 2011). It is thought that this decrease in glucose metabolism is associated with brain insulin resistance (Talbot et al., 2012). Because ketones are the principal alternative fuel for the brain during fasting or starvation, elevating blood ketone levels in AD patients would theoretically bypass the deficiencies in glucose metabolism and provide energy to the starving neurons. Data to support this hypothesis were recently reported by Cunnane and colleagues, who demonstrated that while brain glucose uptake is impaired in AD, ketone uptake remains unaffected (Croteau et al., 2018). Indeed, the authors concluded that supplying ketones to the brains of AD patients could restore the brain fuel supply and serve as a potential therapy (Cunnane et al., 2016). They went on to test this hypothesis in a 6-month trial in which 52 subjects with mild cognitive impairment (MCI) were randomized to receive 30 g/day of a ketogenic MCT drink or placebo (Fortier et al., 2019). Both ketone and glucose metabolism in the brain were quantified using PET, and cognitive performance was also assessed with a battery of neurocognitive tests. Brain ketone metabolism increased by 230% in those receiving the ketogenic drink, while glucose metabolism remained unchanged. And, encouragingly, numerous measures of cognitive performance, including measures of episodic memory, language, executive function, and processing speed, were also improved in the supplement-treated subjects. Thus, exogenous ketone supplementation could be a useful tool for supporting cerebral energy metabolism and cognitive function in individuals with cognitive impairment. Alternatively, novel research also suggests that βHB-induced inhibition of inflammation via the NLRP3 inflammasome may contribute to the therapeutic effects of ketosis in AD (Shippy et al., 2020).

Similarly, there are data to suggest that ketones could protect against AD development or slow its progression (Rusek et al., 2019). The ability of a βHB- and BD-containing KE to suppress AD progression was evaluated in a triple transgenic AD mouse model (3xTgAD; Kashiwaya et al., 2013). Presymptomatic mice were fed a diet with approximately 20% kcal from the KE and were compared to isocaloric standard-diet-fed control animals. KE-treated animals exhibited less anxiety and improved performance on learning and memory tests at 4 and 7 months after initiation of the diet. Immunohistochemical analysis of the brain revealed that the KE-fed mice had less Aβ and hyperphosphorylated tau deposition in the cortex, hippocampus, and amygdala. In a similar study, 3-hydroxybutyrate methyl ester (HBME), a derivative of βHB, was assessed for its therapeutic efficacy in a double transgenic mouse model

of AD (Zhang et al., 2013). HBME-treated mice (40 mg/kg/day via intragastric gavage) exhibited improved spatial learning and working memory and decreased anxiety compared to control mice. MRI analysis revealed that HBME prevented the development of asymmetric ventricular morphology, which was observed in the untreated AD mice. After 2.5 months of treatment, the brains of the animals were analyzed via immunohistochemistry, and in vitro studies were performed to further investigate the mechanism of protection. HBME-treated mice exhibited reduced Aβ plaque deposition in the cortex and hippocampus. The authors reported that HBME supported neuronal survival after glucose deprivation and prevented NaN_3-induced mitochondrial dysfunction by rescuing expression of the respiratory complexes, reducing ROS production, and maintaining mitochondrial membrane potential.

In an encouraging case report by Newport and Veech, supplementation with MCFAs and KME was investigated as a potential therapy for AD (Newport et al., 2015). The patient described was an apolipoprotein E4 (apo E4)-positive 63-year-old Caucasian male with early-onset, sporadic AD diagnosed 12 years prior to the publication of the report. His disease rapidly progressed prior to initiation of ketosis therapy in 2008 and was characterized by increasingly severe memory loss and an inability to carry out normal activities of daily living (ADLs). His Mini-Mental State Examination (MMSE) score declined from 23 to 12 between 2004 and 2008, and his MRI scans revealed diffuse involutional changes of his frontal and parietal lobes, with atrophy of the amygdala and hippocampus. The patient initially began ketosis treatment in May 2008 by consuming sources of MCFAs—MCT oil and coconut oil (CO). His dose and regimen of administration were optimized, and eventually reached 165 ml of a 4:3 mixture of MCT:CO divided into 3 to 4 servings over the course of the day. Within 75 days of treatment, the patient's MMSE score improved from 12 to 20. The patient continued MCFA treatment for 20 months, and during that time he exhibited remarkable cognitive and physical improvements. His Alzheimer's Disease Assessment Scale-Cognitive (ADAS-Cog) rose 6 points and his ADLs score rose 14 points over that time. MRI scans revealed no changes in brain atrophy from June 2008 to April 2010, suggesting stabilization of the disease process. In 2010, the patient also began taking KME (28.7 g KME, three times daily). The patient exhibited many improvements following KME treatment.

Within a few days of initiating KME therapy, the patient regained the ability to recite and write out the alphabet and to dress himself. He began improving in ADLs, such as showering, shaving, and putting away dishes, and he demonstrated improvements in abstract thinking, insight, and sense of humor. The patient himself reported feeling happier and more energetic after beginning treatment with KME. Over time, he exhibited significant improvements in memory retrieval and regained the ability to perform complex tasks, such as vacuuming and yard work. Both MCFA and KME treatment significantly elevated his blood ketones, even while the patient continued to consume a normal diet.

The KME was particularly effective at inducing ketosis, elevating blood ketones up to 7 mM within 1 hr of administration (Figure 33.2), a level approximately 5 to 10 times greater than is possible with the classic KD or MCFA consumption. The patient's caregiver, a physician, noted that his improved cognitive and physical performance seemed to track his plasma ketone concentrations, with the greatest improvements seen during peak elevation in blood ketones. Importantly, there were no adverse effects observed in the patient over this 2-year study, suggesting that prolonged hyperketonemia is likely safe. The authors noted that not all patients may respond to such therapy in a similar manner, but that appropriately designed trials should be conducted to evaluate the percentage of patients with Alzheimer's disease responsive to KE therapy.

An oral ketogenic compound and prescription food product called AC-1202 (trade name Axona) was developed by Accera, Inc., as an AD therapy. AC-1202 elevates blood ketone levels because it contains MCFAs, which are natural

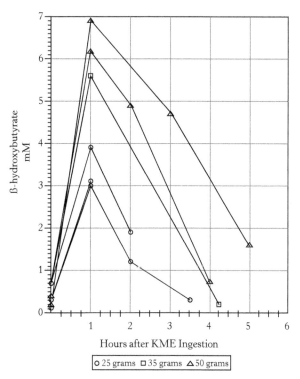

FIGURE 33.2 *Responses of Whole-Blood B-Hydroxybutyrate (βHB) Levels to Different Doses of Ketone Monoester (KME)*

βHB concentrations rose to 3 to 7 mM 1 hr after ingestion of KME in three different doses (25, 35, and 50 g), taken on separate days. The peak levels measured are in the range of those obtained during adherence to the classical KD and are about tenfold the concentrations achievable by MCFA administration. The findings suggest that therapeutic ketosis can be maintained throughout the day if KME is taken every 3 to 4 hr. Precision Xtra Glucose and Ketone Monitoring System (Abbott Diabetes Care, Inc., Alameda, CA, USA) was used to measure βHB levels in capillary blood samples. Acetoacetate (AcAc) was not measured. The figure was reprinted with permission from Newport et al. (2015). *A new way to produce hyperketonemia: Use of a ketone ester in a case of Alzheimer's disease. Alzheimer's and Dementia, 11(1): 99–103* ketogenic precursors. AC-1202 was evaluated in a randomized, double-blind, placebo-controlled, multicenter trial in patients with mild to moderate AD (Henderson et al., 2009). AC-1202 induced a mild level of ketosis in patients (up to 0.3–0.4 mM), which was significantly higher than placebo controls. AC-1202 treatment induced small improvements in ADAS-Cog, MMSE, and ADCS-CGIC (AD Cooperative Study—Clinical Global Impression of Change) scores compared to placebo in some subgroups of AD patients tested. In many of the patient subgroups, AC-1202 did not affect the performance of apo E4-positive patients on these tests. The modest improvements observed in this study may potentially be due to the comparatively low level of ketosis induced by AC-1202, considering what is attainable with KME or similar ketogenic supplements. Furthermore, the lack of effect observed in apo E4-positive patients could also be a result of the mild level of ketosis induced, or alternatively because the study may have lacked the statistical power necessary to reveal a significant effect in this subpopulation (Newport et al., 2015). Indeed, the case report by Newport and colleagues suggests that ketosis can be an effective therapy for AD in some apo E4-positive patients. And more recently, another small trial evaluating Axona in 22 Japanese patients with mild to moderate sporadic AD reported enhanced memory function with no difference between apo E4-positive and apo E4-negative patients (Kimoto et al., 2017). Success was also reported in another Japanese trial where subjects with mild to moderate AD were administered an MCT-containing ketogenic formula called Ketonformula for 12 weeks (Ota et al., 2019). The patients exhibited improvements in verbal memory and processing speed over the course of the study. Taken together, these reports clearly demonstrate the potential utility of exogenous ketone supplementations to confer the therapeutic benefits of ketosis in a population of patients for which severe dietary restrictions would be extremely difficult, if not impossible.

Cancer

Unlike healthy tissues, some cancers do not appear to efficiently metabolize ketone bodies for energy. Some cancer cells lack expression of the ketone-utilization enzymes like succinyl-coenzyme A:3-oxoacid coenzyme A transferase (SCOT; Chang et al., 2013; Sawai et al., 2004; Skinner et al., 2009; Tisdale & Brennan, 1983). Abnormal mitochondrial function and impaired oxidative phosphorylation capacity are other features of some cancers that likely limit their use of ketones, which are metabolized exclusively within the mitochondria, as a fuel. Indeed, a study of five different brain cancer cell lines concluded that glioma cells lack the capacity to metabolize βHB during glucose restriction, unlike healthy brain cells (Fredericks & Ramsey, 1978; Maurer et al., 2011).

The KD, fasting, and caloric restriction are dietary regimens that have been shown to inhibit cancer progression in both preclinical and clinical studies (Fine et al., 2012; Freedland et al., 2008; Khodabakhshi et al., 2020; Mavropoulos et al., 2009; Nebeling et al., 1995; Poff et al., 2013; Rossifanelli et al., 1991; Shelton et al., 2010; Weber, 2019; Wheatley et al., 2008; Zuccoli et al., 2010). Until recently, the generally accepted mechanism of action of these therapies was decreasing glucose availability to the tumor and suppressing the insulin and IGF signaling pathways. However, all three of these therapies also elevate blood ketones, and recent evidence suggests that ketones themselves may possess inherent anticancer properties. One small clinical trial studied the effects of a 28-day KD in patients with late-stage, metastatic cancer (Fine et al., 2012). Prior to beginning the dietary intervention, all patients exhibited progressive disease. Following 1 month of treatment, over 50% of patients showed stable disease or partial remission. Interestingly, there was no significant drop in blood glucose in the patients over the course of the diet; instead, patient response was most strongly correlated with degree of ketosis relative to baseline. In vitro and preclinical studies have confirmed the hypothesis that ketones are damaging to cancer. Magee et al. demonstrated that βHB inhibited proliferation in a dose-dependent manner up to 20 mM in multiple cancer cell lines of varied origin (Magee et al., 1979). Similarly, both AcAc and βHB inhibited viability and induced apoptosis in neuroblastoma cells but had no effect on control fibroblasts (Skinner et al., 2009). Another study demonstrated that 5 mM βHB slows proliferation and decreases viability in VM-M3 glioma cells, even in the presence of excess (25 mM) glucose. Exogenous ketone supplementation with BD or BD-AcAc$_2$ elicited potent anticancer effects in the VM-M3 model of metastatic cancer, slowing tumor growth and prolonging survival by 51% and 69%, respectively (Poff et al., 2014). These observations strongly suggest that exogenous ketone supplements could be used as an effective adjuvant therapy for cancer.

There are multiple mechanisms by which ketones may be damaging to cancer cells. (1) Cancer is particularly reliant on the glycolytic pathway for energy production and biosynthesis (Gillies et al., 2008), and βHB inhibits the first and third enzymatic reactions of glycolysis (Randle et al., 1964). (2) Excess fermentation in cancer cells causes lactate production and a subsequent acidification of the tumor microenvironment, which promotes malignancy. Both lactate and the ketone bodies are transported across the plasma membrane by the monocarboxylic transporter family of transporters (Halestrap & Price, 1999). βHB has been shown to inhibit lactate export from isolated rat hepatocytes in vitro (Metcalfe et al., 1986). It is possible that ketones may damage cancer cells by inhibiting lactate export through competitive inhibition of monocarboxylic transporters, subsequently inducing intracellular acidification and preventing the tumor-promoting effects of lactate in the tumor microenvironment. (3) Inflammation and oxidative stress are both known to promote cancer development and progression (Coussens & Werb, 2002; Wang & Yi, 2008); thus, the inhibitory effects of ketone metabolism on both of these pathways could contribute to its anticancer efficacy. (4) Cancers exhibit widespread differences in epigenetic patterns compared to their normal tissue counterparts, allowing them to increase expression of oncogenes and inhibit the expression of tumor suppressor genes (Hassler & Egger, 2012). HDACIs are being investigated for their use as antineoplastic agents and have been shown to elicit a plethora of anticancer effects in vitro, including activation of apoptosis, induction of ROS generation and DNA damage, and inhibition of DNA repair (Bose et al., 2014). As mentioned, βHB functions as an endogenous HDACI, a mechanism that may underlie its potential use as a cancer treatment. (5) Finally, mitochondrial transfer studies have demonstrated that healthy mitochondria act as tumor suppressors (Seyfried, 2012). The potential for ketone metabolism to support or enhance mitochondrial health could also account for its therapeutic effects and its potential for preventing carcinogenesis.

Insulin Resistance/Type 2 D iabetes Mellitus

As previously described, KE administration simultaneously decreases blood glucose and sometimes blood insulin concentrations (Myette-Cote et al., 2018; Srivastava et al., 2012). These results suggest a potential therapeutic use of exogenous ketone supplementation for insulin resistance and type 2 diabetes mellitus (T2DM; Walsh et al., 2020b). Indeed, exogenous ketones qualitatively mimic the acute metabolic effects of insulin (Kashiwaya et al., 1997). It is known that insulin activates pyruvate dehydrogenase (PDH) to increase the production of acetyl-CoA, and 5-mM ketone administration mimicked this effect, increasing acetyl-CoA production 15-fold in the glucose-perfused isolated rat heart (Kashiwaya et al., 1994). Furthermore, in this model, ketones and insulin increased cardiac hydraulic efficiency to a similar degree, approximately 25% to 35% (Kashiwaya et al., 1994). In another study, mice that were fed a diet formulated with KE (30% kcal) had a 73% increase in the Quantitative Insulin-Sensitivity Check Index (QUICKI), a surrogate marker of insulin sensitivity, compared to control, calorie-matched mice (Srivastava et al., 2012). Fasting plasma glucose levels were not altered in these mice, but fasting plasma insulin levels were reduced by approximately 85% in the KE-fed mice compared to controls. The authors therefore hypothesized that ketones could be therapeutic by correcting metabolic defects of acute insulin deficiency or of the insulin-resistant state (Kashiwaya et al., 1997). A recent study also supported the potential use of ketogenic MCTs in a rat model of T2DM, wherein replacing long-chain triglycerides (LCTs) with medium-chain triglycerides (MCTs) in both a low- and high-fat diet elicited beneficial effects, such as improving blood lipid profiles and lower body weight (Sung et al., 2018). In humans, glycemic response was improved by exogenous KME consumption during an OGTT, further supporting this potential application (Nakagata et al., 2021).

The HDACI activity of βHB could also be beneficial in T2DM by altering the direct regulation of HDAC-dependent glucose metabolism and by inducing resistance to oxidative stress. HDACs regulate the expression of genes encoding many metabolic enzymes, and HDAC3 knockout animals exhibit reduced glucose and insulin. Suberoylanilide hydroxamic acid (SAHA), a class I HDACI, has been shown to improve insulin sensitivity and to increase oxidative metabolism and metabolic rate in a mouse model of diabetes (Galmozzi et al., 2013). Butyrate, a short-chain fatty acid that is structurally similar to βHB and that also acts as an HDACI, lowers blood glucose and insulin levels and improves glucose tolerance and respiratory efficiency (Gao et al., 2009). The vascular dysfunction in T2DM is thought to be caused by oxidative stress (Giacco & Brownlee,

2010). HDAC inhibition prevents renal damage in mouse models of diabetic nephropathy through modulation of redox mechanisms (Advani et al., 2011). Therefore, βHB suppression of oxidative stress through HDAC inhibition may help restore insulin sensitivity and manage complications of diabetes.

Weight Loss

The KD is hypothesized to induce weight loss and/or promote weight-loss maintenance by reducing appetite through the satiety effect of protein and ketone bodies and stabilization of circulating glucose and insulin, by increasing adipose tissue catabolism via reducing de novo lipogenesis and increasing lipolysis, and by altering systemic and adipose tissue metabolic efficiency and hunger hormone profiles (Ebbeling et al., 2018; Ludwig & Ebbeling, 2018; Paoli, 2014). However, the KD can be difficult to maintain in the long term for some individuals (Dansinger et al., 2005; Gardner et al., 2018), and many people regain weight rapidly upon returning to a standard diet (Paoli, 2014). In fact, it has been demonstrated that over 60% of individuals who lost 5% of their initial body weight will fail to maintain the weight loss at 1-year follow-up regardless of dietary choice, with 96% failing to maintain 20% weight loss (Kraschnewski et al., 2010). This has been attributed to a number of powerful counterregulatory responses that attempt to maintain weight homeostasis via reduced thermic effect of food, decreased basal metabolic rate, altered hunger hormones, and increased hyperphagia, among others (Maclean et al., 2011). There is reason to be optimistic that utilizing exogenous ketone supplements can contribute to long-term benefits in weight and body composition. Indeed, studies have shown that exogenous ketone supplementation can also induce and/or assist with weight loss and potentially weight-loss maintenance. However, preliminary studies have shown that exogenous ketone supplementation can also induce weight loss. First, it should be noted that ketone supplements are sources of calories, with each ketone supplement providing on average 5 to 8 kcal/g ingested; therefore, patients would need to decrease dietary caloric intake in order to prevent weight gain.

Our lab has demonstrated that various exogenous ketone supplements contribute to weight loss. In a 28-day oral gavage study, all five ketogenic supplements tested (BD, BD-AcAc$_2$, MCT, KS, KS + MCT) caused a significant reduction in weight gain in supplemented animals compared to controls (Kesl, 2016). Similarly, a 15-week chronic feeding study in which BD-AcAc2, KS, or KS + MCT replaced approximately 20% of the diet by weight, fed ad libitum, led to significant reduction in weight gain in supplemented animals compared to controls (unpublished data). Over a 17-day analysis, BD, BD-AcAc$_2$, MCT, KS, KS + MCT, and caloric restriction all induced weight loss in C57BL6J mice, with various degrees of potency (unpublished data).

In support of these findings, administration of both βHB and BD has been shown to decrease food intake in rats and pygmy goats (Arase et al., 1988; Carpenter & Grossman, 1983; Davis et al., 1981; Langhans et al., 1983; Rossi et al., 2000). Similarly, it is suggested that MCTs increase satiety, resulting in reduced food intake and weight loss as a consequence of their rapid oxidation into ketone bodies (Krotkiewski, 2001; Poppitt et al., 2010; Van Wymelbeke et al., 1998). MCTs may further counteract fat deposition in adipocytes by increasing thermogenesis (Dulloo, 2011). Several studies in animals and humans have revealed increased energy expenditure and lipid oxidation with MCTs compared to LCTs (Baba et al., 1982; Bach & Babayan, 1982; Crozier et al., 1987; Dulloo et al., 1996; Ferreira et al., 2014; Karen & Welma, 2015; Scalfi et al., 1991; Seaton et al., 1986; St-Onge et al., 2003). KEs have also been shown to affect weight in mice, rats, and humans. Mice administered a diet supplemented with KE exhibited reduced voluntary food intake, increased insulin sensitivity, increased resting energy expenditure, and increased brown fat activity, demonstrating the potential utility of the KE as an antiobesity compound (Srivastava et al., 2012). In another study, mice fed a KE diet maintained a body weight of approximately 10% to 12% less than that of control, standard diet-fed animals (Kashiwaya et al., 2013), and in yet another mouse study, KE attenuated weight gain at both standard (23°C) and thermoneutral (30°C) housing temperatures, an effect that was not attributable to increased energy expenditure (Deemer et al., 2020). Kashiwaya et al. suggested that the KE-supplemented diet may benefit obesity because it decreases brain malonyl-CoA, an important metabolic mediator of appetite (Kashiwaya et al., 2010). Stubbs et al. demonstrated that oral administration of a KE in obese patients reduced appetite and circulating ghrelin, an appetite-stimulating hormone (Stubbs et al., 2018a). In a 7-day study, eight humans with T2DM consumed three KE-supplemented drinks a day in conjunction with their normal diet. The group lost an average of 2%

of their body weight (Hashim & VanItallie, 2014). Recent analysis of BD-AcAc$_2$ in a high-fat obese mouse model demonstrated that this KE reduced voluntary food intake and induced greater weight and fat loss than in a pair-fed control group via increased uncoupling protein in adipose tissue (Davis et al., 2019). A follow-up study illustrated the weight- and fat-loss effect of BD-AcAc$_2$ may be dose-dependent (Deemer et al., 2019). Our group has also demonstrated that BD-AcAc$_2$ is a more efficacious weight-loss agent than BD, KS, KS + MCT, and caloric restriction (unpublished data). Together, these findings demonstrate that exogenous ketone molecules may assist in weight loss via appetite regulation, reduced food intake, reduced circulating hunger hormones, and increased adipose tissue mitochondrial energetic inefficiency.

Anticatabolic Effects
Over a century ago, multiple research groups discovered that during prolonged fasting, metrics of skeletal muscle breakdown first increased and then subsequently decreased as fasting prolonged (Benedict, 1915). Fifty years later, George Cahill and colleagues discovered that the elevations of ketone bodies reduced urinary nitrogen excretion and alanine flux from the skeletal muscle, allowing for prolonged survival during fasting by attenuating skeletal muscle catabolism (Cahill, 1970, 2006b; Felig et al., 1969; Owen et al., 1967). From 1973 to 1975, multiple analyses confirmed associations and/or a direct effect between elevations in ketone bodies and reduced metrics of protein breakdown in various populations (Blackburn et al., 1973; Hoover et al., 1975; Kies et al., 1973; Smith et al., 1975). Notably, in 1975, Sherwin et al. were the first to demonstrate that infusion of exogenous ketone bodies directly reduced skeletal muscle alanine flux (6-fold reduction) in a dose-dependent manner without changes in insulin (Sherwin et al., 1975). From 1971 to present, historical and emergent data have demonstrated that ketone bodies can attenuate skeletal muscle catabolism via consistent reductions in blood urea nitrogen (Cahill, 2006b; Maiz et al., 1985; Sherwin et al., 1975), attenuated alanine flux (Beylot et al., 1986; Fearon et al., 1988; Felig et al., 1969; Miles et al., 1981; Sherwin et al., 1975), reduced circulating glucose and glycolysis without obligate insulin (Binkiewicz et al., 1974; Cox et al., 2016; Egan, 2018; Fearon et al., 1988; Kesl et al., 2016; Leckey, 2017; Miles et al., 1981; Nair et al., 1988; Sherwin et al., 1975; Stubbs et al., 2017), augmented ERK/MEK proliferative signaling (Abdelmegeed et

al., 2004; Xia et al., 2017; Zou et al., 2016), and reduced HDAC activity and elevated acetylation status (Roberts et al., 2017; Shimazu et al., 2013), with demonstrated abilities also to reduce leucine oxidation in the fed state (Maiz et al., 1985; Nair et al., 1988), to augment protein synthesis (Nair et al., 1988; Vandoorne et al., 2017), to attenuate inflammation (Kovacs et al., 2019b; Youm et al., 2015), to increase antioxidant production in extramuscular tissues (Kim et al., 2007; Shimazu et al., 2013), and to reduce lactate (Cox et al., 2016; Evans & Egan, 2018; Fearon et al., 1988; Leckey, 2017; Tisdale et al., 1987). Consequently, it was hypothesized by Koutnik et al. that exogenous ketone bodies may attenuate atrophy even in the most devastating multifactorial catabolic diseases, including cancer cachexia and infectious/septic atrophy (Koutnik et al., 2019). Thomsen et al. demonstrated that βHB infusion in septic patients had a more potent anticatabolic effect on skeletal muscle than in controls, including the elevated glucose and hyperinsulinemia group (Thomsen et al., 2018). Koutnik et al. demonstrated that chronic and acute exogenous BD-AcAc$_2$ administration attenuated skeletal muscle catabolism in multifactorial cancer-anorexia cachexia syndrome and septic/inflammatory atrophy environments (Koutnik et al., 2020).

While ketone bodies appear to induce anticatabolic effects in skeletal muscle, they have been demonstrated to reduce catabolic processes and/or pathways, including attenuated glycolysis, lipolysis, and peripheral tissue atrophy. Analysis in muscle preparations demonstrated that ketones reduced glucose oxidation rates but increased glycogen synthesis (Laughlin et al., 1994; Maizels et al., 1977; Randle et al., 1964). Several studies have demonstrated that exogenous ketone administration reduced free fatty acids and glycerol with or without changes in insulin (Beylot et al., 1994; Beylot et al., 1986; Binkiewicz et al., 1974; Cox et al., 2016; Leckey, 2017; Mikkelsen et al., 2015; Myette-Cote et al., 2018; Nair et al., 1988; Tisdale et al., 1987). This effect also appeared to be dose-dependent (Mikkelsen et al., 2015) via βHB's binding of HCAR2/GPR109a and inhibition of lipolysis by inhibiting NF-κB activity in adipose tissue (Taggart et al., 2005). Kripke et al. found that monoacetoacetin induced a positive nitrogen balance and reduced peripheral tissue atrophy (jejunal and colonic atrophy were inhibited; Kripke et al., 1988). Together, ketone bodies appear to regulate multiple catabolic and synthetic processes that contribute to attenuated skeletal muscle breakdown in catabolic environments.

Athletic Performance

Numerous studies have investigated the potential effects of the KD on athletic performance (Ma & Suzuki, 2019; Sherrier & Li, 2019). The KD induces a metabolic transition, upregulating fat and ketone body utilization in lieu of glucose and glycogen and allowing access to a much larger source of calories. A typical 90-kg, well-trained, male athlete will have available more than 40,000 kcal in stored fat, versus just 2,000 kcal in glycogen. In sports that rely on energy from the metabolism of fat and/or ketones (high-endurance/aerobic events), the KD eating strategy could upregulate cellular mechanisms to optimize rapid and efficient access to the more abundant endogenous fuel, thus improving performance. However, maintaining adherence to a KD may be difficult for some, and carbohydrates have demonstrated importance for anaerobic performance. Thus, there is interest in the use of exogenous ketogenic supplements for exercise, which could induce ketosis while still permitting use of dietary carbohydrates to fuel athletic performance.

Early investigation into the potential use of ketogenic agents for enhancing sports performance focused on acutely administered MCTs and led to important findings on fuel usage. One study found that subjects who received a pre-performance test supplement containing either glucose or MCT were able to oxidize both substrates at similar rates and to similar extents during prolonged exercise of modest intensity (Massicotte et al., 1992). MCTs provided as a supplemental drink, either with or without carbohydrates, can provide a rapidly utilized and sustained source of energy for exercise (Angus et al., 2000; Jeukendrup et al., 1995). Having confirmed the potential for MCTs to address the energy demands of endurance sports, several studies investigated how MCTs might affect fuel preference and performance. The consumption of MCTs, either with or without carbohydrates, was postulated to have a glycogen-sparing effect, which has been supported by some studies (Jeukendrup et al., 1998; Van Zyl et al., 1996) but not by others (Angus et al., 2000; Goedecke et al., 1999; Jeukendrup et al., 1995). While acutely administered MCTs are rapidly metabolized after ingestion, to date, their effect on endurance performance has been found to be either negligible, non-existent (Goedecke et al., 1999; Satabin et al., 1987), or negative (Jeukendrup et al., 1998; Van Zyl et al., 1996). Thus, while MCT ingestion has been shown to alter fuel metabolism, it appears that acute dosing of MCT with or without carbohydrates does not augment exercise performance.

However, MCTs could prove useful for athletes, depending upon the desired outcome or performance challenge. Of note, MCTs have been shown to favorably affect body composition (Clegg, 2010), potentially by increasing thermogenesis (Han et al., 2007; Nosaka et al., 2003) and/or altering hunger regulation (Krotkiewski, 2001), which may be useful in activities where an improved power or strength to body weight ratio is desired. Further, in a study investigating the effects of nonacute, 2-week ingestion of food containing MCTs versus LCTs on exercise performance until exhaustion, the MCT group utilized more fat, improved performance, reduced blood lactate, and felt more energetic (Nosaka et al., 2009). Also, there might be very specific cases in sports that may respond favorably to MCT intervention. For instance, a recent tantalizing study (albeit in mice) showed that regular consumption of an MCT-supplemented diet over a 21-day period rescued heat-induced exercise deficit by increasing mitochondrial biogenesis and metabolism (Wang et al., 2018). Future studies will likely include MCT co-administered with other agents, ketogenic or otherwise. Indeed, one such study has already shown that a combination of MCT with vitamin D and the ketogenic amino acid leucine improved muscle strength and function in humans (Abe et al., 2016).

While consumption of MCTs typically elevates blood levels of βHB 0.5 to 1.0 mM, KS and KE have been demonstrated to rapidly and reliably increase circulating ketone levels in humans, increasing D-βHB concentrations approximately 1.0 mM and 2.8 mM, respectively (Stubbs et al., 2017). These compounds have been the focus of studies on exogenous ketones and exercise performance. A seminal work showed that competitive cyclists acutely consuming a drink containing carbohydrates plus KE improved their performance by 2% (Cox et al., 2016). The enhanced exercise performance was attributed in part to altered metabolism, increased substrate availability, and reduced lactate threshold, and it was also marked by subsequent upregulation of glycogen synthesis. Similarly, a glycogen-sparing effect has been shown elsewhere (Holdsworth et al., 2017), but not consistently (Vandoorne et al., 2017).

Not only do KEs rapidly elevate blood ketones about 3 times higher than KSs, they also lack the salt load and are less problematic for the gastrointestinal system. Still GI distress with KEs has been noted as a concern in several studies (Evans

& Egan, 2018; Leckey, 2017). In each of these trials, exercise performance either decreased (Leckey, 2017) or failed to improve (Evans & Egan, 2018). Powdered MCT oils are now commercially available and are reported to be well tolerated. Similarly, development of more tolerable and palatable exogenous ketone formulations is ongoing.

An elevation in central nervous system activity occurs during sports performance (Davis & Bailey, 1997). Since ketones are known to effectively fuel the brain (Owen et al., 1967), several studies have been done to investigate such effects in exercise. One study using a KE showed an improvement in executive function after exhaustive exercise (Evans & Egan, 2018). However, other studies using either KS prior to high-intensity exercise (Prins et al., 2020a; Waldman et al., 2018) or KE prior to moderate-intensity exercise (Evans et al., 2019), showed no cognitive improvement following the task. Other studies investigating the potentially negative effects of KE-induced ketosis have looked at changes in the blood pH and neural signaling accompanying exercise after KE ingestion. A temporary increase in the perception of muscle pain and anxiety (Faull et al., 2019) was experienced, along with a mild decrease in blood pH, which presumably induced an increase in respiration, thereby returning pH to baseline in 15 to 20 min (Dearlove et al., 2019). These findings together suggest that KE-induced acidosis in the performance setting is well compensated for by homeostatic mechanisms.

As mentioned, the duration of treatment and combination of substances are likely crucial. Two published master's dissertations investigated the effect of KS on exercise performance and are worth mention in this regard. In one cross-over study using acute administration of KS + caffeine versus H_2O, an improvement in exercise performance was shown (Short, 2017). In a second longer-term study, twice-a-day administration for 8 days of KS + MCT versus a control with identical salt composition led to exercise improvements (Sonnenburg, 2018). In another long-term 3-week experiment, KE largely prevented the negative effects of overtraining, increased volitional food intake, and enhanced endurance exercise performance (Poffe et al., 2019).

Reportedly, the use of dietary supplements is motivated by the desire to improve either athletic performance, body image, or general state of well-being (Greenwood et al., 2015). Depending on the sport being considered, any or all of these outcomes are desirable. While interest in the use of ketogenic supplements for sports performance

has emerged with promising preclinical data (Ari et al., 2020), results have been mixed (Dearlove et al., 2019; Prins et al., 2020b). Factors underlying the interest include the following: ketone bodies have shown enhanced O_2 to ATP metabolic efficiency over other substrates in cardiac tissue (Kashiwaya et al., 1994), additional and/or alternative fuel types may more efficiently serve specific exercise tasks, exogenous ketones can improve glycogen status and reduce the lactate threshold, and potential multifaceted effects of ketone bodies independent of energetic utilization may influence both acute and chronic exercise performance. Further studies should consider supplementation context, personalized response (Angus et al., 2000), composition, formulation, timing, and dosing protocols.

CONCLUSION

Exogenous ketone supplements are being developed as an alternative or adjuvant method of inducing therapeutic ketosis aside from the classic KD. Emerging evidence has demonstrated that these novel compounds have the potential to offer benefits for both healthy and diseased individuals alike. It is probable that most, if not all, of the conditions that are known to benefit from the KD would receive some benefit from exogenous ketone supplementation through elevation of blood ketones and lowering of blood glucose. Importantly, ketone supplementation provides a tool for achieving ketosis in patients who are unable, unwilling, or uninterested in consuming a KD or low-carbohydrate diet. Ketone supplementation may also help circumvent some of the difficulties associated with KD therapy, because it allows for a rapid, dose-dependent induction of ketosis, which can be sustained with prolonged consumption and monitored precisely with commercially available technologies (e.g., blood ketone meters). Simultaneously, it could provide patients with the opportunity to reap the benefits of ketosis without the practical and social difficulties of a highly restrictive diet. Further research is needed to fully investigate the clinical utility and feasibility of exogenous ketone supplements as a method of inducing therapeutic ketosis.

REFERENCES

Abdelmegeed, M. A., Kim, S. K., Woodcroft, K. J., & Novak, R. F. (2004). Acetoacetate activation of extracellular signal-regulated kinase 1/2 and p38 mitogen-activated protein kinase in primary cultured rat hepatocytes: Role of oxidative stress. *Journal of Pharmacology and Experimental Therapeutics, 310*, 728–736.

Abe, S., Ezaki, O., & Suzuki, M. (2016). Medium-chain triglycerides in combination with leucine and vitamin D increase muscle strength and function in frail elderly adults in a randomized controlled trial. *Journal of Nutrition, 146*, 1017–1026.

Advani, A., Huang, Q., Thai, K., Advani, S. L., White, K. E., Kelly, D. J., Yuen, D. A., Connelly, K. A., Marsden, P. A., & Gilbert, R. E. (2011). Long-term administration of the histone deacetylase inhibitor vorinostat attenuates renal injury in experimental diabetes through an endothelial nitric oxide synthase-dependent mechanism. *American Journal of Pathology, 178*, 2205–2214.

Angus, D. J., Hargreaves, M., Dancey, J., & Febbraio, M. A. (2000). Effect of carbohydrate or carbohydrate plus medium-chain triglyceride ingestion on cycling time trial performance. *Journal of Applied Physiology, 88*, 113–119.

Arase, K., Fisler, J. S., Shargill, N. S., York, D. A., & Bray, G. A. (1988). Intracerebroventricular infusions of 3-OHB and insulin in a rat model of dietary obesity. *American Journal of Physiology, 255*, 81.

Ari, C., D'Agostino, D. P., Diamond, D. M., Kindy, M., Park, C., & Kovacs, Z. (2019a). Elevated Plus Maze Test combined with video tracking software to investigate the anxiolytic effect of exogenous ketogenic supplements. *Journal of Visualized Experiments: JoVE*, (143), 10.3791/58396. https://doi-org.ezproxy.hsc.usf.edu/10.3791/58396

Ari, C., Koutnik, A. P., DeBlasi, J., Landon, C., Rogers, C. Q., Vallas, J., Bharwani, S., Puchowicz, M., Bederman, I., Diamond, D. M., Kindy, M. S., Dean, J. B., & D Agostino, D. P. (2019b). Delaying latency to hyperbaric oxygen-induced CNS oxygen toxicity seizures by combinations of exogenous ketone supplements. *Physiological Reports, 7*(1), e13961. https://doi-org.ezproxy.hsc.usf.edu/10.14814/phy2.13961

Ari, C., Kovacs, Z., Murdun, C., Koutnik, A. P., Goldhagen, C. R., Rogers, C., Diamond, D., & D'Agostino, D. P. (2018). Nutritional ketosis delays the onset of isoflurane induced anesthesia. *BMC Anesthesiology, 18*, 85.

Ari, C., Murdun, C., Goldhagen, C., Koutnik, A. P., Bharwani, S. R., Diamond, D. M., Kindy, M., D'Agostino, D. P., & Kovacs, Z. (2020). Exogenous ketone supplements improved motor performance in preclinical rodent models. *Nutrients, 12*(8), 2459. https://doi-org.ezproxy.hsc.usf.edu/10.3390/nu12082459

Ari, C., Murdun, C., Koutnik, A. P., Goldhagen, C. R., Rogers, C., Park, C., Bharwani, S., Diamond, D. M., Kindy, M. S., D'Agostino, D. P., & Kovács, Z. (2019c). Exogenous ketones lower blood glucose level in rested and exercised rodent models.

Nutrients, 11(10), 2330. https://doi-org.ezproxy.hsc.usf.edu/10.3390/nu11102330

Augustin, K., Khabbush, A., Williams, S., Eaton, S., Orford, M., Cross, J. H., Heales, S. J. R., Walker, M. C., & Williams, R. S. B. (2018). Mechanisms of action for the medium-chain triglyceride ketogenic diet in neurological and metabolic disorders. *Lancet Neurology, 17*, 84–93.

Baba, N., Bracco, E. F., & Hashim, S. A. (1982). Enhanced thermogenesis and diminished deposition of fat in response to overfeeding with diet containing medium chain triglyceride. *The American Journal of Clinical Nutrition, 35*(4), 678–682. https://doi-org.ezproxy.hsc.usf.edu/10.1093/ajcn/35.4.678

Babayan, V. K. (1987). Medium chain triglycerides and structured lipids. *Lipids, 22*(6), 417–420. https://doi-org.ezproxy.hsc.usf.edu/10.1007/BF02537271

Bach, A. C., & Babayan, V. K. (1982). Medium-chain triglycerides: An update. *American Journal of Clinical Nutrition, 36*, 950–962.

Benedict, F. G. (1915). *A study of prolonged fasting.* Carnegie Institute of Washington.

Benjamin, J. S., Pilarowski, G. O., Carosso, G. A., Zhang, L., Huso, D. L., Goff, L. A., Vernon, H. J., Hansen, K. D., & Bjornsson, H. T. (2017). A ketogenic diet rescues hippocampal memory defects in a mouse model of Kabuki syndrome. *Proceedings of the National Academy of Sciences of the United States of America, 114*, 125–130.

Beylot, M., Chassard, D., Chambrier, C., Guiraud, M., Odeon, M., Beaufrere, B., & Bouletreau, P. (1994). Metabolic effects of a D-beta-hydroxybutyrate infusion in septic patients: Inhibition of lipolysis and glucose production but not leucine oxidation. *Critical Care Medicine, 22*, 1091–1098.

Beylot, M., Khalfallah, Y., Riou, J. P., Cohen, R., Normand, S., & Mornex, R. (1986). Effects of ketone bodies on basal and insulin-stimulated glucose utilization in man. *Journal of Clinical Endocrinology and Metabolism, 63*, 9–15.

Binkiewicz, A., Sadeghi-Najad, A., Hochman, H., Loridan, L., & Senior, B. (1974). An effect of ketones on the concentrations of glucose and of free fatty acids in man independent of the release of insulin. *Journal of Pediatrics, 84*, 226–231.

Birkhahn, R. H., & Border, J. R. (1978). Intravenous feeding of the rat with short chain fatty acid esters. II. Monoacetoacetin. *American Journal of Clinical Nutrition, 31*, 436–441.

Birkhahn, R. H., McMenamy, R. H., & Border, J. R. (1977). Intravenous feeding of the rat with short chain fatty acid esters. I. Glycerol monobutyrate. *American Journal of Clinical Nutrition, 30*, 2078–2082.

Birkhahn, R. H., McMenamy, R. H., & Border, J. R. (1979). Monoglyceryl acetoacetate: A ketone body-carbohydrate substrate for parenteral feeding of the rat. *Journal of Nutrition, 109,* 1168–1174.

Bjornsson, H. T., Benjamin, J. S., Zhang, L., Weissman, J., Gerber, E. E., Chen, Y. C., Vaurio, R. G., Potter, M. C., Hansen, K. D., & Dietz, H. C. (2014). Histone deacetylase inhibition rescues structural and functional brain deficits in a mouse model of Kabuki syndrome. *Science Translational Medicine, 6*(256), 256ra135. https://doi-org.ezproxy.hsc.usf. edu/10.1126/scitranslmed.3009278

Blackburn, G. L., Flatt, J. P., Clowes, G. H., Jr., O'Donnell, T. F., & Hensle, T. E. (1973). Protein sparing therapy during periods of starvation with sepsis of trauma. *Annals of Surgery, 177,* 588–594.

Bock, M., Karber, M., & Kuhn, H. (2018). Ketogenic diets attenuate cyclooxygenase and lipoxygenase gene expression in multiple sclerosis. *EBioMedicine, 36,* 293–303.

Borges, K., & Sonnewald, U. (2012). Triheptanoin—A medium chain triglyceride with odd chain fatty acids: A new anaplerotic anticonvulsant treatment? *Epilepsy Research, 100,* 239–244.

Bornfeldt, K. E., & Tabas, I. (2011). Insulin resistance, hyperglycemia, and atherosclerosis. *Cell Metabolism, 14,* 575–585.

Bose, P., Dai, Y., & Grant, S. (2014). Histone deacetylase inhibitor (HDACI) mechanisms of action: Emerging insights. *Pharmacology & Therapeutics, 143*(3), 323–336. https://doi-org.ezproxy.hsc.usf. edu/10.1016/j.pharmthera.2014.04.004

Bough, K. J., & Rho, J. M. (2007). Anticonvulsant mechanisms of the ketogenic diet. *Epilepsia, 48,* 43–58.

Bradshaw, P. C., Seeds, W. A., Miller, A. C., Mahajan, V. R., & Curtis, W. M. (2020). COVID-19: Proposing a ketone-based metabolic therapy as a treatment to blunt the cytokine storm. *Oxidative Medicine and Cellular Longevity, 2020,* 6401341.

Brunengraber, H. (1997). Potential of ketone body esters for parenteral and oral nutrition. *Nutrition, 13,* 233–235.

Budavari, S. E. (1989). The Merck Index: An encyclopedia of chemical, drugs, and biologicals. *Royal Society of Chemistry, 74*(5), 339.

Cahill, G. (2006a). Fuel metabolism in starvation. *Annual Review of Nutrition, 26,* 1–22.

Cahill, G. F., Jr. (1970). Starvation in man. *New England Journal of Medicine, 282,* 668–675.

Cahill, G. F., Jr. (2006b). Fuel metabolism in starvation. *Annual Review of Nutrition, 26,* 1–22.

Cahill, G. F., Jr., & Veech, R. L. (2003). Ketoacids? Good medicine? *Transactions of the American Clinical and Climatological Association, 114,* 149–161; discussion 162–163.

Carpenter, R. G., & Grossman, S. P. (1983). Plasma fat metabolites and hunger. *Physiology & Behavior, 30,* 57–63.

Chang, H. T., Olson, L. K., & Schwartz, K. A. (2013). Ketolytic and glycolytic enzymatic expression profiles in malignant gliomas: Implication for ketogenic diet therapy. *Nutrition & Metabolism, 10,* 47.

Chang, P., Zuckermann, A. M., Williams, S., Close, A. J., Cano-Jaimez, M., McEvoy, J. P., Spencer, J., Walker, M. C., & Williams, R. S. (2015). Seizure control by derivatives of medium chain fatty acids associated with the ketogenic diet show novel branching-point structure for enhanced potency. *Journal of Pharmacology and Experimental Therapeutics, 352,* 43–52.

Chu, C. B., & Jiao, L. D. (2015). (R)-3-Oxobutyl 3-hydroxybutanoate (OBHB) induces hyperketonemia in Alzheimer's disease. *International Journal of Clinical and Experimental Medicine, 8,* 7684–7688.

Ciarlone, S. L., Grieco, J. C., D'Agostino, D. P., & Weeber, E. J. (2016). Ketone ester supplementation attenuates seizure activity and improves behavior and hippocampal synaptic plasticity in an Angelman syndrome mouse model. *Neurobiology of Disease, 96,* 38–46. https://doi-org.ezproxy.hsc. usf.edu/10.1016/j.nbd.2016.08.002

Ciraolo, S. T., Previs, S. F., Fernandez, C. A., Agarwal, K. C., David, F., Koshy, J., Lucas, D., Tammaro, A., Stevens, M. P., & Tserng, K. Y. (1995). Model of extreme hypoglycemia in dogs made ketotic with (R,S)-1,3-butanediol acetoacetate esters. *American Journal of Physiology, 269,* 75.

Clarke, K., Tchabanenko, K., Pawlosky, R., Carter, E., Knight, N., Murray, A., Cochlin, L., King, M., Wong, A., Roberts, A., Robertson, J., & Veech, R. L. (2012a). Oral 28-day and developmental toxicity studies of (R)-3-hydroxybutyl (R)-3-hydroxybutyrate. *Regulatory Toxicology and Pharmacology, 63,* 196–208. https://doi-org. ezproxy.hsc.usf.edu/10.1016/j.yrtph.2012.04.001

Clarke, K., Tchabanenko, K., Pawlosky, R., Carter, E., Todd King, M., Musa-Veloso, K., Ho, M., Roberts, A., Robertson, J., Vanitallie, T. B., & Veech, R. L. (2012b). Kinetics, safety and tolerability of (R)-3-hydroxybutyl (R)-3-hydroxybutyrate in healthy adult subjects. *Regulatory Toxicology and Pharmacology, 63,* 401–408. https://doi-org. ezproxy.hsc.usf.edu/10.1016/j.yrtph.2012.04.008

Clegg, M. E. (2010). Medium-chain triglycerides are advantageous in promoting weight loss although not beneficial to exercise performance. *International Journal of Food Sciences and Nutrition, 61,* 653–679. https://doi-org.ezproxy. hsc.usf.edu/10.3109/09637481003702114

Coussens, L. M., & Werb, Z. (2002). Inflammation and cancer. *Nature, 420,* 860–867.

Cox, P. J., Kirk, T., Ashmore, T., Willerton, K., Evans, R., Smith, A., Murray, A. J., Stubbs, B., West, J., McLure, S. W., King, M. T., Dodd, M. S., Holloway, C., Neubauer, S., Drawer, S., Veech, R. L., Griffin, J. L., & Clarke, K. (2016). Nutritional ketosis alters fuel preference and thereby endurance performance in athletes. *Cell Metabolism, 24*, 256–268.   https://doi-org.ezproxy.hsc.usf.edu/ 10.1016/j.cmet.2016.07.010

Croteau, E., Castellano, C. A., Fortier, M., Bocti, C., Fulop, T., Paquet, N., & Cunnane, S. C. (2018). A cross-sectional comparison of brain glucose and ketone metabolism in cognitively healthy older adults, mild cognitive impairment and early Alzheimer's disease. *Experimental Gerontology, 107*, 18–26. https://doi-org.ezproxy.hsc.usf.edu/ 10.1016/j.exger.2017.07.004

Crozier, G., Bois-Joyeux, B., Chanez, M., Girard, J., & Peret, J. (1987). Metabolic effects induced by long-term feeding of medium-chain triglycerides in the rat. *Metabolism: Clinical and Experimental, 36*(8), 807–814. https://doi-org.ezproxy.hsc.usf. edu/10.1016/0026-0495(87)90122-3

Cunnane, S. C., Courchesne-Loyer, A., St-Pierre, V., Vandenberghe, C., Pierotti, T., Fortier, M., Croteau, E., & Castellano, C. A. (2016). Can ketones compensate for deteriorating brain glucose uptake during aging? Implications for the risk and treatment of Alzheimer's disease. *Annals of the New York Academy of Sciences, 1367*(1), 12–20. https://doi-org.ezproxy.hsc.usf.edu/10.1111/ nyas.12999

D'Agostino, D., Arnold, P., & Kesl, S. (2014). *Compositions and methods for producing elevated and sustained ketosis.* United States Patent. No. US20140350105A1. U.S. Patent and Trademark Office. https://patents.google.com/ patent/US20140350105A1/en

D'Agostino, D., Pilla, R., Held, H., Landon, C., Puchowicz, M., Brunengraber, H., Ari, C., Arnold, P., & Dean, J. (2013). Therapeutic ketosis with ketone ester delays central nervous system oxygen toxicity seizures in rats. *American Journal of Physiology Regulatory, Integrative and Comparative Physiology, 304*, R829–R836.

Dansinger, M. L., Gleason, J. A., Griffith, J. L., Selker, H. P., & Schaefer, E. J. (2005). Comparison of the Atkins, Ornish, Weight Watchers, and Zone diets for weight loss and heart disease risk reduction: A randomized trial. *JAMA, 293*, 43–53.

Davis, J. M., & Bailey, S. P. (1997). Possible mechanisms of central nervous system fatigue during exercise. *Medicine and Science in Sports and Exercise, 29*(1), 45–57. https://doi-org.ezproxy. hsc.usf.edu/10.1097/00005768-199701000-00008

Davis, R. A. H., Deemer, S. E., Bergeron, J. M., Little, J. T., Warren, J. L., Fisher, G., Smith, D. L., Jr., Fontaine, K. R., Dickinson, S. L., Allison, D. B., & Plaisance, E. P. (2019). Dietary R,S-1,3-butanediol diacetoacetate reduces body weight and adiposity in obese mice fed a high-fat diet. *FASEB Journal: Official Publication of the Federation of American Societies for Experimental Biology, 33*(2), 2409–2421. https://doi-org.ezproxy.hsc.usf. edu/10.1096/fj.201800821RR

Davis, R. J., Brand, M. D., & Martin, B. R. (1981). The effect of insulin on plasma-membrane and mitochondrial-membrane potentials in isolated fat-cells. *Biochemical Journal, 196*, 133–147.

de Carvalho Vidigal, F., Guedes Cocate, P., Goncalves Pereira, L., & de Cassia Goncalves Alfenas, R. (2012). The role of hyperglycemia in the induction of oxidative stress and inflammatory process. *Nutricion Hospitalaria, 27*, 1391–1398.

de la Monte, S. M. (2012). Brain insulin resistance and deficiency as therapeutic targets in Alzheimer's disease. *Current Alzheimer Research, 9*, 35–66.

Dearlove, D. J., Faull, O. K., & Clarke, K. (2019). Context is key: Exogenous ketosis and athletic performance. *Current Opinion in Physiology, 10*, 81–89.

Dearlove, D. J., Faull, O. K., Rolls, E., Clarke, K., & Cox, P. J. (2019). Nutritional ketoacidosis during incremental exercise in healthy athletes. *Frontiers in Physiology, 10*, 290.

Deemer, S. E., Davis, R. A. H., Gower, B. A., Koutnik, A. P., Poff, A. M., Dickinson, S. L., Allison, D. B., D'Agostino, D. P., & Plaisance, E. P. (2019). Concentration-dependent effects of a dietary ketone ester on components of energy balance in mice. *Frontiers in Nutrition, 6*, 56. https://doi-org. ezproxy.hsc.usf.edu/10.3389/fnut.2019.00056

Deemer, S. E., Davis, R. A. H., Roberts, B. M., Smith, D. L., Jr., Koutnik, A. P., Poff, A. M., D'Agostino, D. P., & Plaisance, E. P. (2020). Exogenous dietary ketone ester decreases body weight and adiposity in mice housed at thermoneutrality. *Obesity, 28*, 1447–1455.

Desrochers, S., David, F., Garneau, M., Jetté, M., & Brunengraber, H. (1992). Metabolism of R- and S-1,3-butanediol in perfused livers from meal-fed and starved rats. *Biochemical Journal, 285 (Pt 2)*, 647–653.

Desrochers, S., Dubreuil, P., Brunet, J., Jetté, M., David, F., Landau, B. R., & Brunengraber, H. (1995a). Metabolism of (R,S)-1,3-butanediol acetoacetate esters, potential parenteral and enteral nutrients in conscious pigs. *American Journal of Physiology, 268*, 7.

Desrochers, S., Quinze, K., Dugas, H., Dubreuil, P., Bomont, C., David, F., Agarwal, K. C., Kumar, A., Soloviev, M. V., Powers, L., Landau, B., & Brunengraber, H. (1995b). (R,S)-1,3-Butanediol acetoacetate esters, potential alternates to lipid emulsions for total parenteral nutrition. *Journal of Nutritional Biochemistry, 6*, 111–118.

Drackley, J. K., Richard, M. J., & Young, J. W. (1990). In vitro production of beta-hydroxybutyrate from 1,3-butanediol by bovine liver, rumen mucosa, and kidney. *Journal of Dairy Science, 73*, 679–682.

Duewell, P., Kono, H., Rayner, K. J., Sirois, C. M., Vladimer, G., Bauernfeind, F. G., Abela, G. S., Franchi, L., Nunez, G., Schnurr, M., Espevik, T., Lien, E., Fitzgerald, K. A., Rock, K. L., Moore, K.

J., Wright, S. D., Hornung, V., & Latz, E. (2010). NLRP3 inflammasomes are required for atherogenesis and activated by cholesterol crystals. *Nature, 464,* 1357–1361.

Dulloo, A. G. (2011). The search for compounds that stimulate thermogenesis in obesity management: From pharmaceuticals to functional food ingredients. *Obesity Reviews, 12,* 866–883.

Dulloo, A. G., Fathi, M., & Mensi, N. (1996). Twenty-four-hour energy expenditure and urinary catecholamines of humans consuming low-to-moderate amounts of medium-chain triglycerides: A dose-response study in a human respiratory chamber. *European Journal of Clinical Nutrition, 50*(3), 152–158.

Dymsza, H. A. (1975). Nutritional application and implication of 1,3-butanediol. *Federation Proceedings, 34,* 2167–2170.

Ebbeling, C. B., Feldman, H. A., Klein, G. L., Wong, J. M. W., Bielak, L., Steltz, S. K., Luoto, P. K., Wolfe, R. R., Wong, W. W., & Ludwig, D. S. (2018). Effects of a low carbohydrate diet on energy expenditure during weight loss maintenance: Randomized trial. *British Medical Journal, 363,* k4583.

Egan, B. (2018). The glucose-lowering effects of exogenous ketones: Is there therapeutic potential? *Journal of Physiology, 596,* 1317–1318.

Elizabeth, G. N., Hannah, C., Ruby, H. S., Margaret, S. L., Nicole, E., Georgiana, F., Andrea, W., & Cross, J. H. (2009). A randomized trial of classical and medium-chain triglyceride ketogenic diets in the treatment of childhood epilepsy. *Epilepsia, 50,* 1109–1117.

Evans, M., & Egan, B. (2018). Intermittent running and cognitive performance after ketone ester ingestion. *Medicine & Science in Sports & Exercise, 50,* 2330–2338.

Evans, M., McSwiney, F. T., Brady, A. J., & Egan, B. (2019). No benefit of ingestion of a ketone monoester supplement on 10-km running performance. *Medicine & Science in Sports & Exercise, 51*(12), 2506–2515.

Falbe, J., Bahrmann, H., Lipps, W., Mayer, D., & Frey, G. D. (1985). Alcohols, Aliphatic. In Ullmann's Encyclopedia of Industrial Chemistry; Wiley-VCH Verlag GmbH & Co. KgaA: Weinheim, Germany.

Faull, O. K., Dearlove, D. J., Clarke, K., & Cox, P. J. (2019). Beyond RPE: The perception of exercise under normal and ketotic conditions. *Frontiers in Physiology, 10,* 229.

Fearon, K. C., Borland, W., Preston, T., Tisdale, M. J., Shenkin, A., & Calman, K. C. (1988). Cancer cachexia: Influence of systemic ketosis on substrate levels and nitrogen metabolism. *American Journal of Clinical Nutrition, 47,* 42–48.

Felig, P., Owen, O. E., Wahren, J., & Cahill, G. F., Jr. (1969). Amino acid metabolism during prolonged starvation. *Journal of Clinical Investigation, 48,* 584–594.

Ferreira, L., Lisenko, K., Barros, B., Zangeronimo, M., Pereira, L., & Sousa, R. (2014). Influence of medium-chain triglycerides on consumption and weight gain in rats: A systematic review. *Journal of Animal Physiology and Animal Nutrition, 98*(1), 1–8. https://doi-org.ezproxy.hsc.usf.edu/10.1111/jpn.12030

Fine, E., Segal-Isaacson, C., Feinman, R., Herszkopf, S., Romano, M., Tomuta, N., Bontempo, A., Negassa, A., & Sparano, J. (2012). Targeting insulin inhibition as a metabolic therapy in advanced cancer: A pilot safety and feasibility dietary trial in 10 patients. *Nutrition, 28,* 1028–1035.

Fomin, D. A., McDaniel, B., & Crane, J. (2017). The promising potential role of ketones in inflammatory dermatologic disease: A new frontier in treatment research. *The Journal of Dermatological Treatment, 28*(6), 484–487. https://doi-org.ezproxy.hsc.usf.edu/10.1080/09546634.2016.1276259

Forsythe, C. E., Phinney, S. D., Fernandez, M. L., Quann, E. E., Wood, R. J., Bibus, D. M., Kraemer, W. J., Feinman, R. D., & Volek, J. S. (2008). Comparison of low fat and low carbohydrate diets on circulating fatty acid composition and markers of inflammation. *Lipids, 43*(1), 65–77. https://doi-org.ezproxy.hsc.usf.edu/10.1007/s11745-007-3132-7

Fortier, M., Castellano, C. A., Croteau, E., Langlois, F., Bocti, C., St-Pierre, V., Vandenberghe, C., Bernier, M., Roy, M., Descoteaux, M., Whittingstall, K., Lepage, M., Turcotte, É. E., Fulop, T., & Cunnane, S. C. (2019). A ketogenic drink improves brain energy and some measures of cognition in mild cognitive impairment. *Alzheimer's & Dementia, 15,* 625–634.

Fredericks, M., & Ramsey, R. B. (1978). 3-Oxo acid coenzyme A transferase activity in brain and tumors of the nervous system. *Journal of Neurochemistry, 31,* 1529–1531.

Freedland, S., Mavropoulos, J., Wang, A., Darshan, M., Demark-Wahnefried, W., Aronson, W., Cohen, P., Hwang, D., Peterson, B., Fields, T., Pizzo, S. V., & Isaacs, W. B. (2008). Carbohydrate restriction, prostate cancer growth, and the insulin-like growth factor axis. *Prostate, 68,* 11–19.

Fu, S. P., Li, S. N., Wang, J. F., Li, Y., Xie, S. S., Xue, W. J., Liu, H. M., Huang, B. X., Lv, Q. K., Lei, L. C., Liu, G. W., Wang, W., & Liu, J. X. (2014). BHBA suppresses LPS-induced inflammation in BV-2 cells by inhibiting NF-κB activation. *Mediators of Inflammation, 2014,* 983401.

Galmozzi, A., Mitro, N., Ferrari, A., Gers, E., Gilardi, F., Godio, C., Cermenati, G., Gualerzi, A., Donetti, E., Rotili, D., Valente, S., Guerrini, U., Caruso, D., Mai, A., Saez, E., De Fabiani, E., & Crestani, M. (2013). Inhibition of class I histone deacetylases unveils a mitochondrial signature and enhances oxidative metabolism in skeletal muscle and adipose tissue. *Diabetes, 62,* 732–742.

Gambhir, D., Ananth, S., Veeranan-Karmegam, R., Elangovan, S., Hester, S., Jennings, E., Offermanns, S., Nussbaum, J. J., Smith, S. B., Thangaraju, M., Ganapathy, V., & Martin, P. M. (2012). GPR109A as an anti-inflammatory receptor in retinal pigment epithelial cells and its relevance to diabetic retinopathy. *Investigative Ophthalmology & Visual Science, 53*(4), 2208–2217. doi:10.1167/iovs.11-8447. PMID: 22427566; PMCID: PMC4627510.

Gao, Z., Yin, J., Zhang, J., Ward, R. E., Martin, R. J., Lefevre, M., Cefalu, W. T., & Ye, J. (2009). Butyrate improves insulin sensitivity and increases energy expenditure in mice. *Diabetes, 58*, 1509–1517.

Gardner, C. D., Trepanowski, J. F., Del Gobbo, L. C., Hauser, M. E., Rigdon, J., Ioannidis, J. P. A., Desai, M., & King, A. C. (2018). Effect of low-fat vs low-carbohydrate diet on 12-month weight loss in overweight adults and the association with genotype pattern or insulin secretion: The DIETFITS randomized clinical trial. *JAMA, 319*, 667–679.

Giacco, F., & Brownlee, M. (2010). Oxidative stress and diabetic complications. *Circulation Research, 107*, 1058–1070.

Gillies, R., Robey, I., & Gatenby, R. (2008). Causes and consequences of increased glucose metabolism of cancers. *Journal of Nuclear Medicine, 49*(Suppl. 2), 24S–42S. https://doi-org.ezproxy.hsc.usf.edu/10.2967/jnumed.107.047258

Goedecke, J. H., Elmer-English, R., Dennis, S. C., Schloss, I., Noakes, T. D., & Lambert, E. V. (1999). Effects of medium-chain triaclyglycerol ingested with carbohydrate on metabolism and exercise performance. *International Journal of Sport Nutrition, 9*, 35–47.

Goldberg, E. L., Asher, J. L., Molony, R. D., Shaw, A. C., Zeiss, C. J., Wang, C., Morozova-Roche, L. A., Herzog, R. I., Iwasaki, A., & Dixit, V. D. (2017). β-Hydroxybutyrate deactivates neutrophil NLRP3 inflammasome to relieve gout flares. *Cell Reports, 18*, 2077–2087.

Greenwood, M., Cooke, M. B., Ziegenfuss, T., Kalman, D. S., & Antonio, J. (2015). *Nutritional supplements in sports and exercise* (2nd ed.). Springer.

Gross, E. C., Klement, R. J., Schoenen, J., D'Agostino, D. P., & Fischer, D. (2019). Potential protective mechanisms of ketone bodies in migraine prevention. *Nutrients, 11*(4), 811. https://doi-org.ezproxy.hsc.usf.edu/10.3390/nu11040811

Halestrap, A., & Price, N. (1999). The proton-linked monocarboxylate transporter (MCT) family: Structure, function and regulation. *Biochemical Journal, 343*(Part 2), 281–380.

Han, J. R., Deng, B., Sun, J., Chen, C.G., Corkey, B. E., Kirkland, J. L., Ma, J., & Guo, W. (2007). Effects of dietary medium-chain triglyceride on weight loss and insulin sensitivity in a group of moderately overweight free-living type 2 diabetic Chinese subjects. *Metabolism, 56*, 985–991.

Hashim, S. A., & Tantibhedyangkul, P. (1987). Medium chain triglyceride in early life: Effects on growth of adipose tissue. *Lipids, 22*(6), 429–434. https://doi-org.ezproxy.hsc.usf.edu/10.1007/BF02537274

Hashim, S. A., & VanItallie, T. B. (2014). Ketone body therapy: From the ketogenic diet to the oral administration of ketone ester. *Journal of Lipid Research, 55*, 1818–1826.

Hassler, M. R., & Egger, G. (2012). Epigenomics of cancer—Emerging new concepts. *Biochimie, 94*, 2219–2230.

Henderson, S. T., Vogel, J. L., Barr, L. J., Garvin, F., Jones, J. J., & Costantini, L. C. (2009). Study of the ketogenic agent AC-1202 in mild to moderate Alzheimer's disease: A randomized, double-blind, placebo-controlled, multicenter trial. *Nutrition & Metabolism, 6*, 31.

Heneka, M. T., Kummer, M. P., Stutz, A., Delekate, A., Schwartz, S., Vieira-Saecker, A., Griep, A., Axt, D., Remus, A., Tzeng, T. C., Gelpi, E., Halle, A., Korte, M., Latz, E., & Golenbock, D. T. (2013). NLRP3 is activated in Alzheimer's disease and contributes to pathology in APP/PS1 mice. *Nature, 493*, 674–678.

Herber, D. L., Weeber, E. J., D'Agostino, D. P., & Duis, J. (2020). Evaluation of the safety and tolerability of a nutritional Formulation in patients with ANgelman Syndrome (FANS): Study protocol for a randomized controlled trial. *Trials, 21*, 60.

Hess, F. G., Cox, G. E., Bailey, D. E., Parent, R. A., & Becci, P. J. (1981). Reproduction and teratology study of 1,3-butanediol in rats. *Journal of Applied Toxicology, 1*, 202–209.

Holdsworth, D. A., Cox, P. J., Kirk, T., Stradling, H., Impey, S. G., & Clarke, K. (2017). A ketone ester drink increases postexercise muscle glycogen synthesis in humans. *Medicine and Science in Sports and Exercise, 49*, 1789–1795.

Hoover, H. C., Jr., Grant, J. P., Gorschboth, C., & Ketcham, A. S. (1975). Nitrogen-sparing intravenous fluids in postperative patients. *New England Journal of Medicine, 293*, 172–175.

Hove, J. L. K., Grünewald, S., Jaeken, J., & Demaerel, P. (2003). D,L-3-Hydroxybutyrate treatment of multiple acyl-CoA dehydrogenase deficiency (MADD). *Lancet (London, England), 361*(9367), 1433–1435. https://doi-org.ezproxy.hsc.usf.edu/10.1016/S0140-6736(03)13105-4

Huttenlocher, P. R. (1976). Ketonemia and seizures: Metabolic and anticonvulsant effects of two ketogenic diets in childhood epilepsy. *Pediatric Research, 10*, 536–540.

Huttenlocher, P. R., Wilbourn, A. J., & Signore, J. M. (1971). Medium-chain triglycerides as a therapy for intractable childhood epilepsy. *Neurology, 21*, 1097–1103.

Jarrett, S. G., Milder, J. B., Liang, L. P., & Patel, M. (2008). The ketogenic diet increases mitochondrial glutathione levels. *Journal of Neurochemistry, 106*, 1044–1051.

Jensen, N. J., Wodschow, H. Z., Nilsson, M., & Rungby, J. (2020). Effects of ketone bodies on brain metabolism and function in neurodegenerative diseases. *International Journal of Molecular Sciences, 21*(22), 8767. https://doi-org.ezproxy.hsc.usf.edu/10.3390/ijms21228767

Jeukendrup, A. E., Saris, W. H., Schrauwen, P., Brouns, F., & Wagenmakers, A. J. (1995). Metabolic availability of medium-chain triglycerides coingested with carbohydrates during prolonged exercise. *Journal of Applied Physiology, 79*, 756–762.

Jeukendrup, A. E., Thielen, J. J., Wagenmakers, A. J., Brouns, F., & Saris, W. H. (1998). Effect of medium-chain triacylglycerol and carbohydrate ingestion during exercise on substrate utilization and subsequent cycling performance. *American Journal of Clinical Nutrition, 67*, 397–404.

Karen, M., & Welma, S. (2015). Effects of medium-chain triglycerides on weight loss and body composition: A meta-analysis of randomized controlled trials. *Journal of the Academy of Nutrition and Dietetics, 115*(2), 249–263. https://doi-org.ezproxy.hsc.usf.edu/10.1016/j.jand.2014.10.022

Kashiwaya, Y., Bergman, C., Lee, J.-H. H., Wan, R., King, M. T., Mughal, M. R., Okun, E., Clarke, K., Mattson, M. P., & Veech, R. L. (2013). A ketone ester diet exhibits anxiolytic and cognition-sparing properties and lessens amyloid and tau pathologies in a mouse model of Alzheimer's disease. *Neurobiology of Aging, 34*, 1530–1539.

Kashiwaya, Y., King, M. T., & Veech, R. L. (1997). Substrate signaling by insulin: A ketone bodies ratio mimics insulin action in heart. *American Journal of Cardiology, 80*, 50A–64A.

Kashiwaya, Y., Pawlosky, R., Markis, W., King, M. T., Bergman, C., Srivastava, S., Murray, A., Clarke, K., & Veech, R. L. (2010). A ketone ester diet increases brain malonyl-CoA and uncoupling proteins 4 and 5 while decreasing food intake in the normal Wistar rat. *Journal of Biological Chemistry, 285*, 25950–25956.

Kashiwaya, Y., Sato, K., Tsuchiya, N., Thomas, S., Fell, D. A., Veech, R. L., & Passonneau, J. V. (1994). Control of glucose utilization in working perfused rat heart. *Journal of Biological Chemistry, 269*, 25502–25514.

Kesl, S., Poff, A., Ward, N., Fiorelli, T., Ari, C., & D'Agostino, D. (2014). *Methods of sustaining dietary ketosis in Sprague-Dawley rats* [Paper presentation]. Federation of the American Societies for Experimental Biology, San Diego, CA.

Kesl, S. L., Poff, A. M., Ward, N. P., Fiorelli, T. N., Ari, C., Van Putten, A. J., Sherwood, J. W., Arnold, P., & D'Agostino, D. P. (2016). Effects of exogenous ketone supplementation on blood ketone, glucose, triglyceride, and lipoprotein levels in Sprague-Dawley rats. *Nutrition & Metabolism, 13*, 9.

Khodabakhshi, A., Akbari, M. E., Mirzaei, H. R., Mehrad-Majd, H., Kalamian, M., & Davoodi, S. H. (2020). Feasibility, safety, and beneficial effects of MCT-based ketogenic diet for breast cancer treatment: A randomized controlled trial study. *Nutrition and Cancer, 72*(4), 627–634. https://doi-org.ezproxy.hsc.usf.edu/10.1080/01635581.2019.1650942

Kies, C., Tobin, R. B., Fox, H. M., & Mehlman, M. A. (1973). Utilization of 1,3-butanediol and nonspecific nitrogen in human adults. *Journal of Nutrition, 103*, 1155–1163.

Kim, D. Y., Davis, L. M., Sullivan, P. G., Maalouf, M., Simeone, T. A., van Brederode, J., & Rho, J. M. (2007). Ketone bodies are protective against oxidative stress in neocortical neurons. *Journal of Neurochemistry, 101*, 1316–1326.

Kimoto, A., Ohnuma, T., Toda, A., Takebayashi, Y., Higashiyama, R., Tagata, Y., Ito, M., Ota, T., Shibata, N., & Arai, H. (2017). Medium-chain triglycerides given in the early stage of mild-to-moderate Alzheimer's disease enhance memory function. *Psychogeriatrics, 17*, 520–521.

Klein, P., Tyrlikova, I., & Mathews, G. C. (2014). Dietary treatment in adults with refractory epilepsy: A review. *Neurology, 83*, 1978–1985.

Kong, G., Huang, Z., Ji, W., Wang, X., Liu, J., Wu, X., Huang, Z., Li, R., & Zhu, Q. (2017). The ketone metabolite beta-hydroxybutyrate attenuates oxidative stress in spinal cord injury by suppression of class I histone deacetylases. *Journal of Neurotrauma, 34*, 2645–2655.

Koutnik, A. P., D'Agostino, D. P., & Egan, B. (2019). Anticatabolic effects of ketone bodies in skeletal muscle. *Trends in Endocrinology and Metabolism, 30*, 227–229.

Koutnik, A. P., Poff, A. M., Ward, N. P., DeBlasi, J. M., Soliven, M. A., Romero, M. A., Roberson, P. A., Fox, C. D., Roberts, M. D., & D'Agostino, D. P. (2020). Ketone bodies attenuate wasting in models of atrophy. *Journal of Cachexia, Sarcopenia and Muscle, 11*, 973–996.

Kovac, S., Abramov, A. Y., & Walker, M. C. (2013). Energy depletion in seizures: Anaplerosis as a strategy for future therapies. *Neuropharmacology, 69*, 96–104.

Kovacs, Z., Brunner, B., D'Agostino, D. P., & Ari, C. (2020). Inhibition of adenosine A1 receptors abolished the nutritional ketosis-evoked delay in the onset of isoflurane-induced anesthesia in Wistar Albino Glaxo Rijswijk rats. *BMC Anesthesiology, 20*, 30.

Kovacs, Z., D'Agostino, D. P., Diamond, D., Kindy, M. S., Rogers, C., & Ari, C. (2019a). Therapeutic potential of exogenous ketone supplement induced ketosis in the treatment of psychiatric disorders: Review of current literature. *Frontiers in Psychiatry, 10*, 363.

Kovacs, Z., D'Agostino, D. P., Diamond, D. M., & Ari, C. (2019b). Exogenous ketone supplementation decreased the lipopolysaccharide-induced increase in absence epileptic activity in Wistar Albino Glaxo Rijswijk rats. *Frontiers in Molecular Neuroscience, 12*, 45.

Kovacs, Z., D'Agostino, D. P., Dobolyi, A., & Ari, C. (2017). Adenosine A1 receptor antagonism abolished the anti-seizure effects of exogenous ketone supplementation in Wistar Albino Glaxo Rijswijk rats. *Frontiers in Molecular Neuroscience, 10*, 235.

Kraschnewski, J. L., Boan, J., Esposito, J., Sherwood, N. E., Lehman, E. B., Kephart, D. K., & Sciamanna, C. N. (2010). Long-term weight loss maintenance in the United States. *International Journal of Obesity, 34*, 1644–1654.

Kripke, S. A., Fox, A. D., Berman, J. M., DePaula, J., Birkhahn, R. H., Rombeau, J. L., & Settle, R. G. (1988). Inhibition of TPN-associated intestinal mucosal atrophy with monoacetoacetin. *Journal of Surgical Research, 44*, 436–444.

Krotkiewski, M. (2001). Value of VLCD supplementation with medium chain triglycerides. *International Journal of Obesity and Related Metabolic Disorders: Journal of the International Association for the Study of Obesity, 25*, 1393–1400.

Laakso, M., & Kuusisto, J. (2014). Insulin resistance and hyperglycaemia in cardiovascular disease development. *Nature Reviews Endocrinology, 10*, 293–302.

Lan, F., Bayliss, P. E., Rinn, J. L., Whetstine, J. R., Wang, J. K., Chen, S., Iwase, S., Alpatov, R., Issaeva, I., Canaani, E., Roberts, T. M., Chang, H. Y., & Shi, Y. (2007). A histone H3 lysine 27 demethylase regulates animal posterior development. *Nature, 449*, 689–694.

Langhans, W., Wiesenreiter, F., & Scharrer, E. (1983). Different effects of subcutaneous D,L-3-hydroxybutyrate and acetoacetate injections on food intake in rats. *Physiology & Behavior, 31*, 483–486.

Lardy, H. A., & Phillips, P. H. (1945). Studies of fat and carbohydrate oxidation in mammalian spermatozoa. *Archives of Biochemistry, 6*, 53–61.

Laughlin, M. R., Taylor, J., Chesnick, A.S., & Balaban, R. S. (1994). Nonglucose substrates increase glycogen synthesis in vivo in dog heart. *American Journal of Physiology, 267*, H219–223.

Leckey, J. J., Ross, M. L., Qoud, M., Hawley, J. A., & Burke, L. M. (2017). Ketone diester ingestion impairs time-trial performance in professional cyclists. *Frontiers in Physiology, 8*, 806. https://doi-org.ezproxy.hsc.usf.edu/10.3389/fphys.2017.00806

Lennerz, B. S., Koutnik, A. P., Azova, S., Wolfsdorf, J. I., & Ludwig, D. S. (2021). Carbohydrate restriction for diabetes: Rediscovering centuries-old wisdom. *Journal of Clinical Investigation, 131*, e142246. https://doi-org.ezproxy.hsc.usf.edu/10.1172/JCI142246

Levy, R. G., Cooper, P. N., & Giri, P. (2012). Ketogenic diet and other dietary treatments for epilepsy. *Cochrane Database of Systematic Reviews, 3*, CD001903. https://doi-org.ezproxy.hsc.usf.edu/10.1002/14651858.CD001903.pub2

Li, H.-F. F., Zou, Y., & Ding, G. (2013). Therapeutic success of the ketogenic diet as a treatment option for epilepsy: A meta-analysis. *Iranian Journal of Pediatrics, 23*, 613–620.

Ludwig, D. S., & Ebbeling, C. B. (2018). The carbohydrate-insulin model of obesity: Beyond "calories in, calories out." *JAMA Internal Medicine, 178*, 1098–1103.

Ma, S., & Suzuki, K. (2019). Keto-adaptation and endurance exercise capacity, fatigue recovery, and exercise-induced muscle and organ damage prevention: A narrative review. *Sports* (Basel, Switzerland), *7*, 40. https://doi-org.ezproxy.hsc.usf.edu/10.3390/sports7020040

Maalouf, M., Sullivan, P. G., Davis, L., Kim, D. Y., & Rho, J. M. (2007). Ketones inhibit mitochondrial production of reactive oxygen species production following glutamate excitotoxicity by increasing NADH oxidation. *Neuroscience, 145*, 256–264.

Maclean, P. S., Bergouignan, A., Cornier, M. A., & Jackman, M. R. (2011). Biology's response to dieting: The impetus for weight regain. *American Journal of Physiology Regulatory, Integrative and Comparative Physiology, 301*, R581–R600.

Magee, B. A., Potezny, N., Rofe, A. M., & Conyers, R. A. (1979). The inhibition of malignant cell growth by ketone bodies. *Australian Journal of Experimental Biology and Medical Science, 57*, 529–539.

Maiz, A., Moldawer, L. L., Bistrian, B. R., Birkhahn, R. H., Long, C. L., & Blackburn, G. L. (1985). Monoacetoacetin and protein metabolism during parenteral nutrition in burned rats. *Biochemistry Journal, 226*, 43–50.

Maizels, E. Z., Ruderman, N. B., Goodman, M. N., & Lau, D. (1977). Effect of acetoacetate on glucose metabolism in the soleus and extensor digitorum longus muscles of the rat. *Biochemistry Journal, 162*, 557–568.

Mak, S. C., Chi, C. S., & Wan, C. J. (1999). Clinical experience of ketogenic diet on children with refractory epilepsy. *Acta Paediatrica Taiwanica, 40*, 97–100.

Martinon, F., Petrilli, V., Mayor, A., Tardivel, A., & Tschopp, J. (2006). Gout-associated uric acid crystals activate the NALP3 inflammasome. *Nature, 440*, 237–241.

Masino, S. A., & Geiger, J. D. (2009). The ketogenic diet and epilepsy: Is adenosine the missing link? *Epilepsia, 50*, 332–333.

Massicotte, D., Peronnet, F., Brisson, G. R., & Hillaire-Marcel, C. (1992). Oxidation of exogenous medium-chain free fatty acids during prolonged exercise: Comparison with glucose. *Journal of Applied Physiology, 73*, 1334–1339.

Maurer, G., Brucker, D., Bähr, O., Harter, P., Hattingen, E., Walenta, S., Mueller-Klieser, W., Steinbach, J., & Rieger, J. (2011). Differential utilization of ketone bodies by neurons and glioma cell lines: A rationale for ketogenic diet as experimental glioma therapy. *BMC Cancer, 11*, 315.

Mavropoulos, J., Buschemeyer, W., Tewari, A., Rokhfeld, D., Pollak, M., Zhao, Y., Febbo, P., Cohen, P., Hwang, D., Devi, G., Demark-Wahnefried, W., Westman, E. C., Peterson, B. L., Pizzo, S. V., & Freedland, S. J. (2009). The effects of varying dietary carbohydrate and fat content on survival in a murine LNCaP prostate cancer xenograft model. *Cancer Prevention Research, 2*, 557–565.

McDonald, T. J. W., & Cervenka, M. C. (2019). Lessons learned from recent clinical trials of ketogenic diet therapies in adults. *Current Opinion in Clinical Nutrition and Metabolic Care, 22*(6), 418–424. https://doi-org.ezproxy.hsc.usf.edu/10.1097/MCO.0000000000000596

McHenry, L. C., Jr. (1966). Cerebral blood flow. New England Journal of Medicine, 274, 82–91.

Metcalfe, H. K., Monson, J. P., Welch, S. G., & Cohen, R. D. (1986). Inhibition of lactate removal by ketone bodies in rat liver: Evidence for a quantitatively important role of the plasma membrane lactate transporter in lactate metabolism. *Journal of Clinical Investigation, 78*, 743–747.

Mikkelsen, K. H., Seifert, T., Secher, N. H., Grondal, T., & van Hall, G. (2015). Systemic, cerebral and skeletal muscle ketone body and energy metabolism during acute hyper-D-beta-hydroxybutyratemia in post-absorptive healthy males. *Journal of Clinical Endocrinology and Metabolism, 100*, 636–643.

Miles, J. M., Haymond, M. W., & Gerich, J. E. (1981). Suppression of glucose production and stimulation of insulin secretion by physiological concentrations of ketone bodies in man. *Journal of Clinical Endocrinology and Metabolism, 52*, 34–37.

Monzo, L., Sedlacek, K., Hromanikova, K., Tomanova, L., Borlaug, B. A., Jabor, A., Kautzner, J., & Melenovsky, V. (2021). Myocardial ketone body utilization in patients with heart failure: The impact of oral ketone ester. *Metabolism, 115*, 154452.

Mosconi, L., Berti, V., McHugh, P., Pupi, A., & de Leon, M. J. (2011). A tale of two tracers: Glucose metabolism and amyloid positron emission tomography imaging in Alzheimer's disease. *Advances in Alzheimer's Disease, 2*, 219–234.

Myette-Cote, E., Neudorf, H., Rafiei, H., Clarke, K., & Little, J. P. (2018). Prior ingestion of exogenous ketone monoester attenuates the glycaemic response to an oral glucose tolerance test in healthy young individuals. *Journal of Physiology, 596*, 1385–1395.

Nair, K. S., Welle, S. L., Halliday, D., & Campbell, R. G. (1988). Effect of beta-hydroxybutyrate on whole-body leucine kinetics and fractional mixed skeletal muscle protein synthesis in humans. *Journal of Clinical Investigation, 82*, 198–205.

Nagao, K., & Yanagita, T. (2010). Medium-chain fatty acids: functional lipids for the prevention and treatment of the metabolic syndrome. *Pharmacological Research, 61*(3), 208–212. https://doi-org.ezproxy.hsc.usf.edu/10.1016/j.phrs.2009.11.007

Nakagata, T., Tamura, Y., Kaga, H., Sato, M., Yamasaki, N., Someya, Y., Kadowaki, S., Sugimoto, D., Satoh, H., Kawamori, R., & Watada, H. (2021). Ingestion of an exogenous ketone monoester improves the glycemic response during oral glucose tolerance test in individuals with impaired glucose tolerance: A cross-over randomized trial. *Journal of Diabetes Investigation, 12*(5), 756–762. https://doi-org.ezproxy.hsc.usf.edu/10.1111/jdi.13423

Nebeling, L. C., Miraldi, F., Shurin, S. B., & Lerner, E. (1995). Effects of a ketogenic diet on tumor metabolism and nutritional status in pediatric oncology patients: Two case reports. *Journal of the American College of Nutrition, 14*, 202–208.

Neudorf, H., Durrer, C., Myette-Cote, E., Makins, C., O'Malley, T., & Little, J. P. (2019). Oral ketone supplementation acutely increases markers of NLRP3 inflammasome activation in human monocytes. *Molecular Nutrition & Food Research, 63*, e1801171.

Newport, M. T., VanItallie, T. B., Kashiwaya, Y., King, M. T., & Veech, R. L. (2015). A new way to produce hyperketonemia: Use of ketone ester in a case of Alzheimer's disease. *Alzheimer's & Dementia, 11*, 99–103.

Niikawa, N., Kuroki, Y., Kajii, T., Matsuura, N., Ishikiriyama, S., Tonoki, H., Ishikawa, N., Yamada, Y., Fujita, M., & Umemoto, H. (1988). Kabuki make-up (Niikawa-Kuroki) syndrome: A study of 62 patients. *American Journal of Medical Genetics, 31*, 565–589.

Nosaka, N., Maki, H., Suzuki, Y., Haruna, H., Ohara, A., Kasai, M., Tsuji, H., Aoyama, T., Okazaki, M., Igarashi, O., & Kondo, K. (2003). Effects of margarine containing medium-chain triacylglycerols on body fat reduction in humans. *Journal of Atherosclerosis and Thrombosis, 10*, 290–298.

Nosaka, N., Suzuki, Y., Nagatoishi, A., Kasai, M., Wu, J., & Taguchi, M. (2009). Effect of ingestion of medium-chain triacylglycerols on moderate- and high-intensity exercise in recreational athletes. *Journal of Nutritional Science and Vitaminology, 55*, 120–125.

Opitz, K. (1958). Über die glykogenbildende Wirkung von Glykolen [The glycogen-forming effect of glycols]. *Naunyn-Schmiedebergs Archiv fur experimentelle Pathologie und Pharmakologie, 234*(5), 448–454.

Ota, M., Matsuo, J., Ishida, I., Takano, H., Yokoi, Y., Hori, H., Yoshida, S., Ashida, K., Nakamura, K., Takahashi, T., & Kunugi, H. (2019). Effects of a medium-chain triglyceride-based ketogenic formula on cognitive function in patients with mild-to-moderate Alzheimer's disease. *Neuroscience Letters, 690*, 232–236.

Owen, O. E., Morgan, A. P., Kemp, H. G., Sullivan, J. M., Herrera, M. G., & Cahill, G. F., Jr. (1967). Brain metabolism during fasting. *Journal of Clinical Investigation, 46*, 1589–1595.

Paoli, A. (2014). Ketogenic diet for obesity: Friend or foe? *International Journal of Environmental Research and Public Health, 11*, 2092–2107.

Papamandjaris, A. A., MacDougall, D. E., & Jones, P. J. (1998). Medium chain fatty acid metabolism and energy expenditure: Obesity treatment implications. *Life Sciences, 62*, 1203–1215.

Pascual, J. M., Liu, P., Mao, D., Kelly, D. I., Hernandez, A., Sheng, M., Good, L. B., Ma, Q., Marin-Valencia, I., Zhang, X., Park, J. Y., Hynan, L. S., Stavinoha, P., Roe, C. R., & Lu, H. (2014). Triheptanoin for glucose transporter type I deficiency (G1D): Modulation of human ictogenesis, cerebral metabolic rate, and cognitive indices by a food supplement. *JAMA Neurology, 71*, 1255–1265.

Poff, A., Kesl, S., Ward, N., & D'Agostino, D. (2016). *Metabolic effects of exogenous ketone supplementation—An alternative or adjuvant to the ketogenic diet as a cancer therapy?* [Paper presentation]. Keystone Symposia—New Frontiers in Tumor Metabolism, Banff, Alberta, Canada.

Poff, A. M., Ari, C., Arnold, P., Seyfried, T. N., & D'Agostino, D. P. (2014). Ketone supplementation decreases tumor cell viability and prolongs survival of mice with metastatic cancer. *International Journal of Cancer, 135*(7), 1711–1720. https://doi-org.ezproxy.hsc.usf.edu/10.1002/ijc.28809

Poff, A. M., Ari, C., Seyfried, T. N., & D'Agostino, D. P. (2013). The ketogenic diet and hyperbaric oxygen therapy prolong survival in mice with systemic metastatic cancer. *PLOS ONE, 8*, Article e65522.

Poff, A. M., Koutnik, A. P., & Egan, B. (2020). Nutritional ketosis with ketogenic diets or exogenous ketones: Features, convergence, and divergence. *Current Sports Medicine Reports, 19*, 251–259.

Poff, A. M., Rho, J. M., & D'Agostino, D. P. (2019). Ketone administration for seizure disorders: History and rationale for ketone esters and metabolic alternatives. *Frontiers in Neuroscience, 13*, 1041.

Poffe, C., Ramaekers, M., Van Thienen, R., & Hespel, P. (2019). Ketone ester supplementation blunts overreaching symptoms during endurance training overload. *Journal of Physiology, 597*, 3009–3027.

Poppitt, S. D., Strik, C. M., MacGibbon, A. K. H., McArdle, B. H., Budgett, S. C., & McGill, A. T. (2010). Fatty acid chain length, postprandial satiety and food intake in lean men. *Physiology & Behavior, 101*, 161–167.

Prins, P. J., D'Agostino, D. P., Rogers, C. Q., Ault, D. L., Welton, G. L., Jones, D. W., Henson, S. R., Rothfuss, T. J., Aiken, K. G., Hose, J. L., England, E. L., Atwell, A. D., Buxton, J. D., & Koutnik, A. P. (2020a). Dose response of a novel exogenous ketone supplement on physiological, perceptual and performance parameters. *Nutrition & Metabolism, 17*, 81.

Prins, P. J., Koutnik, A. P., D'Agostino, D. P., Rogers, C. Q., Seibert, J. F., Breckenridge, J. A., Jackson, D. S., Ryan, E. J., Buxton, J. D., & Ault, D. L. (2020b). Effects of an exogenous ketone supplement on five-kilometer running performance. *Journal of Human Kinetics, 72*, 115–127.

Puchowicz, M. A., Smith, C. L., Bomont, C., Koshy, J., David, F., & Brunengraber, H. (2000). Dog model of therapeutic ketosis induced by oral administration of R,S-1,3-butanediol diacetoacetate. *Journal of Nutritional Biochemistry, 11*, 281–287.

Rahman, M., Muhammad, S., Khan, M. A., Chen, H., Ridder, D. A., Muller-Fielitz, H., Pokorna, B., Vollbrandt, T., Stolting, I., Nadrowitz, R., Okun, J. G., Offermanns, S., & Schwaninger, M. (2014). The beta-hydroxybutyrate receptor HCA2 activates a neuroprotective subset of macrophages. *Nature Communications, 5*, 3944.

Randle, P. J., Newsholme, E. A., & Garland, P. B. (1964). Regulation of glucose uptake by muscle. 8. Effects of fatty acids, ketone bodies and pyruvate, and of alloxan-diabetes and starvation, on the uptake and metabolic fate of glucose in rat heart and diaphragm muscles. *Biochemical Journal, 93*, 652–665.

Rea, S., Eisenhaber, F., O'Carroll, D., Strahl, B. D., Sun, Z. W., Schmid, M., Opravil, S., Mechtler, K., Ponting, C. P., Allis, C. D., & Jenuwein, T. (2000). Regulation of chromatin structure by site-specific histone H3 methyltransferases. *Nature, 406*, 593–599.

Roberts, M. N., Wallace, M. A., Tomilov, A. A., Zhou, Z., Marcotte, G. R., Tran, D., Perez, G., Gutierrez-Casado, E., Koike, S., Knotts, T. A., Imai, D. M., Griffey, S. M., Kim, K., Hagopian, K., McMackin, M. Z., Haj, F. G., Baar, K., Cortopassi, G. A., Ramsey, J. J., & Lopez-Dominguez, J. A. (2017). A ketogenic diet extends longevity and healthspan in adult mice. *Cell Metabolism, 26*(3), 539–546. e5. https://doi-org.ezproxy.hsc.usf.edu/10.1016/j.cmet.2017.08.005

Rossi, R., Dörig, S., Del Prete, E., & Scharrer, E. (2000). Suppression of feed intake after parenteral administration of ᴅ-beta-hydroxybutyrate in pygmy goats. *Journal of Veterinary Medicine A, Physiology, Pathology, Clinical Medicine, 47*, 9–16.

Rossifanelli, F., Franchi, F., Mulieri, M., Cangiano, C., Cascino, A., Ceci, F., Muscaritoli, M., Seminara, P., & Bonomo, L. (1991). Effect of energy substrate manipulation on tumor-cell proliferation in parenterally fed cancer-patients. *Clinical Nutrition, 10*, 228–232.

Ruby, H. S., Jane, E., Bower, B. D., & Aynsley-Green, A. (1989). Ketogenic diets in the treatment of epilepsy: Short-term clinical effects. *Developmental Medicine & Child Neurology, 31*, 145–151.

Rusek, M., Pluta, R., Ulamek-Koziol, M., & Czuczwar, S. J. (2019). Ketogenic diet in Alzheimer's disease. *International Journal of Molecular Sciences, 20*(16), 3892. https://doi-org.ezproxy.hsc.usf.edu/10.3390/ijms20163892

Ryu, T. Y., Park, J., & Scherer, P. E. (2014). Hyperglycemia as a risk factor for cancer progression. *Diabetes & Metabolism Journal, 38*, 330–336.

Satabin, P., Portero, P., Defer, G., Bricout, J., & Guezennec, C. Y. (1987). Metabolic and hormonal responses to lipid and carbohydrate diets during exercise in man. *Medicine and Science in Sports and Exercise, 19*, 218–223.

Sawai, M., Yashiro, M., Nishiguchi, Y., Ohira, M., & Hirakawa, K. (2004). Growth-inhibitory effects of the ketone body, monoacetoacetin, on human gastric cancer cells with succinyl-CoA:3-oxoacid CoA-transferase (SCOT) deficiency. *Anticancer Research, 24*, 2213–2217.

Scala, R. A., & Paynter, O. E. (1967). Chronic oral toxicity of 1,3-butanediol. *Toxicology and Applied Pharmacology, 10*(1), 160–164. https://doi-org.ezproxy.hsc.usf.edu/10.1016/0041-008x(67)90137-8

Scalfi, L., Coltorti, A., & Contaldo, F. (1991). Postprandial thermogenesis in lean and obese subjects after meals supplemented with medium-chain and long-chain triglycerides. *American Journal of Clinical Nutrition, 53*(5), 1130–1133. https://doi-org.ezproxy.hsc.usf.edu/10.1093/ajcn/53.5.1130

Seaton, T. B., Welle, S. L., & Warenko, M. K. (1986). Thermic effect of medium-chain and long-chain triglycerides in man. *American Journal of Clinical Nutrition, 44*(5), 630–634. https://doi-org.ezproxy.hsc.usf.edu/10.1093/ajcn/44.5.630

Selvaraj, S., & Margulies, K. B. (2021). Exogenous ketones in the healthy heart: The plot thickens. *Cardiovascular Research, 117*(4), 995–996. https://doi-org.ezproxy.hsc.usf.edu/10.1093/cvr/cvaa283

Seyfried, T. N. (2012). *Cancer as a metabolic disease: On the origin, management, and prevention of cancer.* John Wiley & Sons.

Sharman, M., & Volek, J. (2004). Weight loss leads to reductions in inflammatory biomarkers after a very-low-carbohydrate diet and a low-fat diet in overweight men. *Clinical Science, 107*, 365–369.

Shelton, L. M., Huysentruyt, L. C., Mukherjee, P., & Seyfried, T. N. (2010). Calorie restriction as an anti-invasive therapy for malignant brain cancer in the VM mouse. *ASN Neurology, 2*, Article e00038.

Sherrier, M., & Li, H. (2019). The impact of keto-adaptation on exercise performance and the role of metabolic-regulating cytokines. *American Journal of Clinical Nutrition, 110*, 562–573.

Sherwin, R. S., Hendler, R. G., & Felig, P. (1975). Effect of ketone infusions on amino acid and nitrogen metabolism in man. *Journal of Clinical Investigation, 55*, 1382–1390.

Shimazu, T., Hirschey, M. D., Newman, J., He, W., Shirakawa, K., Le Moan, N., Grueter, C. A., Lim, H., Saunders, L. R., Stevens, R. D., Newgard, C. B., Farese, R. V., Jr, de Cabo, R., Ulrich, S., Akassoglou, K., & Verdin, E. (2013). Suppression of oxidative stress by beta-hydroxybutyrate, an endogenous histone deacetylase inhibitor. *Science, 339*, 211–214.

Shippy, D. C., Wilhelm, C., Viharkumar, P. A., Raife, T. J., & Ulland, T. K. (2020). β-Hydroxybutyrate inhibits inflammasome activation to attenuate Alzheimer's disease pathology. *Journal of Neuroinflammation, 17*, 280.

Short, J. (2017). *Effects of a ketone/caffeine supplement on cycling and cognitive performance.* Semantic Scholar [Master's thesis, The Ohio State University].

Sills, M. A., Forsythe, W. I., Haidukewych, D., MacDonald, A., & Robinson, M. (1986). The medium chain triglyceride diet and intractable epilepsy. *Archives of Disease in Childhood, 61*, 1168–1172.

Skinner, R., Trujillo, A., Ma, X., & Beierle, E. (2009). Ketone bodies inhibit the viability of human neuroblastoma cells. *Journal of Pediatric Surgery, 44*, 212.

Smith, R., Fuller, D. J., Wedge, J. H., Williamson, D. H., & Alberti, K. G. (1975). Initial effect of injury on ketone bodies and other blood metabolites. *Lancet, 1*, 1–3.

Sonnenburg, R. (2018). *Examining the effects of exogenous ketones on exercise metabolism and performance in male varsity athletes.* Semantic Scholar [Master's thesis, University of Waterloo].

Srivastava, S., Kashiwaya, Y., King, M., Baxa, U., Tam, J., Niu, G., Chen, X., Clarke, K., & Veech, R. (2012). Mitochondrial biogenesis and increased uncoupling protein 1 in brown adipose tissue of mice fed a ketone ester diet. *FASEB Journal, 26*, 2351–2362.

St-Onge, M. P., Bourque, C., Jones, P. J. H., & Ross, R. (2003). Medium-versus long-chain triglycerides for 27 days increases fat oxidation and energy expenditure without resulting in changes in body composition in overweight. *International Journal of Obesity and Related Metabolic Disorders: Journal of the International Association for the Study of Obesity, 27*(1), 95–102. https://doi-org.ezproxy.hsc.usf.edu/10.1038/sj.ijo.0802169

St-Onge, M. P., Ross, R., & Parsons, W. D. (2003). Medium-chain triglycerides increase energy expenditure and decrease adiposity in overweight men. *Obesity Research, 11*(3), 395–402. https://doi-org.ezproxy.hsc.usf.edu/10.1038/oby.2003.53

Stafstrom, C. E., Ockuly, J. C., Murphree, L., Valley, M. T., Roopra, A., & Sutula, T. P. (2009). Anticonvulsant and antiepileptic actions of 2-deoxy-D-glucose in epilepsy models. *Annals of Neurology, 65*, 435–447.

Stafstrom, C. E., Roopra, A., & Sutula, T. P. (2008). Seizure suppression via glycolysis inhibition with 2-deoxy-D-glucose (2DG). *Epilepsia, 49*(Suppl. 8), 97–100.

Stagey, J. B., Dondeena, B. R., Armour, F., & Bruce, R. B. (1997). The new dietary fats in health and disease. *Journal of the American Dietetic Association, 97*, 280–286.

Stubbs, B. J., Cox, P. J., Evans, R. D., Cyranka, M., Clarke, K., & de Wet, H. (2018a). A ketone ester drink lowers human ghrelin and appetite. *Obesity, 26*, 269–273.

Stubbs, B. J., Cox, P. J., Evans, R. D., Santer, P., Miller, J. J., Faull, O. K., Magor-Elliott, S., Hiyama, S., Stirling, M., & Clarke, K. (2017). On the metabolism of exogenous ketones in humans. *Frontiers in Physiology, 8*, 848.

Stubbs, B. J., Koutnik, A. P., Goldberg, E. L., Upadhyay, V., Turnbaugh, P. J., Verdin, E., & Newman, J. C. (2020). Investigating ketone bodies as immunometabolic countermeasures against respiratory viral infections. *Med (New York, N.Y.), 1*, 43–65.

Stubbs, B. J., Koutnik, A. P., Poff, A. M., Ford, K. M., & D'Agostino, D. P. (2018b). Commentary: Ketone diester ingestion impairs time-trial performance in professional cyclists. *Frontiers in Physiology, 9*, 279.

Stubbs, B. J., Koutnik, A. P., Volek, J. S., & Newman, J. C. (2021). From bedside to battlefield: Intersection of ketone body mechanisms in geroscience with military resilience. *GeroScience, 43*(3), 1071–1081. https://doi-org.ezproxy.hsc.usf.edu/10.1007/s11357-020-00277-y

Sung, M. H., Liao, F. H., & Chien, Y. W. (2018). Medium-chain triglycerides lower blood lipids and body weight in streptozotocin-induced type 2 diabetes rats. *Nutrients, 10*, 963. https://doi-org.ezproxy.hsc.usf.edu/10.3390/nu10080963

Sylvain, D., Khadijah, Q., Hermann, D., Pascal, D., Catherine, B., France, D., Kamlesh, C. A., Alok, K., Maxim, V. S., Lisa, P., Bernard, R. L., & Henri, B. (1995). (R,S)-1,3-Butanediol acetoacetate esters, potential alternates to lipid emulsions for total parenteral nutrition. *Journal of Nutritional Biochemistry, 6*(2), 111–118.

Taggart, A. K., Kero, J., Gan, X., Cai, T. Q., Cheng, K., Ippolito, M., Ren, N., Kaplan, R., Wu, K., Wu, T. J., Jin, L., Liaw, C., Chen, R., Richman, J., Connolly, D., Offermanns, S., Wright, S. D., & Waters, M. G. (2005). D-β-Hydroxybutyrate inhibits adipocyte lipolysis via the nicotinic acid receptor PUMA-G. *Journal of Biological Chemistry, 280*, 26649–26652.

Talbot, K., Wang, H. Y., Kazi, H., Han, L. Y., Bakshi, K. P., Stucky, A., Fuino, R. L., Kawaguchi, K. R., Samoyedny, A. J., Wilson, R. S., Arvanitakis, Z., Schneider, J. A., Wolf, B. A., Bennett, D. A., Trojanowski, J. Q., & Arnold, S. E. (2012). Demonstrated brain insulin resistance in Alzheimer's disease patients is associated with IGF-1 resistance, IRS-1 dysregulation, and cognitive decline. *Journal of Clinical Investigation, 122*, 1316–1338.

Tan, B. T., Jiang, H., Moulson, A. J., Wu, X. L., Wang, W. C., Liu, J., Plunet, W. T., & Tetzlaff, W. (2020). Neuroprotective effects of a ketogenic diet in combination with exogenous ketone salts following acute spinal cord injury. *Neural Regeneration Research, 15*, 1912–1919.

Tate, R. L., Mehlman, M. A., & Tobin, R. B. (1971). Metabolic fate of 1,3-butanediol in the rat: Conversion to β-hydroxybutyrate. *Journal of Nutrition, 101*, 1719–1726.

Thai, P. N., Seidlmayer, L. K., Miller, C., Ferrero, M., Dorn, G. W., II, Schaefer, S., Bers, D. M., & Dedkova, E. N. (2019). Mitochondrial quality control in aging and heart failure: Influence of ketone bodies and mitofusin-stabilizing peptides. *Frontiers in Physiology, 10*, 382.

Thomsen, H. H., Rittig, N., Johannsen, M., Moller, A. B., Jorgensen, J. O., Jessen, N., & Moller, N. (2018). Effects of 3-hydroxybutyrate and free fatty acids on muscle protein kinetics and signaling during LPS-induced inflammation in humans: Anticatabolic impact of ketone bodies. *American Journal of Clinical Nutrition, 108*, 857–867.

Tisdale, M., & Brennan, R. (1983). Loss of acetoacetate coenzyme A transferase activity in tumours of peripheral tissues. *British Journal of Cancer, 47*, 293–297.

Tisdale, M. J., Brennan, R. A., & Fearon, K. C. (1987). Reduction of weight loss and tumour size in a cachexia model by a high fat diet. *British Journal of Cancer, 56*, 39–43.

Tobin, R. B., Mehlman, M. A., & Parker, M. (1972). Effect of 1,3-butanediol and propionic acid on blood ketones, lipids and metal ions in rats. *Journal of Nutrition, 102*, 1001–1008.

Torres-Gonzalez, M., Volek, J. S., Leite, J. O., Fraser, H., & Luz Fernandez, M. (2008). Carbohydrate restriction reduces lipids and inflammation and prevents atherosclerosis in Guinea pigs. *Journal of Atherosclerosis and Thrombosis, 15*, 235–243.

Trauner, D. A. (1985). Medium-chain triglyceride (MCT) diet in intractable seizure disorders. *Neurology, 35*, 237–238.

Turina, M., Fry, D. E., & Polk, H. C., Jr. (2005). Acute hyperglycemia and the innate immune system: Clinical, cellular, and molecular aspects. *Critical Care Medicine, 33*, 1624–1633.

Van Zyl, C. G., Lambert, E. V., Hawley, J. A., Noakes, T. D., & Dennis, S. C. (1996). Effects of medium-chain triglyceride ingestion on fuel metabolism and cycling performance. *Journal of Applied Physiology, 80*, 2217–2225.

Vandanmagsar, B., Youm, Y. H., Ravussin, A., Galgani, J. E., Stadler, K., Mynatt, R. L., Ravussin, E., Stephens, J. M., & Dixit, V. D. (2011). The NLRP3 inflammasome instigates obesity-induced inflammation and insulin resistance. *Nature Medicine, 17*, 179–188.

Vandoorne, T., De Smet, S., Ramaekers, M., Van Thienen, R., De Bock, K., Clarke, K., & Hespel, P. (2017). Intake of a ketone ester drink during recovery from exercise promotes mTORC1 signaling but not glycogen resynthesis in human muscle. *Frontiers in Physiology, 8*, 310.

Veech, R. (2004). The therapeutic implications of ketone bodies: The effects of ketone bodies in pathological conditions; Ketosis, ketogenic diet, redox states, insulin resistance, and mitochondrial metabolism. *Prostaglandins, Leukotrienes, and Essential Fatty Acids, 70*, 309–319.

Veech, R. L. (2014). Ketone ester effects on metabolism and transcription. *Journal of Lipid Research, 55*, 2004–2006.

Viggiano, A., Pilla, R., Arnold, P., Monda, M., D'Agostino, D., & Coppola, G. (2015). Anticonvulsant properties of an oral ketone ester in a pentylenetetrazole-model of seizure. *Brain Research, 1618*, 50–54.

Waldman, H. S., Basham, S. A., Price, F. G., Smith, J. W., Chander, H., Knight, A. C., Krings, B. M., & McAllister, M. J. (2018). Exogenous ketone salts do not improve cognitive responses after a high-intensity exercise protocol in healthy college-aged males. *Applied Physiology, Nutrition, and Metabolism = Physiologie Appliquee, Nutrition et Metabolisme, 43*, 711–717.

Waldman, H. S., & McAllister, M. J. (2020). Exogenous ketones as therapeutic signaling molecules in high-stress occupations: Implications for mitigating oxidative stress and mitochondrial dysfunction in future research. *Nutrition and Metabolic Insights, 13*, 1178638820979029. doi:10.1177/1178638820979029. PMID: 33354110; PMCID: PMC7734540.

Walsh, J. J., Myette-Cote, E., & Little, J. P. (2020a). The effect of exogenous ketone monoester ingestion on plasma BDNF during an oral glucose tolerance test. *Frontiers in Physiology, 11*, 1094.

Walsh, J. J., Myette-Cote, E., Neudorf, H., & Little, J. P. (2020b). Potential therapeutic effects of exogenous ketone supplementation for type 2 diabetes: A review. *Current Pharmaceutical Design, 26*, 958–969.

Wang, J., & Yi, J. (2008). Cancer cell killing via ROS: To increase or decrease, that is the question. *Cancer Biology & Therapy, 7*, 1875–1884.

Wang, X., Wu, X., Liu, Q., Kong, G., Zhou, J., Jiang, J., Wu, X., Huang, Z., Su, W., & Zhu, Q. (2017). Ketogenic metabolism inhibits histone deacetylase (HDAC) and reduces oxidative stress after spinal cord injury in rats. *Neuroscience, 366*, 36–43.

Wang, Y., Liu, Z., Han, Y., Xu, J., Huang, W., & Li, Z. (2018). Medium chain triglycerides enhance exercise endurance through the increased mitochondrial biogenesis and metabolism. *PLOS ONE, 13*, Article e0191182.

Weber, D. D., Aminzadeh-Gohari, S., Tulipan, J., Catalano, L., Feichtinger, R. G., & Kofler, B. (2019). Ketogenic diet in the treatment of cancer–Where do we stand? *Molecular Metabolism, 33*, 102–121.

Wheatley, K. E., Williams, E. A., Smith, N. C., Dillard, A., Park, E. Y., Nunez, N. P., Hursting, S. D., & Lane, M. A. (2008). Low-carbohydrate diet versus caloric restriction: Effects on weight loss, hormones, and colon tumor growth in obese mice. *Nutrition and Cancer, 60*, 61–68.

Wlaz, P., Socala, K., Nieoczym, D., Luszczki, J. J., Zarnowska, I., Zarnowski, T., Czuczwar, S. J., & Gasior, M. (2012). Anticonvulsant profile of caprylic acid, a main constituent of the medium-chain triglyceride (MCT) ketogenic diet, in mice. *Neuropharmacology, 62*, 1882–1889.

Wlaz, P., Socala, K., Nieoczym, D., Zarnowski, T., Zarnowska, I., Czuczwar, S. J., & Gasior, M. (2015). Acute anticonvulsant effects of capric acid in seizure tests in mice. *Progress in Neuropsychopharmacology & Biological Psychiatry, 57*, 110–116.

Van Wymelbeke, V., Himaya, A., Louis-Sylvestre, J., & Fantino, M. (1998). Influence of medium-chain and long-chain triacylglycerols on the control of food intake in men. *American Journal of Clinical Nutrition, 68*(2), 226–234. https://doi-org.ezproxy.hsc.usf.edu/10.1093/ajcn/68.2.226

Xia, S., Lin, R., Jin, L., Zhao, L., Kang, H. B., Pan, Y., Liu, S., Qian, G., Qian, Z., Konstantakou, E., Zhang, B., Dong, J. T., Chung, Y. R., Abdel-Wahab, O., Merghoub, T., Zhou, L., Kudchadkar, R. R., Lawson, D. H., Khoury, H. J., Khuri, F. R., . . . Chen, J. (2017). Prevention of dietary-fat-fueled ketogenesis attenuates BRAF V600E tumor growth. *Cell Metabolism, 25*, 358–373.

Xie, Z., Zhang, D., Chung, D., Tang, Z., Huang, H., Dai, L., Qi, S., Li, J., Colak, G., Chen, Y., Xia, C., Peng, C., Ruan, H., Kirkey, M., Wang, D., Jensen, L. M., Kwon, O. K., Lee, S., Pletcher, S. D., Tan, M., . . . Zhao, Y. (2016). Metabolic regulation of gene expression by histone lysine beta-hydroxy-butyrylation. *Molecular Cell, 62*, 194–206.

Youm, Y. H., Grant, R. W., McCabe, L. R., Albarado, D. C., Nguyen, K. Y., Ravussin, A., Pistell, P., Newman, S., Carter, R., Laque, A., Münzberg, H., Rosen, C. J., Ingram, D. K., Salbaum, J. M., & Dixit, V. D. (2013). Canonical Nlrp3 inflammasome links systemic low-grade inflammation to functional decline in aging. *Cell Metabolism, 18*, 519–532.

Youm, Y. H., Nguyen, K. Y., Grant, R. W., Goldberg, E. L., Bodogai, M., Kim, D., D'Agostino, D., Planavsky, N., Lupfer, C., Kanneganti, T. D., Kang, S., Horvath, T. L., Fahmy, T. M., Crawford, P. A., Biragyn, A., Alnemri, E., & Dixit, V. D. (2015). The ketone metabolite beta-hydroxybutyrate blocks NLRP3 inflammasome-mediated inflammatory disease. *Nature Medicine, 21*, 263–269.

Zhang, J., Cao, Q., Li, S., Lu, X., Zhao, Y., Guan, J. S., Chen, J. C., Wu, Q., & Chen, G. Q. (2013a). 3-Hydroxybutyrate methyl ester as a potential drug against Alzheimer's disease via mitochondria protection mechanism. *Biomaterials, 34*, 7552–7562.

Zhang, Y., Kuang, Y., LaManna, J., & Puchowicz, M. (2013b). Contribution of brain glucose and ketone bodies to oxidative metabolism. *Advances in Experimental Medicine and Biology, 765*, 365–370.

Zou, X., Meng, J., Li, L., Han, W., Li, C., Zhong, R., Miao, X., Cai, J., Zhang, Y., & Zhu, D. (2016). Acetoacetate accelerates muscle regeneration and ameliorates muscular dystrophy in mice. *Journal of Biological Chemistry, 291*, 2181–2195.

Zuccoli, G., Marcello, N., Pisanello, A., Servadei, F., Vaccaro, S., Mukherjee, P., & Seyfried, T. N. (2010). Metabolic management of glioblastoma multiforme using standard therapy together with a restricted ketogenic diet: Case report. *Nutrition & Metabolism, 7*, 33.

Neuroprotective and Behavioral Benefits of Exogenous Ketone Supplementation-Evoked Ketosis

ZSOLT KOVACS, PHD, DOMINIC P. D'AGOSTINO, PHD,
AND CSILLA ARI, PHD

INTRODUCTION

It has been demonstrated that disturbances in different neurotransmitter systems (e.g., in glutamatergic, GABAergic, and monoaminergic systems), the hypothalamic-pituitary-adrenal (HPA) axis, cell metabolism, inflammatory processes (e.g., increased level of pro-inflammatory cytokines, such as interleukin-1β [IL-1β]), and voltage-gated ion channels have a role in the pathophysiology of several central nervous system (CNS) diseases (Craske et al., 2017; Kovács et al., 2019b; Otte et al., 2016; Pérez-Pérez et al., 2021; Terrone et al., 2020; Thijs et al., 2019; Vezzani et al., 2019). Moreover, there is a complex interplay among the different pathologic processes implicated in CNS diseases, such as mitochondrial dysfunction, neuroinflammation, and genetics, as well as environmental factors, in epilepsy, neurodegenerative diseases, and psychiatric diseases (Armada-Moreira et al., 2020; Craske et al., 2017; Lim & Thomas, 2020; Otte et al., 2016; Pérez-Pérez et al., 2021; Thijs et al., 2019; Vezzani et al., 2019). These complex pathophysiologic processes often have interrelated molecular pathways and are present in multiple neurologic and behavioral disorders. Hence, any therapy with the potential to mitigate against such deleterious effects is desirable.

For example, lipopolysaccharide (LPS) binds to Toll-like receptor 4 (TLR4) and induces activation of PI3K/protein kinase B (Akt), mitogen-activated protein kinase (MAPK) and mammalian target of rapamycin (mTOR), leading to NF-κB (nuclear factor κB) activation and production of pro-inflammatory cytokines (e.g., IL-1β and tumor necrosis factor α [TNF-α]), and inducible enzymes (e.g., cyclooxygenase-2 [COX-2] and inducible nitric oxide synthase [iNOS]), prostaglandin E_2 (PGE$_2$), and reactive oxygen species (ROS; Glass et al., 2010; Lugrin et al., 2014;

Shabab et al., 2017; Terrone et al., 2020; van Vliet et al., 2018). TLRs may increase the ROS levels through activation of NOX (NADPH oxidase) and by facilitation of mitochondrial-derived ROS generation (Lugrin et al., 2014). Moreover, mitochondrial stress-associated ROS generation may activate NOD-like receptor pyrin domain 3 (NLRP3), leading to increased IL-1β levels (Lugrin et al., 2014; Tschopp & Schroder, 2010). Overactivation of NOX by, for example, hyperglycemia (e.g., in patients with diabetes) and pro-inflammatory cytokines may evoke excess production of ROS and oxidative stress (Ginnan et al., 2013; Korkmaz et al., 2008; Schramm et al., 2012). Activation of ROS generation may lead to iNOS-evoked increase in nitric oxide (NO), and NO together with an enhanced level of superoxide anion may enhance neuronal cell death (Akbar et al., 2016). Increased release of NO from microglia may block the reuptake of glutamate, leading to increased activation of NMDA receptors and neuronal death (Rao et al., 2012). In addition, glutamate, via NMDA receptors, may mediate activation of NOS and an increase in NO level by Ca^{2+}, which may cause degeneration of neurons (Dawson et al., 1992). Excess NO may evoke inflammation by activation of COX and NF-κB, leading to increased production of TNF-α, as well as promotion of apoptosis (Abramson et al., 2001). It has been demonstrated that COXs have a role in neuroinflammation and neurodegeneration, for example, via COX-2/PGE$_2$/ROS system-generated activation of the NF-κB pathway, leading to activation of pro-inflammatory genes (Glass et al., 2010; Terrone et al., 2020). IL-1β secreted from activated microglial cells/astrocytes can stimulate production of its own and other pro-inflammatory cytokines, COX-2, prostaglandins, iNOS, and ROS, mainly through the IL-1 receptor

(IL-1R1) and TLR4 (Glass et al., 2010; Swaroop et al., 2016), whereas TNF-α may induce apoptosis via its receptor (TNF receptor 1 [TNFR1]) and caspases (Kaushal & Schlichter, 2008; Niquet & Wasterlain, 2004). The metabolism-linked PI3K/Akt pathway can activate mTOR in activated microglial cells, leading to activation of NF-κB and (neuro)inflammatory processes (e.g., by enhanced expression of COX-2, iNOS, and pro-inflammatory cytokines; Glass et al., 2010; Shabab et al., 2017). MAPK pathways play important roles in LPS-generated neuroinflammation (e.g., upregulation of pro-inflammatory genes and expression of pro-inflammatory cytokines), for example, via p38 MAPK (Kheiri et al., 2018; Lee et al., 1994).

All these processes are influenced by metabolic control and can augment inflammatory pathways implicated not only in the pathophysiology of CNS diseases, such as epilepsy, neurodegenerative diseases, and psychiatric diseases, but also in behavior changes (Abg Abd Wahab et al., 2019; García-Bueno et al., 2014; Irwin, 2019; Kim et al., 2012; Shabab et al., 2017; Tan et al., 2013; Terrone et al., 2020). For example, p38 MAPK may be activated by mitochondria-derived oxidative stress/ROS (Robinson et al., 1999) and may be implicated in impaired synaptic plasticity and long-term potentiation (LTP)/memory (Colié et al., 2017). In addition, many brain regions have relatively low levels of endogenous antioxidant enzymes, such as catalase, and are selectively vulnerable to oxidative stress (Coyle & Puttfarcken, 1993).

It has also been demonstrated that mitochondrial dysfunction reduces ATP production, enhances ROS generation, activates the NF-κB pathway, and impairs Ca^{2+} homeostasis. These changes alter not only inflammatory and apoptotic processes, but also neurotransmission, neuronal activity, and synaptic plasticity pathophysiologically linked to treatment-resistant CNS diseases (e.g., Alzheimer's disease and Parkinson's disease; Akbar et al., 2016; Daniels et al., 2020; Glass et al., 2010; Holper et al., 2019; Lim & Thomas, 2020; Lugrin et al., 2014; Wu et al., 2016). Consequently, it is widely accepted that one of the main pathologic changes leading to CNS disorders, such as neurodegenerative diseases, epilepsy, and psychiatric diseases, may be metabolic/mitochondrial dysfunctions (Adzic et al., 2016; Ben-Shachar & Ene, 2018; Daniels et al., 2020; Holper et al., 2019; Joshi & Mochly-Rosen, 2018; Lim & Thomas, 2020; Orth & Schapira, 2001). Based on these observations, metabolic

therapies that can enhance mitochondrial function and suppress ROS and associated neuroinflammation/signaling may alleviate symptoms of several CNS diseases.

Although the pathophysiology, characteristics, and symptoms of many CNS disorders are adequately described and intensively studied, the growing numbers of drugs to treat them remain largely ineffective (e.g., in relation to epilepsy, schizophrenia, and depression; Craske et al., 2017; Dias et al., 2013; Manford, 2017; Pérez-Pérez et al., 2021; Pisanu & Squassina, 2019; Thijs et al., 2019; Werner & Coveñas, 2019). Moreover, some drugs may evoke serious, sometimes life-threatening adverse effects (Burakgazi & French, 2016; Craske et al., 2017; Kahn et al., 2015; Nevitt et al., 2017; Otte et al., 2016). Consequently, metabolic therapies for CNS diseases are eagerly awaited.

The ketogenic diet (KD) is defined by a macronutrient composition that is high-fat, adequate protein, and very low in carbohydrates. If the KD is sustained, it increases blood levels of ketone bodies—D-β-hydroxybutyrate (βHB), acetoacetate (AcAc), and acetone—in a process known as ketogenesis. Ketone bodies can cross the blood–brain barrier and serve as an energy source for brain cells (Achanta & Rae, 2017; Branco et al., 2016; Koppel & Swerdlow, 2018; Newman & Verdin, 2014b; Plecko et al., 2002). It has been demonstrated that KDs (as a metabolism-based therapeutic tool) may have beneficial effects in several CNS diseases, such as epilepsy (Green et al., 2020; Kossoff & Cervenka, 2020; Nathan et al., 2019; Villeneuve et al., 2009; Zupec-Kania & Spellman, 2008), neurodegenerative diseases (Kraeuter et al., 2020b; Neth et al., 2020; Phillips et al., 2018; Vanitallie et al., 2005), cancer (Li et al., 2020; Poff et al., 2015; Seyfried et al., 2020), and psychiatric diseases (Ari et al., 2016; Bostock et al., 2017; Evangeliou et al., 2003; Kovács et al., 2019b; Kraft & Westman, 2009; Spilioti et al., 2013). It has also been demonstrated that amendment of ketone metabolism (e.g., suppressed glycolysis and increased βHB levels) may have neuroprotective effects in the CNS (Camberos-Luna & Massieu, 2020; Koppel & Swerdlow, 2018; Masuda et al., 2005; Newman & Verdin, 2014b; Noh et al., 2008; Pinto et al., 2018; Prins, 2008), with therapeutic effects in several CNS disorders (Kossoff & Rho, 2009; Kovács et al., 2019b; Maalouf et al., 2009; Simeone et al., 2017b, 2018). Nevertheless, achieving KD-evoked therapeutic ketosis, which is marked by blood ketone levels increased from the normal range of 0.1 to 0.2 mM to 1 to 7 mM (Branco et al., 2016; Hashim

& VanItallie, 2014; Veech et al., 2001), requires strict dietary adherence that is challenging for most pediatric and adult patients (Bostock et al., 2017; Lee et al., 2016). In addition, long-term use of a KD may have adverse effects in some patients, causing nephrolithiasis, nausea, growth retardation, constipation, hyperlipidemia, hypoglycemia, hyperuricemia, gastritis, "keto-flu," vascular damage, and ulcerative colitis (Bostock et al., 2017, 2020; Branco et al., 2016; Burkitt, 2020; Hartman & Vining, 2007; Nordli et al., 2001; Zupec-Kania & Spellman, 2008). Consequently, development of a safer method to evoke and maintain therapeutic ketosis and to circumvent dietary restriction is an appealing alternative or adjuvant.

After ingestion, exogenous ketone supplements (EKSs), such as ketone salts (KSs), ketone esters (KEs) and medium-chain triglycerides (MCTs/MCT oils) can be metabolized to their component parts, resulting in increased blood ketone levels. For example, KEs and ketone monoesters (KMEs) are fully hydrolyzed to βHB and R-1,3-butanediol by gut esterases and the latter (R-1,3-butanediol) is further converted to ketone bodies, such as βHB, in the liver by alcohol dehydrogenases (Brownlow et al., 2017; Clarke et al., 2012a, 2012b; Schönfeld & Wojtczak, 2016; Tate et al., 1971). Ketone bodies (e.g., βHB) can enter the bloodstream and the CNS via monocarboxylate transporters and serve the energy/ATP needs of brain cells through the Krebs cycle (Achanta & Rae, 2017; Branco et al., 2016; Koppel & Swerdlow, 2018; Newman & Verdin, 2014b; Plecko et al., 2002; Soto-Mota et al., 2020). It has been demonstrated that not only KDs, but also EKSs, were able to generate and maintain rapid and mild ketosis in both animals and humans (Ari et al., 2016; Clarke et al., 2012b; Kesl et al., 2016; Myette-Côté et al., 2018; Plecko et al., 2002; Stubbs et al., 2017; Veech et al., 2001). Moreover, oral administration of KEs—for example, (R)-3-hydroxybutyl-(R)-3-hydroxybutyrate and R,S-1,3-butanediol AcAc diester—and proper doses of KSs and their combination (e.g., KEKS) may be well-tolerated, safe, and efficient ketogenic agents (Ari et al., 2019b; Clarke et al., 2012b; Gross et al., 2019; Myette-Côté et al., 2018; Newport et al., 2015; Plecko et al., 2002; Soto-Mota et al., 2019). Indeed, as was demonstrated, properly formulated and titrated EKSs may evoke fewer and milder adverse effects (e.g., some gastrointestinal problems) than the KD (Ari et al., 2016; Brunengraber, 1997; Clarke et al., 2012b; D'Agostino et al., 2013; Newport et

al., 2015; Poff et al., 2015; Stubbs et al., 2017). MCTs generate relatively low increases in ketone body levels in the blood and are often not well tolerated (because they cause diarrhea, flatulence, and dyspepsia; Courchesne-Loyer et al., 2013; Henderson, 2008; Vandenberghe et al., 2020). However, combined administration of proper doses of MCTs with other EKSs, such as KE or KS (e.g., KEMCT and KSMCT), can be used with little or no side effects (Ari et al., 2016, 2019b; Kovács et al., 2017, 2018).

It was also demonstrated that EKS administration might be an efficacious alternative way to achieve therapeutic ketosis (Ari et al., 2016; D'Agostino et al., 2013; Poff et al., 2015; Stubbs et al., 2017). Ketosis may be one of the most important factors in the KD-generated beneficial effects in CNS diseases (Camberos-Luna & Massieu, 2020; Gilbert et al., 2000; Kim et al., 2015; Kraeuter et al., 2015; Phelps et al., 2013; Ruskin et al., 2017; Simeone et al., 2018). Consequently, because administration of EKSs rapidly increases and maintains ketone body/βHB levels in a dose-dependent manner in animals and humans (Ari et al., 2016; Courchesne-Loyer et al., 2013; Harvey et al., 2018; Hashim & VanItallie, 2014; Kesl et al., 2016; Myette-Côté et al., 2018; Stubbs et al., 2017), EKSs may provide relief for patients with CNS diseases through ketosis/βHB-evoked neuroprotective effects, such as improved mitochondrial functions, enhanced ATP levels, decreased inflammatory processes, and decreased oxidative stress/ROS production (Koppel & Swerdlow, 2018; Maalouf et al., 2009; Newman & Verdin, 2014b; Norwitz et al., 2019; Pinto et al., 2018; Simeone et al., 2017b; Wu et al., 2020). Moreover, the combination of a KD with EKSs may further augment the therapeutic effects to alleviate symptoms of CNS diseases and behavioral deficits. Indeed, for example, combined administration of a KD with KS can rapidly increase blood ketones and promote motor function recovery in rats with acute spinal cord injury (Tan et al., 2020). In addition, EKSs promote therapeutic ketosis during a normal diet because production of ketone bodies from the supplements is not inhibited by carbohydrates (Brunengraber, 1997). Consequently, EKSs can be used together with normal diet, which eliminates the need for dietary restrictions. Indeed, consumption of diets with standard macronutrient compositions containing ketogenic ingredients (EKSs) may induce and sustain ketosis effectively and with little difficulty (Ari et al., 2016; D'Agostino et al., 2013; Kesl et al., 2016; Kovács et al., 2019a; Myette-Côté et al., 2018; Poff et al., 2015).

Although there has been remarkable progress in knowledge of the physiologic and pathophysiologic influences of EKSs, their exact mechanisms of action in CNS disorders are largely unknown. However, it has been demonstrated that increased levels of ketone bodies may modulate the activity of neurotransmitter systems (Achanta & Rae, 2017; Erecińska et al., 1996; Yudkoff et al., 2007), reduce the hyperexcitability and firing rates of neurons (Achanta & Rae, 2017; D'Agostino et al., 2013; Ma et al., 2007), attenuate neuroinflammatory processes (Achanta & Rae, 2017; Bae et al., 2016; Yamanashi et al., 2017; Youm et al., 2015), decrease oxidative stress (de Ruijter et al., 2003; Gregoretti et al., 2004; Newman & Verdin, 2014a; Shimazu et al., 2013), and improve mitochondrial respiration and increase mitochondrial ATP synthesis (Cantó et al., 2009; Elamin et al., 2017; Newman & Verdin, 2014a; Maalouf et al., 2007; Paoli et al., 2015; Pawlosky et al., 2017). Theoretically, these neuroprotective effects may be also produced by EKS-generated ketosis; thus, EKSs may protect different physiologic processes under pathologic conditions resulting in CNS diseases (Hashim & VanItallie, 2014; Koppel & Swerdlow, 2018; Kovács et al., 2019b; Maalouf et al., 2009; McCarty et al., 2015; Norwitz et al., 2019; Simeone et al., 2017b). Indeed, it has been demonstrated that administration of EKSs is feasible for the treatment of several CNS diseases. For example, KEs, KSs, MCT oils and mixtures of them can evoke antiseizure/antiepileptic effects (Berk et al., 2020; Ciarlone et al., 2016; D'Agostino et al., 2013; Kovács et al., 2017, 2019a), exert alleviating influences on psychiatric disorders (e.g., anxiety; Ari et al., 2016; Kashiwaya et al., 2013; Kovács et al., 2018, 2019b) and neurodegenerative disorders (such as Alzheimer's disease), and improve impaired sleep, learning, memory, and motor functions (Ari et al., 2014, 2015, 2018a; Brownlow et al., 2017; Ciarlone et al., 2016; Newport et al., 2015; Tefera et al., 2016). Moreover, EKS-evoked ketosis may augment the effects of drugs in the treatment of CNS diseases, such as depression (Pan et al., 2020). Consequently, despite limited evidence to support the beneficial effects of EKSs in the treatment of different CNS diseases, we can hypothesize that ketosis generated by exogenous ketone body precursors (EKSs) may be an effective, safe, and adaptable therapeutic tool in the treatment of patients with several CNS diseases. Moreover, EKS administration may be a reasonable alternative or adjuvant to pharmacotherapy in the treatment of different CNS diseases, especially the drug-resistant types.

Ketosis/βHB may also have beneficial effects on tissues/organs other than the nervous system and brain, such as muscle tissue and heart (Abdul Kadir et al., 2020; Cuenoud et al., 2020; Li et al., 2020; Rojas-Morales et al., 2020; Soto-Mota et al., 2020), and have therapeutic potential in the treatment of (CNS) diseases other than epilepsy, neurodegenerative diseases, and psychiatric disorders, such as cancer (Dąbek et al., 2020; Koutnik et al., 2020; Li et al., 2020; Ludwig, 2020; Rojas-Morales et al., 2020; Seyfried et al., 2020), but the rationale behind these approaches is outside the scope of this chapter. Thus, the chapter provides a short overview of both ketosis/βHB-generated neuroprotective influences and the rationale behind the use of ketosis in the treatment of epilepsy, several psychiatric disorders, and neurodegenerative diseases, as well as learning, memory, sleep, and motor function deficiencies/abnormalities.

KETOSIS-EVOKED NEUROPROTECTIVE EFFECTS

Modulation of Mitochondrial Functions, Cell Energetics, and Neurotransmitter Systems

It has been demonstrated that the alterations by βHB adminstration—including a decreased mitochondrial $[NAD^+]:[NADH]$ ratio and increased ratio of coenzyme $[Q]:[QH_2]$—may enhance the difference of redox potentials of the two electron-carrier couples (Mehlman & Veech, 1972; Norwitz et al., 2019; Sato et al., 1995). Consequently, the transfer of electrons from NADH to Q liberates more energy, by which the concentration of protons in the intermembrane space is elevated, and ATP production through ATP synthase enzyme can be increased. Increased ketone-induced mitochondrial ATP production not only can replace glucose as a fuel for brain cells (e.g., under certain circumstances, when the glucose supply is insufficient; Sato et al., 1995; VanItallie & Nufert, 2003), but also supports the repolarization of neuronal membrane after stimulation via Na^+,K^+-ATPase (Simeone et al., 2017b; Figure 34.1). It was also suggested that the KD/EKSs-evoked increase in βHB level may increase both mitochondrial synthesis and release of ATP by brain cells, followed by metabolism of ATP to adenosine extracellularly. Increased levels of adenosine can activate adenosine A_1 receptors (A_1Rs), leading to activation of ATP-sensitive potassium (K_{ATP}) channels and resulting in hyperpolarization

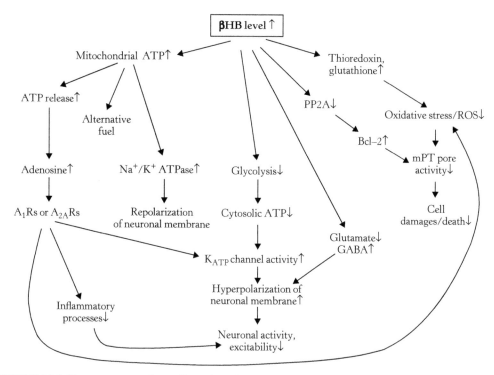

FIGURE 34.1 *Neuroprotective Effects of βHB Through Modulation of Mitochondrial Functions, Cell Energetics, and Several Neurotransmitter Systems*

Abbreviations: $A_1Rs/A_{2A}Rs$ = adenosine receptors; Bcl-2 = B-cell lymphoma-2; βHB = β-hydroxybutyrate; K_{ATP} = ATP-sensitive potassium channel; mPT = mitochondrial permeability transition pore; PP2A = protein phosphatase 2A; ROS = reactive oxygen species.

of neuronal membrane and decreased neuronal activity (Achanta & Rae, 2017; Andoh et al., 2006; Kawamura et al., 2014; Kovács et al., 2013; Simeone et al., 2018; Figure 34.1). Moreover, an increased level of adenosine may decrease oxidative stress and decrease the harmful effects of ROS (Almeida et al., 2003; Hu et al., 2012), decrease the energy demand of brain (Poulsen & Quinn, 1998), and reduce inflammatory processes (van der Putten et al., 2009), likely via A_1Rs and/or the A_{2A} type of adenosine receptor ($A_{2A}R$; Choudhury et al., 2019; Figure 34.1). Moreover, increased levels of ketone bodies, such as βHB, may inhibit glycolysis (Achanta & Rae, 2017), resulting in decreased levels of cytosolic ATP (near the plasma membrane) and increased activity of K_{ATP} channels (Figure 34.1). This process also generates hyperpolarization of neuronal membrane and decreases neuronal activity/excitability (Achanta & Rae, 2017; Ciruela et al., 2006; Haas & Greene, 1984; Kovács et al., 2014; Lund et al., 2015). The flow of electrons from mitochondrial QH_2 to oxygen may generate superoxide (Lugrin et al., 2014; Sato et al., 1995). It has been demonstrated that βHB decreases ROS production by increasing the

Q:QH_2 ratio (oxidizing Q-QH_2 couple), which decreases electron transfer from QH_2 to oxygen (Sato et al., 1995). βHB metabolism enhances antioxidant defenses by decreasing the $NADP^+$:NADPH ratio, reducing $NADP^+$ to NADPH, generating an increase in the reduced levels of different antioxidants, such as thioredoxin and glutathione (Agledal et al., 2010; Kashiwaya et al., 1997; Mehlman & Veech, 1972; Norwitz et al., 2019; Pawlosky et al., 2017; Sato et al., 1995; Veech et al., 2019; Figure 34.1). It was suggested that increased resistance to oxidative stress conferred by βHB may modulate pathomechanisms of type 2 diabetes (Newman & Verdin, 2014a) and protect neurons from hypoglycemic and hypoxic insults (Masuda et al., 2005; Samoilova et al., 2010). In support of this observation, it was reported that βHB reversed insulin-generated hypoglycemic coma in mice (Thurston et al., 1986).

It was suggested that one of the putative downstream effects of oxidative stress-evoked cell damage/death is the opening of the mitochondrial permeability transition (mPT) pore, which may result in activation of the apoptotic cascade and release of pro-apoptotic factors, Ca^{2+}

and cytochrome *c*, into the cytoplasm, as well as uncoupling of the electron transport system from ATP production (Emerit et al., 2004; Sullivan et al., 2005). It was demonstrated that the increase in the ROS level may activate the mPT pore (Emerit et al., 2004; Maalouf et al., 2009). Thus, βHB, which may decrease ROS production (Kim et al., 2007b), can improve mitochondrial respiration and ATP production, which can prevent mPT pore activation and/or alleviate mPT pore activation-generated effects. Indeed, the ketone bodies AcAc and βHB inhibited the activity of protein phosphatase 2A (PP2A); PP2A can inhibit the mPT inhibitor/anti-apoptotic factor B cell lymphoma-2 (Bcl-2) and trigger apoptosis (Kroemer et al., 2007; Maalouf & Rho, 2008; Figure 34.1). Moreover, ketone bodies prevented the mPT activator diamide-evoked neuronal injury/death (Kim et al., 2007b). In this context, it is interesting to note that βHB increased the threshold for Ca^{2+}-induced mPT (Kim et al., 2007b), and ketosis upregulated the Bcl-2 protein level (Puchowicz et al., 2008).

Therapeutic ketosis may enhance the inhibitory GABAergic effects (via increased GABA levels and preserved GABAergic interneurons), elevate both accumulation of GABA in presynaptic vesicles and $GABA_A$ receptor activity (Achanta & Rae, 2017; Cheng et al., 2020; Erecińska et al., 1996; McNally & Hartman, 2012), and increase adenosine levels (Sharma et al., 2015a). Moreover, βHB may inhibit vesicular glutamate transporters, decrease both glutamate loading to vesicles and glutamate release, effects that together suppress glutamate-induced neuronal excitability and toxicity (Juge et al., 2010; McNally & Hartman, 2012; Noh et al., 2008; Simeone et al., 2017b; Figure 34.1). Because GABA is synthesized from glutamate, these results suggest that βHB may shift the inhibitory/excitatory (GABA/glutamate) balance toward inhibition (stabilization), which may alleviate symptoms of CNS disorders like epilepsy. Moreover, it was also suggested that the ketosis/βHB-evoked decrease in the $NADP^+$:NADPH ratio (increased NADPH levels) may increase the levels of dopamine, norepinephrine, epinephrine, serotonin, and melatonin through reduction of dihydrobiopterin (BH_2) to tetrahydrobiopterin (BH_4), a coenzyme needed for the synthesis of transmitters, such as dopamine and serotonin (Tieu et al., 2003; Veech et al., 2019). Indeed, ketosis-evoked enhanced levels of norepinephrine and decreased monoamine dopamine and serotonin metabolite levels were

also demonstrated (Dahlin et al., 2012; Otani et al., 1984).

Inhibition of Histone Deacetylase Activity

Histone acetyl transferases (HATs) attach acetyl groups to histones, thus increasing their positive charge and weakening their interaction with DNA, thereby facilitating DNA transcription. Conversely, histone deacetylases (HDACs) remove the acetyl groups from histones, thus enhancing their interaction with DNA and thereby impeding transcription. So, HDAC antagonism should facilitate DNA transcription (Alageel et al., 2018; de Ruijter et al., 2003).

Increased levels of βHB can inhibit the activity of some members of the classical HDAC family (class I and class IIa HDACs), thereby enhancing acetylation of histone residues and allowing DNA to be accessed by select transcription factors, such as FOXO3A (de Ruijter et al., 2003; Gregoretti et al., 2004; Newman & Verdin, 2014a; Shimazu et al., 2013). Through the downstream activation of FOXO3A, this epigenetic gene regulation process induces expression of various antioxidant genes, including metallothionein 2 (Mt2), manganese superoxide dismutase (MnSOD), and catalase (Shimazu et al., 2013), and decreases oxidative stress (Figure 34.2). Moreover, FOXO3A induces mitochondrial gene expression, leading to protection of mitochondria and cells against oxidative stress and damage by enhancing mitochondrial homeostasis (e.g., regulation of mitochondrial fusion/fission, mitochondrial biogenesis, and ATP production; Tseng et al., 2013; Figure 34.2). It has also been demonstrated that the βHB-evoked inhibition of HDACs may increase brain-derived neurotrophic factor (BDNF) expression (Sleiman et al., 2016). Increased BDNF levels may enhance mitochondrial respiration and ATP levels (Marosi et al., 2016), promote anti-inflammatory effects (via inhibition of NF-κB, and decreased proinflammatory cytokine levels), promote anti-apoptotic effects (Manning & Cantley, 2007; Xu et al., 2017), increase the activity of antioxidant enzymes (such as superoxide dismutase, glutathione reductase, and glutathione peroxidase), and provide protection against glutamate-induced excitotoxicity (Lau et al., 2015; Mattson et al., 1995; Figure 34.2). Moreover, βHB can decrease endoplasmic reticulum (ER) stress-evoked apoptosis and oxidative stress by inhibition of HDACs (Zhao & Ackerman, 2006). βHB can also evoke direct antioxidant effects (Haces et al., 2008) and promote histone, as well as non-histone,

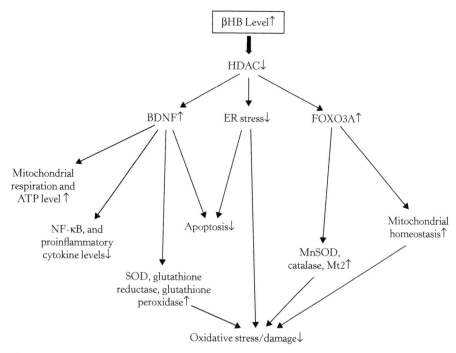

FIGURE 34.2 *Neuroprotective Effects of βHB-Evoked HDAC Inhibition*

Abbreviations: βHB = β-hydroxybutyrate; BDNF = brain-derived neurotrophic factor; FOXO3A = forkhead box O3A; HDAC = histone deacetylase; MnSOD = manganese superoxide dismutase; Mt2 = metallothionein 2; NF-κB = nuclear factor κ-light-chain-enhancer of activated B cells; SOD = superoxide dismutase.

acetylation by histone acetyltransferases, leading to modulation of gene expression (Marosi et al., 2016; Menzies et al., 2016).

Modulation of Hydroxycarboxylic Acid Receptor 2, NLRP3, and Free Fatty Acid Receptor 3 Activity

It has been demonstrated that βHB is a ligand for the $G_{i/o}$-protein-coupled hydroxycarboxylic acid receptor 2 (HCAR2; also known as PUMA-G, niacin receptor 1, or GPR109A receptor; Offermanns, 2006; Offermanns & Schwaninger, 2015) expressed on, for example, microglial cells (Fu et al., 2015; Parodi et al., 2015). βHB can activate HCAR2 (Newman & Verdin, 2014a; Rahman et al., 2014; Taggart et al., 2005). Furthermore, the KD, 3-hydroxybutyrate methyl ester (HBME; a methylated form of βHB), and βHB increased the expression of HCAR2 (Hasan-Olive et al., 2019; Zou et al., 2009). Moreover, it was also suggested that HCAR2 is required for KD/βHB-evoked neuroprotective effects because these influences were lost in HCAR2$^{-/-}$ mice (Rahman et al., 2014).

The Class III HDACs include seven proteins called sirtuins (SIRT1–7). Enzymatic activity of SIRTs requires the cofactor NAD$^+$ (NAD$^+$-dependent protein deacetylases; first described as NAD$^+$-dependent type/class III HDACs; He et al., 2012). Class I SIRTs, such as SIRT1, SIRT2, and SIRT3, localized to nucleus, cytoplasm, and mitochondria (respectively, but the SIRT3 may also be localized to nucleus and cytoplasm), and have deacetylase activity (Frye, 2000; Haigis & Guarente, 2006; He et al., 2012; Kincaid & Bossy-Wetzel, 2013). It was demonstrated that βHB increases NAD$^+$ levels (Elamin et al., 2017, 2018), leading to enhanced activity and expression of SIRTs (e.g., SIRT1 and SIRT3; Elamin et al., 2018; McCarty et al., 2015; Scheibye-Knudsen et al., 2014). HCAR2 may activate AMP-activated protein kinase (AMPK), leading to NAD$^+$ generation (through induction of the rate-limiting enzyme nicotinamide phosphoribosyltransferase of the NAD biosynthesis pathway), so that the increase in NAD$^+$ concentration enhances SIRT1 activity (Parodi et al., 2015; Figure 34.3). It was also demonstrated that KD/βHB can enhance AMPK activity, leading to neuroprotective effects (e.g., through increased NAD$^+$, NAD$^+$:NADH ratio, and SIRT1/SIRT3; Cantó et al., 2009; Elamin et

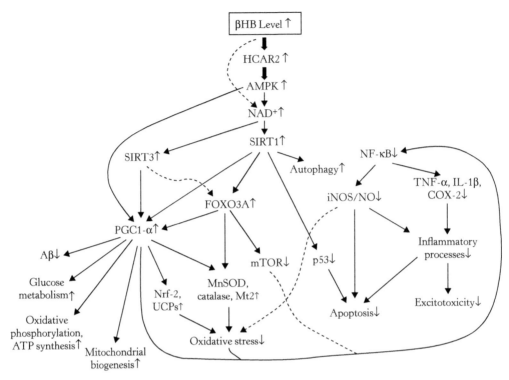

FIGURE 34.3 *Putative Pathways of βHB-Evoked Neuroprotective Effects Through HCAR2*

Abbreviations: Aβ = amyloid β-peptide; AMPK = AMP-activated protein kinase; βHB = β-hydroxybutyrate; COX-2 = cyclooxygenase-2; FOXO3A = forkhead box O3A; HCAR2 = hydroxycarboxylic acid receptor 2; IL1-β = interleukin 1β; iNOS = inducible nitric oxide synthase; MnSOD = manganese superoxide dismutase; Mt2 = metallothionein 2; mTOR = mammalian target of rapamycin; NAD$^+$ = nicotinamide adenine dinucleotide; NF-κB = nuclear factor κ-light-chain-enhancer of activated B cells; NO = nitric oxide; Nrf-2 = nuclear factor erythroid 2-related factor 2; p53 = tumor suppressor protein 53; PGC1-α = peroxisome proliferator-activated receptor gamma (PPARγ) coactivator-1α; SIRT = sirtuin; TNF-α = tumor necrosis factor-α; UCP = uncoupling proteins.

al., 2017; Maalouf et al., 2007; Newman & Verdin, 2014a; Paoli et al., 2015; Pawlosky et al., 2017; Verdin et al., 2010).

Anti-inflammatory, anti-apoptotic, and anti-oxidant influences of KD/βHB were also suggested via HCAR2-evoked inhibitory effects on the pro-inflammatory transcription factor NF-κB (Fu et al., 2015; Offermanns & Schwaninger, 2015; Parodi et al., 2015; Figure 34.3). The KD can decrease expression of pro-apoptotic proteins and increase expression of anti-apoptotic proteins, and consequently it can protect neurons from apoptosis via the HCAR2/SIRT1/transcription factor tumor suppressor protein 53 (p53) pathway (Evan & Littlewood, 1998; Morris, 2005; Norwitz et al., 2019; Scheibye-Knudsen et al., 2014; Figure 34.3). Moreover, SIRT1 can enhance activity of autophagy proteins, such as autophagy-related gene 13, by which it enhances catabolic processes (e.g., degradation and recycling of damaged elements of cells) and facilitates the clearance of

abnormal mitochondria (Herzig & Shaw, 2018; McCarty et al., 2015). It has also been demonstrated that βHB-evoked stimulation of HCAR2 induces expression of genes for antioxidants (e.g., MnSOD, catalase, and Mt2) in a FOXO3A-dependent way (McCarty et al., 2015; Norwitz et al., 2019), leading to protection of cells against oxidative stress (Figure 34.3). βHB can inhibit microglial activation and expression of the pro-inflammatory TNF-α, IL-1β, COX-2, iNOS, and NO, as well as the LPS-induced increase in pro-inflammatory enzymes (e.g., COX-2 and iNOS) and pro-inflammatory cytokines (e.g., TNF-α, IL-1β) via HCAR2 (Digby et al., 2012; Fu et al., 2015; Graff et al., 2016; Shabab et al., 2017; Wu et al., 2020; Yang & Cheng, 2010). The pro-inflammatory molecules may evoke inflammatory processes, excitotoxicity, and apoptosis (e.g., by NO-generated inhibition of glutamate reuptake and by TNF-α via death receptors), and they may induce oxidative stress, such as that caused by

NO (Taylor et al., 2008; Yuste et al., 2015). These effects can be prevented or alleviated by ketosis-evoked influences, likely through, for example, the HCAR2/AMPK/SIRT1/FOXO3A/mTOR/ NF-κB pathway (Finley & Haigis, 2009; Herzig & Shaw, 2018; Morris, 2005; Parodi et al., 2015; Figure 34.3). Moreover, it was suggested that activation of SIRT1 not only decreases levels of pro-inflammatory cytokines, but also enhances insulin sensitivity and action, such as through an increase in insulin signaling and glucose uptake (Luo & Zhang, 2016; Yoshizaki et al., 2009).

Ketone bodies may increase the expression of not only HCAR2, but also SIRTs (e.g., SIRT1 and SIRT3) and peroxisome proliferator-activated receptor gamma (PPARγ) coactivator-1α (PGC1-α; Hasan-Olive et al., 2019; McCarty et al., 2015; Scheibye-Knudsen et al., 2014) suggesting the function of both HCAR2/SIRT1/ PGC1-α pathway and HCAR2/SIRT3/PGC1-α pathway. Indeed, the neuroprotective effects of PGC1-α can be modulated by both SIRT1 and SIRT3 (Hasan-Olive et al., 2019; Houtkooper & Auwerx, 2012; Kong et al., 2010; Shi et al., 2005; St-Pierre et al., 2006; Yeung et al., 2004; Zhu et al., 2011; Figure 34.3). Moreover, FOXO3A also modulates the activity of PGC1-α (Olmos et al., 2009), and antioxidant influence of SIRT3 via the FOXO3A pathway was also demonstrated (Rangarajan et al., 2015; Figure 34.3). In addition, AMPK may also have a role in activation of PGC1-α directly by phosphorylation (before subsequent deacetylation of PGC1-α by SIRT1; Cantó et al., 2009; Cantó & Auwerx, 2009; Figure 34.3). The transcriptional cofactor PGC1-α can bind and coactivate PPARγ (which belongs to the superfamily of nuclear receptors) and promotes/ enhances, among others, glucose metabolism, oxidative phosphorylation, and mitochondrial biogenesis, as well as SOD and catalase activity (Austin & St-Pierre, 2012; Cantó & Auwerx, 2009; Herzig & Shaw, 2018; Kim & Yang, 2013; Puigserver & Spiegelman, 2003). Nevertheless, PGC1-α reduces the level of inflammation/NF-κB/pro-inflammatory cytokines (Scirpo et al., 2015; Tyagi et al., 2011), and decreases amyloid β-peptide (Aβ) generation (Katsouri et al., 2011; Qin et al., 2009; Figure 34.3). Moreover, KD and βHB upregulated the level of mitochondrial uncoupling protein 2 (UCP2; Hasan-Olive et al., 2019); thus, ketosis (evoked by, for example, the KD and KEs) can decrease the production of ROS via enhanced expression of UCPs (Kashiwaya et al., 2010; Koppel & Swerdlow, 2018; Srivastava et al., 2012; Sullivan et al., 2004; Figure 34.3).

Indeed, it has been demonstrated that KD/βHB can rescue mitochondrial functions (e.g., by decreasing oxidative stress) through activation of the SIRT3/PGC1-α/UCP2 pathway (Hasan-Olive et al., 2019) or the SIRT3/PGC1-α/UCP1 pathway (Shi et al., 2005). In addition, increased SIRT3 activity can increase ketone body production (Shimazu et al., 2010) and may suppress mPT pore formation, by which can prevent mitochondrial dysfunction (Hafner et al., 2010). It has been demonstrated that decreased insulin sensitivity may increase inflammation and decrease PGC1-α expression (Handschin & Spiegelman, 2008; Nierenberg et al., 2018). A decrease in PGC1-α level can lead to decreased mitochondrial respiration and increased NF-κB activity/inflammatory processes/ROS levels not only in muscle cells (Eisele et al., 2013, 2015), but also in brain tissue (Agudelo et al., 2014; Phillips & Fahimi, 2018). Moreover, BDNF may stimulate PGC1-α-dependent mitochondrial biogenesis (Cheng et al., 2012), suggesting that a βHB-evoked increase in BDNF level (by HDAC inhibition; Figure 34.2) can modify different mitochondrial functions via PGC1-α.

The KD and βHB can upregulate the expression of PPARs and enhance the activity of the Kelch-like ECH-associated protein-1/Nrf-2 (nuclear factor erythroid 2-related factor 2) system in the brain (Jeong et al., 2011; Morris et al., 2020; Simeone et al., 2017a). It was also suggested that AMPK may enhance the nuclear translocation of the antioxidant transcription factor Nrf-2 (Joo et al., 2016), and both SIRT1 and PGC1-α may increase the expression of Nrf-2 (Choi et al., 2017; Huang et al., 2017b).

The NLRP3 inflammasome may evoke cleavage of pro-IL-1β to its active form (IL-1β) by caspase-1 (Levy et al., 2015; Patel et al., 2017). βHB, as an endogenous NLRP3 inflammasome inhibitor, may decrease inflammatory processes by inhibition of the NLRP3 inflammasome (likely by prevention of K^+ efflux), leading to decreased release of pro-inflammatory cytokines, such as IL-1β (Bae et al., 2016; Thornberry et al., 1995; Yamanashi et al., 2017; Youm et al., 2015). It has been suggested that the NLPRP3-inhibitory effect of βHB was independent of ROS, glycolysis inhibition, autophagy inhibition, AMPK, SIRT2, HCAR2, and UCP2 (Youm et al., 2015). However, others have suggested that βHB may decrease oxidative stress via the AMPK-activated signaling pathway (through the AMPK/FOXO3/MnSOD-catalase pathway and a decrease in oxidative stress; Figure 34.3), resulting in both reduction of

ER stress and, as a consequence, ER stress-induced NLRP3 inflammasome (apoptosis-associated speck-like protein [ASC], caspase-1, and NLRP3) formation (Bae et al., 2016). Nevertheless, it has also been demonstrated that the effects of exogenously increased ketone body levels on inflammatory processes are highly complex (Neudorf et al., 2019, 2020); thus, work is needed to determine the exact effects of ketosis on inflammatory processes under different physiologic and pathologic conditions. Moreover, it is interesting that a high glucose level may also activate the NLRP3 inflammasome, leading to an increase in IL-1β expression/release (Tack et al., 2012) and inflammation (Aeberli et al., 2011; Frazier et al., 2011). Because the KD and EKSs can decrease glucose levels (Ari et al., 2016, 2019b; Kovács et al., 2017), it is possible that ketosis/βHB could decrease the enhancing effect of excessive glucose levels on NLRP3 activity in diabetes (hyperglycemia and insulin resistance).

It was recently demonstrated that βHB can bind to the G-protein-coupled receptor free fatty acid receptor 3 (FFAR3; also known as GPR41) as an agonist (Won et al., 2013). Nevertheless, others have suggested that βHB may antagonize the FFAR3 (Kimura et al., 2011). However, it was concluded that βHB may reduce or control sympathetic tone and body energy expenditure, as well as lower the metabolic rate through both HCAR2 and FFAR3 (Kimura et al., 2011; Newman & Verdin, 2014b).

KETOSIS-EVOKED NEUROPROTECTIVE EFFECTS: BENEFICIAL INFLUENCES ON CNS DISEASES AND BEHAVIOR

Modulation of Mitochondrial Function and Neurotransmitter Systems

It has been suggested that ketosis is necessary, but not sufficient, for the KD's antiseizure effects (Bough & Rho, 2007), and gut microbiota are required for the KD-generated antiseizure effects in a seizure model through mechanisms that do not involve changes in βHB concentrations (Olson et al., 2018). However, ketosis may be an important factor in KD/EKSs-evoked anticonvulsant/antiepileptic effects (Gilbert et al., 2000; Huttenlocher, 1976; Kim et al., 2015; Kossoff et al., 2006; Plecko et al., 2002; Simeone et al., 2018). For example, the KD's alleviating effects on refractory status epilepticus (SE) in FIRES (fever-induced refractory epileptic encephalopathy in school-age

children) may be in connection with increased βHB levels (Nabbout et al., 2010). KE not only delayed occurrence of the CNS oxygen-toxicity-induced seizures, but also increased blood levels of ketone bodies (Ari et al., 2019a; D'Agostino et al., 2013). Similarly, KE supplementation had an anticonvulsant effect and increased levels of ketone bodies in an Angelman syndrome mouse model (Ciarlone et al., 2016). KE and KSMCT (KS + MCT) increased the blood βHB level and decreased absence epileptic activity in an animal model (Wistar Albino Glaxo Rijswijk/WAG/Rij rats; Kovács et al., 2017). Moreover, MCT treatment not only decreased the seizure frequency and severity, but also increased βHB levels (Lambrechts et al., 2015).

Nevertheless, it was also suggested that a decreased glucose level may be a key factor in the antiepileptic effect of KD/EKSs (Freeman et al., 2009; Huttenlocher, 1976; Poff et al., 2019). However, hyperpolarization of the neuronal membrane may reduce cell firing rates and, as a neuroprotective effect, decrease epileptic activity. Indeed, excessive cortical excitation and an increase in glutamate and/or a decrease in GABA levels may cause epileptic activity (Carcak & Ozkara, 2017; Mazarati & Sankar, 2016; Sharma et al., 2015a; Sills & Rogawski, 2020; Werner & Coveñas, 2017). Thus, an increase in synaptic levels of GABA and adenosine may have antiepileptic effects (Figure 34.1) via postsynaptic inhibitory $GABA_A$ receptors and A_1Rs, respectively, by which KD/EKSs-evoked ketosis/βHB may inhibit seizures at the synaptic level in both animal models and humans (D'Alimonte et al., 2009; Effendi et al., 2020; Kovács et al., 2017; Masino et al., 2011; Rho, 2017; Sharma et al., 2015a; Yudkoff et al., 2007).

As was demonstrated, mitochondrial dysfunction can also manifest in seizures/epilepsies (Lim & Thomas, 2020). Impaired mitochondrial respiratory chain activity and/or decreased ATP level, as well as an increase in mitochondrial ROS level/oxidative stress, have a role in the processes (e.g., the cell death) leading to epileptogenesis/epileptic seizures (Kubová et al., 2001; Kudin et al., 2002; Kunz et al., 2000; Rowley & Patel, 2013). Moreover, ROS may mediate cognitive deficits in temporal lobe epilepsy (Pearson et al., 2015). It has been demonstrated that KD/ketosis can decrease epileptic seizures and improve seizure control in patients with Angelman syndrome, among others, via improved mitochondrial function and decreased cortical hyperexcitability (Ben-Shachar & Ene, 2018; Bough & Rho, 2007; Gano et al., 2014; Su et al., 2011; Thibert et al., 2009).

KD/EKSs-evoked ketosis can elevate both the intracellular ATP level and the extracellular adenosine concentration, which generates activation of A_1Rs, opening of K_{ATP} channels, and attenuation of neuronal excitability (Figure 34.1), leading to a decrease in seizure activity (Kawamura et al., 2010; Kovács et al., 2017; Masino et al., 2009, 2011; Tanner et al., 2011). Moreover, it was also demonstrated that the KD may generate antiepileptic/neuroprotective effects by diminishing ROS production via activation of UCPs (Richard et al., 2001) in the hippocampus (Sullivan et al., 2004; Figure 34.1). SE triggers the processes of necrosis- and apoptosis-related cell death. For example, the apoptosis protein Bad dissociates from its chaperone protein 14-3-3; Bad may evoke release of another apoptosis factor, Bax, leading to Bax-generated release of cytochrome *c* from mitochondria to cytosol, which can activate caspases and cell death (Henshall et al., 2000, 2001; Niquet & Wasterlain, 2004). It was suggested that KD-evoked neuroprotective influences may generate antiepileptic/antiseizure effects via inhibition/prevention of dissociation of Bad from protein 14-3-3 and of the ROS/apoptosis cascade at least in kainic acid (KA)-induced seizures (Noh et al., 2003, 2006, 2008). Moreover, βHB blocked spontaneous recurrent seizures by increasing the threshold for mPT (Kim et al., 2015; Figure 34.1). Antiepileptic drugs may have beneficial effects on mitochondrial function, such as beneficial effects on respiratory chain and oxidative phosphorylation (e.g., lamotrigine increased ATP production; Berger et al., 2010), on antioxidative defense (e.g., zonisamide may reduce oxidative stress/ROS level and cell damage; Condello et al., 2013), and on mitochondrial biogenesis (e.g., increased biogenesis of neuronal mitochondria by vigabatrin treatment; Vogel et al., 2015). Nevertheless, antiepileptic drugs may have not only benefits for, but also adverse effects on, mitochondrial function (e.g., increasing ROS production), suggesting that administration of supplementary agents, such as antioxidants, may be needed for successful antiepileptic treatment (Finsterer & Scorza, 2017). These results also suggest that KDs/EKSs may be promising adjuvant agents in the treatment of epilepsy through their ketosis/βHB-evoked improvement in mitochondrial function and decrease in oxidative stress (Figure 34.1).

Impaired mitochondrial function, increased oxidative stress/ROS level, and neuronal injury have been demonstrated not only in epilepsy, but also in other CNS diseases, such as Alzheimer's disease, Parkinson's disease, Huntington's disease, amyotrophic lateral sclerosis (ALS), and psychiatric diseases (Armada-Moreira et al., 2020; Coyle & Puttfarcken, 1993; Gano et al., 2014; Holper et al., 2019; Lin & Beal, 2006; Pathak et al., 2013). For example, complex I dysfunction and complex IV (cytochrome *c* oxidase) dysfunction were demonstrated in Parkinson's disease and Alzheimer's disease, respectively (Greenamyre et al., 2001; Mosconi et al., 2011). A great deal of evidence suggests that microglial activation, neuronal death (e.g., through increased oxidative/nitrosative stress, and ROS), and mitochondrial dysfunctions (e.g., changes in activity of complex I and IV of electron transport chain and decreased ATP production) may have a role in the pathophysiology of schizophrenia (Ben-Shachar & Laifenfeld, 2004; Holper et al., 2019; Kahn et al., 2015; Kim & Na, 2017), anxiety disorders (Einat et al., 2005; Schiavone & Trabace, 2016), bipolar disorders (Berk et al., 2011; Holper et al., 2019; Mertens et al., 2015; Vieta et al., 2018), major depressive disorder (Adzic et al., 2016; Brown et al., 2018; Holper et al., 2019), autism spectrum disorder (Cheng et al., 2017; Filipek et al., 2003; Frye & Rossignol, 2014; Rossignol & Frye, 2014), and attention deficit/hyperactivity disorder (Leffa et al., 2017). Consequently, ketosis/βHB may have beneficial effects in psychiatric diseases through its neuroprotective effects, which improve/preserve mitochondrial function and decrease oxidative stress (Figure 34.1). Indeed, the KD-related increase in the ketone body level may be related to the beneficial effects in schizophrenia (Kraeuter et al., 2015; Kraft & Westman, 2009; Palmer, 2017), anxiety disorder (Ari et al., 2016; Sussman et al., 2015), bipolar disorder (Phelps et al., 2013), depression (Murphy et al., 2004; Sussman et al., 2015), autism spectrum disorder (Ahn et al., 2014; Evangeliou et al., 2003; Mu et al., 2020; Ruskin et al., 2017), and attention deficit/hyperactivity disorder (Murphy & Burnham, 2006; Packer et al., 2016). These results support the benefit of EKSs-evoked ketosis in mental disorders. In fact, for example, administration of KE, KS, and KSMCT had an anxiolytic effect in Sprague-Dawley rats and WAG/Rij rats in correlation with increased levels of βHB (Ari et al., 2016; Kovács et al., 2018). Moreover, βHB decreased anxiety-related and depressive behaviors (Chen et al., 2017; Yamanashi et al., 2017), KE supplementation had anxiolytic effects in an animal model of Alzheimer's disease (Kashiwaya et al., 2013), and an MCT diet had anxiolytic effects and enhanced social competitiveness (Hollis et al., 2018) in animals.

It has been demonstrated that KDs and ketosis are able to improve impaired cognitive functions (Appelberg et al., 2009; Grigolon et al., 2020; Herbert & Buckley, 2013; Krikorian et al., 2012; Maalouf et al., 2009; Xu et al., 2010) and other behavioral changes (e.g., anxious behavior, mood-disturbed behavior, aggression, impaired attention, impaired social functioning/social exploration, decreased alertness, and lowered activity level) under both physiologic and pathophysiologic conditions in animals (Hallböök et al., 2007; IJff et al., 2016; Kasprowska-Liśkiewicz et al., 2017; Kinsman et al., 1992; Nordli et al., 2001; Pulsifer et al., 2001), likely via enhancement of neuroprotective effects. Chronic administration of KDs/βHB alleviated behavioral deficits in an NMDA-receptor hypofunction model of schizophrenia (e.g., MK-801-generated hyperlocomotion, stereotyped behavior, spatial working memory impairment, reduction of sociability, and disruption of prepulse inhibition of startle), possibly via decreased glutamate excitotoxicity as well as improved mitochondrial functions and GABAergic functions (Kraeuter et al., 2015, 2020a; Figure 34.1). It was also suggested that KDs may also improve behavioral disturbances, hyperactivity, attention, interaction, and sleep pattern (e.g., decrease in daytime sleep and increase in night sleep) in patients with Angelman syndrome (Evangeliou et al., 2010; Thibert et al., 2009), likely via supplying ketone bodies as alternative source of energy and/or enhancing GABAergic (inhibitory) effects (Bough & Rho, 2007; Evangeliou et al., 2010). Moreover, as increased glucose level (hyperglycemia; e.g., under diabetic conditions) may be associated with behavior, mood, and sleep problems (Braam et al., 2008; Korkmaz et al., 2008; Leedom et al., 1987; Valdovinos & Weyand, 2006; Warren et al., 2003), KDs/EKSs may generate their beneficial effect on behavior/sleep disturbances not only through increased ketone body level, but also, theoretically, via a decreased glucose level, at least in patients with Angelman syndrome. Furthermore, KD/ketosis decreased total sleep time, but it increased rapid eye movement (REM) sleep time, likely via KD/ketosis-evoked changes in neurotransmitter levels (e.g., GABA and glutamate) and other neuroprotective (e.g., antioxidant) effects (Hallböök et al., 2007, 2012; Figure 34.1). It was also demonstrated that KD/EKS-related ketosis may delay the onset of isoflurane-induced anesthesia in rats via increased adenosine levels and/or a βHB/AMPK signaling system (Ari et al., 2018a; Finley, 2019; Kovács et al., 2020), suggesting neuroprotective

effect against anesthetic gas and potentially against other harmful gases.

It has been demonstrated that mitochondrial dysfunction may result in increased ROS expression in microglial cells, leading to increased expression of pro-inflammatory cytokines and neuroinflammation, which may cause cognitive decline (Lugrin et al., 2014; Wu et al., 2016). Moreover, neuroinflammatory processes may alter the integrity of synapses (e.g., reduce synaptic proteins, such as synaptophysin and debrin), leading to behavioral changes and progressive cognitive decline in patients with neurodegenerative and neuropsychiatric diseases, such as Alzheimer's disease, bipolar disorder, and schizophrenia (Hatanpää et al., 1999; Rao et al., 2012; Scheff et al., 2006; Wingo et al., 2009; Wobrock et al., 2009). In addition, excitotoxicity (e.g., increased iNOS activity) may evoke both synaptic loss and cognitive impairment (e.g., in Alzheimer's disease and bipolar disorders; Kim et al., 2011; Masliah et al., 2001; Rao et al., 2010, 2012). Ketone bodies may prevent oxidative stress-evoked impairment of the major mechanism of learning and memory, LTP. This alleviating effect of ketone bodies was associated with decreased activity of PP2A, likely via an antioxidant mechanism (Maalouf & Rho, 2008; Figure 34.1). In addition, βHB relieved intrinsic impairment of hippocampal LTP and spatial learning-memory defects in Kcna1-null mutant mice (Kim et al., 2015). It was demonstrated that administration of βHB not only enhanced mitochondrial respiration and decreased microglia overactivation/pro-inflammatory cytokine expression, but also improved learning ability and memory in a mouse model of Alzheimer's disease (Wu et al., 2020), and preserved neuronal integrity and stability (Izumi et al., 1998). Moreover, βHB improved working memory performance in patients with type 2 diabetes (Jensen et al., 2020). The improved memory performance with an MCT (triheptanoin)-rich KD in an animal model of Alzheimer's disease (APP/PS1 transgenic mice) may be via improved mitochondrial status, as well as antioxidant and anti-inflammatory influences of the treatment (Figure 34.1; Aso et al., 2013). It was demonstrated that MCT treatment may increase synaptophysin expression, as well as enhance/improve cognitive performance and social recognition through synaptic maintenance (Wang & Mitchell, 2016). Scratch assay on rat primary neuron cell cultures also showed that biomarkers associated with flagellar movement, cytoskeletal functions, axonogenesis, and synaptogenesis were denser in βHB-treated cultures at the regeneration site (Ari et al., 2018b). Moreover, MCT supplementation improved age-related decline in cognitive functions in old dogs (Pan et al., 2010), improved cognition in patients with Alzheimer's disease (Avgerinos et al., 2020; Chatterjee et al., 2020), had positive effects on working memory and executive functions in elderly adults (Ota et al., 2016), and reversed hypoglycemia-evoked impairment in cognitive performance (e.g., in verbal memory and digit symbol coding) in patients with type 1 diabetes (Page et al., 2009). Administration of MCTs and KE increased blood levels of ketone bodies and improved behavioral cognitive functions (e.g., improvements in performance on learning and memory tests) in a mouse model of Alzheimer's disease and patients with Alzheimer's disease (Chintapenta et al., 2017; Fernando et al., 2015; Henderson, 2008; Kashiwaya et al., 2013; Newport et al., 2015; Reger et al., 2004), likely via improved insulin signaling/resistance and glucose hypometabolism-evoked decrease in energy (e.g., because increased levels of ketone bodies served as an alternative energy source/fuel to glucose; Chatterjee et al., 2020; Croteau et al., 2018; DeDea, 2012; Fernando et al., 2015; Steen et al., 2005; Figure 34.1). It is interesting that glucose hypometabolism may contribute to the pathophysiology of not only Alzheimer's disease (Alexander et al., 2002; Reiman et al., 2004), but also several mental disorders, such as bipolar disorders, major depressive disorder, and schizophrenia (Seethalakshmi et al., 2006; Steardo et al., 2019; Su et al., 2014), suggesting therapeutic potential for ketosis in these diseases. Caffeine intake increased plasma ketone levels in humans, which may help to meet the energy demand of the brain (Vandenberghe et al., 2017), for example, under glucose hypometabolism conditions in patients with Alzheimer's disease (DeDea, 2012). It was also revealed that βHB can protect neurons against not only 1-methyl-4-phenylpyridinium (MPP⁺) toxicity (MPP⁺ is the toxic metabolic product of 1-methyl-4-phenyl-1,2,3,6-tetrahydropyridine, MPTP; Singer et al., 1988) in animal models of Parkinson's disease, but also toxicity of Aβ oligomers in models of Alzheimer's disease (Kashiwaya et al., 2000; Wu et al., 2020). Moreover, administration of ketone bodies (βHB + AcAc) reduced oxidative stress, blocked intracellular $A\beta_{42}$ accumulation, and enhanced mitochondrial complex I activity, leading to improved learning, memory, and synaptic plasticity in an Alzheimer's disease mouse model (Yin et al., 2016). Moreover, KE may increase the number of mitochondria and expression of electron transport chain proteins (Srivastava et al., 2012) and normalize behavioral abnormalities (e.g., caused greater exploratory activity) in a mouse model of Alzheimer's disease, likely through improved mitochondrial function (e.g., by overcoming pyruvate dehydrogenase inhibition and restoration of tricarboxylic acid cycle metabolites; Pawlosky et al., 2020). It has also been demonstrated that KE supplementation improved learning, memory, and synaptic plasticity in an Angelman syndrome mouse model (Ciarlone et al., 2016). KS may also improve cognitive functions, likely via enhanced mitochondrial functions and ATP levels (Brownlow et al., 2017; Figure 34.1).

It was demonstrated that βHB protected neurons in models of Alzheimer's disease and Parkinson's disease (Kashiwaya et al., 2000) through improvement of defects in mitochondrial energy generation (Figure 34.1). KDs improved motor function in mouse models of Alzheimer's disease (Beckett et al., 2013; Brownlow et al., 2013) and rodent models of Parkinson's disease (Shaafi et al., 2016; Tieu et al., 2003; Yang & Cheng, 2010). KD and βHB may lead to improvement in Parkinson's disease in humans and animals through activation of neuroprotective mechanism(s) by which ketone bodies can protect against MPTP-induced neurodegeneration and motor deficits, as well as alleviate the tremor/motor dysfunction and impaired cognition/inability to concentrate (Kashiwaya et al., 2000; Tieu et al., 2003; Vanitallie et al., 2005; Veech et al., 2019). Moreover, it has been demonstrated that KDs/ketosis, MCTs, βHB, and the Deanna protocol (containing MCTs) have protective effects on motor performance and/or the number of motor neurons in animal models of ALS through βHB-induced neuroprotective effects, such as increased mitochondrial function and ATP production (Ari et al., 2014; Netzahualcoyotzi & Tapia, 2015; Tefera et al., 2016; Zhao et al., 2006, 2012; Figure 34.1). Moreover, KE supplementation improved motor coordination in an Angelman syndrome mouse model (Ciarlone et al., 2016). Triheptanoin-evoked improvement in motor function was also demonstrated in patients with Huntington's disease, possibly due to improved mitochondrial function (Adanyeguh et al., 2015).

Changes and dysregulation of the glutamatergic and/or monoaminergic, purinergic, and GABAergic systems have a role in the pathophysiology of several neurodegenerative diseases, psychiatric disorders, and behavioral alterations. For example, alterations were demonstrated in animal models and/or patients with impaired motor function/behavior (e.g., dopaminergic dysfunction and GABA/glutamate imbalance; Abg Abd Wahab et al., 2019; Blasco et al., 2014; Brichta et al., 2013; Hauber, 1998; Kumar et al., 2010; Tisch et al., 2004). In sleep disorders, dysregulation of dopaminergic, serotonergic, glutamatergic, GABAergic, cholinergic, and adenosinergic systems were demonstrated (Bollu & Kaur, 2019; Holst et al., 2016; Holst & Landolt, 2018; Jones, 2020; Ma et al., 2018). Impaired learning and memory were associated with dysfunction in glutamatergic, GABAergic, and cholinergic systems (Huang et al., 2017a; Lewis et al., 2004; Ma et al., 2018; Myhrer, 2003; Tisch et al., 2004). In neurodegenerative disorders, for example, decreased serotonin level and enhanced glutamatergic transmission were found in patients with Parkinson's disease, deterioration of cholinergic neurotransmission was found in Alzheimer's disease, and deficits in dopaminergic signaling were demonstrated in both Parkinson's disease and Alzheimer's disease (Abg Abd Wahab et al., 2019; Brichta et al., 2013; D'Amelio et al., 2018; Huang et al., 2017a; Kumar et al., 2010; Martin & Chang, 2012; Stanciu et al., 2019). Several changes/disturbances of neurotransmitter systems were also demonstrated in anxiety disorders (e.g., dysregulation of glutamatergic, serotonergic, purinergic, and GABAergic systems; Li, 2012; Möhler, 2012; Nagy et al., 1979; Tang et al., 2007; Vincenzi et al., 2016), and schizophrenia (e.g., alterations in the GABAergic, glutamatergic, and monoaminergic neurotransmitter systems, such as decrease in GABA, serotonin, and dopamine levels; Brisch et al., 2014; Chiapponi et al., 2016; Kahn & Sommer, 2015; McCullumsmith et al., 2004; Moghaddam & Javitt, 2012; Yoon et al., 2010). It was also suggested that changes in functioning of the glutamatergic system (increased glutamate level), GABAergic system (reduced GABA levels), monoaminergic system (decreased serotonin, norepinephrine, and dopamine level), and purinergic system (overexpression of $A_{2A}R$) may have a role in the pathophysiology of major depressive disorder (Coelho et al., 2014; Dean & Keshavan, 2017; Delgado, 2000; Hashimoto et al., 2007; Krystal et al., 2002; Müller & Schwarz, 2007; Petty, 1995). Several disturbances of neurotransmitter systems were also demonstrated in bipolar disorder (e.g., imbalances in the monoaminergic/serotonergic, dopaminergic, and noradrenergic neurotransmitter systems; Goodwin & Jamison, 2007; Hashimoto et al., 2007; Kurita et al., 2015;

Machado-Vieira et al., 2002; Petty, 1995; Yatham et al., 2018), attention deficit/hyperactivity disorder (e.g., increased glutamatergic tone and changes in the GABAergic system; Courvoisie et al., 2004; Edden et al., 2012; Faraone et al., 2015; Gizer et al., 2009; Oades et al., 2002; Russell, 2003; Sowinski & Karpawich, 2014), and autism spectrum disorder (e.g., decreased GABA receptor expression and GABA-evoked inhibitory effects; Bear et al., 2004; Erickson et al., 2009; Green & Garg, 2018; Lemonnier et al., 2017). These results suggest that ketosis/βHB-evoked neuroprotective effects may be a promising therapeutic tool for the treatment of several CNS diseases and improved behavior via modulation of neurotransmitter systems (Figure 34.1).

Inhibition of Histone Deacetylases

Dysregulation of acetylation/deacetylation activity and changes in histone deacetylation alter the expression of important genes, which may be associated with impaired neuroprotective effects, learning and memory deficits, and CNS diseases (e.g., epilepsy, Alzheimer's disease, Huntington's disease, Parkinson's disease, and schizophrenia; Choong et al., 2016; D'Mello, 2009; Feng et al., 2008; Huang et al., 2012; Lu et al., 2015; Peña-Altamira et al., 2013; Sharma et al., 2008). It was also demonstrated that HDAC inhibitors have beneficial effects on Alzheimer's disease, learning and memory, Parkinson's disease, and Huntington's disease that were mediated by increased expression of neuroprotective factors, such as BDNF (Chuang et al., 2009; Sharma et al., 2015b; Sharma & Taliyan, 2015; Figure 34.2). Moreover, HDACs may have a role in epileptogenesis and ictogenesis; therefore, inhibitors of HDACs may be potential new therapeutic agents for the treatment of epilepsy (Citraro et al., 2017; Huberfeld & Vecht, 2016). Indeed, for example, some therapeutic drugs, such as valproic acid/valproate exert antiepileptic effects through HDAC inhibition (Monti et al., 2009). In addition, valproate (which has not only an antiepileptic effects, but also a mood-stabilizing effect in bipolar disorder, and adjuvant influence in the treatment of schizophrenia; Johannessen, 2000; Phiel et al., 2001) improved the survival of a SOD-mutant mouse model of ALS (Sugai et al., 2004), and improved motor function in a genetic model of Parkinson's disease (Kim et al., 2019).

HDAC inhibitors may have neuroprotective effects (Figure 34.2) in the treatment of psychiatric diseases and related behavioral disturbances (e.g., depression, anxiety, bipolar disorder, autism spectrum disorder, attention deficit/hyperactivity disorder, and schizophrenia, likely via modulation of imbalanced expression of BDNF; Abel & Zukin, 2008; Amiri et al., 2013; Autry & Monteggia, 2012; Saghazadeh & Rezaei, 2017; Schroeder et al., 2007), multiple sclerosis (e.g., via decreased neuroinflammation and demyelination; Camelo et al., 2005; Gray & Dangond, 2006), Huntington's disease (e.g., via increased motor function and decreased neuronal loss; Ferrante et al., 2003; Hockly et al., 2003), ALS (e.g., via promotion of motor neuron survival and motor function; Feng et al., 2008; Rouaux et al., 2007; Ryu et al., 2005), Parkinson's disease (e.g., via decrease in α-synuclein-evoked toxicity and cell death; Choong et al., 2016; Kontopoulos et al., 2006), Alzheimer's disease, and learning/memory functions (Abel and Zukin, 2008; Fischer et al., 2007; Guan et al., 2009; Kilgore et al., 2010; Peleg et al., 2010). It was also suggested that KEs/ketone bodies may exert their neuroprotective effects against MPTP-induced neuronal destruction via HDAC inhibition (Hashim & VanItallie, 2014).

Histone acetylation (as an epigenetic modification) facilitates learning and memory (Fischer et al., 2007; Gräff et al., 2011; Mahgoub & Monteggia, 2014; Peleg et al., 2010). It was demonstrated that cognitive/memory impairment may be associated with decreased histone acetylation, whereas histone acetylation may result in recovery of cognitive abilities; therefore, administration of HDAC inhibitors (likely via inhibition of HDAC2) can restore learning-induced gene expression and memory function in animals (Ganai et al., 2016; Gräff et al., 2011; Kazantsev & Thompson, 2008; Peleg et al., 2010). In addition, HDAC inhibition may evoke protection against sleep deprivation-induced impairment in spatial memory (Duan et al., 2016).

These results suggest that ketosis/βHB may have beneficial effects in epilepsy, neurodegenerative diseases, and psychiatric diseases, as well as may lead to improved learning, memory, and motor function through HDAC inhibition (Figure 34.2).

Modulation of HCAR2 and NLRP3 Activity

It has been suggested that ligands of HCAR2, such as βHB, may have beneficial effects in epilepsy, Parkinson's disease, Alzheimer's disease, Huntington's disease, ALS, traumatic brain injury, multiple sclerosis, impaired learning/memory, and motor impairment through neuroprotective/anti-inflammatory effects (Dupuis et al., 2015; Graff et al., 2016; Kashiwaya et al.,

2013; Lim et al., 2011; Tieu et al., 2003; Wu et al., 2020). Indeed, it was demonstrated that ketosis/βHB may have therapeutic potential in the treatment of epilepsy, multiple sclerosis, Alzheimer's disease, ALS, Parkinson's disease, and behavioral deficits/disturbances through HCAR2-induced anti-inflammatory effects (Alavi et al., 2019; Fu et al., 2015; Graff et al., 2016; Offermanns & Schwaninger, 2015; Rahman et al., 2014; Wakade et al., 2014; Wu et al., 2020). Moreover, it has also been demonstrated that βHB may enhance learning and memory via HCAR2 (Zou et al., 2009).

Activation of microglial cells/astrocytes and the NLRP3 inflammasome, as well as an increase in the expression of pro-inflammatory cytokines, oxidative stress, NO, and ROS (neuroinflammation), participate in the pathophysiology of epilepsy/epileptogenesis (Edye et al., 2014; Kovács et al., 2019a; Swanton et al., 2018; Vezzani et al., 2015, 2019), Alzheimer's disease (Glass et al., 2010; Nunomura et al., 2001; Shabab et al., 2017; Swanton et al., 2018; Swerdlow, 2011; Tan et al., 2013; Yuste et al., 2015), Parkinson's disease (Fu et al., 2015; Glass et al., 2010; Jenner, 2003; Shabab et al., 2017; Swanton et al., 2018; Yuste et al., 2015), multiple sclerosis (Glass et al., 2010; Shabab et al., 2017; Smith & Lassmann, 2002; Swanton et al., 2018; Yuste et al., 2015), and ALS (Glass et al., 2010; Hyun et al., 2003; Swanton et al., 2018; Yuste et al., 2015). Moreover, pathologic changes in function of the HPA axis and inflammatory system (e.g., increased expression of NLRP3 inflammasome, pro-inflammatory cytokines, and ROS) may also be key factors in the pathophysiology of impaired motor functions (Abg Abd Wahab et al., 2019; Lim et al., 2012), sleep disorders (Irwin, 2019; Irwin & Opp, 2017), impaired learning and memory (Hein & O'Banion, 2009; Liu et al., 2012; Lugrin et al., 2014; Rachal Pugh et al., 2001; Wu et al., 2016), anxiety disorders (Hodes et al., 2015; Miller & Raison, 2016), schizophrenia (Kahn et al., 2015; Kim & Na, 2017; Miller et al., 2011; Yegin et al., 2012), depression (Alcocer-Gómez et al., 2014; Dean & Keshavan, 2017; Hodes et al., 2015; Kaufmann et al., 2017; Miller & Raison, 2016; Su et al., 2017; Zhu et al., 2017), bipolar disorder (Berk et al., 2011; Holper et al., 2019; Rao et al., 2010, 2012), and autism spectrum disorder (Bhat et al., 2014; Hughes et al., 2018; Rodriguez & Kern, 2011). Accordingly, KD/EKS-evoked ketosis may improve symptoms of epilepsy and several neurodegenerative and psychiatric diseases, as well as sleep, motor, learning and memory dysfunctions, likely via neuroprotective/anti-inflammatory and antioxidative influences (e.g., by decreasing IL-1β and ROS levels; Bahr et al., 2020; Choi et al., 2016; Kim et al., 2012; Offermanns & Schwaninger, 2015; Figures 34.1–34.3). Indeed, for example, the EKS-related increase in βHB levels decreased not only spontaneous epileptic seizures, but also LPS-generated increase in epileptic activity (Kovács et al., 2019a), likely via inhibition of TLR4/NLRP3/IL-1R/NFκB/COX pathways, as well as decreased the release of IL-1β, COX-2, and ROS (Kovács et al., 2006, 2019a; Menu et al., 2012; Ravizza et al., 2006; Swanton et al., 2018; Terrone et al., 2020; Vezzani et al., 2010). It was also demonstrated that an MCT diet suppressed inflammation by inhibition of NF-κB and p38 MAPK activation in mice (Geng et al., 2016). βHB had antidepressant effects through anti-inflammatory effects in rodent models of depression (e.g., by decreased NLRP3 activity, reduced TNF-α level, and improved HPA axis responses; Kajitani et al., 2020; Pan et al., 2020; Yamanashi et al., 2017). Moreover, βHB improved cognitive functions, likely via HCAR2-generated neuroprotective/anti-inflammatory effects (Wu et al., 2020).

The mTOR signaling pathway inhibitor rapamycin may abolish/reduce not only the development of epilepsy, but also underlying pathophysiologic mechanism(s) and consequences, such as neuronal death/apoptosis in different epilepsy models (Chen et al., 2008; Xu et al., 2011; Zeng et al., 2008, 2009). It was demonstrated that KD (ketosis) may inhibit mTOR pathway signaling in the brain of normal rats, prevent KA/SE-evoked late hippocampal mTOR activation (McDaniel et al., 2011), and evoke anti-apoptotic/neuroprotective effects by inhibition of the mTOR pathway (Zeng et al., 2009; Figure 34.3). However, KDs may exert their antiepileptic effect not only by blocking mTOR (McDaniel et al., 2011; Yamada, 2008), but also, theoretically, by a low glucose level (Thio et al., 2006) resulting from AMPK activation (Hartel et al., 2016; Yamada, 2008). Indeed, it has been demonstrated that βHB may exert its effects via AMPK-activated signaling pathways (Bae et al., 2016), by which it can modulate/inhibit mTOR activity (Herzig & Shaw, 2018; Figure 34.3). Moreover, KDs/EKSs not only increase the level of βHB, but also decrease glucose levels (Ari et al., 2016; Kovács et al., 2017; Myette-Côté et al., 2018). It was demonstrated that decreased mTOR activity may evoke increased autophagy (Laplante & Sabatini, 2009), by which βHB can modulate cell degradation processes, such as clearance of abnormal mitochondria.

Decreased SIRT1 levels were demonstrated in neurodegenerative diseases, such as Alzheimer's disease (in association with the accumulation of Aβ), Parkinson's disease, and Huntington's disease in humans and/or animal models (Julien et al., 2009; Pallàs et al., 2008; Tulino et al., 2016). Thus, it was suggested that activation of SIRT1-modulated pathway(s) may have therapeutic potential in the treatment of neurodegenerative diseases (Herskovits & Guarente, 2014). Indeed, activation of SIRT1 evoked protective effects in mouse models of ALS (e.g., increased mitochondrial biogenesis, suppressed motor neuron degradation, and improved morbidity and mortality; Han et al., 2012; Kim et al., 2007a; Wang et al., 2011), and prevented axonal damage and neuronal loss in a model of multiple sclerosis (Shindler et al., 2010). Moreover, SIRT1 activation protects against Huntington's disease in mice (e.g., improved motor function, and extended survival; Jiang et al., 2014), and plaque formation/neurodegeneration in mouse models of Alzheimer's disease (Karuppagounder et al., 2009; Kim et al., 2007a). Activation of SIRT1 also preserved dopaminergic neurons in an MPTP mouse model of Parkinson's disease (Mudò et al., 2012). It was suggested that these protective influences were modulated likely via the SIRT1/PGC1-α/MnSOD pathway (Parker et al., 2005; Qin et al., 2006; St-Pierre et al., 2006; Watanabe et al., 2014; Figure 34.3). In fact, PGC1-α has a protective role (Figure 34.3) in the neurodegenerative diseases. PGC1-α-deficient mice suffer from neurodegenerative lesions (Lin et al., 2004), and reduced PGC1-α expression/mRNA levels were demonstrated in patients with Huntington's disease and in animal models (Chaturvedi et al., 2009, 2010; Cui et al., 2006; Lloret & Beal, 2019). Moreover, decrease in PGC1-α expression may also have a role in the pathomechanism of Parkinson's disease (Wareski et al., 2009; Zheng et al., 2010), and Alzheimer's disease (Gong et al., 2010; Qin et al., 2009). It was also suggested that a KD-evoked increase in PPARγ may generate alleviating effects not only in epilepsy, but also in neurodegenerative diseases via neuroprotective/anti-inflammatory effects (e.g., by decreased pro-inflammatory cytokine levels and improved mitochondrial function; Simeone et al., 2017a). In relation to ALS, PGC1-α overexpression and administration of the antidiabetic/PPARγ agonist pioglitazone improved motor performance, motor neuron loss, and survival in mouse models (Kiaei et al., 2005; Zhao et al., 2011). Moreover, because Nrf-2 is an important regulator of antioxidant defenses (e.g., by increase in expression of glutathione peroxidase and the thioredoxin system; Banning et al., 2005; Im et al., 2012), and energy production (e.g., by regulation of mitochondrial respiration, enhancement of ATP production and reduction of ROS production; Dinkova-Kostova & Abramov, 2015), the Nrf-2/thioredoxin system may also be a therapeutic target for disorders in which oxidative stress has a role in the pathophysiology, such as Parkinson's disease (Im et al., 2012; Kensler et al., 2007; Figure 34.3). Moreover, activation of SIRT3 may also benefits in Alzheimer's disease, Parkinson's disease, and ALS via neuroprotective effects (e.g., by antioxidant effects and improved mitochondrial function through SIRT3/PGC1-α/MnSOD pathways; Kincaid & Bossy-Wetzel, 2013; Ramesh et al., 2018; Song et al., 2013; Figure 34.3).

It was also demonstrated by genetic studies that the SIRT1 gene might be associated with psychiatric diseases, such as anxiety and depressive disorders (Kishi et al., 2010; Libert et al., 2011). For example, reduced SIRT1 signaling was demonstrated in bipolar disorder, schizophrenia, and depression (Abe-Higuchi et al., 2016; Alageel et al., 2018; Kishi et al., 2011; Lu et al., 2018; Luo & Zhang, 2016; Nivoli et al., 2016). Nevertheless, SIRT1 overexpression caused an increase in anxiety level, whereas a reduced anxiety level was established in SIRT1 knockout mice (Libert et al., 2011). Moreover, others were not able to demonstrate an effect of SIRT1 overexpression on anxiety-like or depression-like behavior (Watanabe et al., 2014). In spite of that, activation of SIRT may generate an antidepressant effect (Hurley et al., 2014), chronic stress increased SIRT1 activity (Ferland & Schrader, 2011). Based on these results, it was concluded that SIRT-mediated effects on depression and anxiety control may depend on the brain region, cell type, and genetic background (Abe-Higuchi et al., 2016). It has also been demonstrated that a decreased PGC-1α level may have a role in the pathophysiology of depression (Agudelo et al., 2014; Phillips & Fahimi, 2018). Furthermore, pioglitazone generated not only a decrease in the severity of depression but also reduction in the insulin resistance and inflammation in patients with major depressive disorder (Kemp et al., 2012). Moreover, behavioral changes, such as hyperactivity, motor abnormalities, and increased anxiety, were also demonstrated in PGC1-α-deficient animals (Cui et al., 2006; Róna-Vörös & Weydt, 2010).

It was demonstrated that SIRT1 also has a role in the modulation of learning and memory. Overexpression of SIRT1 provided protective effects against impairment in learning and memory in animal models of Alzheimer's disease

(Corpas et al., 2017; Wang et al., 2017). Deficits in synaptic plasticity, impaired cognitive abilities (e.g., in spatial learning and short-term memory), and decreased expression of BDNF were demonstrated in SIRT1 knockout animals (Gao et al., 2010; Michán et al., 2010), whereas increased SIRT1 activity may promote plasticity and memory (Gao et al., 2010; Michán et al., 2010). Moreover, ketone bodies are able to improve memory functions (Reger et al., 2004), suggesting a relevant mechanism for ketone body-evoked alleviating effects on memory impairment via SIRT1-dependent pathways (Figure 34.3). In addition, SIRT1 level decreases with age (Quintas et al., 2012), leading to circadian-related deficits in aged mice (Chang & Guarente, 2013). Thus, SIRT1 may have a role in the modulation of circadian rhythms and sleep, for example, in patients with psychiatric diseases, such as depression (Asher et al., 2008; Kudlow et al., 2013).

It was demonstrated that a KD/ketosis-evoked increase in PPARγ expression may contribute to the antiseizure effects of the KD/ketosis (Jeong et al., 2011; Simeone et al., 2017a), likely by anti-inflammatory influence via the TNF-α and PPARγ activation-mediated NFκB-dependent COX-2 signaling pathway and antioxidant effects (Jeong et al., 2011; Knowles et al., 2018; Figure 34.3). Moreover, decreased PPARγ levels/activity and enhanced activity of pro-inflammatory pathways (e.g., increased level of iNOS, COX2, and NF-κB) were found in patients with bipolar disorder and schizophrenia (García-Bueno et al., 2014; Nierenberg et al., 2018). It has also been demonstrated that PPARγ agonists may have beneficial effects in Parkinson's disease, Huntington's disease, Alzheimer's disease, multiple sclerosis, and ALS, as well as on impaired cognitive functions, learning, memory, and social communication in some neurologic diseases, likely via improved mitochondrial function, and decreased oxidative stress/inflammation, and decreased neuronal death (Agarwal et al., 2017; Benedetti et al., 2018; d'Angelo et al., 2019; Ferret-Sena et al., 2018; Tyagi et al., 2011).

Although a regulatory role for FFAR3 in the sympathetic nervous system was demonstrated (Kimura et al., 2011; Newman & Verdin, 2014b), new studies are needed to reveal the therapeutic potential (if any) of βHB on CNS diseases via FFAR3.

Consequently, ketosis/βHB may improve symptoms of epilepsy, neurodegenerative diseases, psychiatric disorders, as well as sleep, motor, learning, and memory dysfunctions not only via improvement of mitochondrial function, changes in functioning of neurotransmitter systems, and HDAC inhibition, but also through HCAR2/SIRT pathway-evoked neuroprotective effects.

CONCLUSION

The effects of EKSs on CNS diseases have not been fully investigated. Consequently, only limited results have demonstrated beneficial effects of EKS-related ketosis in animal models and patients with several CNS diseases. Nevertheless, ketosis/βHB can generate neuroprotective effects (Figures 34.1–34.3), leading to improvement in several pathophysiologic alterations, such as mitochondrial dysfunction, changes in neurotransmitter levels/release, and increased inflammatory processes/oxidative stress through several metabolic/signaling pathways. Thus, ketosis may be one of the primary mediators of the therapeutic effect of the EKSs in different CNS diseases. The neuroprotective effects of ketosis and the pathophysiologic processes implicated in several CNS diseases strongly support the hypothesis that EKS-related ketosis may modulate/alleviate the background pathophysiologic processes of epilepsy, neurodegenerative diseases, and psychiatric diseases. It is unlikely that a single administration of EKSs can alone repair/cure a diseased brain/disorder, but prolonged administration of EKSs supplementing the normal diet or KDs, as well as the therapeutic regimen, may potentially be an effective treatment for epilepsy and several neurodegenerative diseases, as well as psychiatric disorders. Moreover, combining EKSs not only with other therapeutic drugs, but also with lifestyle changes (e.g., stress reduction, exercise, and sleep) may enhance the safety and efficacy of this intervention. However, to estimate clinical benefits and to understand the underlying mechanism behind therapeutic effects, prolonged studies are needed to investigate the efficacy and mechanistic effects of different EKSs in several CNS diseases and behavioral disorders.

The use of EKSs in the treatment of CNS diseases is only in its infancy, and more studies are needed to understand their efficacy and how to employ them. Nevertheless, our increasing knowledge of EKSs/ketosis-evoked neuroprotective effects suggests that EKSs may be ideal and effective adjuvants to drugs used in the treatment of CNS disorders, especially in treatment-resistant cases. Moreover, EKSs modulate endogenous processes that likely augment neuroprotective effects across a range of disease states. Thus, administration of EKSs alone or in combination with therapeutic drugs not only increases the efficacy of the drugs but also may be a safe method for promoting disease-alleviating effects with minimal or no side effects compared to standalone pharmacologic treatments.

The exact mechanisms of action by which EKS-evoked neuroprotective effects alleviate symptoms of different CNS diseases are largely unknown. Thus, future research should explore the physiologic and pathophysiologic processes by which EKS-evoked ketosis can alleviate symptoms of CNS disorders. Moreover, future mechanistic studies are needed to investigate the therapeutic efficacy and exact signaling effects of different types and doses of EKSs, alone or in combination with KDs or different therapeutic drugs, not only on animal models of diseases, but also on patients with CNS disorders. Studies are also needed to reveal factors that can alter the effects of EKSs on CNS diseases, such as age, sex, drugs, lifestyle, and other diseases. Moreover, there is an urgent need to develop both research and therapeutic strategies and broadly accepted protocols guiding the reproducible investigation of EKS formulations. However, better understanding of the mechanisms by which EKSs alleviate symptoms of CNS diseases may promote the development of new, more effective, and safe EKSs, which can be incorporated into ketogenic foods for treatment of CNS disorders, including epilepsy, neurodegenerative diseases, and psychiatric disorders.

REFERENCES

Abdul Kadir, A., Clarke, K., & Evans, R. D. (2020). Cardiac ketone body metabolism. *Biochimica et Biophysica Acta. Molecular Basis of Disease, 1866*(6), 165739.

Abe-Higuchi, N., Uchida, S., Yamagata, H., Higuchi, F., Hobara, T., Hara, K., Kobayashi, A., & Watanabe, Y. (2016). Hippocampal sirtuin 1 signaling mediates depression-like behavior. *Biological Psychiatry, 80*(11), 815–826.

Abel, T., & Zukin, R. S. (2008). Epigenetic targets of HDAC inhibition in neurodegenerative and psychiatric disorders. *Current Opinion in Pharmacology, 8*(1), 57–64.

Abg Abd Wahab, D. Y., Gau, C. H., Zakaria, R., Muthu Karuppan, M. K., A-Rahbi, B. S., Abdullah, Z., Alrafiah, A., Abdullah, J. M., & Muthuraju, S. (2019). Review on cross talk between neurotransmitters and neuroinflammation in striatum and cerebellum in the mediation of motor behaviour. *BioMed Research International, 2019*, 1767203.

Abramson, S. B., Amin, A. R., Clancy, R. M., & Attur, M. (2001). The role of nitric oxide in tissue destruction. *Best Practice & Research Clinical Rheumatology, 15*(5), 831–845.

Achanta, L. B., & Rae, C. D. (2017). β-Hydroxybutyrate in the brain: One molecule, multiple mechanisms. *Neurochemical Research, 42*(1), 35–49.

Adanyeguh, I. M., Rinaldi, D., Henry, P. G., Caillet, S., Valabregue, R., Durr, A., & Mochel, F. (2015). Triheptanoin improves brain energy metabolism in patients with Huntington disease. *Neurology, 84*(5), 490–495.

Adzic, M., Brkic, Z., Bulajic, S., Mitic, M., & Radojcic, M. B. (2016). Antidepressant action on mitochondrial dysfunction in psychiatric disorders. *Drug Development Research, 77*(7), 400–406.

Aeberli, I., Gerber, P. A., Hochuli, M., Kohler, S., Haile, S. R., Gouni-Berthold, I., Berthold, H. K., Spinas, G. A., & Berneis, K. (2011). Low to moderate sugar-sweetened beverage consumption impairs glucose and lipid metabolism and promotes inflammation in healthy young men: A randomized controlled trial. *American Journal of Clinical Nutrition, 94*(2), 479–485.

Agarwal, S., Yadav, A., & Chaturvedi, R. K. (2017). Peroxisome proliferator-activated receptors (PPARs) as therapeutic target in neurodegenerative disorders. *Biochemical and Biophysical Research Communications, 483*(4), 1166–1177.

Agledal, L., Niere, M., & Ziegler, M. (2010). The phosphate makes a difference: Cellular functions of NADP. *Redox Report, 15*(1), 2–10.

Agudelo, L. Z., Femenía, T., Orhan, F., Porsmyr-Palmertz, M., Goiny, M., Martinez-Redondo, V., Correia, J. C., Izadi, M., Bhat, M., Schuppe-Koistinen, I., Pettersson, A. T., Ferreira, D. M. S., Krook, A., Barres, R., Zierath, J. R., Erhardt, S., Lindskog, M., & Ruas, J. L. (2014). Skeletal muscle PGC-1α1 modulates kynurenine metabolism and mediates resilience to stress-induced depression. *Cell, 159*(1), 33–45.

Ahn, Y., Narous, M., Tobias, R., Rho, J. M., & Mychasiuk, R. (2014). The ketogenic diet modifies social and metabolic alterations identified in the prenatal valproic acid model of autism spectrum disorder. *Developmental Neuroscience, 36*(5), 371–380.

Akbar, M., Essa, M. M., Daradkeh, G., Abdelmegeed, M. A., Choi, Y., Mahmood, L, & Song, B. J. (2016). Mitochondrial dysfunction and cell death in neurodegenerative diseases through nitroxidative stress. *Brain Research, 1637*, 34–55.

Alageel, A., Tomasi, J., Tersigni, C., Brietzke, E., Zuckerman, H., Subramaniapillai, M., Lee, Y., Iacobucci, M., Rosenblat, J. D., Mansur, R. B., & McIntyre, R. S. (2018). Evidence supporting a mechanistic role of sirtuins in mood and metabolic disorders. *Progress in Neuro-Psychopharmacology & Biological Psychiatry, 86*, 95–101.

Alavi, M. S., Karimi, G., & Roohbakhsh, A. (2019). The role of orphan G protein-coupled receptors in the pathophysiology of multiple sclerosis: A review. *Life Sciences, 224*, 33–40.

Alcocer-Gómez, E., de Miguel, M., Casas-Barquero, N., Núñez-Vasco, J., Sánchez-Alcazar, J. A., Fernández-Rodríguez, A., & Cordero, M. D. (2014). NLRP3 inflammasome is activated in mononuclear blood cells from patients with major depressive disorder. *Brain, Behavior, and Immunity, 36*, 111–117.

Alexander, G. E., Chen, K., Pietrini, P., Rapoport, S. I., & Reiman, E. M. (2002). Longitudinal PET evaluation of cerebral metabolic decline in dementia: A potential outcome measure in Alzheimer's disease treatment studies. *American Journal of Psychiatry, 159*(5), 738–745.

Almeida, C. G., de Mendonça, A., Cunha, R. A., & Ribeiro, J. A. (2003). Adenosine promotes neuronal recovery from reactive oxygen species induced lesion in rat hippocampal slices. *Neuroscience Letters, 339*(2), 127–130.

Amiri, A., Torabi Parizi, G., Kousha, M., Saadat, F., Modabbernia, M. J., Najafi, K., & Atrkar Roushan, Z. (2013). Changes in plasma brain-derived neurotrophic factor (BDNF) levels induced by methylphenidate in children with attention deficit-hyperactivity disorder (ADHD). *Progress in Neuro-Psychopharmacology & Biological Psychiatry, 47*, 20–24.

Andoh, T., Ishiwa, D., Kamiya, Y., Echigo, N., Goto, T., & Yamada, Y. (2006). A1 adenosine receptor-mediated modulation of neuronal ATP-sensitive K channels in rat substantia nigra. *Brain Research, 1124*(1), 55–61.

Appelberg, K. S., Hovda, D. A., & Prins, M. L. (2009). The effects of a ketogenic diet on behavioral outcome after controlled cortical impact injury in the juvenile and adult rat. *Journal of Neurotrauma, 26*(4), 497–506.

Ari, C., Koutnik, A. P., DeBlasi, J., Landon, C., Rogers, C. Q., Vallas, J., Bharwani, S., Puchowicz, M., Bederman, I., Diamond, D. M., Kindy, M. S., Dean, J. B., & D'Agostino, D. P. (2019a). Delaying latency to hyperbaric oxygen-induced CNS oxygen toxicity seizures by combinations of exogenous ketone supplements. *Physiological Reports, 7*(1), e13961.

Ari, C., Kovács, Z., Juhasz, G., Murdun, C., Goldhagen, C. R., Koutnik, A. P., Poff, A. M., Kesl, S. L., & D'Agostino, D. P. (2016). Exogenous ketone supplements reduce anxiety-related behavior in Sprague-Dawley and Wistar Albino Glaxo/Rijswijk rats. *Frontiers in Molecular Neuroscience, 9*, 137.

Ari, C., Kovács, Z., Murdun, C., Koutnik, A. P., Goldhagen, C. R., Rogers, C., Diamond, D., & D'Agostino, D. P. (2018a). Nutritional ketosis delays the onset of isoflurane induced anesthesia. *BMC Anesthesiology, 18*(1), 85.

Ari, C., Murdun, C., Koutnik, A. P., Goldhagen, C. R., Rogers, C., Park, C., Bharwani, S., Diamond, D. M., Kindy, M. S., D'Agostino, D. P., & Kovács, Z. (2019b). Exogenous ketones lower blood glucose level in rested and exercised rodent models. *Nutrients, 11*(10), pii: E2330.

Ari, C., Pilla, R., & D'Agostino, D. (2015). Nutritional/metabolic therapies in animal models of amyotrophic lateral sclerosis, Alzheimer's disease, and seizures. In R. Watson & V. R. Preedy (Eds.), *Bioactive nutraceuticals and dietary supplements in neurological and brain disease* (pp. 449–459). Academic Press.

Ari, C., Poff, A. M., Held, H. E., Landon, C. S., Goldhagen, C. R., Mavromates, N., & D'Agostino, D. P. (2014). Metabolic therapy with Deanna protocol supplementation delays disease progression and extends survival in amyotrophic lateral sclerosis (ALS) mouse model. *PLOS ONE, 9*(7), Article e103526.

Ari, C., Zippert, M., & D'Agostino, D. P. (2018b). Neuroregeneration improved by ketones. *FASEB Journal, 32*, 545.

Armada-Moreira, A., Gomes, J. I., Pina, C. C., Savchak, O. K., Gonçalves-Ribeiro, J., Rei, N., Pinto, S., Morais, T. P., Martins, R. S., Ribeiro, F. F., Sebastião, A. M., Crunelli, V., & Vaz, S. H. (2020). Going the extra (synaptic) mile: Excitotoxicity as the road toward neurodegenerative diseases. *Frontiers in Cellular Neuroscience, 14*, 90.

Asher, G., Gatfield, D., Stratmann, M., Reinke, H., Dibner, C., Kreppel, F., Mostoslavsky, R., Alt, F. W., & Schibler, U. (2008). SIRT1 regulates circadian clock gene expression through PER2 deacetylation. *Cell, 134*(2), 317–328.

Aso, E., Semakova, J., Joda, L., Semak, V., Halbaut, L., Calpena, A., Escolano, C., Perales, J. C., & Ferrer, I. (2013). Triheptanoin supplementation to ketogenic diet curbs cognitive impairment in APP/PS1 mice used as a model of familial Alzheimer's disease. *Current Alzheimer Research, 10*(3), 290–297.

Austin, S., & St-Pierre, J. (2012). PGC1α and mitochondrial metabolism—Emerging concepts and relevance in ageing and neurodegenerative disorders. *Journal of Cell Science, 125*(Pt 21), 4963–4971.

Autry, A. E., & Monteggia, L. M. (2012). Brain-derived neurotrophic factor and neuropsychiatric disorders. *Pharmacological Reviews, 64*(2), 238–258.

Avgerinos, K. I., Egan, J. M., Mattson, M. P., & Kapogiannis, D. (2020). Medium chain triglycerides induce mild ketosis and may improve cognition in Alzheimer's disease: A systematic review and meta-analysis of human studies. *Ageing Research Reviews, 58*, 101001.

Bae, H. R., Kim, D. H., Park, M. H., Lee, B., Kim, M. J., Lee, E. K., Chung, K. W., Kim, S. M., Im, D. S., & Chung, H. Y. (2016). β-Hydroxybutyrate suppresses inflammasome formation by ameliorating endoplasmic reticulum stress via AMPK activation. *Oncotarget, 7*(41), 66444–66454.

Bahr, L. S., Bock, M., Liebscher, D., Bellmann-Strobl, J., Franz, L., Prüß, A., Schumann, D., Piper, S. K., Kessler, C. S., Steckhan, N., Michalsen, A., Paul, F., & Mähler, A. (2020). Ketogenic diet and fasting diet as Nutritional Approaches in Multiple Sclerosis (NAMS): Protocol of a randomized controlled study. *Trials, 21*(1), 3.

Banning, A., Deubel, S., Kluth, D., Zhou, Z., & Brigelius-Flohé, R. (2005). The GI-GPx gene is a target for Nrf2. *Molecular and Cellular Biology, 25*(12), 4914–4923.

Bear, M. F., Huber, K. M., & Warren, S. T. (2004). The mGluR theory of fragile X mental retardation. *Trends in Neuroscience, 27*(7), 370–377.

Beckett, T. L., Studzinski, C. M., Keller, J. N., Paul Murphy, M., & Niedowicz, D. M. (2013). A ketogenic diet improves motor performance but does not affect β-amyloid levels in a mouse model of Alzheimer's disease. *Brain Research, 1505*, 61–67.

Benedetti, E., Cristiano, L., Antonosante, A., d'Angelo, M., D'Angelo, B., Selli, S., Castelli, V., Ippoliti, R., Giordano, A., & Cimini, A. (2018). PPARs in neurodegenerative and neuroinflammatory pathways. *Current Alzheimer Research, 15*(4), 336–344.

Ben-Shachar, D., & Ene, H. M. (2018). Mitochondrial targeted therapies: Where do we stand in mental disorders? *Biological Psychiatry, 83*(9), 770–779.

Ben-Shachar, D., & Laifenfeld, D. (2004). Mitochondria, synaptic plasticity, and schizophrenia. *International Review of Neurobiology, 59*, 273–296.

Berger, I., Segal, I., Shmueli, D., & Saada, A. (2010). The effect of antiepileptic drugs on mitochondrial activity: A pilot study. *Journal of Child Neurology, 25*(5), 541–545.

Berk, B. A., Law, T. H., Packer, R. M. A., Wessmann, A., Bathen-Nöthen, A., Jokinen, T. S., Knebel, A., Tipold, A., Pelligand, L., Meads, Z., & Volk, H. A. (2020). A multicenter randomized controlled trial of effect of medium-chain triglyceride dietary supplementation on epilepsy in dogs. *Journal of Veterinary Internal Medicine, 34*(3), 1248–1259.

Berk, M., Kapczinski, F., Andreazza, A. C., Dean, O. M., Giorlando, F., Maes, M., Yücel, M., Gama, C. S., Dodd, S., Dean, B., Magalhães, P. V., Amminger, P., McGorry, P., & Malhi, G. S. (2011). Pathways underlying neuroprogression in bipolar disorder: Focus on inflammation, oxidative stress and neurotrophic factors. *Neuroscience and Biobehavioral Reviews, 35*(3), 804–817.

Bhat, S., Acharya, U. R., Adeli, H., Bairy, G. M., & Adeli, A. (2014). Autism: Cause factors, early diagnosis and therapies. *Reviews in the Neurosciences, 25*(6), 841–850.

Blasco, H., Mavel, S., Corcia, P., & Gordon, P. H. (2014). The glutamate hypothesis in ALS: Pathophysiology and drug development. *Current Medical Chemistry, 21*(31), 3551–3575.

Bollu, P. C., & Kaur, H. (2019). Sleep medicine: Insomnia and sleep. *Missouri Medicine, 116*(1), 68–75.

Bostock, E. C., Kirkby, K. C., & Taylor, B. V. (2017). The current status of the ketogenic diet in psychiatry. *Frontiers in Psychiatry, 8*, 43.

Bostock, E. C. S., Kirkby, K. C., Taylor, B. V., & Hawrelak, J. A. (2020). Consumer reports of "keto flu" associated with the ketogenic diet. *Frontiers in Nutrition, 7*, 20.

Bough, K. J., & Rho, J. M. (2007). Anticonvulsant mechanisms of the ketogenic diet. *Epilepsia, 48*(1), 43–58.

Braam, W., Didden, R., Smits, M. G., & Curfs, L. M. (2008). Melatonin for chronic insomnia in Angelman syndrome: A randomized placebo-controlled trial. *Journal of Child Neurology, 23*(6), 649–654.

Branco, A. F., Ferreira, A., Simões, R. F., Magalhães-Novais, S., Zehowski, C., Cope, E., Silva, A. M., Pereira, D., Sardão, V. A., & Cunha-Oliveira, T. (2016). Ketogenic diets: From cancer to mitochondrial diseases and beyond. *European Journal of Clinical Investigation, 46*(3), 285–298.

Brichta, L., Greengard, P., & Flajolet, M. (2013). Advances in the pharmacological treatment of Parkinson's disease: Targeting neurotransmitter systems. *Trends in Neuroscience, 36*(9), 543–554.

Brisch, R., Saniotis, A., Wolf, R., Bielau, H., Bernstein, H. G., Steiner, J., Bogerts, B., Braun, K., Jankowski, Z., Kumaratilake, J., Henneberg, M., & Gos, T. (2014). The role of dopamine in schizophrenia from a neurobiological and evolutionary perspective: Old fashioned, but still in vogue. *Frontiers in Psychiatry, 5*, 47.

Brown, G. M., McIntyre, R. S., Rosenblat, J., & Hardeland, R. (2018). Depressive disorders: Processes leading to neurogeneration and potential novel treatments. *Progress in Neuro-Psychopharmacology & Biological Psychiatry, 80*(Pt C), 189–204.

Brownlow, M. L., Benner, L., D'Agostino, D., Gordon, M. N., & Morgan, D. (2013). Ketogenic diet improves motor performance but not cognition in two mouse models of Alzheimer's pathology. *PLOS ONE, 8*(9), Article e75713.

Brownlow, M. L., Jung, S. H., Moore, R. J., Bechmann, N., & Jankord, R. (2017). Nutritional ketosis affects metabolism and behavior in Sprague-Dawley rats in both control and chronic stress environments. *Frontiers in Molecular Neuroscience, 10*, 129.

Brunengraber, H. (1997). Potential of ketone body esters for parenteral and oral nutrition. *Nutrition, 13*(3), 233–235.

Burakgazi, E., & French, J. A. (2016). Treatment of epilepsy in adults. *Epileptic Disorders, 18*(3), 228–239.

Burkitt, M. J. (2020). An overlooked danger of ketogenic diets: Making the case that ketone bodies induce vascular damage by the same mechanisms as glucose. *Nutrition, 75-76*, 110763.

Camberos-Luna, L., & Massieu, L. (2020). Therapeutic strategies for ketosis induction and their potential efficacy for the treatment of acute brain injury and neurodegenerative diseases. *Neurochemistry International, 133*, 104614.

Camelo, S., Iglesias, A. H., Hwang, D., Due, B., Ryu, H., Smith, K., Gray, S. G., Imitola, J., Duran, G., Assaf, B., Langley, B., Khoury, S. J., Stephanopoulos, G., De Girolami, U., Ratan, R. R., Ferrante, R. J., & Dangond, F. (2005). Transcriptional therapy with the histone deacetylase inhibitor trichostatin A ameliorates experimental autoimmune encephalomyelitis. *Journal of Neuroimmunology, 164*(1–2), 10–21.

Cantó, C., & Auwerx, J. (2009). PGC-1α, SIRT1 and AMPK, an energy sensing network that controls energy expenditure. *Current Opinion in Lipidology, 20*(2), 98–105.

Cantó, C., Gerhart-Hines, Z., Feige, J. N., Lagouge, M., Noriega, L., Milne, J. C., Elliott, P. J., Puigserver, P., & Auwerx, J. (2009). AMPK regulates energy expenditure by modulating NAD$^+$ metabolism and SIRT1 activity. *Nature, 458*(7241), 1056–1060.

Carcak, N., & Ozkara, C. (2017). Seizures and antiepileptic drugs: From pathophysiology to clinical practice. *Current Pharmaceutical Design, 23*(42), 6376–6388.

Chang, H. C., & Guarente, L. (2013). SIRT1 mediates central circadian control in the SCN by a mechanism that decays with aging. *Cell, 153*(7), 1448–1460.

Chatterjee, P., Fernando, M., Fernando, B., Dias, C. B., Shah, T., Silva, R., Williams, S., Pedrini, S., Hillebrandt, H., Goozee, K., Barin, E., Sohrabi, H. R., Garg, M., Cunnane, S., & Martins, R. N. (2020). Potential of coconut oil and medium chain triglycerides in the prevention and treatment of Alzheimer's disease. *Mechanisms of Ageing and Development, 186*, 111209.

Chaturvedi, R. K., Adhihetty, P., Shukla, S., Hennessy, T., Calingasan, N., Yang, L., Starkov, A., Kiaei, M., Cannella, M., Sassone, J., Ciammola, A., Squitieri, F., & Beal, M. F. (2009). Impaired PGC-1α function in muscle in Huntington's disease. *Human Molecular Genetics, 18*(16), 3048–3065.

Chaturvedi, R. K., Calingasan, N. Y., Yang, L., Hennessey, T., Johri, A., & Beal, M. F. (2010). Impairment of PGC-1α expression, neuropathology and hepatic steatosis in a transgenic mouse model of Huntington's disease following chronic energy deprivation. *Human Molecular Genetics, 19*(16), 3190–3205.

Chen, L., Liu, L., Luo, Y., & Huang, S. (2008). MAPK and mTOR pathways are involved in cadmium-induced neuronal apoptosis. *Journal of Neurochemistry, 105*(1), 251–261.

Chen, L., Miao, Z., & Xu, X. (2017). β-Hydroxybutyrate alleviates depressive behaviors in mice possibly by increasing the histone3-lysine9-β-hydroxybutyrylation. *Biochemical and Biophysical Research Communications, 490*(2), 117–122.

Cheng, A., Wang, J., Ghena, N., Zhao, Q., Perone, I., King, T. M., Veech, R. L., Gorospe, M., Wan, R., & Mattson, M. P. (2020). SIRT3 haploinsufficiency aggravates loss of GABAergic interneurons and neuronal network hyperexcitability in an Alzheimer's disease model. *Journal of Neuroscience, 40*(3), 694–709.

Cheng, A., Wan, R., Yang, J. L., Kamimura, N., Son, T. G., Ouyang, X., Luo, Y., Okun, E., & Mattson, M. P. (2012). Involvement of PGC-1α in the formation and maintenance of neuronal dendritic spines. *Nature Communications, 3*, 1250.

Cheng, N., Rho, J. M., & Masino, S. A. (2017). Metabolic dysfunction underlying autism spectrum disorder and potential treatment approaches. *Frontiers in Molecular Neuroscience, 10*, 34.

Chiapponi, C., Piras, F., Piras, F., Caltagirone, C., & Spalletta, G. (2016). GABA system in schizophrenia and mood disorders: A mini review on third-generation imaging studies. *Frontiers in Psychiatry, 7*, 61.

Chintapenta, M., Spence, J., Kwon, H. I., & Blaszczyk, A. T. (2017). A brief review of caprylidene (Axona) and coconut oil as alternative fuels in the fight against Alzheimer's disease. *The Consultant Pharmacist, 32*(12), 748–751.

Choi, H. I., Kim, H. J., Park, J. S., Kim, I. J., Bae, E. H., Ma, S. K., & Kim, S. W. (2017). PGC-1α attenuates hydrogen peroxide-induced apoptotic cell death by upregulating Nrf-2 via GSK3β inactivation mediated by activated p38 in HK-2 Cells. *Scientific Reports, 7*(1), 4319.

Choi, I. Y., Piccio, L., Childress, P., Bollman, B., Ghosh, A., Brandhorst, S., Suarez, J., Michalsen, A., Cross, A. H., Morgan, T. E., Wei, M., Paul, F., Bock, M., & Longo, V. D. (2016). A diet mimicking fasting promotes regeneration and reduces autoimmunity and multiple sclerosis symptoms. *Cell Reports, 15*(10), 2136–2146.

Choong, C. J., Sasaki, T., Hayakawa, H., Yasuda, T., Baba, K., Hirata, Y., Uesato, S., & Mochizuki, H. (2016). A novel histone deacetylase 1 and 2 isoform-specific inhibitor alleviates experimental Parkinson's disease. *Neurobiology of Aging, 37*, 103–116.

Choudhury, H., Chellappan, D. K., Sengupta, P., Pandey, M., & Gorain, B. (2019). Adenosine receptors in modulation of central nervous system disorders. *Current Pharmaceutical Design, 25*(26), 2808–2827.

Chuang, D. M., Leng, Y., Marinova, Z., Kim, H. J., & Chiu, C. T. (2009). Multiple roles of HDAC inhibition in neurodegenerative conditions. *Trends in Neuroscience, 32*(11), 591–601.

Ciarlone, S. L., Grieco, J. C., D'Agostino, D. P., & Weeber, E. J. (2016). Ketone ester supplementation attenuates seizure activity, and improves behavior and hippocampal synaptic plasticity in an Angelman syndrome mouse model. *Neurobiology of Disease, 96*, 38–46.

Ciruela, F., Casadó, V., Rodrigues, R. J., Luján, R., Burgueño, J., Canals, M., Borycz, J., Rebola, N., Goldberg, S. R., Mallol, J., Cortés, A., Canela, E. I., López-Giménez, J. F., Milligan, G., Lluis, C., Cunha, R. A., Ferré, S., & Franco, R. (2006). Presynaptic control of striatal glutamatergic neurotransmission by adenosine A_1-A_{2A} receptor heteromers. *Journal of Neuroscience, 26*(7), 2080–2087.

Citraro, R., Leo, A., Santoro, M., D'Agostino, G., Constanti, A., & Russo, E. (2017). Role of histone deacetylases (HDACs) in epilepsy and epileptogenesis. *Current Pharmaceutical Design, 23*(37), 5546–5562.

Clarke, K., Tchabanenko, K., Pawlosky, R., Carter, E., Knight, N. S., Murray, A. J., Cochlin, L. E., King, M. T., Wong, A. W., Roberts, A., Robertson, J., & Veech, R. L. (2012a). Oral 28-day and developmental toxicity studies of (R)-3-hydroxybutyl (R)-3-hydroxybutyrate. *Regulatory Toxicology and Pharmacology, 63*(2), 196–208.

Clarke, K., Tchabanenko, K., Pawlosky, R., Carter, E., Todd King, M., Musa-Veloso, K., Ho, M., Roberts, A., Robertson, J., Vanitallie, T. B., & Veech, R. L. (2012b). Kinetics, safety and tolerability of (R)-3-hydroxybutyl (R)-3-hydroxybutyrate in healthy adult subjects. *Regulatory Toxicology and Pharmacology, 63*(3), 401–408.

Coelho, J. E., Alves, P., Canas, P. M., Valadas, J. S., Shmidt, T., Batalha, V. L., Ferreira, D. G., Ribeiro, J. A., Bader, M., Cunha, R. A., do Couto, F. S., & Lopes, L. V. (2014). Overexpression of adenosine A_{2A} receptors in rats: Effects on depression, locomotion, and anxiety. *Frontiers in Psychiatry, 5*, 67.

Colié, S., Sarroca, S., Palenzuela, R., Garcia, I., Matheu, A., Corpas, R., Dotti, C. G., Esteban, J. A., Sanfeliu, C., & Nebreda, A. R. (2017). Neuronal p38α mediates synaptic and cognitive dysfunction in an Alzheimer's mouse model by controlling β-amyloid production. *Scientific Reports, 7,* 45306.

Condello, S., Currò, M., Ferlazzo, N., Costa, G., Visalli, G., Caccamo, D., Pisani, L. R., Costa, C., Calabresi, P., Ientile, R., & Pisani, F. (2013). Protective effects of zonisamide against rotenone-induced neurotoxicity. *Neurochemical Research, 38*(12), 2631–2639.

Corpas, R., Revilla, S., Ursulet, S., Castro-Freire, M., Kaliman, P., Petegnief, V., Giménez-Llort, L., Sarkis, C., Pallàs, M., & Sanfeliu, C. (2017). SIRT1 overexpression in mouse hippocampus induces cognitive enhancement through proteostatic and neurotrophic mechanisms. *Molecular Neurobiology, 54*(7), 5604–5619.

Courchesne-Loyer, A., Fortier, M., Tremblay-Mercier, J., Chouinard-Watkins, R., Roy, M., Nugent, S., Castellano, C. A., & Cunnane, S. C. (2013). Stimulation of mild, sustained ketonemia by medium-chain triacylglycerols in healthy humans: Estimated potential contribution to brain energy metabolism. *Nutrition, 29*(4), 635–640.

Courvoisie, H., Hooper, S. R., Fine, C., Kwock, L., & Castillo, M. (2004). Neurometabolic functioning and neuropsychological correlates in children with ADHD-H: Preliminary findings. *The Journal of Neuropsychiatry and Clinical Neurosciences, 16*(1), 63–69.

Coyle, J. T., & Puttfarcken, P. (1993). Oxidative stress, glutamate, and neurodegenerative disorders. *Science, 262*(5134), 689–695.

Craske, M. G., Stein, M. B., Eley, T. C., Milad, M. R., Holmes, A., Rapee, R. M., & Wittchen, H. U. (2017). Anxiety disorders. *Nature Reviews Disease Primers, 3,* 17024.

Croteau, E., Castellano, C. A., Richard, M. A., Fortier, M., Nugent, S., Lepage, M., Duchesne, S., Whittingstall, K., Turcotte, É. E., Bocti, C., Fülöp, T., & Cunnane, S. C. (2018). Ketogenic medium chain triglycerides increase brain energy metabolism in Alzheimer's disease. *Journal of Alzheimer's Disease, 64*(2), 551–561.

Cuenoud, B., Hartweg, M., Godin, J. P., Croteau, E., Maltais, M., Castellano, C. A., Carpentier, A. C., & Cunnane, S. C. (2020). Metabolism of exogenous D-β-hydroxybutyrate, an energy substrate avidly consumed by the heart and kidney. *Frontiers in Nutrition, 7,* 13.

Cui, L., Jeong, H., Borovecki, F., Parkhurst, C. N., Tanese, N., & Krainc, D. (2006). Transcriptional repression of PGC-1α by mutant huntingtin leads to mitochondrial dysfunction and neurodegeneration. *Cell, 127*(1), 59–69.

Dąbek, A., Wojtala, M., Pirola, L., & Balcerczyk, A. (2020). Modulation of cellular biochemistry, epigenetics and metabolomics by ketone bodies: Implications of the ketogenic diet in the physiology of the organism and pathological states. *Nutrients, 12*(3), pii: E788.

D'Agostino, D. P., Pilla, R., Held, H. E., Landon, C. S., Puchowicz, M., Brunengraber, H., Ari, C., Arnold, P., & Dean, J. B. (2013). Therapeutic ketosis with ketone ester delays central nervous system oxygen toxicity seizures in rats. *American Journal of Physiology. Regulatory, Integrative and Comparative Physiology, 304*(10), 829–836.

Dahlin, M., Månsson, J. E., & Åmark, P. (2012). CSF levels of dopamine and serotonin, but not norepinephrine, metabolites are influenced by the ketogenic diet in children with epilepsy. *Epilepsy Research, 99*(1–2), 132–138.

D'Alimonte, I., D'Auro, M., Citraro, R., Biagioni, F., Jiang, S., Nargi, E., Buccella, S., Di Iorio, P., Giuliani, P., Ballerini, P., Caciagli, F., Russo, E., De Sarro, G., & Ciccarelli, R. (2009). Altered distribution and function of A$_{2A}$ adenosine receptors in the brain of WAG/Rij rats with genetic absence epilepsy, before and after appearance of the disease. *European Journal of Neuroscience, 30*(6), 1023–1035.

D'Amelio, M., Puglisi-Allegra, S., & Mercuri, N. (2018). The role of dopaminergic midbrain in Alzheimer's disease: Translating basic science into clinical practice. *Pharmacological Research, 130,* 414–419.

d'Angelo, M., Castelli, V., Catanesi, M., Antonosante, A., Dominguez-Benot, R., Ippoliti, R., Benedetti, E., & Cimini, A. (2019). PPARγ and cognitive performance. *International Journal of Molecular Sciences, 20*(20), pii: E5068.

Daniels, T. E., Olsen, E. M., & Tyrka, A. R. (2020). Stress and psychiatric disorders: The role of mitochondria. *Annual Review of Clinical Psychology, 16,* 165–186.

Dawson, T. M., Dawson, V. L., & Snyder, S. H. (1992). A novel neuronal messenger molecule in brain: The free radical, nitric oxide. *Annals of Neurology, 32*(3), 297–311.

Dean, J., & Keshavan, M. (2017). The neurobiology of depression: An integrated view. *Asian Journal of Psychiatry, 27,* 101–111.

DeDea, L. (2012). Can coconut oil replace caprylidene for Alzheimer disease? *Journal of the American Academy of Physician Assistants, 25*(8), 19.

Delgado, P. L. (2000). Depression: The case for a monoamine deficiency. *The Journal of Clinical Psychiatry, 61,* 7–11.

de Ruijter, A. J., van Gennip, A. H., Caron, H. N., Kemp, S., & van Kuilenburg, A. B. (2003). Histone deacetylases (HDACs): Characterization of the classical HDAC family. *The Biochemical Journal, 370*(Pt 3), 737–749.

Dias, B. G., Banerjee, S. B., Goodman, J. V., & Ressler, K. J. (2013). Towards new approaches to disorders of fear and anxiety. *Current Opinion in Neurobiology, 23*(3), 346–352.

Digby, J. E., Martinez, F., Jefferson, A., Ruparelia, N., Chai, J., Wamil, M., Greaves, D. R., & Choudhury, R. P. (2012). Anti-inflammatory effects of nicotinic acid in human monocytes are mediated by GPR109A dependent mechanisms. *Arteriosclerosis, Thrombosis, and Vascular Biology, 32*(3), 669–676.

Dinkova-Kostova, A. T., & Abramov, A. Y. (2015). The emerging role of Nrf2 in mitochondrial function. *Free Radical Biology & Medicine, 88*(Pt B), 179–188.

D'Mello, S. R. (2009). Histone deacetylases as targets for the treatment of human neurodegenerative diseases. *Drug News & Perspectives, 22*(9), 513–524.

Duan, R., Liu, X., Wang, T., Wu, L., Gao, X., & Zhang, Z. (2016). Histone acetylation regulation in sleep deprivation-induced spatial memory impairment. *Neurochemical Research, 41*(9), 2223–2232.

Dupuis, N., Curatolo, N., Benoist, J. F., & Auvin, S. (2015). Ketogenic diet exhibits anti-inflammatory properties. *Epilepsia, 56*(7), e95–e98.

Edden, R. A., Crocetti, D., Zhu, H., Gilbert, D. L., & Mostofsky, S. H. (2012). Reduced GABA concentration in attention-deficit/hyperactivity disorder. *Archives of General Psychiatry, 69*(7), 750–753.

Edye, M. E., Walker, L. E., Sills, G. J., Allan, S. M., & Brough, D. (2014). Epilepsy and the inflammasome: Targeting inflammation as a novel therapeutic strategy for seizure disorders. *Inflammasome, 1*(1), 36–43.

Effendi, W. I., Nagano, T., Kobayashi, K., & Nishimura, Y. (2020). Focusing on adenosine receptors as a potential targeted therapy in human diseases. *Cells, 9*(3), pii: E785.

Einat, H., Yuan, P., & Manji, H. K. (2005). Increased anxiety-like behaviors and mitochondrial dysfunction in mice with targeted mutation of the Bcl-2 gene: Further support for the involvement of mitochondrial function in anxiety disorders. *Behavioural Brain Research, 165*(2), 172–180.

Eisele, P. S., Furrer, R., Beer, M., & Handschin, C. (2015). The PGC-1 coactivators promote an anti-inflammatory environment in skeletal muscle in vivo. *Biochemical and Biophysical Research Communications, 464*(3), 692–697.

Eisele, P. S., Salatino, S., Sobek, J., Hottiger, M. O., & Handschin, C. (2013). The peroxisome proliferator-activated receptor γ coactivator 1α/β (PGC-1) coactivators repress the transcriptional activity of NF-κB in skeletal muscle cells. *The Journal of Biological Chemistry, 288*(4), 2246–2260.

Elamin, M., Ruskin, D. N., Masino, S. A., & Sacchetti, P. (2017). Ketone-based metabolic therapy: Is increased NAD$^+$ a primary mechanism? *Frontiers in Molecular Neuroscience, 10*, 377.

Elamin, M., Ruskin, D. N., Masino, S. A., & Sacchetti, P. (2018). Ketogenic diet modulates NAD$^+$-dependent enzymes and reduces DNA damage in hippocampus. *Frontiers in Cellular Neuroscience, 12*, 263.

Emerit, J., Edeas, M., & Bricaire, F. (2004). Neurodegenerative diseases and oxidative stress. *Biomedicine & Pharmacotherapy, 58*(1), 39–46.

Erecińska, M., Nelson, D., Daikhin, Y., & Yudkoff, M. (1996). Regulation of GABA level in rat brain synaptosomes: Fluxes through enzymes of the GABA shunt and effects of glutamate, calcium, and ketone bodies. *Journal of Neurochemistry, 67*(6), 2325–2334.

Erickson, C. A., Mullett, J. E., & McDougle, C. J. (2009). Open-label memantine in fragile X syndrome. *Journal of Autism and Developmental Disorders, 39*(12), 1629–1635.

Evan, G., & Littlewood, T. (1998). A matter of life and cell death. *Science, 281*(5381), 1317–1322.

Evangeliou, A., Doulioglou, V., Haidopoulou, K., Aptouramani, M., Spilioti, M., & Varlamis, G. (2010). Ketogenic diet in a patient with Angelman syndrome. *Pediatrics International, 52*(5), 831–834.

Evangeliou, A., Vlachonikolis, I., Mihailidou, H., Spilioti, M., Skarpalezou, A., Makaronas, N., Prokopiou, A., Christodoulou, P., Liapi-Adamidou, G., Helidonis, E., Sbyrakis, S., & Smeitink, J. (2003). Application of a ketogenic diet in children with autistic behavior: Pilot study. *Journal of Child Neurology, 18*(2), 113–118.

Faraone, S. V., Asherson, P., Banaschewski, T., Biederman, J., Buitelaar, J. K., Ramos-Quiroga, J. A., Rohde, L. A., Sonuga-Barke, E. J., Tannock, R., & Franke, B. (2015). Attention-deficit/hyperactivity disorder. *Nature Reviews Disease Primers, 1*, 15020.

Feng, H. L., Leng, Y., Ma, C. H., Zhang, J., Ren, M., & Chuang, D. M. (2008). Combined lithium and valproate treatment delays disease onset, reduces neurological deficits and prolongs survival in an amyotrophic lateral sclerosis mouse model. *Neuroscience, 155*(3), 567–572.

Ferland, C. L., & Schrader, L. A. (2011). Regulation of histone acetylation in the hippocampus of chronically stressed rats: A potential role of sirtuins. *Neuroscience, 174*, 104–114.

Fernando, W. M., Martins, I. J., Goozee, K. G., Brennan, C. S., Jayasena, V., & Martins, R. N. (2015). The role of dietary coconut for the prevention and treatment of Alzheimer's disease: Potential mechanisms of action. *British Journal of Nutrition, 114*(1), 1–14.

Ferrante, R. J., Kubilus, J. K., Lee, J., Ryu, H., Beesen, A., Zucker, B., Smith, K., Kowall, N. W., Ratan, R. R., Luthi-Carter, R., & Hersch, S. M. (2003). Histone deacetylase inhibition by sodium butyrate chemotherapy ameliorates the neurodegenerative phenotype in Huntington's disease mice. *Journal of Neuroscience, 23*(28), 9418–9427.

Ferret-Sena, V., Capela, C., & Sena, A. (2018). Metabolic dysfunction and peroxisome proliferator-activated receptors (PPAR) in multiple sclerosis. *International Journal of Molecular Sciences, 19*(6), pii: E1639.

Filipek, P. A., Juranek, J., Smith, M., Mays, L. Z., Ramos, E. R., Bocian, M., Masser-Frye, D., Laulhere, T. M., Modahl, C., Spence, M. A., & Gargus, J. J. (2003). Mitochondrial dysfunction in autistic patients with 15q inverted duplication. *Annals of Neurology, 53*(6), 801–804.

Finley, J. (2019). Cellular stress and AMPK links metformin and diverse compounds with accelerated emergence from anesthesia and potential recovery from disorders of consciousness. *Medical Hypotheses, 124*, 42–52.

Finley, L. W., & Haigis, M. C. (2009). The coordination of nuclear and mitochondrial communication during aging and calorie restriction. *Ageing Research Reviews, 8*(3), 173–188.

Finsterer, J., & Scorza, F. A. (2017). Effects of anti-epileptic drugs on mitochondrial functions, morphology, kinetics, biogenesis, and survival. *Epilepsy Research, 136*, 5–11.

Fischer, A., Sananbenesi, F., Wang, X., Dobbin, M., & Tsai, L. H. (2007). Recovery of learning and memory is associated with chromatin remodelling. *Nature, 447*(7141), 178–182.

Frazier, T. H., DiBaise, J. K., & McClain, C. J. (2011). Gut microbiota, intestinal permeability, obesity-induced inflammation, and liver injury. JPEN. *Journal of Parenteral and Enteral Nutrition, 35*(5 Suppl), 14–20.

Freeman, J. M., Vining, E. P., Kossoff, E. H., Pyzik, P. L., Ye, X., & Goodman, S. N. (2009). A blinded, crossover study of the efficacy of the ketogenic diet. *Epilepsia, 50*(2), 322–325.

Frye, R. A. (2000). Phylogenetic classification of prokaryotic and eukaryotic Sir2-like proteins. *Biochemical and Biophysical Research Communications, 273*(2), 793–798.

Frye, R. E., & Rossignol, D. A. (2014). Treatments for biomedical abnormalities associated with autism spectrum disorder. *Frontiers in Pediatrics, 2*, 66.

Fu, S. P., Wang, J. F., Xue, W. J., Liu, H. M., Liu, B. R., Zeng, Y. L., Li, S. N., Huang, B. X., Lv, Q. K., Wang, W., & Liu, J. X. (2015). Anti-inflammatory effects of BHBA in both in vivo and in vitro Parkinson's disease models are mediated by GPR109A-dependent mechanisms. *Journal of Neuroinflammation, 12*, 9.

Ganai, S. A., Ramadoss, M., & Mahadevan, V. (2016). Histone deacetylase (HDAC) inhibitors—Emerging roles in neuronal memory, learning, synaptic plasticity and neural regeneration. *Current Neuropharmacology, 14*(1), 55–71.

Gano, L. B., Patel, M., & Rho, J. M. (2014). Ketogenic diets, mitochondria, and neurological diseases. *Journal of Lipid Research, 55*(11), 2211–2228.

Gao, J., Wang, W. Y., Mao, Y. W., Gräff, J., Guan, J. S., Pan, L., Mak, G., Kim, D., Su, S. C., & Tsai, L. H. (2010). A novel pathway regulates memory and plasticity via SIRT1 and miR-134. *Nature, 466*(7310), 1105–1109.

García-Bueno, B., Bioque, M., Mac-Dowell, K. S., Barcones, M. F., Martínez-Cengotitabengoa, M., Pina-Camacho, L., Rodríguez-Jiménez, R., Sáiz, P. A., Castro, C., Lafuente, A., Santabárbara, J., González-Pinto, A., Parellada, M., Rubio, G., García-Portilla, M. P., Micó, J. A., Bernardo, M., & Leza, J. C. (2014). Pro-/anti-inflammatory dysregulation in patients with first episode of psychosis: toward an integrative inflammatory hypothesis of schizophrenia. *Schizophrenia Bulletin, 40*(2), 376–387.

Geng, S., Zhu, W., Xie, C., Li, X., Wu, J., Liang, Z., Xie, W., Zhu, J., Huang, C., Zhu, M., Wu, R., & Zhong, C. (2016). Medium-chain triglyceride ameliorates insulin resistance and inflammation in high fat diet-induced obese mice. *European Journal of Nutrition, 55*(3), 931–940.

Gilbert, D. L., Pyzik, P. L., & Freeman, J. M. (2000). The ketogenic diet: Seizure control correlates better with serum beta-hydroxybutyrate than with urine ketones. *Journal of Child Neurology, 15*(12), 787–790.

Ginnan, R., Jourd'heuil, F. L., Guikema, B., Simons, M., Singer, H. A., & Jourd'heuil, D. (2013). NADPH oxidase 4 is required for interleukin-1β-mediated activation of protein kinase Cδ and downstream activation of c-jun N-terminal kinase signaling in smooth muscle. *Free Radical Biology & Medicine, 54*, 125–134.

Gizer, I. R., Ficks, C., & Waldman, I. D. (2009). Candidate gene studies of ADHD: A meta-analytic review. *Human Genetics, 126*(1), 51–90.

Glass, C. K., Saijo, K., Winner, B., Marchetto, M. C., & Gage, F. H. (2010). Mechanisms underlying inflammation in neurodegeneration. *Cell, 140*(6), 918–934.

Gong, B., Chen, F., Pan, Y., Arrieta-Cruz, I., Yoshida, Y., Haroutunian, V., & Pasinetti, G. M. (2010). SCFFbx2-E3-ligase-mediated degradation of BACE1 attenuates Alzheimer's disease amyloidosis and improves synaptic function. *Aging Cell, 9*(6), 1018–1031.

Goodwin, F. K., & Jamison, K. R. (2007). *Manic-depressive illness: Bipolar disorders and recurrent depression.* Oxford University Press.

Graff, E. C., Fang, H., Wanders, D., & Judd, R. L. (2016). Anti-inflammatory effects of the hydroxy-carboxylic acid receptor 2. *Metabolism, 65*(2), 102–113.

Gräff, J., Kim, D., Dobbin, M. M., & Tsai, L. H. (2011). Epigenetic regulation of gene expression in physiological and pathological brain processes. *Physiological Reviews, 91*(2), 603–649.

Gray, S. G., & Dangond, F. (2006). Rationale for the use of histone deacetylase inhibitors as a dual therapeutic modality in multiple sclerosis. *Epigenetics, 1*(2), 67–75.

Green, J., & Garg, S. (2018). Annual research review: The state of autism intervention science; Progress, target psychological and biological mechanisms and future prospects. *Journal of Child Psychology and Psychiatry, 59*(4), 424–443.

Green, S. F., Nguyen, P., Kaalund-Hansen, K., Rajakulendran, S., & Murphy, E. (2020). Effectiveness, retention, and safety of modified ketogenic diet in adults with epilepsy at a tertiary-care centre in the UK. *Journal of Neurology, 267*(4), 1171–1178.

Greenamyre, J. T., Sherer, T. B., Betarbet, R., & Panov, A. V. (2001). Complex I and Parkinson's disease. *IUBMB Life, 52*(3–5), 135–141.

Gregoretti, I. V., Lee, Y. M., & Goodson, H. V. (2004). Molecular evolution of the histone deacetylase family: Functional implications of phylogenetic analysis. *Journal of Molecular Biology, 338*(1), 17–31.

Grigolon, R. B., Gerchman, F., Schöffel, A. C., Hawken, E. R., Gill, H., Vazquez, G. H., Mansur, R. B., McIntyre, R. S., & Brietzke, E. (2020). Mental, emotional, and behavioral effects of ketogenic diet for non-epileptic neuropsychiatric conditions. *Progress in Neuro-Psychopharmacology and Biological Psychiatry, 102*, 109947.

Gross, E., Putananickal, N., Orsini, A. L., Schmidt, S., Vogt, D. R., Cichon, S., Sandor, P., & Fischer, D. (2019). Efficacy and safety of exogenous ketone bodies for preventive treatment of migraine: A study protocol for a single-centred, randomised, placebo-controlled, double-blind crossover trial. *Trials, 20*(1), 61.

Guan, J. S., Haggarty, S. J., Giacometti, E., Dannenberg, J. H., Joseph, N., Gao, J., Nieland, T. J., Zhou, Y., Wang, X., Mazitschek, R., Bradner, J. E., DePinho, R. A., Jaenisch, R., & Tsai, L. H. (2009). HDAC2 negatively regulates memory formation and synaptic plasticity. *Nature, 459*(7243), 55–60.

Haas, H. L., & Greene, R. W. (1984). Adenosine enhances afterhyperpolarization and accommodation in hippocampal pyramidal cells. *Pflugers Archiv, 402*(3), 244–247.

Haces, M. L., Hernández-Fonseca, K., Medina-Campos, O. N., Montiel, T., Pedraza-Chaverri, J., & Massieu, L. (2008). Antioxidant capacity contributes to protection of ketone bodies against oxidative damage induced during hypoglycemic conditions. *Experimental Neurology, 211*(1), 85–96.

Hafner, A. V., Dai, J., Gomes, A. P., Xiao, C. Y., Palmeira, C. M., Rosenzweig, A., & Sinclair, D. A. (2010). Regulation of the mPTP by SIRT3-mediated deacetylation of CypD at lysine 166 suppresses age-related cardiac hypertrophy. *Aging, 2*(12), 914–923.

Haigis, M. C., & Guarente, L. P. (2006). Mammalian sirtuins—Emerging roles in physiology, aging, and calorie restriction. *Genes & Development, 20*(21), 2913–2921.

Hallböök, T., Ji, S., Maudsley, S., & Martin, B. (2012). The effects of the ketogenic diet on behavior and cognition. *Epilepsy Research, 100*(3), 304–309.

Hallböök, T., Köhler, S., Rosén, I., & Lundgren, J. (2007). Effects of ketogenic diet on epileptiform activity in children with therapy resistant epilepsy. *Epilepsy Research, 77*(2–3), 134–140.

Han, S., Choi, J. R., Soon Shin, K., & Kang, S. J. (2012). Resveratrol upregulated heat shock proteins and extended the survival of G93A-SOD1 mice. *Brain Research, 1483*, 112–117.

Handschin, C., & Spiegelman, B. M. (2008). The role of exercise and PGC1α in inflammation and chronic disease. *Nature, 454*(7203), 463–469.

Hartel, I., Ronellenfitsch, M., Wanka, C., Wolking, S., Steinbach, J. P., & Rieger, J. (2016). Activation of AMP-activated kinase modulates sensitivity of glioma cells against epidermal growth factor receptor inhibition. *International Journal of Oncology, 49*(1), 173–180.

Hartman, A. L., & Vining, E. P. (2007). Clinical aspects of the ketogenic diet. *Epilepsia, 48*(1), 31–42.

Harvey, C. J. D. C., Schofield, G. M., & Williden, M. (2018). The use of nutritional supplements to induce ketosis and reduce symptoms associated with keto-induction: A narrative review. *PeerJ, 6*, e4488.

Hasan-Olive, M. M., Lauritzen, K. H., Ali, M., Rasmussen, L. J., Storm-Mathisen, J., & Bergersen, L. H. (2019). A ketogenic diet improves mitochondrial biogenesis and bioenergetics via the PGC1α-SIRT3-UCP2 axis. *Neurochemical Research, 44*(1), 22–37.

Hashim, S. A., & VanItallie, T. B. (2014). Ketone body therapy: From the ketogenic diet to the oral administration of ketone ester. *Journal of Lipid Research, 55*(9), 1818–1826.

Hashimoto, K., Sawa, A., & Iyo, M. (2007). Increased levels of glutamate in brains from patients with mood disorders. *Biological Psychiatry, 62*(11), 1310–1316.

Hatanpää, K., Isaacs, K. R., Shirao, T., Brady, D. R., & Rapoport, S. I. (1999). Loss of proteins regulating synaptic plasticity in normal aging of the human brain and in Alzheimer disease. *Journal of Neuropathology and Experimental Neurology, 58*(6), 637–643.

Hauber, W. (1998). Involvement of basal ganglia transmitter systems in movement initiation. *Progress in Neurobiology, 56*(5), 507–540.

He, W., Newman, J. C., Wang, M. Z., Ho, L., & Verdin, E. (2012). Mitochondrial sirtuins: Regulators of protein acylation and metabolism. *Trends in Endocrinology and Metabolism, 23*(9), 467–476.

Hein, A. M., & O'Banion, M. K. (2009). Neuroinflammation and memory: The role of prostaglandins. *Molecular Neurobiology, 40*(1), 15–32.

Henderson, S. T. (2008). Ketone bodies as a therapeutic for Alzheimer's disease. *Neurotherapeutics, 5*(3), 470–480.

Henshall, D. C., Bonislawski, D. P., Skradski, S. L., Lan, J. Q., Meller, R., & Simon, R. P. (2001). Cleavage of bid may amplify caspase-8-induced neuronal death following focally evoked limbic seizures. *Neurobiology of Disease, 8*(4), 568–580.

Henshall, D. C., Chen, J., & Simon, R. P. (2000). Involvement of caspase-3-like protease in the mechanism of cell death following focally evoked limbic seizures. *Journal of Neurochemistry, 74*(3), 1215–1223.

Herbert, M. R., & Buckley, J. A. (2013). Autism and dietary therapy: Case report and review of the literature. *Journal of Child Neurology, 28*(8), 975–982.

Herskovits, A. Z., & Guarente, L. (2014). SIRT1 in neurodevelopment and brain senescence. *Neuron, 81*(3), 471–483.

Herzig, S., & Shaw, R. J. (2018). AMPK: Guardian of metabolism and mitochondrial homeostasis. *Nature Reviews Molecular Cell Biology, 19*(2), 121–135.

Hockly, E., Richon, V. M., Woodman, B., Smith, D. L., Zhou, X., Rosa, E., Sathasivam, K., Ghazi-Noori, S., Mahal, A., Lowden, P. A., Steffan, J. S., Marsh, J. L., Thompson, L. M., Lewis, C. M., Marks, P. A., & Bates, G. P. (2003). Suberoylanilide hydroxamic acid, a histone deacetylase inhibitor, ameliorates motor deficits in a mouse model of Huntington's disease. *Proceedings of the National Academy of Sciences of the United States of America, 100*(4), 2041–2046.

Hodes, G. E., Kana, V., Menard, C., Merad, M., & Russo, S. J. (2015). Neuroimmune mechanisms of depression. *Nature Neuroscience, 18*(10), 1386–1393.

Hollis, F., Mitchell, E. S., Canto, C., Wang, D., & Sandi, C. (2018). Medium chain triglyceride diet reduces anxiety-like behaviors and enhances social competitiveness in rats. *Neuropharmacology, 138*, 245–256.

Holper, L., Ben-Shachar, D., & Mann, J. J. (2019). Multivariate meta-analyses of mitochondrial complex I and IV in major depressive disorder, bipolar disorder, schizophrenia, Alzheimer disease, and Parkinson disease. *Neuropsychopharmacology, 44*(5), 837–849.

Holst, S. C., & Landolt, H. P. (2018). Sleep-wake neurochemistry. *Sleep Medicine Clinics, 13*(2), 137–146.

Holst, S. C., Valomon, A., & Landolt, H. P. (2016). Sleep pharmacogenetics: Personalized sleep-wake therapy. *Annual Review of Pharmacology and Toxicology, 56*, 577–603.

Houtkooper, R. H., & Auwerx, J. (2012). Exploring the therapeutic space around NAD$^+$. *The Journal of Cell Biology, 199*(2), 205–209.

Hu, S., Dong, H., Zhang, H., Wang, S., Hou, L., Chen, S., Zhang, J., & Xiong, L. (2012). Noninvasive limb remote ischemic preconditioning contributes neuroprotective effects via activation of adenosine A_1 receptor and redox status after transient focal cerebral ischemia in rats. *Brain Research, 1459*, 81–90.

Huang, D., Liu, D., Yin, J., Qian, T., Shrestha, S., & Ni, H. (2017a). Glutamate-glutamine and GABA in brain of normal aged and patients with cognitive impairment. *European Radiology, 27*(7), 2698–2705.

Huang, K., Gao, X., & Wei, W. (2017b). The crosstalk between Sirt1 and Keap1/Nrf2/ARE anti-oxidative pathway forms a positive feedback loop to inhibit FN and TGF-β1 expressions in rat glomerular mesangial cells. *Experimental Cell Research, 361*(1), 63–72.

Huang, Y., Zhao, F., Wang, L., Yin, H., Zhou, C., & Wang, X. (2012). Increased expression of histone deacetylases 2 in temporal lobe epilepsy: A study of epileptic patients and rat models. *Synapse, 66*(2), 151–159.

Huberfeld, G., & Vecht, C. J. (2016). Seizures and gliomas—Towards a single therapeutic approach. *Nature Reviews Neurology, 12*(4), 204–216.

Hughes, H. K., Mills Ko, E., Rose, D., & Ashwood, P. (2018). Immune dysfunction and autoimmunity as pathological mechanisms in autism spectrum disorders. *Frontiers in Cellular Neuroscience, 12*, 405.

Hurley, L. L., Akinfiresoye, L., Kalejaiye, O., & Tizabi, Y. (2014). Antidepressant effects of resveratrol in an animal model of depression. *Behavioural Brain Research, 268*, 1–7.

Huttenlocher, P. R. (1976). Ketonemia and seizures: Metabolic and anticonvulsant effects of two ketogenic diets in childhood epilepsy. *Pediatric Research, 10*(5), 536–540.

Hyun, D. H., Lee, M., Halliwell, B., & Jenner, P. (2003). Proteasomal inhibition causes the formation of protein aggregates containing a wide range of proteins, including nitrated proteins. *Journal of Neurochemistry, 86*(2), 363–373.

IJff, D. M., Postulart, D., Lambrechts, D. A. J. E., Majoie, M. H. J. M., de Kinderen, R. J. A., Hendriksen, J. G. M., Evers, S. M. A. A., & Aldenkamp, A. P. (2016). Cognitive and behavioral impact of the ketogenic diet in children and adolescents with refractory epilepsy: A randomized controlled trial. *Epilepsy & Behavior, 60,* 153–157.

Im, J. Y., Lee, K. W., Woo, J. M., Junn, E., & Mouradian, M. M. (2012). DJ-1 induces thioredoxin 1 expression through the Nrf2 pathway. *Human Molecular Genetics, 21*(13), 3013–3024.

Irwin, M. R. (2019). Sleep and inflammation: Partners in sickness and in health. *Nature Reviews Immunology, 19*(11), 702–715.

Irwin, M. R., & Opp, M. R. (2017). Sleep health: Reciprocal regulation of sleep and innate immunity. *Neuropsychopharmacology, 42*(1), 129–155.

Izumi, Y., Ishii, K., Katsuki, H., Benz, A. M., & Zorumski, C. F. (1998). β-Hydroxybutyrate fuels synaptic function during development: Histological and physiological evidence in rat hippocampal slices. *Journal of Clinical Investigation, 101*(5), 1121–1132.

Jenner, P. (2003). Oxidative stress in Parkinson's disease. *Annals of Neurology, 53,* 26–38.

Jensen, N. J., Nilsson, M., Ingerslev, J. S., Olsen, D. A., Fenger, M., Svart, M., Møller, N., Zander, M., Miskowiak, K. W., & Rungby, J. (2020). Effects of β-hydroxybutyrate on cognition in patients with type 2 diabetes. *European Journal of Endocrinology, 182*(2), 233–242.

Jeong, E. A., Jeon, B. T., Shin, H. J., Kim, N., Lee, D. H., Kim, H. J., Kang, S. S., Cho, G. J., Choi, W. S., & Roh, G. S. (2011). Ketogenic diet-induced peroxisome proliferator-activated receptor-γ activation decreases neuroinflammation in the mouse hippocampus after kainic acid-induced seizures. *Experimental Neurology, 232*(2), 195–202.

Jiang, M., Zheng, J., Peng, Q., Hou, Z., Zhang, J., Mori, S., Ellis, J. L., Vlasuk, G. P., Fries, H., Suri, V., & Duan, W. (2014). Sirtuin 1 activator SRT2104 protects Huntington's disease mice. *Annals of Clinical and Translational Neurology, 1*(12), 1047–1052.

Johannessen, C. U. (2000). Mechanisms of action of valproate: a commentary. *Neurochemistry International, 37*(2–3), 103–110.

Jones, B. E. (2020). Arousal and sleep circuits. *Neuropsychopharmacology, 45*(1), 6–20.

Joo, M. S., Kim, W. D., Lee, K. Y., Kim, J. H., Koo, J. H., & Kim, S. G. (2016). AMPK facilitates nuclear accumulation of Nrf2 by phosphorylating at serine 550. *Molecular and Cellular Biology, 36*(14), 1931–1942.

Joshi, A. U., & Mochly-Rosen, D. (2018). Mortal engines: Mitochondrial bioenergetics and dysfunction in neurodegenerative diseases. *Pharmacological Research, 138,* 2–15.

Juge, N., Gray, J. A., Omote, H., Miyaji, T., Inoue, T., Hara, C., Uneyama, H., Edwards, R. H., Nicoll, R. A., & Moriyama, Y. (2010). Metabolic control of vesicular glutamate transport and release. *Neuron, 68*(1), 99–112.

Julien, C., Tremblay, C., Emond, V., Lebbadi, M., Salem, N., Jr., Bennett, D. A., & Calon, F. (2009). Sirtuin 1 reduction parallels the accumulation of tau in Alzheimer disease. *Journal of Neuropathology and Experimental Neurology, 68*(1), 48–58.

Kahn, R. S., & Sommer, I. E. (2015). The neurobiology and treatment of first-episode schizophrenia. *Molecular Psychiatry, 20*(1), 84–97.

Kahn, R. S., Sommer, I. E., Murray, R. M., Meyer-Lindenberg, A., Weinberger, D. R., Cannon, T. D., O'Donovan, M., Correll, C. U., Kane, J. M., van Os, J., & Insel, T. R. (2015). Schizophrenia. *Nature Reviews Disease Primers, 1,* 15067.

Kajitani, N., Iwata, M., Miura, A., Tsunetomi, K., Yamanashi, T., Matsuo, R., Nishiguchi, T., Fukuda, S., Nagata, M., Shibushita, M., Yamauchi, T., Pu, S., Shirayama, Y., Watanabe, K., & Kaneko, K. (2020). Prefrontal cortex infusion of beta-hydroxybutyrate, an endogenous NLRP3 inflammasome inhibitor, produces antidepressant-like effects in a rodent model of depression. *Neuropsychopharmacology Reports, 40*(2), 157–165.

Karuppagounder, S. S., Pinto, J. T., Xu, H., Chen, H. L., Beal, M. F., & Gibson, G. E. (2009). Dietary supplementation with resveratrol reduces plaque pathology in a transgenic model of Alzheimer's disease. *Neurochemistry International, 54*(2), 111–118.

Kashiwaya, Y., Bergman, C., Lee, J. H., Wan, R., King, M. T., Mughal, M. R., Okun, E., Clarke, K., Mattson, M. P., & Veech, R. L. (2013). A ketone ester diet exhibits anxiolytic and cognition-sparing properties, and lessens amyloid and tau pathologies in a mouse model of Alzheimer's disease. *Neurobiology of Aging, 34*(6), 1530–1539.

Kashiwaya, Y., King, M. T., & Veech, R. L. (1997). Substrate signaling by insulin: A ketone bodies ratio mimics insulin action in heart. *American Journal of Cardiology, 80*(3A), 50–64.

Kashiwaya, Y., Pawlosky, R., Markis, W., King, M. T., Bergman, C., Srivastava, S., Murray, A., Clarke, K., & Veech, R. L. (2010). A ketone ester diet increases brain malonyl-CoA and uncoupling proteins 4 and 5 while decreasing food intake in the normal Wistar rat. *The Journal of Biological Chemistry, 285*(34), 25950–25956.

Kashiwaya, Y., Takeshima, T., Mori, N., Nakashima, K., Clarke, K., & Veech, R. L. (2000). D-β-Hydroxybutyrate protects neurons in models of Alzheimer's and Parkinson's disease. *Proceedings of the National Academy of Sciences of the United States of America, 97*(10), 5440–5444.

Kasprowska-Liśkiewicz, D., Liśkiewicz, A. D., Nowacka-Chmielewska, M. M., Nowicka, J., Małecki, A., & Barski, J. J. (2017). The ketogenic diet affects the social behavior of young male rats. *Physiology & Behavior, 179,* 168–177.

Katsouri, L., Parr, C., Bogdanovic, N., Willem, M., & Sastre, M. (2011). PPARγ co-activator-1α (PGC-1α) reduces amyloid-β generation through a PPARγ-dependent mechanism. *Journal of Alzheimer's Disease, 25*(1), 151–162.

Kaufmann, F. N., Costa, A. P., Ghisleni, G., Diaz, A. P., Rodrigues, A. L. S., Peluffo, H., & Kaster, M. P. (2017). NLRP3 inflammasome-driven pathways in depression: Clinical and preclinical findings. *Brain, Behavior, and Immunity, 64*, 367–383.

Kaushal, V., & Schlichter, L. C. (2008). Mechanisms of microglia-mediated neurotoxicity in a new model of the stroke penumbra. *Journal of Neuroscience, 28*(9), 2221–2230.

Kawamura, M., Jr., Ruskin, D. N., Geiger, J. D., Boison, D., & Masino, S. A. (2014). Ketogenic diet sensitizes glucose control of hippocampal excitability. *Journal of Lipid Research, 55*(11), 2254–2260.

Kawamura, M., Jr., Ruskin, D. N., & Masino, S. A. (2010). Metabolic autocrine regulation of neurons involves cooperation among pannexin hemichannels, adenosine receptors, and K_{ATP} channels. *Journal of Neuroscience, 30*(11), 3886–3895.

Kazantsev, A. G., & Thompson, L. M. (2008). Therapeutic application of histone deacetylase inhibitors for central nervous system disorders. *Nature Reviews Drug Discovery, 7*(10), 854–868.

Kemp, D. E., Ismail-Beigi, F., Ganocy, S. J., Conroy, C., Gao, K., Obral, S., Fein, E., Findling, R. L., & Calabrese, J. R. (2012). Use of insulin sensitizers for the treatment of major depressive disorder: A pilot study of pioglitazone for major depression accompanied by abdominal obesity. *Journal of Affective Disorders, 136*(3), 1164–1173.

Kensler, T. W., Wakabayashi, N., & Biswal, S. (2007). Cell survival responses to environmental stresses via the Keap1-Nrf2-ARE pathway. *Annual Review of Pharmacology and Toxicology, 47*, 89–116.

Kesl, S. L., Poff, A. M., Ward, N. P., Fiorelli, T. N., Ari, C., Van Putten, A. J., Sherwood, J. W., Arnold, P., & D'Agostino, D. P. (2016). Effects of exogenous ketone supplementation on blood ketone, glucose, triglyceride, and lipoprotein levels in Sprague-Dawley rats. *Nutrition & Metabolism, 13*, 9.

Kheiri, G., Dolatshahi, M., Rahmani, F., & Rezaei, N. (2018). Role of p38/MAPKs in Alzheimer's disease: Implications for amyloid beta toxicity targeted therapy. *Reviews in the Neurosciences, 30*(1), 9–30.

Kiaei, M., Kipiani, K., Chen, J., Calingasan, N. Y., & Beal, M. F. (2005). Peroxisome proliferator-activated receptor-gamma agonist extends survival in transgenic mouse model of amyotrophic lateral sclerosis. *Experimental Neurology, 191*(2), 331–336.

Kilgore, M., Miller, C. A., Fass, D. M., Hennig, K. M., Haggarty, S. J., Sweatt, J. D., & Rumbaugh, G. (2010). Inhibitors of class 1 histone deacetylases reverse contextual memory deficits in a mouse model of

Alzheimer's disease. *Neuropsychopharmacology, 35*(4), 870–880.

Kim, D., Nguyen, M. D., Dobbin, M. M., Fischer, A., Sananbenesi, F., Rodgers, J. T., Delalle, I., Baur, J. A., Sui, G., Armour, S. M., Puigserver, P., Sinclair, D. A., & Tsai, L. H. (2007a). SIRT1 deacetylase protects against neurodegeneration in models for Alzheimer's disease and amyotrophic lateral sclerosis. *EMBO Journal, 26*(13), 3169–3179.

Kim, D. Y., Davis, L. M., Sullivan, P. G., Maalouf, M., Simeone, T. A., van Brederode, J., & Rho, J. M. (2007b). Ketone bodies are protective against oxidative stress in neocortical neurons. *Journal of Neurochemistry, 101*(5), 1316–1326.

Kim, D. Y., Hao, J., Liu, R., Turner, G., Shi, F. D., & Rho, J. M. (2012). Inflammation-mediated memory dysfunction and effects of a ketogenic diet in a murine model of multiple sclerosis. *PLOS ONE, 7*(5), Article e35476.

Kim, D. Y., Simeone, K. A., Simeone, T. A., Pandya, J. D., Wilke, J. C., Ahn, Y., Geddes, J. W., Sullivan, P. G., & Rho, J. M. (2015). Ketone bodies mediate antiseizure effects through mitochondrial permeability transition. *Annals of Neurology, 78*(1), 77–87.

Kim, H. W., Rapoport, S. I., & Rao, J. S. (2011). Altered arachidonic acid cascade enzymes in postmortem brain from bipolar disorder patients. *Molecular Psychiatry, 16*(4), 419–428.

Kim, T., Song, S., Park, Y., Kang, S., & Seo, H. (2019). HDAC inhibition by valproic acid induces neuroprotection and improvement of PD-like behaviors in LRRK2 R1441G transgenic mice. *Experimental Neurobiology, 28*(4), 504–515.

Kim, T., & Yang, Q. (2013). Peroxisome-proliferator-activated receptors regulate redox signaling in the cardiovascular system. *World Journal of Cardiology, 5*(6), 164–174.

Kim, Y. K., & Na, K. S. (2017). Neuroprotection in schizophrenia and its therapeutic implications. *Psychiatry Investigation, 14*(4), 383–391.

Kimura, I., Inoue, D., Maeda, T., Hara, T., Ichimura, A., Miyauchi, S., Kobayashi, M., Hirasawa, A., & Tsujimoto, G. (2011). Short-chain fatty acids and ketones directly regulate sympathetic nervous system via G protein-coupled receptor 41 (GPR41). *Proceedings of the National Academy of Sciences of the United States of America, 108*(19), 8030–8035.

Kincaid, B., & Bossy-Wetzel, E. (2013). Forever young: SIRT3 a shield against mitochondrial meltdown, aging, and neurodegeneration. *Frontiers in Aging Neuroscience, 5*, 48.

Kinsman, S. L., Vining, E. P., Quaskey, S. A., Mellits, D., & Freeman, J. M. (1992). Efficacy of the ketogenic diet for intractable seizure disorders: Review of 58 cases. *Epilepsia, 33*(6), 1132–1136.

Kishi, T., Fukuo, Y., Kitajima, T., Okochi, T., Yamanouchi, Y., Kinoshita, Y., Kawashima, K.,

Inada, T., Kunugi, H., Kato, T., Yoshikawa, T., Ujike, H., Ozaki, N., & Iwata, N. (2011). *SIRT1* gene, schizophrenia and bipolar disorder in the Japanese population: an association study. *Genes, Brain, and Behavior, 10*(3), 257–263.

Kishi, T., Yoshimura, R., Kitajima, T., Okochi, T., Okumura, T., Tsunoka, T., Yamanouchi, Y., Kinoshita, Y., Kawashima, K., Fukuo, Y., Naitoh, H., Umene-Nakano, W., Inada, T., Nakamura, J., Ozaki, N., & Iwata, N. (2010). *SIRT1* gene is associated with major depressive disorder in the Japanese population. *Journal of Affective Disorders, 126*(1–2), 167–173.

Knowles, S., Budney, S., Deodhar, M., Matthews, S. A., Simeone, K. A., & Simeone, T. A. (2018). Ketogenic diet regulates the antioxidant catalase via the transcription factor PPARγ2. *Epilepsy Research, 147*, 71–74.

Kong, X., Wang, R., Xue, Y., Liu, X., Zhang, H., Chen, Y., Fang, F., & Chang, Y. (2010). Sirtuin 3, a new target of PGC-1α, plays an important role in the suppression of ROS and mitochondrial biogenesis. *PLOS ONE, 5*(7), Article e11707.

Kontopoulos, E., Parvin, J. D., & Feany, M. B. (2006). Alpha-synuclein acts in the nucleus to inhibit histone acetylation and promote neurotoxicity. *Human Molecular Genetics, 15*(20), 3012–3023.

Koppel, S. J., & Swerdlow, R. H. (2018). Neuroketotherapeutics: A modern review of a century-old therapy. *Neurochemistry International, 117*, 114–125.

Korkmaz, A., Topal, T., Oter, S., Tan, D. X., & Reiter, R. J. (2008). Hyperglycemia-related pathophysiologic mechanisms and potential beneficial actions of melatonin. *Mini Reviews in Medicinal Chemistry, 8*(11), 1144–1153.

Kossoff, E., & Cervenka, M. (2020). Ketogenic dietary therapy controversies for its second century. *Epilepsy Currents, 20*(3), 125–129.

Kossoff, E. H., McGrogan, J. R., Bluml, R. M., Pillas, D. J., Rubenstein, J. E., & Vining, E. P. (2006). A modified Atkins diet is effective for the treatment of intractable pediatric epilepsy. *Epilepsia, 47*(2), 421–424.

Kossoff, E. H., & Rho, J. M. (2009). Ketogenic diets: Evidence for short- and long-term efficacy. *Neurotherapeutics, 6*(2), 406–414.

Koutnik, A. P., Poff, A. M., Ward, N. P., DeBlasi, J. M., Soliven, M. A., Romero, M. A., Roberson, P. A., Fox, C. D., Roberts, M. D., & D'Agostino, D. P. (2020). Ketone bodies attenuate wasting in models of atrophy. *Journal of Cachexia, Sarcopenia and Muscle, 11*(4), 973–996.

Kovács, Z., Brunner, B., D'Agostino, D. P., & Ari, C. (2020). Inhibition of adenosine A_1 receptors abolished the nutritional ketosis-evoked delay in the onset of isoflurane-induced anesthesia in Wistar Albino Glaxo Rijswijk rats. *BMC Anesthesiology, 20*(1), 30.

Kovács, Z., D'Agostino, D. P., & Ari, C. (2018). Anxiolytic effect of exogenous ketone supplementation is abolished by adenosine A_1 receptor inhibition in Wistar Albino Glaxo/Rijswijk rats. *Frontiers in Behavioral Neuroscience, 12*, 29.

Kovács, Z., D'Agostino, D. P., Diamond, D. M., & Ari, C. (2019a). Exogenous ketone supplementation decreased the lipopolysaccharide-induced increase in absence epileptic activity in Wistar Albino Glaxo Rijswijk rats. *Frontiers in Molecular Neuroscience, 12*, 45.

Kovács, Z., D'Agostino, D. P., Diamond, D., Kindy, M. S., Rogers, C., & Ari, C. (2019b). Therapeutic potential of exogenous ketone supplement induced ketosis in the treatment of psychiatric disorders: Review of current literature. *Frontiers in Psychiatry, 10*, 363.

Kovács, Z., D'Agostino, D. P., Dobolyi, A., & Ari, C. (2017). Adenosine A_1 receptor antagonism abolished the anti-seizure effects of exogenous ketone supplementation in Wistar Albino Glaxo Rijswijk rats. *Frontiers in Molecular Neuroscience, 10*, 235.

Kovács, Z., Dobolyi, A., Kékesi, K. A., & Juhász, G. (2013). 5′-Nucleotidases, nucleosides and their distribution in the brain: Pathological and therapeutic implications. *Current Medicinal Chemistry, 20*(34), 4217–4240.

Kovács, Z., Kékesi, K. A., Juhász, G., & Dobolyi, A. (2014). The antiepileptic potential of nucleosides. *Current Medicinal Chemistry, 21*(6), 788–821.

Kovács, Z., Kékesi, K. A., Szilágyi, N., Abrahám, I., Székács, D., Király, N., Papp, E., Császár, I., Szego, E., Barabás, K., Péterfy, H., Erdei, A., Bártfai, T., & Juhász, G. (2006). Facilitation of spike-wave discharge activity by lipopolysaccharides in Wistar Albino Glaxo/Rijswijk rats. *Neuroscience, 140*(2), 731–742.

Kraeuter, A. K., Loxton, H., Lima, B. C., Rudd, D., & Sarnyai, Z. (2015). Ketogenic diet reverses behavioral abnormalities in an acute NMDA receptor hypofunction model of schizophrenia. *Schizophrenia Research, 169*(1–3), 491–493.

Kraeuter, A. K., Mashavave, T., Suvarna, A., van den Buuse, M., & Sarnyai, Z. (2020a). Effects of beta-hydroxybutyrate administration on MK-801-induced schizophrenia-like behaviour in mice. *Psychopharmacology, 237*(5), 1397–1405.

Kraeuter, A. K., Phillips, R., & Sarnyai, Z. (2020b). Ketogenic therapy in neurodegenerative and psychiatric disorders: From mice to men. *Progress in Neuro-Psychopharmacology & Biological Psychiatry, 101*, 109913.

Kraft, B. D., & Westman, E. C. (2009). Schizophrenia, gluten, and low-carbohydrate, ketogenic diets: A case report and review of the literature. *Nutrition & Metabolism, 6*, 10.

Krikorian, R., Shidler, M. D., Dangelo, K., Couch, S. C., Benoit, S. C., & Clegg, D. J. (2012). Dietary ketosis enhances memory in mild cognitive impairment. *Neurobiology of Aging. 33*(2), 425. e19–e27.

Kroemer, G., Galluzzi, L., & Brenner, C. (2007). Mitochondrial membrane permeabilization in cell death. *Physiological Reviews, 87*(1), 99–163.

Krystal, J. H., Sanacora, G., Blumberg, H., Anand, A., Charney, D. S., Marek, G., Epperson, C. N., Goddard, A., & Mason, G. F. (2002). Glutamate and GABA systems as targets for novel antidepressant and mood-stabilizing treatments. *Molecular Psychiatry, 7*, 71–80.

Kubová, H., Druga, R., Lukasiuk, K., Suchomelová, L., Haugvicová, R., Jirmanová, I., & Pitkänen, A. (2001). Status epilepticus causes necrotic damage in the mediodorsal nucleus of the thalamus in immature rats. *Journal of Neuroscience, 21*(10), 3593–3599.

Kudin, A. P., Kudina, T. A., Seyfried, J., Vielhaber, S., Beck, H., Elger, C. E., & Kunz, W. S. (2002). Seizure-dependent modulation of mitochondrial oxidative phosphorylation in rat hippocampus. *European Journal of Neuroscience, 15*(7), 1105–1114.

Kudlow, P. A., Cha, D. S., Lam, R. W., & McIntyre, R. S. (2013). Sleep architecture variation: A mediator of metabolic disturbance in individuals with major depressive disorder. *Sleep Medicine, 14*(10), 943–949.

Kumar, P., Kalonia, H., & Kumar, A. (2010). Huntington's disease: Pathogenesis to animal models. *Pharmacological Reports, 62*(1), 1–14.

Kunz, W. S., Kudin, A. P., Vielhaber, S., Blümcke, I., Zuschratter, W., Schramm, J., Beck, H., & Elger, C. E. (2000). Mitochondrial complex I deficiency in the epileptic focus of patients with temporal lobe epilepsy. *Annals of Neurology, 48*(5), 766–773.

Kurita, M., Nishino, S., Numata, Y., Okubo, Y., & Sato, T. (2015). The noradrenaline metabolite MHPG is a candidate biomarker between the depressive, remission, and manic states in bipolar disorder I: Two long-term naturalistic case reports. *Neuropsychiatric Disease and Treatment, 11*, 353–358.

Lambrechts, D. A., de Kinderen, R. J., Vles, H. S., de Louw, A. J., Aldenkamp, A. P., & Majoie, M. J. (2015). The MCT-ketogenic diet as a treatment option in refractory childhood epilepsy: A prospective study with 2-year follow-up. *Epilepsy & Behavior, 51*, 261–266.

Laplante, M., & Sabatini, D. M. (2009). mTOR signaling at a glance. *Journal of Cell Science, 122*(Pt 20), 3589–3594.

Lau, D., Bengtson, C. P., Buchthal, B., & Bading, H. (2015). BDNF reduces toxic extrasynaptic NMDA receptor signaling via synaptic NMDA receptors and nuclear-calcium-induced transcription of inhba/activin A. *Cell Reports, 12*(8), 1353–1366.

Lee, E., Kang, H. C., & Kim, H. D. (2016). Ketogenic diet for children with epilepsy: A practical meal plan in a hospital. *Clinical Nutrition Research, 5*(1), 60–63.

Lee, J. C., Laydon, J. T., McDonnell, P. C., Gallagher, T. F., Kumar, S., Green, D., McNulty, D., Blumenthal, M. J., Heys, J. R., Landvatter, S. W., Strickler, J. E., McLaughlin, M. M., Siemens, I. R., Fisher, S. M., Livi, G. P., White, J. R., Adams, J. L., & Young, P. R. (1994). A protein kinase involved in the regulation of inflammatory cytokine biosynthesis. *Nature, 372*(6508), 739–746.

Leedom, L. J., Meehan, W. P., & Zeidler, A. (1987). Avoidance responding in mice with diabetes mellitus. *Physiology & Behavior, 40*(4), 447–451.

Leffa, D. T., Bellaver, B., de Oliveira, C., de Macedo, I. C., de Freitas, J. S., Grevet, E. H., Caumo, W., Rohde, L. A., Quincozes-Santos, A., & Torres, I. L. S. (2017). Increased oxidative parameters and decreased cytokine levels in an animal model of attention-deficit/hyperactivity disorder. *Neurochemical Research, 42*(11), 3084–3092.

Lemonnier, E., Villeneuve, N., Sonie, S., Serret, S., Rosier, A., Roue, M., Brosset, P., Viellard, M., Bernoux, D., Rondeau, S., Thummler, S., Ravel, D., & Ben-Ari, Y. (2017). Effects of bumetanide on neurobehavioral function in children and adolescents with autism spectrum disorders. *Translational Psychiatry, 7*(3), e1056.

Levy, M., Thaiss, C. A., & Elinav, E. (2015). Taming the inflammasome. *Nature Medicine, 21*(3), 213–215.

Lewis, D. A., Volk, D. W., & Hashimoto, T. (2004). Selective alterations in prefrontal cortical GABA neurotransmission in schizophrenia: A novel target for the treatment of working memory dysfunction. *Psychopharmacology, 174*(1), 143–150.

Li, R. J., Liu, Y., Liu, H. Q., & Li, J. (2020). Ketogenic diets and protective mechanisms in epilepsy, metabolic disorders, cancer, neuronal loss, and muscle and nerve degeneration. *Journal of Food Biochemistry, 44*(3), e13140.

Li, X. (2012). Using the conditioned fear stress (CFS) animal model to understand the neurobiological mechanisms and pharmacological treatment of anxiety. *Shanghai Archives of Psychiatry, 24*(5), 241–249.

Libert, S., Pointer, K., Bell, E. L., Das, A., Cohen, D. E., Asara, J. M., Kapur, K., Bergmann, S., Preisig, M., Otowa, T., Kendler, K. S., Chen, X., Hettema, J. M., van den Oord, E. J., Rubio, J. P., & Guarente, L. (2011). SIRT1 activates MAO$_A$ in the brain to mediate anxiety and exploratory drive. *Cell, 147*(7), 1459–1472.

Lim, A., & Thomas, R. H. (2020). The mitochondrial epilepsies. *European Journal of Paediatric Neurology, 24*, 47–52.

Lim, J. E., Song, M., Jin, J., Kou, J., Pattanayak, A., Lalonde, R., & Fukuchi, K. (2012). The effects of MyD88 deficiency on exploratory activity, anxiety, motor coordination, and spatial learning in

C57BL/6 and APPswe/PS1dE9 mice. *Behavioural Brain Research, 227*(1), 36–42.

Lim, S., Chesser, A. S., Grima, J. C., Rappold, P. M., Blum, D., Przedborski, S., & Tieu, K. (2011). D-β-Hydroxybutyrate is protective in mouse models of Huntington's disease. *PLOS ONE, 6*(9), e24620.

Lin, J., Wu, P. H., Tarr, P. T., Lindenberg, K. S., St-Pierre, J., Zhang, C. Y., Mootha, V. K., Jäger, S., Vianna, C. R., Reznick, R. M., Cui, L., Manieri, M., Donovan, M. X., Wu, Z., Cooper, M. P., Fan, M. C., Rohas, L. M., Zavacki, A. M., Cinti, S., Spiegelman, B. M. (2004). Defects in adaptive energy metabolism with CNS-linked hyperactivity in PGC-1α null mice. *Cell, 119*(1), 121–135.

Lin, M. T., & Beal, M. F. (2006). Mitochondrial dysfunction and oxidative stress in neurodegenerative diseases. *Nature, 443*(7113), 787–795.

Liu, X., Wu, Z., Hayashi, Y., & Nakanishi, H. (2012). Age-dependent neuroinflammatory responses and deficits in long-term potentiation in the hippocampus during systemic inflammation. *Neuroscience, 216*, 133–142.

Lloret, A., & Beal, M. F. (2019). PGC-1α, sirtuins and PARPs in Huntington's disease and other neurodegenerative conditions: NAD$^+$ to rule them all. *Neurochemical Research, 44*(10), 2423–2434.

Lu, G., Li, J., Zhang, H., Zhao, X., Yan, L. J., & Yang, X. (2018). Role and possible mechanisms of SIRT1 in depression. *Oxidative Medicine and Cellular Longevity, 2018*, 8596903.

Lu, X., Wang, L., Yu, C., Yu, D., & Yu, G. (2015). Histone acetylation modifiers in the pathogenesis of Alzheimer's disease. *Frontiers in Cellular Neuroscience, 9*, 226.

Ludwig, D. S. (2020).The ketogenic diet: Evidence for optimism but high-quality research needed. *Journal of Nutrition, 150*(6), 1354–1359.

Lugrin, J., Rosenblatt-Velin, N., Parapanov, R., & Liaudet, L. (2014). The role of oxidative stress during inflammatory processes. *Biological Chemistry, 395*(2), 203–230.

Lund, T. M., Ploug, K. B., Iversen, A., Jensen, A. A., & Jansen-Olesen, I. (2015). The metabolic impact of β-hydroxybutyrate on neurotransmission: Reduced glycolysis mediates changes in calcium responses and KATP channel receptor sensitivity. *Journal of Neurochemistry, 132*(5), 520–531.

Luo, X. J., & Zhang, C. (2016). Down-regulation of SIRT1 gene expression in major depressive disorder. *American Journal of Psychiatry, 173*(10), 1046.

Ma, S., Hangya, B., Leonard, C. S., Wisden, W., & Gundlach, A. L. (2018). Dual-transmitter systems regulating arousal, attention, learning and memory. *Neuroscience and Biobehavioral Reviews, 85*, 21–33.

Ma, W., Berg, J., & Yellen, G. (2007). Ketogenic diet metabolites reduce firing in central neurons by opening K$_{ATP}$ channels. *Journal of Neuroscience, 27*(14), 3618–3625.

Maalouf, M., & Rho, J. M. (2008). Oxidative impairment of hippocampal long-term potentiation involves activation of protein phosphatase 2A and is prevented by ketone bodies. *Journal of Neuroscience Research, 86*(15), 3322–3330.

Maalouf, M., Rho, J. M., & Mattson, M. P. (2009). The neuroprotective properties of calorie restriction, the ketogenic diet, and ketone bodies. *Brain Research Reviews, 59*(2), 293–315.

Maalouf, M., Sullivan, P. G., Davis, L., Kim, D. Y., & Rho, J. M. (2007). Ketones inhibit mitochondrial production of reactive oxygen species production following glutamate excitotoxicity by increasing NADH oxidation. *Neuroscience, 145*(1), 256–264.

Machado-Vieira, R., Lara, D. R., Souza, D. O., & Kapczinski, F. (2002). Purinergic dysfunction in mania: An integrative model. *Medical Hypotheses, 58*(4), 297–304.

Mahgoub, M., & Monteggia, L. M. (2014). A role for histone deacetylases in the cellular and behavioral mechanisms underlying learning and memory. *Learning & Memory, 21*(10), 564–568.

Manford, M. (2017). Recent advances in epilepsy. *Journal of Neurology, 264*(8), 1811–1824.

Manning, B. D., & Cantley, L. C. (2007). AKT/PKB signaling: Navigating downstream. *Cell, 129*(7), 1261–1274.

Marosi, K., Kim, S. W., Moehl, K., Scheibye-Knudsen, M., Cheng, A., Cutler, R., Camandola, S., & Mattson, M. P. (2016). 3-Hydroxybutyrate regulates energy metabolism and induces BDNF expression in cerebral cortical neurons. *Journal of Neurochemistry, 139*(5), 769–781.

Martin, L. J., & Chang, Q. (2012). Inhibitory synaptic regulation of motoneurons: A new target of disease mechanisms in amyotrophic lateral sclerosis. *Molecular Neurobiology, 45*(1), 30–42.

Masino, S. A., Kawamura, M., Wasser, C. D., Pomeroy, L. T., & Ruskin, D. N. (2009). Adenosine, ketogenic diet and epilepsy: The emerging therapeutic relationship between metabolism and brain activity. *Current Neuropharmacology, 7*(3), 257–268.

Masino, S. A., Li, T., Theofilas, P., Sandau, U. S., Ruskin, D. N., Fredholm, B. B., Geiger, J. D., Aronica, E., & Boison, D. (2011). A ketogenic diet suppresses seizures in mice through adenosine A$_1$ receptors. *Journal of Clinical Investigation, 121*(7), 2679–2683.

Masliah, E., Mallory, M., Alford, M., DeTeresa, R., Hansen, L. A., McKeel, D. W., Jr., & Morris, J. C. (2001). Altered expression of synaptic proteins occurs early during progression of Alzheimer's disease. *Neurology, 56*(1), 127–129.

Masuda, R., Monahan, J. W., & Kashiwaya, Y. (2005). D-β-Hydroxybutyrate is neuroprotective against hypoxia in serum-free hippocampal primary cultures. *Journal of Neuroscience Research, 80*(4), 501–509.

Mattson, M. P., Lovell, M. A., Furukawa, K., & Markesbery, W. R. (1995). Neurotrophic factors attenuate glutamate-induced accumulation of peroxides, elevation of intracellular Ca²⁺ concentration, and neurotoxicity and increase antioxidant enzyme activities in hippocampal neurons. *Journal of Neurochemistry, 65*(4), 1740–1751.

Mazarati, A., & Sankar, R. (2016). Common mechanisms underlying epileptogenesis and the comorbidities of epilepsy. *Cold Spring Harbor Perspectives in Medicine, 6*(7), pii: a022798.

McCarty, M. F., DiNicolantonio, J. J., & O'Keefe, J. H. (2015). Ketosis may promote brain macroautophagy by activating SIRT1 and hypoxia-inducible factor-1. *Medical Hypotheses, 85*(5), 631–639.

McCullumsmith, R. E., Clinton, S. M., & Meador-Woodruff, J. H. (2004). Schizophrenia as a disorder of neuroplasticity. *International Review of Neurobiology, 59*, 19–45.

McDaniel, S. S., Rensing, N. R., Thio, L. L., Yamada, K. A., & Wong, M. (2011). The ketogenic diet inhibits the mammalian target of rapamycin (mTOR) pathway. *Epilepsia, 52*(3), e7–11.

McNally, M. A., & Hartman, A. L. (2012). Ketone bodies in epilepsy. *Journal of Neurochemistry, 121*(1), 28–35.

Mehlman, M. A., & Veech, R. L. (1972). Redox and phosphorylation states and metabolite concentrations in frozen clamped livers of rats fed diets containing 1,3-butanediol and DL-carnitine. *Journal of Nutrition, 102*(1), 45–51.

Menu, P., Mayor, A., Zhou, R., Tardivel, A., Ichijo, H., Mori, K., & Tschopp, J. (2012). ER stress activates the NLRP3 inflammasome via an UPR-independent pathway. *Cell Death & Disease, 3*(1), e261.

Menzies, K. J., Zhang, H., Katsyuba, E., & Auwerx, J. (2016). Protein acetylation in metabolism—Metabolites and cofactors. *Nature Reviews Endocrinology, 12*(1), 43–60.

Mertens, J., Wang, Q. W., Kim, Y., Yu, D. X., Pham, S., Yang, B., Zheng, Y., Diffenderfer, K. E., Zhang, J., Soltani, S., Eames, T., Schafer, S. T., Boyer, L., Marchetto, M. C., Nurnberger, J. I., Calabrese, J. R., Ødegaard, K. J., McCarthy, M. J., Zandi, P. P., & Yao, J. (2015). Differential responses to lithium in hyperexcitable neurons from patients with bipolar disorder. *Nature, 527*(7576), 95–99.

Michán, S., Li, Y., Chou, M. M., Parrella, E., Ge, H., Long, J. M., Allard, J. S., Lewis, K., Miller, M., Xu, W., Mervis, R. F., Chen, J., Guerin, K. I., Smith, L. E., McBurney, M. W., Sinclair, D. A., Baudry, M., de Cabo, R., & Longo, V. D. (2010). SIRT1 is essential for normal cognitive function and synaptic plasticity. *Journal of Neuroscience, 30*(29), 9695–9707.

Miller, A. H., & Raison, C. L. (2016). The role of inflammation in depression: From evolutionary imperative to modern treatment target. *Nature Reviews Immunology, 16*(1), 22–34.

Miller, B. J., Buckley, P., Seabolt, W., Mellor, A., & Kirkpatrick, B. (2011). Meta-analysis of cytokine alterations in schizophrenia: Clinical status and antipsychotic effects. *Biological Psychiatry, 70*(7), 663–671.

Moghaddam, B., & Javitt, D. (2012). From revolution to evolution: The glutamate hypothesis of schizophrenia and its implication for treatment. *Neuropsychopharmacology, 37*(1), 4–15.

Monti, B., Polazzi, E., & Contestabile, A. (2009). Biochemical, molecular and epigenetic mechanisms of valproic acid neuroprotection. *Current Molecular Pharmacology, 2*(1), 95–109.

Morris, B. J. (2005). A forkhead in the road to longevity: The molecular basis of lifespan becomes clearer. *Journal of Hypertension, 23*(7), 1285–1309.

Morris, G., Puri, B. K., Carvalho, A., Maes, M., Berk, M., Ruusunen, A., & Olive, L. (2020). Induced ketosis as a treatment for neuroprogressive disorders: Food for thought? *The International Journal of Neuropsychopharmacology, 23*(6), 366–384.

Mosconi, L., de Leon, M., Murray, J, E, L., Lu, J., Javier, E., McHugh, P., & Swerdlow, R. H. (2011). Reduced mitochondria cytochrome oxidase activity in adult children of mothers with Alzheimer's disease. *Journal of Alzheimer's Disease, 27*(3), 483–490.

Möhler, H. (2012). The GABA system in anxiety and depression and its therapeutic potential. *Neuropharmacology, 62*(1), 42–53.

Mu, C., Corley, M. J., Lee, R. W. Y., Wong, M., Pang, A., Arakaki, G., Miyamoto, R., Rho, J. M., Mickiewicz, B., Dowlatabadi, R., Vogel, H. J., Korchemagin, Y., & Shearer, J. (2020). Metabolic framework for the improvement of autism spectrum disorders by a modified ketogenic diet: A pilot study. *Journal of Proteome Research, 19*(1), 382–390.

Mudò, G., Mäkelä, J., Di Liberto, V., Tselykh, T. V., Olivieri, M., Piepponen, P., Eriksson, O., Mälkiä, A., Bonomo, A., Kairisalo, M., Aguirre, J. A., Korhonen, L., Belluardo, N., & Lindholm, D. (2012). Transgenic expression and activation of PGC-1α protect dopaminergic neurons in the MPTP mouse model of Parkinson's disease. *Cellular and Molecular Life Sciences, 69*(7), 1153–1165.

Murphy, P., & Burnham, W. M. (2006). The ketogenic diet causes a reversible decrease in activity level in Long-Evans rats. *Experimental Neurology, 201*(1), 84–89.

Murphy, P., Likhodii, S., Nylen, K., & Burnham, W. M. (2004). The antidepressant properties of the ketogenic diet. *Biological Psychiatry, 56*(12), 981–983.

Müller, N., & Schwarz, M. J. (2007). The immune-mediated alteration of serotonin and glutamate: Towards an integrated view of depression. *Molecular Psychiatry, 12*(11), 988–1000.

Myette-Côté, É., Neudorf, H., Rafiei, H., Clarke, K., & Little, J. P. (2018). Prior ingestion of exogenous ketone monoester attenuates the glycaemic response to an oral glucose tolerance test in healthy young individuals. *The Journal of Physiology, 596*(8), 1385–1395.

Myhrer, T. (2003). Neurotransmitter systems involved in learning and memory in the rat: A meta-analysis based on studies of four behavioral tasks. *Brain Research Brain Research Reviews, 41*(2–3), 268–287.

Nabbout, R., Mazzuca, M., Hubert, P., Peudennier, S., Allaire, C., Flurin, V., Aberastury, M., Silva, W., & Dulac, O. (2010). Efficacy of ketogenic diet in severe refractory status epilepticus initiating fever induced refractory epileptic encephalopathy in school age children (FIRES). *Epilepsia, 51*(10), 2033–2037.

Nagy, J., Zámbó, K., & Decsi, L. (1979). Anti-anxiety action of diazepam after intra-amygdaloid application in the rat. *Neuropharmacology, 18*(6), 573–576.

Nathan, J., Bailur, S., Datay, K., Sharma, S., & Khedekar Kale, D. (2019). A switch to polyunsaturated fatty acid based ketogenic diet improves seizure control in patients with drug-resistant epilepsy on the mixed fat ketogenic diet: A retrospective open label trial. *Cureus, 11*(12), e6399.

Neth, B. J., Mintz, A., Whitlow, C., Jung, Y., Solingapuram Sai, K., Register, T. C., Kellar, D., Lockhart, S. N., Hoscheidt, S., Maldjian, J., Heslegrave, A. J., Blennow, K., Cunnane, S. C., Castellano, C. A., Zetterberg, H., & Craft, S. (2020). Modified ketogenic diet is associated with improved cerebrospinal fluid biomarker profile, cerebral perfusion, and cerebral ketone body uptake in older adults at risk for Alzheimer's disease: A pilot study. *Neurobiology of Aging, 86*, 54–63.

Netzahualcoyotzi, C., & Tapia, R. (2015). Degeneration of spinal motor neurons by chronic AMPA-induced excitotoxicity in vivo and protection by energy substrates. *Acta Neuropathologica Communications, 3*, 27.

Neudorf, H., Durrer, C., Myette-Cote, E., Makins, C., O'Malley, T., & Little, J. P. (2019). Oral ketone supplementation acutely increases markers of NLRP3 inflammasome activation in human monocytes. *Molecular Nutrition and Food Research, 63*(11), Article e1801171.

Neudorf, H., Myette-Côté, É., & Little, J. P. (2020). The impact of acute ingestion of a ketone monoester drink on LPS-stimulated NLRP3 activation in humans with obesity. *Nutrients, 12*(3), pii: E854.

Nevitt, S. J., Sudell, M., Weston, J., Tudur Smith, C., & Marson, A. G. (2017). Antiepileptic drug monotherapy for epilepsy: A network meta-analysis of individual participant data. *Cochrane Database of Systematic Reviews, 12*(12), CD011412.

Newman, J. C., & Verdin, E. (2014a). β-Hydroxybutyrate: Much more than a metabolite. *Diabetes Research and Clinical Practice, 106*(2), 173–181.

Newman, J. C., & Verdin, E. (2014b). Ketone bodies as signaling metabolites. *Trends in Endocrinology and Metabolism, 25*(1), 42–52.

Newport, M. T., VanItallie, T. B., Kashiwaya, Y., King, M. T., & Veech, R. L. (2015). A new way to produce hyperketonemia: Use of ketone ester in a case of Alzheimer's disease. *Alzheimer's & Dementia, 11*(1), 99–103.

Nierenberg, A. A., Ghaznavi, S. A., Sande Mathias, I., Ellard, K. K., Janos, J. A., & Sylvia, L. G. (2018). Peroxisome proliferator-activated receptor gamma coactivator-1α as a novel target for bipolar disorder and other neuropsychiatric disorders. *Biological Psychiatry, 83*(9), 761–769.

Niquet, J., & Wasterlain, C. G. (2004). Bim, Bad, and Bax: A deadly combination in epileptic seizures. *Journal of Clinical Investigation, 113*(7), 960–962.

Nivoli, A., Porcelli, S., Albani, D., Forloni, G., Fusco, F., Colom, F., Vieta, E., & Serretti, A. (2016). Association between sirtuin 1 gene rs10997870 polymorphism and suicide behaviors in bipolar disorder. *Neuropsychobiology, 74*(1), 1–7.

Noh, H. S., Kim, Y. S., & Choi, W. S. (2008). Neuroprotective effects of the ketogenic diet. *Epilepsia, 49*, 120–123.

Noh, H. S., Kim, Y. S., Kim, Y. H., Han, J. Y., Park, C. H., Kang, A. K., Shin, H. S., Kang, S. S., Cho, G. J., & Choi, W. S. (2006). Ketogenic diet protects the hippocampus from kainic acid toxicity by inhibiting the dissociation of bad from 14-3-3. *Journal of Neuroscience Research, 84*(8), 1829–1836.

Noh, H. S., Kim, Y. S., Lee, H. P., Chung, K. M., Kim, D. W., Kang, S. S., Cho, G. J., & Choi, W. S. (2003). The protective effect of a ketogenic diet on kainic acid-induced hippocampal cell death in the male ICR mice. *Epilepsy Research, 53*(1–2), 119–128.

Nordli, D. R. Jr., Kuroda, M. M., Carroll, J., Koenigsberger, D. Y., Hirsch, L. J., Bruner, H. J., Seidel, W. T., & De Vivo, D. C. (2001). Experience with the ketogenic diet in infants. *Pediatrics, 108*(1), 129–133.

Norwitz, N. G., Hu, M. T., & Clarke, K. (2019). The mechanisms by which the ketone body D-β-hydroxybutyrate may improve the multiple cellular pathologies of Parkinson's disease. *Frontiers in Nutrition, 6*, 63.

Nunomura, A., Perry, G., Aliev, G., Hirai, K., Takeda, A., Balraj, E. K., Jones, P. K., Ghanbari, H., Wataya, T., Shimohama, S., Chiba, S., Atwood, C. S., Petersen, R. B., & Smith, M. A. (2001). Oxidative damage is the earliest event in Alzheimer disease. *Journal of Neuropathology and Experimental Neurology, 60*(8), 759–767.

Oades, R. D., Slusarek, M., Velling, S., & Bondy, B. (2002). Serotonin platelet-transporter measures in childhood attention-deficit/hyperactivity disorder (ADHD): Clinical versus experimental measures of impulsivity. *The World Journal of Biological Psychiatry, 3*(2), 96–100.

Offermanns, S. (2006). The nicotinic acid receptor GPR109A (HM74A or PUMA-G) as a new therapeutic target. *Trends in Pharmacological Sciences, 27*(7), 384–390.

Offermanns, S., & Schwaninger, M. (2015). Nutritional or pharmacological activation of HCA$_2$ ameliorates neuroinflammation. *Trends in Molecular Medicine, 21*(4), 245–255.

Olmos, Y., Valle, I., Borniquel, S., Tierrez, A., Soria, E., Lamas, S., & Monsalve, M. (2009). Mutual dependence of Foxo3a and PGC-1α in the induction of oxidative stress genes. *The Journal of Biological Chemistry, 284*(21), 14476–14484.

Olson, C. A., Vuong, H. E., Yano, J. M., Liang, Q. Y., Nusbaum, D. J., & Hsiao, E. Y. (2018). The gut microbiota mediates the anti-seizure effects of the ketogenic diet. *Cell, 173*(7), 1728–1741.

Orth, M., & Schapira, A. H. (2001). Mitochondria and degenerative disorders. *American Journal of Medical Genetics, 106*(1), 27–36.

Ota, M., Matsuo, J., Ishida, I., Hattori, K., Teraishi, T., Tonouchi, H., Ashida, K., Takahashi, T., & Kunugi, H. (2016). Effect of a ketogenic meal on cognitive function in elderly adults: Potential for cognitive enhancement. *Psychopharmacology, 233*(21–22), 3797–3802.

Otani, K., Yamatodani, A., Wada, H., Mimaki, T., & Yabuuchi, H. (1984). Effect of ketogenic diet on the convulsive threshold and brain amino acid and monoamine levels in young mice. *No To Hattatsu, 16*(3), 196–204.

Otte, C., Gold, S. M., Penninx, B. W., Pariante, C. M., Etkin, A., Fava, M., Mohr, D. C., & Schatzberg, A. F. (2016). Major depressive disorder. *Nature Reviews Disease Primers, 2*, 16065.

Packer, R. M., Law, T. H., Davies, E., Zanghi, B., Pan, Y., & Volk, H. A. (2016). Effects of a ketogenic diet on ADHD-like behavior in dogs with idiopathic epilepsy. *Epilepsy & Behavior, 55*, 62–68.

Page, K. A., Williamson, A., Yu, N., McNay, E. C., Dzuira, J., McCrimmon, R. J., & Sherwin, R. S. (2009). Medium-chain fatty acids improve cognitive function in intensively treated type 1 diabetic patients and support in vitro synaptic transmission during acute hypoglycemia. *Diabetes, 58*(5), 1237–1244.

Pallàs, M., Pizarro, J. G., Gutierrez-Cuesta, J., Crespo-Biel, N., Alvira, D., Tajes, M., Yeste-Velasco, M., Folch, J., Canudas, A. M., Sureda, F. X., Ferrer, I., & Camins, A. (2008). Modulation of SIRT1 expression in different neurodegenerative models and human pathologies. *Neuroscience, 154*(4), 1388–1397.

Palmer, C. M. (2017). Ketogenic diet in the treatment of schizoaffective disorder: Two case studies. *Schizophrenia Research, 189*, 208–209.

Pan, S., Hu, P., You, Q., Chen, J., Wu, J., Zhang, Y., Cai, Z., Ye, T., Xu, X., Chen, Z., et al. (2020). Evaluation of the antidepressive property of β-hydroxybutyrate in mice. *Behavioural Pharmacology, 31*(4), 322–332.

Pan, Y., Larson, B., Araujo, J. A., Lau, W., de Rivera, C., Santana, R., Gore, A., & Milgram, N. W. (2010). Dietary supplementation with medium-chain TAG has long-lasting cognition-enhancing effects in aged dogs. *British Journal of Nutrition, 103*(12), 1746–1754.

Paoli, A., Bosco, G., Camporesi, E. M., & Mangar, D. (2015). Ketosis, ketogenic diet and food intake control: A complex relationship. *Frontiers in Psychology, 6*, 27.

Parker, J. A., Arango, M., Abderrahmane, S., Lambert, E., Tourette, C., Catoire, H., & Néri, C. (2005). Resveratrol rescues mutant polyglutamine cytotoxicity in nematode and mammalian neurons. *Nature Genetics, 37*(4), 349–350.

Parodi, B., Rossi, S., Morando, S., Cordano, C., Bragoni, A., Motta, C., Usai, C., Wipke, B. T., Scannevin, R. H., Mancardi, G.L., Centonze, D., Kerlero de Rosbo, N., & Uccelli, A. (2015). Fumarates modulate microglia activation through a novel HCAR2 signaling pathway and rescue synaptic dysregulation in inflamed CNS. *Acta Neuropathologica, 130*(2), 279–295.

Patel, M. N., Carroll, R. G., Galván-Peña, S., Mills, E. L., Olden, R., Triantafilou, M., Wolf, A. I., Bryant, C. E., Triantafilou, K., & Masters, S. L. (2017). Inflammasome priming in sterile inflammatory disease. *Trends in Molecular Medicine, 23*(2), 165–180.

Pathak, D., Berthet, A., & Nakamura, K. (2013). Energy failure: Does it contribute to neurodegeneration? *Annals of Neurology, 74*(4), 506–516.

Pawlosky, R. J., Kashiwaya, Y., King, M. T., & Veech, R. L. (2020). A dietary ketone ester normalizes abnormal behavior in a mouse model of Alzheimer's disease. *International Journal of Molecular Sciences, 21*(3), pii: E1044.

Pawlosky, R. J., Kemper, M. F., Kashiwaya, Y., King, M. T., Mattson, M. P., & Veech, R. L. (2017). Effects of a dietary ketone ester on hippocampal glycolytic and tricarboxylic acid cycle intermediates and amino acids in a 3xTgAD mouse model of Alzheimer's disease. *Journal of Neurochemistry, 141*(2), 195–207.

Pearson, J. N., Rowley, S., Liang, L. P., White, A. M., Day, B. J., & Patel, M. (2015). Reactive oxygen species mediate cognitive deficits in experimental temporal lobe epilepsy. *Neurobiology of Disease, 82*, 289–297.

Peleg, S., Sananbenesi, F., Zovoilis, A., Burkhardt, S., Bahari-Javan, S., Agis-Balboa, R. C., Cota,

P., Wittnam, J. L., Gogol-Doering, A., Opitz, L., Salinas-Riester, G., Dettenhofer, M., Kang, H., Farinelli, L., Chen, W., & Fischer, A. (2010). Altered histone acetylation is associated with age-dependent memory impairment in mice. *Science, 328*(5979), 753–756.

Peña-Altamira, L. E., Polazzi, E., & Monti, B. (2013). Histone post-translational modifications in Huntington's and Parkinson's diseases. *Current Pharmaceutical Design, 19*(28), 5085–5092.

Petty, F. (1995). GABA and mood disorders: a brief review and hypothesis. *Journal of Affective Disorders, 34*(4), 275–281.

Pérez-Pérez, D., Frías-Soria, C. L., & Rocha, L. (2021). Drug-resistant epilepsy: From multiple hypotheses to an integral explanation using preclinical resources. *Epilepsy & Behavior, 121*(Pt B), 106430.

Phelps, J. R., Siemers, S. V., & El-Mallakh, R. S. (2013). The ketogenic diet for type II bipolar disorder. *Neurocase, 19*(5), 423–426.

Phiel, C. J., Zhang, F., Huang, E. Y., Guenther, M. G., Lazar, M. A., & Klein, P. S. (2001). Histone deacetylase is a direct target of valproic acid, a potent anticonvulsant, mood stabilizer, and teratogen. *The Journal of Biological Chemistry, 276*(39), 36734–36741.

Phillips, C., & Fahimi, A. (2018). Immune and neuroprotective effects of physical activity on the brain in depression. *Frontiers in Neuroscience, 12*, 498.

Phillips, M. C. L., Murtagh, D. K. J., Gilbertson, L. J., Asztely, F. J. S., & Lynch, C. D. P. (2018). Low-fat versus ketogenic diet in Parkinson's disease: A pilot randomized controlled trial. *Movement Disorders, 33*(8), 1306–1314.

Pinto, A., Bonucci, A., Maggi, E., Corsi, M., & Businaro, R. (2018). Anti-oxidant and anti-inflammatory activity of ketogenic diet: New perspectives for neuroprotection in Alzheimer's disease. *Antioxidants, 7*(5), pii: E63.

Pisanu, C., & Squassina, A. (2019). Treatment-resistant schizophrenia: Insights from genetic studies and machine learning approaches. *Frontiers in Pharmacology, 10*, 617.

Plecko, B., Stoeckler-Ipsiroglu, S., Schober, E., Harrer, G., Mlynarik, V., Gruber, S., Moser, E., Moeslinger, D., Silgoner, H., & Ipsiroglu, O. (2002). Oral beta-hydroxybutyrate supplementation in two patients with hyperinsulinemic hypoglycemia: Monitoring of beta-hydroxybutyrate levels in blood and cerebrospinal fluid, and in the brain by in vivo magnetic resonance spectroscopy. *Pediatric Research, 52*(2), 301–306.

Poff, A. M., Rho, J. M., & D'Agostino, D. P. (2019). Ketone administration for seizure disorders: History and rationale for ketone esters and metabolic alternatives. *Frontiers in Neuroscience, 13*, 1041.

Poff, A. M., Ward, N., Seyfried, T. N., Arnold, P., & D'Agostino, D. P. (2015). Non-toxic metabolic management of metastatic cancer in VM mice: Novel combination of ketogenic diet, ketone supplementation, and hyperbaric oxygen therapy. *PLOS ONE, 10*(6), Article e0127407.

Poulsen, S. A., & Quinn, R. J. (1998). Adenosine receptors: New opportunities for future drugs. *Bioorganic & Medicinal Chemistry, 6*(6), 619–641.

Prins, M. L. (2008). Cerebral metabolic adaptation and ketone metabolism after brain injury. *Journal of Cerebral Blood Flow and Metabolism, 28*(1), 1–16.

Puchowicz, M. A., Zechel, J. L., Valerio, J., Emancipator, D. S., Xu, K., Pundik, S., LaManna, J. C., & Lust, W. D. (2008). Neuroprotection in diet-induced ketotic rat brain after focal ischemia. *Journal of Cerebral Blood Flow and Metabolism, 28*(12), 1907–1916.

Puigserver, P., & Spiegelman, B. M. (2003). Peroxisome proliferator-activated receptor-gamma coactivator 1α (PGC-1α): Transcriptional coactivator and metabolic regulator. *Endocrine Reviews, 24*(1), 78–90.

Pulsifer, M. B., Gordon, J. M., Brandt, J., Vining, E. P., & Freeman, J. M. (2001). Effects of ketogenic diet on development and behavior: Preliminary report of a prospective study. *Developmental Medicine and Child Neurology, 43*(5), 301–306.

Qin, W., Haroutunian, V., Katsel, P., Cardozo, C. P., Ho, L., Buxbaum, J. D., & Pasinetti, G. M. (2009). PGC-1α expression decreases in the Alzheimer disease brain as a function of dementia. *Archives of Neurology, 66*(3), 352–361.

Qin, W., Yang, T., Ho, L., Zhao, Z., Wang, J., Chen, L., Zhao, W., Thiyagarajan, M., MacGrogan, D., Rodgers, J. T., Puigserver, P., Sadoshima, J., Deng, H., Pedrini, S., Gandy, S., Sauve, A. A., & Pasinetti, G. M. (2006). Neuronal SIRT1 activation as a novel mechanism underlying prevention of Alzheimer disease amyloid neuropathology by calorie restriction. *The Journal of Biological Chemistry, 281*(31), 21745–21754.

Quintas, A., de Solís, A. J., Díez-Guerra, F. J., Carrascosa, J. M., & Bogónez, E. (2012). Age-associated decrease of SIRT1 expression in rat hippocampus: Prevention by late onset caloric restriction. *Experimental Gerontology, 47*(2), 198–201.

Rachal Pugh, C., Fleshner, M., Watkins, L. R., Maier, S. F., & Rudy, J. W. (2001). The immune system and memory consolidation: A role for the cytokine IL-1β. *Neuroscience and Biobehavioral Reviews, 25*(1), 29–41.

Rahman, M., Muhammad, S., Khan, M. A., Chen, H., Ridder, D. A., Müller-Fielitz, H., Pokorná, B., Vollbrandt, T., Stölting, I., Nadrowitz, R., Okun, J. G., Offermanns, S., & Schwaninger, M. (2014). The β-hydroxybutyrate receptor HCA2 activates a neuroprotective subset of macrophages. *Nature Communications, 5*, 3944.

Ramesh, S., Govindarajulu, M., Lynd, T., Briggs, G., Adamek, D., Jones, E., Heiner, J., Majrashi, M., Moore, T., Amin, R., Suppiramaniam, V., & Dhanasekaran, M. (2018). SIRT3 activator Honokiol attenuates β-amyloid by modulating amyloidogenic pathway. *PLOS ONE, 13*(1), Article e0190350.

Rangarajan, P., Karthikeyan, A., Lu, J., Ling, E. A., & Dheen, S. T. (2015). Sirtuin 3 regulates Foxo3a-mediated antioxidant pathway in microglia. *Neuroscience, 311*, 398–414.

Rao, J. S., Harry, G. J., Rapoport, S. I., & Kim, H. W. (2010). Increased excitotoxicity and neuro-inflammatory markers in postmortem frontal cortex from bipolar disorder patients. *Molecular Psychiatry, 15*(4), 384–392.

Rao, J. S., Kellom, M., Kim, H. W., Rapoport, S. I., & Reese, E. A. (2012). Neuroinflammation and synaptic loss. *Neurochemical Research, 37*(5), 903–910.

Ravizza, T., Lucas, S. M., Balosso, S., Bernardino, L., Ku, G., Noé, F., Malva, J., Randle, J. C., Allan, S., & Vezzani, A. (2006). Inactivation of caspase-1 in rodent brain: A novel anticonvulsive strategy. *Epilepsia, 47*(7), 1160–1168.

Reger, M. A., Henderson, S. T., Hale, C., Cholerton, B., Baker, L. D., Watson, G. S., Hyde, K., Chapman, D., & Craft, S. (2004). Effects of beta-hydroxybutyrate on cognition in memory-impaired adults. *Neurobiology of Aging, 25*(3), 311–314.

Reiman, E. M., Chen, K., Alexander, G. E., Caselli, R. J., Bandy, D., Osborne, D., Saunders, A. M., & Hardy, J. (2004). Functional brain abnormalities in young adults at genetic risk for late-onset Alzheimer's dementia. *Proceedings of the National Academy of Sciences of the United States of America, 101*(1), 284–289.

Rho, J. M. (2017). How does the ketogenic diet induce anti-seizure effects? *Neuroscience Letters, 637*, 4–10.

Richard, D., Clavel, S., Huang, Q., Sanchis, D., & Ricquier, D. (2001). Uncoupling protein 2 in the brain: Distribution and function. *Biochemical Society Transactions, 29*(Pt 6), 812–817.

Robinson, K. A., Stewart, C. A., Pye, Q. N., Nguyen, X., Kenney, L., Salzman, S., Floyd, R. A., & Hensley, K. (1999). Redox-sensitive protein phosphatase activity regulates the phosphorylation state of p38 protein kinase in primary astrocyte culture. *Journal of Neuroscience Research, 55*(6), 724–732.

Rodriguez, J. I., & Kern, J. K. (2011). Evidence of microglial activation in autism and its possible role in brain underconnectivity. *Neuron Glia Biology, 7*(2–4), 205–213.

Rojas-Morales, P., Pedraza-Chaverri, J., & Tapia, E. (2020). Ketone bodies, stress response, and redox homeostasis. *Redox Biology, 29*, 101395.

Rossignol, D. A., & Frye, R. E. (2014). Evidence linking oxidative stress, mitochondrial dysfunction, and inflammation in the brain of individuals with autism. *Frontiers in Physiology, 5*, 150.

Rouaux, C., Panteleeva, I., René, F., Gonzalez de Aguilar, J. L., Echaniz-Laguna, A., Dupuis, L., Menger, Y., Boutillier, A. L., & Loeffler, J. P. (2007). Sodium valproate exerts neuroprotective effects in vivo through CREB-binding protein-dependent mechanisms but does not improve survival in an amyotrophic lateral sclerosis mouse model. *Journal of Neuroscience, 27*(21), 5535–5545.

Rowley, S., & Patel, M. (2013). Mitochondrial involvement and oxidative stress in temporal lobe epilepsy. *Free Radical Biology & Medicine, 62*, 121–131.

Róna-Vörös, K., & Weydt, P. (2010). The role of PGC-1α in the pathogenesis of neurodegenerative disorders. *Current Drug Targets, 11*(10), 1262–1269.

Ruskin, D. N., Fortin, J. A., Bisnauth, S. N., & Masino, S. A. (2017). Ketogenic diets improve behaviors associated with autism spectrum disorder in a sex-specific manner in the EL mouse. *Physiology & Behavior, 168*, 138–145.

Russell, V. A. (2003). Dopamine hypofunction possibly results from a defect in glutamate-stimulated release of dopamine in the nucleus accumbens shell of a rat model for attention deficit hyperactivity disorder—The spontaneously hypertensive rat. *Neuroscience and Biobehavioral Reviews, 27*(7), 671–682.

Ryu, H., Smith, K., Camelo, S. I., Carreras, I., Lee, J., Iglesias, A. H., Dangond, F., Cormier, K. A., Cudkowicz, M. E., Brown, R. H., Jr., & Ferrante, R. J. (2005). Sodium phenylbutyrate prolongs survival and regulates expression of anti-apoptotic genes in transgenic amyotrophic lateral sclerosis mice. *Journal of Neurochemistry, 93*(5), 1087–1098.

Saghazadeh, A., & Rezaei, N. (2017). Brain-derived neurotrophic factor levels in autism: A systematic review and meta-analysis. *Journal of Autism and Developmental Disorders, 47*(4), 1018–1029.

Samoilova, M., Weisspapir, M., Abdelmalik, P., Velumian, A. A., & Carlen, P. L. (2010). Chronic in vitro ketosis is neuroprotective but not anticonvulsant. *Journal of Neurochemistry, 113*(4), 826–835.

Sato, K., Kashiwaya, Y., Keon, C. A., Tsuchiya, N., King, M. T., Radda, G. K., Chance, B., Clarke, K., & Veech, R. L. (1995). Insulin, ketone bodies, and mitochondrial energy transduction. *FASEB Journal, 9*(8), 651–658.

Scheff, S. W., Price, D. A., Schmitt, F. A., & Mufson, E. J. (2006). Hippocampal synaptic loss in early Alzheimer's disease and mild cognitive impairment. *Neurobiology of Aging, 27*(10), 1372–1384.

Scheibye-Knudsen, M., Mitchell, S. J., Fang, E. F., Iyama, T., Ward, T., Wang, J., Dunn, C. A., Singh,

N., Veith, S., Hasan-Olive, M. M., Mangerich, A., Wilson, M. A., Mattson, M. P., Bergersen, L. H., Cogger, V. C., Warren, A., Le Couteur, D. G., Moaddel, R., Wilson, D. M. 3rd, & Bohr, V. A. (2014). A high-fat diet and NAD$^+$ activate SIRT1 to rescue premature aging in Cockayne syndrome. *Cell Metabolism, 20*(5), 840–855.

Schiavone, S., & Trabace, L. (2016). Pharmacological targeting of redox regulation systems as new therapeutic approach for psychiatric disorders: A literature overview. *Pharmacological Research, 107*, 195–204.

Schönfeld, P., & Wojtczak, L. (2016). Short- and medium-chain fatty acids in energy metabolism: The cellular perspective. *Journal of Lipid Research, 57*(6), 943–954.

Schramm, A., Matusik, P., Osmenda, G., & Guzik, T. J. (2012). Targeting NADPH oxidases in vascular pharmacology. *Vascular Pharmacology, 56*(5–6), 216–231.

Schroeder, F. A., Lin, C. L., Crusio, W. E., & Akbarian, S. (2007). Antidepressant-like effects of the histone deacetylase inhibitor, sodium butyrate, in the mouse. *Biological Psychiatry, 62*(1), 55–64.

Scirpo, R., Fiorotto, R., Villani, A., Amenduni, M., Spirli, C., & Strazzabosco, M. (2015). Stimulation of nuclear receptor peroxisome proliferator-activated receptor-γ limits NF-κB-dependent inflammation in mouse cystic fibrosis biliary epithelium. *Hepatology, 62*(5), 1551–1562.

Seethalakshmi, R., Parkar, S. R., Nair, N., Adarkar, S. A., Pandit, A. G., Batra, S. A., Baghel, N. S., & Moghe, S. H. (2006). Regional brain metabolism in schizophrenia: An FDG-PET study. *Indian Journal of Psychiatry, 48*(3), 149–153.

Seyfried, T. N., Mukherjee, P., Iyikesici, M. S., Slocum, A., Kalamian, M., Spinosa, J. P., & Chinopoulos, C. (2020). Consideration of ketogenic metabolic therapy as a complementary or alternative approach for managing breast cancer. *Frontiers in Nutrition, 7*, 21.

Shaafi, S., Najmi, S., Aliasgharpour, H., Mahmoudi, J., Sadigh-Etemad, S., Farhoudi, M., & Baniasadi, N. (2016). The efficacy of the ketogenic diet on motor functions in Parkinson's disease: A rat model. *Iranian Journal of Neurology, 15*(2), 63–99.

Shabab, T., Khanabdali, R., Moghadamtousi, S. Z., Kadir, H. A., & Mohan, G. (2017). Neuroinflammation pathways: A general review. *The International Journal of Neuroscience, 127*(7), 624–633.

Sharma, A. K., Rani, E., Waheed, A., & Rajput, S. K. (2015a). Pharmacoresistant epilepsy: A current update on non-conventional pharmacological and non-pharmacological interventions. *Journal of Epilepsy Research, 5*(1), 1–8.

Sharma, R. P., Grayson, D. R., & Gavin, D. P. (2008). Histone deactylase 1 expression is increased in the prefrontal cortex of schizophrenia subjects: Analysis of the National Brain Databank microarray collection. *Schizophrenia Research, 98*(1–3), 111–117.

Sharma, S., & Taliyan, R. (2015). Targeting histone deacetylases: A novel approach in Parkinson's disease. *Parkinson's Disease, 2015*, 303294.

Sharma, S., Taliyan, R., & Ramagiri, S. (2015b). Histone deacetylase inhibitor, trichostatin A, improves learning and memory in high-fat diet-induced cognitive deficits in mice. *Journal of Molecular Neuroscience, 56*(1), 1–11.

Shi, T., Wang, F., Stieren, E., & Tong, Q. (2005). SIRT3, a mitochondrial sirtuin deacetylase, regulates mitochondrial function and thermogenesis in brown adipocytes. *The Journal of Biological Chemistry, 280*(14), 13560–13567.

Shimazu, T., Hirschey, M. D., Hua, L., Dittenhafer-Reed, K. E., Schwer, B., Lombard, D. B., Li, Y., Bunkenborg, J., Alt, F. W., Denu, J. M., Jacobson, M. P., & Verdin, E. (2010). SIRT3 deacetylates mitochondrial 3-hydroxy-3-methylglutaryl CoA synthase 2 and regulates ketone body production. *Cell Metabolism, 12*(6), 654–661.

Shimazu, T., Hirschey, M. D., Newman, J., He, W., Shirakawa, K., Le Moan, N., Grueter, C. A., Lim, H., Saunders, L. R., Stevens, R. D., Newgard, C. B., Farese, R. V. Jr, de Cabo, R., Ulrich, S., Akassoglou, K., & Verdin, E. (2013). Suppression of oxidative stress by β-hydroxybutyrate, an endogenous histone deacetylase inhibitor. *Science, 339*(6116), 211–214.

Shindler, K. S., Ventura, E., Dutt, M., Elliott, P., Fitzgerald, D. C., & Rostami, A. (2010). Oral resveratrol reduces neuronal damage in a model of multiple sclerosis. *Journal of Neuro-Ophthalmology, 30*(4), 328–339.

Sills, G. J., & Rogawski, M. A. (2020). Mechanisms of action of currently used antiseizure drugs. *Neuropharmacology, 168*, 107966.

Simeone, T. A., Matthews, S. A., Samson, K. K., & Simeone, K. A. (2017a). Regulation of brain PPARγ2 contributes to ketogenic diet anti-seizure efficacy. *Experimental Neurology, 287*(Pt 1), 54–64.

Simeone, T. A., Simeone, K. A., & Rho, J. M. (2017b). Ketone bodies as anti-seizure agents. *Neurochemical Research, 42*(7), 2011–2018.

Simeone, T. A., Simeone, K. A., Stafstrom, C. E., & Rho, J. M. (2018). Do ketone bodies mediate the anti-seizure effects of the ketogenic diet? *Neuropharmacology, 133*, 233–241.

Singer, T. P., Ramsay, R. R., McKeown, K., Trevor, A., & Castagnoli, N. E., Jr. (1988). Mechanism of the neurotoxicity of 1-methyl-4-phenylpyridinium (MPP$^+$), the toxic bioactivation product of 1-methyl-4-phenyl-1,2,3,6-tetrahydropyridine (MPTP). *Toxicology, 49*(1), 17–23.

Sleiman, S. F., Henry, J., Al-Haddad, R., El Hayek, L., Abou Haidar, E., Stringer, T., Ulja, D.,

Karuppagounder, S. S., Holson, E. B., Ratan, R. R., Ninan, I., & Chao, M. V. (2016). Exercise promotes the expression of brain derived neurotrophic factor (BDNF) through the action of the ketone body β-hydroxybutyrate. *Elife, 5*, pii: e15092.

Smith, K. J., & Lassmann, H. (2002). The role of nitric oxide in multiple sclerosis. *Lancet Neurology, 1*(4), 232–241.

Song, W., Song, Y., Kincaid, B., Bossy, B., & Bossy-Wetzel, E. (2013). Mutant SOD1G93A triggers mitochondrial fragmentation in spinal cord motor neurons: Neuroprotection by SIRT3 and PGC-1α. *Neurobiology of Disease, 51*, 72–81.

Soto-Mota, A., Norwitz, N. G., & Clarke, K. (2020). Why a D-β-hydroxybutyrate monoester? *Biochemical Society Transactions, 48*(1), 51–59.

Soto-Mota, A., Vansant, H., Evans, R. D., & Clarke, K. (2019). Safety and tolerability of sustained exogenous ketosis using ketone monoester drinks for 28 days in healthy adults. *Regulatory Toxicology and Pharmacology, 109*, 104506.

Sowinski, H., & Karpawich, P. P. (2014). Management of a hyperactive teen and cardiac safety. *Pediatric Clinics of North America, 61*(1), 81–90.

Spilioti, M., Evangeliou, A. E., Tramma, D., Theodoridou, Z., Metaxas, S., Michailidi, E., Bonti, E., Frysira, H., Haidopoulou, A., Asprangathou, D., Tsalkidis, A. J., Kardaras, P., Wevers, R. A., Jakobs, C., & Gibson, K. M. (2013). Evidence for treatable inborn errors of metabolism in a cohort of 187 Greek patients with autism spectrum disorder (ASD). *Frontiers in Human Neuroscience, 7*, 858.

Srivastava, S., Kashiwaya, Y., King, M. T., Baxa, U., Tam, J., Niu, G., Chen, X., Clarke, K., & Veech, R. L. (2012). Mitochondrial biogenesis and increased uncoupling protein 1 in brown adipose tissue of mice fed a ketone ester diet. *FASEB Journal, 26*(6), 2351–2362.

Stanciu, G. D., Luca, A., Rusu, R. N., Bild, V., Beschea Chiriac, S. I., Solcan, C., Bild, W., & Ababei, D. C. (2019). Alzheimer's disease pharmacotherapy in relation to cholinergic system involvement. *Biomolecules, 10*(1), pii: E40.

Steardo, L., Jr., Fabrazzo, M., Sampogna, G., Monteleone, A. M., D'Agostino, G., Monteleone, P., & Maj, M. (2019). Impaired glucose metabolism in bipolar patients and response to mood stabilizer treatments. *Journal of Affective Disorders, 245*, 174–179.

Steen, E., Terry, B. M., Rivera, E. J., Cannon, J. L., Neely, T. R., Tavares, R., Xu, X. J., Wands, J. R., & de la Monte, S. M. (2005). Impaired insulin and insulin-like growth factor expression and signaling mechanisms in Alzheimer's disease—Is this type 3 diabetes? *Journal of Alzheimer's Disease, 7*(1), 63–80.

St-Pierre, J., Drori, S., Uldry, M., Silvaggi, J. M., Rhee, J., Jäger, S., Handschin, C., Zheng, K., Lin, J., Yang, W., Simon, D. K., Bachoo, R., & Spiegelman, B. M. (2006). Suppression of reactive oxygen species and neurodegeneration by the PGC-1 transcriptional coactivators. *Cell, 127*(2), 397–408.

Stubbs, B. J., Cox, P. J., Evans, R. D., Santer, P., Miller, J. J., Faull, O. K., Magor-Elliott, S., Hiyama, S., Stirling, M., & Clarke, K. (2017). On the metabolism of exogenous ketones in humans. *Frontiers in Physiology, 8*, 848.

Su, H., Fan, W., Coskun, P. E., Vesa, J., Gold, J. A., Jiang, Y. H., Potluri, P., Procaccio, V., Acab, A., Weiss, J. H., Wallace, D. C., & Kimonis, V. E. (2011). Mitochondrial dysfunction in CA1 hippocampal neurons of the UBE3A deficient mouse model for Angelman syndrome. *Neuroscience Letters, 487*(2), 129–133.

Su, L., Cai, Y., Xu, Y., Dutt, A., Shi, S., & Bramon, E. (2014). Cerebral metabolism in major depressive disorder: A voxel-based meta-analysis of positron emission tomography studies. *BMC Psychiatry, 14*, 321.

Su, W. J., Zhang, Y., Chen, Y., Gong, H., Lian, Y. J., Peng, W., Liu, Y. Z., Wang, Y. X., You, Z. L., Feng, S. J., Zong, Y., Lu, G. C., & Jiang, C. L. (2017). NLRP3 gene knockout blocks NF-κB and MAPK signaling pathway in CUMS-induced depression mouse model. *Behavioural Brain Research, 322*(Pt A), 1–8.

Sugai, F., Yamamoto, Y., Miyaguchi, K., Zhou, Z., Sumi, H., Hamasaki, T., Goto, M., & Sakoda, S. (2004). Benefit of valproic acid in suppressing disease progression of ALS model mice. *European Journal of Neuroscience, 20*(11), 3179–3183.

Sullivan, P. G., Rabchevsky, A. G., Waldmeier, P. C., & Springer, J. E. (2005). Mitochondrial permeability transition in CNS trauma: Cause or effect of neuronal cell death? *Journal of Neuroscience Research, 79*(1–2), 231–239.

Sullivan, P. G., Rippy, N. A., Dorenbos, K., Concepcion, R. C., Agarwal, A. K., & Rho, J. M. (2004). The ketogenic diet increases mitochondrial uncoupling protein levels and activity. *Annals of Neurology, 55*(4), 576–580.

Sussman, D., Germann, J., & Henkelman, M. (2015). Gestational ketogenic diet programs brain structure and susceptibility to depression and anxiety in the adult mouse offspring. *Brain and Behavior, 5*(2), e00300.

Swanton, T., Cook, J., Beswick, J. A., Freeman, S., Lawrence, C. B., & Brough, D. (2018). Is targeting the inflammasome a way forward for neuroscience drug discovery? *SLAS Discovery, 23*(10), 991–1017.

Swaroop, S., Sengupta, N., Suryawanshi, A. R., Adlakha, Y. K., & Basu, A. (2016). HSP60 plays a regulatory role in IL-1β-induced microglial inflammation via TLR4-p38 MAPK axis. *Journal of Neuroinflammation, 13*, 27.

Swerdlow, R. H. (2011). Brain aging, Alzheimer's disease, and mitochondria. *Biochimica et Biophysica Acta, 1812*(12), 1630–1639.

Tack, C. J., Stienstra, R., Joosten, L. A., & Netea, M. G. (2012). Inflammation links excess fat to insulin resistance: the role of the interleukin-1 family. *Immunological Reviews, 249*(1), 239–252.

Taggart, A. K., Kero, J., Gan, X., Cai, T. Q., Cheng, K., Ippolito, M., Ren, N., Kaplan, R., Wu, K., Wu, T. J., Jin, L., Liaw, C., Chen, R., Richman, J., Connolly, D., Offermanns, S., Wright, S. D., & Waters, M. G. (2005). D-β-Hydroxybutyrate inhibits adipocyte lipolysis via the nicotinic acid receptor PUMA-G. *The Journal of Biological Chemistry, 280*(29), 26649–26652.

Tan, B. T., Jiang, H., Moulson, A. J., Wu, X. L., Wang, W. C., Liu, J., Plunet, W. T., & Tetzlaff, W. (2020). Neuroprotective effects of a ketogenic diet in combination with exogenous ketone salts following acute spinal cord injury. *Neural Regeneration Research, 15*(10), 1912–1919.

Tan, M. S., Yu, J. T., Jiang, T., Zhu, X. C., & Tan, L. (2013). The NLRP3 inflammasome in Alzheimer's disease. *Molecular Neurobiology, 48*(3), 875–882.

Tang, H. H., McNally, G. P., & Richardson, R. (2007). The effects of FG7142 on two types of forgetting in 18-day-old rats. *Behavioral Neuroscience, 121*(6), 1421–1425.

Tanner, G. R., Lutas, A., Martínez-François, J. R., & Yellen, G. (2011). Single K_{ATP} channel opening in response to action potential firing in mouse dentate granule neurons. *Journal of Neuroscience, 31*(23), 8689–8696.

Tate, R. L., Mehlman, M. A., & Tobin, R. B. (1971). Metabolic fate of 1,3-butanediol in the rat: Conversion to -hydroxybutyrate. *Journal of Nutrition, 101*(12), 1719–1726.

Taylor, R. C., Cullen, S. P., & Martin, S. J. (2008). Apoptosis: Controlled demolition at the cellular level. *Nature Reviews Molecular Cell Biology, 9*(3), 231–241.

Tefera, T. W., Wong, Y., Barkl-Luke, M. E., Ngo, S. T., Thomas, N. K., McDonald, T. S., & Borges, K. (2016). Triheptanoin protects motor neurons and delays the onset of motor symptoms in a mouse model of amyotrophic lateral sclerosis. *PLOS ONE, 11*(8), Article e0161816.

Terrone, G., Balosso, S., Pauletti, A., Ravizza, T., & Vezzani, A. (2020). Inflammation and reactive oxygen species as disease modifiers in epilepsy. *Neuropharmacology, 167*, 107742.

Thibert, R. L., Conant, K. D., Braun, E. K., Bruno, P., Said, R. R., Nespeca, M. P., & Thiele, E. A. (2009). Epilepsy in Angelman syndrome: A questionnaire-based assessment of the natural history and current treatment options. *Epilepsia, 50*(11), 2369–2376.

Thijs, R. D., Surges, R., O'Brien, T. J., & Sander, J. W. (2019). Epilepsy in adults. *Lancet, 393*(10172), 689–701.

Thio, L. L., Erbayat-Altay, E., Rensing, N., & Yamada, K. A. (2006). Leptin contributes to slower weight gain in juvenile rodents on a ketogenic diet. *Pediatric Research, 60*(4), 413–417.

Thornberry, N. A., Miller, D. K., & Nicholson, D. W. (1995). Interleukin-1β-converting enzyme and related proteases as potential targets in inflammation and apoptosis. *Perspectives in Drug Discovery and Design, 2*, 389–399.

Thurston, J. H., Hauhart, R. E., & Schiro, J. A. (1986). Beta-hydroxybutyrate reverses insulin-induced hypoglycemic coma in suckling-weanling mice despite low blood and brain glucose levels. *Metabolic Brain Disease, 1*(1), 63–82.

Tieu, K., Perier, C., Caspersen, C., Teismann, P., Wu, D. C., Yan, S. D., Naini, A., Vila, M., Jackson-Lewis, V., Ramasamy, R., & Przedborski, S. (2003). D-β-Hydroxybutyrate rescues mitochondrial respiration and mitigates features of Parkinson disease. *Journal of Clinical Investigation, 112*(6), 892–901.

Tisch, S., Silberstein, P., Limousin-Dowsey, P., & Jahanshahi, M. (2004). The basal ganglia: Anatomy, physiology, and pharmacology. *The Psychiatric Clinics of North America, 27*(4), 757–799.

Tschopp, J., & Schroder, K. (2010). NLRP3 inflammasome activation: The convergence of multiple signalling pathways on ROS production? *Nature Reviews Immunology, 10*(3), 210–215.

Tseng, A. H., Shieh, S. S., & Wang, D. L. (2013). SIRT3 deacetylates FOXO3 to protect mitochondria against oxidative damage. *Free Radical Biology & Medicine, 63*, 222–234.

Tulino, R., Benjamin, A. C., Jolinon, N., Smith, D. L., Chini, E. N., Carnemolla, A., & Bates, G. P. (2016). SIRT1 activity is linked to its brain region-specific phosphorylation and is impaired in Huntington's disease mice. *PLOS ONE, 11*(1), Article e0145425.

Tyagi, S., Gupta, P., Saini, A. S., Kaushal, C., & Sharma, S. T. (2011). The peroxisome proliferator-activated receptor: A family of nuclear receptors role in various diseases. *Journal of Advanced Pharmaceutical Technology & Research, 2*(4), 236–240.

Valdovinos, M. G., & Weyand, D. (2006). Blood glucose levels and problem behavior. *Research in Developmental Disabilities, 27*(2), 227–231.

Vandenberghe, C., St-Pierre, V., Courchesne-Loyer, A., Hennebelle, M., Castellano, C. A., & Cunnane, S. C. (2017). Caffeine intake increases plasma ketones: An acute metabolic study in humans. *Canadian Journal of Physiology and Pharmacology, 95*(4), 455–458.

Vandenberghe, C., St-Pierre, V., Fortier, M., Castellano, C. A., Cuenoud, B., & Cunnane, S. C.

(2020). Medium chain triglycerides modulate the ketogenic effect of a metabolic switch. *Frontiers in Nutrition, 7*, 3.

van der Putten, C., Zuiderwijk-Sick, E. A., van Straalen, L., de Geus, E. D., Boven, L. A., Kondova, I., IJzerman, A. P., & Bajramovic, J. J. (2009). Differential expression of adenosine A$_3$ receptors controls adenosine A$_{2A}$ receptor-mediated inhibition of TLR responses in microglia. *Journal of Immunology, 182*(12), 7603–7612.

Vanitallie, T. B., Nonas, C., Di Rocco, A., Boyar, K., Hyams, K., & Heymsfield, S. B. (2005). Treatment of Parkinson disease with diet-induced hyperketonemia: A feasibility study. *Neurology, 64*(4), 728–730.

VanItallie, T. B., & Nufert, T. H. (2003). Ketones: Metabolism's ugly duckling. *Nutrition Reviews, 61*(10), 327–341.

van Vliet, E. A., Aronica, E., Vezzani, A., & Ravizza, T. (2018). Review: Neuroinflammatory pathways as treatment targets and biomarker candidates in epilepsy; Emerging evidence from preclinical and clinical studies. *Neuropathology and Applied Neurobiology, 44*(1), 91–111.

Veech, R. L., Chance, B., Kashiwaya, Y., Lardy, H. A., & Cahill, G. F., Jr. (2001). Ketone bodies, potential therapeutic uses. *IUBMB Life, 51*(4), 241–247.

Veech, R. L., Todd King, M., Pawlosky, R., Kashiwaya, Y., Bradshaw, P. C., & Curtis, W. (2019). The "great" controlling nucleotide coenzymes. *IUBMB Life, 71*(5), 565–579.

Verdin, E., Hirschey, M. D., Finley, L. W., & Haigis, M. C. (2010). Sirtuin regulation of mitochondria: Energy production, apoptosis, and signaling. *Trends in Biochemical Sciences, 35*(12), 669–675.

Vezzani, A., Balosso, S., Maroso, M., Zardoni, D., Noé, F., & Ravizza, T. (2010). ICE/caspase 1 inhibitors and IL-1β receptor antagonists as potential therapeutics in epilepsy. *Current Opinion in Investigational Drugs, 11*(1), 43–50.

Vezzani, A., Balosso, S., & Ravizza, T. (2019). Neuroinflammatory pathways as treatment targets and biomarkers in epilepsy. *Nature Reviews Neurology, 15*(8), 459–472.

Vezzani, A., Lang, B., & Aronica, E. (2015). Immunity and inflammation in epilepsy. *Cold Spring Harbor Perspectives in Medicine, 6*(2), a022699.

Vieta, E., Berk, M., Schulze, T. G., Carvalho, A. F., Suppes, T., Calabrese, J. R., Gao, K., Miskowiak, K. W., & Grande, I. (2018). Bipolar disorders. *Nature Reviews Disease Primers, 4*, 18008.

Villeneuve, N., Pinton, F., Bahi-Buisson, N., Dulac, O., Chiron, C., & Nabbout, R. (2009). The ketogenic diet improves recently worsened focal epilepsy. *Developmental Medicine and Child Neurology, 51*(4), 276–281.

Vincenzi, F., Ravani, A., Pasquini, S., Merighi, S., Gessi, S., Romagnoli, R., Baraldi, P. G., Borea,

P. A., & Varani, K. (2016). Positive allosteric modulation of A$_1$ adenosine receptors as a novel and promising therapeutic strategy for anxiety. *Neuropharmacology, 111*, 283–292.

Vogel, K. R., Ainslie, G. R., Jansen, E. E., Salomons, G. S., & Gibson, K. M. (2015). Torin 1 partially corrects vigabatrin-induced mitochondrial increase in mouse. *Annals of Clinical and Translational Neurology, 2*(6), 699–706.

Wakade, C., Chong, R., Bradley, E., Thomas, B., & Morgan, J. (2014). Upregulation of GPR109A in Parkinson's disease. *PLOS ONE, 9*(10), Article e109818.

Wang, D., & Mitchell, E. S. (2016). Cognition and synaptic-plasticity related changes in aged rats supplemented with 8- and 10-carbon medium chain triglycerides. *PLOS ONE, 11*(8), Article e0160159.

Wang, J., Zhang, Y., Tang, L., Zhang, N., & Fan, D. (2011). Protective effects of resveratrol through the up-regulation of SIRT1 expression in the mutant hSOD1-G93A-bearing motor neuron-like cell culture model of amyotrophic lateral sclerosis. *Neuroscience Letters, 503*(3), 250–255.

Wang, R., Zhang, Y., Li, J., & Zhang, C. (2017). Resveratrol ameliorates spatial learning memory impairment induced by Aβ$_{1-42}$ in rats. *Neuroscience, 344*, 39–47.

Wareski, P., Vaarmann, A., Choubey, V., Safiulina, D., Liiv, J., Kuum, M., & Kaasik, A. (2009). PGC-1α and PGC-1β regulate mitochondrial density in neurons. *The Journal of Biological Chemistry, 284*(32), 21379–21385.

Warren, R. E., Deary, I. J., & Frier, B. M. (2003). The symptoms of hyperglycaemia in people with insulin-treated diabetes: Classification using principal components analysis. *Diabetes Metabolism Research and Reviews, 19*(5), 408–414.

Watanabe, S., Ageta-Ishihara, N., Nagatsu, S., Takao, K., Komine, O., Endo, F., Miyakawa, T., Misawa, H., Takahashi, R., Kinoshita, M., & Yamanaka, K. (2014). SIRT1 overexpression ameliorates a mouse model of SOD1-linked amyotrophic lateral sclerosis via HSF1/HSP70i chaperone system. *Molecular Brain, 7*, 62.

Werner, F. M., & Coveñas, R. (2017). Classical neurotransmitters and neuropeptides involved in generalized epilepsy in a multi-neurotransmitter system: How to improve the antiepileptic effect? *Epilepsy & Behavior, 71*(Pt B), 124–129.

Werner, F. M., & Coveñas, R. (2019). Therapeutic effect of novel antidepressant drugs acting at specific receptors of neurotransmitters and neuropeptides. *Current Pharmaceutical Design, 25*(4), 388–395.

Wingo, A. P., Harvey, P. D., & Baldessarini, R. J. (2009). Neurocognitive impairment in bipolar disorder patients: Functional implications. *Bipolar Disorders, 11*(2), 113–125.

Wobrock, T., Ecker, U. K., Scherk, H., Schneider-Axmann, T., Falkai, P., & Gruber, O. (2009). Cognitive impairment of executive function as a core symptom of schizophrenia. *The World Journal of Biological Psychiatry, 10*(4 Pt 2), 442–451.

Won, Y. J., Lu, V. B., Puhl, H. L., III, & Ikeda, S. R. (2013). β-Hydroxybutyrate modulates N-type calcium channels in rat sympathetic neurons by acting as an agonist for the G-protein-coupled receptor FFA3. *Journal of Neuroscience, 33*(49), 19314–19325.

Wu, Y., Gong, Y., Luan, Y., Li, Y., Liu, J., Yue, Z., Yuan, B., Sun, J., Xie, C., Li, L., Zhen, J., Jin, X., Zheng, Y., Wang, X., Xie, L., & Wang, W. (2020). BHBA treatment improves cognitive function by targeting pleiotropic mechanisms in transgenic mouse model of Alzheimer's disease. *FASEB Journal, 34*(1), 1412–1429.

Wu, Z., Yu, J., Zhu, A., & Nakanishi, H. (2016). Nutrients, microglia aging, and brain aging. *Oxidative Medicine and Cellular Longevity, 2016*, 7498528.

Xu, B., Chen, S., Luo, Y., Chen, Z., Liu, L., Zhou, H., Chen, W., Shen, T., Han, X., Chen, L., & Huang, S. (2011). Calcium signaling is involved in cadmium-induced neuronal apoptosis via induction of reactive oxygen species and activation of MAPK/mTOR network. *PLOS ONE, 6*(4), Article e19052.

Xu, D., Lian, D., Wu, J., Liu, Y., Zhu, M., Sun, J., He, D., & Li, L. (2017). Brain-derived neurotrophic factor reduces inflammation and hippocampal apoptosis in experimental *Streptococcus pneumoniae* meningitis. *Journal of Neuroinflammation, 14*(1), 156.

Xu, K., Sun, X., Eroku, B. O., Tsipis, C. P., Puchowicz, M. A., & LaManna, J. C. (2010). Diet-induced ketosis improves cognitive performance in aged rats. *Advances in Experimental Medicine and Biology, 662*, 71–75.

Yamada, K. A. (2008). Calorie restriction and glucose regulation. *Epilepsia, 49*, 94–96.

Yamanashi, T., Iwata, M., Kamiya, N., Tsunetomi, K., Kajitani, N., Wada, N., Iitsuka, T., Yamauchi, T., Miura, A., Pu, S., Shirayama, Y., Watanabe, K., Duman, R. S., & Kaneko, K. (2017). Beta-hydroxybutyrate, an endogenic NLRP3 inflammasome inhibitor, attenuates stress-induced behavioral and inflammatory responses. *Scientific Reports, 7*(1), 7677.

Yang, X., & Cheng, B. (2010). Neuroprotective and anti-inflammatory activities of ketogenic diet on MPTP-induced neurotoxicity. *Journal of Molecular Neuroscience, 42*(2), 145–153.

Yatham, L. N., Kennedy, S. H., Parikh, S. V., Schaffer, A., Bond, D. J., Frey, B. N., Sharma, V., Goldstein, B. I., Rej, S., Beaulieu, S., Alda, M., MacQueen, G., Milev, R. V., Ravindran, A., O'Donovan, C., McIntosh, D., Lam, R. W., Vazquez, G., Kapczinski, F., & Berk M. (2018). Canadian Network for Mood and Anxiety Treatments (CANMAT) and International Society for Bipolar Disorders (ISBD) 2018 guidelines for the management of patients with bipolar disorder. *Bipolar Disorders, 20*(2), 97–170.

Yegin, A., Ay, N., Aydin, O., Yargici, N., Eren, E., & Yilmaz, N. (2012). Increased oxidant stress and inflammation in patients with chronic schizophrenia. *International Journal of Clinical Medicine, 3*(5), 368–376.

Yeung, F., Hoberg, J. E., Ramsey, C. S., Keller, M. D., Jones, D. R., Frye, R. A., & Mayo, M. W. (2004). Modulation of NF-κB-dependent transcription and cell survival by the SIRT1 deacetylase. *EMBO Journal, 23*(12), 2369–2380.

Yin, J. X., Maalouf, M., Han, P., Zhao, M., Gao, M., Dharshaun, T., Ryan, C., Whitelegge, J., Wu, J., Eisenberg, D., Reiman, E. M., Schweizer, F. E., & Shi, J. (2016). Ketones block amyloid entry and improve cognition in an Alzheimer's model. *Neurobiology of Aging, 39*, 25–37.

Yoon, J. H., Maddock, R. J., Rokem, A., Silver, M. A., Minzenberg, M. J., Ragland, J. D., & Carter, C. S. (2010). GABA concentration is reduced in visual cortex in schizophrenia and correlates with orientation-specific surround suppression. *Journal of Neuroscience, 30*(10), 3777–3781.

Yoshizaki, T., Milne, J. C., Imamura, T., Schenk, S., Sonoda, N., Babendure, J. L., Lu, J. C., Smith, J. J., Jirousek, M. R., & Olefsky, J. M. (2009). SIRT1 exerts anti-inflammatory effects and improves insulin sensitivity in adipocytes. *Molecular and Cellular Biology, 29*(5), 1363–1374.

Youm, Y. H., Nguyen, K. Y., Grant, R. W., Goldberg, E. L., Bodogai, M., Kim, D., D'Agostino, D., Planavsky, N., Lupfer, C., Kanneganti, T. D., Kang, S., Horvath, T. L., Fahmy, T. M., Crawford, P. A., Biragyn, A., Alnemri, E., & Dixit, V. D. (2015). The ketone metabolite β-hydroxybutyrate blocks NLRP3 inflammasome-mediated inflammatory disease. *Nature Medicine, 21*(3), 263–269.

Yudkoff, M., Daikhin, Y., Melø, T. M., Nissim, I., Sonnewald, U., & Nissim, I. (2007). The ketogenic diet and brain metabolism of amino acids: Relationship to the anticonvulsant effect. *Annual Review of Nutrition, 27*, 415–430.

Yuste, J. E., Tarragon, E., Campuzano, C. M., & Ros-Bernal, F. (2015). Implications of glial nitric oxide in neurodegenerative diseases. *Frontiers in Cellular Neuroscience, 9*, 322.

Zeng, L. H., Rensing, N. R., & Wong, M. (2009). The mammalian target of rapamycin signaling pathway mediates epileptogenesis in a model of temporal lobe epilepsy. *Journal of Neuroscience, 29*(21), 6964–6972.

Zeng, L. H., Xu, L., Gutmann, D. H., & Wong, M. (2008). Rapamycin prevents epilepsy in a mouse model of tuberous sclerosis complex. *Annals of Neurology, 63*(4), 444–453.

Zhao, L., & Ackerman, S. L. (2006). Endoplasmic reticulum stress in health and disease. *Current Opinion in Cell Biology, 18*(4), 444–452.

Zhao, W., Varghese, M., Vempati, P., Dzhun, A., Cheng, A., Wang, J., Lange, D., Bilski, A., Faravelli, I., & Pasinetti, G. M. (2012). Caprylic triglyceride as a novel therapeutic approach to effectively improve the performance and attenuate the symptoms due to the motor neuron loss in ALS disease. *PLOS ONE, 7*(11), Article e49191.

Zhao, W., Varghese, M., Yemul, S., Pan, Y., Cheng, A., Marano, P., Hassan, S., Vempati, P., Chen, F., Qian, X., & Pasinetti, G. M. (2011). Peroxisome proliferator activator receptor gamma coactivator-1α (PGC-1α) improves motor performance and survival in a mouse model of amyotrophic lateral sclerosis. *Molecular Neurodegeneration, 6*(1), 51.

Zhao, Z., Lange, D. J., Voustianiouk, A., MacGrogan, D., Ho, L., Suh, J., Humala, N., Thiyagarajan, M., Wang, J., & Pasinetti, G. M. (2006). A ketogenic diet as a potential novel therapeutic intervention in amyotrophic lateral sclerosis. *BMC Neuroscience, 7*, 29.

Zheng, B., Liao, Z., Locascio, J. J., Lesniak, K. A., Roderick, S. S., Watt, M. L., Eklund, A. C., Zhang-James, Y., Kim, P. D., Hauser, M. A., Grünblatt, E., Moran, L. B., Mandel, S. A., Riederer, P., Miller, R. M., Federoff, H. J., Wüllner, U., Papapetropoulos, S., Youdim, M. B., & Scherzer, C. R. (2010). PGC-1α, a potential therapeutic target for early intervention in Parkinson's disease. *Science Translational Medicine, 2*(52), 52ra73.

Zhu, W., Cao, F. S., Feng, J., Chen, H. W., Wan, J. R., Lu, Q., & Wang, J. (2017). NLRP3 inflammasome activation contributes to long-term behavioral alterations in mice injected with lipopolysaccharide. *Neuroscience, 343*, 77–84.

Zhu, X., Liu, Q., Wang, M., Liang, M., Yang, X., Xu, X., Zou, H., & Qiu, J. (2011). Activation of Sirt1 by resveratrol inhibits TNF-α induced inflammation in fibroblasts. *PLOS ONE, 6*(11), Article e27081.

Zou, X. H., Li, H. M., Wang, S., Leski, M., Yao, Y. C., Yang, X. D., Huang, Q. J., & Chen, G. Q. (2009). The effect of 3-hydroxybutyrate methyl ester on learning and memory in mice. *Biomaterials, 30*(8), 1532–1541.

Zupec-Kania, B. A., & Spellman, E. (2008). An overview of the ketogenic diet for pediatric epilepsy. *Nutrition in Clinical Practice, 23*(6), 589–596.

Amino Acids in the Treatment of Neurologic Disorders

ADAM L. HARTMAN, MD

INTRODUCTION

Studies of the mechanisms of action of nutrient-based therapies mainly focus on fats and carbohydrates (Masino & Rho, 2012). The role of protein, the third major diet component, has not been studied as thoroughly as fats and carbohydrates, yet dietary protein and amino acid management are important in the treatment of neurologic disorders. As an example, protein must be restricted for systemic ketosis to occur in the ketogenic diet (KD; Laeger et al., 2014; Yudkoff et al., 2007). In a related but nuanced finding, the lack of threonine in either control diets or KDs worsens various aspects of seizure activity in multiple seizure models (Gietzen et al., 2018). Together, these findings point to the importance of selective, rather than global, amino acid restriction for the KD to treat seizures. This chapter focuses on the therapeutic use of naturally occurring proteinogenic amino acids (and some of their D-enantiomers) for two model neurologic disorders, epilepsy and traumatic brain injury. Organic acids (e.g., taurine) and modified/synthetic amino acids are not discussed.

Generally, the L-enantiomers of most amino acids are more biologically active than their D-enantiomers. However, increased attention is being paid to the D-enantiomers in mammals (Genchi, 2017; Weatherly et al., 2017). D-Amino acids are considered by some to be "unnatural," but the extant literature shows that they have biologic functions (Genchi, 2017). One example is D-leucine, which is produced by bacteria and is found in food products, particularly those that are plant-based (Ekborg-Ott & Armstrong, 1996; Mutaguchi et al., 2013). D-Leucine has been isolated from rat and mouse hippocampus, mouse neocortex, pineal gland, and other areas of the brain at lower concentrations, but not much is known about its physiologic function (Hamase et al., 1997, 2001; Weatherly et al., 2017).

SEIZURES AND EPILEPSY

L-Amino Acids

An extended discussion of seizures and epilepsy can be found elsewhere in this book (Zack & Kobau, 2017). Nearly one third of patients have seizures that are not successfully treated by currently used medicines, prompting the need for novel treatments (Berg & Rychlik, 2015; Chen et al., 2018; Choi et al., 2016; French et al., 2013; Kwan & Brodie, 2000; Schmidt & Schachter, 2014). Amino acids have been explored as an option. A limited number of L-amino acids have been studied in the treatment of seizures and epilepsy (for an excellent review of the topic, see Gruenbaum et al., 2019a). Specific amino acids are discussed here.

Administration of L-leucine and L-isoleucine (300 mg/kg, a high dose) prior to seizure induction protects against seizure onset by prolonging the latency to onset of spike-wave discharges and clinical tonic-clonic seizures induced by the $GABA_A$ receptor antagonist pentylenetetrazol (PTZ). L-Leucine also decreases the duration of spike-wave discharges, but neither amino acid affects seizure duration (Dufour et al., 1999). Interestingly, α-ketoisocaproic acid, a metabolite of L-leucine that results from a transamination reaction that also produces L-glutamate, is inactive against PTZ, suggesting that the parent amino acid, not its metabolite, is responsible for these effects. Each of the branched-chain amino acids (L-leucine, L-isoleucine, and L-valine) also increased the latency to onset of seizures induced by another $GABA_A$ receptor antagonist, picrotoxin (Skeie et al., 1994). Conversely, the branched-chain amino acids increased the number of spike-and-wave discharges in the GAERS (Genetic Absence Epilepsy Rats from Strasbourg) Wistar rat, possibly due to a perturbation in the glutamate/GABA balance (Dufour et al., 2001a, 2001b). Given the variable findings in both different acute seizure tests and in different aspects of epileptiform activity, the antiseizure effect does not appear to be a general property of this class of amino acids. Although it is tempting to say that the findings are dependent on the seizure model or organism studied, the data indicate that this effect remains poorly understood.

Our laboratory set out further investigate amino acids in our studies of ketogenic compounds, including the ketogenic-only (i.e., not glucogenic) amino acid L-leucine. It is tempting to speculate that part of the KD's seizure protection is due to L-leucine, a ketogenic-only amino acid. However, cerebrospinal fluid levels of L-leucine (and the other branched-chain amino acids) in patients consuming a KD were unchanged from baseline (as a cross-reference to comments in the introduction, threonine concentration correlated positively with responsiveness to treatment in patients consuming a KD; Dahlin et al., 2005). Another study showed no differences in cerebrospinal fluid levels of leucine between responders and nonresponders to the KD (Sariego-Jamardo et al., 2015). Despite these findings, the preclinical data discussed previously suggested that treatment with branched-chain L-amino acids might be a fruitful line of investigation.

Using a different seizure test and dosing paradigms, we showed that pretreatment with L-leucine terminates seizures induced by the excitotoxin kainic acid, while L-valine was ineffective, again suggesting that in this test, there is not a class effect of branched-chain amino acids (Hartman et al., 2015). Interestingly, L-leucine was ineffective in terminating kainic acid-induced seizures when injected after seizure onset, suggesting that it affected seizure initiation more than propagation. However, another group showed that in a chronic model of mesial temporal lobe epilepsy (methionine sulfoximine intrahippocampal infusion), supplementation of drinking water with a 4% branched-chain amino acid solution (both pre- and post-convulsant) had no impact on number of seizures/week, but rats treated with 4% branched-chain amino acids had a lower hippocampal hilar neuron count, and treatment appeared to facilitate seizure spread, both of which are adverse outcomes (Gruenbaum et al., 2019b). Therefore, caution is needed when translating the findings noted here into humans.

Other amino acids have been studied in the context of seizures. Glycine is somewhat unique among amino acids in that it can have either excitatory or inhibitory effects, depending on which receptor is involved: glycine binding to N-methyl-D-aspartate (NMDA) receptors in the brain is excitatory but binding to glycine receptors in the spinal cord is inhibitory (Johnson & Ascher, 1987; Werman et al., 1968), although there are exceptions to this general rule. The glycine transporter (GlyT1) is overexpressed in the hippocampus in some preclinical models of epilepsy (mice and rats) and humans with epilepsy (surgical specimens), although in the human samples, there were some important potential confounders: there was a statistically significant difference in age between postsurgical samples and autopsy controls, and all of the postsurgical samples had been treated with antiseizure medicines, compared to none of the controls (Shen et al., 2015). Inhibition of the GlyT1 protects against acute and chronic seizures in rodents (Kalinichev et al., 2010; Shen et al., 2015). However, binding of glycine to the NMDA receptor likely does not mediate this effect (Zellinger et al., 2014), and in fact, inhibitors of this site have acute antiseizure effects (Bristow et al., 1996; Nichols & Yielding, 1998). The exact role of glycine in seizure initiation versus the progression or propagation of seizure activity remains unclear. Treatment using inhibitors of amino acid transporters would need to be done, with significant attention paid to safety, given their important role in normal physiologic function and brain development.

A number of potential mechanisms might be responsible for an antiseizure effect of amino acids. First, amino acids may be working through either cell-surface transporters or receptors, as in the case of glycine and the GlyT1 transporter. Alternatively, they may activate intracellular amino acid "sensors," with downstream effects on signaling pathways. For example, L-leucine activates the master integrator of cellular metabolism, mammalian target of rapamycin complex 1 (mTORC1) via Sestrin2 (Bar-Peled et al., 2012; Cota et al., 2006; Sancak et al., 2008; Wolfson et al., 2016). However, data suggest that mTORC1 activation is not the mechanism for seizure control with L-leucine because pathologically increased mTORC1 activity has been measured in both humans and rodent models of tuberous sclerosis complex (Orlova & Crino, 2010; Zeng et al., 2008), as well as some chemoconvulsant rodent models of temporal lobe epilepsy. Similarly, pharmacologic inhibition of mTORC1 decreases seizures in some models (Buckmaster & Lew, 2011; Huang et al., 2010; Sosanya et al., 2015; Zeng et al., 2009). This effect is weak and inconsistent across seizure tests, however (Chachua et al., 2012; Hartman et al., 2012). Therefore, the data indicate that it is unlikely that L-leucine, an mTORC1 activator, protects against seizures by increasing activity in this particular pathway. Nonetheless, the role of L-leucine in mTORC1-related disorders is unknown. This mechanism also does not explain the limited antiseizure effects of L-isoleucine and L-valine.

Another potential mechanism for the action of L-leucine (and other amino acids) on seizure activity is activation via amino acid transporters. Examples include LAT1/SLC7A5, which has implications for transport of other small molecules into the brain (Geier et al., 2013) and B⁰AT2/SLC6A15 (Bröer et al., 2006; Hägglund et al., 2013). LAT1/SLC7A5 also transports aromatic acid precursors (e.g., tryptophan) of other neurotransmitters (e.g., serotonin), so L-leucine transport may impact neurotransmission via this mechanism (Gruenbaum et al., 2019a). (Interestingly, LAT1/SLC7A5 is expressed in pathologic balloon cells in tissue from patients with tuberous sclerosis, supporting the role of this transporter in cell growth, one of the cardinal abnormal features in this disease [Lim et al., 2011].) An antiseizure mechanism may also involve countertransport of other amino acids, which would in turn lead to decreased synaptic concentration of the excitatory amino acid glutamate and a resulting decrease in seizure activity (Yudkoff et al., 2005, 2007). Several other amino acid transporters also may transport leucine (Box 35.1). Further testing of these transporters (either using pharmacologic inhibitors or genetically modified organisms) is needed to determine their importance in chronic epilepsy.

L-Serine is less well known for a role in neurotransmission than its D-enantiomer. Mice lacking the ASC1 transporter (alanine-serine-cysteine) have seizures (Xie et al., 2005). Indicating stereospecific requirements, L-serine does not potentiate NMDA-induced seizures, although D-serine, an endogenous ligand of this receptor, does (Singh et al., 1990a). D-Serine is discussed in the D-amino acid section below.

L-Arginine is important because it is the metabolic precursor of nitric oxide, which itself has shown mixed results in seizure and epilepsy studies (Banach et al., 2011). Not surprisingly, mixed results have been shown with L-arginine. In an electrical kindling paradigm of epilepsy, L-arginine did not affect acquisition of kindling or seizure severity in rats (Herberg et al., 1995). In a developmental model of seizures, L-arginine prolonged PTZ-induced EEG-recorded seizure duration in Postnatal Day 10 (P10) rat pups, although somewhat paradoxically, P21 rats had increased survival (with no change in seizure duration; de Vasconcelos et al., 2000). The type of seizure (i.e., tonic versus tonic-clonic) also was different in L-arginine-treated P21 pups compared to controls, suggesting a form of neuromodulation that needs further clarification (and as the authors note, that may have an impact on survival).

D-Amino Acids

The paradoxical results in our studies of L-leucine led us to consider transporter-mediated effects or contaminants in commercial preparations of L-leucine. The most abundant other amino acid "species" in this preparation was D-leucine, which represented up to 0.5% of the leucine in our commercial source (Sigma-Aldrich technical information).

Surprisingly, D-leucine terminates the behavioral manifestations of kainic acid-induced seizures, even when administered after seizure onset, at doses similar to, or lower than, those in the L-leucine experiments (Hartman et al., 2015). As mentioned previously, L-leucine was ineffective when given after seizure onset in this test. D-Leucine (administered in drinking water for 14 days) also protects against seizures in the 6-Hz electroshock test, which models focal-onset seizures, demonstrating seizure protection in a different assay. However, D-leucine does not protect against spontaneous recurrent seizures after kainic acid-induced status epilepticus (Holden & Hartman, 2018). In an exploratory analysis, D-leucine protected against spontaneous recurrent

---

BOX 35.1

NEUROLOGICALLY IMPORTANT
L-LEUCINE TRANSPORTERS

SLC3A2 (ATA2)
SLC6A14
SLC6A15
SLC7A5 (LAT1)
SLC7A6 (y+LAT2)
SLC7A7 (y+LAT1)
SLC7A9

Note. Transporters are listed in numerical order. Table modified from gallus.reactome.org.

seizures in the dark cycle, which is interesting because D-leucine is highly concentrated in the pineal gland, a key organ in regulation of the circadian cycle (Hamase et al., 1997).

Although D-leucine is more ketogenic than L-leucine (i.e., its degradation results in the production of ketone bodies but not glucose; Embden, 1908), D-leucine treatment does not induce systemic ketosis; therefore, the antiseizure effect is not medicated via ketone bodies (Hartman et al., 2015). D-Leucine does not bind to the kainic acid receptor (thus eliminating competition on the receptor as a mechanism of seizure protection), nor does it bind to a panel of other CNS receptors or transporters.

However, D-leucine is a known ligand of the taste receptors Tas1R2/R3 (which are expressed in the hippocampus, a major seizure-generating region of the brain), but it is unclear whether this represents the mechanism of D-leucine antiseizure action (Bassoli et al., 2014; Shin et al., 2010). Mice lacking the Tas1R2/R3 receptors are protected against seizures in the maximal electroshock test (not the 6-Hz seizure test), but other ligands of this receptor also have limited antiseizure activity in this test (Holden & Hartman, 2018; Talevi et al., 2012). These data supporting a potential role for Tas1R2/R3 receptors in epilepsy, but the nature of that role is unclear and may relate to receptor physiology in different background strains of mice.

The only other data on therapeutic use of D-leucine were from analgesia studies, some of which also included use of D-phenylalanine in combination with D-leucine (Cheng & Pomeranz, 1980; McKibbin & Cheng, 1982; Ninomiya et al., 1990). Importantly, the doses required of each amino acid in the analgesia studies were ~ 80 times greater than the lowest effective dose in our seizure studies, suggesting a different receptor physiology (and possibly even a different mechanism) for D-leucine in terminating seizures.

Other D-amino acids may play a role in seizure activity, although the literature has shown mixed results in terms of efficacy (Box 35.2). D-Serine binds to the glycine site on the NMDA receptor, and decreased endogenous concentrations have been shown to be partly responsible for cognitive dysfunction in rats with epilepsy induced by pilocarpine status epilepticus (Klatte et al., 2013; Schell et al., 1995). Results of studies on the anticonvulsant effects of D-serine are mixed. D-Serine protects weakly in the maximal electroshock test, where it also potentiates the effects of some antiseizure drugs (Kalinichev

---

BOX 35.2
D-AMINO ACIDS WITH ANTISEIZURE EFFECTS

D-Leucine
D-Serine
D-Arginine

---

et al., 2010; Peterson, 1991). D-Serine increases after-discharge thresholds in amygdala-kindled rats (Löscher et al., 1994). Conversely, serine racemase knockout mice, which have decreased extracellular levels of D-serine in the dentate gyrus, are relatively protected against seizures induced by PTZ (Harai et al., 2012; Singh et al., 1990a). Similarly, exogenously administered D-serine potentiates seizures induced by PTZ, and it potentiates seizures induced by NMDA, as might be expected (Singh et al., 1990a). D-Serine does not affect spike-wave discharges in GAERS rats (Koerner et al., 1996). In studies designed to test the efficacy of antiseizure medicines at the D-serine/glycine binding site on the NMDA receptor, D-serine decreased the antiseizure effect of the clinical medicine felbamate, the experimental compound L-687,414, and the opioid κ-receptor agonist CI-977, among others (De Sarro et al., 1994; Singh et al., 1990b; Tricklebank et al., 1994; White et al., 1995). Notably, the latter experiments were not designed to directly test the antiseizure efficacy of D-serine but to use it as a coactivator of NMDA receptors.

D-Alanine binds to the D-serine/glycine site on the NMDA receptor and may play a role in circadian endocrine function (Kleckner & Dingledine, 1988; Morikawa et al., 2008). Treatment with D-alanine does not change seizure-related parameters in fully amygdala-kindled rats (Croucher & Bradford, 1991). High doses (1400 mg/kg) of exogenously administered D-arginine has CNS depressant effects and increases the latency to onset of PTZ-induced convulsions (but 700 mg/kg was ineffective; Navarro et al., 2005).

Other D-amino acids are discussed briefly here for the sake of interest and completeness, although they do not have a direct role in epilepsy. D-Aspartate has neurotransmitter properties and may play a role in neurodevelopment, learning, and neuroendocrine function (D'Aniello et al., 2000, 2011); it also decreases chemically induced schizophrenia-associated symptoms in rodents

(Errico et al., 2008, 2011). The brain concentration of D-proline is highest in pineal and pituitary tissue, but its endogenous function has not been reported (Hamase et al., 2005). D-Glutamate has been detected by immunohistochemical techniques in subsets of neuronal cell bodies in the mesencephalon and thalamus, but its role is unknown (Mangas et al., 2007). D-Methionine (1 mM) protects cultured auditory neurons against cisplatin-induced neurotoxicity (Gopal et al., 2012). A role for these D-amino acids in seizures has not been reported. Interestingly, plasma concentrations of D-serine, D-aspartate, D-alanine, D-leucine, and D-proline are reduced in the rat β-amyloid hippocampus injection model of Alzheimer's disease (Xing et al., 2016). Further work should clarify whether D-amino acid detection will be useful as a biomarker for either identifying the disease or monitoring disease progression.

TRAUMATIC BRAIN INJURY

Branched-chain amino acids (particularly leucine) represent a major source of glutamate in the central nervous system (Sakai et al., 2004). In the mouse lateral fluid percussion model of traumatic brain injury (TBI), hippocampal concentrations of each of the branched-chain amino acids (total levels, i.e., L- and D-amino acids) are decreased; supplementation of these amino acids for 5 or 10 days (but not shorter durations) reverses injury-induced deficits in both anterograde and retrograde memory (Cole et al., 2010; Elkind et al., 2015). In human trials, supplementation of all three branched-chain amino acids led to a substantial improvement in Disability Rating Scale scores (which evaluate factors like self-care and employability) in patients with severe TBI or in a posttraumatic vegetative state (in both studies, mean Glasgow Coma Scale scores were in the 5.5–5.9 range; Aquilani et al., 2005, 2008).

L-Serine is neuroprotective in a mouse weight-drop model in the acute phase of TBI (measured morphologically) and the mechanism may involve activation of glycine receptors (Zhai et al., 2015). L-Serine also decreases astrocytosis, microglial activation, and concentrations of inflammatory cytokines in the later phases of this model of TBI (Zhai et al., 2015). Similar findings were noted in the same test when mice were treated 24 hr after the weight drop using 6-chloro-1,2-benzisoxazol-3(2H)-one, an inhibitor of D-amino acid oxidase, which leads to an increase in select D-amino acids, including D-serine (Liraz-Zaltsman et al., 2018). For reasons that remain unclear, treatment with exogenous D-serine did not consistently lead to the same results, nor did combined treatment with the inhibitor plus D-serine. One potential explanation is that inhibition of the enzyme leads to a decrease in oxidative stress, which may have led to neuroprotection (Liraz-Zaltsman et al., 2018), rather than a specific effect of the amino acid. Because of potential nephrotoxicity, additional safety studies are indicated for these compounds.

CONCLUSIONS

Select amino acids protect against seizure activity and the sequelae of TBI. Interestingly, these compounds have a variety of different potential mechanisms in these disorders, including receptor binding, transporter effects, and as metabolic intermediates for other signaling molecules. They also may affect intracellular signaling pathways, although evidence for the latter is scant at this point. Preclinical studies show variability in therapeutic response and highlight potential safety concerns, indicating the need for well-designed early clinical studies in humans. Further research will elucidate additional roles for these amino acids in the treatment of neurologic disorders.

DISCLAIMER

The content is solely the responsibility of the author and does not necessarily represent the official views of the National Institute of Neurological Disorders and Stroke, National Institutes of Health, Department of Health and Human Services, or the U.S. Government.

REFERENCES

Aquilani, R., Boselli, M., Boschi, F., Viglio, S., Iadarola, P., Dossena, M., Pastoris, O., & Verri, M. (2008). Branched-chain amino acids may improve recovery from a vegetative or minimally conscious state in patients with traumatic brain injury: A pilot study. *Archives of Physical Medicine and Rehabilitation*, 89, 1642–1647.

Aquilani, R., Iadarola, P., Contardi, A., Boselli, M., Verri, M., Pastoris, O., Boschi, F., Arcidiaco, P., & Viglio, S. (2005). Branched-chain amino acids enhance the cognitive recovery of patients with severe traumatic brain injury. *Archives of Physical Medicine and Rehabilitation*, 86, 1729–1735.

Banach, M., Piskorska, B., Czuczwar, S. J., & Borowicz, K. K. (2011). Nitric oxide, epileptic seizures, and action of antiepileptic drugs. *CNS & Neurological Disorders—Drug Targets*, 10, 808–819.

Bar-Peled, L., Schweitzer, L. D., Zoncu, R., & Sabatini, D. M. (2012). Ragulator is a GEF for the rag GTPases that signal amino acid levels to mTORC1. *Cell, 150*, 1196–1208.

Bassoli, A., Borgonovo, G., Caremoli, F., & Mancuso, G. (2014). The taste of D- and L-amino acids: In vitro binding assays with cloned human bitter (TAS2Rs) and sweet (TAS1R2/TAS1R3) receptors. *Food Chemistry, 150*, 27–33.

Berg, A. T., & Rychlik, K. (2015). The course of childhood-onset epilepsy over the first two decades: A prospective, longitudinal study. *Epilepsia, 56*, 40–48.

Bristow, L. J., Hutson, P. H., Kulagowski, J. J., Leeson, P. D., Matheson, S., Murray, F., Rathbone, D., Saywell, K. L., Thorn, L., Watt, A. P., & Tricklebank, M. D. (1996). Anticonvulsant and behavioral profile of L-701,324, a potent, orally active antagonist at the glycine modulatory site on the *N*-methyl-D-aspartate receptor complex. *Journal of Pharmacology and Experimental Therapeutics, 279*, 492–501.

Bröer, A., Tietze, N., Kowalczuk, S., Chubb, S., Munzinger, M., Bak, L. K., & Bröer, S. (2006). The orphan transporter v7-3 (slc6a15) is a Na$^+$-dependent neutral amino acid transporter (B^{0}AT2). *Biochemistry Journal, 393*, 421–430.

Buckmaster, P. S., & Lew, F. H. (2011). Rapamycin suppresses mossy fiber sprouting but not seizure frequency in a mouse model of temporal lobe epilepsy. *Journal of Neuroscience, 31*, 2337–2347.

Chachua, T., Poon, K.-L., Yum, M.-S., Nesheiwat, L., DeSantis, K., Velíšková, J., & Velíšek, L. (2012). Rapamycin has age-, treatment paradigm-, and model-specific anticonvulsant effects and modulates neuropeptide Y expression in rats. *Epilepsia, 53*, 2015–2025.

Chen, Z., Brodie, M. J., Liew, D., & Kwan, P. (2018). Treatment outcomes in patients with newly diagnosed epilepsy treated with established and new antiepileptic drugs: A 30-year longitudinal cohort study. *JAMA Neurology, 75*, 279–286.

Cheng, R. S., & Pomeranz, B. (1980). A combined treatment with D-amino acids and electroacupuncture produces a greater analgesia than either treatment alone: Naloxone reverses these effects. *Pain, 8*, 231–236.

Choi, H., Hayat, M. J., Zhang, R., Hirsch, L. J., Bazil, C. W., Mendiratta, A., Kato, K., Javed, A., Legge, A. W., Buchsbaum, R., Resor, S., & Heiman, G. A. (2016). Drug-resistant epilepsy in adults: Outcome trajectories after failure of two medications. *Epilepsia, 57*, 1152–1160.

Cole, J. T., Mitala, C. M., Kundu, S., Verma, A., Elkind, J. A., Nissim, I., & Cohen, A. S. (2010). Dietary branched chain amino acids ameliorate injury-induced cognitive impairment. *Proceedings of the National Academy of Sciences of the U S A, 107*, 366–371.

Cota, D., Proulx, K., Smith, K. A. B., Kozma, S. C., Thomas, G., Woods, S. C., & Seeley, R. J. (2006). Hypothalamic mTOR signaling regulates food intake. *Science, 312*, 927–930.

Croucher, M. J., & Bradford, H. F. (1991). The influence of strychnine-insensitive glycine receptor agonists and antagonists on generalized seizure thresholds. *Brain Research, 543*, 91–96.

D'Aniello, A., Di Fiore, M. M., Fisher, G. H., Milone, A., Seleni, A., D'Aniello, S., Perna, A. F., & Ingrosso, D. (2000). Occurrence of D-aspartic acid and *N*-methyl-D-aspartic acid in rat neuroendocrine tissues and their role in the modulation of luteinizing hormone and growth hormone release. *FASEB Journal, 14*, 699–714.

D'Aniello, S., Somorjai, I., Garcia-Fernàndez, J., Topo, E., & D'Aniello, A. (2011). D-Aspartic acid is a novel endogenous neurotransmitter. *FASEB Journal, 25*, 1014–1027.

Dahlin, M., Elfving, A., Ungerstedt, U., & Amark, P. (2005). The ketogenic diet influences the levels of excitatory and inhibitory amino acids in the CSF in children with refractory epilepsy. *Epilepsy Research, 64*, 115–125.

De Sarro, G., Ongini, E., Bertorelli, R., Aguglia, U., & De Sarro, A. (1994). Excitatory amino acid neurotransmission through both NMDA and non-NMDA receptors is involved in the anticonvulsant activity of felbamate in DBA/2 mice. *European Journal of Pharmacology, 262*, 11–19.

De Vasconcelos, A. P., Gizard, F., Marescaux, C., & Nehlig, A. (2000). Role of nitric oxide in pentylenetetrazol-induced seizures: Age-dependent effects in the immature rat. *Epilepsia, 41*, 363–371.

Dufour, F., Nalecz, K. A., Nalecz, M. J., & Nehlig, A. (1999). Modulation of pentylenetetrazol-induced seizure activity by branched-chain amino acids and alpha-ketoisocaproate. *Brain Research, 815*, 400–404.

Dufour, F., Nalecz, K. A., Nalecz, M. J., & Nehlig, A. (2001a). Metabolic approach of absence seizures in a genetic model of absence epilepsy, the GAERS: Study of the leucine-glutamate cycle. *Journal of Neuroscience Research, 66*, 923–930.

Dufour, F., Nalecz, K. A., Nalecz, M. J., & Nehlig, A. (2001b). Modulation of absence seizures by branched-chain amino acids: Correlation with brain amino acid concentrations. *Neuroscience Research, 40*, 255–263.

Ekborg-Ott, K. H., & Armstrong, D. W. (1996). Evaluation of the concentration and enantiomeric purity of selected free amino acids in fermented malt beverages (beers). *Chirality, 8*, 49–57.

Elkind, J. A., Lim, M. M., Johnson, B. N., Palmer, C. P., Putnam, B. J., Kirschen, M. P., & Cohen, A. S. (2015). Efficacy, dosage, and duration of action of branched chain amino acid therapy for traumatic brain injury. *Frontiers in Neurology, 6*, 73.

Embden, G. (1908). Uber das Verhalten der optish-isomeren leucine in der Leber [On the behavior of the optic-isomeric leucine in the liver]. *Beiträge zur chemisch Physiologie und Pathologie, 11*, 348–355.

Errico, F., Rossi, S., Napolitano, F., Catuogno, V., Topo, E., Fisone, G., D'Aniello, A., Centonze, D., & Usiello, A. (2008). D-Aspartate prevents corticostriatal long-term depression and attenuates schizophrenia-like symptoms induced by amphetamine and MK-801. *Journal of Neuroscience, 28*, 10404–10414.

Errico, F., Nisticò, R., Napolitano, F., Mazzola, C., Astone, D., Pisapia, T., Giustizieri, M., D'Aniello, A., Mercuri, N. B., & Usiello, A. (2011). Increased D-aspartate brain content rescues hippocampal age-related synaptic plasticity deterioration of mice. *Neurobiology of Aging, 32*, 2229–2243.

French, J. A., White, H. S., Klitgaard, H., Holmes, G. L., Privitera, M. D., Cole, A. J., Quay, E., Wiebe, S., Schmidt, D., Porter, R. J., Arzimanoglou, A., Trinka, E., & Perucca, E. (2013). Development of new treatment approaches for epilepsy: Unmet needs and opportunities. *Epilepsia, 54*(Suppl. 4), 3–12.

Geier, E. G., Schlessinger, A., Fan, H., Gable, J. E., Irwin, J. J., Sali, A., & Giacomini, K. M. (2013). Structure-based ligand discovery for the large-neutral amino acid transporter 1, LAT-1. *Proceedings of the National Academy of Sciences of the U S A, 110*, 5480–5485.

Genchi, G. (2017). An overview on D-amino acids. *Amino Acids, 49*, 1521–1533.

Gietzen, D. W., Lindström, S. H., Sharp, J. W., Teh, P. S., & Donovan, M. J. (2018). Indispensable amino acid-deficient diets induce seizures in ketogenic diet-fed rodents, demonstrating a role for amino acid balance in dietary treatments for epilepsy. *Journal of Nutrition, 148*, 480–489.

Gopal, K. V., Wu, C., Shrestha, B., Campbell, K. C. M., Moore, E. J., & Gross, G. W. (2012). D-Methionine protects against cisplatin-induced neurotoxicity in cortical networks. *Neurotoxicology and Teratology, 34*, 495–504.

Gruenbaum, S. E., Chen, E. C., Sandhu, M. R. S., Deshpande, K., Dhaher, R., Hersey, D., & Eid, T. (2019a). Branched-chain amino acids and seizures: A systematic review of the literature. *CNS Drugs, 33*, 755–770.

Gruenbaum, S. E., Dhaher, R., Rapuano, A., Zaveri, H. P., Tang, A., de Lanerolle, N., & Eid, T. (2019b). Effects of branched-chain amino acid supplementation on spontaneous seizures and neuronal viability in a model of mesial temporal lobe epilepsy. *Journal of Neurosurgery and Anesthesiology, 31*, 247–256.

Hägglund, M. G. A., Roshanbin, S., Löfqvist, E., Hellsten, S. V., Nilsson, V. C. O., Todkar, A., Zhu, Y., Stephansson, O., Drgonova, J., Uhl, G. R., Schiöth, H. B., & Fredriksson, R. (2013). B⁰AT2 (SLC6A15) is localized to neurons and astrocytes, and is involved in mediating the effect of leucine in the brain. *PLOS ONE, 8*, Article e58651.

Hamase, K., Homma, H., Takigawa, Y., Fukushima, T., Santa, T., & Imai, K. (1997). Regional distribution and postnatal changes of D-amino acids in rat brain. *Biochimica et Biophysica Acta, 1334*, 214–222.

Hamase, K., Inoue, T., Morikawa, A., Konno, R., & Zaitsu, K. (2001). Determination of free D-proline and D-leucine in the brains of mutant mice lacking D-amino acid oxidase activity. *Analytical Biochemistry, 298*, 253–258.

Hamase, K., Konno, R., Morikawa, A., & Zaitsu, K. (2005). Sensitive determination of D-amino acids in mammals and the effect of D-amino-acid oxidase activity on their amounts. *Biological and Pharmaceutical Bulletin, 28*, 1578–1584.

Harai, T., Inoue, R., Fujita, Y., Tanaka, A., Horio, M., Hashimoto, K., Hongou, K., Miyawaki, T., & Mori, H. (2012). Decreased susceptibility to seizures induced by pentylenetetrazole in serine racemase knockout mice. *Epilepsy Research, 102*, 180–187.

Hartman, A. L., Santos, P., Dolce, A., & Hardwick, J. M. (2012). The mTOR inhibitor rapamycin has limited acute anticonvulsant effects in mice. *PLOS ONE, 7*, Article e45156.

Hartman, A. L., Santos, P., O'Riordan, K. J., Stafstrom, C. E., & Marie Hardwick, J. (2015). Potent anti-seizure effects of D-leucine. *Neurobiology of Disease, 82*, 46–53.

Herberg, L. J., Grottick, A., & Rose, I. C. (1995). Nitric oxide synthesis, epileptic seizures and kindling. *Psychopharmacology, 119*, 115–123.

Holden, K., & Hartman, A. L. (2018). D-Leucine: Evaluation in an epilepsy model. *Epilepsy & Behavior, 78*, 202–209.

Huang, X., Zhang, H., Yang, J., Wu, J., McMahon, J., Lin, Y., Cao, Z., Gruenthal, M., & Huang, Y. (2010). Pharmacological inhibition of the mammalian target of rapamycin pathway suppresses acquired epilepsy. *Neurobiology of Disease, 40*, 193–199.

Johnson, J. W., & Ascher, P. (1987). Glycine potentiates the NMDA response in cultured mouse brain neurons. *Nature, 325*, 529–531.

Kalinichev, M., Starr, K. R., Teague, S., Bradford, A. M., Porter, R. A., & Herdon, H. J. (2010). Glycine transporter 1 (GlyT1) inhibitors exhibit anticonvulsant properties in the rat maximal electro-shock threshold (MEST) test. *Brain Research, 1331*, 105–113.

Klatte, K., Kirschstein, T., Otte, D., Pothmann, L., Müller, L., Tokay, T., Kober, M., Uebachs, M., Zimmer, A., & Beck, H. (2013). Impaired D-serine-mediated cotransmission mediates cognitive dysfunction in epilepsy. *Journal of Neuroscience, 33*, 13066–13080.

Kleckner, N. W., & Dingledine, R. (1988). Requirement for glycine in activation of NMDA-receptors expressed in *Xenopus* oocytes. *Science, 241*, 835–837.

Koerner, C., Danober, L., Boehrer, A., Marescaux, C., & Vergnes, M. (1996). Thalamic NMDA transmission in a genetic model of absence epilepsy in rats. *Epilepsy Research, 25*, 11–19.

Kwan, P., & Brodie, M. J. (2000). Early identification of refractory epilepsy. *New England Journal of Medicine, 342*, 314–319.

Laeger, T., Henagan, T. M., Albarado, D. C., Redman, L. M., Bray, G. A., Noland, R. C., Münzberg, H., Hutson, S. M., Gettys, T. W., Schwartz, M. W., & Morrison, C. D. (2014). FGF21 is an endocrine signal of protein restriction. *Journal of Clinical Investigation, 124*, 3913–3922.

Lim, B.-C., Cho, K.-Y., Lim, J.-S., Lee, R.-S., Kim, H.-S., Kim, M.-K., Kim, J.-H., Woo, Y.-J., Kim, J.-K., Kim, D. K., Kim, H.-I., Lee, K.-W., & Lee, M. C. (2011). Increased expression of L-amino acid transporters in balloon cells of tuberous sclerosis. *Childs Nervous System, 27*, 63–70.

Liraz-Zaltsman, S., Slusher, B., Atrakchi-Baranes, D., Rosenblatt, K., Friedman Levi, Y., Kesner, E., Silva, A. J., Biegon, A., & Shohami, E. (2018). Enhancement of brain D-serine mediates recovery of cognitive function after traumatic brain injury. *Journal of Neurotrauma, 35*, 1667–1680.

Löscher, W., Wlaź, P., Rundfeldt, C., Baran, H., & Hönack, D. (1994). Anticonvulsant effects of the glycine/NMDA receptor ligands D-cycloserine and D-serine but not R-(+)-HA-966 in amygdala-kindled rats. *British Journal of Pharmacology, 112*, 97–106.

Mangas, A., Coveñas, R., Bodet, D., Geffard, M., Aguilar, L. A., & Yajeya, J. (2007). Immunocytochemical visualization of D-glutamate in the rat brain. *Neuroscience, 144*, 654–664.

Masino, S. A., & Rho, J. M. (2012). Mechanisms of ketogenic diet action. In J. L. Noebels, M. Avoli, M. A. Rogawski, R. W. Olsen, & A. V. Delgado-Escueta (Eds.), *Jasper's basic mechanisms of the epilepsies*. National Center for Biotechnology Information [Internet]. 4th ed. Bethesda (MD): National Center for Biotechnology Information (US); 2012. PMID: 22787591.

McKibbin, L. S., & Cheng, R. S. (1982). Systemic D-phenylalanine and D-leucine for effective treatment of pain in the horse. *Canadian Veterinary Journal, 23*, 39–40.

Morikawa, A., Hamase, K., Miyoshi, Y., Koyanagi, S., Ohdo, S., & Zaitsu, K. (2008). Circadian changes of D-alanine and related compounds in rats and the effect of restricted feeding on their amounts. *Journal of Chromatography B Analytical Technologies in the Biomedical and Life Sciences, 875*, 168–173.

Mutaguchi, Y., Ohmori, T., Wakamatsu, T., Doi, K., & Ohshima, T. (2013). Identification, purification, and characterization of a novel amino acid racemase, isoleucine 2-epimerase, from *Lactobacillus* species. *Journal of Bacteriology, 195*, 5207–5215.

Navarro, E., Alonso, S. J., Martín, F. A., & Castellano, M. A. (2005). Toxicological and pharmacological effects of D-arginine. *Basic and Clinical Pharmacology and Toxicology, 97*, 149–154.

Nichols, A. C., & Yielding, K. L. (1998). Anticonvulsant activity of 4-urea-5,7-dichlorokynurenic acid derivatives that are antagonists at the NMDA-associated glycine binding site. *Molecular and Chemical Neuropathology, 35*, 1–12.

Ninomiya, Y., Kawamura, H., Nomura, T., Uebayashi, H., Sabashi, K., & Funakoshi, M. (1990). Analgesic effects of D-amino acids in four inbred strains of mice. *Comparative Biochemistry and Physiology Part C, Comparative Pharmacology and Toxicology, 97*, 341–343.

Orlova, K. A., & Crino, P. B. (2010). The tuberous sclerosis complex. *Annals of the New York Academy of Sciences, 1184*, 87–105.

Peterson, S. L. (1991). Anticonvulsant drug potentiation by glycine in maximal electroshock seizures is mimicked by D-serine and antagonized by 7-chlorokynurenic acid. *European Journal of Pharmacology, 199*, 341–348.

Sakai, R., Cohen, D. M., Henry, J. F., Burrin, D. G., & Reeds, P. J. (2004). Leucine-nitrogen metabolism in the brain of conscious rats: Its role as a nitrogen carrier in glutamate synthesis in glial and neuronal metabolic compartments. *Journal of Neurochemistry, 88*, 612–622.

Sancak, Y., Peterson, T. R., Shaul, Y. D., Lindquist, R. A., Thoreen, C. C., Bar-Peled, L., & Sabatini, D. M. (2008). The Rag GTPases bind raptor and mediate amino acid signaling to mTORC1. *Science, 320*, 1496–1501.

Sariego-Jamardo, A., García-Cazorla, A., Artuch, R., Castejón, E., García-Arenas, D., Molero-Luis, M., Ormazábal, A., & Sanmartí, F. X. (2015). Efficacy of the ketogenic diet for the treatment of refractory childhood epilepsy: Cerebrospinal fluid neurotransmitters and amino acid levels. *Pediatric Neurology, 53*, 422–426.

Schell, M. J., Molliver, M. E., & Snyder, S. H. (1995). D-Serine, an endogenous synaptic modulator: Localization to astrocytes and glutamate-stimulated release. *Proceedings of the National Academy of Sciences of the U S A, 92*, 3948–3952.

Schmidt, D., & Schachter, S. C. (2014). Drug treatment of epilepsy in adults. *BMJ, 348*, g254.

Shen, H.-Y., van Vliet, E. A., Bright, K.-A., Hanthorn, M., Lytle, N. K., Gorter, J., Aronica, E., & Boison, D. (2015). Glycine transporter 1 is a target for the treatment of epilepsy. *Neuropharmacology, 99*, 554–565.

Shin, Y.-J., Park, J.-H., Choi, J.-S., Chun, M.-H., Moon, Y. W., & Lee, M.-Y. (2010). Enhanced expression of the sweet taste receptors and alpha-gustducin in reactive astrocytes of the rat hippocampus following ischemic injury. *Neurochemistry Research, 35,* 1628–1634.

Singh, L., Oles, R. J., & Tricklebank, M. D. (1990a). Modulation of seizure susceptibility in the mouse by the strychnine-insensitive glycine recognition site of the NMDA receptor/ion channel complex. *British Journal of Pharmacology, 99,* 285–288.

Singh, L., Vass, C. A., Hunter, J. C., Woodruff, G. N., & Hughes, J. (1990b). The anticonvulsant action of CI-977, a selective κ-opioid receptor agonist: A possible involvement of the glycine/NMDA receptor complex. *European Journal of Pharmacology, 191,* 477–480.

Skeie, B., Petersen, A. J., Manner, T., Askanazi, J., & Steen, P. A. (1994). Effects of valine, leucine, isoleucine, and a balanced amino acid solution on the seizure threshold to picrotoxin in rats. *Pharmacology Biochemistry Behavior, 48,* 101–103.

Sosanya, N. M., Brager, D. H., Wolfe, S., Niere, F., & Raab-Graham, K. F. (2015). Rapamycin reveals an mTOR-independent repression of Kv1.1 expression during epileptogenesis. *Neurobiology of Disease, 73,* 96–105.

Talevi, A., Enrique, A. V., & Bruno-Blanch, L. E. (2012). Anticonvulsant activity of artificial sweeteners: A structural link between sweet-taste receptor T1R3 and brain glutamate receptors. *Bioorganic & Medicinal Chemistry Letters, 22,* 4072–4074.

Tricklebank, M. D., Bristow, L. J., Hutson, P. H., Leeson, P. D., Rowley, M., Saywell, K., Singh, L., Tattersall, F. D., Thorn, L., & Williams, B. J. (1994). The anticonvulsant and behavioural profile of L-687,414, a partial agonist acting at the glycine modulatory site on the N-methyl-D-aspartate (NMDA) receptor complex. *British Journal of Pharmacology, 113,* 729–736.

Weatherly, C. A., Du, S., Parpia, C., Santos, P. T., Hartman, A. L., & Armstrong, D. W. (2017). D-Amino acid levels in perfused mouse brain tissue and blood: A comparative study. *ACS Chemical Neuroscience, 8,* 1251–1261.

Werman, R., Davidoff, R. A., & Aprison, M. H. (1968). Inhibitory of glycine on spinal neurons in the cat. *Journal of Neurophysiology, 31,* 81–95.

White, H. S., Harmsworth, W. L., Sofia, R. D., & Wolf, H. H. (1995). Felbamate modulates the strychnine-insensitive glycine receptor. *Epilepsy Research, 20,* 41–48.

Wolfson, R. L., Chantranupong, L., Saxton, R. A., Shen, K., Scaria, S. M., Cantor, J. R., & Sabatini, D. M. (2016). Sestrin2 is a leucine sensor for the mTORC1 pathway. *Science, 351,* 43–48.

Xie, X., Dumas, T., Tang, L., Brennan, T., Reeder, T., Thomas, W., Klein, R. D., Flores, J., O'Hara, B. F., Heller, H. C., & Franken P. (2005). Lack of the alanine-serine-cysteine transporter 1 causes tremors, seizures, and early postnatal death in mice. *Brain Research, 1052,* 212–221.

Xing, Y., Li, X., Guo, X., & Cui, Y. (2016). Simultaneous determination of 18 D-amino acids in rat plasma by an ultrahigh-performance liquid chromatography-tandem mass spectrometry method: Application to explore the potential relationship between Alzheimer's disease and D-amino acid level alterations. *Analytical Bioanalytical Chemistry, 408,* 141–150.

Yudkoff, M., Daikhin, Y., Melø, T. M., Nissim, I., Sonnewald, U., & Nissim, I. (2007). The ketogenic diet and brain metabolism of amino acids: Relationship to the anticonvulsant effect. *Annual Review of Nutrition, 27,* 415–430.

Yudkoff, M., Daikhin, Y., Nissim, I., Horyn, O., Lazarow, A., Luhovyy, B., Wehrli, S., & Nissim, I. (2005). Response of brain amino acid metabolism to ketosis. *Neurochemistry International, 47,* 119–128.

Zack, M. M., & Kobau, R. (2017). National and state estimates of the numbers of adults and children with active epilepsy—United States, 2015. *Morbidity and Mortality Weekly Report, 66,* 821–825.

Zellinger, C., Salvamoser, J. D., Soerensen, J., van Vliet, E. A., Aronica, E., Gorter, J., & Potschka, H. (2014). Pre-treatment with the NMDA receptor glycine-binding site antagonist L-701,324 improves pharmacosensitivity in a mouse kindling model. *Epilepsy Research, 108,* 634–643.

Zeng, L.-H., Xu, L., Gutmann, D. H., & Wong, M. (2008). Rapamycin prevents epilepsy in a mouse model of tuberous sclerosis complex. *Annals of Neurology, 63,* 444–453.

Zeng, L.-H., Rensing, N. R., & Wong, M. (2009). The mammalian target of rapamycin signaling pathway mediates epileptogenesis in a model of temporal lobe epilepsy. *Journal of Neuroscience, 29,* 6964–6972.

Zhai, P.-P., Xu, L.-H., Yang, J.-J., Jiang, Z.-L., Zhao, G.-W., Sun, L., Wang, G.-H., & Li, X. (2015). Reduction of inflammatory responses by L-serine treatment leads to neuroprotection in mice after traumatic brain injury. *Neuropharmacology, 95,* 1–11.

Identifying the Molecular Mechanism of the MCT (Ketogenic) Diet

MATTHEW C. WALKER, MA, FRCP, PHD AND
ROBIN S. B. WILLIAMS, BSC, PHD

INTRODUCTION

The medium-chain triglyceride (MCT) ketogenic diet (KD) was first introduced as a more palatable alternative to the classic KD for the treatment of refractory epilepsy by Huttenlocher et al. (1971). It now provides a key therapeutic approach for the treatment of children with drug-resistant epilepsy (Levy et al., 2012; Liu, 2008; Neal & Cross, 2010; Neal et al., 2009). The diet involves a stringent reduction in carbohydrate intake, with an elevated consumption of medium-chain fatty acids (MCFA) within a triglyceride backbone. Typically, the fats in this diet provide 65% to 75% of the total daily energy requirement. These fats comprise two medium, straight-chain fats; octanoic acid (comprising 8 carbons) and decanoic acid (comprising 10 carbons). Of the MCT intake, 60% to 80% is octanoic acid and the remainder is mostly decanoic acid (Sills et al., 1986b). Both fats are rapidly hydrolyzed off the triglyceride backbone in the gut and are absorbed as free fatty acids (Bach & Babayan, 1982) and are metabolized into ketones (β-hydroxybutryate, acetone, and acetoacetate) and carbon dioxide, or they are catabolized into long-chain fatty acids. The diet results in an elevation of the concentration of both fatty acids in peripheral blood: octanoic acid increase from 104 to 859 µM and averages around 306 µM, and decanoic acid increases from 87 to 552 µM, with an average of 157 µM (Dean et al., 1989; Haidukewych et al., 1982; Sills et al., 1986a). In animal models, decanoic acid has been found to penetrate the blood–brain barrier and to be present in brain at 60% to 80% of serum levels (Wlaz et al., 2012).

The dietary restrictions and high fat intake of the MCT KD can cause a variety of gastrointestinal side effects, such as cramps, bloating, diarrhea, and vomiting (Liu, 2008). Use of the diet has also been limited by poor tolerability, especially in adults, resulting in a high attrition rate (Levy et al., 2012). Due to its adverse effects and a desire to increase the efficacy of the MCT KD, many studies have sought to identify the therapeutic mechanism of the diet. Because the diet was based on the classic KD, it was thought that it acted through the generation of ketones (Bough & Rho, 2007; Rho & Stafstrom, 2011). However, the presence of ketones poorly correlates with anti-seizure efficacy, and the ketone-based mechanism has not been widely supported in animal studies (Likhodii et al., 2000; Thavendiranathan et al., 2000). Furthermore, ketones do not directly alter hippocampal synaptic transmission (Thio et al., 2000), nor do they affect epileptiform activity induced by 4-aminopyridine in ex vivo seizure models (Thio et al., 2000). Thus, the therapeutic mechanism of the MCT KD has, until recently, been unclear.

MCFA IN SEIZURE CONTROL

A clinical role for MCFA in direct seizure control was proposed over 30 years ago (Dean et al., 1989; Haidukewych et al., 1982; Sills et al., 1986a), but due to limited study sizes, a direct correlation between plasma concentrations and seizure control was not established. Recently, however, an unbiased screen for MCFA and short-chain fatty acids related to valproate (Chang et al., 2012) in a simple cellular model identified a number of fatty acids as potential seizure-control treatments. In this study, where valproate had been shown to regulate phosphoinositide turnover (Cunliffe et al., 2015; Xu et al., 2007), over 60 compounds were screened for an inhibitory effect on rapid phosphoinositide turnover. Interestingly, this inhibitory effect has since been confirmed as a therapeutic mechanism for valproate in animal seizure models *in vitro* and *in vivo* (Chang et al., 2014). Thus, using this phosphoinositide screen, Chang et al. (2012) were able to investigate a wide range of fatty acids and related compounds, with some structures producing little effect, and some structures showing enhanced activity over valproate. The potent compounds included decanoic acid, nonanoic acid, and the branched 8-carbon backbone 4-methyloctanoic acid. In this simple model, these compounds did not act by regulating inositol levels, which was previously suggested as a mechanism of valproate (Shaltiel et al., 2007; Vaden et al., 2001; Williams, 2005; Williams et al., 2002). The compounds were then tested in a well-established *ex vivo* mammalian model for drug-resistant epilepsy, the low-magnesium hippocampal-entorhinal cortex model (Chang et al., 2012). Here, brain slices are kept "alive" in a bath perfused with oxygenated artificial cerebrospinal fluid (aCSF), and seizure-like activity is induced by reducing magnesium levels, enhancing NMDA receptor currents. In these experiments, equimolar concentrations of a range of fatty acids were more potent than valproate, within 10 min of compound addition (the time for the compounds to perfuse the bath and penetrate the slice); thus, significant levels of ketosis in these experiments are unlikely. These experiments therefore suggested a direct role for MCFA in seizure control.

Further studies pursued the analysis of the activity of the MCFA in seizure control and related effects (Chang et al., 2013), and decanoic acid and nonanoic acid were shown to provide protection against an *ex vivo* model of epileptiform activity generated by decreasing GABAergic inhibition (pentylenetetrazol, PTZ; Figure 36.1). In these studies, decanoic acid completely blocks seizure activity 35 min after its addition. Interestingly, octanoic acid, also prescribed in the MCT KD, did not reduce seizure activity in this model. However, branched derivatives of octanoic acid show variable efficacy, with some compounds providing strong seizure control (e.g., 4-methyloctanoic acid) and some showing no activity (3,7-dimethyloctanoic acid). These results confirmed earlier studies (Chang et al., 2012) but extended these findings to establish a wide chemical space showing potential efficacy in seizure control. This study also examined these chemicals for inhibition of histone deacetylase activity (HDAC), an effect associated with teratogenicity (Gottlicher et al., 2001; Gurvich et al., 2004; Phiel et al., 2001), and thus limiting their use during pregnancy (Jentink et al., 2010; Koren et al., 2006). Of the compounds analyzed in the study, only valproate and 2-proplyoctanoic acid caused significant inhibition of HDAC activity at 1 mM, a concentration considerably higher than that of MCFA found during MCT KD treatment (Sills et al., 1986a). This suggests

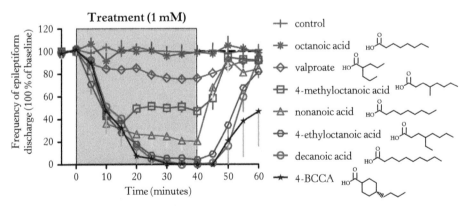

FIGURE 36.1 *Structurally Specific Medium-Chain Fatty Acids Strongly Reduce Frequency of in Vitro Epileptiform Activity*

In these experiments, an ex vivo hippocampal slice model was used, with seizurelike activity induced by application of PTZ. Compounds were added (gray box) at 1 mM and were removed after 40 min. The frequency of epileptiform activity is plotted against time after control (DMSO). Straight medium-chain fatty acids decanoic (10-carbon), nonanoic acid (9-carbon), two branched-chain derivatives (4-methyloctanoic acid and 4-ethyloctanoic acid), and a cyclic congener (*trans*-4-butylcyclocarboxylic acid; 4-BCCA) were able to strongly reduce seizurelike activity. In contrast, octanoic acid showed no inhibitory activity. The widely used, established epilepsy treatment, valproate, showed weak activity in this seizure model. Data derived from Chang et al. (2014, 2015, 2016).

that the MCFA are unlikely to exhibit the teratogenic effects found with valproate treatment. This study also showed that MCFA (4-methyloctanoic acid and nonanoic acid) provide control against self-sustaining status epilepticus (SSSE), induced by perforant pathway stimulation, in an *in vivo* rat model (Walker & Williams, 2015). Analysis of neuronal cell death in these animals as a result of SSSE showed that 2 months after seizure induction, nonanoic acid significantly reduced cell death in the hilus of the hippocampus, suggesting a neuroprotective effect. This therapeutic effect is also unlikely to be related to ketosis, since these compounds rapidly reduced seizure activity within 10 min of treatment. For nonanoic acid, the effects were also unlikely to occur due to sedation, since sedative effects were not shown even at high concentrations (600 mg/ kg). Together, these studies provide strong evidence for the direct activity of a range of MCFA in seizure control and neuroprotection.

One further study has been reported, investigating the breadth of chemical space for MCFA in seizure control (Chang et al., 2015). This study specifically investigated octanoic acid-related compounds, including a systematic analysis of methyloctanoic acid derivatives. Using an *ex vivo* model of seizure activity, induced in rat hippocampal slices by the application of PTZ, a clear structure–activity relationship was seen in seizure control, provided by the position of branching on the octanoic acid backbone. The most potent compounds branched around the fifth carbon. This study also examined these compounds for protection against excitotoxic cell death, an effect that is similar to that resulting from status epilepticus (DeLorenzo et al., 2005). In these experiments, exposure of hippocampal neurons in culture to low magnesium for 4 hr triggered cell death (Deshpande et al., 2008), and consistent with the seizure-control experiments, neuroprotection was seen with the addition of compounds with methyl branching from the fourth to the seventh carbon (Chang et al., 2015). Based on these results, three related compounds were then examined: 4-ethyloctanoic acid, containing a longer side chain; 4-methylnonanoic acid, containing a longer backbone, and *trans*-4-butylcyclohexane carboxylic acid (4-BCCA), a related cyclic compound. All three compounds also showed strong seizure control in the PTZ model (Figure 36.1) and were not active against HDAC activity. These compounds were further screened in a range of *in vivo* seizure models (Table 36.1), providing promising activity for 4-BCCA in multiple models. In a related study, mice treated with decanoic acid by gastric gavage (30 mmol/kg) also showed seizure control in the 6-Hz seizure and maximal electroshock seizure threshold (MEST) models (Wlaz et al., 2012). These data provide evidence that MCFA

TABLE 36.1 IN VIVO SEIZURE CONTROL DATA FOR ACTIVE COMPOUNDS

Compound	Species	Seizure model	Dose (mg/kg)	Animals (protected/ tested)	Animals (toxic/ tested)	ED_{50} (mg/kg)
4-EOA[a]	Mice	6 Hz	150	7/8	—	110
	Rats	MES	125	12/16	4/15†	100
	Mice	scMET	200	8/8	4/8¥	142
	Mice	CKM	110	6/8	0/8	71
4-BCCA[a]	Mice	6-Hz	100	3/4	0/4	81
	Rats	MES	100	4/8	1/8†	~ 100*
	Mice	scMET	150	4/8	0/8	~ 150*
	Mice	CKM	80	8/8	0/8	44
VPA	Mice	6-Hz				263[b]
	Rats	MES				485[c]
	Mice	scMET				191[d]
	Mice	CKM				174[e]

Note. Summary of *in vivo* seizure control in multiple models, with data provided by collaborative research with [a] NINDS; or previously determined by [b] Barton et al. (2001); [c] Loscher (1999); [d] Rowley and White (2010); [e] by NINDS. * = based upon single-dose data; — = not determined; † = unable to grasp rotorod; ¥ = ataxia/loss of righting reflex. Partially reproduced from Chang et al. (2015), with permission. MES = maximal electric shock, scMET = subcutaneous Metrazol, CKM = Corneal Kindling Model.

of defined structures show activity in a range of *in vivo* seizure models.

MCFA ARE AMPA RECEPTOR ANTAGONISTS

The molecular mechanism of decanoic acid in direct seizure control has recently been established (Chang et al., 2016). In this study, decanoic acid (1 mM) was shown to abolish seizure activity *in vitro* in both the PTZ and low-magnesium-induced drug-resistant seizure models. As previously described, decanoic acid blocks seizure activity within 15 min of addition to each model, strongly suggesting that the effect is directly related to the fatty acid, and not to ketone generation. Moreover, acetone and β-hydroxybutyrate (two ketone bodies) have no effect in either model at high concentrations (10 mM). The mechanism of decanoic acid for this effect was then shown using whole-cell patch-clamp recordings of evoked AMPA receptor-mediated excitatory postsynaptic currents (EPSCs) from CA1 pyramidal neurons, where decanoic acid reduced EPSC amplitude by $17.0 \pm 5.6\%$ at a concentration comparable to its steady-state level in children on the MCT diet (100 μM; Sills et al., 1986a). These data, for the first time, provided evidence of a direct mechanism of the MCT ketogenic diet in seizure control through inhibition of AMPA receptor currents.

To investigate a direct effect of decanoic acid on AMPA receptor activity, a range of experiments were carried out using a *Xenopus* heterologous expression system (Chang et al., 2016). Here, AMPA receptor subunits (GluA1–3) were expressed in oocytes individually or in pairs to produce homotetramers (GluA1) or heterotetramers (GluA1/2 and GluA2/3), and glutamate was applied, resulting in inward currents, on which direct application of decanoic acid and related compounds was tested. This approach allowed the quantification of the direct inhibition of AMPA receptor-mediated currents by MCFA (Table 36.2). From these experiments, decanoic acid was shown to be an AMPA receptor antagonist, with efficacy across all subunit compositions, and greatest potency against GluA2/3 heterotetramers ($IC_{50} = 0.52$ mM). Decreasing the length of the backbone reduced potency, such that nonanoic acid and octanoic acid were increasingly less potent ($IC_{50} = 1.48$ and 3.82 mM, respectively), although addition of a side chain to octanoic acid to produce 4-methyloctanoic acid-enhanced potency ($IC_{50} = 0.84$ mM). These data indicate a direct action of decanoic acid and specific related structures in inhibition of AMPA receptors to regulate neuronal function.

TABLE 36.2 SUMMARY OF MEDIUM-CHAIN FATTY ACIDS' INHIBITORY EFFECTS ON AMPA RECEPTORS

Subunit specificity: IC_{50} (mM)			
	GluA2/3	GluA1/2	GluA1
Decanoic acid	0.52	1.16	2.09
Nonanoic acid	1.48		1.79
4-Methyloctanoic acid	0.84		
Octanoic acid	3.82		

Voltage dependence (IC_{50} mM, Decanoic acid, GluA2/3)	
–80 mV	1.11
–40 mV	0.43

Kinetics
Decanoic acid is noncompetitive toward glutamate

Data were derived from heterologous expression of rat glutamate receptors in a *Xenopus* oocyte model, activated with 100 μM glutamate. Data derived from Chang et al. (2016).

This study also investigated some kinetic aspects of MCFA-dependent AMPA receptor inhibition (Chang et al., 2016). First, since membrane depolarization occurs during seizure activity, and this may alter inhibitory activity at AMPA receptors, the effect of decanoic acid was analyzed at varying membrane potentials. The studies identified that under depolarized membrane potentials, decanoic acid showed enhanced inhibitory activity, thus providing more potent inhibition of AMPA receptors during seizure activity. Second, since AMPA receptors are activated by glutamate, and glutamate levels increase during seizure activity (Van Den Pol et al., 1996), competition assays were used to explore if altered glutamate levels modulate decanoic acid-dependent AMPA receptor inhibition. The experiments indicated that decanoic acid is a noncompetitive AMPA receptor antagonist (Table 36.2), so its inhibitory activity is independent of glutamate concentrations.

These studies have suggested that MCFA function in seizure control through inhibition of AMPA receptors. However, it remained possible that these compounds gave rise to seizure control through alternative mechanisms. To address this, Chang et al. (2016) employed the hippocampal/PTZ seizure model, treated with the well-characterized AMPA receptor antagonist GYKI 52466 (Arai, 2001), to provide a similar level of AMPA receptor inhibition as decanoic acid (1 mM). Under these conditions, GYKI

52466 blocked seizure activity. These results are strongly supportive of a role for decanoic acid in seizure control through direct AMPA inhibition. Moreover, AMPA receptors are widely recognized as targets for seizure control (Meldrum & Rogawski, 2007; Russo et al., 2012; Szenasi et al., 2008). Perampanel, a selective AMPA receptor antagonist, has been introduced for the treatment of refractory partial epilepsy (Rektor, 2013), confirming the relevance of this mechanism to patient treatment. Chang et al. (2016) also showed that inhibition of AMPA receptors by decanoic acid at therapeutically relevant concentrations provided inhibitory effects similar to those resulting from perampanel at blood levels found during clinical use (Ceolin et al., 2012; Rogawski & Hanada, 2013). It is interesting to note, however, that the use of perampanel is limited by neuropsychiatric side effects, particularly aggression (Rugg-Gunn, 2014; Steinhoff et al., 2014). This effect is not seen during the MCT KD and suggests that the side effects may be peculiar to perampanel, perhaps due to off-target effects rather than an action at AMPA receptors; ideally, the development of pharmaceutical reagents based upon the mechanisms of decanoic acid will not cause similar side effects.

Finally, the binding site for decanoic acid on AMPA receptors was investigated by *in silico* modeling (Chang et al., 2016). Using the transmembrane domains of GluA2, a putative decanoic acid binding region was identified in the M3 helix, thought to be involved in regulating and gating inward currents. This site is distinct from that reported for perampanel (Szenasi et al., 2008), suggesting potential differences in the effects of decanoic acid and perampanel on AMPA receptor function. This binding site is consistent with the results from electrophysiological experiments described here, and similar mechanism has also been identified for novel decanoic acid analogs (Yelshanskaya et al., 2020).

IS THERE STILL A ROLE FOR KETONES IN SEIZURE CONTROL?

Over the last 30 years, many studies have suggested a role for ketones in seizure control and neuroprotection (Bough & Rho, 2007; Rho & Stafstrom, 2011). In some types of epilepsy, ketones may provide an alternative energy source for the brain (Kim et al., 2015; Masino et al., 2011)—for example, in GLUT1 deficiency when glucose is poorly transported across the blood–brain barrier. Ketones have also been demonstrated to alter

transcriptional regulation relevant to a putative disease-modifying role (Kim et al., 2015; Masino et al., 2011) and to have indirect effects on ion channels (Sada et al., 2015). Thus, ketones may still provide some beneficial effects related to specific causes of epilepsy and in protection against long-term epileptogenic changes.

IMPLICATIONS

Understanding the mechanism of action of the KD is essential for the development of diets or treatments that are less restrictive and that do not produce the same diet-associated side effects. The recent data outlined here provide a strong case for the antiseizure effects of the MCT KD resulting from increases in plasma fatty acid concentrations rather than through the production of ketones. Thus, despite the potential beneficial roles of ketones, due to the burgeoning evidence that fatty acids play a primary role in the diet's therapeutic effect, it would perhaps be more appropriate to call it the MCT diet.

Decanoic acid may have beneficial effects beyond its action at AMPA receptors. A study has identified a role for decanoic acid in regulating mitochondrial proliferation (Hughes et al., 2014). Here, decanoic acid acts through regulation of a fatty acid receptor, PPARγ (Malapaka et al., 2012; Zuckermann et al., 2015), at therapeutically relevant concentrations (250 μM) over a 6-day period in a neuronal cell line and in human fibroblasts. Interestingly, this effect was not shown by octanoic acid. The consequent increase in mitochondrial load has been suggested to protect against seizure induction (Bough et al., 2006) and to protect against mitochondrial dysfunction in epilepsy, which has been clearly demonstrated in animal models of status epilepticus (Cock et al., 2002) and in patients (Kunz et al., 2000). It has also been shown to function through reducing activity of the mTORC1 complex (Warren et al., 2020), where increased activation of this complex is associated with a range of disorders, including cancer and epilepsy.

MCFA are rapidly metabolized *in vivo* (Bach & Babayan, 1982). Therefore, a key consideration in the design and management of seizure-control treatments based upon decanoic aid is to ensure maintenance of therapeutic fatty acid levels. Early studies of MCFA showed considerable variation in plasma fatty acid levels over a 24-hr period (Sills et al., 1986b). More recently, in a 12 week study of adults and children with drug-resistant epilepsy using a novel MCT containing elevated levels of decanoic acid ('K.vita') and a mostly unrestricted diet, ketosis was not induced in >90% of individuals, but plasma decanoic acid increased, and provided a 50% reduction in seizures (Schoeler et al., 2021). This suggests that decanoic acid is likely to function directly in seizure control, and that clinicians using the MCT diet should focus on monitoring blood fatty acids rather than just ketone levels.

The discovery of a molecular target for the MCT diet also opens the possibility of a pharmaceutical approach to replace the diet. Several considerations are germane here. Due to the rapid metabolism of decanoic acid, a chemical that provides similar inhibitory activity against AMPA receptors but is resistant to metabolic degradation may overcome the need for a stringent dietary regime. Developing novel chemical structures that show enhanced binding to the target site on the receptor may also reduce the amount of compound needing consumption. This would additionally help to reduce the side effects associated with high fatty acid intake, in particular gastric irritation. Studies outlined here have provided some evidence for the efficacy of decanoic acid congeners in seizure control and in direct inhibition of AMPA receptors. Further studies will be necessary to identify suitable candidates for clinical testing, but they may result in the "diet in a pill."

REFERENCES

Arai, A. C. (2001). GYKI 52466 has positive modulatory effects on AMPA receptors. *Brain Research*, *892*, 396–400.

Bach, A. C. & Babayan, V. K. (1982). Medium-chain triglycerides: An update. *American Journal of Clinical Nutrition*, *36*, 950–962.

Barton, M. E., Klein, B. D., Wolf, H. H., & White, H. S. (2001). Pharmacological characterization of the 6 Hz psychomotor seizure model of partial epilepsy. *Epilepsy Research*, *47*, 217–227.

Bough, K. J., & Rho, J. M. (2007). Anticonvulsant mechanisms of the ketogenic diet. *Epilepsia*, *48*, 43–58.

Bough, K. J., Wetherington, J., Hassel, B., Pare, J. F., Gawryluk, J. W., Greene, J. G., Shaw, R., Smith, Y., Geiger, J. D., & Dingledine, R. J. (2006). Mitochondrial biogenesis in the anticonvulsant mechanism of the ketogenic diet. *Annals of Neurology*, *60*, 223–235.

Ceolin, L., Bortolotto, Z. A., Bannister, N., Collingridge, G. L., Lodge, D., & Volianskis, A. (2012). A novel anti-epileptic agent, perampanel, selectively inhibits AMPA receptor-mediated synaptic transmission in the hippocampus. *Neurochemistry International*, *61*, 517–522.

Chang, P., Orabi, B., Deranieh, R. M., Dham, M., Hoeller, O., Shimshoni, J. A., Yagen, B., Bialer, M., Greenberg, M. L., Walker, M. C., & Williams, R. S. (2012). The antiepileptic drug valproic acid and other medium-chain fatty acids acutely reduce phosphoinositide levels independently of inositol in *Dictyostelium*. *Disease, Models, and Mechanisms*, *5*, 115–124.

Chang, P., Terbach, N., Plant, N., Chen, P. E., Walker, M. C., & Williams, R. S. (2013). Seizure control by ketogenic diet-associated medium chain fatty acids. *Neuropharmacology*, *69*, 105–114.

Chang, P., Walker, M. C., & Williams, R. S. (2014). Seizure-induced reduction in PIP$_3$ levels contributes to seizure-activity and is rescued by valproic acid. *Neurobiology of Disease*, *62*, 296–306.

Chang, P., Zuckermann, A. M., Williams, S., Close, A. J., Cano-Jaimez, M., McEvoy, J. P., Spencer, J., Walker, M. C., & Williams, R. S. (2015). Seizure control by derivatives of medium chain fatty acids associated with the ketogenic diet show novel branching-point structure for enhanced potency. *Journal of Pharmacology Experimental Therapeutics*, *352*, 43–52.

Chang, P., Augustin, A. M., Boddum, K., Williams, S., Sun, M., Terschak, J. A., Hardege, J. D., Chen, P. E., Walker, M. C., & Williams, R. S. B. (2016). Seizure control by decanoic acid through direct AMPA receptor inhibition. *Brain*, *139*, 431–443.

Cock, H. R., Tong, X., Hargreaves, I. P., Heales, S. J., Clark, J. B., Patsalos, P. N., Thom, M., Groves, M., Schapira, A. H., Shorvon, S. D., & Walker, M. C. (2002). Mitochondrial dysfunction associated with neuronal death following status epilepticus in rat. *Epilepsy Research*, *48*, 157–168.

Cunliffe, V. T., Baines, R. A., Giachello, C. N., Lin, W. H., Morgan, A., Reuber, M., Russell, C., Walker, M. C., & Williams, R. S. (2015). Epilepsy research methods update: Understanding the causes of epileptic seizures and identifying new treatments using non-mammalian model organisms. *Seizure*, *24*, 44–51.

Dean, H. G., Bonser, J. C., & Gent, J. P. (1989). HPLC analysis of brain and plasma for octanoic and decanoic acids. *Clinical Chemistry*, *35*, 1945–1948.

DeLorenzo, R. J., Sun, D. A., & Deshpande, L. S. (2005). Cellular mechanisms underlying acquired epilepsy: The calcium hypothesis of the induction and maintenance of epilepsy. *Pharmacology & Therapeutics*, *105*, 229–266.

Deshpande, L. S., Lou, J. K., Mian, A., Blair, R. E., Sombati, S., Attkisson, E., & DeLorenzo, R. J. (2008). Time course and mechanism of hippocampal neuronal death in an in vitro model of status epilepticus: Role of NMDA receptor activation and NMDA dependent calcium entry. *European Journal of Pharmacology*, *583*, 73–83.

Gottlicher, M., Minucci, S., Zhu, P., Kramer, O. H., Schimpf, A., Giavara, S., Sleeman, J. P., Lo, C. F., Nervi, C., Pelicci, P. G., & Heinzel, T. (2001). Valproic acid defines a novel class of HDAC inhibitors inducing differentiation of transformed cells. *EMBO Journal, 20*, 6969–6978.

Gurvich, N., Tsygankova, O. M., Meinkoth, J. L., & Klein, P. S. (2004). Histone deacetylase is a target of valproic acid-mediated cellular differentiation. *Cancer Research, 64*, 1079–1086.

Haidukewych, D., Forsythe, W. I., & Sills, M. (1982). Monitoring octanoic and decanoic acids in plasma from children with intractable epilepsy treated with medium-chain triglyceride diet. *Clinical Chemistry, 28*, 642–645.

Hughes, S. D., Kanabus, M., Anderson, G., Hargreaves, I. P., Rutherford, T., O'Donnell, M., Cross, J. H., Rahman, S., Eaton, S., & Heales, S. J. (2014). The ketogenic diet component decanoic acid increases mitochondrial citrate synthase and complex I activity in neuronal cells. *Journal of Neurochemistry, 129*, 426–433.

Huttenlocher, P. R., Wilbourn, A. J., & Signore, J. M. (1971). Medium-chain triglycerides as a therapy for intractable childhood epilepsy. *Neurology, 21*, 1097–1103.

Jentink, J., Loane, M. A., Dolk, H., Barisic, I., Garne, E., Morris, J. K., & de Jong-van den Berg, L. T. (2010). Valproic acid monotherapy in pregnancy and major congenital malformations. *New England Journal of Medicine, 362*, 2185–2193.

Kim, D. Y., Simeone, K. A., Simeone, T. A., Pandya, J. D., Wilke, J. C., Ahn, Y., Geddes, J. W., Sullivan, P. G., & Rho, J. M. (2015). Ketone bodies mediate anti-seizure effects through mitochondrial permeability transition. *Annals of Neurology, 78*(1), 77–87.

Koren, G., Nava-Ocampo, A. A., Moretti, M. E., Sussman, R., & Nulman, I. (2006). Major malformations with valproic acid. *Canadian Family Physician, 52*, 441–447.

Kunz, W. S., Kudin, A. P., Vielhaber, S., Blumcke, I., Zuschratter, W., Schramm, J., Beck, H., & Elger, C. E. (2000). Mitochondrial complex I deficiency in the epileptic focus of patients with temporal lobe epilepsy. *Annals of Neurology, 48*, 766–773.

Levy, R. G., Cooper, P. N., & Giri, P. (2012). Ketogenic diet and other dietary treatments for epilepsy. *Cochrane Database of Systematic Reviews, 3*, CD001903.

Likhodii, S. S., Musa, K., Mendonca, A., Dell, C., Burnham, W. M., & Cunnane, S. C. (2000). Dietary fat, ketosis, and seizure resistance in rats on the ketogenic diet. *Epilepsia, 41*, 1400–1410.

Liu, Y. M. (2008). Medium-chain triglyceride (MCT) ketogenic therapy. *Epilepsia, 49*(Suppl. 8), 33–36.

Loscher, W. (1999). Animal models of epilepsy and epileptic seizures. In M. J.Eadie & F. J. E. Vajda (Eds.), *Antiepileptic drugs, pharmacology and therapeutics* (pp. 19–62). Springer-Verlag.

Malapaka, R. R., Khoo, S., Zhang, J., Choi, J. H., Zhou, X. E., Xu, Y., Gong, Y., Li, J., Yong, E. L., Chalmers, M. J., Chang, L., Resau, J. H., Griffin, P. R., Chen, Y. E., & Xu, H. E. (2012). Identification and mechanism of 10-carbon fatty acid as modulating ligand of peroxisome proliferator-activated receptors. *Journal of Biological Chemistry, 287*, 183–195.

Masino, S. A., Li, T., Theofilas, P., Sandau, U. S., Ruskin, D. N., Fredholm, B. B., Geiger, J. D., Aronica, E., & Boison, D. (2011). A ketogenic diet suppresses seizures in mice through adenosine A_1 receptors. *Journal of Clinical Investigation, 121*, 2679–2683.

Meldrum, B. S., & Rogawski, M. A. (2007). Molecular targets for antiepileptic drug development. *Neurotherapeutics, 4*, 18–61.

Neal, E. G., Chaffe, H., Schwartz, R. H., Lawson, M. S., Edwards, N., Fitzsimmons, G., Whitney, A., & Cross, J. H. (2009). A randomized trial of classical and medium-chain triglyceride ketogenic diets in the treatment of childhood epilepsy. *Epilepsia, 50*, 1109–1117.

Neal, E. G., & Cross, J. H. (2010). Efficacy of dietary treatments for epilepsy. *Journal of Human Nutrition and Dietetics, 23*, 113–119.

Phiel, C. J., Zhang, F., Huang, E. Y., Guenther, M. G., Lazar, M. A., & Klein, P. S. (2001). Histone deacetylase is a direct target of valproic acid, a potent anticonvulsant, mood stabilizer, and teratogen. *Journal of Biological Chemistry, 276*, 36734–36741.

Rektor, I. (2013). Perampanel, a novel, noncompetitive, selective AMPA receptor antagonist as adjunctive therapy for treatment-resistant partial-onset seizures. *Expert Opinion on Pharmacotherapy, 14*, 225–235.

Rho, J. M., & Stafstrom, C. E. (2011). The ketogenic diet: What has science taught us? *Epilepsy Research, 100*(3), 210–217.

Rogawski, M. A., & Hanada, T. (2013). Preclinical pharmacology of perampanel, a selective noncompetitive AMPA receptor antagonist. *Acta Neurologica Scandinavica, 197*, 19–24.

Rowley, N. M., & White, H. S. (2010). Comparative anticonvulsant efficacy in the corneal kindled mouse model of partial epilepsy: Correlation with other seizure and epilepsy models. *Epilepsy Research, 92*, 163–169.

Rugg-Gunn, F. (2014). Adverse effects and safety profile of perampanel: A review of pooled data. *Epilepsia, 55*(Suppl. 1), 13–15.

Russo, E., Gitto, R., Citraro, R., Chimirri, A., & De, S. G. (2012). New AMPA antagonists in epilepsy.

Expert Opinion on Investigational Drugs, 21, 1371–1389.

Sada, N., Lee, S., Katsu, T., Otsuki, T., & Inoue, T. (2015). Epilepsy treatment: Targeting LDH enzymes with a stiripentol analog to treat epilepsy. *Science, 347,* 1362–1367.

Schoeler, N. E., Orford, M., Vivekananda, U., Simpson, Z., Van de Bor, B., Smith, H., Balestrini, S., Rutherford, T., Brennan, E., McKenna, J., et al. (2021). K.Vita®: A feasibility study of a blend of medium chain triglycerides to manage drug-resistant epilepsy. *Brain Communications,* fcab160.

Shaltiel, G., Mark, S., Kofman, O., Belmaker, R. H., & Agam, G. (2007). Effect of valproate derivatives on human brain myo-inositol-1-phosphate (MIP) synthase activity and amphetamine-induced rearing. *Pharmacological Reports, 59,* 402–407.

Sills, M. A., Forsythe, W. I., & Haidukewych, D. (1986a). Role of octanoic and decanoic acids in the control of seizures. *Archives of Disease in Childhood, 61,* 1173–1177.

Sills, M. A., Forsythe, W. I., Haidukewych, D., MacDonald, A., & Robinson, M. (1986b). The medium chain triglyceride diet and intractable epilepsy. *Archives of Disease in Childhood, 61,* 1168–1172.

Steinhoff, B. J., Hamer, H., Trinka, E., Schulze-Bonhage, A., Bien, C., Mayer, T., Baumgartner, C., Lerche, H., & Noachtar, S. (2014). A multicenter survey of clinical experiences with perampanel in real life in Germany and Austria. *Epilepsy Research, 108,* 986–988.

Szenasi, G., Vegh, M., Szabo, G., Kertesz, S., Kapus, G., Albert, M., Greff, Z., Ling, I., Barkoczy, J., Simig, G., Spedding, M., & Harsing, L. G., Jr. (2008). 2,3-Benzodiazepine-type AMPA receptor antagonists and their neuroprotective effects. *Neurochemistry International, 52,* 166–183.

Thavendiranathan, P., Mendonca, A., Dell, C., Likhodii, S. S., Musa, K., Iracleous, C., Cunnane, S. C., & Burnham, W. M. (2000). The MCT ketogenic diet: Effects on animal seizure models. *Experimental Neurology, 161,* 696–703.

Thio, L. L., Wong, M., & Yamada, K. A. (2000). Ketone bodies do not directly alter excitatory or inhibitory hippocampal synaptic transmission. *Neurology, 54,* 325–331.

Vaden, D. L., Ding, D., Peterson, B., & Greenberg, M. L. (2001). Lithium and valproate decrease inositol mass and increase expression of the yeast *INO1* and *INO2* genes for inositol biosynthesis. *Journal of Biological Chemistry, 276,* 15466–15471.

Van Den Pol, A. N., Obrietan, K., & Belousov, A. (1996). Glutamate hyperexcitability and seizure-like activity throughout the brain and spinal cord upon relief from chronic glutamate receptor blockade in culture. *Neuroscience, 74,* 653–674.

Walker, M. C., & Williams, R. S. (2015). New experimental therapies for status epilepticus in preclinical development. *Epilepsy & Behavior, 49,* 290–293.

Warren, E. C., Dooves, S., Lugarà, E., Damstra-Oddy, J., Schaf, J., Heine, V. M., Walker, M. C., & Williams, R. S. B. (2020). Decanoic acid inhibits mTORC1 activity independent of glucose and insulin signaling. *Proceedings of the National Academy of Sciences USA, 117* (38), 23617–23625.

Williams, R. S. B. (2005). Pharmacogenetics in model systems: Defining a common mechanism of action for mood stabilisers. *Progress in Neuropsychopharmacology and Biological Psychiatry, 29,* 1029–1037.

Williams, R. S. B., Cheng, L., Mudge, A. W., & Harwood, A. J. (2002). A common mechanism of action for three mood-stabilizing drugs. *Nature, 417,* 292–295.

Wlaz, P., Socala, K., Nieoczym, D., Luszczki, J. J., Zarnowska, I., Zarnowski, T., Czuczwar, S. J., & Gasior, M. (2012). Anticonvulsant profile of caprylic acid, a main constituent of the medium-chain triglyceride (MCT) ketogenic diet, in mice. *Neuropharmacology, 62,* 1882–1889.

Xu, X., Muller-Taubenberger, A., Adley, K. E., Pawolleck, N., Lee, V. W., Wiedemann, C., Sihra, T. S., Maniak, M., Jin, T., & Williams, R. S. (2007). Attenuation of phospholipid signaling provides a novel mechanism for the action of valproic acid. *Eukaryotic Cell, 6,* 899–906.

Yelshanskaya, M. V., Singh, A. K., Narangoda, C., Williams, R. S. B., Kurnikova, M. G., & Sobolevsky, A. I. (2020). Structural basis of AMPA receptor inhibition by 4-BCCA. *British Journal of Pharmacology,* 1–17.

Zuckermann, A. M., La Ragione, R. M., Baines, D. L., & Williams, R. S. (2015). Valproic acid protects against haemorrhagic shock-induced signalling changes via PPARγ activation in an in vitro model. *British Journal of Pharmacology, 172* (22), 5306–5317.

Triheptanoin in Epilepsy and Beyond

KARIN BORGES, PHD

INTRODUCTION TO ANAPLEROSIS AND TRIHEPTANOIN

Under nonfasting conditions, glucose is usually the main fuel for the CNS, and glycogen can provide extra energy when the brain is stimulated (Dienel, 2019). Glycolysis, which occurs in cytosol, is the main pathway of metabolic breakdown of glucose as well as glucose-6-phosphate derived from glucose and glycogen into pyruvate. During brain stimulation and also when there is limited oxygen, glycolysis produces lactate, which can leave the brain or potentially be used as further fuel for brain cells (Dienel, 2019). Also, pyruvate produces acetyl-CoA via the pyruvate dehydrogenase pathway for further oxidation in the tricarboxylic acid (TCA) cycle in mitochondria

(Figure 37.1). In aerobic metabolism, after citrate synthase transfers the acetyl-group onto oxaloacetate, forming citrate, the TCA cycle oxidizes acetyl-CoA to two carbon dioxide molecules in a series of chemical reactions. At the same time, the TCA cycle provides the electron transport chain with reducing equivalents, which then together produce the majority of ATP during aerobic conditions (Figure 37.2). The TCA cycle is also part of many other key metabolic pathways. TCA cycle intermediates containing four or five carbons not only are part of the cycle involved in energy production, but also are used for other metabolic pathways, such as synthesis of various amino acids and neurotransmitters, such as glutamate and γ-aminobutyric acid (GABA). It is therefore important that C4 intermediates

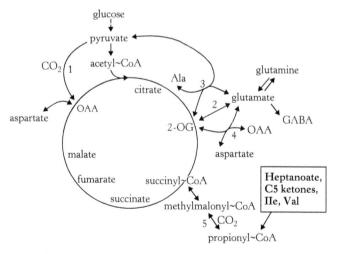

FIGURE 37.1 *The TCA Cycle and Anaplerotic Pathways*

Numbers indicate five different anaplerotic pathways. 1: Pyruvate carboxylase forms oxaloactetate by carboxylation of pyruvate. 2: The activity of glutamate dehydrogenase, which metabolizes glutamate into 2-oxoglutarate and ammonia and vice versa. 3: The reversible reaction catalyzed by glutamic pyruvic transaminases (also called alanine aminotransferases): pyruvate + glutamate ↔ 2-oxoglutarate + alanine. 4: Aspartate transaminase (also called glutamic oxaloacetic transaminase) produces oxaloacetate from aspartate, while transferring the amino group onto 2-oxoglutarate, forming glutamate, and vice versa. 5: The activity of the propionyl-CoA carboxylation pathway forming succinyl-CoA. 2-OG = 2-oxoglutarate

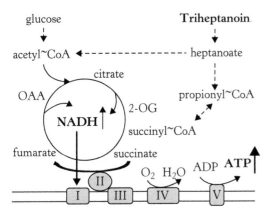

FIGURE 37.2 *Boosting the TCA Cycling Capacity via the Propionyl-CoA Carboxylation Pathway Can Increase ATP Production*

This schematic includes the reduction of NAD⁺ to NADH by the TCA cycle, which then feeds electrons into complex I of the mitochondrial electron transport chain, while succinate directly feeds electrons into complex II. Ultimately, ATP is produced by ATP synthase.

of the TCA cycle get "refilled," which is anaplerosis (Brunengraber & Roe, 2006; Hassel, 2000; Kornberg, 1966). Anaplerosis is required for TCA cycling to occur because it enhances acetyl-CoA entry into the TCA cycle by providing oxaloacetate, thus increasing TCA cycling and ATP production. Moreover, with increased amounts of TCA cycle metabolites, more substrate for complex II can be produced and reduction of NAD⁺ will be enhanced, which again will contribute to ATP production. Please note that the TCA cycle can also be short-circuited and still produce ATP, for example with 2-oxoglutarate or succinate as substrates. In many different models of disease, there is evidence of reduced amounts of TCA cycle metabolites, such as in epilepsy (Alvestad et al., 2008; Melo et al., 2005; Smeland et al., 2013; Willis et al., 2010), stroke (Haberg et al., 2009), and amyotrophic lateral sclerosis (ALS; Niessen et al., 2007). This is expected to lead to low oxaloacetate levels, which then can reduce the binding of acetyl-CoA by citrate synthase, reduce its oxidation, and ultimately decrease ATP production.

Various enzymes partake in the refilling of the TCA cycle. In the CNS, carboxylation of pyruvate to oxaloacetate (number 1 in Figure 37.1) is the main refilling pathway, thought to be taking place mainly in astrocytes (Patel, 1974). Also, several enzymes facilitate the formation of 2-oxoglutarate (also called α-ketoglutarate) from glutamate. This includes glutamate dehydrogenase, which

forms 2-oxoglutarate and ammonia from glutamate and vice versa (2 in Figure 37.1). The reaction catalyzed by glutamic pyruvic transaminases (alanine aminotransferases), pyruvate + glutamate ↔ 2-oxoglutarate + alanine, refills the cycle with 2-oxoglutarate (3 in Figure 37.1). In addition, aspartate transaminase (also called glutamic oxaloacetic transaminase) can bypass part of the TCA cycle to produce oxaloacetate from 2-oxoglutarate in the reaction: Asp + 2-OG ↔ OAA + Glu (4 in Figure 37.1).

Another anaplerotic pathway, the propionyl-CoA carboxylation pathway (5 in Figure 37.1) has largely been studied in peripheral tissues (Deng et al., 2009; Martini et al., 2003; Nuutinen et al., 1981; Owen et al., 2002; Reszko et al., 2003). It involves the carboxylation of propionyl-CoA to methylmalonyl-CoA by propionyl-CoA carboxylase (EC 6.4.1.3). Methylmalonyl-CoA epimerase (EC 5.1.99.1) and methylmalonyl-CoA mutase (EC 5.4.99.2) then produce succinyl-CoA. The branched-chain amino acids, isoleucine and valine, as well as uneven fatty acids, are anaplerotic via this pathway, all providing propionyl-CoA (Figure 37.1). Treatment with triheptanoin, the triglyceride of heptanoate (C7 fatty acid), appears to currently be the least toxic treatment when fueling this pathway to a large extent. Unlike the branched-chain amino acids, triheptanoin does not overload the body with nitrogen. In addition, providing the uneven medium-chain fat as a triglyceride avoids excessive levels of sodium or acid, which otherwise could challenge physiologic homeostasis.

Triheptanoin is a tasteless oil and can be mixed with various foods or made into an emulsion. As a medium-chain triglyceride, it is hydrolyzed in the gastrointestinal tract, and due to its lipophilicity the free medium-chain heptanoate is thought to diffuse directly into blood and mitochondria of all tissues. This is unlike long-chain fatty acids, which are much more slowly metabolized, because they first enter the lymph and require various transport proteins in the blood and for final transport into mitochondria for β-oxidation. Similar to even medium-chain fats, heptanoate is bound to albumin in the blood and is converted by the liver to ketones bodies. While even-chain fats octanoate and decanoate (C8 and C10) are turned into C4 ketone bodies, β-hydroxybutyrate and acetoacetate, heptanoate is metabolized to C5 ketone bodies, β-hydroxypentanoate and β-keto-pentanoate (Brunengraber & Roe, 2006; Gu et al., 2010; Kinman et al., 2006; Roe & Mochel, 2006; Roe et al., 2002). After release into the blood, C4 and C5 ketone bodies are taken up into cells by monocarboxylate transporters. For crossing the blood–brain barrier, monocarboxylate transporters of the MCT1 type (Broer et al., 1998; Meredith & Christian, 2008) are thought to transport C5 ketone bodies into the brain, while heptanoate is more likely to enter the brain via diffusion (Oldendorf, 1973). Once in cells, both heptanoate and C5 ketone molecules are metabolized to their CoA adducts via medium-chain acyl-CoA synthetases or 3-oxoacid CoA transferase, respectively, and then are converted into the main TCA cycle fuels acetyl-CoA and propionyl-CoA. After carboxylation, the latter can refill the TCA cycle with succinyl-CoA (see above) and thus promote acetyl-CoA oxidation and ATP production (Figure 37.2).

ENERGY METABOLISM IN EPILEPSY

An epileptic seizure or hypersynchronous activation of neuronal networks can be initiated by imbalances between excitation and inhibition. In addition, impairments in energy metabolism can also cause seizures and contribute to epilepsy. Numerous studies have attempted to shed light on energy metabolism in brains of patients with epilepsy and rodent epilepsy models. Assessments of metabolic functions or metabolite levels have revealed dysfunction in energy metabolism in patients with temporal lobe epilepsy (TLE) and extra-temporal lobe epilepsy (Burneo et al., 2015; Pan et al., 2008; Portnow et al., 2013; Sarikaya, 2015). Similar changes have been found in rodent epilepsy models (Alvestad et al., 2008; Melo et al., 2005, 2010; Smeland et al., 2013; Willis et al., 2010; reviewed in McDonald et al., 2018, Figure 37.3). Furthermore, mitochondrial dysfunction and mutations in mitochondrial constituents have been described (Kann & Kovacs, 2007; Kudin et al., 2009; Waldbaum & Patel, 2010), which can also contribute to energetic imbalances contributing to seizures.

Many studies in the literature discuss interictal glucose hypometabolism in patients with TLE, which is a common epilepsy type in adults that is largely treatment-resistant. Local cerebral glucose utilization (CMR_{GLC}) was first quantified using [^{14}C]deoxyglucose (Sokoloff et al., 1977), which is similar to FDG (radioactive [^{18}F]fluoro-2-deoxyglucose). Later, FDG-positron emission tomography (PET) was developed as a tool for imaging glucose utilization in vivo (Portnow et al., 2013). FDG and 2-deoxyglucose (2DG) are structural glucose analogs and enter brain cells via facilitative glucose transporters. They are then phosphorylated by the glycolysis rate-limiting enzyme hexokinase to FDG-6-phosphate and 2DG-6-phosphate. These metabolites are considered to be trapped, because they do not undergo any further steps of glycolysis. Because glucose transport through facilitative glucose transporters is reversible, the method mostly indicates the rates of hexokinase and glycolysis. Thus, low signals seen when using ^{14}C-DG or FDG-PET are interpreted as low glucose utilization or "hypometabolism" (Chassoux et al., 2004; Sokoloff et al., 1977), as interictally in TLE (Arnold et

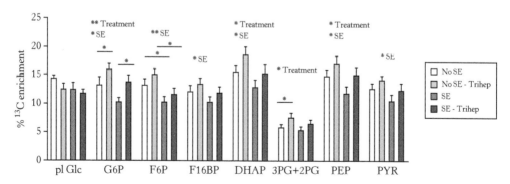

FIGURE 37.3 *Reduced Glucose Metabolism in the Hippocampus in the Chronic Stage of the Pilocarpine Epilepsy Model*

Results of [^{13}C]glucose injections in mice (SE and no-SE controls). Interictally in the chronic epileptic stage (SE), the plasma percentage ^{13}C-enrichment of glucose (pl GLC) is similar, but hippocampal percentage ^{13}C-enrichment in most glycolytic metabolites is reduced compared to control mice. G6P = glucose-6-phosphate, F6P = fructose-6-phosphate, DHAP = dihydroxyacetone phosphate, F16BP = fructose-1,6-bisphosphate, PEP = phosphoenolpyruvate, PYR = pyruvate. ($N = 9–12$, $M \pm SEM$). ANOVA $p < 0.001$; * posttests $p < 0.05$. Data from McDonald et al., 2020.

al., 1996; Henry et al., 1993; Henry et al., 1990). Originally, brain damage was believed to correlate with hypometabolism in epilepsy. However, the severity of hippocampal sclerosis or atrophy often did not correlate with the topography of hypometabolism (Chassoux et al., 2004; O'Brien et al., 1997). In the lithium pilocarpine rat model of TLE, FDG-PET showed normal metabolism in the silent period before spontaneous seizures occurred, but limbic hypometabolic areas in the chronic "epileptic" period (Lee et al., 2012). This indicates that altered energy metabolism may be a cause for seizures. Also, decreased metabolism of ^{14}C-DG was found in the chronic phase of the lithium-pilocarpine rat model of TLE (Dube et al., 2001; Melo et al., 2005).

Note that, when using FDG or ^{14}C-DG, one cannot fully assess metabolism beyond hexokinase as well as oxidative glucose metabolism, because after phosphorylation of FDG or ^{14}C-DG, there is no further metabolism via glycolysis. Therefore, it is important that our recent studies confirmed reduced glucose metabolism via glycolysis by following the metabolism of [^{13}C]glucose (Figure 37.3). We injected [^{13}C]glucose (intraperitoneally) into awake mice between seizures in the chronic stage of the pilocarpine model to track the metabolism of [^{13}C]glucose (McDonald et al., 2017). The percentage enrichment of [^{13}C]glucose-derived glycolytic metabolites relative to total metabolites was reduced in epileptogenic hippocampus compared to healthy tissue (Figure 37.3), while the overall levels of all measured hippocampal glycolytic metabolites and the plasma percent enrichment of [^{13}C]glucose versus total glucose levels were similar to those in healthy mice. The reduced percentage of ^{13}C-enrichment in glucose-6-phosphate (Figure 37.3) is similar to the findings with FDG-PET in people with epilepsy (Chassoux et al., 2004; O'Brien et al., 1997) and chronic rat epilepsy models (Di Liberto et al., 2018; Lee et al., 2012). In a parallel cohort of status epilepticus (SE) mice, there was no obvious hippocampal damage, except for some hilar neuronal loss, indicating that the results are not due to neuronal loss. In summary, decreased glucose metabolism via glycolysis appears to be common in some "epileptic" tissues, but little is known about the further oxidative metabolism of this major fuel. Given the anticonvulsant efficacy of dietary treatments, such as the ketogenic and modified Atkins diets, there is a critical need for more knowledge about the fate of major metabolites in epilepsy.

Intermediates of the TCA cycle, such as 2-oxogluarate and oxaloacetate, are precursors of the amino acids and neurotransmitters glutamate, GABA, and aspartate. Decreased levels of TCA cycle intermediates and amino acids have been found in the chronic seizure stage of rat and mouse epilepsy models that display recurrent spontaneous seizures (Alvestad et al., 2008; McDonald et al., 2018; Melo et al., 2005; Smeland et al., 2013; Willis et al., 2010). For example, in the CF1 mouse pilocarpine epilepsy model, animals sacrificed during the day (when mice are in their sleep phase) had lower forebrain levels of malate, aspartate, and acetyl- and propionyl-CoA during the chronic epileptic stage compared to mice without seizures (Willis et al., 2010). Our recent work in the chronic epileptic stage in the CD1 mouse pilocarpine model did not show reduced total levels of TCA cycle intermediates when mice were killed in the evening after they had started feeding (McDonald et al., 2017). However, we reported evidence that there was reduced entry of [^{13}C]glucose-derived pyruvate into the TCA cycle, both by demonstrating reduced maximal activity of pyruvate dehydrogenase and lack of correlation between the percentage of ^{13}C-enrichment in citrate versus pyruvate in hippocampal extracts of the epileptic mice (McDonald et al., 2017, 2018). Taken together, several lines of evidence point to decreased oxidative phosphorylation.

Providing additional alternative anaplerotic fuel that can increase the amounts of C4 intermediates of the TCA cycle in the brain is a biochemically valid approach to improve energy metabolism in epilepticbrains (Brunengraber & Roe, 2006). Thus, we tested the metabolic effects and anticonvulsant profile of triheptanoin treatment as an anaplerotic approach, which at that time had already been explored in a few animal models and in patients with various genetic metabolic disorders. The reader is also referred to three reviews on the effects of other approaches to supplementing TCA cycle substrates (Kovac et al., 2013; McDonald et al., 2018; Tan et al., 2015).

TRIHEPTANOIN ALTERS BRAIN ENERGY METABOLISM IN VARIOUS SETTINGS, INCLUDING EPILEPSY MODELS

Few publications shed light on the metabolic effects of triheptanoin or its metabolite heptanoate in the brain. An elegant study by the Pascual's group (Marin-Valencia et al., 2013) infused ^{13}C-labeled 5,6,7-heptanoate into the jugular vein of mice. The ^{13}C-carbons were largely found in brain glutamine, but not glutamate, indicating that astrocytes primarily metabolize heptanoate and its C5 ketone metabolites. McDonald et al. (2014) compared the amounts of various hippocampal metabolites within energy metabolism pathways (adenosine nucleotides, NAD$^+$, NADH, and NADPH), glycolysis, the pentose phosphate pathway, and the TCA cycle in healthy mice after feeding the mice triheptanoin and trioctanoin (the triglyceride of octanoate) for 3 weeks. While the even medium-chain triglyceride altered the levels of various metabolites, no significant changes were found with triheptanoin, indicating that it would have few metabolic side effects.

A recent study in patients with Huntington's disease found that 1-month triheptanoin treatment corrected the energetic response to brain activation (Adanyeguh et al., 2015). In patients with untreated Huntington's disease, a visual stimulus failed to alter the ratio of inorganic phosphate to phosphocreatine, while healthy control and treated patients showed an increase in this ratio, indicating that triheptanoin could restore metabolism of high-energy phosphates.

Several studies (Hadera et al., 2014; McDonald et al., 2020; Willis et al., 2010) aimed to increase the understanding of the metabolic effects of triheptanoin treatment in mouse "epileptic" brain tissue. In the pilocarpine model, mice that experience SE have one motor seizure per day on average in the chronic stage of the model, while mice without SE (no-SE mice) do not show any seizure activity or neuropathologic changes (Benson et al., 2015; Borges et al., 2003). Please note that we do not know to what extent triheptanoin treatment decreased seizure frequencies in these mice, although preliminary data indicate that seizure frequency is lowered and mice are not seizure-free (James Stoll, personal communication). Willis et al. (2010) compared the levels of various forebrain metabolites related to the TCA cycle in the chronic stage of this model. Forebrain levels of malate and propionyl-CoA were reduced in SE versus no-SE mice on control diet, but this was prevented by triheptanoin feeding, indicating that triheptanoin can improve a low capacity of the TCA cycle. Hadera et al. (2014) followed the metabolism of [1,2-^{13}C]glucose in the same mouse model to be able to evaluate the activities of pyruvate dehydrogenase and pyruvate carboxylase, the latter of which provides C4 carbons to the TCA cycle. The analyses of ^{13}C-label incorporation into TCA cycle intermediates showed that in control diet-fed SE mice, the percentage of

enrichment for two ^{13}C atoms in malate, citrate, succinate, and GABA was reduced compared to control diet-fed no-SE mice. Except for succinate, triheptanoin feeding alleviated these reductions, which provides additional evidence that triheptanoin can increase the metabolism of glucose via the TCA cycle. Similar results were found recently when we evaluated the metabolism of [^{13}C]glucose via glycolysis and the TCA cycle (McDonald et al., 2018, 2020). The reductions in ^{13}C-enrichments in glycolytic and TCA cycle intermediates in the epileptogenic hippocampi were mostly reversed with triheptanoin (McDonald et al., 2020; Figure 37.3). In addition, the activities of pyruvate and 2-oxoglutarate dehydrogenases were restored. However, because seizure frequencies were probably reduced in the triheptanoin-treated mice, we cannot distinguish between the direct metabolic versus anticonvulsant effects of triheptanoin. If metabolic changes are due to seizure activity, the anticonvulsant effects of triheptanoin may ultimately be responsible for the improvements in metabolism. However, it is likely that an adequate energy supply is very important in epileptic tissue to keep neuronal membrane potentials stable and to prevent seizure generation, and therefore the metabolic improvements likely underlie the anticonvulsant effects. Also, the finding that, in the no-SE mice, triheptanoin increased the percentage of ^{13}C-enrichment of glucose-6-phosphate (McDonald et al., 2020) indicates that triheptanoin increases glucose metabolism. Taken together, all studies are consistent with the brain's ability to metabolize heptanoate or C5 ketone bodies, and improvements in several signs of impaired energy metabolism could be detected.

ANTICONVULSANT EFFECTS OF TRIHEPTANOIN AND CLINICAL TRIALS

Triheptanoin has a unique anticonvulsant profile. It was found to be anticonvulsant in various mouse seizure models (McDonald et al., 2014; Thomas et al., 2012; Willis et al., 2010; Figure 37.4), with efficacy in three chronic mouse seizure models. In the chronic corneal kindling model, we found a reproducible delay in the kindling process in CF1 mice, which is similar to effects found with established anticonvulsant drugs in the rat kindling model, namely phenobarbital and low concentrations of valproate (Brandt et al., 2006; Matagne et al., 2008; Silver et al., 1991). Protective effects of various compounds in kindling models correlate well with efficacy in humans against absence seizures. In chronically epileptic mice after

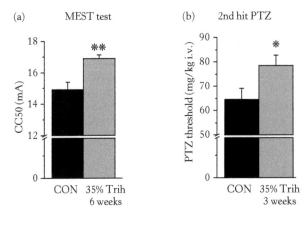
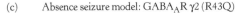
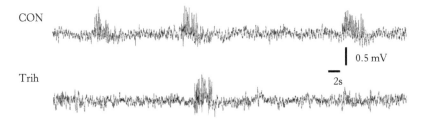

FIGURE 37.4 *Anticonvulsant Effects of Oral Triheptanoin in Three Models*

(a) Triheptanoin increased the critical current at which 50% of mice seize (CC50) in the maximal electroshock threshold test (Thomas et al., 2012). (b) It also increased the threshold to PTZ-induced tonic seizures in chronically epileptic mice (Willis et al., 2010), and (c) decreased spike-wave discharges in a mouse model of absence seizures (Kim et al., 2013).

pilocarpine-induced SE, triheptanoin reproducibly increased the pentylenetetrazole (PTZ) seizure threshold (Figure 37.4b). Efficacy in this model suggests efficacy against drug-resistant seizures, based on the finding that a similar second-hit rat model is resistant to valproate, phenytoin, and phenobarbital (Blanco et al., 2009; Borges & Sonnewald, 2011). In a mouse model for genetic absence seizures (Tan et al., 2007), namely mice with a missense (R43Q) mutation in the GABA_A receptor γ2 subunit, triheptanoin decreased the number and duration of spike-wave discharges (SWD), resulting in a halved time with seizures (Kim et al., 2013; Figure 37.4c). In the acute maximal electroshock threshold test (MEST), a test for the efficacy against generalized seizures, we observed a reproducible increase of the critical current at which 50% of mice seize (Thomas et al., 2012; CC50, Figure 37.4a). Also, triheptanoin improved seizures in *Drosophila* with mutations in genes involved in mitochondrial function, the citric acid cycle, and glycolytic activities (Fogle et al., 2019).

Effects in other acute seizure mouse models have been variable; for example, in the 6-Hz model, the threshold to motor seizures was elevated only in some experiments, and not in others (McDonald et al., 2014; Thomas et al., 2012). Similarly, anticonvulsant effects in models using the GABA_A receptor channel blockers, fluorothyl or PTZ, have been inconsistent. Moreover, triheptanoin treatment did not prevent pilocarpine-induced SE or epileptic behavior during SE (Tan et al., 2018b). This lack of consistent effects in acute mouse models is not surprising, because energy metabolism in healthy mice is likely to be optimal and unlikely to require additional fuel and/or anaplerosis.

In summary, triheptanoin's anticonvulsant profile suggests efficacy against a variety of seizure types, including focal and general motor seizures, absence seizures, and possibly pharmacoresistant motor seizures (Smith et al., 2007; White, 2003).

There have been three clinical trials of triheptanoin in adults and children with medically refractory epilepsy in Australia (Borges et al., 2019; Calvert et al., 2018). The first phase IIa randomized double-blind controlled study to evaluate the safety and tolerability of oral triheptanoin as an add-on treatment for adolescent and adult patients with medically refractory epilepsy showed that food-grade triheptanoin and "regular" even medium-chain triglyceride oil, containing 55% octanoate and 45% decanoate were equally tolerated in adults with refractory epilepsy, with about two thirds of participants finishing the study in each treatment arm (Borges et al., 2019). Side effects were mostly expected and consisted of abdominal issues, such as diarrhea, bloating, and nausea, which could be minimized by titrating up doses slowly, mixing the oils into food, and reducing doses. The study was underpowered to investigate anticonvulsant effects; however, only one participant (out of nine) had more than 50% reduction in seizure frequency during triheptanoin treatment, while five out of 11 people showed > 50% seizure frequency reductions with even medium-chain triglycerides. All the participants who responded well to treatment had focal unaware seizures. In each treatment arm, there was one person with doubling of seizure frequency.

People who participated in this first randomized trial were invited to continue in an open-label extension study of oral pharmaceutical grade triheptanoin (UX007) as an add-on treatment for 48 weeks (Borges et al., 2020). The 10 participants were able to tolerate an addition of 0.49 to 1.1 ml/kg triheptanoin per day (40–100 ml/day) for 27 to 513 days (median 247 days). Eight people left the study early, due to perceived lack of efficacy or other reasons independent from tolerability. The only adverse effects deemed possibly related to treatment were diarrhea in two people and bloating in one person. Efficacy with over 50% reduction in seizure frequency was found in five of the participants, including two who finished the treatment period and extended their treatment. Again, the five participants showing efficacy all had focal seizures, mostly with loss of awareness. In the previous study, they had either shown seizure reductions or no effect when taking triheptanoin or even medium-chain triglycerides. The lack of 100% consistent effects of similar treatments can be explained by natural changes in seizure frequencies over time. On the other hand, some participants showed consistent efficacy or no efficacy with the treatments, indicating that certain seizure or epilepsy types may respond better to metabolic treatment. However, due to the scarce data and the effects of even medium-chain triglycerides in the randomized study, it is unclear if the two treatments are similar or different.

In addition, the effects of pharmaceutical grade triheptanoin (UX007) were evaluated in children age 3 to 18 with medically refractory epilepsy (Calvert et al., 2018). Eight out of 12 children tolerated between 30 and 100 ml of triheptanoin per day. Adverse effects were mostly limited to gastrointestinal effects, but there were also problems with endoscopic gastrostomy buttons, which became leaky or infected in two children. Five out of eight children who tolerated the treatment showed > 50% reduction in seizure frequency, including one child who was seizure-free for more than half a year. Four children went into the extension phase, and the longest treatment with triheptanoin was for 2.5 years. Seizures eventually returned in all patients, for unknown reasons, but there were no serious interactions with antiepileptic medications during the trial or the extension phase. Taken together with the studies in adults, this indicates that triheptanoin is very likely safe as an add-on treatment to existing antiseizure medications in children and adults and may be efficacious in certain types of epilepsies.

TRIHEPTANOIN AND OTHER DISORDERS

Metabolic Disorders: Glucose Transporter Type 1 Deficiency, Long-Chain Fatty Acid Oxidation Disorders, and Pyruvate Decarboxylase Deficiency

Although this chapter has been focused on epilepsies of various or unknown etiologies, triheptanoin is also being developed as a treatment for glucose transporter type 1 deficiency (Pascual et al., 2014). In this genetic disorder, glucose is not efficiently taken up into the brain, which results in epileptic seizures around age 3 to 4 and later in paroxysmal exercise-induced dyskinesias, which can be very disabling (Klepper & Leiendecker, 2007; Suls et al., 2009). A standard treatment for this disorder is ketogenic diet.

Originally, triheptanoin was given to patients with rare inborn metabolic disorders, including long-chain fatty acid oxidation disorders due to deficiencies in different enzymes, namely carnitine palmitoyltransferase I or II, very-long-chain acyl-CoA dehydrogenase, long-chain 3-hydroxy acyl-CoA dehydrogenase, and mitochondrial trifunctional protein (Roe et al., 2002, 2008; Wehbe & Tucci, 2020). The use of dietary and body fat as energy sources is pre-empted in these disorders, which can result in severe clinical problems, such as cardiomyopathy, intermittent rhabdomyolysis, hypoglycemia, and sudden death. Treatment with traditional medium-chain triglycerides has been unsatisfactory in the past, while triheptanoin, as an alternatively medium-chain and anaplerotic fuel that is also gluconeogenic, could decrease hospitalizations due to major clinical manifestations and hypoglycemia (Roe & Brunengraber, 2015; Roe & Mochel, 2006; Roe et al., 2002; Vockley et al., 2015). The latest published studies are summarized here.

As of 2020, triheptanoin has been FDA-approved as a source of calories and fatty acids for the treatment of people with molecularly confirmed long-chain fatty acid oxidation disorders. Moderate or severe cardiomyopathy associated with long-chain fatty acid oxidation disorders appears to respond well to triheptanoin in humans (Mahapatra et al., 2018; Vockley et al., 2016), but not in a mouse model (Tucci et al., 2017). A case report series describes 10 children with long-chain fatty acid oxidation disorders (mostly infants, a 5-year-old, and a 20-year-old) who suffered cardiomyopathy and/or heart failure requiring hospitalization while being treated with standard treatment, which includes medium-chain triglycerides (Vockley et al., 2016). Cardiac function measured by echocardiography showed that the ejection fraction was moderately to severely impaired, ranging between 12% and 45%. In response, even medium-chain triglycerides were discontinued, and triheptanoin treatment was initiated and was followed by improvements in ejection fraction starting 2 and 21 days thereafter. Nine of the 10 patients subsequently achieved a normalization of their ejection fraction (ranging from 33% to 71%) and longer-term stabilization of clinical signs of cardiomyopathy while continuing triheptanoin. Adverse events were gastrointestinal problems, similar to those found with even medium-chain triglycerides, mostly diarrhea. In another case report, triheptanoin reversed cardiogenic shock in an infant with carnitine-acylcarnitine translocase deficiency who had suffered severe metabolic crisis developing into acute heart failure (Mahapatra et al., 2018). The girl continued treatment for over 2 years.

In 2017, interim results were provided about a safety and efficacy phase 2 open-label trial in 29 children and adults with severe long-chain fatty acid oxidation deficiencies, including deficiencies in carnitine palmitoyltransferase II, very-long-chain acyl-CoA dehydrogenase, long-chain 3-hydroxy acyl-CoA dehydrogenase, and mitochondrial trifunctional protein, after 24 weeks of UX007 triheptanoin treatment (25% to 35% of total daily caloric intake; Vockley et al., 2017). Treatment-related mild to moderate gastrointestinal side effects were reported in 62% of study participants, and one person developed gastroenteritis. Participants eligible for the exercise tests (N = 5 to 8) improved their exercise endurance and tolerance compared to those for their 4-week baseline period. Positive changes were found in self-reported health-related quality of life. Most participants continued the trial (25 out of 29). In 2019, the full data were published after 78 weeks of UX007 treatment (average 27.5% of total daily caloric intake; Vockley et al., 2019). The annualized frequency and duration of major clinical events occurring during 78 weeks of UX007 treatment was compared to events captured retrospectively from medical records for 78 weeks before UX007 initiation while patients were being treated with even medium-chain triglycerides. The events included hospitalizations and emergency interventions due to rhabdomyolysis, hypoglycemia, and cardiomyopathy. The annualized mean event numbers and durations were halved after UX007 initiation (both p = 0.02). Specifically, hospitalizations due to rhabdomyolysis, the most common event, decreased by about 40%, and cardiomyopathy events by two thirds. Treatment-related mild to moderate gastrointestinal side effects were managed with smaller and more frequent doses of triheptanoin and mixing it with food. Taken together, the findings show safety and promising efficacy in these severely affected patients.

More data regarding efficacy of triheptanoin were reported in a double-blind trial from 2017 (Gillingham et al., 2017), comparing the clinical effects of 20% daily caloric intake triheptanoin versus trioctanoin (the triglyceride of octanoate) for treatment of long-chain fatty acid oxidation deficiencies, with 16 participants in each treatment arm. After 4 months with triheptanoin, there was a significant improvement in cardiac structure and function at rest and during exercise and improved cardiorespiratory fitness.

It has been known for some time that propionate is an anaplerotic substrate for the heart, (Martini et al., 2003). Recently, the effects of triheptanoin in a rat model of cardiac hypertrophy were assessed. A 30% triheptanoin diet reduced left ventricular hypertrophy and improved diastolic function and myocardial glucose oxidation (Nguyen et al., 2015), indicating that anaplerotic actions of heptanoate or C5 ketones can benefit the ailing heart.

In contrast to the data from people and rats, a study by Tucci and colleagues (Tucci et al., 2017) found no improvement of cardiac dysfunction when mice with very-long-chain acyl-CoA dehydrogenase deficiency were treated with triheptanoin for up to 1 year. Comparisons of expression and activity levels of enzymes indicated an increase in glucose oxidation in heart and increased activity of the citric acid cycle in the liver mediated via higher activities of liver citrate acid synthase and α-ketoglutarate dehydrogenase. However, anaplerotic effects were not measured via metabolite analysis, which makes it difficult to assess to what extent anaplerosis was improved in tissues. Moreover, triheptanoin increased the amount of lipids, including uneven long-chain fatty acids, in the liver, which suggests that medium-chain fatty acids can be elongated.

Another metabolic disorder that may benefit from triheptanoin is pyruvate carboxylase deficiency, although so far studies have reported mixed success (Breen et al., 2014; Mochel et al., 2005).

Other Disorders: Neurologic Conditions, Muscle Disorders, and Cardiac Hypertrophy

Triheptanoin appears to be a promising treatment for other neurologic disorders, including Canavan disease, stroke, ALS, Alzheimer's disease, Huntington's disease, autism, and glycogenosis (Wehbe & Tucci, 2020). In four models of neurologic conditions, triheptanoin treatment was found to prevent neuronal cell death, and it is conceivable that increased energy levels can protect cells from degeneration. This includes models of Canavan disease, stroke, ALS, and SE.

The pediatric leukodystrophy Canavan disease is caused by mutations in aspartoacylase, an enzyme that is largely found in oligodendrocytes and that catalyzes the hydrolysis of neuronally derived N-acetylaspartate to provide acetyl groups for lipid synthesis. In *nur7* mutant mice containing a nonsense mutation in the aspartoacylase gene, early triheptanoin treatment prevented the loss of oligodendrocytes, dysmyelination, and impairments in motor function (Francis et al., 2014). The early loss of various brain metabolites, such as ATP and acetyl-, malonyl- and propionyl-CoA, was largely prevented in this model, indicating that triheptanoin can rescue metabolic deficits in oligodendrocytes.

The brain infarct area after middle cerebral artery occlusion (MCAO), a mouse model of stroke, was smaller when mice were fed triheptanoin before the insult (Schwarzkopf et al., 2015). In addition, mitochondrial functions were preserved in mitochondria isolated from brains 1 hr after onset of MCAO (Schwarzkopf et al., 2015), indicating that improved mitochondrial energetic functions contribute to triheptanoin's neuroprotective effects. Our recent study was underpowered to find neuroprotective effects in a rat MCAO model (Tan et al., 2018a). However, we found that pretreatment with small amounts of heptanoate (50 µM) protected cultured mouse neurons against cell death induced by oxygen and glucose deprivation or exposure to N-methyl-D-aspartate or hydrogen peroxide (Tan et al., 2018b). In cultured mouse astrocytes, basal respiration and ATP turnover were higher with 200 µM heptanoate than with 1-mM sodium pyruvate (Tan et al., 2018a). This suggests that, like octanoate and decanoate (Tan et al., 2017, Anderson et al. 2021), heptanoate is oxidized directly by astrocytes.

Triheptanoin also was neuroprotective in an ALS model overexpressing the human SOD1 G93A mutation. Treatment with 35% triheptanoin resulted in 33% less motor neuron loss in the L4–L5 spinal cord, and loss of motor functions was significantly delayed (Tefera et al., 2016). A pilot clinical trial by Rick Bedlack (NCT03506425) showed that triheptanoin was poorly tolerated and did not slow progression of disease or biomarkers (personal communication).

In mice, 10-day pretreatment with triheptanoin (35%) did not affect the induction and severity of SE (Tan et al., 2018b). However, we demonstrated improvements in SE-induced hippocampal mitochondrial impairments, lipid peroxidation, and neuronal degeneration. Isolated hippocampal mitochondria-enriched extracts from triheptanoin-treated mice showed protection of the activities of pyruvate and oxoglutarate dehydrogenase complexes against the oxidative attack by the Fenton reaction, further supporting and adding to the antioxidant effects of triheptanoin.

A study in an Alzheimer's disease model indicated that triheptanoin in the context of a ketogenic diet increased the expression of the mRNA levels of *Sirt1*, *Pparg*, *Sod1*, and *Sod2* (Aso et al., 2013). Because sirtuin 1 and PPARγ are involved in the regulation of lipid and glucose metabolism as well as mitochondrial respiration and oxidative stress, this suggests that the neuroprotective effects of triheptanoin may also include other mechanisms that can improve energy metabolism, such as reduced oxidative stress and preserved mitochondrial function. Overall, it still needs to be investigated to what extent the neuroprotective effects of triheptanoin are mediated via its antioxidant effects or via the preservation of energy metabolism, or both.

There is increasing hope that Huntington's disease patients might benefit from long-term triheptanoin therapy, as there is evidence that triheptanoin improves energy metabolism in the CNS (see above) and skeletal muscle (Adanyeguh et al., 2015; Mochel et al., 2010). Moreover, improvements in muscle function were found in skeletal muscle in a Rett syndrome model (Park et al., 2014) and rat heart (Nguyen et al., 2015). In Sydney, a pilot clinical study took place with a handful of patients with inclusion body myositis and Pompe's disease (http://www.anzctr.org.au/; Corbett et al., 2015). The study showed feasibility but no significant improvement; however, treatment duration was short and treatment initiation may have been too late.

Adult polyglucosan body disease (APBD) is a rare autosomal recessive disorder due to partial deficiency of the glycogen brancher enzyme (GBE) and leads to deposition of polyglucosan bodies in neurons and glia. As in other glycogenoses (e.g., Pompe's disease) in which glycogen cannot be metabolized, in APBD the progressive deposition of polysaccharides is thought to cause cells to be disrupted. APBD patients show gradual progression, with difficulty walking, impaired balance, neurogenic bladder, weakness, and, in about half of cases, dementia. Five APBD patients treated with triheptanoin experienced stabilization of disease progression or some functional improvement (Roe et al., 2010). However, a recent double-blind placebo-controlled crossover trial comparing the effects of 6 months of triheptanoin versus vegetable oil in 23 participants with APBD did not find any improvements in motor functions (Schiffmann et al., 2018). While triheptanoin was safe and generally well tolerated, the patient population was heterogeneous and other problems of the disease, such as neurogenic bladder, peripheral nerve deficit, and cognitive decline, were not studied.

A 12-week triheptanoin versus safflower oil treatment (30% of caloric intake) was tested in 10 patients with alternating hemiplegia of childhood due to mutations in the α3 catalytic subunit of a transmembrane sodium-potassium pump (ATP1A3) gene in a randomized, double-blind, placebo-controlled crossover study. The disease is a neurodevelopmental disorder manifesting in paroxysmal motor deficits, which were not prevented by triheptanoin (Hainque et al., 2017).

Among the autism spectrum disorders, Rett syndrome is a genetic disorder largely caused by mutations in the X-linked gene for the transcription factor methyl-CpG binding protein 2 (MeCP2), resulting in severe disability in cognitive and motor function. In male MeCP2-deficient mice, triheptanoin increased life span and improved social interaction and motor function as well as mitochondrial morphology in skeletal muscle (Park et al., 2014). The mutant mice also showed increased adiposity and lower glucose tolerance and insulin sensitivity, which all improved with triheptanoin treatment, indicating that this medium-chain triglyceride can counteract obesity and normalize glucose metabolism.

Studies of the effect of triheptanoin on alterations in fatty acid composition have just begun. Traditionally, it was thought that medium-chain fats do not get elongated and subsequently stored. However, in mice, feeding of even and uneven medium-chain triglycerides for 1 year altered the fatty acid profile of liver and heart significantly, with unusual fatty acids becoming detectable, such as C15, C17:1, and C22:1 with triheptanoin and C22:5n3 with trioctanoin (Tucci et al., 2015, 2017). The potential impacts of these changes remain to be explored.

CONCLUSIONS

Triheptanoin was first used as a novel alternative approach to satisfy energy needs in patients with rare metabolic enzyme deficiencies, and many patients with fatty acid oxidation disorders depend on its availability. New research has indicated the safety and shown promising effects of triheptanoin in some other human disorders and their animal models, including epilepsy. Large-scale controlled clinical trials are now needed to prove triheptanoin's safety, tolerability, and efficacy and to identify which disorders respond best.

DISCLOSURE/CONFLICT OF INTEREST
None.

ACKNOWLEDGMENTS
The author is grateful for funding by the American Epilepsy Foundation, Parents against Childhood Epilepsy, UniQuest, The Thrasher Research Fund, and Ultragenyx Pharmaceuticals Inc. for clinical trials of triheptanoin in adults and children with treatment-resistant epilepsy. The Australian National Health and Medical Research Council (grants 1044407, 1186025) and the Australian

Brain Foundation are thanked for funding the author's laboratory research.

REFERENCES

Adanyeguh, I. M., Rinaldi, D., Henry, P. G., Caillet, S., Valabregue, R., Durr, A., & Mochel, F. (2015). Triheptanoin improves brain energy metabolism in patients with Huntington disease. *Neurology, 84,* 490–495.

Alvestad, S., Hammer, J., Eyjolfsson, E., Qu, H., Ottersen, O. P., & Sonnewald, U. (2008). Limbic structures show altered glial-neuronal metabolism in the chronic phase of kainate induced epilepsy. *Neurochemical Research, 33,* 257–266.

Anderson, J. V., Westi, E. W., Jakobsen, E., Urruticoecha, N., Borges, K. & Aldana, B. I. (2021). Astrocyte metabolism of the medium-chain fatty acids octanoic acid and decanoic acids promote GABA synthesis in neurons via elevated glutamine supply. *Molecular Brain, 14,* 132.

Arnold, S., Schlaug, G., Niemann, H., Ebner, A., Luders, H., Witte, O. W., & Seitz, R. J. (1996). Topography of interictal glucose hypometabolism in unilateral mesiotemporal epilepsy. *Neurology, 46,* 1422–1430.

Aso, E., Semakova, J., Joda, L., Semak, V., Halbaut, L., Calpena, A., Escolano, C., Perales, J. C., & Ferrer, I. (2013). Triheptanoin supplementation to ketogenic diet curbs cognitive impairment in APP/PS1 mice used as a model of familial Alzheimer's disease. *Current Alzheimer Research, 10,* 290–297.

Benson, M. J., Thomas, N. K., Talwar, S., Hodson, M. P., Lynch, J. W., Woodruff, T. M., & Borges, K. (2015). A novel anticonvulsant mechanism via inhibition of complement receptor C5ar1 in murine epilepsy models. *Neurobiology of Disease, 76,* 87–97.

Blanco, M. M., dos Santos, J. G., Jr., Perez-Mendes, P., Kohek, S. R., Cavarsan, C. F., Hummel, M., Albuquerque, C., & Mello, L. E. (2009). Assessment of seizure susceptibility in pilocarpine epileptic and nonepileptic Wistar rats and of seizure reinduction with pentylenetetrazole and electroshock models. *Epilepsia, 50,* 824–831.

Borges, K., Gearing, M., McDermott, D. L., Smith, A. B., Almonte, A. G., Wainer, B. H., & Dingledine, R. (2003). Neuronal and glial pathological changes during epileptogenesis in the mouse pilocarpine model. *Experimental Neurology, 182,* 21–34.

Borges, K., Kaul, N., Germaine, J., Carrasco-Pozo, C., Kwan, P., & O'Brien, T. J. (2020). Open-label long-term treatment of add-on triheptanoin in adults with drug-resistant epilepsy. *Epilepsia Open, 5,* 1–10.

Borges, K., Kaul, N., Germaine, J., Kwan, P., & O'Brien, T. (2019). Randomised trial of add-on triheptanoin vs. medium chain triglycerides in adults with refractory epilepsy. *Epilepsia Open, 4,* 153–163.

Borges, K., & Sonnewald, U. (2011). Triheptanoin—A medium chain triglyceride with odd chain fatty acids: A new anaplerotic anticonvulsant treatment? *Epilepsy Research, 100,* 239–244.

Brandt, C., Heile, A., Potschka, H., Stoehr, T., & Loscher, W. (2006). Effects of the novel antiepileptic drug lacosamide on the development of amygdala kindling in rats. *Epilepsia, 47,* 1803–1809.

Breen, C., White, F. J., Scott, C. A., Heptinstall, L., Walter, J. H., Jones, S. A., & Morris, A. A. (2014). Unsuccessful treatment of severe pyruvate carboxylase deficiency with triheptanoin. *European Journal of Pediatrics, 173,* 361–366.

Broer, S., Schneider, H. P., Broer, A., Rahman, B., Hamprecht, B., & Deitmer, J. W. (1998). Characterization of the monocarboxylate transporter 1 expressed in *Xenopus laevis* oocytes by changes in cytosolic pH. *Biochemical Journal, 333*(Part 1), 167–174.

Brunengraber, H., & Roe, C. R. (2006). Anaplerotic molecules: Current and future. *Journal of Inherited Metabolic Disease, 29,* 327–331.

Burneo, J. G., Poon, R., Kellett, S., & Snead, O. C. (2015). The utility of positron emission tomography in epilepsy. *Canadian Journal of Neurological Science, 42,* 360–371.

Calvert, S., Barwick, K., Par, M., Ni Tan, K., & Borges, K. (2018). A pilot study of add-on oral triheptanoin treatment for children with medically refractory epilepsy. *European Journal of Paediatric Neurology, 22,* 1074–1080.

Chassoux, F., Semah, F., Bouilleret, V., Landre, E., Devaux, B., Turak, B., Nataf, F., & Roux, F. X. (2004). Metabolic changes and electro-clinical patterns in mesio-temporal lobe epilepsy: A correlative study. *Brain, 127,* 164–174.

Corbett, A., Garg, N., Crosbie, A., & Borges, K. (2015). A pilot study of triheptanoin treatment in sporadic inclusion body myositis (sIBM). *Annals of Neurology, 78,* S102.

Deng, S., Zhang, G. F., Kasumov, T., Roe, C. R., & Brunengraber, H. (2009). Interrelations between C4 ketogenesis, C5 ketogenesis, and anaplerosis in the perfused rat liver. *Journal of Biological Chemistry, 284,* 27799–27807.

Di Liberto, V., van Dijk, R. M., Brendel, M., Waldron, A. M., Moller, C., Koska, I., Seiffert, I., Gualtieri, F., Gildehaus, F. J., von Ungern-Sternberg, B., Lindner, M., Ziegler, S., Palme, R., Hellweg, R., Gass, P., Bartenstein, P., & Potschka, H. (2018). Imaging correlates of behavioral impairments: An experimental PET study in the rat pilocarpine epilepsy model. *Neurobiology of Disease, 118,* 9–21.

Dienel, G. A. (2019). Brain glucose metabolism: Integration of energetics with function. *Physiological Reviews, 99,* 949–1045.

Dube, C., Boyet, S., Marescaux, C., & Nehlig, A. (2001). Relationship between neuronal loss and interictal glucose metabolism during the chronic phase of the lithium-pilocarpine model of epilepsy in the immature and adult rat. *Experimental Neurology, 167*, 227–241.

Fogle, K. J., Smith, A. R., Satterfield, S. L., Gutierrez, A. C., Hertzler, J. I., McCardell, C. S., Shon, J. H., Barile, Z. J., Novak, M. O., & Palladino, M.J. (2019). Ketogenic and anaplerotic dietary modifications ameliorate seizure activity in *Drosophila* models of mitochondrial encephalomyopathy and glycolytic enzymopathy. *Molecular Genetics and Metabolism, 126*, 439–447.

Francis, J. S., Markov, V., & Leone, P. (2014). Dietary triheptanoin rescues oligodendrocyte loss, dysmyelination and motor function in the nur7 mouse model of Canavan disease. *Journal of Inherited Metabolic Disease, 37*, 369–381.

Gillingham, M. B., Heitner, S. B., Martin, J., Rose, S., Goldstein, A., El-Gharbawy, A. H., Deward, S., Lasarev, M. R., Pollaro, J., DeLany, J. P., Burchill, J. P., Goodpaster, B., Shoemaker, J., Matern, D., Harding, C. O., & Vockley, J. (2017). Triheptanoin versus trioctanoin for long-chain fatty acid oxidation disorders: A double blinded, randomized controlled trial. *Journal of Inherited Metabolic Disease, 40*, 831–843.

Gu, L., Zhang, G. F., Kombu, R. S., Allen, F., Kutz, G., Brewer, W. U., Roe, C. R., & Brunengraber, H. (2010). Parenteral and enteral metabolism of anaplerotic triheptanoin in normal rats. II. Effects on lipolysis, glucose production, and liver acyl-CoA profile. *American Journal of Physiology Endocrinology Metabolism, 298*, E362–371.

Haberg, A. K., Qu, H., & Sonnewald, U. (2009). Acute changes in intermediary metabolism in cerebellum and contralateral hemisphere following middle cerebral artery occlusion in rat. *Journal of Neurochemistry, 109*(Suppl. 1), 174–181.

Hadera, M. G., Smeland, O. B., McDonald, T. S., Tan, K. N., Sonnewald, U., & Borges, K. (2014). Triheptanoin partially restores levels of tricarboxylic acid cycle intermediates in the mouse pilocarpine model of epilepsy. *Journal of Neurochemistry, 129*, 107–119.

Hainque, E., Caillet, S., Leroy, S., Flamand-Roze, C., Adanyeguh, I., Charbonnier-Beaupel, F., Retail, M., Le Toullec, B., Atencio, M., Rivaud-Pechoux, S., Brochard, V., Habarou, F., Ottolenghi, C., Cormier, F., Méneret, A., Ruiz, M., Doulazmi, M., Roubergue, A., Corvol, J, C., . . . Roze, E. (2017). A randomized, controlled, double-blind, crossover trial of triheptanoin in alternating hemiplegia of childhood. *Orphanet Journal of Rare Diseases, 12*, 160.

Hassel, B. (2000). Carboxylation and anaplerosis in neurons and glia. *Molecular Neurobiology, 22*, 21–40.

Henry, T. R., Mazziotta, J. C., & Engel, J., Jr. (1993). Interictal metabolic anatomy of mesial temporal lobe epilepsy. *Archives of Neurology, 50*, 582–589.

Henry, T. R., Mazziotta, J. C., Engel, J., Jr., Christenson, P. D., Zhang, J. X., Phelps, M. E., & Kuhl, D. E. (1990). Quantifying interictal metabolic activity in human temporal lobe epilepsy. *Journal of Cerebral Blood Flow and Metabolism, 10*, 748–757.

Kann, O., & Kovacs, R. (2007). Mitochondria and neuronal activity. *American Journal of Physiology Cell Physiology, 292*, C641–C657.

Kim, T. H., Borges, K., Petrou, S., & Reid, C. A. (2013). Triheptanoin reduces seizure susceptibility in a syndrome-specific mouse model of generalized epilepsy. *Epilepsy Research, 103*, 101–105.

Kinman, R. P., Kasumov, T., Jobbins, K. A., Thomas, K. R., Adams, J. E., Brunengraber, L. N., Kutz, G., Brewer, W. U., Roe, C. R., & Brunengraber, H. (2006). Parenteral and enteral metabolism of anaplerotic triheptanoin in normal rats. *American Journal of Physiology- Endocrinology and Metabolism, 291*, E860–E866.

Klepper, J., & Leiendecker, B. (2007). GLUT1 deficiency syndrome—2007 update. *Developmental Medicine Child Neurology, 49*, 707–716.

Kornberg, H. L. (1966). Anaplerotic sequences and their role in metabolism. *Essays Biochemistry, 2*, 1–31.

Kovac, S., Abramov, A. Y., & Walker, M. C. (2013). Energy depletion in seizures: Anaplerosis as a strategy for future therapies. *Neuropharmacology, 69*, 96–104.

Kudin, A. P., Zsurka, G., Elger, C. E., & Kunz, W. S. (2009). Mitochondrial involvement in temporal lobe epilepsy. *Experimental Neurology, 218*, 326–332.

Lee, E. M., Park, G. Y., Im, K. C., Kim, S. T., Woo, C. W., Chung, J. H., Kim, K. S., Kim, J. S., Shon, Y. M., Kim, Y. I., & Kang, J. K. (2012). Changes in glucose metabolism and metabolites during the epileptogenic process in the lithium-pilocarpine model of epilepsy. *Epilepsia, 53*, 860–869.

Mahapatra, S., Ananth, A., Baugh, N., Damian, M., & Enns, G. M. (2018). Triheptanoin: A rescue therapy for cardiogenic shock in carnitine-acylcarnitine translocase deficiency. *Journal of Inherited Metabolic Disease Reports, 39*, 19–23.

Marin-Valencia, I., Good, L. B., Ma, Q., Malloy, C. R., & Pascual, J. M. (2013). Heptanoate as a neural fuel: Energetic and neurotransmitter precursors in normal and glucose transporter I-deficient (G1D) brain. *Journal of Cerebral Blood Flow and Metabolism, 33*, 175–182.

Martini, W. Z., Stanley, W. C., Huang, H., Rosiers, C. D., Hoppel, C. L., & Brunengraber, H. (2003). Quantitative assessment of anaplerosis from propionate in pig heart in vivo. *American Journal of*

Physiology-Endocrinology and Metabolism, 284, E351–356.

Matagne, A., Margineanu, D. G., Kenda, B., Michel, P., & Klitgaard, H. (2008). Anti-convulsive and anti-epileptic properties of brivaracetam (UCB 34714), a high-affinity ligand for the synaptic vesicle protein, SV2A. *British Journal of Pharmacology, 154,* 1662–1671.

McDonald, T., Hodson, M. P., Bederman, I., Puchowicz, M., & Borges, K. (2020). Triheptanoin alters [U-^{13}C$_6$]-glucose incorporation into glycolytic intermediates and increases TCA cycling normalizing the activities of pyruvate dehydrogenase and oxoglutarate dehydrogenase in a chronic epilepsy mouse model. *Journal of Cerebral Blood Flow and Metabolism, 60,* 678–691.

McDonald, T., Puchowicz, M., & Borges, K. (2018). Impairments in oxidative glucose metabolism in epilepsy and metabolic treatments thereof. *Frontiers in Cellular Neuroscience, 12,* 274

McDonald, T. S., Carrasco-Pozo, C., Hodson, M. P., & Borges, K. (2017). Alterations in cytosolic and mitochondrial [U-^{13}C]glucose metabolism in a chronic epilepsy mouse model. *eNeuro, 4,* 1–11.

McDonald, T. S., Tan, K. N., Hodson, M. P., & Borges, K. (2014). Alterations of hippocampal glucose metabolism by even versus uneven medium chain triglycerides. *Journal of Cerebral Blood Flow and Metabolism, 34,* 153–160.

Melo, T., Bigini, P., Sonnewald, U., Balosso, S., Cagnotto, A., Barbera, S., Uboldi, S., Vezzani, A., & Mennini, T. (2010). Neuronal hyperexcitability and seizures are associated with changes in glial-neuronal interactions in the hippocampus of a mouse model of epilepsy with mental retardation. *Journal of Neurochemistry, 115,* 1445–1454.

Melo, T. M., Nehlig, A., & Sonnewald, U. (2005). Metabolism is normal in astrocytes in chronically epileptic rats: A ^{13}C NMR study of neuronal-glial interactions in a model of temporal lobe epilepsy. *Journal of Cerebral Blood Flow and Metabolism, 25,* 1254–1264.

Meredith, D., & Christian, H. C. (2008). The SLC16 monocaboxylate transporter family. *Xenobiotica, 38,* 1072–1106.

Mochel, F., DeLonlay, P., Touati, G., Brunengraber, H., Kinman, R. P., Rabier, D., Roe, C. R., & Saudubray, J. M. (2005). Pyruvate carboxylase deficiency: Clinical and biochemical response to anaplerotic diet therapy. *Molecular Genetics Metabolism, 84,* 305–312.

Mochel, F., Duteil, S., Marelli, C., Jauffret, C., Barles, A., Holm, J., Sweetman, L., Benoist, J. F., Rabier, D., Carlier, P. G., & Durr, A. (2010). Dietary anaplerotic therapy improves peripheral tissue energy metabolism in patients with Huntington's disease. *European Journal of Human Genetics, 18,* 1057–1060.

Nguyen, T. D., Shingu, Y., Amorim, P. A., Schwarzer, M., & Doenst, T. (2015). Triheptanoin alleviates ventricular hypertrophy and improves myocardial glucose oxidation in rats with pressure overload. *Journal of Cardiac Failure, 21,* 906–915.

Niessen, H. G., Debska-Vielhaber, G., Sander, K., Angenstein, F., Ludolph, A. C., Hilfert, L., Willker, W., Leibfritz, D., Heinze, H. J., Kunz, W. S., & Vielhaber, S. (2007). Metabolic progression markers of neurodegeneration in the transgenic G93A-SOD1 mouse model of amyotrophic lateral sclerosis. *European Journal of Neuroscience, 25,* 1669–1677.

Nuutinen, E. M., Peuhkurinen, K. J., Pietilainen, E. P., Hiltunen, J. K., & Hassinen, I. E. (1981). Elimination and replenishment of tricarboxylic acid-cycle intermediates in myocardium. *Biochemical Journal, 194,* 867–875.

O'Brien, T. J., Newton, M. R., Cook, M. J., Berlangieri, S. U., Kilpatrick, C., Morris, K., & Berkovic, S. F. (1997). Hippocampal atrophy is not a major determinant of regional hypometabolism in temporal lobe epilepsy. *Epilepsia, 38,* 74–80.

Oldendorf, W. H. (1973). Carrier-mediated blood-brain barrier transport of short-chain monocarboxylic organic acids. *American Journal of Physiology, 224,* 1450–1453.

Owen, O. E., Kalhan, S. C., & Hanson, R. W. (2002). The key role of anaplerosis and cataplerosis for citric acid cycle function. *Journal of Biological Chemistry, 277,* 30409–30412.

Pan, J. W., Williamson, A., Cavus, I., Hetherington, H. P., Zaveri, H., Petroff, O. A., & Spencer, D. D. (2008). Neurometabolism in human epilepsy. *Epilepsia, 49*(Suppl. 3), 31–41.

Park, M. J., Aja, S., Li, Q., Degano, A. L., Penati, J., Zhuo, J., Roe, C. R., & Ronnett, G. V. (2014). Anaplerotic triheptanoin diet enhances mitochondrial substrate use to remodel the metabolome and improve lifespan, motor function, and sociability in MeCP2-null mice. *PLOS ONE, 9,* Article e109527.

Pascual, J. M., Liu, P., Mao, D., Kelly, D. I., Hernandez, A., Sheng, M., Good, L. B., Ma, Q., Marin-Valencia, I., Zhang, X., Park, J. J., Hynan, L. S., Stavinoha, P., Roe, C. R., & Lu, H. (2014). Triheptanoin for glucose transporter type I deficiency (G1D): Modulation of human ictogenesis, cerebral metabolic rate, and cognitive indices by a food supplement. *JAMA Neurology, 71,* 1255–1265.

Patel, M. S. (1974). The relative significance of CO2-fixing enzymes in the metabolism of rat brain. *Journal of Neurochemistry, 22,* 717–724.

Portnow, L. H., Vaillancourt, D. E., & Okun, M. S. (2013). The history of cerebral PET scanning: From physiology to cutting-edge technology. *Neurology, 80,* 952–956.

Reszko, A. E., Kasumov, T., Pierce, B. A., David, F., Hoppel, C. L., Stanley, W. C., Des Rosiers, C., & Brunengraber, H. (2003). Assessing the reversibility of the anaplerotic reactions of the propionyl-CoA pathway in heart and liver. *Journal of Biological Chemistry, 278*, 34959–34965.

Roe, C. R., Bottiglieri, T., Wallace, M., Arning, E., & Martin, A. (2010). Adult polyglucosan body disease (APBD): Anaplerotic diet therapy (triheptanoin) and demonstration of defective methylation pathways. *Molecular Genetics Metabolism, 101*, 246–252.

Roe, C. R., & Brunengraber, H. (2015). Anaplerotic treatment of long-chain fat oxidation disorders with triheptanoin: Review of 15 years experience. *Molecular Genetics Metabolism, 116*, 260–268.

Roe, C. R., & Mochel, F. (2006). Anaplerotic diet therapy in inherited metabolic disease: Therapeutic potential. *Journal of Inherited Metabolic Disease, 29*, 332–340.

Roe, C. R., Sweetman, L., Roe, D. S., David, F., & Brunengraber, H. (2002). Treatment of cardiomyopathy and rhabdomyolysis in long-chain fat oxidation disorders using an anaplerotic odd-chain triglyceride. *Journal of Clinical Investigation, 110*, 259–269.

Roe, C. R., Yang, B. Z., Brunengraber, H., Roe, D.S., Wallace, M., & Garritson, B. K. (2008). Carnitine palmitoyltransferase II deficiency: Successful anaplerotic diet therapy. *Neurology, 71*, 260–264.

Sarikaya, I. (2015). PET studies in epilepsy. *American Journal of Nuclear Imaging, 5*, 416–430.

Schiffmann, R., Wallace, M. E., Rinaldi, D., Ledoux, I., Luton, M. P., Coleman, S., Akman, H. O., Martin, K., Hogrel, J. Y., Blankenship, D., Turner, J., & Mochel, F. (2018). A double-blind, placebo-controlled trial of triheptanoin in adult polyglucosan body disease and open-label, long-term outcome. *Journal of Inherited Metabolic Disease, 41*, 877–883.

Schwarzkopf, T. M., Koch, K., & Klein, J. (2015). Reduced severity of ischemic stroke and improvement of mitochondrial function after dietary treatment with the anaplerotic substance triheptanoin. *Neuroscience, 300*, 201–209.

Silver, J. M., Shin, C., & McNamara, J. O. (1991). Antiepileptogenic effects of conventional anticonvulsants in the kindling model of epilepsy. *Annals of Neurology, 29*, 356–363.

Smeland, O. B., Hadera, M. G., McDonald, T. S., Sonnewald, U., & Borges, K. (2013). Brain mitochondrial metabolic dysfunction and glutamate level reduction in the pilocarpine model of temporal lobe epilepsy in mice. *Journal of Cerebral Blood Flow and Metabolism, 33*, 1090–1097.

Smith, M., Wilcox, K.S., & White, H.S. (2007). Discovery of antiepileptic drugs. *Neurotherapeutics, 4*, 12–17.

Sokoloff, L., Reivich, M., Kennedy, C., Des Rosiers, M. H., Patlak, C. S., Pettigrew, K. D., Sakurada, O., & Shinohara, M. (1977). The [^{14}C] deoxyglucose method for the measurement of local cerebral glucose utilization: Theory, procedure, and normal values in the conscious and anesthetized albino rat. *Journal of Neurochemistry, 28*, 897–916.

Suls, A., Mullen, S. A., Weber, Y. G., Verhaert, K., Ceulemans, B., Guerrini, R., Wuttke, T. V., Salvo-Vargas, A., Deprez, L., Claes, L. R., Jordanova, A., Berkovic, S. F., Lerche, H., De Jonge, P., & Scheffer, I. E. (2009). Early-onset absence epilepsy caused by mutations in the glucose transporter GLUT1. *Annals of Neurology, 66*, 415–419.

Tan, H. O., Reid, C. A., Single, F. N., Davies, P. J., Chiu, C., Murphy, S., Clarke, A. L., Dibbens, L., Krestel, H., Mulley, J. C., Jones, M. V., Seeburg, P. H., Sakmann, B., Berkovic, S. F., Sprengel, R., & Petrou, S. (2007). Reduced cortical inhibition in a mouse model of familial childhood absence epilepsy. *Proceedings of the National Academy of Sciences of the United States of America, 104*, 17536–17541.

Tan, K. N., Carrasco-Pozo, C., McDonald, T. S., Puchowicz, M., & Borges, K. (2017). Tridecanoin is anticonvulsant, antioxidant, and improves mitochondrial function. *Journal of Cerebral Blood Flow and Metabolism, 37*, 2035–2048.

Tan, K. N., Hood, R., Warren, K., Pepperall, D., Carrasco-Pozo, C., Manzanero, S., Borges, K., & Spratt, N. J. (2018a). Heptanoate is neuroprotective in vitro but triheptanoin post-treatment did not protect against middle cerebral artery occlusion in rats. *Neuroscience Letters, 683*, 207–214.

Tan, K. N., McDonald, T. S., & Borges, K. (2015). Metabolic dysfunctions in epilepsy and novel metabolic treatment approaches. In W. R. Preedy (Ed.), *Bioactive nutraceuticals and dietary supplements in neurological and brain disease: prevention and therapy* (pp. 461–470). Elsevier.

Tan, K. N., Simmons, D., Carrasco-Pozo, C., & Borges, K. (2018b). Triheptanoin protects against status epilepticus-induced hippocampal mitochondrial dysfunctions, oxidative stress and neuronal degeneration. *Journal of Neurochemistry, 144*, 431–442.

Tefera, T. W., Wong, Y., Ngo, S. T., Thomas, N. K., McDonald, T. S., & Borges, K. (2016). Triheptanoin protects motor neurons and delays the onset of motor symptoms in a mouse model of amyotrophic lateral sclerosis. *PLOS ONE, 11*, Article e0161816.

Thomas, N. K., Willis, S., Sweetman, L., & Borges, K. (2012). Triheptanoin in acute mouse seizure models. *Epilepsy Research, 99*, 312–317.

Tucci, S., Behringer, S., & Spiekerkoetter, U. (2015). De novo fatty acid biosynthesis and elongation in very long-chain acyl-CoA dehydrogenase-deficient mice supplemented with odd or even medium-chain fatty acids. *FEBS Journal, 282*, 4242–4253.

Tucci, S., Floegel, U., Beermann, F., Behringer, S., & Spiekerkoetter, U. (2017). Triheptanoin: Long-term effects in the very long-chain acyl-CoA dehydrogenase-deficient mouse. *Journal of Lipid Research, 58,* 196–207.

Vockley, J., Burton, B., Berry, G. T., Longo, N., Phillips, J., Sanchez-Valle, A., Tanpaiboon, P., Grunewald, S., Murphy, E., Bowden, A., Chen, W., Chen, C. Y., Cataldo, J., Marsden, D., & Kakkis, E. (2019). Results from a 78-week, single-arm, open-label phase 2 study to evaluate UX007 in pediatric and adult patients with severe long-chain fatty acid oxidation disorders (LC-FAOD). *Journal of Inherited Metabolic Disease, 42,* 169–177.

Vockley, J., Burton, B., Berry, G. T., Longo, N., Phillips, J., Sanchez-Valle, A., Tanpaiboon, P., Grunewald, S., Murphy, E., Humphrey, R., Mayhew, J., Bowden, A., Zhang, L., Cataldo, J., Marsden, D. L., & Kakkis, E. (2017). UX007 for the treatment of long chain-fatty acid oxidation disorders: Safety and efficacy in children and adults following 24 weeks of treatment. *Molecular Genetics and Metabolism, 120,* 370–377.

Vockley, J., Charrow, J., Ganesh, J., Eswara, M., Diaz, G. A., McCracken, E., Conway, R., Enns, G. M., Starr, J., Wang, R., Abdenur, J. E., Sanchez-de-Toledo, J., & Marsden, D. L. (2016). Triheptanoin treatment in patients with pediatric cardiomyopathy associated with long chain-fatty acid oxidation disorders. *Molecular Genetics and Metabolism, 119,* 223–231.

Vockley, J., Marsden, D., McCracken, E., DeWard, S., Barone, A., Hsu, K., & Kakkis, E. (2015). Long-term major clinical outcomes in patients with long chain fatty acid oxidation disorders before and after transition to triheptanoin treatment—A retrospective chart review. *Molecular Genetics and Metabolism, 116,* 53–60.

Waldbaum, S., & Patel, M. (2010). Mitochondria, oxidative stress, and temporal lobe epilepsy. *Epilepsy Research, 88,* 23–45.

Wehbe, Z., & Tucci, S. (2020). Therapeutic potential of triheptanoin in metabolic and neurodegenerative diseases. *Journal of Inherited Metabolic Disease, 43,* 385–391.

White, H. S. (2003). Preclinical development of antiepileptic drugs: Past, present, and future directions. *Epilepsia, 44*(Suppl. 7), 2–8.

Willis, S., Stoll, J., Sweetman, L., & Borges, K. (2010). Anticonvulsant effects of a triheptanoin diet in two mouse chronic seizure models. *Neurobiology of Disease, 40,* 565–572.

38

Antiseizure and Antiepileptic Effects of Glycolysis Inhibition with 2-Deoxyglucose

CARL E. STAFSTROM, MD, PHD, LI-RONG SHAO, MD,
AND THOMAS P. SUTULA, MD, PHD

INTRODUCTION

Conventional anticonvulsant medications reduce neuronal excitability through effects on ion channels or synaptic function. In recent years, it has become clear that metabolic factors also play a role in the modulation of neuronal excitability (Reid et al., 2014). This volume contains many examples of potentially beneficial metabolic treatments for epilepsy and other neurologic disorders. Figure 38.1 illustrates the pathway of

glucose metabolism with sites of potential metabolic regulation of excitability. The best known available metabolic treatment is the high-fat, low-carbohydrate ketogenic diet (KD), which effectively controls seizures in many children whose seizures are refractory to anticonvulsant medications (Neal et al., 2008). However, the mechanisms of action of the KD and its variants (e.g., medium-chain triglyceride [MCT] diet, modified Atkins diet [MAD], low glycemic index treatment

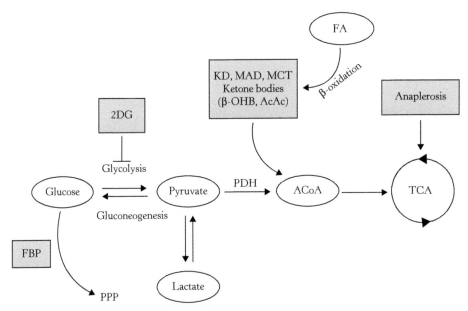

FIGURE 38.1 *Glucose Metabolism (ovals) and Points at Which Interventions (gray boxes) Could Affect Neuronal Excitability and Seizure Control*

Glucose can be diverted to the pentose phosphate shunt (PPP) via fructose-1,6-bisphosphate (FBP). 2-Deoxyglucose (2DG) inhibits glycolysis by blocking the phosphoglucose isomerase step. Via ketone body production from fatty acid (FA) breakdown, the ketogenic diet (KD), modified Atkins diet (MAD), and medium-chain triglyceride (MCT) diet bypass glycolysis by providing acetyl-CoA (ACoA) to the TCA (tricarboxylic acid cycle). Anaplerosis refers to the "refilling" of intermediate compounds depleted from the TCA cycle. Other abbreviations: β-OHB = β-hydroxybutyrate; AcAc = acetoacetate; PDH = pyruvate dehydrogenase. Reprinted in modified form with permission from Rho and Stafstrom (2012).

[LGIT]) are very complex and are not fully characterized (Gano et al., 2014; Lutas & Yellen, 2013; Rho & Stafstrom, 2012). Possible mechanisms include reduction of excitability by ketone bodies or fatty acids, altered neurotransmitter synthesis or action, improved mitochondrial function, or a combination of these and other factors. The key observation that ingestion of small amounts of carbohydrate by children on the KD results in loss of seizure control (Huttenlocher, 1976) led to the idea that carbohydrate restriction could exert a protective effect against seizures (Greene et al., 2003). In addition to limiting carbohydrate intake, restricting calorie intake also suppresses seizures and affords neuroprotection (Greene et al., 2003; Ingram & Roth, 2011; Pani, 2015; Yuen & Sander, 2014), and in fact, the KD was initially formulated to mimic the physiologic effects of fasting. Although some data support intermittent fasting for seizure control (Hartman et al., 2013), fasting is not a feasible long-term treatment option.

As an alternative to fasting, the KD restricts dietary carbohydrates and generates ketone bodies as the proximate energy source. Owing to the reduction of carbohydrate availability, the glycolytic pathway is less active. The observation that carbohydrate intake can abolish seizure control achieved by the KD suggests that inhibitors of glycolysis may mimic some of the favorable therapeutic effects of the diet. Among compounds that inhibit glycolysis, the glucose analog 2-deoxy-D-glucose (2DG) is a promising novel agent for seizure protection. 2DG differs from glucose by removal of a single oxygen atom from the 2 position (Figure 38.2). 2DG is taken up by cells and undergoes phosphorylation at the 6 position to 2DG-6P, but glycolytic flux is reduced because 2DG-6P cannot undergo isomerization by phosphoglucose isomerase. Uptake of glucose and 2DG is enhanced in energetically active cells. 2DG has been used for decades as a fluorinated positron emitted tracer (^{18}F-2DG) for measurement and imaging of regional glucose utilization

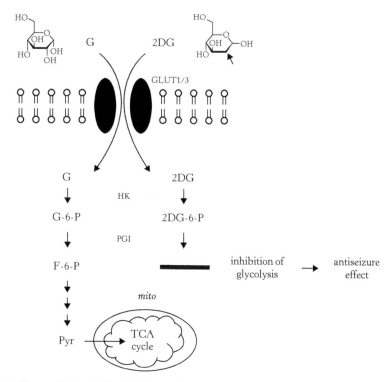

FIGURE 38.2 *Glucose, 2DG, and the Glycolytic Pathway*

Glucose (G) and 2-deoxyglucose (2DG) gain entry into cells via the glucose transporters GLUT1 and GLUT3. Glucose is phosphorylated to glucose-6-phosphate, then to fructose-6-phosphate, followed by further steps in glycolysis, eventually producing energy in the form of ATP; pyruvate is utilized by the tricarboxylic acid cycle to produce additional ATP. Phosphorylation of 2DG yields 2DG-6P, which cannot undergo isomerization by glucose-6-phosphate (glucose-6-P) isomerase (PGI) to fructose-6-phosphate (fructose-6-P), thereby preventing subsequent steps of glycolysis (black bar). Through unclear mechanisms, inhibition of glycolysis leads to an antiseizure effect (see text). Arrow pointing to 2DG chemical structure indicates the 2-carbon position, which lacks a hydroxyl group.

by positron emission tomography (PET; Wree, 1990). 2DG has also been investigated as an adjuvant chemotherapeutic agent for several types of cancer, since rapidly dividing, metabolically hyperactive neoplastic cells with enhanced glucose uptake are vulnerable to glycolytic inhibition by 2DG (Pelicano et al., 2006).

ANTICONVULSANT ACTIONS OF 2DG

The effects of 2DG have been tested in several models of acute seizures in vivo and in vitro (Stafstrom et al., 2009). When exposed to elevated extracellular potassium (K_o^+, 7.5 mM), hippocampal CA3 neurons in slices from adult rats developed high-frequency interictal (epileptiform) bursts at a frequency of about 30 per minute. Addition of 2DG (10 mM) to the bathing medium reversibly reduced the burst frequency by about 50% (Stafstrom et al., 2009). Similarly, 2DG reduced epileptiform bursts induced by bath application of the chemical convulsants bicuculline, a γ-aminobutyric acid (GABA) receptor antagonist, or 4-aminopyridine (4-AP), a potassium channel blocker. In slices from young animals (P10–13), 7.5 mM K_o^+ induced prolonged ictal discharges in area CA3 for 10 to 30 s; 2DG decreased the occurrence of these ictal bursts. More recently, we tested 2DG effects in a different model (Mg^{2+}-free plus 4-AP, 50 μM) in area CA3 of the developing hippocampus. 2DG ceased spontaneous intrinsic firing in two thirds of the immature CA3 neurons under normal conditions and abolished epileptiform network bursts induced by 0 Mg^{2+}/4-AP in a dose-dependent manner (Shao & Stafstrom, 2017), consistent with previous data (Stafstrom et al., 2009). Moreover, 2DG decreases neuronal excitability of naïve animals and rapidly attenuates epileptiform activity in neocortical slices examined 3 to 5 weeks after traumatic brain injury (Koenig et al., 2019). Therefore, 2DG exhibits an anticonvulsant effect on both interictal and ictal epileptiform activity, in both hippocampus and neocortex, and in both naïve and posttraumatic brain-injured animals.

An anticonvulsant effect of 2DG has also been demonstrated in in vivo seizure models. Kindling refers to the progressive decrease in seizure threshold in response to repeated subconvulsive electrical stimuli. Kindled seizures can be elicited by stimulation of many brain pathways. We assessed the effect of 2DG on kindling development by stimulation of the perforant path or the olfactory bulb (Garriga-Canut et al., 2006; Stafstrom et al., 2009). 2DG was administered at a dose of 250 mg/kg intraperitoneally (IP) 30 min prior to daily kindling stimulation of either pathway. In response to kindling of the perforant path, but not the olfactory bulb, 2DG-pretreated rats displayed an increase in mean afterdischarge (AD) threshold over time, defining a region-specific anticonvulsant effect.

In addition, an anticonvulsant effect of 2DG was seen in four other acute seizure models in animals. First, in the 6-Hz stimulation model (Barton et al., 2001), psychomotor seizures were induced by corneal stimulation using electrical pulses at a frequency of 6 Hz. Pretreatment with 2DG resulted in seizure protection in 75% of rats tested (Stafstrom et al., 2009). Second, in Fring's mice with audiogenic seizures, 50% of mice were protected from sound-induced seizures after pretreatment with 2DG (Stafstrom et al., 2009). Third, in mice with 4-AP induced neocortical seizures, 2DG (200 mg/kg, IP) effectively diminished seizures in ~ 20 min (Bazzigaluppi et al., 2017). Fourth, in pilocarpine-induced status epilepticus in neonatal rats, 2DG (50, 100, 500 mg/kg, IP) completely stopped seizures in all animals, and 2DG was as effective as the two first-line drugs for neonatal seizures, phenobarbital and levetiracetam (Janicot et al., 2020). However, 2DG did not protect against pentylenetetrazole- or maximal electroshock-induced seizures in rats. Therefore, anticonvulsant effects of 2DG could be demonstrated in several but not all in vivo seizure models, with a pattern of effectiveness unlike that afforded by any currently available antiseizure medicine. For example, no conventional antiseizure medication exhibits region-specific activity, as indicated by 2DG's differential action on perforant path versus olfactory bulb kindling. Thus, 2DG's mechanisms of action are likely to be broad, affecting seizure-induced plasticity across many seizure types and syndromes, but an exact correlation with human epilepsies is not yet possible (Holmes & Zhao, 2008).

Not all studies have confirmed that 2DG exerts an anticonvulsant effect. In the presence of 2DG, latency to seizure onset was slightly decreased in mice when chemoconvulsants (pentylenetetrazole, kainic acid) were co-administered intravenously with 2DG (Gasior et al., 2010). While this outcome has been interpreted as a possible proconvulsant effect, an alternative explanation is that the well-documented acute increase in cerebral blood flow induced by 2DG enhances brain delivery of parenteral convulsants like pentylenetetrazole and kainic acid, thereby shortening the latency to initial seizure manifestations as a threshold outcome measure. In another in vitro model in hippocampal slices with blocking of K+ currents, $GABA_A$ receptors, and NMDA receptors (with Cs+, bicuculline, and MK-801, respectively), 2DG had two opposing actions: it reduced interictal-like discharges, but it also induced ictal-like epileptiform bursts (Nedergaard & Andreasen, 2018), further complicating the issue.

It is worth mentioning that the KD and 2DG both suppress seizure activity, but our studies with 2DG were not intended to investigate KD mechanisms. For instance, 2DG does not cause ketosis. Both 2DG and the KD suppress seizures in Fring's mice and in the 6-Hz model (Hartman et al., 2008); the KD is effective in the maximal electroshock (MES) model but 2DG is not. The former two models are used to model focal onset seizures, whereas the MES is considered to mimic generalized tonic-clonic seizures. Kindling is abrogated by both the KD and 2DG, although exact kindling protocols differ widely among studies (Hori et al., 1997; Garriga-Canut et al., 2006; Stafstrom et al., 2009). Therefore, 2DG and the KD are not comparable directly, although both modify seizure susceptibility by altering metabolic pathways involved in energy regulation (Shao et al., 2018a). Therefore, potentially useful clinical information can be gained from studies of both compounds (2DG and ketones).

ANTIEPILEPTIC ACTIONS OF 2DG

An antiepileptic (or antiepileptogenic) effect is defined as the slowing or prevention of epilepsy development. Antiepileptogenesis is "disease-modifying," meaning that the process of epilepsy development is hindered. Using the kindling model, with stimulation of either the olfactory bulb or perforant path, we investigated whether 2DG mediates an antiepileptogenic effect. Kindling progression was quantified by the number of ADs required to elicit specific stages of seizure severity, using the Racine scoring scale (Racine, 1972). Pretreatment with 2DG at doses ranging from 37.5 mg/kg IP (we found this to be the minimally effective dose) up to 250 mg/kg IP, given 30 min before each kindling stimulation, resulted in an approximately two-fold increase in the number of ADs required to achieve class III, IV, or V kindled seizures in both regions

(Garriga-Canut et al., 2006; Stafstrom et al., 2009; Sutula & Franzoso, 2008). These results indicate a disease-modifying antiepileptic action. Note that the olfactory bulb kindling experiments described in the preceding paragraph, testing the anticonvulsant effects of 2DG, showed no significant effect of this compound on kindled seizure threshold. Therefore, 2DG has different anticonvulsant effects in different brain regions, whereas its antiepileptic effects were similar in hippocampus and olfactory bulb. Furthermore, 2DG retarded kindled seizure progression when administered immediately after, or 10 min after, a kindled seizure, suggesting that 2DG can be used as a "postseizure" interventional treatment (e.g., for clusters of seizures or even status epilepticus; Sutula & Franzoso, 2008) to mitigate the progress of epileptogenesis. A recent study using 6-Hz corneal kindling in outbred NMRI (Naval Medical Research Institute) mice showed that 2DG (250 mg/kg, IP) given 1 min after stimulation attenuated kindling progression (Leiter et al., 2019), further supporting 2DG's disease-modifying role. Moreover, in an animal model of post-traumatic epilepsy (controlled cortical impact, CCI), Dulla and colleagues showed that chronic treatment with 2DG (250 mg/kg, IP) immediately after injury for 1 week prevented the development of epileptiform activity, restored synaptic activity, and attenuated the loss of GABAergic interneurons (Koenig et al., 2019). 2DG also has acute anticonvulsant actions against chemoconvulsant-induced status epilepticus evoked by pilocarpine in adult mice (Yang et al., 2013) and in neonatal rats (Janicot et al., 2020), and in status epilepticus evoked by kainic acid in rats (Lian et al., 2007). The findings of robust acute anticonvulsant action against chemoconvulsant-induced status epilepticus are promising for a novel metabolic treatment for status epilepticus, particularly given the energy needs and high glycolytic flux of neurons generating status epilepticus, as well as focal enhanced delivery of 2DG into neural circuitry generating status epilepticus by neurovascular coupling. Furthermore, in the neonatal pilocarpine model, 2DG effectively stopped neonatal seizures when given 30 min into pilocarpine-induced status epilepticus (a widely used model to develop spontaneous chronic seizures when lasting for > 90 min; Janicot et al., 2020). These data raise the possibility of using 2DG to prevent status epilepticus-induced or posttraumatic epilepsy, although the long-term effects of 2DG on epileptogenesis in these two models are yet to be assessed by chronic seizure monitoring at later stages.

Consistent with the clinical observation that recurrent hypoglycemia may be associated with seizures, chronic treatment of 2DG (daily intracerebroventricular administration for 4 weeks) has been reported to be possibly proepileptogenic (Samokhina et al., 2017). In that study, two of ten rats treated with chronic high concentrations of 2DG administered intraventricularly developed spontaneous seizures with extremely high frequency (26 to 42 per hour, lasting up to a minute), while the other eight 2DG-treated rats had no spontaneous seizures at all. It is unclear why such a dichotomous all-or-none result occurs if 2DG is inherently proconvulsant. Also, in that study, evoked excitatory synaptic potentials in chronically treated rats were reduced, which is not consistent with the reported proconvulsant effects. It should also be cautioned that chronic implantation of the intraventricular cannula (for 2DG injection) is an invasive approach that could cause brain injury and potentially lead to posttraumatic epilepsy in some animals.

2DG exerts neuroprotective actions in several other models as well. In hippocampal cell cultures, 2DG increased neuronal resistance to oxidative and metabolic insults by inducing stress proteins, and in rats, 2DG allayed kainic acid seizure-induced memory deficits and hippocampal neuron loss (Lee et al., 1999). In another model, 2DG pretreatment protected against the delayed emergence of postischemic seizures in mice after bilateral carotid artery occlusion (Redjak et al., 2001). In the traumatic brain injury model, 2DG reduced the loss of parvalbumin-expressing GABAergic neurons after injury (Koenig et al., 2019). Numerous mechanisms of 2DG-mediated neuroprotection have been hypothesized, including activation of adenosine monophosphate (AMP)-activated protein kinase (Park et al., 2009), reduction in oxidative stress (Yao et al., 2011), and disruption of glycosylation causing protein unfolding (Zhang et al., 2014), to name a few.

POSSIBLE MECHANISMS OF 2DG EFFECTS

The acute and chronic actions of 2DG probably involve different cellular and molecular mechanisms. The chronic antiepileptic effects of 2DG have been associated with decreased expression of brain-derived neurotrophic factor (BDNF) and its receptor, tyrosine kinase B (trkB), which

are required for kindling progression (He et al., 2004). 2DG suppression of seizure-induced increases in BDNF and trkB is mediated by the transcriptional repressor neuron- restrictive silencing factor (NRSF) and its nicotinamide adenine dinucleotide hydride (NADH)-sensitive corepressor carboxy-terminal binding protein (CtBP) acting at the promoter regions of *BDNF* and *trkB* genes. In pathologic conditions like seizures, glycolysis is enhanced to meet the energy demands of activated neurons. The increase in glycolysis elevates NADH, which in turn causes dissociation of CtBP from NRSF, thus decreasing transcriptional repression and resulting in increased expression of BDNF and trkB. In the presence of 2DG, which reduces NADH levels by glycolytic inhibition, the NRSF-CtBP complex maintains repression of *BDNF* and *trkB*, and kindling progression is slowed (Garriga-Canut et al., 2006).

Compared to its pivotal role in mediating chronic 2DG effects, NRSF is not required for the antiepileptic effect of the KD (Hu et al., 2011). The antiepileptic effect of 2DG was abolished in mice with conditional knockout of NRSF, but the KD continued to afford protection against kindling progression in these transgenic animals.

Others have reported evidence that the effect of 2DG is mediated by activation of K_{ATP} channels (Forte et al., 2016; Zhao et al., 1997), through upregulation of K_{ATP} channel subunits Kir6.1 and Kir6.2 (Long et al., 2019; Yang et al., 2013). K_{ATP} channels are closed in the presence of intracellular ATP and open when intracellular ATP is depleted. Open K_{ATP} channels export K^+, hyperpolarizing the cell and decreasing its excitability. It has been hypothesized that ketones, by decreasing glycolysis and thus ATP production, may lower cellular excitability (Ma et al., 2007). Decreased ATP levels, perhaps restricted to submembrane compartments adjacent to K_{ATP} channels, might lead to enhanced K^+ efflux and hyperpolarization. Such effects could be limited to certain neuron types (e.g., substantia nigra, dentate gyrus) that function as a gate for pathologic discharges (Forte et al., 2016; Lutas & Yellen, 2013; Tanner et al., 2011). Similar to K_{ATP}, several membrane-bound ATP-dependent pumps are also dependent on submembrane glycolysis-derived "local" ATP production, including the Na^+,K^+ pump (Na^+,K^+-ATPase) and H^+ pump (V-ATPase), which are important for neuronal firing and transmitter release (Moriyama & Futai, 1990). Thus, it is possible that the reduced local ATP production caused by 2DG may impair the function of these pumps and disrupt epileptiform activity; this hypothesis remains to be tested experimentally.

The rapid onset of anticonvulsant effects of 2DG in vitro and in vivo suggests that 2DG may be exerting direct actions at the synaptic or membrane levels. The effects of 2DG on excitatory synaptic transmission were investigated in experiments using hippocampal slices (Pan et al., 2019). In hippocampal area CA3, there was no effect of 10 mM 2DG on the frequency or amplitude of spontaneous excitatory postsynaptic currents (sEPSCs). However, after the induction of epileptiform bursting in this region by application of elevated (7.5 mM) K_o^+, 2DG reduced sEPSC frequency and amplitude, suggesting that the effects of 2DG are activity-dependent—2DG is taken up by actively firing cells and works preferentially in conditions of intense neuronal activity, such as seizures. The same dose of 2DG had no effect on miniature EPSCs isolated by exposure to tetrodotoxin, which blocks sodium channels and thus neuronal activity-mediated synaptic release of neurotransmitters, but miniature EPSCs were significantly reduced by 10 mM 2DG in the elevated K_o^+ condition. These effects are not a general consequence of glycolysis inhibition, since other glycolysis blockers depress sEPSCs in both normal and epileptic slices (Devinney et al., 2009; Pan et al., 2009). 2DG also reduces spontaneous inhibitory postsynaptic current (sIPSC) frequency in conditions of elevated K_o^+ (7.5 mM), but to a lesser extent than sEPSCs, resulting in a net reduction in excitatory transmission (Pan et al., 2019). 2DG has no significant effects on intrinsic membrane properties (Pan et al., 2019; Shao & Stafstrom, 2017), and its acute effects on synaptic transmission appear to be presynaptic based on analysis of miniature EPSCs (Pan et al., 2019). In addition, 2-DG has been reported to enhance tonic GABAergic current (Forte et al., 2016). This slow and persistent current is caused by the spillover of GABA into synaptic cleft and is mediated by extrasynaptic $GABA_A$ receptors (Farrant & Nusser, 2005); this tonic GABA current hyperpolarizes neurons and reduces excitation. 2DG potentiates tonic GABAergic current by shunting glycolysis to the pentose phosphate pathway, increasing the production of neurosteroids (Forte et al., 2016), which may directly activate extrasynaptic $GABA_A$ receptors (Reddy et al., 2013).

Therefore, one of the unique features of 2DG is its use-dependence. That is, 2DG is taken up only by neurons that are metabolically active, as occurs in areas of circuitry involved in seizure activity. This represents a distinct advantage when considering the goal of a medication in targeting only brain areas displaying pathologic seizure activity.

The acute anticonvulsant effects of 2DG may be influenced by other, yet undetermined metabolic or electrophysiologic consequences of glycolytic inhibition. For example, 2DG's effects might be spatially limited to certain submembrane compartments, it might alter systemic lipid metabolism, or it might modify mitochondrial metabolism in a manner that subsequently influences neuronal excitability.

Another compound in the glycolytic pathway, fructose-1,6-bisphosphate (FBP), has been shown to exert acute anticonvulsant activity in several seizure models in adult rats, including models with seizures caused by kainic acid, pilocarpine, and pentylenetetrazole (Lian et al., 2007). In that study, the effectiveness of FBP as an anticonvulsant surpassed that of 2DG, KD, and valproate. The mechanism of FBP's anticonvulsant effect is unclear. FBP increases glucose flux from glycolysis to the pentose phosphate pathway (PPP; Figure 38.1). NADPH generated in the PPP increases glutathione, which has anticonvulsant activity. Therefore, FBP may exert an endogenous anticonvulsant action (Stringer & Xu, 2008). Subsequent studies have established that FBP retards kindling progression by attenuating BDNF and trkB expression (Ding et al., 2010), like 2DG. Furthermore, during the kindling process, FBP inhibits the kindling-induced downregulation of the expression of potassium-chloride cotransporter 2 (KCC2) and decreases the expression of sodium-potassium-chloride cotransporter 1 (NKCC1), suggesting that FBP might alter the switch between GABAergic excitation and inhibition (Ding et al., 2013). In addition to these mechanisms, we found that FBP can block epileptiform activity through an extracellular mechanism by reducing voltage-gated Ca^{2+} currents (Shao et al., 2018b). These findings remain to be verified, but together, results from several laboratories have identified modification of glycolysis as a possible novel mechanism for treatment of seizures.

2DG AS A POTENTIAL CLINICAL AGENT

Preclinical studies to evaluate the safety and toxicity of 2DG have demonstrated that 2DG is well tolerated in rats and dogs at doses associated with anticonvulsant and antiepileptic effects. We tested the effects of 2DG on spatial learning and memory in the Morris water maze using both acute and chronic protocols (Ockuly et al., 2012). For acute testing, 2DG was injected 15 min prior to the water maze trial each testing day. For chronic testing, 2DG (250 mg/kg or 500 mg/kg IP, twice daily) was injected daily for 14 days before water maze testing began. Neither protocol caused a difference in the latency to platform acquisition (spatial learning) or retention of platform location (probe test) by either dose of 2DG, suggesting that 2DG has no obvious deleterious effect on spatial memory or learning.

Rats were also tested on the open-field test, which assesses exploratory activity and is regarded as a measure of anxiety (Ockuly et al., 2012). Rats were pretreated (30 min prior to open-field testing) IP with saline, 50 mg/kg 2DG, or 250 mg/kg 2DG in a crossover design. The exploratory activity (number of lines crossed in the open-field arena) did not differ between the saline- and 50 mg/kg 2DG-treated groups, but the rats receiving 250 mg/kg 2DG had decreased motor activity (fewer lines crossed). When the saline group was crossed over to receive 2DG 250 mg/kg and the prior 250 mg/kg group was crossed over to saline, the results reversed—rats receiving 250 mg/kg 2DG had diminished open-field activity and the group now receiving saline had increased motor activity. Therefore, the 250 mg/kg dose of 2DG caused a transient, reversible decrease in exploratory activity. Taken together, these findings suggest that 2DG has no permanent adverse behavioral effects on spatial learning and memory, exploratory activity, or anxiety at doses that suppress seizures and retard epilepsy progression, supporting its potential for clinical use.

Some animal studies have shown that repeated administration of 2DG at high doses is associated with adverse cardiac effects. Oral or intravenous doses of 2DG of 250 to 2,000 mg/kg given to rats or mice over 7 days caused a dose-dependent fall in mean arterial pressure, decreased respiratory rate, and increased mortality (Vijayaraghavan et al., 2006). Detailed pathologic evaluation of cardiac tissue after chronic oral 2DG ingestion in two rat strains revealed cardiotoxic effects, with vacuolization of cardiac myocytes, increased incidence of pheochromocytomas, and reduced lifespans (Minor et al., 2010). Cardiac effects of 2DG in rats had features consistent with autophagy, a process by which a cell degrades unnecessary cellular components in response to nutrient stress. Comprehensive preclinical safety and toxicology studies have subsequently demonstrated reversible species-specific cardiac toxicity at high doses in F344 rats but not in Beagle dogs; this toxicity was detectable by monitoring plasma N-terminal pro-brain natriuretic peptide (Nt-proBNP; Terse et al., 2016).

Experience regarding human safety of 2DG has been obtained in cancer trials (Pelicano et al., 2006). Tumor cells are dependent on glycolysis to support their metabolic requirements. By reducing glycolysis, 2DG deprives rapidly growing cells of their required cellular fuel (Cheong et al., 2011). For example, 2DG inhibits breast cancer cell growth in a dose-dependent manner and causes cell death through apoptosis (Aft et al., 2002). In combination with adriamycin, 2DG slows the growth of solid tumors, such as osteosarcoma (Maschek et al., 2004). In patients with advanced prostate cancer, a 2-week dose-escalation study revealed dose-limiting toxicity of grade 3 asymptomatic QTc prolongation at a dose of 60 mg/kg, but doses of 45 mg/kg were well tolerated (Stein et al., 2010).

CONCLUSIONS

The inhibition of glycolysis with compounds like 2DG represents a novel therapeutic approach to epilepsy. The effects of 2DG in animal models are summarized in Table 38.1. 2DG exerts acute anticonvulsant effects in vitro that are independent of the method of seizure induction. 2DG has acute anticonvulsant effects in vivo in several models of seizure induction and possesses novel chronic antiepileptic effects against progression of seizures and the adverse consequences of seizure-induced plasticity that are associated with alterations in neuronal gene expression. Because the dose-dependent, fully reversible cardiac toxicity observed in rats with repeated administration of 2DG is not observed after single doses or limited repetitive dosing, and acute administration is well tolerated, potential clinical therapeutic applications for 2DG include brief treatment to abort status epilepticus, to interrupt acute repetitive seizures, and to prevent delayed complications of TBI. Trials to determine the pharmacokinetics, safety, and tolerability of 2DG in patients with epilepsy are planned. The detailed anticonvulsant and antiepileptic mechanisms of 2DG actions remain to be clarified.

ACKNOWLEDGMENTS

This work was supported by The Malcolm and Sandra Berman Fund, the Paine Foundation, The Charlie Foundation (CES), NIH RO1 25020,

TABLE 38.1 EFFECTS OF 2DG IN MODELS OF SEIZURES AND EPILEPSY

Anticonvulsant Effects

In Vitro

High K$_o^+$	Decreased interictal and ictal bursting (CA3)	Stafstrom et al., 2009
	Reduced EPSC and IPSC bursts (CA3)	Pan et al., 2019
Bicuculline	Decreased interictal bursting (CA3)	Stafstrom et al., 2009
4-Aminopyridine	Decreased interictal bursting (CA3)	Stafstrom et al., 2009
	Decreased interictal bursting (dentate gyrus)	Forte et al., 2016
0 Mg^{2+}/4-Aminopyridine	Abolished interictal bursting (immature CA3)	Shao and Stafstrom, 2017
Cs$^+$/bicuculline/MK-801	Decreased interictal bursts but induced ictal bursts	Nedergaard & Andreasen, 2018
Traumatic brain injury (CCI)	Acute application of 2DG decreased injury-induced epileptiform activity (neocortex)	Koenig et al., 2019

In Vivo

6-Hz corneal stimulation in mice	Seizure protection	Stafstrom et al., 2009; Gasior et al., 2010
Audiogenic seizures in Fring's mice	Seizure protection	Stafstrom et al., 2009
Kindling of perforant path	Increased afterdischarge threshold	Garriga-Canut et al., 2006
Pilocarpine (adult rats)	Decreased seizure severity and duration; increased seizure latency	Lian et al., 2007
4-Aminopyridine in mice	Minimized neocortical seizures	Bazzigaluppi et al., 2017
Pilocarpine (neonatal rats)	Stopped status epilepticus	Janicot et al., 2020
Kainic acid IP	No effect	Lian et al., 2007
Kainic acid IV	Decreased seizure threshold	Gasior et al., 2010
Pentylenetetrazole IV or SC	Decreased seizure threshold	Gasior et al., 2010
	Shortened seizures	Lian et al., 2007
	No effect	Stafstrom et al., 2009
Maximum electroshock	No effect	Stafstrom et al., 2009
	Decreased seizure threshold	Gasior et al., 2010

Antiepileptic Effects

Kindling of perforant path	Greater number of afterdischarges required to reach class III, IV, and V seizures	Garriga-Canut et al., 2006
Kindling of olfactory bulb	Greater number of afterdischarges required to reach class III, IV, and V seizures	Stafstrom et al., 2009
Amygdala kindling	No effect	Gasior et al., 2010
Traumatic brain injury (CCI)	Chronic administration of 2DG prevented injury-induced hyperexcitability in neocortex	Koenig et al., 2019
6 Hz-corneal kindling (NMRI mice)	Attenuated kindling progression	Leiter et al., 2019
Chronic intracerebroventricular-administration (4 weeks)	Reported to be proepileptogenic	Samokhina et al., 2017

Behavioral Effects

Morris water maze	No adverse effect on spatial learning or memory	Ockuly et al., 2012
Open field test	No lasting effect on exploratory activity	Ockuly et al., 2012

Note. CCI = controlled cortical impact; IP = intraperitoneal; IV = intravenous; K$_o^+$ = extracellular potassium; NMRI = Naval Medical Research Institute; SC = subcutaneous; EPSP = excitatory postsynaptic potential; IPSP = inhibitory postsynaptic potential.

NIH NCATS BrIDGs X01 NS066866, the Epilepsy Research Foundation New Therapy Development Project, Citizens United for Research in Epilepsy (CURE), the U.S. Department of Defense (TPS), and the Wisconsin Alumni Research Foundation (CES, TPS).

REFERENCES

Aft, R. L., Zhang, F. W., & Gius, D. (2002). Evaluation of 2-deoxy-D-glucose as a chemotherapeutic agent: Mechanism of cell death. *British Journal of Cancer, 87*, 805–812.

Barton, M. E., Klein, B. D., Wolf, H. H., & White, H. S. (2001). Pharmacological characterization of the 6 Hz psychomotor seizure model of partial epilepsy. *Epilepsy Research, 47*, 217–227.

Bazzigaluppi, P., Ebrahim Amini, A., Weisspapir, I., Stefanovic, B., & Carlen, P. L. (2017). Hungry neurons: *Metabolic insights on seizure dynamics. International Journal of Molecular Sciences, 18*(11), 2269.

Cheong, J. H., Park, E. S., Liang, J., Dennison, J. B., Tsavachidou, D., Nguyen-Charles, C., Wa Cheng, K., Hall, H., Zhang, D., Lu, Y., Ravoori, M., Kundra, V., Ajani, J., Lee, J.-S., Hong, W. K., & Mills, G. B. (2011). Dual inhibition of tumor energy pathway by 2-deoxyglucose and metformin is effective against a broad spectrum of preclinical cancer models. *Molecular Cancer Therapeutics, 10*, 2350–2362.

Devinney, M. J., Pan, Y.-Z., Rutecki, P. A., & Sutula, T. P. (2009). Differential effects of glycolytic and mitochondrial metabolism on epileptic network synchronization in the CA3 subfield of the hippocampus. *Society for Neuroscience Abstracts, 331*, 9–15.

Ding, Y., Wang, S., Jiang, Y., Yang, Y., Zhang, M., Guo, Y., Wang, S., & Ding, M. P. (2013). Fructose-1,6-diphosphate protects against epileptogenesis by modifying cation-chloride co-transporters in a model of amygdaloid-kindling temporal epilepticus. *Brain Research, 1539*, 87–94.

Ding, Y., Wang, S., Zhang, M. M., Guo, Y., Yang, Y., Weng, S. Q., Wu, J. M., Qiu, X., & Ding, M. P. (2010). Fructose-1,6-diphosphate inhibits seizure acquisition in fast hippocampal kindling. *Neuroscience Letters, 477*, 33–36.

Farrant, M., & Nusser, Z. (2005). Variations on an inhibitory theme: Phasic and tonic activation of GABA$_A$ receptors. *Nature Reviews Neuroscience, 6*, 215–229.

Forte, N., Medrihan, L., Cappetti, B., Baldelli, P., & Benfenati, F. (2016). 2-Deoxy-D-glucose enhances tonic inhibition through the neurosteroid-mediated activation of extrasynaptic GABA$_A$ receptors. *Epilepsia, 57*, 1987–2000.

Gano, L. B., Patel, M., & Rho, J. M. (2014). Ketogenic diets, mitochondria, and neurological diseases. *Journal of Lipid Research, 55*, 2211–2228.

Garriga-Canut, M., Schoenike, B., Qazi, R., Bergendahl, K., Daley, T. J., Pfender, R. M., Morrison, J. F., Ockuly, J., Stafstrom, C., Sutula, T., & Roopra, A. (2006). 2-Deoxy-D-glucose reduces epilepsy progression by NRSF-CtBP-dependent metabolic regulation of chromatin structure. *Nature Neuroscience, 9*, 1382–1387.

Gasior, M., Yankura, J., Hartman, A. L., French, A., & Rogawski, M. A. (2010). Anticonvulsant and proconvulsant actions of 2-deoxy-D-glucose. *Epilepsia, 5*, 1385–1394.

Greene, A. E., Todorova, M. T., & Seyfried, T. N. (2003). Perspectives on the metabolic management of epilepsy through dietary reduction of glucose and elevation of ketone bodies. *Journal of Neurochemistry, 86*, 529–537.

Hartman, A. L., Rubenstein, J. E., & Kossoff, E. H. (2013). Intermittent fasting: A "new" historical strategy for controlling seizures? *Epilepsy Research, 104*, 275–279.

He, X. P., Kotloski, R., Nef, S., Luikart, B. W., Parada, L. F., & McNamara, J. O. (2004). Conditional deletion of TrkB but not BDNF prevents epileptogenesis in the kindling model. *Neuron, 43*, 31–42.

Holmes, G. L., & Zhao, Q. (2008). Choosing the correct antiepileptic drugs: From animal studies to the clinic. *Pediatric Neurology, 38*, 151–162.

Hori, A., Tandon, P., Holmes, G. L., & Stafstrom, C. E. (1997). Ketogenic diet: Effects on expression of kindled seizures and behavior in adult rats. *Epilepsia, 38*, 750–758.

Hu, X. L., Cheng, X., Fei, J., & Xiong, Z. Q. (2011). Neuron-restrictive silencer factor is not required for the antiepileptic effect of the ketogenic diet. *Epilepsia, 52*, 1609–1616.

Huttenlocher, P. R. (1976). Ketonemia and seizures: Metabolic and anticonvulsant effects of two ketogenic diets in childhood epilepsy. *Pediatric Research, 10*, 536–540.

Ingram, D. K., & Roth, G. S. (2011). Glycolytic inhibition as a strategy for developing calorie restriction mimetics. *Experimental Gerontology, 46*, 148–154.

Janicot, R., Stafstrom, C. E., & Shao, L. R. (2020). 2-Deoxyglucose terminates pilocarpine-induced status epilepticus in neonatal rats. *Epilepsia, 61*, 1528–1537.

Koenig, J. B., Cantu, D., Low, C., Sommer, M., Noubary, F., Croker, D., Whalen, M., Kong, D., & Dulla, C. G. (2019). Glycolytic inhibitor 2-deoxyglucose prevents cortical hyperexcitability after traumatic brain injury. *Journal of Clinical Investigation Insight, 5*(11), e126506.

Lee, J., Bruce-Keller, A. J., Kruman, Y., Chan, S. L., & Mattson, M.P. (1999). 2-Deoxy-D-glucose protects hippocampal neurons against excitotoxic and oxidative injury: Evidence for the involvement of stress proteins. *Journal of Neuroscience Research, 57*, 48–61.

Leiter, I., Bascunana, P., Bengel, F. M., Bankstahl, J. P., & Bankstahl, M. (2019). Attenuation of epileptogenesis by 2-deoxy-D-glucose is accompanied by increased cerebral glucose supply, microglial activation and reduced astrocytosis. *Neurobiology of Disease, 130*, 104510.

Lian, X. Y., Khan, F. A., & Stringer, J. L. (2007). Fructose-1,6-bisphosphate has anticonvulsant activity in models of acute seizures in adult rats. *Journal of Neuroscience, 27*, 12007–12011.

Long, Y., Zhuang, K., Ji, Z., Han, Y., Fei, Y., Zheng, W., Song, Z., & Yang, H. (2019). 2-Deoxy-D-glucose exhibits anti-seizure effects by mediating the netrin-G1-KATP signaling pathway in epilepsy. *Neurochemical Research, 44*, 994–1004.

Lutas, A., & Yellen, G. (2013). The ketogenic diet: Metabolic influences on brain excitability and epilepsy. *Trends in Neuroscience, 36*, 32–40.

Ma, W., Berg, J., & Yellen, G. (2007). Ketogenic diet metabolites reduce firing in central neurons by opening K_{ATP} channels. *Journal of Neuroscience, 27*, 3618–3625.

Maschek, G., Savaraj, N., Priebe, W., Braunschweiger, P., Hamilton, K., Tidmarsh, G. F., DeYoung, L. R., & Lampidis, T. J. (2004). 2-Deoxy-D-glucose increases the efficacy of adriamycin and paclitaxel in human osteosarcoma and non-small cell lung cancers in vivo. *Cancer Research, 64*, 31–34.

Minor, R. K., Smith, D. L., Jr., Sossong, A. M., Kaushik, S., Poosala, S., Spangler, E. L., Roth, G. S., Lane, M., Allison, D. B., deCabo, R., Ingram, D. K., & Mattison, J. A. (2010). Chronic ingestion of 2-deoxy-D-glucose induces cardiac vacuolization and increases mortality in rats. *Toxicology and Applied Pharmacology, 243*, 332–339.

Moriyama, Y., & Futai, M. (1990). H^+-ATPase, a primary pump for accumulation of neurotransmitters, is a major constituent of brain synaptic vesicles. *Biochemical and Biophysical Research Communications, 173*, 443–448.

Neal, E. G., Chaffe, H., Schwartz, R. H., Lawson, M. S., Edwards, N., Fitzsimmons, G., Whitney, A., & Cross, J. H. (2008). The ketogenic diet for the treatment of childhood epilepsy: A randomised controlled trial. *Lancet Neurology, 7*, 500–506.

Nedergaard, S., & Andreasen, M. (2018). Opposing effects of 2-deoxy-D-glucose on interictal- and ictal-like activity when K^+ currents and $GABA_A$ receptors are blocked in rat hippocampus in vitro. *Journal of Neurophysiology, 119*, 1912–1923.

Ockuly, J. C., Gielissen, J. M., Levenick, C. V., Zeal, C., Groble, K., Munsey, K., Sutula, T. P., & Stafstrom, C. E. (2012). Behavioral, cognitive, and safety profile of 2-deoxy-D-glucose (2DG) in adult rats. *Epilepsy Research, 101*, 246–252.

Pan, Y. Z., Devinney, M. J., Rutecki, P. A., & Sutula, T. P. (2009). Effect of glycolytic metabolism on synaptic currents in CA3 pyramidal neurons. *Society for Neuroscience Abstracts, 331*, 10/16.

Pan, Y. Z., Sutula, T. P., & Rutecki, P. A. (2019). 2-Deoxy-D-glucose reduces epileptiform activity by presynaptic mechanisms. *Journal of Neurophysiology, 121*, 1092–1101.

Pani, G. (2015). Neuroprotective effects of dietary restriction: Evidence and mechanisms. *Seminars in Cell and Developmental Biology, 40*, 106–114.

Park, M., Song, K. S., Kim, H. K., Park, Y. J., Kim, H. S., Bae, M. I., & Lee, J. (2009). 2-Deoxy-D-glucose protects neural progenitor cells against oxidative stress through the activation of AMP-activated protein kinase. *Neuroscience Letters, 449*, 201–206.

Pelicano, H., Martin, D. S., Xu, R.-H., & Huang, P. (2006). Glycolysis inhibition for anticancer treatment. *Oncogene, 25*, 4633–4646.

Racine, R. J. (1972). Modification of seizure activity by electrical stimulation: II. Motor seizure. *Electroencephalography and Clinical Neurophysiology, 32*, 281–294.

Reddy, K., Reife, R., & Cole, A. J. (2013). SGE-102: A novel therapy for refractory status epilepticus. *Epilepsia, 54*(Suppl. 6), 81–83.

Redjak, K., Redjak, R., Sieklucka-Dziuba, M., Stelmasiak, Z., & Grieb, P. (2001). 2-Deoxyglucose enhances epileptic tolerance evoked by transient incomplete brain ischemia in mice. *Epilepsy Research, 43*, 271–278.

Reid, C. A., Mullen, S., Kim, T. H., & Petrou, S. (2014). Epilepsy, energy deficiency and new therapeutic approaches including diet. *Pharmacology and Therapeutics, 144*, 192–201.

Rho, J. M., & Stafstrom, C. E. (2012). The ketogenic diet: What has science taught us? *Epilepsy Research, 100*, 210–217.

Samokhina, E., Popova, I., Malkov, A., Ivanov, A. I., Papadia, D., Osypov, A., Molchanov, M., Paskevich, S., Fisahn, A., Zilberter, M., & Zilberter, Y. (2017). Chronic inhibition of brain glycolysis initiates epileptogenesis. *Journal of Neuroscience Research, 95*, 2195–2206.

Shao, L. R., Rho, J. M., & Stafstrom, C. E. (2018a). Glycolytic inhibition: A novel approach toward controlling neuronal excitability and seizures. *Epilepsia Open, 3*, 191–197.

Shao, L. R., & Stafstrom, C. E. (2017). Glycolytic inhibition by 2-deoxy-D-glucose abolishes both neuronal and network bursts in an in vitro seizure model. *Journal of Neurophysiology, 118*, 103–113.

Shao, L. R., Wang, G., & Stafstrom, C. E. (2018b). The glycolytic metabolite, fructose-1,6-bisphosphate, blocks epileptiform bursts by attenuating voltage-activated calcium currents in hippocampal slices. *Frontiers in Cellular Neuroscience, 12*, 168.

Stafstrom, C. E., Ockuly, J. C., Murphree, L., Valley, M. T., Roopra, A., & Sutula, T. P. (2009). Anticonvulsant and antiepileptic actions of 2-deoxy-D-glucose in epilepsy models. *Annals of Neurology, 65*, 435–447.

Stein, M., Lin, H., Jeyamohan, C., Dvorzhinski, D., Gounder, M., Bray, K., Eddy, S., Goodin, S., White, E., & Dipaola, R. S. (2010). Targeting tumor metabolism with 2-deoxyglucose in patients with castrate-resistant prostate cancer and advanced malignancies. *The Prostate, 70*, 1388–1394.

Stringer, J. L., & Xu, K. (2008). Possible mechanisms for the anticonvulsant activity of fructose-1,6-diphosphate. *Epilepsia, 49*(Suppl. 8), 101–103.

Sutula, T., & Franzoso, S. (2008). Dose-response and time course of action of disease-modifying effects of 2DG on kindling progression: effectiveness of administration after seizures. *Epilepsia, 49*(Suppl. 7), 382.

Tanner, G. R., Lutas, A., Martínez-François, J. R., & Yellen, G. (2011). Single K_{ATP} channel opening in response to action potential firing in mouse dentate granule neurons. *Journal of Neuroscience, 31*, 8689–8696.

Terse, P. S., Joshi, P. S., Bordelon, N. R., Brys, A. M., Patton, K. M., Arndt, T. P., & Sutula, T. P. (2016). 2-Deoxy-D-glucose (2-DG)-induced cardiac toxicity in rat: NT-proBNP and BNP as potential early cardiac safety biomarkers. *International Journal of Toxicology, 35*, 284–293.

Vijayaraghavan, R., Kumar, D., Dube, S. N., Singh, R., Pandey, K. S., Bag, B.C., Kaushik, M. P., Sekhar, K., Dwarakanath, B. S., & Ravindranath, T. (2006). Acute toxicity and cardio-respiratory effects of 2-deoxy-2-glucose: A promising radio sensitiser. *Biomedical and Environmental Sciences, 19*, 96–103.

Wree, A. (1990). Principles of the 2-deoxyglucose method for the determination of the local cerebral glucose utilization. *European Journal of Morphology, 28*, 132–138.

Yang, H., Guo, R., Wu, J., Peng, Y., Xie, D., Zheng, W., Huang, X., Liu, D., Liu, W., Huang, L., & Song, Z. (2013). The antiepileptic effect of the glycolytic inhibitor 2-deoxy-D-glucose is mediated by upregulation of K_{ATP} channel subunits Kir6.1 and Kir6.2. *Neurochemical Research, 38*, 677–685.

Yao, J., Chen, S., Mao, Z., Cadenas, E., & Brinton, R. D. (2011). 2-Deoxy-D-glucose treatment induces ketogenesis, sustains mitochondrial function, and reduces pathology in female mouse model of Alzheimer's disease. *PLOS ONE, 6*, Article e21788.

Yuen, A. W. C., & Sander, J. W. (2014). Rationale for using intermittent calorie restriction as a dietary treatment for drug resistant epilepsy. *Epilepsy & Behavior, 33*, 110–114.

Zhang, D., Li, J., Wang, F., Hu, J., Wang, S., & Sun, Y. (2014). 2-Deoxy-D-glucose targeting of glucose metabolism in cancer cells as a potential therapy. *Cancer Letters, 355*, 176–183.

Zhao, Y. T., Tekkok, S., & Krnjevic, K. (1997). 2-Deoxy-D-glucose-induced changes in membrane potential, input resistance, and excitatory postsynaptic potentials of CA1 hippocampal neurons. *Canadian Journal of Physiology and Pharmacology, 75*, 368–374.

Low-Carbohydrate, Ketogenic Diets for the Treatment of Type 2 Diabetes and Obesity

ERIC C. WESTMAN, MD, MHS, JUSTIN TONDT, MD,
AND WILLIAM S. YANCY, JR., MD, MHS

INTRODUCTION

The prevalence of metabolic disorders like overweight, obesity, prediabetes, and type 2 diabetes mellitus (T2DM) has dramatically increased in the past 40 years, with levels now reaching epidemic proportions in both developed and developing countries (Emerging Risk Factors Collaboration et al., 2010). Obesity itself carries an increased risk for premature mortality, but it is also a significant contributor to the comorbidities of hypertension, dyslipidemia, and T2DM (Flegal et al., 2013). The excessive fat mass of obesity leads to insulin resistance, and insulin resistance is a major component of the pathophysiology of T2DM (Reaven, 2005).

T2DM is present in approximately 9.1% of adults 20 to 79 years old, affecting 463 million people worldwide. It is estimated that $760 billion were spent on T2DM in 2019 alone (International Diabetes Federation, 2019). Obesity has been shown to be one of the main etiologic factors in the development of T2DM, and modest weight loss of 5% to 10% can lead to significant improvements in cardiovascular disease risk factors (Wing et al., 2011). So, clearly, a treatment that addresses obesity and T2DM simultaneously would be of particular interest in the treatment of T2DM, and a low-carbohydrate diet can treat obesity and T2DM simultaneously.

A low-carbohydrate diet was first described for the treatment of obesity in 1863 by William Banting in his publication *A Letter on Corpulence* (Banting, 1864). Leaders in the medical world in the early 20th century, Frederick Allen and Elliot P. Joslin, also recommended low-carbohydrate diets for the treatment of diabetes (Allen, 1920; Joslin, 1928). This chapter reviews the mechanisms of action and recent clinical research supporting the use of a carbohydrate-restricted diet for individuals with obesity and T2DM.

DEFINITION OF CARBOHYDRATE RESTRICTION

Over the last 15 years, several independent groups have examined low-carbohydrate diets in human clinical trials and have given them the name "carbohydrate-restricted diets" (Westman et al., 2007). A low-carbohydrate diet is defined as having 50 to 150 g of carbohydrate per day. If the dietary carbohydrate is sufficiently low to cause an increase in blood or urine ketone bodies, typically less than 50 g of total dietary carbohydrate per day, then the diet is a low-carbohydrate, ketogenic diet. Various iterations of a low-carbohydrate diet have been incorporated into popular diet books, so the diet is best known for its use in weight loss.

While there were no formal studies published about the effect of low-carbohydrate diets until after 2002, it was commonly known that both hunger and calorie intake were reduced if carbohydrates were limited. It is important to highlight that experts who were unfamiliar with low-carbohydrate diets thought that weight loss without explicitly limiting calories was impossible. In a low-calorie diet, the caloric intake is explicitly limited, and the caloric-restriction approach was studied and used extensively by academic researchers and practitioners, with limited success.

Mechanisms of Carbohydrate Restriction: Reduced Hunger and Caloric Intake

There may be several mechanisms whereby low-carbohydrate diets lead to weight loss, due to the changes in metabolism that occur. Several studies have now shown that a low-carbohydrate diet enhances satiety, leading to a spontaneous reduction in hunger and ad libitum caloric intake

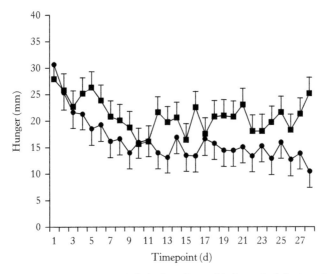

FIGURE 39.1 *Reduction in Hunger on a Low-Carbohydrate Versus Medium-Carbohydrate Diet*

Plot of mean (*SEM*) daily hunger (mm), as assessed with the Visual Analogue Scale, with consumption of the high-protein, low-carbohydrate (ketogenic) diet and the high-protein, medium-carbohydrate (nonketogenic) diet. Over the 4-week period, hunger was significantly lower (*p* = 0.014) with the low-carbohydrate diet than with the medium-carbohydrate diet in the 17 subjects (ANOVA). Reprinted with permission from Johnstone (2008).

(Boden et al., 2005; Hu et al., 2016; Johnstone et al., 2008; Figure 39.1). The research includes studies with the close monitoring of metabolic wards, as well as outpatient "real-world" studies. In studies of the treatment of obesity, the caloric intake is reduced to the level of a low-calorie diet, without explicitly limiting calories—typically, it ranges from 1,200 to 1,500 kcal/day (Yancy et al., 2004).

Two recent studies have examined the metabolic adaptations that occur with weight loss, and they have found that there is a small, but clinically significant, "metabolic advantage" to using a low-carbohydrate diet as compared to a low-fat, low-calorie diet for weight loss. This "metabolic advantage" appears to be about 200 kcal per day on average and is attributed to the thermogenic effect of food, and a lesser reduction in metabolic rate compared to other diets during the weight-loss process (Ebbeling et al., 2018; Hall et al., 2016).

Mechanisms of Carbohydrate Restriction: Glycemic Control

The consumption of carbohydrates (sugars and starches) raises the blood glucose more than consumption of proteins, and fats don't raise the blood glucose at all. Because diets that are restricted in carbohydrate have less of an impact on the glycemic response to a meal, it is logical

to restrict carbohydrate to treat a disease that, by definition, is an abnormal elevation in blood glucose (Figure 39.2; Nuttall et al., 2015). There is a recurring theme that low-carbohydrate diets lead to a greater improvement in T2DM than diets containing higher levels of carbohydrate. The reduction in blood glucose can occur on the first day of lowering dietary carbohydrate, so medical monitoring is needed if the patient is taking anti-diabetes medication.

Mechanisms of Carbohydrate Restriction: Metabolic Syndrome

Although different diets may be effective for weight loss, it is important to note that the metabolic effects of low-carbohydrate and low-fat diets are different. When compared to low-fat diets, low-carbohydrate ketogenic diets improve serum triglyceride and HDL levels to a greater degree. In the DIETFITS trial, the carbohydrate-restricted group saw a greater improvement in triglycerides and HDL, even though their carbohydrate intake was not restricted to the point of ketosis, and both groups eliminated refined grains and added sugars (Gardner et al., 2018). These studies are notable in that, despite the higher fat content of the low-carbohydrate diet, the adverse changes in serum cholesterol that were predicted from other diet studies did not occur. The low-carbohydrate diet improves

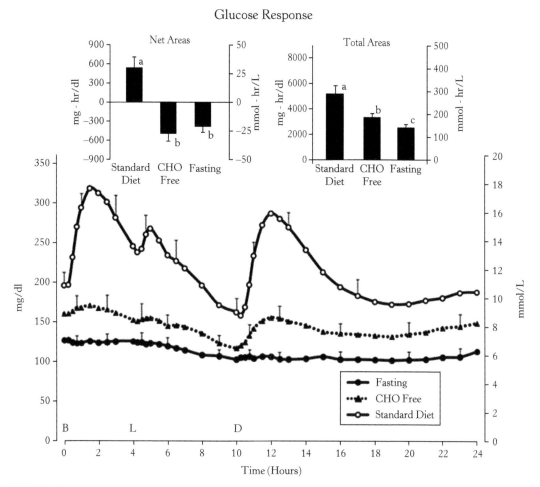

FIGURE 39.2 *Effect of a Ketogenic Diet on Fasting and Postprandial Glucose*

Twenty-four-hour glucose response. The open circle–solid line trace represents the mean glucose concentration at several times during the first 24 hr of both days during which the standard diet was ingested (i.e., day 1 of each arm of the study). The triangle–dotted line represents the mean glucose concentration during the last 24 hr on a carbohydrate-free diet. The closed circle–solid line represents the mean glucose concentration during the last 24 hr of the fast (energy-free) diet. B, L, D, indicate the times at which breakfast, lunch, and dinner were ingested. The net area response (left insert) indicates the area under the curve using the fasting concentration as baseline. Different letters on bars indicate statistically significant differences (Friedman $p < 0.0012$). The total area response (right insert) indicates the area under the curve, using zero as baseline. Different letters on bars indicate statistically significant differences (Friedman $p < 0.0001$). Reprinted with permission from Nuttall et al., (2015).

cardiometabolic risk factors by lowering serum triglycerides, raising HDL cholesterol levels, reducing abdominal circumference, improving blood glucose, and lowering blood pressure—that is, improving the major components of the metabolic syndrome (Volek & Feinman, 2005; Volek et al., 2008; Figure 39.3).

There are very few dietary intervention studies with "hard" clinical endpoints (such as myocardial infarction or mortality), but a low-carbohydrate diet was one of the intervention arms in the Workplace Diet Trial, a study that measured body weight and carotid intimal thickness after 2 years (Shai et al., 2008, 2010). In this study, all diet interventions, including the low-carbohydrate diet, led to significant regression of carotid intimal thickness. The effect appeared to be mediated by weight loss and a reduction in blood pressure. How a ketogenic diet reduces cardiovascular disease risk may be related to its effect on the metabolic syndrome—improvements in abdominal circumference, blood glucose, blood pressure, serum triglycerides, and HDL cholesterol levels.

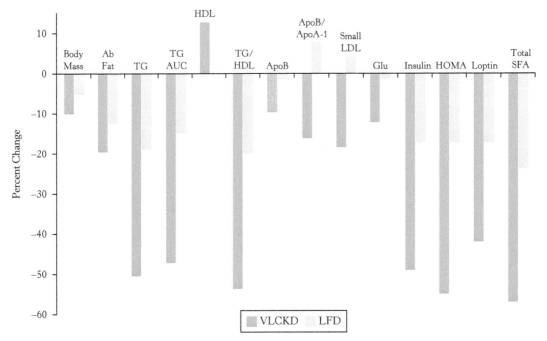

FIGURE 39.3 *Effect of Carbohydrate Restriction on Metabolic Syndrome*

Summary of changes in subjects who consumed a very-low-carbohydrate ketogenic diet (VLCKD) or a low-fat diet (LFD) for 12 weeks. Mean changes were all significantly different between the VLCKD and LFD. Ab Fat = abdominal fat; HOMA = Homeostasis Model Assessment; TG AUC = area under (time) curve. Reprinted with permission from Volek et al., (2008).

CLINICAL TRIALS OF CARBOHYDRATE RESTRICTION FOR THE TREATMENT OF OBESITY

Numerous studies were performed from 2002 to 2010 comparing low-carbohydrate diets to low-fat diets, because the low-fat diet was the recommended "one-size-fits-all" approach for many years. These studies (over 10 of which lasted 12 months or more) have been summarized in several meta-analyses (Bueno et al., 2013; Churuangsuk et al., 2018; Hession et al., 2009; Nordmann et al., 2006; Santos et al., 2012). The meta-analyses found that low-carbohydrate diets led to greater weight loss than low-fat diets and should be considered an alternative tool for treating obesity.

CARBOHYDRATE RESTRICTION FOR T2DM

The use of a carbohydrate-restricted diet for T2DM is sensible because it leads to an immediate reduction in blood glucose and then a reduction in insulin resistance and T2DM over time as weight loss progresses. A carbohydrate-restricted dietary approach may be a preferred lifestyle approach because of its mechanisms of hunger and calorie reduction.

Randomized, Controlled Trials of Carbohydrate Restriction for T2DM

There has been increasing interest in use of low-carbohydrate diets for the treatment of T2DM. In the majority of studies, the diets containing fewer carbohydrates led to a greater improvement in T2DM and weight than the diets containing higher levels of carbohydrate (Daly et al., 2006; Guldbrand et al., 2012; Mayer et al., 2014; Michalczyk et al., 2020; Saslow et al., 2014; Tay et al., 2014; Westman et al., 2008; Yamada et al., 2014; Yancy et al., 2019; Table 39.1). In other words, there is a dose-dependency of carbohydrates: lower amounts of carbohydrate will lead to less of a glycemic response. If a higher carbohydrate level still leads to a reduction in caloric intake and weight loss, then there still may be improvements in diabetes despite a higher carbohydrate level. (Recall that high-carbohydrate diets that are low in calories can lead to weight loss and improvement in diabetes, as well.)

One study is worth highlighting because it used carbohydrate restriction within the

TABLE 39.1 OUTPATIENT RANDOMIZED, CONTROLLED TRIALS OF
CARBOHYDRATE RESTRICTION FOR HYPERGLYCEMIC DISORDERS

Reference	N	BMI (kg/m²)	Carbohydrates (g/day)	Duration (months)	Start HbA$_{1c}$ (percent)	End HbA$_{1c}$ (percent)	Difference HbA$_{1c}$ (percent)	Weight difference (kg)
Daly et al. (2006)	102	36	170	3	9.0	8.8	−0.2	−0.9
			110		9.0	8.5	−0.5	−3.6
Westman et al. (2008)	49	38	100	6	8.3	7.8	−0.5*	−6.9
			20		8.8	7.3	−1.5*	−11.0
Guldbrand et al. (2012)	61	32	225	24	7.2	7.4	+0.2	−4.0
			90		7.5	7.5	−0.0	−4.0
Saslow et al. (2014)	34	36	138	3	6.9	6.9	0*	−2.6
			58		6.6	6.0	−0.6*	−5.5
Tay et al. (2014)	115	34	205	6	7.3	6.6	−0.7*	−12
			57		7.4	6.2	−0.6*	−12
Yamada et al. (2014)	24	25	203	6	7.7	7.5	−0.2*	−1.4
			126		7.6	7.0	−0.6*	−2.6
Mayer et al. (2014)	46	40	156 + O	12	7.6	7.7	+0.1*	−8.1
			76		7.6	6.9	−0.7*	−7.5
Yancy et al. (2019)	261	35	hi	12	9.1	8.3	−0.8	−3.7
			lo		9.1	8.2	−0.9	−5.5
Michalczyk et al. (2020)**	91	33	286	12	5.9	5.9	0.0*	−1.0
			36		5.9	5.4	−0.5*	−14.0

Note. *$p < 0.1$. ** Inclusion criteria: glucose > 5.5 mmol/L and insulin > 10 uU/ml. N = sample size, O = Orlistat.

established healthcare system (Yancy et al., 2019). The study was conducted within the Veterans Affairs system; 263 medical patients with T2DM and overweight/obesity were randomized to a usual care group (control group) or a group that included instruction about a carbohydrate-restricted diet (CR group). Group visits occurred every 2 to 4 weeks for 16 weeks, then every 8 weeks over a 48-week period. For the instruction on the carbohydrate-restricted diet, the methods read, "A dietitian provided the nutritional counseling using a book [*The New Atkins for a New You*] and handouts. Initially, carbohydrate intake was restricted to approximately 20 to 30 g per day with no specified caloric restriction. Participants were taught how to add to daily carbohydrate intake gradually as they approached their weight goal or if adherence was threatened." After 48 weeks, the hemoglobin A1c (HbA$_{1c}$) went down in both groups (from 9.1% to 8.2% in the CR group, and to 8.3% in the control group), with no between-group difference. The CR group had greater weight loss

and a reduction in medication use, and they had 50% fewer hypoglycemic events.

Looking at this study in greater detail, in the supplementary materials, the estimated actual nutritional intake was reported (Yancy et al., 2019). At baseline, both groups consumed about 190 g of carbohydrate per day. For the control group, the carbohydrate intake at 16, 32, and 48 weeks was 179, 166, and 176 g/day. For the CR group, the carbohydrate intake at 16, 32, and 48 weeks was 90, 106, and 114 g/day. While the initial teaching was "20 to 30 g per day" of carbohydrate, this level of restriction was not actually achieved at any point in the study. So a reduction of carbohydrate to about 100 g/day led to a 0.9% reduction in HbA$_{1c}$ from 9.1 to 8.2, compared to a 1.5% reduction in HbA$_{1c}$ in a study where subjects achieved 20 g/day.(Westman et al., 2008)

Nonrandomized Trials Using Carbohydrate-restricted Diets in T2DM

The best study yet to thoroughly examine the details of the metabolic and therapeutic effects of nutritional ketosis in T2DM, known as the Virta Health Study, has a planned follow-up duration of 5 years. The results over the first 2 years have been published in a series of papers (Athinarayanan et al., 2020; Bhanpuri et al., 2018; Hallberg et al., 2018; McKenzie et al., 2017; Siegmann et al., 2019). This nonrandomized study gives insight into the effects of nutritional ketosis in 262 participants with T2DM compared to 83 control participants who received usual care (UC). The Virta Clinic Continuous Care Intervention (CCI) was a remote care intervention involving an outpatient protocol providing intensive, well-formulated, ketogenic diet instruction, behavioral counseling, home digital coaching and monitoring, and physician-guided medication management. The home monitoring included body weight, blood glucose level, and blood ketone level to document adherence to the diet and to assist in medication de-prescribing.

Many novel findings resulted from this study. At 10 weeks, most of the blood ketone levels (βHB, β-hydroxybutyrate) of those in nutritional ketosis ranged from 0 to 2.0 mmol/L, with the βHB observed in patients using SGLT-2 inhibitors. After 10 weeks, the HbA_{1c} level was reduced by 1.0%, from 7.6% to 6.6%, and the percentage of individuals with an HbA_{1c} level of < 6.5% increased to 56.1. At baseline, 89.3% of participants were taking at least one diabetes medication, and by 10 weeks, 56.8% of individuals had one or more diabetes medications reduced or eliminated. There was also 7.2% weight loss. An important feature of this study was the daily monitoring of blood βHB, which may have contributed to the excellent adherence to the diet, including nutritional ketosis. The improvements in glycemic control and weight were sustained at 1 year and 2

years (Athinarayanan et al., 2020; Hallberg et al., 2018; Table 39.2). After 2 years, resolution of T2DM (reversal, 53.5%, remission, 17.6%) was achieved. An extensive evaluation of cardiometabolic risk factors after 1 year showed that all risk factors improved except the LDL cholesterol level (Bhanpuri et al., 2018).

Another study involved a digitally delivered, carbohydrate-restricted intervention for T2DM using behavioral support (Saslow et al., 2018). While the levels of carbohydrate restriction taught and achieved were not reported, it clearly was possible for health improvements to occur with this type of intervention. For example, participants with elevated baseline HbA_{1c} (≥ 7.5%) who engaged with all 10 weekly modules reduced their HbA_{1c} from 9.2% to 7.1% and lost an average of 6.9% of their body weight.

CONCLUSION

In summary, lifestyle modification that uses carbohydrate restriction is effective in the treatment of obesity and T2DM. This dietary intervention combines two approaches that, on their own, improve blood glucose control: weight loss and reduction of glycemic index/load in the dietary intake.

As for any lifestyle change program, research efforts to improve adherence are needed. Adherence may be improved by changing the frequency of follow-up visits, monitoring of weight and ketones, modifying the level of carbohydrate restriction, and providing better behavioral support (individually, in groups, or digitally).

The history of using the low-carbohydrate diet for treating obesity and T2DM and the new research regarding the mechanisms and safety of carbohydrate restriction suggest that the low-carbohydrate diet may be an important

TABLE 39.2 NONRANDOMIZED STUDIES OF CARBOHYDRATE RESTRICTION FOR TYPE 2 DIABETES MELLITUS > 12 MONTHS

Reference	N	Baseline weight (kg)	Carbohydrates (% kcal/day)	Duration (months)	Pre HbA_{1c} (percent)	Post HBA_{1c} (percent)	Weight difference (percent)
Athinarayanan et al. (2018)	262	114.6	30 g/d advised	24	7.6	6.7	−10.9
	87	111.1	Usual care	24	7.6	7.9	0.0
Saslow et al. (2018)	528	88.9	Completers	12	7.4	6.2	−8.4
	144	87.8	Partial completers	12	7.0	6.4	−2.4
	328	91.7	Noncompleters	12	8.8	8.6	0.0

nonpharmacologic approach for reversing the current epidemics of obesity and T2DM.

CONFLICTS OF INTEREST

Dr. Westman receives royalties from the sale of popular books and is founder of Adapt Your Life, an educational and product company based on low-carbohydrate principles.

REFERENCES

Allen, F. (1920). Protein diets and undernutrition in treatment of diabetes. *Journal of the American Medical Association, 74,* 571–577.

Athinarayanan, S. J., Hallberg, S. J., McKenzie, A. L., Lechner, K., King, S., McCarter, J. P., Volek, J. S., Phinney, S. D., & Krauss, R. M. (2020). Impact of a 2-year trial of nutritional ketosis on indices of cardiovascular disease risk in patients with type 2 diabetes. *Cardiovascular Diabetology, 19,* 208.

Banting, W. (1864). *Letter on corpulence, addressed to the public.* Harrison.

Bhanpuri, N. H., Hallberg, S. J., Williams, P. T., McKenzie, A. L., Ballard, K. D., Campbell, W. W., McCarter, J. P., Phinney, S. D., & Volek, J. S. (2018). Cardiovascular disease risk factor responses to a type 2 diabetes care model including nutritional ketosis induced by sustained carbohydrate restriction at 1 year: An open label, non-randomized, controlled study. *Cardiovascular Diabetology, 17,* 56.

Boden, G., Sargrad, K., Homko, C., Mozzoli, M., & Stein, T. P. (2005). Effect of a low-carbohydrate diet on appetite, blood glucose levels, and insulin resistance in obese patients with type 2 diabetes. *Annals of Internal Medicine, 142,* 403–411.

Bueno, N. B., de Melo, I. S. V., de Oliveira, S. L., & da Rocha Ataide, T. (2013). Very-low-carbohydrate ketogenic diet v. low-fat diet for long-term weight loss: A meta-analysis of randomised controlled trials. *British Journal of Nutrition, 110,* 1178–1187.

Churuangsuk, C., Kherouf, M., Combet, E., & Lean, M. (2018). Low-carbohydrate diets for overweight and obesity: A systematic review of the systematic reviews. *Obesity Reviews, 19,* 1700–1718.

Daly, M. E., Paisey, R., Paisey, R., Millward, B. A., Eccles, C., Williams, K., Hammersley, S., MacLeod, K. M., & Gale, T. J. (2006). Short-term effects of severe dietary carbohydrate-restriction advice in type 2 diabetes—A randomized controlled trial. *Diabetic Medicine, 23,* 15–20.

Ebbeling, C. B., Feldman, H. A., Klein, G. L., Wong, J. M. W., Bielak, L., Steltz, S. K., Luoto, P. K., Wolfe, R. R., Wong, W. W., & Ludwig, D. S. (2018). Effects of a low carbohydrate diet on energy expenditure during weight loss maintenance: Randomized trial. *British Medical Journal, 363,* k4583.

Emerging Risk Factors Collaboration. (2010). Diabetes mellitus, fasting blood glucose concentration, and risk of vascular disease: A collaborative meta-analysis of 102 prospective studies. *Lancet, 375,* 2215–2222.

Flegal, K. M., Kit, B. K., Orpana, H., & Graubard, B. I. (2013). Association of all-cause mortality with overweight and obesity using standard body mass index categories: A systematic review and meta-analysis. *Journal of the American Medical Association, 309,* 71–82.

Gardner, C. D., Trepanowski, J. F., Del Gobbo, L. C., Hauser, M. E., Rigdon, J., Ioannidis, J. P. A., Desai, M., & King, A. C. (2018). Effect of low-fat vs low-carbohydrate diet on 12-month weight loss in overweight adults and the association with genotype pattern or insulin secretion: The DIETFITS randomized clinical trial. *Journal of the American Medical Association, 319,* 667–679.

Guldbrand, H., Dizdar, B., Bunjaku, B., Lindström, T., Bachrach-Lindström, M., Fredrikson, M., Ostgren, C. J., & Nystrom, F. H. (2012). In type 2 diabetes, randomisation to advice to follow a low-carbohydrate diet transiently improves glycaemic control compared with advice to follow a low-fat diet producing a similar weight loss. *Diabetologia, 55,* 2118–2127.

Hall, K. D., Chen, K. Y., Guo, J., Lam, Y. Y., Leibel, R. L., Mayer, L. E., Reitman, M. L., Rosenbaum, M., Smith, S. R., Walsh, B. T., & Ravussin, E. (2016). Energy expenditure and body composition changes after an isocaloric ketogenic diet in overweight and obese men. *American Journal of Clinical Nutrition, 104,* 324–333.

Hallberg, S. J., McKenzie, A. L., Williams, P. T., Bhanpuri, N. H., Peters, A. L., Campbell, W. W., Hazbun, T. L., Volk, B. M., McCarter, J. P., Phinney, S. D., & Volek, J.S. (2018). Effectiveness and safety of a novel care model for the management of type 2 diabetes at 1 year: An open-label, non-randomized, controlled study. *Diabetes Therapy, 9,* 583–612.

Hession, M., Rolland, C., Kulkarni, U., Wise, A., & Broom, J. (2009). Systematic review of randomized controlled trials of low-carbohydrate vs. low-fat/low-calorie diets in the management of obesity and its comorbidities. *Obesity Reviews, 10,* 36–50.

Hu, T., Yao, L., Reynolds, K., Niu, T., Li, S., Whelton, P., He, J., & Bazzano, L. (2016). The effects of a low-carbohydrate diet on appetite: A randomized controlled trial. *Nutrition, Metabolism, and Cardiovascular Diseases, 26,* 476–488.

International Diabetes Federation. (2019). *IDF diabetes atlas* (9th ed.). International Diabetes Federation.

Johnstone, A. M., Horgan, G. W., Murison, S. D., Bremner, D. M., & Lobley, G. E. (2008). Effects of a high-protein ketogenic diet on hunger, appetite, and weight loss in obese men feeding ad libitum. *American Journal of Clinical Nutrition, 87*, 44–55.

Joslin, E. (1928). Ideals in the treatment of diabetes and methods for their realization. *New England Journal of Medicine, 198*, 379–382.

Mayer, S. B., Jeffreys, A. S., Olsen, M. K., McDuffie, J. R., Feinglos, M. N., & Yancy, W. S. (2014). Two diets with different haemoglobin A1c and anti-glycaemic medication effects despite similar weight loss in type 2 diabetes. *Diabetes, Obesity & Metabolism, 16*, 90–93.

McKenzie, A. L., Hallberg, S. J., Creighton, B. C., Volk, B. M., Link, T. M., Abner, M. K., Glon, R. M., McCarter, J. P., Volek, J. S., & Phinney, S. D. (2017). A novel intervention including indi-vidualized nutritional recommendations reduces hemoglobin A1c level, medication use, and weight in type 2 diabetes. *JMIR Diabetes, 2*, e5.

Michalczyk, M. M., Klonek, G., Maszczyk, A., & Zajac, A. (2020). The effects of a low calorie ketogenic diet on glycaemic control variables in hyperinsulinemic overweight/obese females. *Nutrients, 12*.

Nordmann, A. J., Nordmann, A., Briel, M., Keller, U., Yancy, W. S., Brehm, B. J., & Bucher, H. C. (2006). Effects of low-carbohydrate vs low-fat diets on weight loss and cardiovascular risk factors: A meta-analysis of randomized controlled trials. *Archives of Internal Medicine, 166*, 285–293.

Nuttall, F. Q., Almokayyad, R. M., & Gannon, M. C. (2015). Comparison of a carbohydrate-free diet vs. fasting on plasma glucose, insulin and gluca-gon in type 2 diabetes. *Metabolism, 64*, 253–262.

Reaven, G. (2005). Insulin resistance, type 2 diabetes mellitus, and cardiovascular disease: The end of the beginning. *Circulation, 112*, 3030–3032.

Santos, F. L., Esteves, S. S., da Costa Pereira, A., Yancy, W. S., & Nunes, J. P. L. (2012). Systematic review and meta-analysis of clinical trials of the effects of low carbohydrate diets on cardiovascu-lar risk factors. *Obesity Reviews, 13*, 1048–1066.

Saslow, L. R., Kim, S., Daubenmier, J. J., Moskowitz, J. T., Phinney, S. D., Goldman, V., Murphy, E. J., Cox, R. M., Moran, P., & Hecht, F. M. (2014). A randomized pilot trial of a moderate carbohy-drate diet compared to a very low carbohydrate diet in overweight or obese individuals with type 2 diabetes mellitus or prediabetes. *PLos One, 9*, e91027.

Saslow, L. R., Summers, C., Aikens, J. E., & Unwin, D. J. (2018). Outcomes of a digitally delivered low-carbohydrate type 2 diabetes self-management program: 1-year results of a single-arm longitu-dinal study. *JMIR Diabetes, 3*, e12.

Shai, I., Schwarzfuchs, D., Henkin, Y., Shahar, D. R., Witkow, S., Greenberg, I., Golan, R., Fraser, D., Bolotin, A., Vardi, H., Tangi-Rozental, O., Zuk-Ramot, R., Sarusi, B., Brickner, D., Schwartz, Z., Sheiner, E., Marko, R., Katorza, E., Thiery, J., . . . Stampfer, M. J. (2008). Weight loss with a low-carbohydrate, Mediterranean, or low-fat diet. *New England Journal of Medicine, 359*, 229–241.

Shai, I., Spence, J. D., Schwarzfuchs, D., Henkin, Y., Parraga, G., Rudich, A., Fenster, A., Mallett, C., Liel-Cohen, N., Tirosh, A., Bolotin, A., Thiery, J., Fiedler, G. M., Blüher, M., Stumvoll, M., & Stampfer, M. J. (2010). Dietary intervention to reverse carotid atherosclerosis. *Circulation, 121*, 1200–1208.

Siegmann, M. J., Athinarayanan, S. J., Hallberg, S. J., McKenzie, A. L., Bhanpuri, N. H., Campbell, W. W., McCarter, J. P., Phinney, S. D., Volek, J. S., & Van Dort, C. J. (2019). Improvement in patient-reported sleep in type 2 diabetes and prediabetes participants receiving a continuous care inter-vention with nutritional ketosis. *Sleep Medicine, 55*, 92–99.

Tay, J., Luscombe-Marsh, N. D., Thompson, C. H., Noakes, M., Buckley, J. D., Wittert, G. A., Yancy, W. S., & Brinkworth, G. D. (2014). A very low-car-bohydrate, low-saturated fat diet for type 2 dia-betes management: A randomized trial. *Diabetes Care, 37*, 2909–2918.

Volek, J. S., & Feinman, R. D. (2005). Carbohydrate restriction improves the features of metabolic syndrome: Metabolic syndrome may be defined by the response to carbohydrate restriction. *Nutrition & Metabolism, 2*, 31.

Volek, J. S., Fernandez, M. L., Feinman, R. D., & Phinney, S. D. (2008). Dietary carbohydrate restriction induces a unique metabolic state positively affecting atherogenic dyslipidemia, fatty acid partitioning, and metabolic syndrome. *Progress in Lipid Research, 47*, 307–318.

Westman, E. C., Feinman, R. D., Mavropoulos, J. C., Vernon, M. C., Volek, J. S., Wortman, J. A., Yancy, W. S., & Phinney, S. D. (2007). Low-carbohydrate nutrition and metabolism. *American Journal of Clinical Nutrition, 86*, 276–284.

Westman, E. C., Yancy, W. S., Mavropoulos, J. C., Marquart, M., & McDuffie, J. R. (2008). The effect of a low-carbohydrate, ketogenic diet versus a low-glycemic index diet on glycemic control in type 2 diabetes mellitus. *Nutrition & Metabolism, 5*, 36.

Wing, R. R., Lang, W., Wadden, T. A., Safford, M., Knowler, W. C., Bertoni, A. G., Hill, J. O., Brancati, F. L., Peters, A., Wagenknecht, L., Look AHEAD Research Group. (2011). Benefits of mod-est weight loss in improving cardiovascular risk factors in overweight and obese individuals with type 2 diabetes. *Diabetes Care, 34*, 1481–1486.

Yamada, Y., Uchida, J., Izumi, H., Tsukamoto, Y., Inoue, G., Watanabe, Y., Irie, J., & Yamada, S. (2014). A non-calorie-restricted low-carbohy-drate diet is effective as an alternative therapy for patients with type 2 diabetes. *Internal Medicine, 53*, 13–19.

Yancy, W. S., Crowley, M. J., Dar, M. S., Coffman, C. J., Jeffreys, A. S., Maciejewski, M. L., Voils, C. I., Bradley, A. B., & Edelman, D. (2019). Comparison of group medical visits combined with intensive weight management vs group medical visits alone for glycemia in patients with type 2 diabetes: A noninferiority randomized clinical trial. *JAMA Internal Medicine, 180*, 70–79.

Yancy, W. S., Olsen, M. K., Guyton, J. R., Bakst, R. P., & Westman, E. C. (2004). A low-carbohydrate, ketogenic diet versus a low-fat diet to treat obesity and hyperlipidemia: A randomized, controlled trial. *Annals of Internal Medicine, 140*, 769.

Intermittent Exogenous Ketosis for Athletic Performance, Recovery, and Adaptation

BRIANNA J. STUBBS, DPHIL AND PETER HESPEL, PHD

INTRODUCTION TO SPORTS PERFORMANCE NUTRITION

Since the dawn of competitive sport, athletes have manipulated diet to optimize performance. The evolution of sports nutrition science has taken us from the figs and cheese eaten by the first Olympians in ancient Greece (Sweet, 1987) to our modern, highly sophisticated understanding of fueling elite performance (Burke et al., 2019). It is impossible to have one dietary solution that fulfills the metabolic demands of all athletes, given the disparities between competitive events. This is demonstrated by comparing a world-class sprinter to an elite marathon runner—to excel in power events lasting seconds requires a different approach to training and nutrition than the approach for endurance events, which often last several hours.

The fundamental biochemical reaction that powers performance is the capture and release of chemical potential energy in the phosphate bonds of adenosine triphosphate (ATP). ATP acts as a transducer between energy stored in bonds of metabolic substrates (carbohydrates [CHO], fats, protein, and ketones) and release of energy as kinetic work by muscle. In short, all-out exercise (< 30 s), muscle ATP can be replenished through substrate-level phosphorylation: the breakdown of phosphocreatine and the conversion of stored CHO (muscle glycogen) into lactate. Physical efforts lasting minutes to hours are fueled primarily by mitochondrial oxidative metabolism of intramuscular substrates—glycogen and triglycerides—as well as extramuscular substrates—glucose generated in the liver or consumed in the diet and fatty acids from adipocytes (Milou et al., 2010).

In athletes on a mixed diet, utilization of plasma and muscle fatty acids predominates at low exercise intensities, and muscle glycogen and plasma glucose utilization increase with intensity (Romijn et al., 1993; van Loon et al., 2001). This has been taken to indicate an obligate requirement for CHO to fuel high-intensity competitive performance. As a result, the recommendation to endurance athletes is to ensure adequate dietary CHO intake to maximize muscle glycogen concentrations ahead of key performances and to ingest CHO at a high rate during exercise to maintain CHO supply and thereby prevent premature fatigue (Burke et al., 2019). Endogenous triglyceride stores represent a greater source of energy than stored glycogen. Therefore, adaptation to a low-carbohydrate, high-fat diet (LCHF; < 50 g/day) has been suggested as a tool to improve endurance by increasing reliance on fatty acid oxidation (FAO). However, while substantial increases in fat oxidation have been described in well-trained athletes habituated to a LCHF diet (Volek et al., 2016), no consistent changes in performance (positive or negative) have been demonstrated (Burke, 2015). By comparison, for elite athletes competing in high-intensity events, a LCHF diet may decrease oxygen efficiency and prevent improved performance after intensified training (Burke et al., 2017, 2020).

While sports nutrition focuses heavily on physical performance and the needs of the working muscle, there is an inescapable interplay between physical and cognitive fatigue, as well as between cognitive function and performance. Like muscle, the brain is sensitive to fuel availability (i.e., hypoglycemia), hydration status, and body temperature; these must all be maintained within homeostatic limits to maintain optimal function (Nybo & Rasmussen, 2007; Nybo & Secher, 2004). Thus, strategies like CHO fueling and hydration protect against both peripheral fatigue and central fatigue. Other ergogenic strategies that are believed to act centrally include caffeine (Goldstein et al., 2010) and oral CHO mouthwash (Chambers et al., 2009).

Another area of nutrition that has gained more attention with the increasing professionalization of sport is the role of diet in recovery and adaptation. Post-exercise nutrition recommendations typically focus on replenishing fuel stores, facilitating muscle repair by improving muscle protein balance, and rehydration, all aiming to restore readiness to perform as quickly as possible (Milou et al., 2010). However, recovery practices may differ according to sport or training phase. As an example, in training, when performance is less of a focus, endurance athletes might deliberately withhold CHO in order to promote adaptation to fat oxidative metabolism in the muscle (Impey et al., 2018).

Nutrition is a critical factor in peak physical and cognitive performance. Differences between sports and between individual athletes mean that dietary recommendations vary, but an underpinning feature is the obligate requirement for fuel availability for muscle and brain function. Therefore, a long-term focus of sports science has been exploring novel fueling strategies and their effects on performance, and one such strategy is the induction of a state of ketosis.

ENDOGENOUS VERSUS EXOGENOUS KETOSIS

One hallmark of a LCHF diet is the endogenous increase in circulating ketones, known as hyperketonemia or ketosis (Volek et al., 2016). Low glucose availability and low circulating insulin during a LCHF diet or prolonged fasting trigger increased fatty acid mobilization (lipolysis). Some of the fatty acids are converted in the liver into ketones (β-hydroxybutyrate [βHB], acetoacetate [AcAc], and acetone, via mitochondrial β-oxidation and ketogenesis), and the ketones are released into the circulation (Robinson & Williamson, 1980). Ketosis also occurs in some less common scenarios, such as during poorly controlled type 1 diabetes (Laffel, 1999) or immediately after prolonged exercise (Koeslag et al., 1980).

Exogenous ketones are a class of compounds that can be consumed to elevate blood ketones without further dietary interventions. This creates a novel physiologic state of "fed ketosis," where the body is not limited in its choice of available substrates and could oxidize CHO, fats,

and ketones to meet energy demands. Exogenous ketones typically aim to deliver R-βHB, which is the most abundant of the circulating ketone bodies, although some products co-deliver significant amounts of the nonnatural optical isoform S-βHB, which does not appear to be as readily oxidized as R-βHB (Stubbs et al., 2017; Webber & Edmond, 1977). By strategically using intermittent exogenous ketosis (IEK), athletes could support their training and competition without the perceived trade-offs that accompany the ketogenic diet.

Despite the common feature of hyperketonemia, there are many differences between endogenous and exogenous ketosis (Figure 40.1). Endogenous ketosis occurs in the context of low insulin, increased lipolysis, and low glycogen concentrations in liver and muscle. Circulating D-βHB concentrations usually rise over days to weeks and range between 0.5 and 5 mM (Hallberg et al., 2018). Over this time, it is believed that adaptations occur that increase ketone production and utilization (Volek et al., 2015). By contrast, exogenous ketosis can elevate R-βHB within minutes, with increases in S-βHB also seen when racemic sources of βHB are consumed. Concentration of βHB attained can range from 0.3 to 1 mM with a racemic ketone salt (Stubbs et al., 2017), and up to > 5 mM with some ketone esters (Cox et al., 2016; Stubbs et al., 2017). However, these compounds only transiently deliver ketosis for ~ 2 to 3 hr, as βHB is cleared by both oxidative metabolism and urinary excretion (Cox et al., 2016). Importantly, exogenous ketones directly inhibit endogenous ketone production, because βHB reduces lipolysis and blood free fatty acid (FFA) concentrations (Mikkelsen et al., 2015; Stubbs et al., 2017) through direct binding to a G-protein-coupled receptor on adipose tissue (HCAR1; Taggart et al., 2005). Consumption of exogenous ketones also appears to acutely lower blood glucose concentrations (Gormsen Lars et al., 2017; Myette-Cote et al., 2018). To summarize, exogenous ketones create a novel state, whereby blood ketone concentrations are elevated in the presence of normal muscle and liver CHO stores.

Several types of exogenous ketones exist, all aiming to elevate blood βHB concentrations. However, there are substantial differences between the physiologic effects of different exogenous ketone compounds that are important to consider when considering the application of IEK for athletic performance.

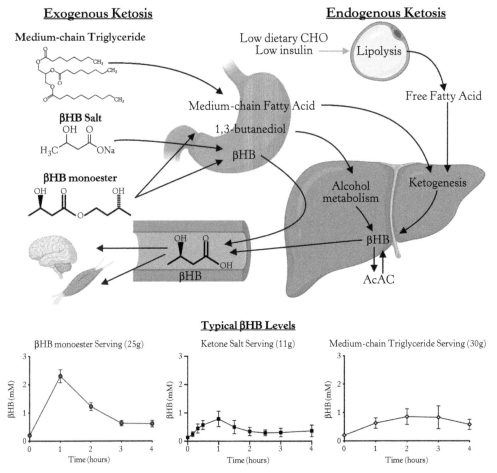

FIGURE 40.1 *Metabolism of Exogenous Ketones and Typical Blood Ketones Following Standard Servings of Common Ketone Supplements*

Subjects were healthy adults at rest (N = 10). Data are $M \pm SEM$. Abbreviations: βHB = β-hydroxybutyrate; AcAc = acetoacetate.

Ketone Esters

Ketone esters (KEs) are a class of exogenous ketones consisting of ketogenic components joined by ester bonds. The ketogenic components can be ketone bodies (i.e., βHB or AcAc) or ketogenic precursors, such as (R)-1,3-butanediol (BD), medium-chain fatty acids, and glycerol. Because there are several possible ketogenic components, and the possibility of joining them in mono-, di-, or even tri- ester forms, the KE family includes many possible compositions. The specific combination and number of components likely has important implications for the physical characteristics and physiologic effects of each KE; thus, all KEs cannot be considered equal.

Broadly speaking, a class advantage of KEs is that they provide highly bioavailable ketones (βHB between 1 and 5 mM), with no free acid or mineral load (Clarke et al., 2012). A disadvantage of the KE family is that they are typically expensive to synthesize and have a strong bitter taste, which can be aversive and lead to acute feelings of nausea (Stubbs et al., 2019). Most KE research to date has used two compounds: a monoester of βHB and (R)-BD (βHB monoester) and a diester of AcAc and (R/S)-BD (AcAc diester), although other KE compounds have been described in studies dating back to the 1960s (Birkhahn & Border, 1978).

Ketone Salts

Ketone salts (KSs) are a family of compounds that consist of a ketone anion bound to a mineral cation. Because AcAc is unstable, usually βHB is the ketone body found in KS products. The accompanying mineral ion is typically sodium, potassium, calcium, or magnesium. The advantages of KSs are that they are generally more palatable, more widely available, and cheaper than KEs. However, disadvantages include a high mineral load that, especially in case of sodium, could limit daily use levels; a high incidence of lower GI issues, increasing with dose (Stubbs et al., 2019); and relatively poor delivery of R-βHB (βHB between 0.5 and 1 mM; Evans et al., 2018; O'Malley et al., 2017; Prins et al., 2020; Rodger et al., 2017; Stubbs et al., 2017; Waldman et al., 2018). In part, this is because most products are racemic mixtures of both R- and S-enantiomers of βHB. Some of these issues can be mitigated by including multiple minerals, or by purification to give R-only βHB salts, but this is uncommon in typical consumer products.

Others

Two other classes of compound are used as a low-potency source of exogenous ketones. First are medium-chain triglycerides (MCT), which are rapidly metabolized in the liver via β-oxidation

to generate ketones (Bhavsar & St-Onge, 2016). Ingestion of MCT modestly raises blood ketones to ~ 0.4 to 0.8 mM (Ivy et al., 1980; St-Pierre et al., 2019); however, consumption of high doses can result in GI distress (Ivy et al., 1980). Second is BD, a widely available nontoxic di-alcohol. Following ingestion, BD undergoes hepatic conversion via the alcohol metabolism pathway to βHB (Desrochers et al., 1992). Ingestion of BD increases blood βHB concentrations to ~ 0.8 mM in athletes (David et al., 2019; Scott et al., 2019).

EFFECTS OF ACUTE EXOGENOUS KETOSIS ON EXERCISE PHYSIOLOGY

Interest in the application of IEK for athletes began recently; therefore, the small number of completed, comparable studies means that no conclusive recommendations can be made at this time. The following mechanisms may be implicated in the effect of IEK on athletic performance (Figure 40.2). These are primarily based on the use of ketones as an alternative energy substrate,

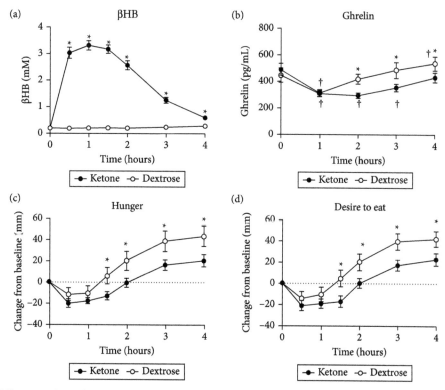

FIGURE 40.2 *Effects of calorie-matched ketone and glucose drinks in healthy young individuals*

Changes in blood βHB (A), ghrelin (B), and subjective appetite scores in healthy young individuals (*N* = 15) consuming calorie-matched βHB monoester and dextrose (glucose) drinks after an overnight fast. Data are *M* ± *SEM*. *p < 0.05 difference between KE and dextrose. †p < 0.05 difference from baseline value. Adapted from Stubbs et al. (2018).

competing with fat and CHO in skeletal muscle, and possibly substituting for glucose in the brain.

βHB May Offer an Oxidizable Substrate

At a fundamental metabolic level, oxidation of ketones is hypothesized to offer several advantages over CHO and fat oxidation. First, ketones are readily transported to the mitochondria in a concentration-dependent manner via a ubiquitously expressed, nonspecific monocarboxylate transporter (Halestrap & Price, 1999). This is in contrast to the regulated uptake of CHO via cell-surface membrane GLUT4 and fat by the carnitine palmitoyl transferase system in the mitochondrial membrane (Jeppesen & Kiens, 2012). Second, the oxidation of ketones has just two metabolic intermediates (AcAc and acetoacetyl-CoA) prior to acetyl-CoA formation, and thus fewer possible sites of regulation or substrate inhibition, compared to CHO and fats. By comparison, glucose must undergo glycolysis, which consists of nine intermediates with three tightly regulated steps prior to the formation of acetyl-CoA. Similarly, β-oxidation of FFAs is relatively complex, requiring ATP-driven activation of the fatty acid, a multi-intermediate translocation into the mitochondria, and four steps (oxidation, hydration, oxidation, thiolysis) for each acetyl-CoA produced. Third, the intrinsic combustion enthalpy (ΔH° kcal/mol per 2 carbon units) of βHB and the fatty acid palmitate is higher than that of pyruvate, the end product of glycolysis. This is inherently important to determine the maximum potential energy that a substrate can transfer to ATP as a result of complete oxidation (Veech, 2004). Finally, the oxidation of βHB itself is believed to result in advantageous thermodynamic conditions within the mitochondria (reviewed in Cox & Clarke, 2014). In brief, the oxidation of βHB increases the redox span across the inner mitochondrial membrane. The energy stored in the high-energy phosphate bonds of ATP is not fixed and can vary slightly according to intracellular conditions. Increasing the redox span across the inner mitochondrial membrane leads to a greater free energy of hydrolysis of ATP ($\Delta G'$ ATP). In a seminal study using an isolated heart perfused with βHB, the increase in $\Delta G'$ ATP was reported to increase cardiac efficiency by 28% compared to glucose perfusion (Sato et al., 1995). Notably, because the ketone body AcAc requires NADH for its reduction to βHB, it is not believed to offer the same metabolic advantage. Taking these mechanisms together, one might expect measurable changes in muscle efficiency during IEK (i.e., same power output with lower O_2 consumption). However, data describing the effect of IEK on VO_2 thus far are inconsistent, showing no changes (Cox et al., 2016), small increases (Poffé et al., 2020, 2021), and small decreases (Dearlove et al., 2019; Evans et al., 2019).

While ketone levels do fall during exercise (Balasseet al., 1978) in an intensity-dependent manner (Cox et al., 2016), estimated βHB oxidation rates (0.3–0.5 g/min) are fairly low compared to oxidation rates of CHO (~ 1–3 g/min) and fat (0.5–1.5 g/min; Burke et al., 2017; van Loon et al., 2001; Volek et al., 2016). Stable isotope studies are required to definitively determine the contribution of ketones to the energy requirements of exercise. Furthermore, if ketone oxidation were a key mediator of an ergogenic effect, there would be a relationship between βHB and performance. It was hypothesized that βHB levels should be elevated > 2 mM to achieve an ergogenic effect (Evans et al., 2017). This was based on studies of KSs that raised βHB by ~ 1 mM (O'Malley et al., 2017; Prins et al., 2020; Rodger et al., 2017; Waldman et al., 2018) and ketone mono- and diesters raising βHB < 1.5 mM (Evans et al., 2019; Leckey et al., 2017; Poffé et al., 2020b) in which no changes in performance were seen, whereas a βHB monoester study that achieved βHB > 2 mM did report slightly improved performance (Cox et al., 2016). This hypothesis was challenged by a study of the βHB monoester given with the acid buffer, bicarbonate, showing a 5% increase in performance of a 15-min time trial after a 3-hr simulated cycling race. Blood ketone levels were > 3 mM early in the protocol but had returned to < 1 mM during the time trial; thus, ketone oxidation was not a likely cause of the observed ergogenic effect (Poffé et al., 2021).

Available evidence does not support a pivotal role for ketone oxidation in the potential ergogenic effect of IEK where optimal evidence-based nutrition strategies are applied. However, the importance of ketones in energy provision conceivably might increase when CHO availability is impaired, for instance during exercise in the fasted state.

IEK May Regulate Carbohydrate Metabolism

Given the importance of CHO availability for prolonged exercise, and of rapid energy production from glycolysis for short, high-intensity exercise, the following effects of IEK on CHO metabolism could be of relevance to athletes.

Blood Glucose

Exogenous ketones reliably lower blood glucose at rest (Balasse & Ooms, 1968; Mikkelsen et al., 2015; Myette-Côté et al., 2018, 2019; Stubbs et al., 2017), and a glucose-lowering effect of IEK has also been seen in some (Bleeker et al., 2020; Cox et al., 2016; Dearlove et al., 2019; Evans et al., 2018; Evans & Egan, 2018; Leckey et al., 2017; O'Malley et al., 2017), but not all (David et al., 2019; Evans et al., 2019; Poffé et al., 2020; 2021; Prins et al., 2020; Rodger et al., 2017; Scott et al., 2019) exercise studies. The likely mechanism for reduced blood glucose is inhibition of hepatic glucose output driven by ketones (Balasse & Ooms, 1968; Mikkelsen et al., 2015), although it cannot be excluded that a reduction in plasma FFAs also contributes to increased peripheral glucose uptake (Spriet, 2014). During exercise, maintenance of glycemia is important to delay fatigue of both muscle (Coyle et al., 1983) and the central nervous system (Christensen & Hansen, 1939). The presence of ketosis in conjunction with hypoglycemia can protect cognitive function (Page et al., 2009), and during intense exercise, βHB monoester consumption was found to preserve executive function in spite of reduced blood glucose (Evans & Egan, 2018). Therefore, one might speculate that IEK could exert an ergogenic effect by maintain CNS substrate supply during exercise, particularly in the setting of limited CHO availability. Current data do not indicate an interaction between blood concentration of ketones and glucose with muscle function.

Blood Lactate

In several studies of both the βHB monoester and the AcAc diester, blood lactate concentrations were lower during ketosis at both submaximal and maximal intensities (Cox et al., 2016; Evans & Egan, 2018; Poffe et al., 2019), leading to a shift in the lactate threshold determined during an incremental exercise test (Dearlove et al., 2019). However, this effect was not seen in all KE studies (Evans et al., 2019; Poffé et al., 2020b) nor in studies of KS or BD (David et al., 2019; Evans et al., 2018; O'Malley et al., 2017; Prins et al., 2020; Scott et al., 2019; Waldman et al., 2018). The acute "lactate-lowering" effect of IEK does not appear to be consistently linked to pretest feeding state (fasted vs. fed), nor to level of βHB delivered by the ketone supplement. Despite concern that attenuation of

lactate production could impair high-intensity performance, studies of sprint exercise have not yet shown a consistent inhibitory effect of ketones on maximal exercise (Dearlove et al., 2019; Evans & Egan, 2018; O'Malley et al., 2017; Poffé et al., 2020b; Rodger et al., 2017; Waldman et al., 2018), but this cannot be excluded. The mechanisms underlying a possible lactate-lowering effect of IEK, as well as any link to performance in specific exercise contexts, remains to be fully elucidated.

Muscle Glycogen

Exhaustion of muscle glycogen correlates with fatigue in prolonged endurance exercise (Burke et al., 2011). Therefore, strategies that delay glycogen depletion could be ergogenic. Two studies to date have examined the effect of exogenous ketosis on muscle glycogen use during exercise. First, Cox et al. (2016) studied the βHB monoester taken after an overnight fast, before exercise, and along with CHO, finding that IEK had a profound sparing effect on glycogen breakdown compared with isocaloric CHO feeding alone. This observation, in conjunction with the decreased muscle glycolytic intermediates seen here and in another exercise study (Bleeker et al., 2020; Cox et al., 2016), as well as the lower blood lactate concentrations during exercise with IEK, reinforced the view that exogenous ketones triggered a switch away from CHO metabolism during exercise. This view was recently challenged when a second study by Poffé et al. (2020b) used a CHO-rich pretest meal and matched CHO intake during exercise along with the βHB monoester. In this study, there was no difference in muscle glycogen utilization between ketosis and control conditions over ~ 3 hr of exercise. There are several possible explanations for the discrepancy between the results, including the feeding state of the athletes and the absolute rate of CHO co-delivered with the βHB monoester. Further studies are required to expand on these findings and to determine the interaction between exogenous ketones, CHO feeding before and during exercise, and muscle glycogen utilization.

IEK May Regulate Lipid Metabolism

At rest, exogenous ketones reliably reduce lipolysis and lower circulating FFA concentrations (Balasse & Ooms, 1968; Mikkelsen et al., 2015; Stubbs et al., 2017), and studies have shown suppression of circulating fatty acid concentrations (< 1 mM) during exercise with IEK (Cox et al., 2016; Dearlove et al., 2019; Leckey et al., 2017; Poffé et al., 2020b). This is likely due to direct inhibition of lipolysis by βHB on the G-protein-coupled receptor HCAR2 (Taggart et al., 2005). During endogenous ketosis, where fatty acid mobilization is dramatically increased, this would function as a negative feedback loop to modulate fatty acid availability and prevent excessively high levels of blood ketones. In exogenous ketosis, however, lipolytic inhibition causes a dramatic drop in circulating FFA concentrations, because there is less opposing stimulus for fatty acid mobilization. Plasma fatty acid oxidation provides a substantial contribution to energy provision during exercise (van Loon et al., 2001), and the rate of FFA oxidation is at least partly regulated by FFA availability (i.e., circulating blood FFA concentration), thus one might hypothesize that this effect might be more pronounced in athletes who have high rates of fat oxidation, such as keto-adapted athletes (Volek et al., 2016).

The effect of IEK on intramuscular triglyceride (IMTG) utilization is poorly understood. Cox et al. described an increase in IMTG disappearance during IEK with steady-state exercise; notably, niacin (which decreases lipolysis without providing βHB as an oxidizable fuel source) did not increase IMTG oxidation, instead causing a heavier reliance on glycolysis (Cox et al., 2016). This study also found higher intramuscular acylcarnitine concentrations during IEK, indicating greater fat or ketone oxidation. However, these findings were not replicated in the study by Poffé et al., where ketosis had no effect on IMTG use during a ~ 3-hr simulated cycling race (Poffé et al., 2020b).

IEK May Alter the Respiratory Exchange Ratio

The respiratory exchange ratio (RER) is commonly used to infer the relative oxidation of CHO and fat during exercise. If βHB were to play a significant role in oxidative ATP production, coincident ketone oxidation alongside fat and glucose would confound the conventional interpretation of RER (Frayn, 1983). The stoichiometry of ketone body oxidation yields RQ values of 1.0 for AcAc and 0.89 for βHB (Frayn, 1983), so IEK should increase the RER for exercise that is dependent on fat oxidation (RER = 0.7) and decrease the RER for exercise that is dependent on aerobic CHO oxidation (RER = 1.0) Furthermore, one might hypothesize that increasing ketone levels could drive increased ketone oxidation and thus larger RER changes. However, there are no clear patterns in the existing data to confirm that IEK alters RER in a βHB-concentration or exercise-intensity-dependent manner.

IEK Alters Acid–Base Balance and Blood Electrolyte Levels

At rest, exogenous ketones can alter blood pH, with KS alkalinizing (Stubbs et al., 2017; Fery & Balasse, 1988; Müller et al., 1984) and KE acidifying, the plasma (Stubbs et al., 2017). Furthermore, this may be accompanied by changes in the intra- and extracellular balance of strong ions, such as sodium, potassium, and chloride (Stubbs et al., 2017). Such changes are all the more important to consider during exercise, as blood pH and strong-ion balance both contribute to skeletal muscle excitability and contractile function (Cairns & Lindinger, 2008; McKenna, 1992). Exercise perturbs acid–base and strong-ion homeostasis; thus, if IEK has effects during exercise similar to those seen at rest, there may be an interaction. Existing data are limited but strongly suggestive of an important interaction between exogenous ketones and regulation of pH and strong ions. Dearlove et al. (2019) demonstrated that ingestion of the βHB monoester during an incremental exercise test raised βHB > 3 mM, decreased blood bicarbonate, and caused a mild metabolic acidosis, which induced respiratory compensation. In this study, there was no difference in maximal power output between IEK and control conditions. Similarly, Poffé et al. (2020b) described a decrease in blood pH and bicarbonate when the βHB monoester was ingested ahead of 3 hr of mixed-intensity cycling. In a follow-up study, βHB monoester was co-administered with sodium bicarbonate (300 mg/kg); this attenuated acidosis, caused a fall in bicarbonate, and led to ~ 5% increased performance in a 15-min time trial (Poffé et al., 2021). This was accompanied by changes in plasma calcium and chloride, but not in sodium and potassium. Given that potassium is the strong ion most implicated in fatigue during exercise (Cairns & Lindinger, 2008), existing data do not fully explain how ketosis, protons, and strong ions interact to modulate muscle function. Nonetheless, the strong ergogenic effect of βHB monoester combined with bicarbonate suggests that this is an important area for future investigation.

BHB May Maintain or Improve Cognitive Performance

The evolutionary role of ketones is thought to be as an alternative fuel for the brain when glucose is in short supply (Owen et al., 1967). The brain plays a central role in perceiving and modulating the response to increasing physical fatigue as well as decision-making and tactics in skill or team sports. Given the established capacity of the brain to take up and oxidize ketones (Courchesne-Loyer et al., 2016), the positive effects of IEK during hypoglycemia (Page et al., 2009) and in individuals with mild cognitive impairment (Fortier et al., 2019), as well as the importance of substrate availability for cognitive performance (Dalsgaard et al., 2004), it has been hypothesized that ketones might maintain or even improve cognitive performance during depletive exercise. Evidence for a cognitive effect of ketones during exercise thus far is limited and inconclusive. A low level of ketosis during exercise after a KS drink did not lead to any changes in cognitive performance (Waldman et al., 2018). In contrast, Evans et al. found that supplementation with βHB monoester better maintained performance on an executive multitasking test during exercise compared to CHO (Evans & Egan, 2018). However, they found no effect with the same battery of cognitive tests after a 10-km running time trial with βHB monoester consumption (Evans et al., 2019). Thus, the possible role of exogenous ketones to help delay central fatigue or to maintain cognitive function during exercise requires further exploration.

EFFECTS OF ACUTE EXOGENOUS KETOSIS ON PERFORMANCE

The literature describing the effects of IEK on performance is in its infancy, so it is too early to conclude if, and how, IEK may be ergogenic (studies summarized in Table 40.1). There are many questions relating to the ketone supplement and to the athletic use case that must be answered to determine the optimal context for use of ketones. To define the optimal supplementation strategy, further studies should address the dose-response for different ketone supplements, as well as the relationship to exercise duration and intensity, and the interaction with other nutrition or supplements. Thus far, studies have focused on young, trained male athletes who consume a mixed diet; future studies should address responses to IEK in female athletes, less well-trained athletes, and athletes who follow a low-carbohydrate diet. Furthermore, there may be other important physiologic effects of exogenous ketones that have not yet been fully examined. For example, two recent studies using the βHB monoester reported

a decrease in urine output of ~ 200 ml on average (Poffé et al., 2020, 2021); an antidiuretic effect of IEK could be relevant to athletes who compete in the heat. Also, infusions of ketones reliably cause vasodilation (Gormsen Lars et al., 2017; Hasselbalch et al., 1996; Nielsen et al., 2019; Svart et al., 2018), which could alter muscle or cerebral function in athletes. Because some individuals in the published studies responded more strongly to ketones, these athletes may be ahead of the science for some time, devising and testing protocols for use of exogenous ketones. Lessons from the field can provide feedback to inform research study design, which will expedite the development of evidence-based guidelines for use of exogenous ketones.

EFFECTS OF CHRONIC EXOGENOUS KETOSIS ON TRAINING AND ADAPTATION

As well as its possible role as an acute ergogenic aid, chronic ketone supplementation may yield diverse beneficial training adaptations that accumulate and improve exercise performance. While ketones can act as an energy substrate, they can also act as signaling metabolites that may impact manifold cellular processes, at the level of skeletal muscle, the brain, and other tissues (Newman & Verdin, 2017; Puchalska & Crawford, 2017).

Endogenous ketosis is known to trigger multiple, long-term physiologic adaptations. As discussed above, the effects of adaptation to chronic endogenous ketosis on athletic training and performance have been extensively researched over the last decade (Burke, 2015). Additionally, several recent studies have examined adaptation to chronic ketosis achieved through ketogenic diet or ketone supplementation in patient populations, as a strategy to manage conditions like epilepsy, neurodegenerative diseases, and diabetes (Puchalska & Crawford, 2017). By contrast, research addressing the effects of chronic exogenous ketosis is in its infancy, with just a small number of studies to date investigating effects of relatively short-term (2 to 4 weeks) exogenous ketosis in healthy adults in resting or exercise contexts (Poffé et al., 2019; Soto-Mota et al., 2019). Extrapolation between studies of endogenous and exogenous ketosis in athletes are confounded, because IEK allows athletes to adhere to their habitual, CHO-sufficient diet, delivering tailored amounts of macro- and micronutrients to optimally support athletic performance. Equally, extrapolations from studies

TABLE 40.1 SUMMARY OF STUDY DESIGN AND RESULTS WHERE THE EFFECTS OF EXOGENOUS KETONES BEFORE EXERCISE HAVE BEEN INVESTIGATED

Participants	Study Design	Exercise Protocol	Ketone Source	βHB (mM)	CHO Metabolism	Lipid Metabolism	Other	Performance
Cox et al. (2016)								
Highly trained cyclists ($N = 8$; $M = 6$, $F = 2$)	KME + CHO vs. isocaloric CHO control drinks after overnight fast	60-min SS cycling at 75% W_{max} followed by a 30-min maximal performance test on bicycle ergometer	Three servings of KME, total 573 mg/kg, 50% before exercise, 25% servings after both 30 and 60 min of exercise	~ 2 mM	Lower BG and BLa with KE. Decreased glycolytic intermediates, no change in TCA intermediates. Glycogen sparing.	Lower blood FFA. Increased acyl-carnitine species. Increased IMTG oxidation.	Lower levels of ketones with increasing exercise intensity. Low (< 0.5 g) urinary βHB excretion. RER similar between conditions.	Significantly greater distance during performance test; With KE + CHO, athletes cycled ($M \pm SEM$) 411 $\pm$ 162 m (+ 2%) further than with CHO control
O'Malley et al. (2017)								
Healthy adult males ($N = 10$)	KS vs. low-calorie control drinks (matched for electrolytes) after overnight fast	15-min incremental cycling (5 min at 30%, 60%, and 80% power at VT) followed by a 150-kJ (10 km) TT (10–14 min) on bicycle ergometer	One serving racemic sodium and potassium KS taken before exercise, delivering 0.3 g/kg βHB	< 1 mM	Lower BG, no difference in BLa	ND	Lower RER in KS	Significantly slower TT performance with KS ($M \pm SD$); KS, 711 $\pm$ 137 s; control, 665 $\pm$ 120 s
Rodger et al. (2017)								
Highly trained male cyclists ($N = 12$)	KS vs. calorie-free control drinks following 2.5-hr fast	90-min SS cycling at 80% of second ventilatory threshold followed by 4-min maximal performance test on a bicycle ergometer	Two servings of racemic KS, taken 20 min before and halfway through (45 min) exercise, each delivering 11.7 g βHB	0.6 mM	Similar BLa and BG	ND	Moderate increase in RER with KS, no difference in submaximal VO_2, small increase in VO_2 in performance test	No difference

Study / Participants	Intervention	Exercise test		Blood ketone	BG / BLa	FFA	HR / RPE	Performance
Leckey et al. (2017) Elite male cyclists ($N = 11$)	KDE vs. calorie-free control, with matched CHO during exercise and after high-CHO pre-exercise meal	31-km cycling TT on a bicycle ergometer	Two servings of KDE, total 500 mg/kg as two 250 mg/kg doses 50 and 30 min before TT	~ 0.4 mM	Lower BG, lower post-exercise BLa	Lower plasma FFA	No difference in RER. Lower HR. No difference in RPE. All participants experienced moderate to severe GI issues with KDE.	Significantly slower TT performance and power output ($M \pm SEM$); KE, 339 ± 37 W; PLACEBO, 352 ± 35 W
Evans et al. (2018a) Trained cyclists ($N = 19$; M = 12, F = 7)	KS vs. calorie-free control after 10-hr overnight fast	Incremental cycling exercise test (8-min steps at 30%, 40%, 50%, 60%, 70%, and 80% of VO_2 peak) on a bicycle ergometer	Two servings of racemic KS, each 0.38 g/kg, each providing ~ 18.5 g βHB, 60 min and 15 min before exercise	~ 1.2 mM	Lower BG, no difference in BLa	ND	RER higher with KS. 13 of 19 participants had GI distress.	ND
Evans et al., (2018b) Trained team sport athletes ($N = 11$)	KME + CHO vs. isocaloric CHO after 2 standard high-CHO meals	Loughborough intermittent running shuttle test (part A, 5 x 15 min intermittent running; part B, shuttle run to exhaustion)	Three servings of KME, total 750 mg/kg, 50% 20 min before exercise, 25% servings after both 30 and 60 min of exercise	2.6 mM	Lower BG and BLa.	ND	No change in HR or RPE during part A. Lower HR in TTE shuttle run. Executive function multitasking performance maintained with KE.	No difference
Waldman et al. (2018) Healthy adult males ($N = 15$)	KS vs. low-calorie control drinks after 10-hr fast	Cycling: 5-min warm-up at 100 W, 4 x 15 s maximal sprint with 4 min recovery on a bicycle ergometer	One serving of racemic KS, providing 11.38 g βHB, taken 30 min before the test	0.5 mM	Similar BLa and BG	ND	Higher fatigue; lower HR with KS; no difference in cognitive performance	No difference

(continued)

TABLE 40.1 CONTINUED

Participants	Study Design	Exercise Protocol	Ketone Source	βHB (mM)	CHO Metabolism	Lipid Metabolism	Other	Performance
Scott et al. (2019) Trained male runners (N = 11)	1,3-BD + CHO vs. isocaloric CHO after an overnight fast	60-min SS running followed by 5-km TT on treadmill	One serving of R,S-1,3-BD 0.5 g/kg	~ 0.9 mM	Similar BLa and BG	ND	No difference in HR, VO₂, RER, or RPE	No difference
Shaw et al., 2019 Trained male cyclists (N = 9)	1,3-BD vs. calorie-free control after a 4-hr fast	85-min SS cycling at 85% of second ventilatory threshold followed by 7 kJ/kg TT (25–35 min) on a bicycle ergometer	Two servings of R,S-1,3-BD as 0.35 g/kg boluses	0.7 mM	Similar BLa and BG	ND	No difference in VO₂, VCO₂, RER, HR, or RPE	No difference
Evans et al. (2019) Trained runners (N = 8; M = 7, F = 1)	KME + CHO vs non-isocaloric CHO, following a high-CHO pre-exercise meal.	60-min SS running at 65% VO₂max followed by 10-km TT treadmill run	Three servings of KME, total 573 mg/kg, 50% 30 min before exercise, 25% servings at 20-min intervals during 60-min SS	1–1.3 mM	Similar BLa and BG	ND	No differences in VO₂, running economy, RER, HR, and RPE. No difference in cognitive performance.	No difference
Dearlove et al. (2019) Trained endurance athletes (N =12; M = 9, F = 3)	KME vs. calorie-free control after overnight fast	Incremental cycling exercise test to exhaustion (3-min steps, 25-W increases) on bicycle ergometer	One serving of KME, total 330 mg/kg, taken 30 min before exercise	3.7 mM	Lower BG and BLa	Lower FFA	Lower pH and bicarbonate, higher anion gap. Higher VE at max. Lower PET CO₂, small decrease in VO₂ at one point. RPE same with KE (Faull et al., 2019).	No difference

Study (population)	Intervention	Exercise protocol	Dosing	βHB	BG / BLa	IMTG / Glycogen	Other effects	Performance
Prins et al. (2020) Male recreational endurance runners (N = 10)	KS + MCT vs. calorie-free control after a 3-hr fast	5-km running TT on treadmill	One serving of racemic KS + MCT- delivering 0.3 g/kg of supplement (~ 9 g βHB salt, 7 g MCT) taken 60 min before test	0.6 mM	Similar BLa and BG	ND	No difference in HR, RPE, VO$_2$, VCO$_2$, RER	No difference
Poffé et al. (2020b) Highly trained male cyclists and triathletes (N = 12)	KME + low-calorie control, both with 60 g/hr CHO, during exercise and after a high- CHO breakfast	3-hr intermittent cycling, 15-min performance test, maximal sprint on bicycle ergometer	Three servings of KME, total 65 g, 25 g 60 min before exercise, 20 g 20 min before exercise, and 20 g 30 min into 3-hr cycling exercise	2–3 mM	Slight decrease in BG (early), similar BLa. No difference in muscle glycogen.	No difference in IMTG breakdown	RPE higher halfway through 3-hr cycling with KME. Lower blood pH and bicarbonate. Similar GDF15. Lower ghrelin and appetite with KE. Slightly lower norepinephrine with KME.	No difference
Poffé et al. (2021) Well-trained male cyclists N = 9	1. KME 2. Low-calorie control 3. Bicarbonate (300 mg/kg) 4. KME + bicarbonate. All with 60 g/hr CHO during exercise and after a high- CHO breakfast.	3-hr intermittent cycling, 15-min performance test, maximal sprint on bicycle ergometer	Three servings of KME, total 65 g, 25 g 60 min before exercise, 20 g 20 min before exercise, and 20 g 30 min into 3-hr cycling exercise	2–4 mM	Slight reduction in BG in both KE arms. bicarbonate increased BLa with and without KME.	ND	Bicarbonate increased βHB levels (0.5–0.8 mM). KE induced acidosis and bicarbonate attenuated KE- induced acidosis. KE increased plasma Ca^{2+}, Na$^+$, Cl$^-$. RPE was similar between trials.	5% higher power with KE + bicarbonate in 15-min TT

Abbreviations: 1,3-BD = 1,3-butanediol; BG = blood glucose; βHB = β-hydroxybutyrate; BLa = blood lactate; CHO = carbohydrate; F = female; FFA = free fatty acids; HR = heart rate; IMTG = intramuscular triglyceride; KDE = ketone diester; KME = ketone monoester; KS = ketone salt; M = male; MCT = medium-chain triglyceride; ND = not done; RER = respiratory exchange ratio; RPE = rating of perceived exertion; SD = standard deviation; SEM = standard error of the mean; SS = steady state; TCA = tricarboxylic acid cycle; TT = time trial; VCO$_2$ = carbon dioxide expiration; VO$_2$ = oxygen uptake; VT = ventilatory threshold; W$_{max}$ = maximal wattage.

of patients, who may be older and sedentary, to young athletes participating in strenuous exercise training are often invalid. Thus, while knowledge of adaptation to endogenous ketosis can generate hypotheses to be tested in IEK, conclusions cannot be formed on the basis of endogenous ketone research. Caution is warranted in interpreting the limited IEK data, pending further studies of chronic exogenous ketosis in exercise training.

IEK May Stimulate Post-Exercise Muscle Repair

Adaptation to training results from manifold tissue changes at the level of gene expression, translation, and posttranslational protein modifications occurring in response to repeated exercise bouts. It is well established that post-exercise protein intake stimulates net muscle protein synthesis, which is not only crucial for muscle repair but also to enhance adaptive training responses (Jäger et al., 2017) and to stimulate muscle hypertrophy (Morton et al., 2018; Stokes et al., 2018). While it seems intuitive that this would lead to improved functional capacity, such an effect remains to be definitively demonstrated.

Data from non-athlete model systems support the hypothesis that ketone bodies could induce muscle anabolism in humans, or at least prevent muscle catabolism (Koutnik et al., 2019). This hypothesis fits with the teleologic role of ketones as a survival substrate, whereby elevation of βHB actively spares muscle catabolism during starvation (Cahill, 2006; Owen, 2005). Several ketone-infusion studies support this notion; βHB infusion reduced whole-body protein degradation during starvation in obese individuals (Pawan & Semple, 1983; Sherwin et al., 1975) and during inflammation in healthy young men (Thomsen et al., 2018), and stimulated muscle protein synthesis in fasted healthy volunteers (Nair et al., 1988). However, the physiologic context of starvation-induced catabolism may be irrelevant in conditions of net muscle anabolism produced by exercise combined with protein intake. Thus, a recent study in athletes investigated the effect of ingestion of a standard post-exercise recovery beverage delivering optimal protein and CHO doses, alone or in combination with βHB monoester (Vandoorne et al., 2017). The βHB monoester enhanced post-exercise activation of mTORC1, which plays a pivotal role in activation of muscle protein synthesis and maintenance of muscle mass (Yoon, 2017). Follow-up experiments in myotubes in vitro confirmed that ketone bodies directly potentiated leucine-induced mTORC1 activation and protein synthesis (Vandoorne et al., 2017).

Muscle-supportive effects may not be exclusive to βHB. The ketone body AcAc can directly stimulate muscle satellite-cell activation and proliferation in mice, thereby counteracting muscular dystrophy in X-linked muscular dystrophy (mdx) mice, while stimulating regeneration of tibialis anterior muscle after cardiotoxin-induced injury (Zou et al., 2016). Satellite-cell activation and proliferation also have an important role in muscle repair after exercise-induced muscle damage (Bazgir et al., 2017; Blaauw & Reggiani, 2014; Snijders et al., 2015). Furthermore, inducing ketosis with the AcAc diester was profoundly anticatabolic in a multifaceted inflammatory model (Koutnik et al., 2020).

Ultimately, whether chronic IEK during recovery from exercise can facilitate training-induced muscle anabolism or prevent muscle wasting caused by exercise-specific catabolic stress requires further investigation.

IEK May Stimulate Post-Exercise Muscle Glycogen Resynthesis

Muscle glycogen provides the primary substrate for high-intensity muscle contractions. Hence initial muscle glycogen level is a key determinant of performance in endurance exercise events lasting > 60 min (Bergström et al., 1967), and ability to replenish glycogen between repeated bouts is crucial to maintain endurance performance. In addition to its role as an energy source, muscle glycogen availability might also play a role in training-induced adaptation of muscular oxidative capacity, possibly by regulation of AMPK activity (Derave et al., 2000; Viollet et al., 2003).

Early experiments in dogs and rats demonstrated that ketosis could stimulate muscle glucose uptake (Mebane & Madison, 1964) as well as glycogen storage (Maizels et al., 1977). More recently, experiments by Cox et al. (2016) in healthy volunteers provided circumstantial evidence of a pro-glycogen effect of IEK, showing that βHB monoester intake elevated muscle glucose-6-phosphate concentration, this being a potent stimulator of the glycogen synthase when occurring in conjunction with low muscle glycogen content (Jensen & Richter, 2012). The first direct support of IEK-mediated increase in glycogen synthesis in athletes came from a study showing that oral βHB monoester ingestion during a hyperglycemic intravenous clamp stimulated muscle glycogen resynthesis after exercise through increasing insulin secretion (Holdsworth et al., 2016). However, there was no effect on muscle glycogen when the βHB monoester was ingested after exercise in combination with gold-standard oral CHO + protein (Vandoorne et al., 2017), designed to maximally stimulate muscle glycogen regeneration after exercise (Burke et al., 2011). Similarly, a study employing consistent post-exercise βHB monoester intake in combination with a protein–CHO mixture did not alter basal muscle glycogen content at the end of a 3-week endurance training period involving two training sessions per day, 6 days per week, in young healthy volunteers (Poffe et al., 2019). Thus, it appears that the synergistic action of glucose and amino acids on pancreatic insulin release in the context of ample oral CHO + protein intake (Floyd et al., 1970) negates the potential of ketones to further stimulate muscle glycogen synthase activity, although this may still occur at lower circulating insulin levels.

IEK Impacts Food Intake and Hormonal Appetite Regulation During Training

Optimal body weight and body composition are cornerstones of elite performance. For example, reducing body weight helps to improve running economy (Morgan et al., 1989), and in cycling, lower weight boosts performance in uphill racing by virtue of elevated power output per kg body weight (W/kg). In weight-class sports, athletes often undertake periods of extreme dietary restriction to achieve arbitrary competition weight targets. Thus, extreme pressure for low body weight likely explains the high incidence of eating disorders in athletic populations (Joy et al., 2016; Mountjoy et al., 2018). It is tempting to speculate that nutritional ketosis, by promoting the advantageous muscle-sparing aspects of starvation ketosis (Cahill, 2006; Owen, 2005), could play a role in "functional"" weight management and lean mass maintenance in athletic populations, by stimulating muscle protein synthesis and preventing muscle wasting (Vandoorne et al., 2017). Although there is still debate about the long-term health outcomes, a ketogenic diet clearly can generate short-term weight loss in overweight individuals (Joshi et al., 2019). This weight loss is probably at least partly linked to decreased ghrelin secretion, which results in appetite and hunger suppression (Deemer et al., 2020; Joshi et al., 2019; Sumithran et al., 2013).

In athletes, matching food intake to energy expenditure in training and competition (energy balance) is a complex, multifactorial process, which involves both psychologic and physiologic factors. From the physiologic perspective, appetite/hunger-regulating hormones play an important role in modulating the response to energy balance shifts. The hormones leptin and insulin are primarily implicated in long-term regulation of energy intake (Perry & Wang, 2012; Stensel, 2010). Shorter-term regulation is thought to be mediated by the concerted actions of ghrelin, GLP1, peptide YY, and GDF15 in response to altered energy expenditure due to changes in exercise or dietary intake (Dorling et al., 2018; Stensel, 2010). Importantly, ketone bodies, predominantly βHB, are believed to modulate appetite directly at the level of the central nervous system, or indirectly by regulation of gut hormone secretion by enteroendocrine cells (Deemer et al., 2020; Newman & Verdin, 2017; Puchalska & Crawford, 2017). Recent findings indicate that ketone bodies directly modulate hormonal responses to food intake or energy stress; for example, βHB monoester intake in young healthy individuals elicited a lower ghrelin response and reduced both hunger and desire to eat compared to the ingestion of an isocaloric glucose dose (Stubbs et al., 2018; Figure 40.2). Furthermore, βHB monoester and CHO co-administration before and during a ~ 3-hr simulated cycling race resulted in lower circulating ghrelin levels (Poffé et al., 2020b). Importantly, in both cases, IEK suppressed subjective feelings of hunger and the desire to eat (Poffé et al., 2020b; Stubbs et al., 2018). While this would be beneficial for people with obesity who were trying to lose weight, by contrast, suppression of appetite during periods of strenuous training could result in a concerning negative energy balance for athletes, and thereby potentially impair recovery and training adaptation. However, this was not seen in a study of daily post-exercise βHB monoester intake during a 3-week intensified training period (Poffé et al., 2019). In fact, IEK was found to stimulate spontaneous food intake, which in turn prevented the development of energy deficit as training load was gradually increased (Poffé et al., 2019). This protective effect occurred independently of ghrelin but was associated with blunted rise in serum GDF15 throughout the training period (Poffé et al., 2019). Therefore, use of IEK during training may contribute to better matching of energy intake to energy expenditure by suppressing exercise-induced upregulation of GDF15, which is a well-established marker of cellular stress (Patel et al., 2019; Starling, 2019).

Further studies are needed to elucidate the effects of IEK on central and hormonal regulation of appetite and hunger regulation during exercise and training, and the potential impact on body composition to stimulate athletic performance.

IEK May Impact Training Adaptation by Suppression of Exercise-Induced Inflammation or Oxidative Stress, or by Regulation of Gene Expression

Multiple lines of basic science data indicate that βHB could modulate inflammation and oxidative stress, both processes that play a key role in exercise recovery and training adaptation. βHB at physiologic concentrations has been found to possesses numerous signaling roles, of which the most relevant are its ability to inhibit histone deacetylases (HDACs), the NOD-like receptor protein 3 (NLRP3) inflammasome (Youm et al., 2015), and the G-protein-coupled receptor 41 (GPR41; Kimura et al., 2011; Newman & Verdin, 2017; Puchalska & Crawford, 2017). Inhibition of HDACs by βHB counteracts histone deacetylation and thereby stimulates gene expression, which in turn restricts oxidative stress (Shimazu et al., 2013). Moreover, because the activity of class IIa HDACs in skeletal muscle is responsive to endurance exercise, βHB may also affect the adaptations to exercise and training (Egan & Zierath, 2013). βHB also functions as a direct antioxidant, can suppress mitochondrial ROS production, and promotes transcriptional activity of antioxidant defenses via FOXO1, FOXO3a, and NRF2 (Rojas-Morales et al., 2020). Besides upregulation of the capacity for redox homeostasis, βHB has also been shown to counteract inflammation by decreasing the activity of the NLRP3 inflammasome (Youm et al., 2015). Finally, experiments in different animal models have shown βHB to suppress sympathetic nervous system activity, energy expenditure, and heart rate via inhibition of GPR41 (Kimura et al., 2011).

As yet, there is no direct evidence that exogenous ketosis may stimulate beneficial training adaptations or counteract exercise-induced degenerative events, via one or more of the aforementioned mechanisms. But based on studies addressing the cellular and physiologic responses to caloric restriction, fasting, or ketogenic diet, it is reasonable to assume that such regulation might occur (Dąbek et al., 2020; Miller et al., 2018). For instance, data from mouse studies robustly demonstrate that a ketogenic diet can significantly alter the epigenetic regulation of genes implicated in regulation of energy substrate metabolism, oxidative capacity, and mitochondrial biogenesis (Ahola-Erkkilä et al., 2010; Jornayvaz et al., 2010; Miller et al., 2018; Srivastava et al., 2012). Whether such beneficial effects can also be produced by IEK, alone or in conjunction with exercise training, remains to be established.

Only one study to date has directly addressed the possible cumulative benefit of signaling effects of IEK for recovery and adaptation. This study demonstrated that IEK during a 3-week period of endurance training overload blunted the development of overreaching symptoms (Poffe et al., 2019). Specifically, IEK prevented the overload training-induced drop in resting and maximal heart rate, as well as suppressed the levels of the "stress signal" GDF15 (Figure 40.3). An interesting observation in this study was that the protective effect in the test group, compared with a control group receiving isocaloric, low-ketogenic-potency MCT supplements, occurred early in the training process, against the background of identical energy intakes and exercise training loads and, importantly, in the absence of elevated blood ketone concentrations (Poffe et al., 2019). Indeed, most measurements were done after an overnight fast and at least 10 hr after the dose of KE intake, when blood ketones were fully normalized (< 0.5 mM). The data suggest that IEK can induce short-term regulation of physiologic adaptations to training, even beyond the short episodes of acute exogenous ketosis caused by ketone supplement intake. The cellular and molecular mechanism underlying these adaptations are currently unknown. However, effects of IEK on exercise-induced inflammation, oxidative stress, and regulation of gene expression might play a role. Future studies need to extend the findings of this first study (Poffe et al., 2019) and investigate the dose-response relationship between IEK, training adaptation, and exercise performance and the underlying mechanisms in different exercise contexts.

IEK Impacts the Central and Peripheral Nervous System During Training

Increasingly, evidence indicates that ketone bodies exert both neuroprotective and neuromodulatory effects (Newman & Verdin, 2017; Norwitz et al., 2019; Puchalska & Crawford, 2017; Yang et al., 2019), and IEK can acutely alter neuronal function. For example, a recent study showed that the βHB monoester can increase brain activity and stabilize functional neuronal

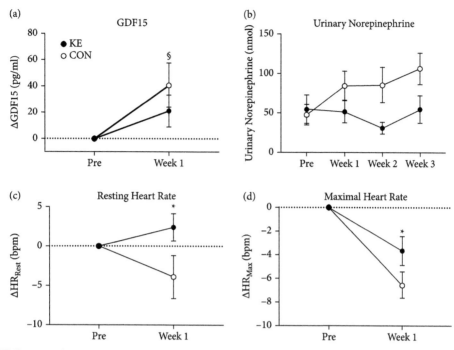

FIGURE 40.3 *Effects of endurance training in healthy young individuals*

Changes in GDF15, urinary norepinephrine, and heart rate after 1 week of endurance training overload in healthy young individuals ($N = 12$), consuming three servings (25 g) of βHB monoester (KE, λ) or an isocaloric control drink (CON, Υ) per day. (A) serum GDF15; (B) urinary nocturnal epinephrine excretion; (C) resting heart rate; (D) maximal heart rate. Data are $M \pm SEM$. *$p < 0.05$ difference between KE and CON. Adapted from Poffé et al. (2019).

networks (Mujica-Parodi et al., 2020). The underlying mechanisms of these actions remain to be established, but in vitro studies indicate that improved neuronal energy status, reduction of oxidative stress and inflammation, and suppression of apoptosis could be implicated in the neuroprotective effect of ketones (Newman & Verdin, 2017; Norwitz et al., 2019; Puchalska & Crawford, 2017). Support for a neuroprotective effect of ketones comes from animal studies showing that a ketogenic diet reduces neuronal loss and infarct size in experimental rat models of ischemia (Puchowicz et al., 2008; Tai et al., 2008) and exogenous ketone provision reduces traumatic brain injury in multiple animal models (Prins 2008; Prins et al., 2004; Zhang et al., 2016). It is tempting to speculate that the latter indication could be relevant to combat sports, such as boxing, with a high incidence of head injuries (Bernick & Banks, 2013; Clausen et al., 2005) and is deserving of further investigation. Apart from their neuroprotective actions, there is also evidence to prove that ketones can directly modulate neuronal function via binding to GPR41 to decrease sympathetic outflow (Kimura

et al., 2011), or via the G-protein-coupled adenosine A_1 receptor (Kovács et al., 2017).

The interaction of ketosis, acute exercise, and chronic training and its effect on neuronal stress or neurohormonal activity remain largely unknown. However, observations from our 3-week training-overload study (Poffe et al., 2019) indicate that IEK may modulate autonomic nervous system output during strenuous training. It is the prevailing opinion that increased sympathetic tone occurs as an initial stress response to intensified training and may underlie subsequent physiologic alterations (Fry et al., 1994; Meeusen et al., 2013). Overnight urinary epinephrine and norepinephrine excretion rates are known surrogate measures that reflect basal sympathetic activity (Bosker et al., 2012; Esler et al., 1988). We found that 3 weeks of endurance training overload markedly increased nocturnal catecholamine excretion, predominantly of norepinephrine, in the absence, but not in the presence, of IEK during the training period (Figure 40.3; Poffe et al., 2019). Concomitantly with suppression of basal sympathetic activity, IEK also negated the training-induced attenuation of resting and exercise heart rates (Figure 40.3). Further studies need to elucidate the effects of IEK on nervous system adaptation in response to different exercise training loads and contexts.

CONCLUSION AND FUTURE DIRECTIONS

In conclusion, exogenous ketones provide a promising tool to manipulate manifold processes implicated in exercise performance, recovery, and training adaptation. Given the relative infancy of this field of research, it is impossible to make definitive recommendations on the optimal use of IEK. Evidence to date does not support an acute ergogenic effect of IEK during exercise in addition to current best practice sports nutrition; however, the role of IEK across a broader range of athletic requirements remains unknown (i.e., female athletes, different training states, different habitual diets, ultra-endurance events) and should be addressed. Similarly, only limited data exist describing the effect of IEK used as a recovery and adaptation strategy, but work to date is encouraging. Just as the research supporting the use of IEK must continue to evolve, commercial exogenous ketone supplements also require development to improve their palatability and cost-effectiveness so that they can be a viable nutritional strategy for athletes. Ketone bodies' manifold roles as a substrate and a signaling metabolite have yet to be investigated in the context of exercise and training; therefore, research into the use of IEK to support athletic performance remains full of tantalizing opportunities for discovery.

REFERENCES

Ahola-Erkkilä, S., Carroll, C. J., Peltola-Mjösund, K., Tulkki, V., Mattila, I., Seppänen-Laakso, T., Oresic, M., Tyynismaa, H., & Suomalainen, A. (2010). Ketogenic diet slows down mitochondrial myopathy progression in mice. *Human Molecular Genetics*, 19, 1974–1984.

Balasse, E. O., Fery, F., & Neef, M. A. (1978). Changes induced by exercise in rates of turnover and oxidation of ketone bodies in fasting man. *Journal of Applied Physiology: Respiratory, Environmental & Exercise Physiology*, 44, 5–11.

Balasse, E., & Ooms, H. A. (1968). Changes in the concentrations of glucose, free fatty acids, insulin and ketone bodies in the blood during sodium β-hydroxybutyrate infusions in man. *Diabetologia*, 4, 133–135.

Bazgir, B., Fathi, R., Valojerdi, M. R., Mozdziak, P., & Asgari, A. (2017). Satellite cells contribution to exercise mediated muscle hypertrophy and repair. *Cell Journal*, 18, 473–484.

Bergström, J., Hermansen, L., Hultman, E., & Saltin, B. (1967). Diet, muscle glycogen and physical performance. *Acta Physiologica Scandinavica*, 71, 140–150.

Bernick, C., & Banks, S. (2013). What boxing tells us about repetitive head trauma and the brain. *Alzheimer's Research & Therapy*, 5, 23.

Bhavsar, N., & St-Onge, M. P. (2016). The diverse nature of saturated fats and the case of medium-chain triglycerides: How one recommendation may not fit all. *Current Opinion in Clinical Nutrition and Metabolic Care*, 19, 81–87.

Birkhahn, R. H., & Border, J. R. (1978). Intravenous-feeding of rat with short chain fatty-acid esters. 2. Monoacetoacetin. *American Journal of Clinical Nutrition*, 31, 436–441.

Blaauw, B., & Reggiani, C. (2014). The role of satellite cells in muscle hypertrophy. *Journal of Muscle Research and Cell Motility*, 35, 3–10.

Bleeker, J. C., Visser, G., Clarke, K., Ferdinandusse, S., de Haan, F. H., Houtkooper, R. H., Ijlst, L., Kok, I. L., Langeveld, M., van der Pol, W. L., de Sain-van der Velden, M. G. M., Sibeijn-Kuiper, A., Takken, T., Wanders, R. J. A., van Weeghel, M., Wijburg, F. A., van der Woude, L. H., Wüst, R. C. I., Cox, P. J., & Jeneson, J. A. L. (2020). Nutritional ketosis improves exercise metabolism in patients with very long-chain acyl-CoA dehydrogenase deficiency. *Journal of Inherited Metabolic Disease*, 43(4), 787–799.

Bosker, F. J., Wu, T., Gladkevich, A., Ge, D., Treiber, F. A., & Snieder, H. (2012). Urinary norepinephrine and epinephrine excretion rates are heritable, but not associated with office and ambulatory blood pressure. *Hypertension Research*, 35, 1164–1170.

Burke, L. M. (2015). Re-examining high-fat diets for sports performance: Did we call the "nail in the coffin" too soon? *Sports Medicine*, 45(Suppl. 1), S33–S49.

Burke, L. M., Castell, L. M., Casa, D. J., Close, G. L., Costa, R. J. S., Desbrow, B., Halson, S. L., Lis, D. M., Melin, A. K., Peeling, P., Saunders, P. U., Slater, G. J., Sygo, J., Witard, O. C., Bermon, S., & Stellingwerff, T. (2019). International Association of Athletics Federations consensus statement 2019: Nutrition for athletics. *International Journal of Sport Nutrition and Exercise Metabolism*, 29, 73–84.

Burke, L. M., Hawley, J. A., Wong, S. H. S., & Jeukendrup, A. E. (2011). Carbohydrates for training and competition. *Journal of Sports Sciences*, 29, S17–S27.

Burke, L. M., Ross, M. L., Garvican-Lewis, L. A., Welvaert, M., Heikura, I. A., Forbes, S. G., Mirtschin, J. G., Cato, L. E., Strobel, N., Sharma, A. P., & Hawley, J. A. (2017). Low carbohydrate, high fat diet impairs exercise economy and negates the performance benefit from intensified training in elite race walkers. *Journal of Physiology, 595,* 2785–2807.

Burke, L. M., Sharma, A. P., Heikura, I. A., Forbes, S. F., Holloway, M., McKay, A. K. A., Bone, J. L., Leckey, J. J., Welvaert, M., & Ross, M. L. (2020). Crisis of confidence averted: Impairment of exercise economy and performance in elite race walkers by ketogenic low carbohydrate, high fat (LCHF) diet is reproducible. *PLOS ONE, 15,* Article e0234027.

Cahill, G. F., Jr. (2006). Fuel metabolism in starvation. *Annual Review of Nutrition, 26,* 1–22.

Cairns, S. P., & Lindinger, M. I. (2008). Do multiple ionic interactions contribute to skeletal muscle fatigue? *Journal of Physiology, 586,* 4039–4054.

Chambers, E. S., Bridge, M. W., & Jones, D. A. (2009). Carbohydrate sensing in the human mouth: Effects on exercise performance and brain activity. *Journal of Physiology, 587,* 1779–1794.

Christensen, E. H., & Hansen, O. (1939). Ability to work and nutrition. *Skandinavisches Archiv Für Physiologie, 81,* 160–171.

Clarke, K., Tchabanenko, K., Pawlosky, R., Carter, E., Todd King, M., Musa-Veloso, K., Ho, M., Roberts, A., Robertson, J., Vanitallie, T. B., & Veech, R. L. (2012). Kinetics, safety and tolerability of (R)-3-hydroxybutyl (R)-3-hydroxybutyrate in healthy adult subjects. *Regulatory Toxicology and Pharmacology, 63,* 401–408.

Clausen, H., McCrory, P., & Anderson, V. (2005). The risk of chronic traumatic brain injury in professional boxing: Change in exposure variables over the past century. *British Journal of Sports Medicine, 39,* 661.

Courchesne-Loyer, A., Croteau, E., Castellano, C.-A., St-Pierre, V., Hennebelle, M., & Cunnane, S. C. (2016). Inverse relationship between brain glucose and ketone metabolism in adults during short-term moderate dietary ketosis: A dual tracer quantitative positron emission tomography study. *Journal of Cerebral Blood Flow & Metabolism, 37,* 2485–2493.

Cox, P., & Clarke, K. (2014). Acute nutritional ketosis: Implications for exercise performance and metabolism. *Extreme Physiology & Medicine, 3,* 17.

Cox, P. J., Kirk, T., Ashmore, T., Willerton, K., Evans, R., Smith, A., Murray, A. J., Stubbs, B., West, J., McLure, S. W., King, M. T., Dodd, M. S., Holloway, C., Neubauer, S., Drawer, S., Veech, R. L., Griffin, J. L., & Clarke, K. (2016). Nutritional ketosis alters fuel preference and thereby endurance performance in athletes. *Cell Metabolism, 24,* 1–13.

Coyle, E. F., Hagberg, J. M., Hurley, B. F., Martin, W. H., Ehsani, A. A., & Holloszy, J. O. (1983). Carbohydrate feeding during prolonged strenuous exercise can delay fatigue. *Journal of Applied Physiology, 55,* 230–235.

Dąbek, A., Wojtala, M., Pirola, L., & Balcerczyk, A. (2020). Modulation of cellular biochemistry, epigenetics and metabolomics by ketone bodies: Implications of the ketogenic diet in the physiology of the organism and pathological states. *Nutrients, 12,* 788.

Dalsgaard, M. K., Ogoh, S., Dawson, E. A., Yoshiga, C. C., Quistorff, B., & Secher, N. H. (2004). Cerebral carbohydrate cost of physical exertion in humans. *American Journal of Physiology: Regulatory, Integrative and Comparative Physiology, 287,* R534–R540.

Dearlove, D. J., Faull, O. K., Rolls, E., Clarke, K., & Cox, P. J. (2019). Nutritional ketoacidosis during incremental exercise in healthy athletes. *Frontiers in Physiology, 10,* 290.

Deemer, S. E., Plaisance, E. P., & Martins, C. (2020). Impact of ketosis on appetite regulation—A review. *Nutrition Research, 77,* 1–11.

Derave, W., Ai, H., Ihlemann, J., Witters, L. A., Kristiansen, S., Richter, E. A., & Ploug, T. (2000). Dissociation of AMP-activated protein kinase activation and glucose transport in contracting slow-twitch muscle. *Diabetes, 49,* 1281.

Desrochers, S., David, F., Garneau, M., Jette, M., & Brunengraber, H. (1992). Metabolism of R-1,3-butanediol and S-1,3-butanediol in perfused livers from meal-fed and starved rats. *Biochemical Journal, 285,* 647–653.

Dorling, J., Broom, D. R., Burns, S. F., Clayton, D. J., Deighton, K., James, L. J., King, J. A., Miyashita, M., Thackray, A. E., Batterham, R. L., & Stensel, D. J. (2018). Acute and chronic effects of exercise on appetite, energy intake, and appetite-related hormones: The modulating effect of adiposity, sex, and habitual physical activity. *Nutrients, 10,* 1140.

Egan, B., & Zierath, J. R. (2013). Exercise metabolism and the molecular regulation of skeletal muscle adaptation. *Cell Metabolism, 17,* 162–184.

Esler, M., Jennings, G., Korner, P., Willett, I., Dudley, F., Hasking, G., Anderson, W., & Lambert, G. (1988). Assessment of human sympathetic nervous system activity from measurements of norepinephrine turnover. *Hypertension, 11,* 3–20.

Evans, M., & Egan, B. (2018). Intermittent running and cognitive performance after ketone ester ingestion. *Medicine & Science in Sports & Exercise, 50,* 2330–2338.

Evans, M., Cogan, K. E., & Egan, B. (2017). Metabolism of ketone bodies during exercise and training: Physiological basis for exogenous supplementation. *Journal of Physiology, 595,* 2857–2871.

Evans, M., McSwiney, F. T., Brady, A. J., & Egan, B. (2019). No benefit of ingestion of a ketone monoester supplement on 10-km running performance. *Medicine & Science in Sports & Exercise, 51*(12), 2506–2515.

Evans, M., Patchett, E., Nally, R., Kearns, R., Larney, M., & Egan, B. (2018). Effect of acute ingestion of β-hydroxybutyrate salts on the response to graded exercise in trained cyclists. *European Journal of Sport Science, 18*(3), 376–386.

Faull, O. K., Dearlove, D. J., Clarke, K., & Cox, P. J. (2019). Beyond RPE: The perception of exercise under normal and ketotic conditions. *Frontiers in Physiology, 10*, 229.

Fery, F., & Balasse, E. O. (1988). Effect of exercise on the disposal of infused ketone-bodies in humans. *Journal of Clinical Endocrinology & Metabolism, 67*, 245–250.

Floyd, J. C., Fajans, S. S., Pek, S., Thiffault, C. A., Knopf, R. F., & Conn, J. W. (1970). Synergistic effect of essential amino acids and glucose upon insulin secretion in man. *Diabetes, 19*, 109–115.

Fortier, M., Castellano, C.-A., Croteau, E., Langlois, F., Bocti, C., St-Pierre, V., Vandenberghe, C., Bernier, M., Roy, M., Descoteaux, M., Whittingstall, K., Lepage, M., Turcotte, E. E., Fulop, T., & Cunnane, S. C. (2019). A ketogenic drink improves brain energy and some measures of cognition in mild cognitive impairment. *Alzheimer's & Dementia, 15*, 625–634.

Frayn, K. N. (1983). Calculation of substrate oxidation rates in vivo from gaseous exchange. *Journal of Applied Physiology, 55*, 628–634.

Fry, A. C., Kraemer, W. J., Van Borselen, F., Lynch, J. M., Triplett, N. T., Koziris, L. P., & Fleck, S. J. (1994). Catecholamine responses to short-term high-intensity resistance exercise overtraining. *Journal of Applied Physiology, 77*, 941–946.

Goldstein, E. R., Ziegenfuss, T., Kalman, D., Kreider, R., Campbell, B., Wilborn, C., Taylor, L., Willoughby, D., Stout, J., Graves, B. S., Wildman, R., Ivy, J. L., Spano, M., Smith, A. E., & Antonio, J. (2010). International society of sports nutrition position stand: Caffeine and performance. *Journal of the International Society of Sports Nutrition, 7*, 5.

Gormsen L. C., Svart, M., Thomsen, H. H., Søndergaard, E., Vendelbo, M. H., Christensen, N., Tolbod, L. P., Harms, H. J., Nielsen, R., Wiggers, H., Jessen, N., Hansen, J., Bøtker, H. E., & Møller, N. (2017). Ketone body infusion with 3-hydroxybutyrate reduces myocardial glucose uptake and increases blood flow in humans: A positron emission tomography study. *Journal of the American Heart Association, 6*, e005066.

Halestrap, A. P., & Price, N. T. (1999). The proton-linked monocarboxylate transporter (MCT) family: Structure, function and regulation. *Biochemical Journal, 343*(Part 2), 281–299.

Hallberg, S. J., McKenzie, A. L., Williams, P. T., Bhanpuri, N. H., Peters, A. L., Campbell, W. W., Hazbun, T. L., Volk, B. M., McCarter, J. P., Phinney, S. D., & Volek, J. S. (2018). Effectiveness and safety of a novel care model for the management of type 2 diabetes at 1 year: An open-label, non-randomized, controlled study. *Diabetes Therapy, 9*, 583–612.

Hasselbalch, S. G., Madsen, P. L., Hageman, L. P., Olsen, K. S., Justesen, N., Holm, S., & Paulson, O. B. (1996). Changes in cerebral blood flow and carbohydrate metabolism during acute hyperketonemia. *American Journal of Physiology, 270*, E746–E751.

Holdsworth, D. A., Cox, P. J., Kirk, T., Stradling, H., Impey, S. G., & Clarke, K. (2017). A ketone ester drink increases postexercise muscle glycogen synthesis in humans. *Medicine & Science in Sports & Exercise, 49*(9), 1789–1795.

Impey, S. G., Hearris, M. A., Hammond, K. M., Bartlett, J. D., Louis, J., Close, G. L., & Morton, J. P. (2018). Fuel for the work required: A theoretical framework for carbohydrate periodization and the glycogen threshold hypothesis. *Sports Medicine, 48*, 1031–1048.

Ivy, J. L., Costill, D. L., Fink, W. J., & Maglischo, E. (1980). Contribution of medium and long chain triglyceride intake to energy metabolism during prolonged exercise. *International Journal of Sports Medicine, 1*, 15–20.

Jäger, R., Kerksick, C. M., Campbell, B. I., Cribb, P. J., Wells, S. D., Skwiat, T. M., Purpura, M., Ziegenfuss, T. N., Ferrando, A. A., Arent, S. M., Smith-Ryan, A. E., Stout, J. R., Arciero, P. J., Ormsbee, M. J., Taylor, L. W., Wilborn, C. D., Kalman, D. S., Kreider, R. B., Willoughby, D. S., . . . Antonio, J. (2017). International Society of Sports Nutrition position stand: Protein and exercise. *Journal of the International Society of Sports Nutrition, 14*, 20.

Jensen, T. E., & Richter, E. A. (2012). Regulation of glucose and glycogen metabolism during and after exercise. *Journal of Physiology, 590*, 1069–1076.

Jeppesen, J., & Kiens, B. (2012). Regulation and limitations to fatty acid oxidation during exercise. *Journal of Physiology, 590*, 1059–1068.

Jornayvaz, F. R., Jurczak, M. J., Lee, H.-Y., Birkenfeld, A. L., Frederick, D. W., Zhang, D., Zhang, X.-M., Samuel, V. T., & Shulman, G. I. (2010). A high-fat, ketogenic diet causes hepatic insulin resistance in mice, despite increasing energy expenditure and preventing weight gain. *American Journal of Physiology, Endocrinology and Metabolism, 299*, E808–E815.

Joshi, S., Ostfeld, R. J., & McMacken, M. (2019). The ketogenic diet for obesity and diabetes—Enthusiasm outpaces evidence. *JAMA Internal Medicine, 179*, 1163–1164.

Joy, E., Kussman, A., & Nattiv, A. (2016). 2016 update on eating disorders in athletes: A comprehensive narrative review with a focus on clinical assessment and management. *British Journal of Sports Medicine, 50*, 154.

Kimura, I., Inoue, D., Maeda, T., Hara, T., Ichimura, A., Miyauchi, S., Kobayashi, M., Hirasawa, A., & Tsujimoto, G. (2011). Short-chain fatty acids and ketones directly regulate sympathetic nervous system via G protein-coupled receptor 41 (GPR41). *Proceedings of the National Academy of Sciences of the United States of America, 108*, 8030–8035.

Koeslag, J. H., Noakes, T. D., & Sloan, A. W. (1980). Post-exercise ketosis. *Journal of Physiology-London, 301*, 79–90.

Koutnik, A. P., D'Agostino, D. P., & Egan, B. (2019). Anticatabolic effects of ketone bodies in skeletal muscle. *Trends in Endocrinology and Metabolism, 30*, 227–229.

Koutnik, A. P., Poff, A. M., Ward, N. P., DeBlasi, J. M., Soliven, M. A., Romero, M. A., Roberson, P. A., Fox, C. D., Roberts, M. D., & D'Agostino, D. P. (2020). Ketone bodies attenuate wasting in models of atrophy. *Journal of Cachexia, Sarcopenia and Muscle, 11*(4), 973–996.

Kovács, Z., D'Agostino, D. P., Dobolyi, A., & Ari, C. (2017). Adenosine A_1 receptor antagonism abolished the anti-seizure effects of exogenous ketone supplementation in Wistar Albino Glaxo Rijswijk rats. *Frontiers in Molecular Neuroscience, 10*, 235.

Laffel, L. (1999). Ketone bodies: A review of physiology, pathophysiology and application of monitoring to diabetes. *Diabetes/Metabolism Research and Reviews, 15*, 412–426.

Leckey, J. J., Ross, M. L., Quod, M., Hawley, J. A., & Burke, L. M. (2017). Ketone diester ingestion impairs time-trial performance in professional cyclists. *Frontiers in Physiology, 8*, 806.

Maizels, E. Z., Ruderman, N. B., Goodman, M. N., & Lau, D. (1977). Effect of acetoacetate on glucose metabolism in the soleus and extensor digitorum longus muscles of the rat. *Biochemical Journal, 162*, 557–568.

McKenna, M. J. (1992). The roles of ionic processes in muscular fatigue during intense exercise. *Sports Medicine, 13*, 134–145.

Mebane, D., & Madison, L. L. (1964). Hypoglycemic action of ketones. I. Effects of ketones on hepatic glucose output and peripheral glucose utilization. *The Journal of Laboratory and Clinical Medicine, 63*, 177–192.

Meeusen, R., Duclos, M., Foster, C., Fry, A., Gleeson, M., Nieman, D., Raglin, J., Rietjens, G., Steinacker, J., & Urhausen, A. (2013). Prevention, diagnosis, and treatment of the overtraining syndrome: Joint consensus statement of the European College of Sport Science and the American College of Sports Medicine. *Medicine & Science in Sports & Exercise, 45*, 186–205.

Mikkelsen, K. H., Seifert, T., Secher, N. H., Grondal, T., & van Hall, G. (2015). Systemic, cerebral and skeletal muscle ketone body and energy metabolism during acute hyper-D-beta-hydroxybutyratemia in post-absorptive healthy males. *Journal of Clinical Endocrinology and Metabolism, 100*, 636–643.

Miller, V. J., Villamena, F. A., & Volek, J. S. (2018). Nutritional ketosis and mitohormesis: Potential implications for mitochondrial function and human health. *Journal of Nutrition and Metabolism, 2018*: 5157645.

Milou, B., Burke, L. M., Gibala, M. J., & van Loon, L. J. C. (2010). Nutritional strategies to promote postexercise recovery. *International Journal of Sport Nutrition and Exercise Metabolism, 20*, 515–532.

Morgan, D. W., Martin, P. E., & Krahenbuhl, G. S. (1989). Factors affecting running economy. *Sports Medicine, 7*, 310–330.

Morton, R. W., Murphy, K. T., McKellar, S. R., Schoenfeld, B. J., Henselmans, M., Helms, E., Aragon, A. A., Devries, M. C., Banfield, L., Krieger, J. W., & Phillips, S. M. (2018). A systematic review, meta-analysis and meta-regression of the effect of protein supplementation on resistance training-induced gains in muscle mass and strength in healthy adults. *British Journal of Sports Medicine, 52*, 376.

Mountjoy, M., Sundgot-Borgen, J. K., Burke, L. M., Ackerman, K. E., Blauwet, C., Constantini, N., Lebrun, C., Lundy, B., Melin, A. K., Meyer, N. L., Sherman, R. T., Tenforde, A. S., Torstveit, M. K., & Budgett, R. (2018). IOC consensus statement on relative energy deficiency in sport (RED-S): 2018 update. *British Journal of Sports Medicine, 52*, 687.

Mujica-Parodi, L. R., Amgalan, A., Sultan, S. F., Antal, B., Sun, X., Skiena, S., Lithen, A., Adra, N., Ratai, E.-M., Weistuch, C., Govindarajan, S. T., Strey, H. H., Dill, K. A., Stufflebeam, S. M., Veech, R. L., & Clarke, K. (2020). Diet modulates brain network stability, a biomarker for brain aging, in young adults. *Proceedings of the National Academy of Sciences of the United States of America, 117*, 6170.

Müller, M. J., Paschen, U., & Seitz, H. J. (1984). Effect of ketone bodies on glucose production and utilization in the miniature pig. *Journal of Clinical Investigation, 74*, 249–261.

Myette-Côté, É., Caldwell, H. G., Ainslie, P. N., Clarke, K., & Little, J. P. (2019). A ketone monoester drink reduces the glycemic response to an oral glucose challenge in individuals with obesity: A randomized trial. *The American Journal of Clinical Nutrition, 110*, 1491–1501.

Myette-Cote, E., Neudorf, H., Rafiei, H., Clarke, K., & Little, J. P. (2018). Prior ingestion of exogenous ketone monoester attenuates the glycaemic response to an oral glucose tolerance test in healthy young individuals. *Journal of Physiology, 596*(8), 1385–1395.

Nair, K. S., Welle, S. L., Halliday, D., & Campbell, R. G. (1988). Effect of beta-hydroxybutyrate on whole-body leucine kinetics and fractional mixed skeletal muscle protein synthesis in humans. *Journal of Clinical Investigation, 82,* 198–205.

Newman, J. C., & Verdin, E. (2017). Ketone bodies as signaling metabolites. *Trends in Endocrinology and Metabolism, 25,* 42–52.

Nielsen, R., Møller, N., Gormsen, L. C., Tolbod, L. P., Hansson, N. H., Sorensen, J., Harms, H. J., Frøkiær, J., Eiskjaer, H., Jespersen, N. R., Mellemkjaer, S., Lassen, T. R., Pryds, K., Bøtker, H. E., & Wiggers, H. (2019). Cardiovascular effects of treatment with the ketone body 3-hydroxybutyrate in chronic heart failure patients. *Circulation, 139,* 2129–2141.

Norwitz, N. G., Hu, M. T., & Clarke, K. (2019). The mechanisms by which the ketone body D-β-hydroxybutyrate may improve the multiple cellular pathologies of Parkinson's disease. *Frontiers in Nutrition, 6,* 63.

Nybo, L., & Rasmussen, P. (2007). Inadequate cerebral oxygen delivery and central fatigue during strenuous exercise. *Exercise and Sport Sciences Reviews, 35,* 110–118.

Nybo, L., & Secher, N. H. (2004). Cerebral perturbations provoked by prolonged exercise. *Progress in Neurobiology, 72,* 223–261.

O'Malley, T., Myette-Cote, E., Durrer, C., & Little, J. P. (2017). Nutritional ketone salts increase fat oxidation but impair high-intensity exercise performance in healthy adult males. *Applied Physiology, Nutrition, and Metabolism, 42*(10), 1031–1035.

Owen, O. E. (2005). Ketone bodies as a fuel for the brain during starvation. *Biochemistry and Molecular Biology Education, 33,* 246–251.

Owen, O. E., Morgan, A. P., Kemp, H. G., Sullivan, J. M., Herrera, M. G., & Cahill, G. F. (1967). Brain metabolism during fasting. *Journal of Clinical Investigation, 46,* 1589.

Page, K. A., Williamson, A., Yu, N., McNay, E. C., Dzuira, J., McCrimmon, R. J., & Sherwin, R. S. (2009). Medium-chain fatty acids improve cognitive function in intensively treated type 1 diabetic patients and support in vitro synaptic transmission during acute hypoglycemia. *Diabetes, 58,* 1237–1244.

Patel, S., Alvarez-Guaita, A., Melvin, A., Rimmington, D., Dattilo, A., Miedzybrodzka, E. L., Cimino, I., Maurin, A. C., Roberts, G. P., Meek, C. L., Virtue, S., Sparks, L. M., Parsons, S. A., Redman, L. M., Bray, G. A., Liou, A. P., Woods, R. M., Parry, S. A., Jeppesen, P. B., . . . O'Rahilly, S. (2019). GDF15 provides an endocrine signal of nutritional stress in mice and humans. *Cell Metabolism, 29,* 707–718.

Pawan, G. L., & Semple, S. J. (1983). Effect of 3-hydroxybutyrate in obese subjects on very-low-energy diets and during therapeutic starvation. *Lancet, 1,* 15–17.

Perry, B., & Wang, Y. (2012). Appetite regulation and weight control: The role of gut hormones. *Nutrition & Diabetes, 2,* e26.

Poffé, C., Ramaekers, M., Bogaerts, S., & Hespel, P. (2020). Exogenous ketosis impacts neither performance nor muscle glycogen breakdown in prolonged endurance exercise. *Journal of Applied Physiology, 128,* 1643–1653.

Poffé, C., Ramaekers, M., Bogaerts, S., & Hespel, P. (2021). Bicarbonate unlocks the ergogenic action of ketone monoester intake in endurance exercise. *Medicine & Science in Sports & Exercise, 53*(2), 431–441.

Poffe, C., Ramaekers, M., Van Thienen, R., & Hespel, P. (2019). Ketone ester supplementation blunts overreaching symptoms during endurance training overload. *Journal of Physiology, 597,* 3009–3027.

Prins, M. L. (2008). Cerebral metabolic adaptation and ketone metabolism after brain injury. *Journal of Cerebral Blood Flow and Metabolism, 28,* 1–16.

Prins, M. L., Lee, S. M., Fujima, L. S., & Hovda, D. A. (2004). Increased cerebral uptake and oxidation of exogenous βHB improves ATP following traumatic brain injury in adult rats. *Journal of Neurochemistry, 90,* 666–672.

Prins, P. J., Koutnik, A. P., D'Agostino, D. P., Rogers, C. Q., Seibert, J. F., Breckenridge, J. A., Jackson, D. S., Ryan, E. J., Buxton, J. D., & Ault, D. L. (2020). Effects of an exogenous ketone supplement on five-kilometer running performance. *Journal of Human Kinetics, 72,* 115–127.

Puchalska, P., & Crawford, P. A. (2017). Multi-dimensional roles of ketone bodies in fuel metabolism, signaling, and therapeutics. *Cell Metabolism, 25,* 262–284.

Puchowicz, M. A., Zechel, J. L., Valerio, J., Emancipator, D. S., Xu, K., Pundik, S., LaManna, J. C., & Lust, W. D. (2008). Neuroprotection in diet-induced ketotic rat brain after focal ischemia. *Journal of Cerebral Blood Flow and Metabolism, 28,* 1907–1916.

Robinson, A. M., & Williamson, D. H. (1980). Physiological roles of ketone-bodies as substrates and signals in mammalian-tissues. *Physiological Reviews, 60,* 143–187.

Rodger, S., Plews, D., Laursen, P., & Driller, M. (2017). The effects of an oral β-hydroxybutyrate supplement on exercise metabolism and cycling performance. *Journal of Science and Cycling, 6*(1).

Rojas-Morales, P., Pedraza-Chaverri, J., & Tapia, E. (2020). Ketone bodies, stress response, and redox homeostasis. *Redox Biology, 29,* 101395.

Romijn, J. A., Coyle, E. F., Sidossis, L. S., Gastaldelli, A., Horowitz, J. F., Endert, E., & Wolfe, R. R. (1993). Regulation of endogenous fat and carbohydrate metabolism in relation to exercise intensity and duration. *American Journal of Physiology, Endocrinology and Metabolism, 265,* E380–E391.

Sato, K., Kashiwaya, Y., Keon, C. A., Tsuchiya, N., King, M. T., Radda, G. K., Chance, B., Clarke,

K., & Veech, R. L. (1995). Insulin, ketone bodies, and mitochondrial energy transduction. *FASEB Journal, 9*, 651–658.

Scott, B. E., Laursen, P. B., James, L. J., Boxer, B., Chandler, Z., Lam, E., Gascoyne, T., Messenger, J., & Mears, S. A. (2019). The effect of 1,3-butanediol and carbohydrate supplementation on running performance. *Journal of Science and Medicine in Sport, 22*, 702–706.

Shaw, D. M., Fabrice, M., Andrea, B., Daniel, P., Paul, L., & Dulson Deborah, K. (2019). The effect of 1,3-butanediol on cycling time-trial performance. *International Journal of Sport Nutrition and Exercise Metabolism, 29*, 466–473.

Sherwin, R. S., Hendler, R. G., & Felig, P. (1975). Effect of ketone infusions on amino acid and nitrogen metabolism in man. *Journal of Clinical Investigation, 55*, 1382–1390.

Shimazu, T., Hirschey, M. D., Newman, J., He, W., Shirakawa, K., Le Moan, N., Grueter, C. A., Lim, H., Saunders, L. R., Stevens, R. D., Newgard, C. B., Farese, R. V., Jr., De Cabo, R., Ulrich, S., Akassoglou, K., & Verdin, E. (2013). Suppression of oxidative stress by β-hydroxybutyrate, an endogenous histone deacetylase inhibitor. *Science, 339*, 211–214.

Snijders, T., Nederveen, J. P., McKay, B. R., Joanisse, S., Verdijk, L. B., van Loon, L. J. C., & Parise, G. (2015). Satellite cells in human skeletal muscle plasticity. *Frontiers in Physiology, 6*, 283.

Soto-Mota, A., Vansant, H., Evans, R. D., & Clarke, K. (2019). Safety and tolerability of sustained exogenous ketosis using ketone monoester drinks for 28 days in healthy adults. *Regulatory Toxicology and Pharmacology, 109*, 104506.

Spriet, L. L. (2014). New insights into the interaction of carbohydrate and fat metabolism during exercise. *Sports Medicine, 44*(Suppl. 1), S87–S96.

Srivastava, S., Kashiwaya, Y., Todd King, M., Baxa, U., Tam, J., Niu, G., Chen, X., Clarke, K., & Veech, R. L. (2012). Mitochondrial biogenesis and increased uncoupling protein 1 in brown adipose tissue of mice fed a ketone ester diet. *FASEB Journal, 26*, 2351–2362.

St-Pierre, V., Vandenberghe, C., Lowry, C.-M., Fortier, M., Castellano, C.-A., Wagner, R., & Cunnane, S. C. (2019). Plasma ketone and medium chain fatty acid response in humans consuming different medium chain triglycerides during a metabolic study day. *Frontiers in Nutrition, 6*(46), 46.

Starling, S. (2019). GDF15 signals nutritional stress. *Nature Reviews Endocrinology, 15*, 130.

Stensel, D. (2010). Exercise, appetite and appetite-regulating hormones: Implications for food intake and weight control. *Annals of Nutrition and Metabolism, 57*(Suppl. 2), 36–42.

Stokes, T., Hector, A. J., Morton, R. W., McGlory, C., & Phillips, S. M. (2018). Recent perspectives regarding the role of dietary protein for the promotion of muscle hypertrophy with resistance exercise training. *Nutrients, 10*, 180.

Stubbs, B. J., Cox, P. J., Evans, R. D., Santer, P., Miller, J. J., Faull, O. K., Magor-Elliott, S., Hiyama, S., Stirling, M., & Clarke, K. (2017). On the metabolism of exogenous ketones in humans. *Frontiers in Physiology, 8*, 848.

Stubbs, B. J., Cox, P. J., Evans, R. D., Cyranka, M., Clarke, K., & de Wet, H. (2018). A ketone ester drink lowers human ghrelin and appetite. *Obesity, 26*, 269–273.

Stubbs, B. J., Cox, P. J., Kirk, T., Evans, R. D., & Clarke, K. (2019). Gastrointestinal effects of exogenous ketone drinks are infrequent, mild and vary according to ketone compound and dose. *International Journal of Sport Nutrition and Exercise Metabolism, 29*(6), 596–603.

Sumithran, P., Prendergast, L. A., Delbridge, E., Purcell, K., Shulkes, A., Kriketos, A., & Proietto, J. (2013). Ketosis and appetite-mediating nutrients and hormones after weight loss. *European Journal of Clinical Nutrition, 67*, 759–764.

Svart, M., Gormsen, L. C., Hansen, J., Zeidler, D., Gejl, M., Vang, K., Aanerud, J., & Moeller, N. (2018). Regional cerebral effects of ketone body infusion with 3-hydroxybutyrate in humans: Reduced glucose uptake, unchanged oxygen consumption and increased blood flow by positron emission tomography; A randomized, controlled trial. *PLOS ONE, 13*, Article e0190556.

Sweet, W. E. (1987). *Sport and recreation in ancient Greece: A sourcebook with translations.* Oxford University Press.

Taggart, A. K., Kero, J., Gan, X., Cai, T. Q., Cheng, K., Ippolito, M., Ren, N., Kaplan, R., Wu, K., Wu, T. J., Jin, L., Liaw, C., Chen, R., Richman, J., Connolly, D., Offermanns, S., Wright, S. D., & Waters, M. G. (2005). (D)-β-Hydroxybutyrate inhibits adipocyte lipolysis via the nicotinic acid receptor PUMA-G. *Journal of Biological Chemistry, 280*, 26649–26652.

Tai, K. K., Nguyen, N., Pham, L., & Truong, D. D. (2008). Ketogenic diet prevents cardiac arrest-induced cerebral ischemic neurodegeneration. *Journal of Neural Transmission (Vienna), 115*, 1011–1107.

Thomsen, H. H., Jørgensen, J. O., Møller, N., Rittig, N., Johannsen, M., Møller, A. B., & Jessen, N. (2018). Effects of 3-hydroxybutyrate and free fatty acids on muscle protein kinetics and signaling during LPS-induced inflammation in humans: Anticatabolic impact of ketone bodies. *The American Journal of Clinical Nutrition, 108*, 857–867.

van Loon, L. J., Greenhaff, P. L., Constantin-Teodosiu, D., Saris, W. H., & Wagenmakers. A. J. (2001). The effects of increasing exercise intensity on muscle fuel utilisation in humans. *Journal of Physiology, 536*, 295–304.

Vandoorne, T., De Smet, S., Ramaekers, M., Van Thienen, R., De Bock, K., Clarke, K., & Hespel, P. (2017). Intake of a ketone ester drink during recovery from exercise promotes mTORC1 signaling but not glycogen resynthesis in human muscle. *Frontiers in Physiology, 8*, 310.

Veech, R. L. (2004). The therapeutic implications of ketone bodies: The effects of ketone bodies in pathological conditions; Ketosis, ketogenic diet, redox states, insulin resistance, and mitochondrial metabolism. *Prostaglandins, Leukotrienes and Essential Fatty Acids, 70*, 309–319.

Viollet, B., Andreelli, F., Jørgensen, S. B., Perrin, C., Flamez, D., Mu, J., Wojtaszewski, J. F. P., Schuit, F. C., Birnbaum, M., & Richter, E. (2003). Physiological role of AMP-activated protein kinase (AMPK): Insights from knockout mouse models. *Biochemical Society Transactions, 31*(Pt 1), 216–219. doi:10.1042/bst0310216

Volek, J. S., Freidenreich, D. J., Saenz, C., Kunces, L. J., Creighton, B. C., & Bartley, J. M. (2016). Metabolic characteristics of keto-adapted ultra-endurance runners. *Metabolism, 65*(3), 100–110.

Volek, J. S., Noakes, T., & Phinney, S. D. (2015). Rethinking fat as a fuel for endurance exercise. *European Journal of Sport Science, 15*, 13–20.

Waldman, H. S., Basham, S. A., Price, F. G., Smith, J. W., Chander, H., Knight, A. C., Krings, B. M., & McAllister, M. J. (2018). Exogenous ketone salts do not improve cognitive responses after a high-intensity exercise protocol in healthy college-aged males. *Applied Physiology, Nutrition, and Metabolism, 43*(7), 711–717.

Webber, R. J., & Edmond, J. (1977). Utilization of L(+)-3-hydroxybutyrate, D(–)-3-hydroxybutyrate, acetoacetate, and glucose for respiration and lipid-synthesis in 18-day-old rat. *Journal of Biological Chemistry, 252*, 5222–5226.

Yang, H., Shan, W., Zhu, F., Wu, J., & Wang, Q. (2019). Ketone bodies in neurological diseases: Focus on neuroprotection and underlying mechanisms. *Frontiers in Neurology, 10*, 585–585.

Yoon, M.-S. (2017). mTOR as a key regulator in maintaining skeletal muscle mass. *Frontiers in Physiology, 8*, 788.

Youm, Y.-H., Nguyen, K. Y., Grant, R. W., Goldberg, E. L., Bodogai, M., Kim, D., D'Agostino, D., Planavsky, N., Lupfer, C., Kanneganti, T. D., Kang, S., Horvath, T. L., Fahmy, T. M., Crawford, P. A., Biragyn, A., Alnemri, E., & Dixit, V. D. (2015). The ketone metabolite β-hydroxybutyrate blocks NLRP3 inflammasome-mediated inflammatory disease. *Nature Medicine, 21*, 263–269.

Zhang, Y., Cao, R. Y., Jia, X., Li, Q., Qiao, L., Yan, G., & Yang, J. (2016). Treadmill exercise promotes neuroprotection against cerebral ischemia-reperfusion injury via downregulation of pro-inflammatory mediators. *Neuropsychiatric Disease and Treatment, 12*, 3161–3173.

Zou, X., Meng, J., Li, L., Han, W., Li, C., Zhong, R., Miao, X., Cai, J., Zhang, Y., & Zhu, D. (2016). Acetoacetate accelerates muscle regeneration and ameliorates muscular dystrophy in mice. *Journal of Biological Chemistry, 291*, 2181–2195.

41

Advancing the Awareness and Application of Ketogenic Therapies Globally

The Charlie Foundation for Ketogenic Therapies and Matthew's Friends

BETH ZUPEC-KANIA, RD, CD, JIM ABRAHAMS, EMMA WILLIAMS,
MBE, SUSAN A. MASINO, PHD, AND JONG M. RHO, MD

OVERVIEW

The Charlie Foundation for Ketogenic Therapies was formed out of the desire to spare children the unnecessary suffering that Charlie Abrahams endured before achieving seizure freedom with the ketogenic diet (KD). Jim and Nancy Abrahams shared their story in 1994 on *Dateline NBC* and later in a 1997 television movie called *First Do No Harm*. Across the Atlantic in the United Kingdom, Matthew Williams suffered for 6 years with a devastating seizure disorder before becoming practically seizure-free within 2 weeks of starting the KD. Based on this experience, Matthew's Friends was founded in 2004 by Emma Williams, Matthew's mother, with a mission similar to that of the Charlie Foundation. Despite dramatic testimonials and these dedicated foundations, the KD remained underutilized. Several key breakthroughs came in 2008: the Charlie Foundation commissioned medical professionals with KD experience to collaborate on guidelines for prescribing the diet. This culminated in a consensus guideline published in *Epilepsia*, a prestigious international medical journal, and written by internationally recognized leaders in the field. At the same time, a Class I clinical study was published in *Lancet Neurology* confirming the diet's efficacy as a treatment for medically intractable epilepsy; more positive Class I studies followed, cementing the scientific evidence for KD use. Use of KD therapy spread rapidly worldwide, and with increased use came a broader understanding of its potential benefits for other neurologic disorders. Less restrictive versions of the diet were developed to meet the needs of older children and adults. In 2012, the Charlie Foundation also began educating all people with epilepsy to

eliminate sugar, to reduce refined carbohydrates, and to choose a predominantly whole-foods diet. In addition, both foundations have expanded efforts to address other conditions that can benefit from ketogenic therapies, including neurologic and neurodegenerative disorders and certain forms of cancer.

GENESIS OF THE CHARLIE FOUNDATION

Charlie Abrahams, the youngest in a family of three children, had no apparent health problems until his first birthday in March 1993, when he experienced his first seizure. This was followed by a series of tumultuous events that changed his life as well as the lives of his siblings, Joseph and Jamie, his parents, Jim and Nancy, and ultimately thousands (possibly millions) of others. Jim Abrahams described those months as follows:

> After thousands of epileptic seizures, an incredible array of drugs, dozens of blood draws, eight hospitalizations, a mountain of EEGs, MRIs, CST scans and PET scans, one fruitless brain surgery, five pediatric neurologists in three cities, two homeopaths, one faith healer, and countless prayers, Charlie's seizures were unchecked, his development "delayed," and he had a prognosis of continued seizures and "progressive retardation."

Charlie lived that period in his bed, on a blanket, or in an infant seat, where he was safely padded during the violent seizures that caused him to thrash uncontrollably. The adverse effects of the antiseizure medications were nearly as destructive as the seizures themselves. Between seizures, he was groggy, chronically constipated, and in the words of his father, seemingly "drunk." Charlie also underwent a high-risk brain surgery to attempt to remove the area of the brain suspected to be the source of his seizures. He experienced zero improvement, and the seizures continued unabated.

Exhausted by the failure of the medical community to provide an effective therapy and reeling from the severe disruption inflicted on the rest of the family, Jim began looking for another option. He spent countless hours in the medical library at UCLA reading through literature on epilepsy, and it was there that he came across an epilepsy book containing a chapter on KD as a treatment for epilepsy. He subsequently discovered a 1992 study from Johns Hopkins University that had been published in *Epilepsia* documenting 29% seizure freedom with an additional 30% significant improvement in 58 consecutive cases of children who were placed on a KD (Kinsman et al., 1992). Notably, these children were as compromised by their disease as Charlie. Jim brought this book and the study to Charlie's pediatric neurologist. Although Charlie's neurologist was aware of the diet, he immediately dismissed it as a treatment that "he had never seen work." Despite this discouragement, Jim and Nancy made the fateful decision to take Charlie to Johns Hopkins Hospital in Baltimore, Maryland. (At the time, Johns Hopkins was one of the few hospitals in the United States that had provided the KD continuously since its discovery in 1921.) Dr. John Freeman and the dietitian Millicent Kelly formed the hospital team that implemented Charlie's KD.

Within 3 days of starting this treatment, Charlie was seizure-free. Over the course of the following month, he was weaned off the four failed antiseizure medications. Free from the sedating effects of the drugs, Charlie could finally hold his head up and once again interact with his family. Although the diet required careful measurements of specific foods, Jim described this as a "walk on the beach" in comparison to their previous circumstances. This abrupt and almost incomprehensible reversal left the Abrahams with a diverse range of emotions; exhilaration and gratitude for Charlie's sudden recovery were mixed with anger about the 9 months of unnecessary suffering that Charlie had endured.

Jim and Nancy appeared on *Dateline NBC* in 1994 to recap those months. They soon found their mailbox overflowing with letters from other families, thanking them for bringing the diet out into the light of day. Each letter described a similar journey to the one the Abrahams family experienced with Charlie. The names and ages of the kids were different, but the stories were the same: uncontrolled seizures, multiple medications, trips to the emergency department, mounting medical bills, and a drugged, poorly functioning child experiencing a rapid decline. Adoption of the KD was the common denominator, and, for some, their lifesaver.

One letter came from a family who had to mortgage their farm to pay their son's medical bills. The child was admitted to a hospital for treatment of uncontrollable seizures and was placed under heavy sedation. The family requested a trial of the KD, but the treating physicians refused to consider it. Instead, they wanted to add more medications and had recommended surgery. With the help of a compassionate nurse, the family made the difficult decision to leave without medical authorization. They flew directly to Johns Hopkins Hospital. Several days later, their child, like Charlie, became seizure-free.

Jim was compelled to use his professional skills as a movie producer/director and his connections in the industry to find ways to help more families learn about the diet. He wrote, directed, and produced a dramatization of the devastating impact epilepsy can have, and the potential for the diet to stop seizures when nothing else has helped. In 1997, this story aired in a made-for-TV film called *First Do No Harm*. The film starred Meryl Streep (who received a Humanitas Award for her performance), and the movie became a conduit for spreading the word about the KD worldwide. More than two decades later, the Charlie Foundation continues to hear from people who learned about the diet through this movie. Furthermore, despite the diet's now 100-year history, many physicians first learn about the diet from the families of their patients.

The Abrahams founded what was originally termed the Charlie Foundation to Cure Pediatric Epilepsy in 1994. Funding was provided for public awareness and research in animal models. Videos were developed for families and medical professionals, and the Johns Hopkins team received financial support for a book, *The Ketogenic Diet: A Treatment for Epilepsy* (now in its 6th edition). Over the last two decades, the Charlie Foundation has organized educational conferences, maintained a website, and trained medical teams at countless hospitals worldwide.

GENESIS OF MATTHEW'S FRIENDS

Matthew Williams was born in 1994. He suffered from a catastrophic form of epilepsy called Dravet syndrome, and his seizures started when he was 9 months old. Like Charlie, he had severe seizures that were frequent and uncontrolled by medications. Emma, his mother, asked if Matthew could try the KD when he was 2 years old; she was told the diet "didn't work." As none of the medications had helped, she continued to ask periodically about the KD and was given a variety of responses; she was told the diet was "too hard" and caused "terrible side effects." Like the Abrahams family, Emma battled on, trying many medications that did not help Matthew's seizures and themselves caused devastating side effects. Neither family was told that it has long been known that once the first medication fails, the chance of seizure control with another medication or an added medication is much lower, and even lower with successively added drugs (down to 2.7% seizure control at the third round; Mohanraj & Brodie, 2006). There is even evidence that polypharmacy can aggravate seizures (Perucca et al., 1998; Shorvon & Reynolds, 1979). Matthew continued to suffer from thousands of seizures, and his situation did not improve on what Emma termed the "merry-go-round" of medications. Emma was told that if Matthew lived to age 12, he would likely be confined to a residential home.

When Matthew was 7, at a routine appointment Emma insisted on trying the KD—the only other option was new combinations of drugs that had already been proven ineffective and shown to cause terrible side effects in Matthew. Emma said, "The side effects of the medications were awful. He was on a considerable amount of medication and his quality of life was so poor already that it really could not have got any worse for any of us."

Fortunately, there was a new option. Six years after Emma first asked about the KD, Matthew and 144 other children with severe epilepsy were enrolled in a clinical research trial of the KD spearheaded by Dr. Helen Cross at Great Ormond Street Hospital (GOSH) in London, England (Neal et al., 2008). Within 2 weeks of his starting the diet, Matthew's seizures had decreased by 90%, and within 8 months he was off all medication. His behavior improved dramatically. Unfortunately for Matthew, the damage had been done. Years of his experiencing thousands of seizures had caused tremendous brain damage and had broken his family apart, and Emma was now a single mum to Matthew and his younger sister, Alice.

Inspired by Matthew and hoping she could spare other families from what they had endured, and especially to prevent others from lifelong disabilities, Emma started Matthew's Friends in 2004—initially running the charity out of her kitchen. She, like Jim and Nancy Abrahams, was shocked at, and angry about, the lack of information about, and the underutilization of, the KD—even when Emma had asked about it years earlier! She was determined to raise awareness of, and access to, the KD.

TEN YEARS OF ACCELERATING AND COMPLEMENTARY EFFORTS

The years since the foundations' formation have been a period of enormous growth and revitalization for the field of metabolic therapy and for both foundations. Beth Zupec-Kania, a registered dietitian and nutritionist, joined the Charlie Foundation in 2006 to develop resources and trainings for ketogenic therapies. She designed an online ketogenic diet calculator program (KetoDietCalculator.org), which allows nutritionists to efficiently create diets, including meal plans, special recipes, and infant and feeding tube formulas. A help line in the program supports clinicians by answering daily questions. KetoDietCalculator is provided without cost to licensed nutritionists, who can choose to extend access to their patients or clients. It receives regular updates and additions and has been used by over 50,000 people worldwide.

In 2007, the Charlie Foundation estimated that fewer than 15 of the 200 children's hospitals in the United States had a KD therapy program. Frustrated by this lack of progress, the Charlie Foundation commissioned a group of physicians and dietitians to collaborate on methods of providing ketogenic diets. Their report, published in 2009 in *Epilepsia*, and updated in 2018 in *Epilepsia Open* is titled "Optimal Clinical Management of Children Receiving the Ketogenic Diet: Updated Recommendations of the International Ketogenic Diet Study Group" (Kossoff et al., 2018). This consensus statement became the cornerstone for developing new programs worldwide. The report identified which patients were most likely to benefit, outlined methods for starting the diet, and provided monitoring guidelines. The group summarized its conclusions as follows:

> The ketogenic diet (KD) should be strongly considered in a child who has failed two to three anticonvulsant therapies, regardless of age or gender, and particularly in those with symptomatic generalized epilepsies. It can be considered the treatment of choice for two distinct disorders of brain metabolism, GLUT-1 deficiency syndrome and pyruvate dehydrogenase deficiency disorder. In the particular epilepsy syndromes of Dravet syndrome, infantile spasms, myoclonic-astatic epilepsy, [and] tuberous sclerosis complex, the KD could be offered earlier.

In the same year as this collaborative report, a randomized controlled study of children receiving the classic and medium-chain triglyceride-supplemented KDs was published in *Lancet Neurology* (Neal et al., 2008). This is the clinical trial that Matthew Williams participated in. Children between the ages of 2 and 16 with medically intractable epilepsy continued their current treatment and were randomized to either a KD or standard of care for 3 months. The results were clear: children treated with the diet showed significant improvement compared with baseline and with the control group; some had over a 90% reduction in their seizures or were seizure-free. Seizure frequency in children who continued to receive the standard of care worsened compared with baseline, and none had over a 90% reduction or were seizure-free. This Class I study is considered the highest level of conclusive evidence and was the affirmation that doctors and advocates had been waiting for. At the time, it had been nearly 90 years since the ketogenic diet was developed, and finally a comparison of the diet as treatment for difficult-to-control epilepsy against multiple antiseizure medications proved that the diet was superior in effectiveness. More recently, another Class I study found similar results (Lambrechts et al., 2016).

The combination of the *Epilepsia* and *Lancet Neurology* publications gave further credence to the diet, and in 2010 they led to the requirement for inclusion of KD therapies in Level 3 and 4 Epilepsy Centers in the United States. The Level 3 and Level 4 distinction is granted by the NAEC (National Association of Epilepsy Centers) to centers that provide medically approved epilepsy treatments.

A SPECTRUM OF KD THERAPIES

Expanding use of the KD for epilepsy paved the way to variations in the diet, particularly for adults and for older children who find it difficult to adhere to a restrictive diet. Eric Kossoff at Johns Hopkins developed a modified version of the KD known as the modified Atkins diet (Kossoff et al., 2003). At about the same time, Heidi Pfeifer, a Massachusetts General Hospital dietitian, developed the low-glycemic-index treatment (LGIT; Pfeiffer & Thiele, 2005). These two newer diets are similar to the classic KD in their high-fat, low-carbohydrate content, but they are different in that they could be initiated outside of the hospital and do not require careful weighing of each food item. The modified Atkins diet was shown to be effective in a Class I study (Sharma et al., 2013). Clinical reviews began to indicate that the efficacy of the modified Atkins and LGIT diets was "nearly as effective" as the classic KD (Coppola et al., 2011; Karimzadeh et al., 2014; Thibert et al., 2012). These two diets are often easier for older children and adults to manage and are sometimes used as alternatives to the classic KD.

For now, the classic KD remains the most effective diet therapy based on current scientific evidence. However, less strict versions may be more realistic for certain individuals, especially older children and adults. These metabolic diet treatments are referred to collectively as "ketogenic therapies." The Charlie Foundation published a chart (Table 41.1) that outlines the differences between the therapies to assist families and health professionals in selecting the best option.

Both the Charlie Foundation and Matthew's Friends offer a wealth of recipes and expertise, including demonstration videos. Their tireless dedication to developing and sharing recipes has helped make the diet much more palatable and more accessible to patients and their families throughout the world.

OTHER CONDITIONS THAT MAY BENEFIT

A study published in 2008 in *Lipids* laid the groundwork for an entirely new application of KD therapy. Metabolic syndrome is a diagnosis that includes three or more of the following abnormalities: abdominal obesity, elevated blood pressure, elevated fasting blood glucose, and elevated lipids or triglycerides. This syndrome is currently an epidemic in many areas of the

TABLE 41.1

QUESTIONS	Ketogenic Therapies	MCT OII	Low Glycemic Index Treatment	Modified Atkins
Is Medical supervision required	Yes	Yes	Yes	Yes
Is diet high in fat?	Yes	Yes	Yes	Yes
Is diet low in carbohydrate?	Yes	Yes	Yes	Yes
What is the ratio of fat to carbohydrate & protein?	4:1, 3:1, 2:1, 1:1	Approximately 1:1	Approximately 1:1	Approximately 2:1
How much carbohydrate is allowed on a 1000 Calorie diet?	8gm carb on a4:1 16gm carb on a3:1 30gm carb on a 2:1 40-60gm carb on a 1:1	40-50gm	40-60gm	10:gm adolescents or 15gm adults for 1 month 20gm afterwards
How are foods measured?	Weighed	Weighed or measured	Weighed or estimated	Estimated
Are meal plans used?	Yes	Yes	Yes	Optional
Where is the diet started?	Hospital	Hospital	Home	Home
Are calories controlled?	Yes	Yes	Yes	No
Are vitamin and mineral supplements required?	Yes	Yes	Yes	Yes
Are liquids (fluids) restricted?	No	No	No	No
Is a pre-diet laboratory evaluation required?	Yes	Yes	Yes	Yes
Can there be side-effects?	Yes	Yes	Yes	Yes
What is the overall difference in design of these diets?	This is an individualized and structured diet that provides specific meal plans. Foods are weighed and meals should be consumed in their entirety for best results. The ratio of this diet can be adjusted to effect better seizure-control and also liberalized for better tolerance. This diet is also considered a low glycermic therapy and results in steady glucose levels.	An individualized and structured diet containing Medium Chain Triglycerides (MCT) which are highly ketogenic. This allows more carbohydrate and protein than the classic ketogenic diet. A 2008 study showed that both diets are equal in eliminating seizures. A source of essential fatty acids must be included with this diet.	This is individualized but less structured diet than the ketogenic diet. It uses exchange lists for planning meal and emphasize complex carbohydrates. The balance of low glycemic carbohydrates in combination with fat result in steady glucose levels. It is not intended to promote ketosis.	This diet focuses on limiting the amount of carbohydrate while encouraging fat. Carbohydrate may be consumed at any time during the day as long as it is within limits and should be consumed with fat. Suggested meal plans are used us a guide. Protein is not limited but too much is docouraged

world, including the United States and the United Kingdom. Improvements in metabolic syndrome were significantly better in a group who followed a modified KD versus those who followed a low-fat, high-carbohydrate diet (Volek et al., 2008). Due in part to the appetite-suppressing effect of ketosis, fewer calories are consumed—resulting in weight and adipose tissue loss along with lowered blood glucose, triglycerides, and saturated fatty acids.

People inquiring about ketogenic therapy for brain cancer have become the second-largest group (next to epilepsy sufferers and their families) requesting information about the KD from both organizations. Individuals with brain cancer often experience seizures; therefore, the role that the KD plays as an antiseizure, anti-inflammatory, and antitumor therapy offers multifaceted benefits (Seyfried & Mukherjee, 2005; Veech, 2004). Several studies are currently in progress through the National Institutes of Health (NIH) investigating the KD's effects on cancer. Recently, Matthews Friends has partnered with the Astro Brain Tumour Fund to help adults and children with brain cancer.

Additional applications of KD therapies for other conditions have grown exponentially in recent years. Benefits have been reported in a multitude of neurologic disorders and animal models of disorders, including autism spectrum disorder, certain mitochondrial diseases, diabetes, migraine, Prader-Willi syndrome, neurodegenerative diseases (including Alzheimer's disease and Parkinson's disease), multiple sclerosis, traumatic brain injury, and stroke. New research may expand the mission of the Charlie Foundation and Matthew's Friends—or it may bring new partners who support metabolic therapies for diverse applications.

In response to the increasing demands for adult resources, the Charlie Foundation produced a guide in 2014 titled *Modified Ketogenic Therapy for Neurologic and Other Conditions*. Intended for use under medical supervision, it describes portion sizes for protein, fat, and carbohydrate and offers advice for optimal nutrition. The Charlie Foundation has shared resources with oncology medical professionals and expanded its website information to include this new population of users. A new link on the charliefoundation.org landing page has been added for studies conducted through the NIH on KD for cancer, epilepsy, and other disorders.

Medical supervision for ketogenic therapies and choosing the appropriate diet therapy for each patient is an evolving focus. The spectrum of therapies enables selection of the optimum diet for individuals, while accounting for their overall health, diagnosis, age, and ability to comply. To enhance the likelihood of success, Matthew's Friends developed a support system to help families before and during use of the diet. Adjusting the therapy during treatment to optimize effectiveness is often necessary. Discontinuing the diet is usually the goal in childhood epilepsy: 2 to 3 years is the typical course of treatment. However, in some cases of epilepsy and other neurologic disorders, it may be necessary to continue with a modified version of the diet indefinitely. These discussions are frequently addressed at the Charlie Foundation and have become the topics of collaborative journal articles and professional guidelines spearheaded by nutritionists.

News of KD therapies has spread quickly through social media and the popular press. Thousands of copies of the Charlie Foundation's *Parent's Guide to the Ketogenic Diet* have been distributed in English and Spanish. Consultant chef Dawn Martenz and nutritionist Beth Zupec-Kania have collaborated on a new cookbook, *Keto Cookbook II* (Demos Publications). Videos of cooks preparing the most popular keto recipes have been added to the charliefoundation.org website, and posts of creative snacks and meals are added to the Facebook page regularly. In addition, an app is under development for the modified KD. Similarly, Matthew's Friends is dedicated to developing and publishing delicious keto-friendly meals and has produced a wealth of information for both parents and professionals by way of printed booklets, information films and national and international conferences.

Both the Charlie Foundation and Matthew's Friends have been continuously supportive of research and have partnered in funding global symposia on KDs. They stay abreast of new research related to KD therapies. A study in the journal *Obesity* (2015) showed dramatic improvements in the health of obese children just 10 days after eliminating sugar in their diets (Lustig et al., 2016). The metabolic impact of a sugar-free foods is one element of KDs that can be undertaken by anyone without the need for medical supervision. Eliminating sugar can be a difficult task for most people and requires strong motivation. A 2007 study published in *Neuroscience and Behavioral Reviews* showed that rats that were fed sugar intermittently had behavior and neurochemical changes that resembled the effects of substance abuse

(Avena et al., 2008). Eliminating refined (processed) foods is a second step that can be taken to improve one's diet.

The Charlie Foundation has translated these and other similar research findings into pragmatic guidelines. A new publication, *Does What I Eat Affect My Epilepsy?*, outlines steps that can be taken to eliminate sugar and refined foods and to consume a mostly whole-foods diet. This publication has been distributed widely (in English and Spanish) for all people with epilepsy regardless of their interest in KD therapy.

For conditions that may benefit from ketogenic therapies, the Charlie Foundation wrote an informational publication, *Pre-Ketogenic Diet*. This document is distributed (free) to health professionals to provide to their patients or clients who are potential candidates for KD therapy. It recommends the elimination of gluten and sugar, in keeping with the classic KD; however, it is not intended to induce ketosis. Instead, it can be described as a whole-foods, Mediterranean-style diet that prepares the user for the transition to ketogenic therapy and helps determine which diet in the spectrum is best suited for their needs and preferences. In addition, healthcare professionals can use the pre-ketogenic diet as a screening tool to identify individuals who are able to adhere to the lifestyle changes required for the KD.

THE CHARLIE FOUNDATION AND MATTHEW'S FRIENDS—LOOKING TO THE FUTURE

In 2013, the Charlie Foundation renamed itself the Charlie Foundation for Ketogenic Therapies to better define its mission for the future: advocacy, awareness, and education for epilepsy and beyond (Figure 41.1). Its expansion of educational efforts includes adult-focused media and training. Development of new resources in both English and Spanish remains a goal. A list of current resources is shown in Box 41.1.

Throughout the more than two decades of its existence, the Charlie Foundation has continued to receive daily e-mails and letters from families and health professionals requesting assistance. Jim Abrahams has responded to most of these requests himself, while triaging some to support staff. Although Charlie has been seizure-free and drug-free and completely off the diet since 1999, Charlie's family continues to represent ketogenic therapies in their Los Angeles community and on a national level through partnerships with other nonprofits and with supportive commercial organizations. Over 160 medical centers have been trained in the spectrum of ketogenic therapies in the United States and elsewhere, including Canada, Portugal, Austria, Jamaica, Slovenia, Kuwait, Saudi Arabia, and the Republic

---

BOX 41.1
CHARLIE FOUNDATION EDUCATIONAL RESOURCES

Parent's Guide to the Ketogenic Diet
Modified Ketogenic Diet Therapy: 1:1 and 2:1 Prescriptions
Does What I Eat Affect My Epilepsy?
Pre-Ketogenic Diet; Low-Carb, Gluten-Free, High-Fat
KetoDietCalculator Guide for the Nutritionist and the User
Professional's Guide to the Ketogenic Diet
Frequently Asked Questions about Ketogenic Diets
Comparison of Ketogenic Diet Therapies
Ketogenic Diet Primer for Health Professionals

MATTHEW'S FRIENDS EDUCATIONAL RESOURCES
A Guide to Medical Ketogenic Dietary Therapies (KDT)
Keto Therapies—Keto Introduction
Colour and Shine starter book for young people and adults on KDT (dietician request)
I am going on a Ketogenic Diet (A booklet and video aimed at children)
Electronic Ketogenic Manager (EKM) meal planner guide and filmed tutorials

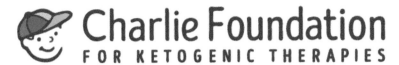

FIGURE 41.1 *Logo, Charlie Foundation for Ketogenic Therapies*

of Georgia. Beginning in 2008, the Charlie Foundation has also sponsored and organized global symposia that have brought together leading scientists and medical professionals with the intent of advancing research and clinical use of ketogenic therapies. Plans for future symposia are currently in progress. As new clinical and scientific research continues to emerge, the Charlie Foundation will respond with further resources to promote safe and effective use of ketogenic therapy and to make it less daunting for the user to manage.

Matthew's Friends grew rapidly from Emma's kitchen table, and in 2011 it opened its own clinic (Figure 41.2). The charity has continued to grow rapidly, and it has expanded into New Zealand and Canada and more recently to the Netherlands, Flanders, and South Africa. In 2016, it embarked on a new program, called KetoCollege, that offers training for teams around the globe, adding to and complementing the efforts of the Charlie Foundation to train KD teams at their home institutions worldwide.

Now seizure-free young adults—no longer on a special diet—Charlie Abrahams and Matthew Williams are two clear examples of evidence that even catastrophic epilepsy can be cured by a KD. A question frequently asked about Charlie, Matthew, and others who have become seizure-free or nearly so on a ketogenic therapy is, "How is it possible that they can retain the benefits after weaning from the diet?" At the present time, there

is no clear answer to this question. Emerging scientific research may soon clarify whether early application of ketogenic therapy may either ameliorate the disease or even cure it. For example, the field of nutritional genomics examines the effect of nutritional changes on genes and suggests that maladaptive epigenetic changes can be altered by diet. Targeted diet therapies are already being prescribed, along with genetic testing, for certain metabolic disorders.

Implementation of a restrictive diet is easiest in infants and children (given their reliance on their parents and caregivers) and becomes more challenging as children gain independence. Early initiation of ketogenic therapies is better tolerated in young children—which may result in improved compliance and outcomes. Nevertheless, the diet has been shown to work in adults, and so in this light, future potential applications will continue to expand.

EPILOGUE

As this current volume amply demonstrates, diet and nutrition can profoundly influence brain development and function. Indeed, from a medical perspective, dietary and metabolic therapies have been, and continue to be, explored in a wide variety of neurologic diseases, including epilepsy, autism spectrum disorder, traumatic brain and spinal cord injury, Alzheimer's disease, Parkinson's disease, sleep disorders, malignant brain cancer, headache, and chronic pain

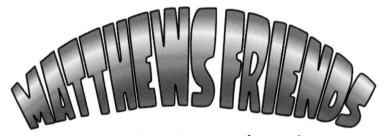

FIGURE 41.2 *Logo, Matthew's Friends*

syndromes, as well as multiple sclerosis. More recently, a parallel approach has been taken to treat mental disorders, such as depression, anxiety, bipolar disorder, and even schizophrenia. The impetus for using various diets to treat these disorders stems from both a relative lack of effectiveness of existing pharmacologic therapies for many medical conditions and the intrinsic appeal of implementing nonpharmacologic treatments.

Over the past 25 years, the metabolic underpinnings of diseases that affect highly energy-dependent organs like the brain have garnered widespread global interest and scientific validation. The catalyst for this exponential surge of activity was the KD, a high-fat and low-carbohydrate treatment for pharmacoresistant epilepsy that was created a century ago to mirror the biochemical changes induced by fasting—a strategy to control seizures that had been applied for over two millennia. While there have been great advances in our scientific understanding of how the KD works, one of the more noteworthy observations has been that this metabolism-based approach affords neuroprotective and potentially disease-modifying effects—not simply symptom relief. Thus, there is now a timely opportunity to fully exploit these advances for the benefit of patients across the lifespan.

Since 2017, medical professionals and non-profit organizations representing six continents on Earth have convened regularly to create a new global society devoted to the advancement of metabolism-based therapies for neurologic disorders—from clinical, educational, research, training, community outreach, and advocacy perspectives. This professional organization has been named the International Neurological Ketogenic Society, or INKS, and its formal inauguration during the October 2021 Brighton (United Kingdom) Ketogenic Therapies Symposium coincides with the 100th Anniversary of the birth of the KD. In parallel, regional INKS chapters will be created to establish a truly global network of centers and organizations whose mission will be to promote metabolism-based therapies for neurologic and mental disorders. While not all metabolism-based treatments result in prominent ketone body production, the term *ketogenic* has been retained to honor the historic origins of the rapidly growing fields fully embraced and supported by INKS.

For further information, please visit: https://globalketo.com/ and https://neuroketo.org/

REFERENCES

Avena, N. M., Rada, P., & Hoebel, B. G. (2008). Evidence for sugar addiction: Behavioral and neurochemical effects of intermittent, excessive sugar intake. *Neuroscience & Biobehavioral Reviews, 32,* 20–39.

Coppola, G., D'Aniello, A., Messana, T., Di Pasquale, F., della Corte, R., Pascotto, A., & Verrotti, A. (2011). Low glycemic index diet in children and young adults with refractory epilepsy: First Italian experience. *Seizure, 20,* 526–528.

Karimzadeh, P., Sedighi, M., Beheshti, M., Azargashb, E., Ghofrani, M., & Abdollahe-Gorgi, F. (2014). Low glycemic index treatment in pediatric refractory epilepsy: The first Middle East report. *Seizure, 23,* 570–572.

Kinsman, S. L., Vining, E. P., Quaskey, S. A., Mellits, D., & Freeman, J. M. (1992). Efficacy of the ketogenic diet for intractable seizure disorders: Review of 58 cases. *Epilepsia, 33,* 1132–1136.

Kossoff, E. H., Krauss, G. L., McGrogan, J. R., & Freeman, J. M. (2003). Efficacy of the Atkins diet as therapy for intractable epilepsy. *Neurology, 61,* 1789–1791.

Kossoff, E. H., Zupec-Kania, B. A., Auvin, S., Ballaban-Gil, K. R., Bergqvist, A. G. C., Blackford, R., Buchhalter, J. R., Caraballo, R. H., Cross, J. H., Dahlin, M. G., Donner, E. J., Guzel, O., Jehle, R. S., Klepper, J., Kang, H. C., Lambrechts, D. A., Liu, Y. M. C., Nathan, J. K., Nordli, D. R., Jr., Pfeifer, H. H., . . . Practice Committee of the Child Neurology, S. (2018). Optimal clinical management of children receiving dietary therapies for epilepsy: Updated recommendations of the International Ketogenic Diet Study Group. *Epilepsia Open, 3*(2), 175–192.

Lambrechts, D. A. J. E., de Kinderen, R. J. A., Vles, J. S. H., de Louw, A. J. A., Aldenkamp, A. P., & Majoie, H. J. M. (2016). A randomized controlled trial of the ketogenic diet in refractory childhood epilepsy. *Acta Neurologica Scandinavica, 135*(2), 231–239.

Lustig, R. H., Mulligan, K., Noworolski, S. M., Tai, V. W., Wen, M. J., Erkin-Cakmak, A., Gugliucci, A., & Schwarz, J. M. (2016). Isocaloric fructose restriction and metabolic improvement in children with obesity and metabolic syndrome. *Obesity, 24,* 453–460.

Mohanraj, R., & Brodie, M. J. (2006). Diagnosing refractory epilepsy: Response to sequential treatment schedules. *European Journal of Neurology, 13,* 277–282.

Neal, E. G., Chaffe, H., Schwartz, R. H., Lawson, M. S., Edwards, N., Fitzsimmons, G., Whitney, A., & Cross, J. H. (2008). The ketogenic diet for the treatment of childhood epilepsy: A randomised controlled trial. *Lancet Neurology, 7,* 500–506.

Perucca, E., Gram, L., Avanzini, G., & Dulac, O. (1998). Antiepileptic drugs as a cause of worsening seizures. *Epilepsia, 39*, 5–17.

Pfeiffer, H. H., & Thiele, E. A. (2005). Low-glycemic-index treatment: A liberalized ketogenic diet for treatment of intractable epilepsy. *Neurology, 65*, 1810–1812.

Seyfried, T. N., & Mukherjee, P. (2005). Targeting energy metabolism in brain cancer: Review and hypothesis. *Nutrition & Metabolism, 2*, 30.

Sharma, S., Sankhyan, N., Gulati, S., & Agarwala, A. (2013). Use of the modified Atkins diet for treatment of refractory childhood epilepsy: A randomized controlled trial. *Epilepsia, 54*, 481–486.

Shorvon, S. D., & Reynolds, E. H. (1979). Reduction in polypharmacy in epilepsy. *British Journal of Clinical Pharmacology, 7*, 413P.

Thibert, R. L., Pfeifer, H. H., Larson, A. M., Raby, A. R., Reynolds, A. A., Morgan, A. K., & Thiele, E. A. (2012). Low glycemic index treatment for seizures in Angelman syndrome. *Epilepsia, 53*, 1498–1502.

Veech, R. L. (2004). The therapeutic implications of ketone bodies: The effects of ketone bodies in pathological conditions; Ketosis, ketogenic diet, redox states, insulin resistance, and mitochondrial metabolism. *Prostaglandins, Leukotrienes and Essential Fatty Acids, 70*, 309–319.

Volek, J. S., Fernandez, M. L., Feinman, R. D., & Phinney, S. D. (2008). Dietary carbohydrate restriction induces a unique metabolic state positively affecting atherogenic dyslipidemia, fatty acid partitioning, and metabolic syndrome. *Progress in Lipid Research, 47*, 307–318.

INDEX

Boxes, figures, and tables are indicated by *b, f,* and *t* following the page numbers.